PHOTOGRAPHIC REGIONAL ATLAS OF NON-METRIC TRAITS AND ANATOMICAL VARIANTS IN THE HUMAN SKELETON

PHOTOGRAPHIC REGIONAL ATLAS OF NON-METRIC TRAITS AND ANATOMICAL VARIANTS IN THE HUMAN SKELETON

By

ROBERT W. MANN, Ph.D.
DAVID R. HUNT, Ph.D.
SCOTT LOZANOFF, Ph.D.

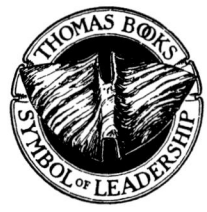

CHARLES C THOMAS • PUBLISHER, LTD.
Springfield • Illinois • U.S.A.

Published and Distributed Throughout the World by

CHARLES C THOMAS • PUBLISHER, LTD.
2600 South First Street
Springfield, Illinois 62704-9265

This book is protected by copyright. No part of
it may be reproduced in any manner without written
permission from the publisher. All rights reserved.

© 2016 by CHARLES C THOMAS • PUBLISHER, LTD.

ISBN 978-0-398-09103-3 (Hard)
ISBN 978-0-398-09104-0 (Ebook)

Library of Congress Catalog Card Number: 2015050126

With THOMAS BOOKS *careful attention is given to all details of manufacturing and design. It is the Publisher's desire to present books that are satisfactory as to their physical qualities and artistic possibilities and appropriate for their particular use.* THOMAS BOOKS *will be true to those laws of quality that assure a good name and good will.*

Printed in the United States of America
UBC-R-*3*

Library of Congress Cataloging-in-Publication Data

Names: Mann, Robert W., 1949- , author. | Hunt, David R., author. | Lozanoff, Scott, author.
Title: Photographic regional atlas of non-metric traits and anatomical variants in the human skeleton / by Robert W. Mann, David R. Hunt, Scott Lozanoff.
Description: Springfield, Illinois, U.S.A. : Charles C Thomas, Publisher, Ltd., [2016] | Includes bibliographical references and index.
Identifiers: LCCN 2015050126 (print) | LCCN 2016000092 (ebook) | ISBN 9780398091033 (hard) | ISBN 9780398091040 (pdf)
Subjects: | MESH: Bone and Bones--anatomy & histology | Atlases
Classification: LCC QM101 (print) | LCC QM101 (ebook) | NLM WE 17 | DDC 611/.710222--dc23
LC record available at http://lccn.loc.gov/2015050126

SPECIAL CONTRIBUTORS

Anna Dhody, MA. Curator of Collections, Mütter Museum, College of Physicians of Philadelphia, Philadelphia, Pennsylvania

Prof. Dr. Katerina Harvati, PhD, Director Paleoanthropology, University of Tübingen, Tübingen, Germany

Joseph T. Hefner, PhD, Forensic Anthropologist and Assistant Professor, Michigan State University (formerly at the Joint POW/MIA Accounting Command, Central Identification Laboratory, Joint Base Pearl Harbor-Hickam, Hawaii)

Pap I. Ildikó, PhD, Natural History Museum of Hungary (Magyar Termeszettudományi Múzeum), Budapest, Hungary

Ericka L'Abbe, PhD, Curator of the Bone Collection, Department of Anatomy, University of Pretoria, Pretoria, South Africa

Steven Labrash, Director Willed Body Program, Department of Anatomy, John A. Burns School of Medicine, University of Hawai`i, Hawai`i

Beth Lozanoff, Medical Illustrator, Department of Anatomy, John A. Burns School of Medicine, University of Hawai`i, Hawai`i

Pasuk Mahakkanukrauh, MD, Rehabilitation Medicine, Professor of Anatomy, Department of Anatomy, Chiang Mai University School of Medicine, Chiang Mai, Thailand

Janet Monge, PhD, Professor, Department of Anthropology, University of Pennsylvania Museum of Archaeology and Anthropology, Philadelphia, Pennsylvania

Cortland Sciotto, (Retired Master Chief Petty Office) Forensic Science Academy, Joint POW/MIA Accounting Command, Hawaii

Professor Dr. Dr. Michael Schultz, Department of Anatomy, (Universitätsmedizin Göttingen), School of Medicine University of Göttingen, Göttingen, Germany

Barbara Straßmann, M.A., Curator for the Berliner Gesellschaft für Anthropologie, Ethnologie and Urgenschichte (BGAEU), Berlin, Germany

Panya Tuamsuk, MD, Professor of Anatomy, Curator Osteology Collection, Department of Anatomy, Khon Kaen University School of Medicine, Khon Kaen, Thailand

Hugh H. Tuller, MA, Anthropologist, Joint POW/MIA Accounting Command (JPAC), Central Identification Laboratory (CIL), Hawaii

This book is dedicated to my wife Vara. My best friend and love of my life.
                                        RWM

To my lovely wife Kim and my daughter Hannah, and the continuous love and support of my parents.
                                        DRH

To Alexandra, Natasha, Nicholas, and most of all, Beth.
                                        SL

INTRODUCTION

The impetus for this book was the first author's interest in skeletons, libraries and vintage textbooks. This passion led him down a sometimes poorly lit path searching the medical and anatomical literature going back to the 1700s in order to learn more about the human skeleton and, more precisely, to gain a better understanding of our past, through the eyes of our anatomical, anthropological and medical predecessors. It was this personal journey and revival of bringing what had been found, often in obscure and mostly forgotten articles, to the present, and to incorporate them into a teaching regimen for students. This book is a result of that journey, one that incorporates physical anthropology with medicine, anatomy, biomechanics, chemistry, and biology in one text.

It was based on this endeavor that the book took roots and the authors combined their experience, skills and knowledge as anthropologists and anatomists. Wherever possible, the authors have sought to cover these skeletal traits as best they can and to show the range of variation of traits along a continuum from small to large, single and multiple, divided and undivided, left and right, and so forth. The goal in compiling this book was not to show only the most unusual expression of a trait, its smallest or largest form, or its most unusual shape, but to show its typical ("expected") and rare ("unexpected") expressions. Showing only the most extreme examples of traits and variants, they believe, ignores the range of variation and can lead to a bias in reported frequencies, geographical distributions and appearance of traits. These differences in trait expression in this book, therefore, reflect significant variation in size, shape, location and frequencies of many, perhaps even most, traits that an observer may encounter in examining one or a thousand skeletons.

To better understand how scientists perceive, classify and categorize anatomical variants of the human skeleton, the authors reviewed the literature and noted nearly 300 features that scientists have identified or classified as non-metric traits, discrete traits and dichotomous traits, among others, in the human skeleton (see Table 1). Interestingly, when considered more closely, many of these features appear to suffer from misidentification or interpretation. For example, some "non-metric" traits are the result of abnormal or pathological growth leading to pathological symptoms while many have yet to be shown to have a genetic basis. Other variant features, such as nasal and chin shape, are shared by all of us and might more accurately be classified as morphoscopic characteristics.

The question, therefore, one that is not easily answered, is how do we define normal from pathological, non-metric traits, typical and atypical? For example, a parietal foramen, commonly classified as a non-metric trait or anatomical variant is a normal and occasionally occurring feature that transmits an emissary vessel (Santorini's vein) connecting veins of the scalp with the superior sagittal sinus. This hypostotic feature is the result of a normal developmental process where an emissary vessel penetrates the outer table into the diploe or through the inner table. The formation of this vein is typical, as is the concomitant formation of a foramen housing it in the vault; not having this foramen, however, is clearly a "normal" condition that is present in many people.

An enlarged parietal foramen, in comparison, is an atypical or pathological feature resulting in faulty ossification in the region of Obelion that may or may not transmit an emissary vessel. A small, normally occurring parietal foramen and an enlarged parietal foramen are not merely features that differ in size along a continuum of "normal," but by the developmental processes that produce them. A parietal foramen, therefore, is a feature that may or may not be present in one or both parietal bones, may be double or triple on one side, or may be considered pathological if larger than 5 mm in maximum diameter. Here we see a feature or anatomical variant that can be viewed as normal or pathological, based on size alone. Other "normal" variants and non-metric traits include the supraorbital notch and foramen, nasal bone foramen, accessory frontal grooves, occipital foramen exsutural (the expressed non-metric trait), and rhomboid fossa for attachment of the costoclavicular ligament, to name a few. Surprisingly, it is difficult to discern whether it is the presence or absence of some traits that represents the "norm." One feature that most non-metric traits share, however, is that they seem to be "unexpectedly" present.

There are, of course, variants and features included in some non-metric trait lists that reflect abnormal or pathological development. Examples of what the authors would call "abnormal" non-metric traits and anatomical variants include the external auditory exostosis, tertiary occipital condyle, bone spur, exostosis in the trochanteric fossa and palatal exostosis (torus palatinus), the latter, if large enough, becomes symptomatic. Still other variants, such as a bipartite parietal bone that is formed by an accessory (subsagittal) suture, is such a rare feature that it is sometimes viewed as pathological in comparison to the normally and commonly occurring ossicles often present along the lambdoidal and sagittal sutures. While both conditions develop through the same process, one is common (lambdoidal ossicle) while the other is exceedingly rare (subsagittal suture). When discussing the bipartite parietal bone, the rarity of the trait makes it a significant finding, one worthy of reporting in the literature. Researchers have, of course, been aware that some non-metric traits are pathological in origin, but they often include these features in their parameter trait lists of normal or non-metric traits. Still other traits fall within a gray area where their origin and development is either unknown or debated. Some "gray area" examples include the ossified trochlear pulley, vastus notch and bipartite patella, distal femoral cortical excavation, cervical fossa of Allen, Walmsley's facet, third trochanter, os trigonum and calcaneus secundarius, to name a few.

Considering the extensive research and many thousands of human skeletons and cadavers that have been dissected and studied long before the days of Albinus and Vesalius, it is perhaps surprising that variation of the human skeleton has not been better documented and more easily available in a single reference book. This compartmentalization of non-metric traits and anatomical variants of the skeleton in books, scientific articles, poster presentations, abstracts, and public discussions is evident when one attempts to find an example of a trait, variant, or unusual osseous or dental feature. Searching the literature to identify a skeletal feature can take weeks or months and, at the end of a search, one may still remain confused regarding its name, frequency and rarity, etiology, range of expression and whether anyone has published a description. Exacerbating this issue is the fact that many traits and features that some view as anecdotal and not "worthy of mention" would likely help explain human diversity and development, if described and reported. Unfortunately, many subtle traits and variants go unreported and, as a result, so do their existence, frequency and range of variation. This book is intended to alleviate some of these mysteries, although it cannot address or answer all of them.

As previously mentioned, non-metric traits and anatomical variants are often identified based on their frequency of expression/presence in an osteology collection or a geographical group. Typically, the most common expression of a trait is viewed as typical or normal while unusual, uncommon, atypical, or rare traits are viewed as variants along a size and shape continuum. While some researchers choose to view non-metric traits merely as features that are either present or absent, these traits actually vary in size, shape, number and location, and not merely their presence or absence.

Choosing the appropriate terms to identify or describe a non-metric trait or anatomical variant, therefore, can sometimes be alleviated or, at the very least, reconsidered, by the choice of terms. For example, dichotomous terms such as normal or abnormal lead us to believe there are only two states for a particular feature – one is the result of normal developmental processes, while the other is pathological in origin, expression, or symptoms. The dilemma of how to view and interpret variability of the human body and which terms to use, however, is one of antiquity and in fact, was a topic of great concern to Andreas Vesalius (1514-1564), the Father of Anatomy (Straus and Temkin 1943). To avoid having to identify or label anatomical traits as normal or abnormal, Vesalius referred to them based on their frequency as "always," "usually," "frequently," "more frequently," "most frequently," "sometimes," "not always," rarely," relatively rarely," much more rarely," and "very rarely." What Vesalius did was remove the "finality" and "diagnosis" of normal or abnormal by using qualitative terms to quantify features according to how often he found them in his own research. While contemporary statisticians and researchers typically rely more on quantitative methods such as frequencies, intra- and inter-observer variability and multivariate statistics to report frequencies of traits and anatomical variants, steadfast qualitative terms such as "rare" and "common" maintain their place in scientific research and reporting. The current authors utilized quantitative, semi-quantitative and qualitative frequencies when reporting traits and anatomical variants in this book.

This atlas is the culmination of more than 75 combined years' of skeletal research and analysis by the authors and is intended to:

1) Utilize large, color photographs and a regional skeletal approach, to provide as many examples as we could of anatomical variants and non-metric traits in the human skeleton.
2) Identify and describe the widest possible range of anatomical variants and non-metric traits in the human skeleton in a single source.

3) Impart information on anatomical variants and non-metric traits spanning diverse temporal and geographical regions.
4) Provide clarity or, at the very least, stimulate discussion on the difference between an anatomical variant, non-metric trait, anomaly and morphoscopic trait.
5) Provide descriptions, relative frequencies, and references for anatomical variants and non-metric traits in the human skeleton.
6) Increase our knowledge of the intra- and inter-variability of the human skeleton.

Some recommended anatomy and skeletal reference texts and databases that the authors have found especially helpful include, but are not restricted to the following:

Anderson, S. *A Comparative Study of the Human Skeletal Material from Late First and Early Second Millennium Sites in the North-East of England.* Unpublished Thesis, University of Durham, 1991.

Anson, B. J. and McVay, C. B. *Surgical Anatomy*, Fifth Edition. W. B. Saunders Company, Philadelphia, 1971.

Barker, L. F. *A Laboratory Manual of Human Anatomy.* J. B. Lippincott Company, Philadelphia, 1904.

Corruccini, R. S. An examination of the meaning of cranial discrete traits for human skeletal biological studies. *American Journal of Physical Anthropology* 40:425-446, 1974.

Gerrish, F. H. (editor). *A Textbook of Anatomy by American Authors.* Lea Brothers and Company, Philadelphia, 1902.

Grant, J. C. Boileau. *A Method of Anatomy: Descriptive and Deductive*, Fourth Edition. The Williams and Wilkins Company, Baltimore, 1948.

Gray, H. T. *Anatomy, Descriptive and Surgical ("Gray's Anatomy")*, T. Pickering Pick (editor), Thirteenth English Edition, Lea Brothers and Company, Philadelphia, 1897.

Hefner, J. T. *The statistical determination of ancestry using cranial non-metric traits.* Doctoral Dissertation, the University of Florida, Gainesville, 2007.

Holden, L. and Langton, J. (editors). *Holden's Manual of the Dissection of the Human Body.* J. & A. Churchill, London, 1879.

Jantz, R. L. *Change and variation in skeletal populations of Arikara Indians.* Ph.D. dissertation, University of Kansas, Lawrence, 1970.

Kopsch, F. *Rauber-Kopsch Lehrbuch der Anatomie Abteilung 2:* Knochen, Bänder. Verlag von Georg Thieme, Leipzig, 1914.

Khudaverdyan, A. Yu. Non-metric cranial variation in human skeletal remains from Armenia. *Acta Biological Szegediensis* 56(1):13-24, 2012.

Leidy, J. *An Elementary Treatise on Human Anatomy.* J. B. Lippincott and Company, Philadelphia, 1861.

Morris' Human Anatomy: A Complete Systematic Treatise by English and American Authors (Part 1 Morphogenesis, Osteology, Articulations), C. M. Jackson (editor). P. Blakiston's Son and Company, Philadelphia, 1914.

Ossenberg, N. S. *Discontinuous Morphological Variation in the Human Cranium.* Ph.D. Thesis. University of Toronto: Toronto, Ontario, 1969.

Ossenberg, N. S. *Cranial Non-metric Trait Data Base User Guide* (available on-line at http://hdl.handle.net/1974/7870). Data and Government Information Centre, Queen's University Library, Canada, 2013.

Perizonius, W. R. K. Non-metrical Cranial Traits: Sex Difference and Age Dependence. *Journal of Human Evolution* 8:679-684, 1979.

Pernkopf, E. *Topographical and Applied Human Anatomy* (Volumes I and II).H. Ferner and H. Monsen (editors). W. B. Saunders Company, Philadelphia, 1963.

Piersol, G. A. (editor) *Human Anatomy Including Structure and Development and Practical Considerations*, Eighth Edition. Thomas Dwight, J. Playfair McMurrich, Carl A. Hamann, George A. Piersol and J. William White. J. B. Lippincott Company, Philadelphia, 1923.

Sappey, P. C. *Traite D'Anatomie Descriptive* (Four Volumes). Adreien Delahaye et Emile Lecrosnier, Editeurs. Paris, 1888.
Schafer, E. A. and Thane, G. D. (editors). *Quain's Elements of Anatomy*. Longmans, Green, and Company, London, 1891.
Sobotta, J. and McMurrich, J. P. *Atlas of Human Anatomy*, Volume 1. G. E. Stechert and Company, New York, 1936.
Sobotta, J. and Figge, F. H. J. *Atlas of Human Anatomy*, Volume 1. Urban and Schwarzenberg, Baltimore-Munich, 1977.
Spalteholz, W. *Hand Atlas of Human Anatomy, Volume 1*. Leipzig, S. Hirzel, 1900.
Toldt, C. *An Atlas of Human Anatomy for Students and Physicians*, 2nd edition, Volume 1. The Macmillan Company, New York, 1928.
Ward, F. O. *Outlines of Human Osteology*. Henry Renshaw, London, 1876.
Wood, C. C. E. *The Influence of Growth and Development in the Expression of Human Morphological Variation*. Doctoral thesis, University of Toronto, 2012. Available on-line at http://hdl.handle.net/1807/
Yavornitzky, V. N. *A Test of Non-metric Ancestry Determination in Forensic Anthropology: Should the Current Categorization of Individuals of European Descent be Reconsidered?* Master's thesis, Michigan State University, Ann Arbor, 2002.

ACKNOWLEDGMENTS

This book would not have been possible without the contributions of many professionals. The authors would like to thank the following people.

Prof. and Dr. Professor Cristina Cattaneo of the University of Milan (Laboratorio di Antropologia e Odontologia Forense, Sezione di Medicina Legale, Dipartimento di Scienze Biomediche per la Salute, Università degli Studi di Milano, LABANOF) provided access to the osteology collection. Special thanks to Dr. Pasquale Poppa, Dr Daniele Gibelli, Dr. Daniel Gaudio, and Labanof's technicians, academic staff, graduate and post graduate students and forensic medicine trainees Annalisa Cappella, Elisa Castoldi, Elisa Baldini, Enrico Muccino, Debora Mazzarelli, Davide Porta, Danilo De Angelis, Federica Collini, Maria Carlotta Gorio, Francesca Magli, Francesca Cornacchia, Mirko Mattia, Lara Olivieri, Emanuela Sguazza, Matteo Palombelli, Ivana Fusco, Valentina Caruso, Giulia Caccia, Zuzana Caplova and Marco Cummaudo and other medical faculty and staff at the University of Milan, Italy and at the Municipality of Milano for providing access, assistance, examination space, and historical information on their osteology collection. The first author was privileged to visit the historic crypt and burial chamber of the Ospedale Maggiore di Milano Ca Granda for which I thank Dr. Paolo Galimberti. Thanks also to the wonderful people of Pontestura who hosted the "Summer Bone Camp" and made the first author's visit so pleasant and memorable. Special thanks to Gianni and Francesca Pasino and Vicky Cattaneo.

Prof. Dr. Katerina Harvati, Director of Paleoanthropology, University of Tübingen and Senckenberg Center for Human Evolution and Paleoecology, Tübingen, Germany for allowing access to their extensive osteological collection. The authors also thank the collection manager Michael Francken and the anthropology students at Tübingen University, especially Judith Beier for hosting and facilitating the first author's visit to the osteology collection.

Ms. Anna Dhody and Dr. Robert D. Hicks of the Mütter Museum of the College of Physicians of Philadelphia, Pennsylvania provided access to the vast anatomical, pathological and medical collection, as well as guidance and opinion on many of the Mütter Museum specimens. Thanks to Emily Yates for helping coordinate the construction of a special photographic stand for one of the cover images. The cover image of the skull with an elongated styloid process was provided courtesy of Evi Numen who does spectacular photography. RWM also enjoyed many fascinating and lively lunches with Anna, Robert and others on the staff at the Mütter.

Dr. Pap I. Ildikó of the Natural History Museum of Hungary (Magyar Termeszettudományi Múzeum), Budapest, Hungary allowed access to the vast osteological collection and provided information on several of the specimens.

Dr. Gerhard Hotz of the Anthropologe bei Naturhistorisches Museum Basel (Natural History Museum) in Basel, Switzerland hosted the first author's visit and provided access, expertise and opinion on many specimens in the extensive osteological collection.

Ms. Beth Lozanoff of the John A. Burns School of Medicine (JABSOM) at the University of Hawaii skillfully rendered some of the medical illustrations and provided insight on variation of the human body. Mr. Steven Labrash, curator of Willed Body Program at JABSOM provided access to the osteological and cadaver collection. Steven was always on the lookout for unusual pathological conditions and anatomical variants during the preparation of this book and brought many to our attention when he encountered them. We are delighted and thankful to have Beth and Steven at JABSOM.

Prof. Dr. Pasuk Mahakkanukrauh graciously provided access to the Osteology Collection at the Department of Anatomy, Chiang Mai University Medical School, Thailand, as well as offered background and medical information on many of the specimens. Several graduate students at Chiang Mai University who assisted by laying out skeletons for examination included Mr. Phuwadon Duangto, Ms. Sithee (Praneatpolgrang) Yodnin ("Beer"), Ms. Phruksachat Singsuwan ("Doi"), Mr. Sitthiporn Ruengdit (Neu), and Ms. Orawan Kumplien (Ning Nong). Ajarn Apichat Sinthubua, M. Sc., Anatomy instructor, was very helpful on many of the first author's visits to Chiang Mai. "Khob khun mahk khrub" to each of you.

Dr. Janet Monge graciously allowed access to and provided historical information about many of the specimens in the University of Pennsylvania Archaeological and Anthropological Museum, Philadelphia.

Prof. Dr. Dr. Michael Schultz provided access to the anatomy collection at Göttingen University in Göttingen, Germany. The first author is indebted to Michael for allowing access and providing background information on the Johann Friedrich Blumenbach Skull Collection in the Department of Anatomy. It was an honor meeting and working with Professor Dr. Dr. Schultz and having the opportunity to examine Blumenbach's "Five Famous Skulls" used as the prototypes for establishing the five ancestral groups in the 1700s.

Ms. Barbara Straßmann, Curator, allowed access to the BGAEU collection (Berliner Gesellschaft für Anthropologie, Ethnologie und Urgeschichte) in Berlin, Germany.

Prof. Dr. Maria Teschler-Nicola, Director, Department of Archaeological Biology and Anthropology of the Museum of Natural History of Vienna for hosting the first author's visit, as well as providing access, expertise and opinion on several specimens in the extensive osteological collection in Vienna.

Prof. Dr. Panya Tuamsuk of the Department of Anatomy, Faculty of Medicine, Khon Kaen University Medical School, Thailand allowed access to the

Osteology Collection and patient records, as well as provided insight and opinion on many of the Thai specimens.

The authors thank Prof. Dr. Ursula Wittwer-Backofen, anthropology and medical faculty and staff, anthropology graduate students, and Universitätsarchive staff at Freiburg University, Germany for providing access, assistance and historical information on their osteology collection.

Mr. Hugh H. Tuller provided photographs and information on specimens from Chiba University, Japan. Mr. Christopher C. Sciotto took several photographs and cleaned up the background in a few others. Thanks also to CIL anthropologists Dr. Mary Megyesi, Dr. Megan-Tomasita J. Cosgriff-Hernandez and Ms. Alexandra Wink for their casework contribution. Retired Master Chief Petty Officer and Chief of the Boat (COB) Cortland Sciotto provided an abundance of expertise, insight, inspiration, and guidance to RWM as the latter's assistant at the Forensic Science Academy in Hawaii. Thank you for always keeping the FSA "on course."

Dr. Ivett Kövári, Herman Otto Museum, Hungary provided the photograph of the bipartite parietal bone, one of the rarest skeletal anomalies one might expect to encounter in a lifetime. Mr. Nunto Sartprasit of the Missing Persons Center (MPIC) in Thailand provided two photographs of excellent quality and detail. Dr. Christine Pink and Dr. Rebecca Taylor of the University of Tennessee, Knoxville and Dr. Laurel Freas of the University of Florida provided comments on some of the specimens when they were Forensic Science Academy Fellows. Mr. Paul Mitchell, Mr. Sergio Guerra and Ms. Katie Rubin, anthropology students at the University of Pennsylvania, helped pull specimens for examination and provided assistance and opinion on some specimens in the Samuel G. Morton Collection. The anthropology faculty and staff at the University of Tennessee, Knoxville, especially Dr. William M. Bass, Dr. Richard L. Jantz, Dr. Lee Meadows-Jantz, Dr. Murray K. Marks and Dr. Dawnie Steadman deserve special thanks for their years of devoted teaching and research as pioneers in the field of physical and forensic anthropology and taphonomy.

Captain Teunis M. Briers of the South African Police Service assisted with the examination of specimens at the University of Pretoria, South Africa. Mr. Johan du Plooy of "forensicworx" (South Africa) was instrumental in helping the first author get access to the Ditsong Museum and the Department of Anatomy at the University of Pretoria. Mr. Frank Teichert and Dr. Johnny van Schalkwyk provided access and information on the skeletal collection at the Ditsong Museum in Pretoria, South Africa. Dr. Ethne Barnes, friend and colleague whom RWM first met at the Smithsonian Institution in the 1980s, provided much helpful insight into vertebral anomalies and defects.

We would like to extend our gratitude and appreciation to all of the altruistic body donors, Ajarn Yai or "Great Teacher" as they are known in Thailand, without whom this study and book could not have been undertaken and completed. Their unique contributions to the advancement of the discipline of osteology, anatomy and medicine will be remembered for many lifetimes to come.

Robert W. Mann and David R. Hunt would like to extend a special debt of gratitude to renowned forensic anthropologist and professor, Dr. William M. Bass of the University of Tennessee for sparking their interest in forensic anthropology and for allowing RWM to be his forensic anthropology teaching assistant and for RWM and DRH to participate in forensic investigations in the early 1980s. We want to also thank friend and colleague Dr. Douglas Owsley of the Smithsonian Institution for getting RWM interested in paleopathology and skeletal variation and for providing RWM and DRH the opportunity and guidance to pursue their interests in bone disease and human variation both at the University of Tennessee, Knoxville and later at the Smithsonian Institution as assistant (RWM) and field and laboratory work (RWM & DRH). Doug always supported RWM's research and inspired him with his knowledge, wisdom and vision. It was at his side that RWM learned much of what it takes to become a dedicated researcher, and through our collaborative work have built a strong friendship. RWM and DRH also thank Dr. Douglas Ubelaker for his friendship, expertise and inspiration for more than two decades. The authors would also wish to thank Dr. T. Dale Stewart (whom we both were able to get to know at the SI in his later years) for his vision and many contributions to physical and forensic anthropology, and medicine.

RWM and DRH thank their instructors, friends and classmates at the University of Tennessee and the Smithsonian Institution where they both were in graduate school and worked.

RWM acknowledges and thanks the College of William and Mary and then-instructor Dr. Edwin S. Dethlefsen and visiting archaeologist Mr. Bill Buchanan where he was introduced to anthropology and the human skeleton.

DRH would also like to extend a personal thanks to University of Illinois (Urbana) professors Dr. Linda Klepinger, Dr. Gene Giles and Diane Mann for their influence in leading DRH to the facinating study of human osteology, paleopathology and human variation. DRH is also indebted to Dr. James Dengate, in the Classics Department, for his guidance and training in literature and historical research and the opportunity to learn conservation methods at the World Heritage Museum at the University of Illinois. And DRH also must identify Dr. Donald Ortner as an influential mentor at the Smithsonian Institution; and Dr. Lucile St. Hoyme as a "quiet voice in the wilderness" in his formative years at the Smithsonian—to be cautious and methodical in analysis and interpretation.

Scott Lozanoff was fortunate to have an undergraduate educational experience that fostered his interest in anatomical variation of the human skeleton made possible by Dr. Seamus Metress and the late Dr. Dave Stothers at the University of Toledo as well as a cadre of passionate students, especially Dr. Bill Baden who eventually introduced SL to the dynamic environment at the University of Tennessee. SL also acknowledges Drs. John Negulesco and Ken Jones from The Ohio State University who provided critical insights into the discipline of Gross Anatomy and mechanisms of variation as well as Dr. Paul Sciulli at the same institution that motivated SL to embrace morphometric assessment for the study of anatomical variation. Finally, SL would like to acknowledge Dr. Virginia Diewert, at the University of British Columbia whose thoughtful, engaged, and inspirational mentorship provided the foundation for his academic career.

Most of all, we thank our families.

The authors extend their sincerest thanks to Michael Thomas for his never ending support, encouragement and editorial skills for helping to transform this from a manuscript to a book.

RWM extends special thanks to the many dedicated men and women at the Central Identification Laboratory (CIL) for their dedicated service to the mission of finding, recovering and identifying America's missing heroes. Last, but certainly not least, the first author extends special thanks to Dr. Thomas D. Holland for his support, mentorship and friendship over the years and for providing the scientific vision, leadership and inspiration to the CIL staff for more than 23 years.

The views expressed in this book are those of the authors and do not reflect the official policy or position of the Department of the Army, Department of Defense, or the U.S. Government.

CONTENTS

	Page
Special Contributors	v
Introduction	xi
Abbreviations and Names of Skeletal Collections Used in This Book	xvi
Acknowledgments	xvii

Chapter

1. Frontal View of the Skull. 3
2. Right Lateral View of the Skull 119
3. Left Lateral View of the Skull 155
4. Superior View of the Skull. 189
5. Occipital View of the Skull 216
6. Endocranial View of the Skull 266
7. Basilar (Inferior) View of the Skull. 301
8. Mandible and Teeth, Hyoid, Maxilla and Teeth. 451
9. Shoulder, Arm and Hand (Clavicle, Scapula, Humerus, Radius, Ulna, Carpal) 521
10. Sternum, Spine and Pelvis (Sternum, Vertebra, Hip and Sacrum) . 542
11. Leg and Foot (Femur, Tibia, Fibula, Patella, Tarsal, Metatarsal, Phalanx) 607
12. A Method for Removing Soft Tissue from a Human Rib Cage with Bleach 642
13. Unusual Combination of Skeletal Variants in an Adult Thai Male (KKU): A Photographic Case Report 647

Appendix: Non-metric Trait List 655
References 663
Name Index 683
Subject Index 697

PHOTOGRAPHIC REGIONAL ATLAS OF NON-METRIC TRAITS AND ANATOMICAL VARIANTS IN THE HUMAN SKELETON

Abbreviations and Names of Skeletal Collections Used in This Book

CIL = Central Identification Laboratory, Hickam Air Force Base, Hawaii.

CSC = CIL Study Collection, Central Identification Laboratory, Joint POW/MIA Accounting Command, Joint Base Pearl Harbor-Hickam, Hawaii.

CMU = Chiang Mai University, Department of Anatomy, Faculty of Medicine, Chiang Mai, Thailand.

CU = Chiba University, Chiba, Japan.

FSA = Forensic Science Academy, Central Identification Laboratory, Joint POW/MIA Accounting Command, Joint Base Pearl Harbor-Hickam, Hawaii.

Freiburg University, Freiburg, Germany.

GU = Göttingen University, Georg-August University of Göttingen, Göttingen, Germany.

HNHM = Hungarian Natural History Museum (Magyar Termeszettudományi Múzeum), Budapest, Hungary.

JABSOM = John A. Burns School of Medicine, University of Hawaii School of Medicine, Hawaii.

KKU = Khon Kaen University, Department of Anatomy, Faculty of Medicine, Khon Kaen University Medical School, Khon Kaen, Thailand.

LABANOF = Laboratorio di Antropologia e Odontologia Forense, University of Milano.

MM = Mütter Museum, College of Physicians of Philadelphia, Pennsylvania.

PAVN = Peoples Army of Vietnam Forensic Institute, Vietnam.

RV = Rudolf Virchow Skull Collection, Berliner Gesellschaft für Anthropologie, Ethnologie und Urgeschichte (BGAEU), Berlin, Germany.

SI = Smithsonian Institution, National Museum of Natural History, Washington, DC.

UPenn = University of Pennsylvania Museum of Archaeology and Anthropology, Philadelphia, Pennsylvania.

University of Pretoria, Department of Anatomy, Pretoria, South Africa.

UTK = University of Tennessee, William M. Bass Osteology Collection, Knoxville.

University of Tübingen (Eberhard Karls Universität Tübingen), Institute for Archaeological Sciences, Tübingen, Germany.

Chapter 1

FRONTAL VIEW OF THE SKULL

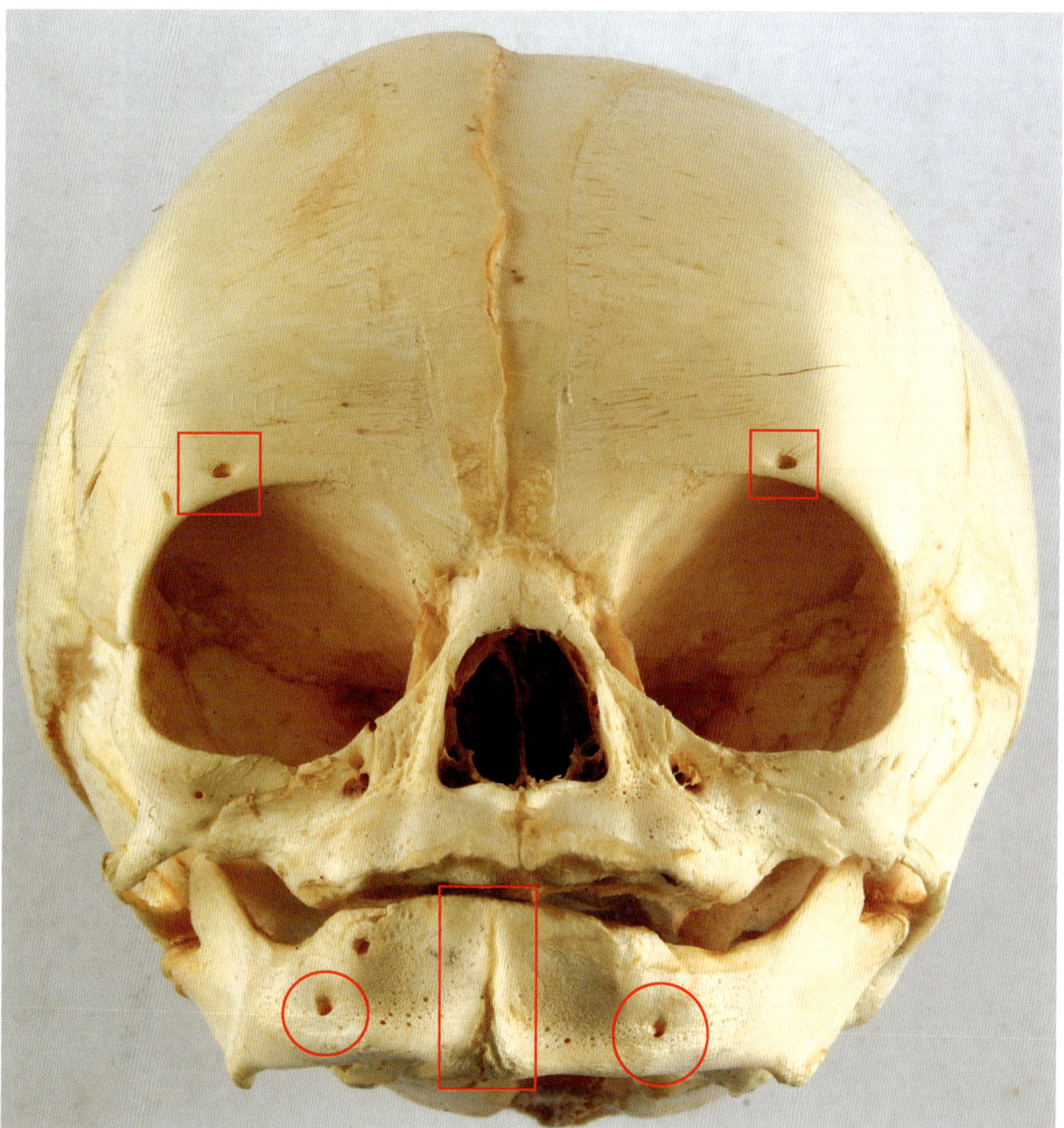

Figure 1. Anatomy of a newborn skull showing bilateral supraorbital foramina (squares), patent/open metopic (frontal, interfrontal, median frontal) suture, partially fused mental symphysis (rectangle) and mental foramina (circles). Note the horizontal growth lines (striae) in the frontal bone (CSC). The metopic, in comparison to other sutures, contributes little to growth of the cranium (Massler and Schour 1951). The approximately 110 centers of ossification typically result in 45 bones in the neonate and 22 in the adult skull (Sperber et al. 2010). See Apinhasmit et al. (2006); Berge and Bergman (2001); Chung et al. (1995); Dutton (2011); Hauser and DeStefano (1989); Schaefer et al. (2009); Scheuer and Black (2000, 2004).

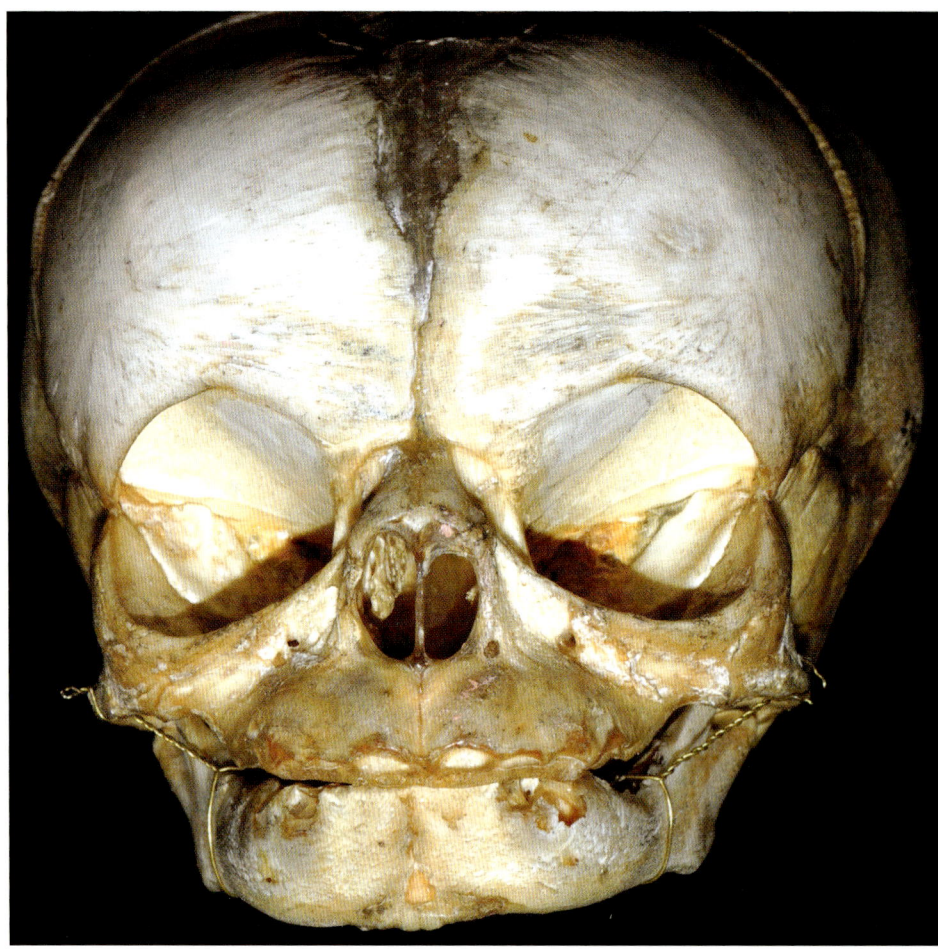

Figure 2. Normal morphology of a fetal skull. Note the wide metopic/interfrontal/frontal/median frontal suture that widens as it approaches the coronal suture, "sunburst" growth lines in the frontal bones, presence of a bony nasal septum and nasal bones, and "V" or "kite-shaped" anterior fontanelle covered by thin but tough membrane (dura mater) that later becomes replaced by bone (cf. Basmajian 1964). The anterior fontanelle usually closes between 10 and 18 months, but as early as 3 months or as late as 28 months (Segall et al. 1973). Although the cranial bones of a newborn and infant are eggshell thin, they are pliable, flexible, and can withstand considerable force. The heraldic shape of the anterior fontanelle and sagittal suture when viewed from above gives the sagittal suture its name: sagitta = an arrow (Brash 1953). Cf. Schaefer et al. (2009); Scheuer and Black (2000, 2004). The ectocranial surface of sutures is predominately under tension, resulting in bone deposition, while the endocranial surface is predominately under compression, resulting in bone resorption.

Frontal View of the Skull

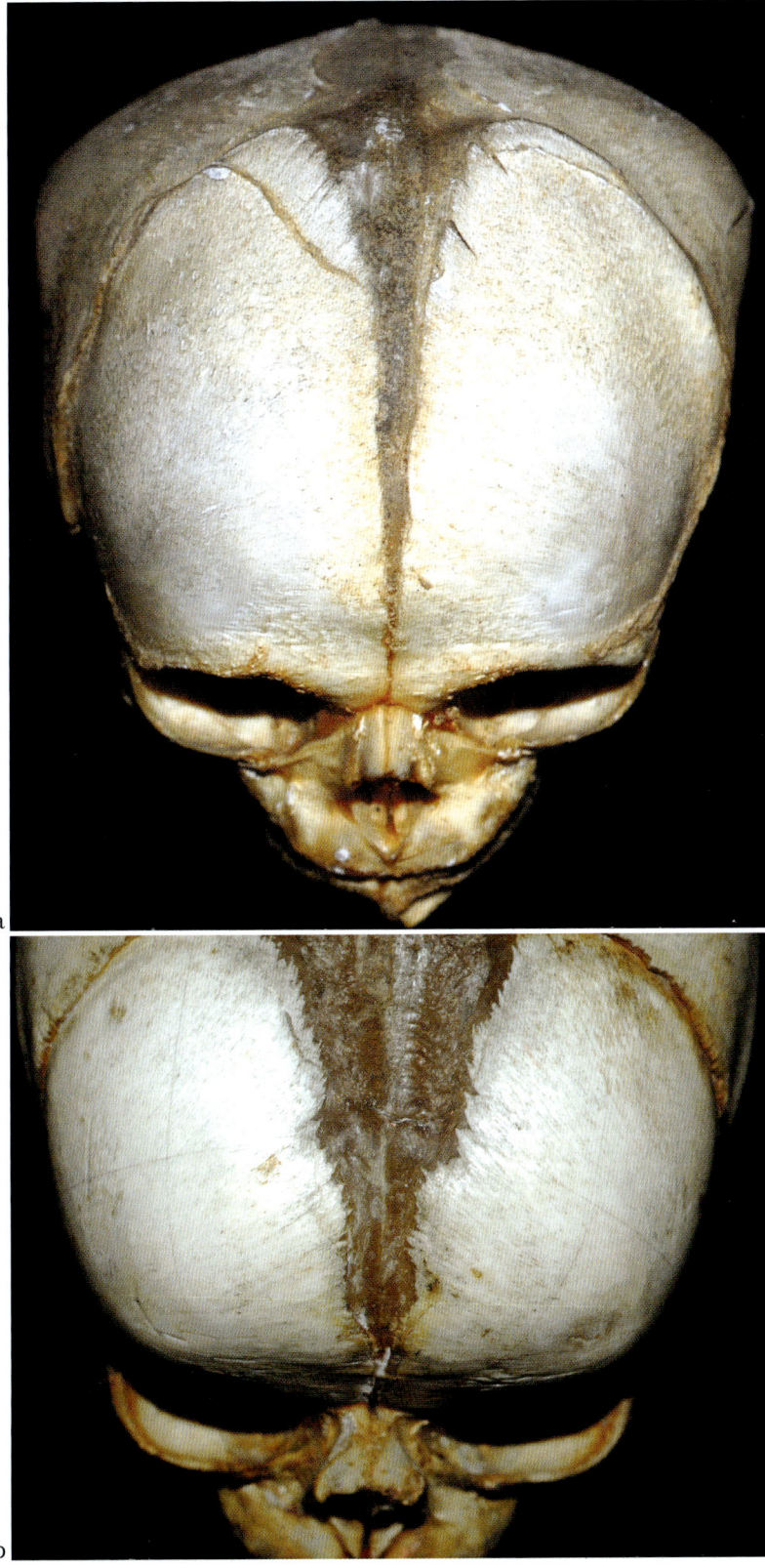

Figure 3a-b. Comparison of the anterior fontanelle in two fetuses. (a) The dura mater, a translucent membrane (dura mater or "tough mother") spanning the bones. (b) Close-up of the irregular, scalloped margins forming the metopic suture in one of the fetuses.

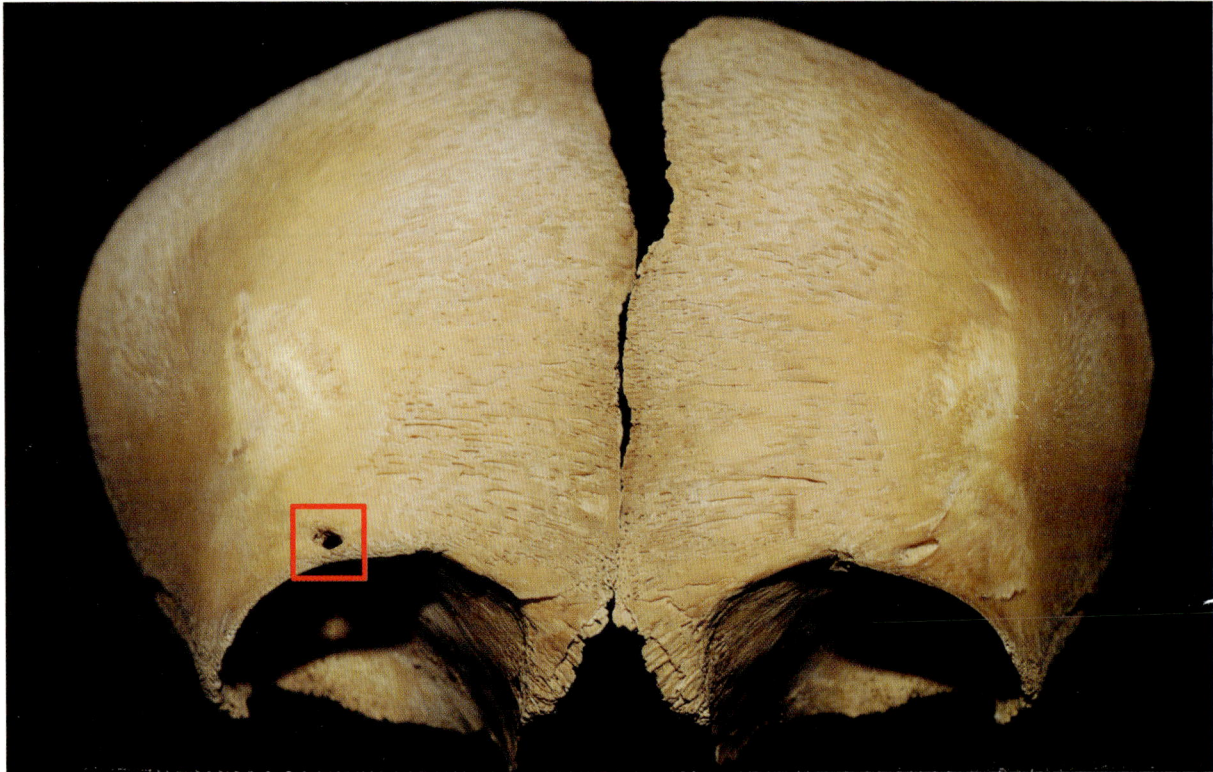

Figure 4. Beginning closure i.e., fusion, obliteration, of the metopic/frontal/interfrontal/median frontal suture in an approximately 1-year-old child (KKU). Note the presence of a lateral supraorbital foramen (square) and normal horizontal striae along either side of the metopic suture. Normal anatomy. Cf. Bryce (1917) for early research on metopism and Weinzweig et al. (2003) for discussion of normal and abnormal synostosis; Vu et al. (2001). Note: The frontal bone may exhibit both a metopic and supranasal suture, making it difficult to distinguish between the two.

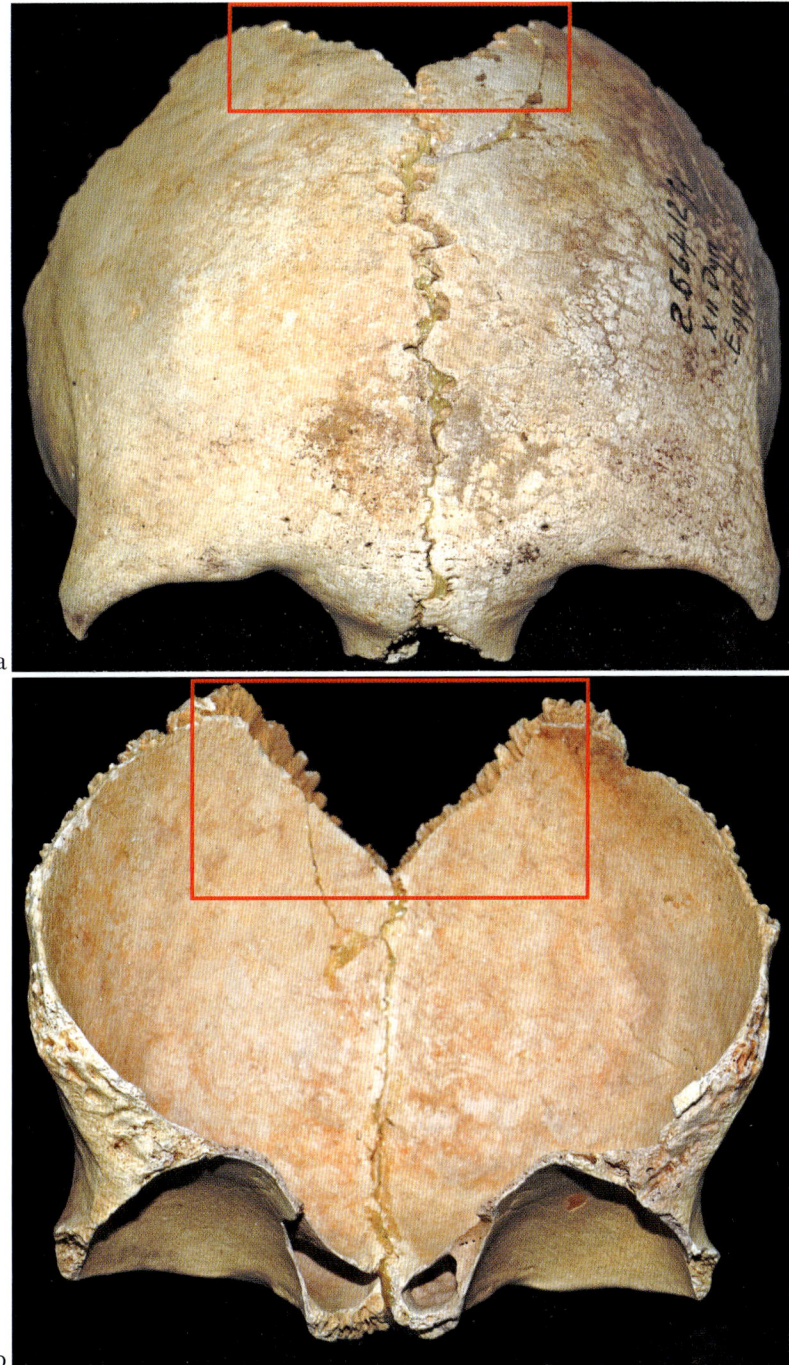

Figure 5a-b. Metopism and large V-shaped bregmatic fontanelle bone. (a) Ectocranial and (b) endocranial views of a bregmatic fontanelle, missing the ossicle, also known as an anterior fontanelle suture bone in an adult ancient Egyptian (SI 256412). While small bregmatic bones/ossicles at Bregma are common findings, large fontanelle bones such as this are uncommon or rare in osteological collections. Although not present for examination, it is likely that the parietal bones would have exhibited a defect similar in size and shape to the one in the frontal bone. Anterior fontanelle bones may be present at birth or develop several months to a few years after birth. Cf. Girdany and Blank (1965) and Barberini et al. (2008).

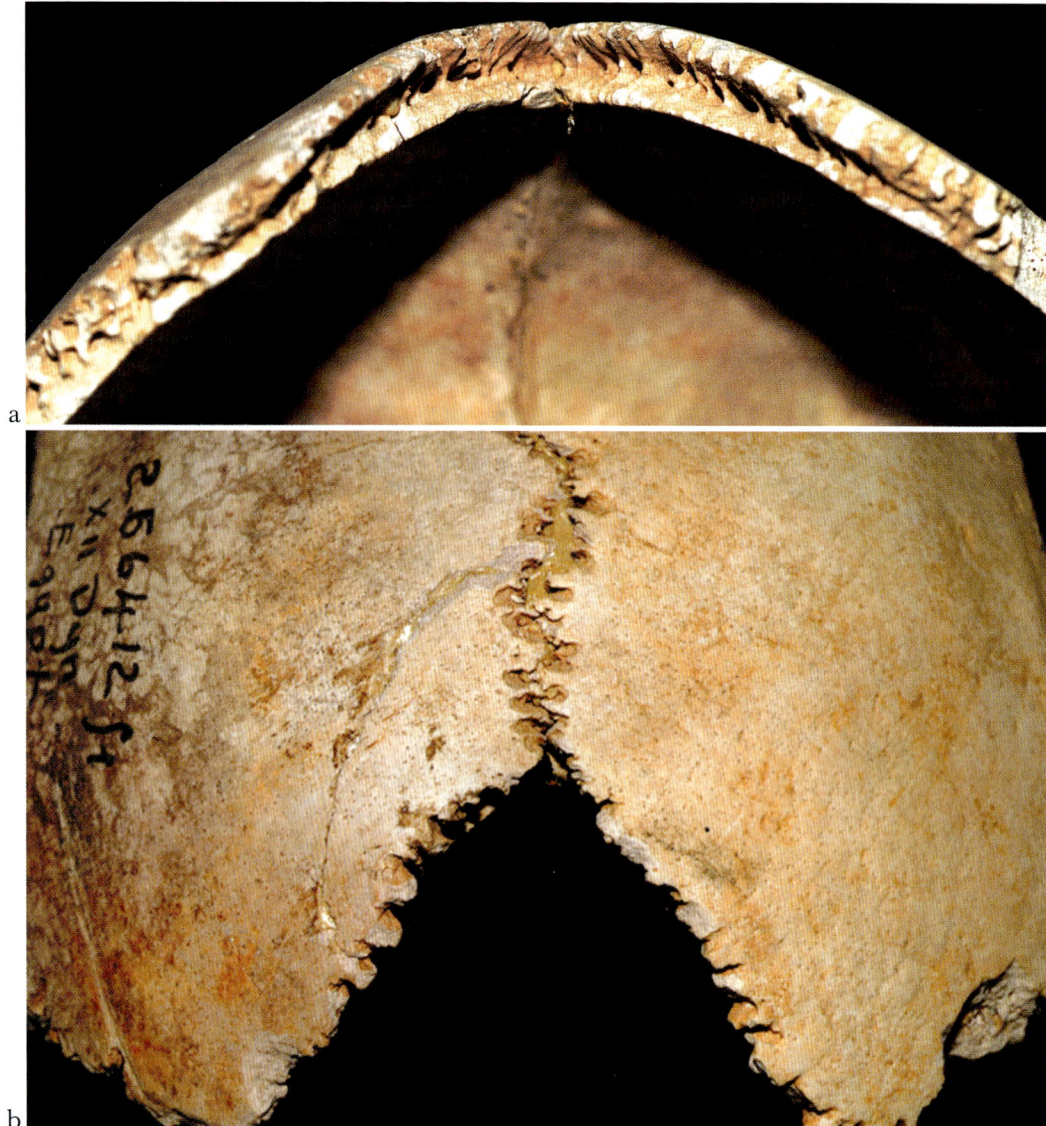

Figure 6a-b. Close-up of a bregmatic fontanelle. (a) Coronal and (b) superior views of the V-shaped bregmatic fontanelle bone suture, showing its resemblance (i.e., interlocking bony projections) to the sagittal suture in an ancient Egyptian (SI 256412). Uncommon to rare finding in dry bone specimens. The anterior fontanelle usually closes between 10 and 18 months after birth (Segall et al. 1973). See Girdany and Blank (1965) for radiographic examples of anterior fontanel bones.

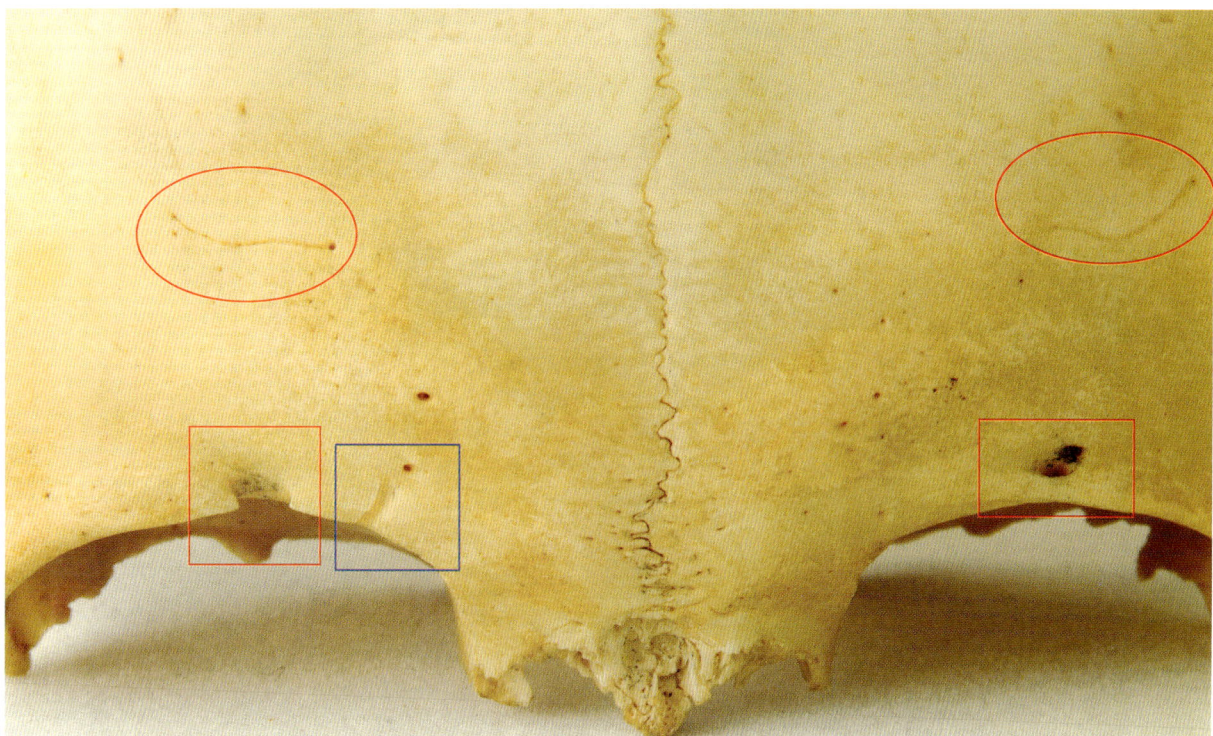

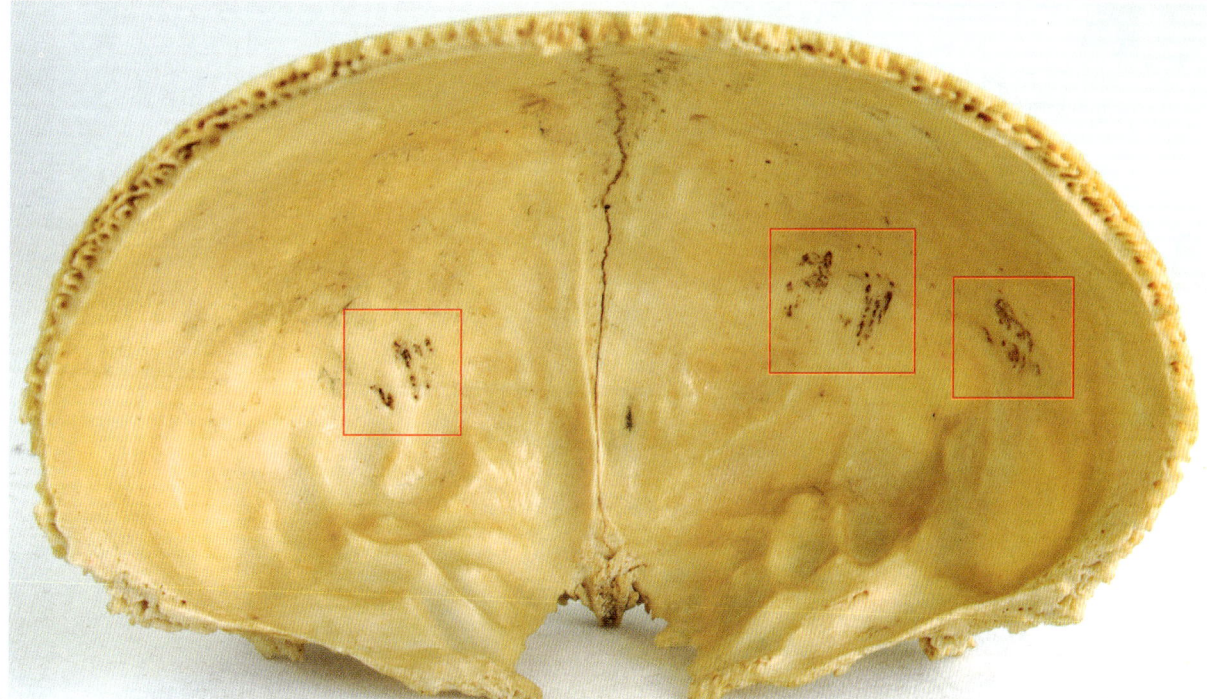

Figure 7a-b. Patent/open metopic suture, vessel grooves, Pacchionian pits and "frozen waves" of the orbital plates in a child. (a) Right supraorbital notch (red square), left supraorbital foramina (red rectangle), right supraorbital groove (blue square) and small frontal grooves (red ovals). (b) Note normal endocranial "frozen waves" of the orbital plates for the frontal/cerebral gyri, Pacchionian pits/arachnoid granulations (red squares) and differences in complexity of the metopic suture ectocranially and endocranially. Suture complexity reflects the combined effect of the predominant stress applied to each suture. Higher tensile stresses sustained by the ectocranium, a convex surface, results in a complex outer suture, while compressive stresses resulting predominantly in bone resorption endocranially (concave surface) result in a simpler endocranial suture. Normal anatomy. Cf. Apinhasmit et al. (2006); Chung et al. (1995); Le Gros Clark (1920); Vu et al. (2001); Weinzweig et al. (2003).

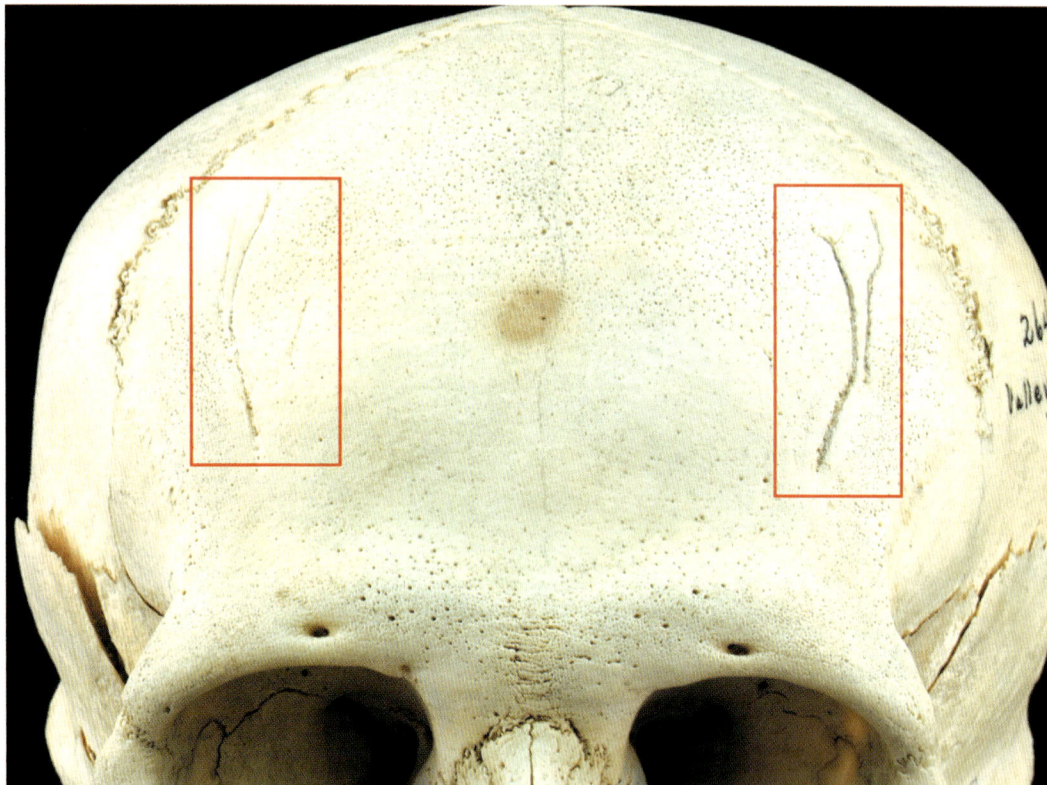

Figure 8. Frontal grooves/accessory frontal/sulci/supra-orbital grooves in an ancient Peruvian (SI). The frontal grooves may carry an artery, vein or nerve. Common findings. Cf. Dixon (1904, 1937); Hauser and DeStefano (1989). Note: the diffuse frontal pitting reflects porotic hyperostosis.

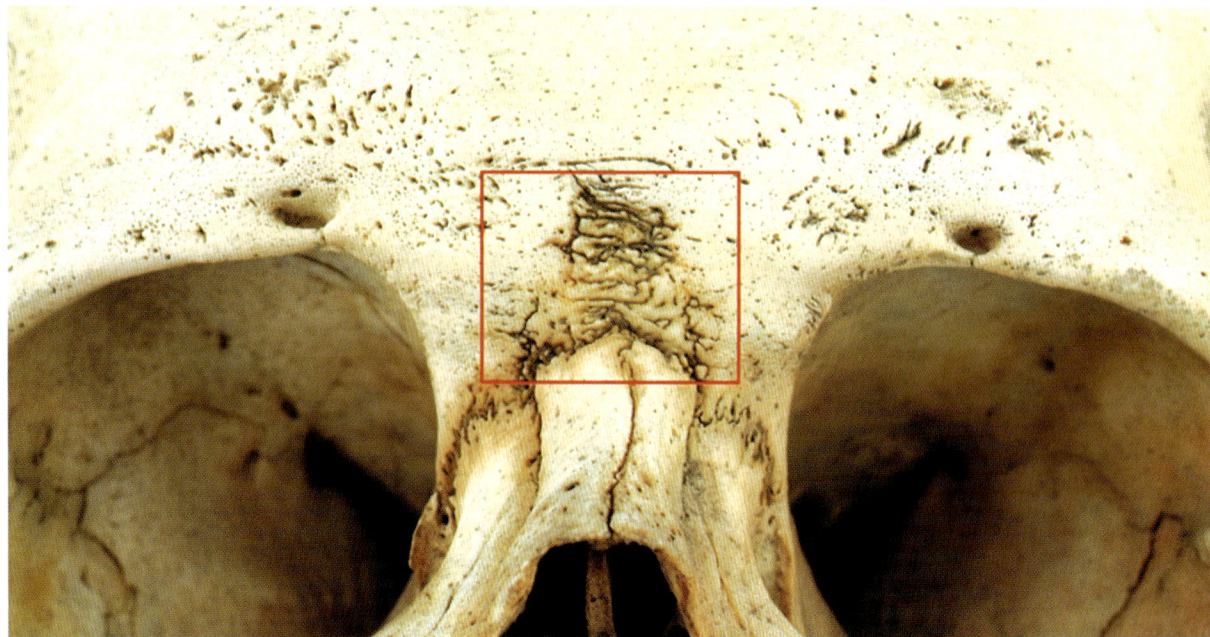

Figure 9. Prominent supranasal suture (rectangle) and male vermiculate pattern in the form of pits and lines above the orbits (KKU). Common to uncommon findings. Cf. Hauser and DeStefano (1989).

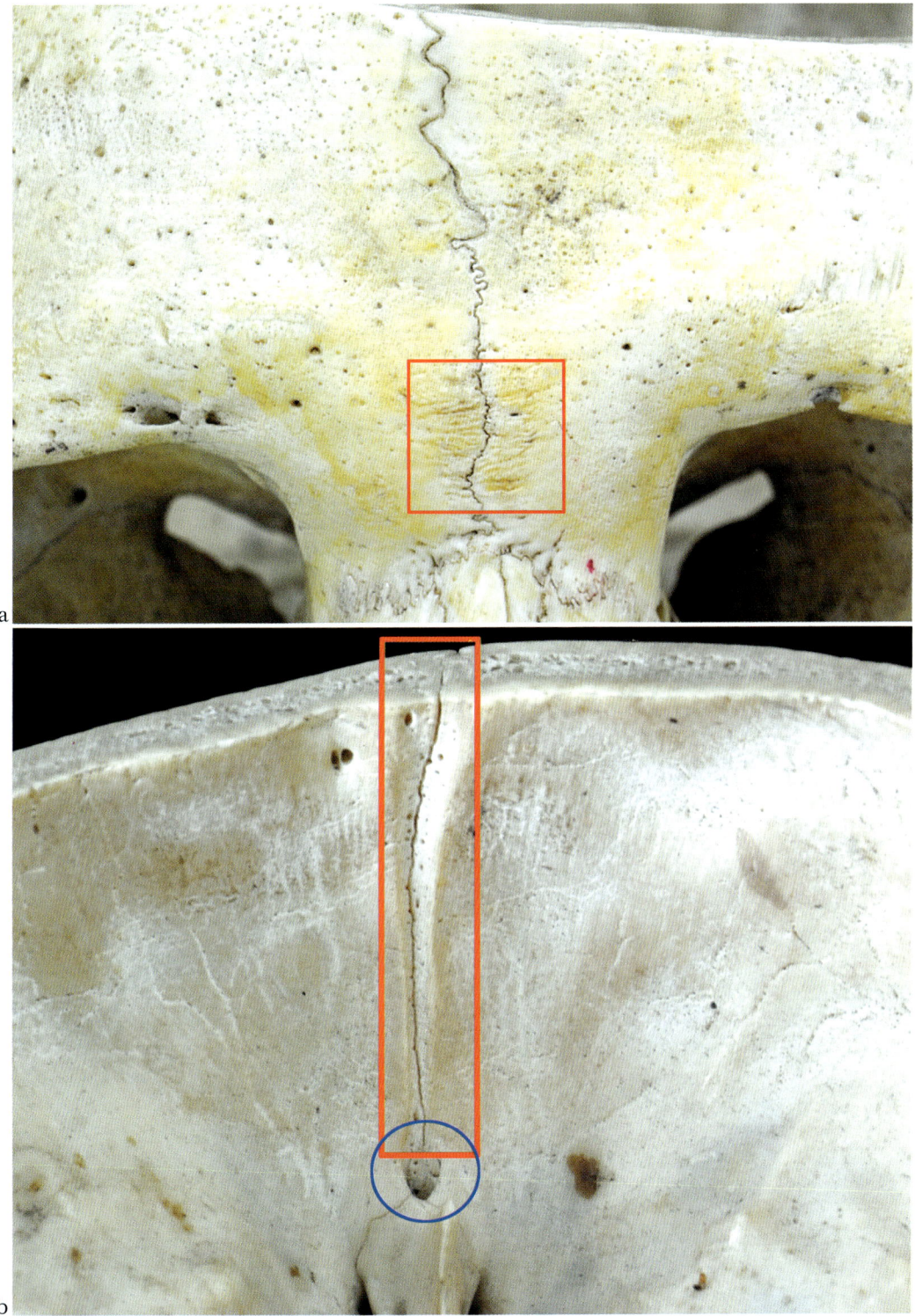

a

b

Figure 10a-b. Metopic and supranasal sutures in an adult Asian male. (a) Metopic suture through the middle of a jagged ectocranial remnant of supranasal suture (square) (KKU). (b) Note the unfused and much simpler endocranial portion of the metopic suture (rectangle) and leading into the foramen caecum (blue circle). The metopic suture, also known as the frontal or interfrontal suture, usually closes by two years of age. Metopism is a common finding. Normal anatomy. Cf. Vu et al. (2001).

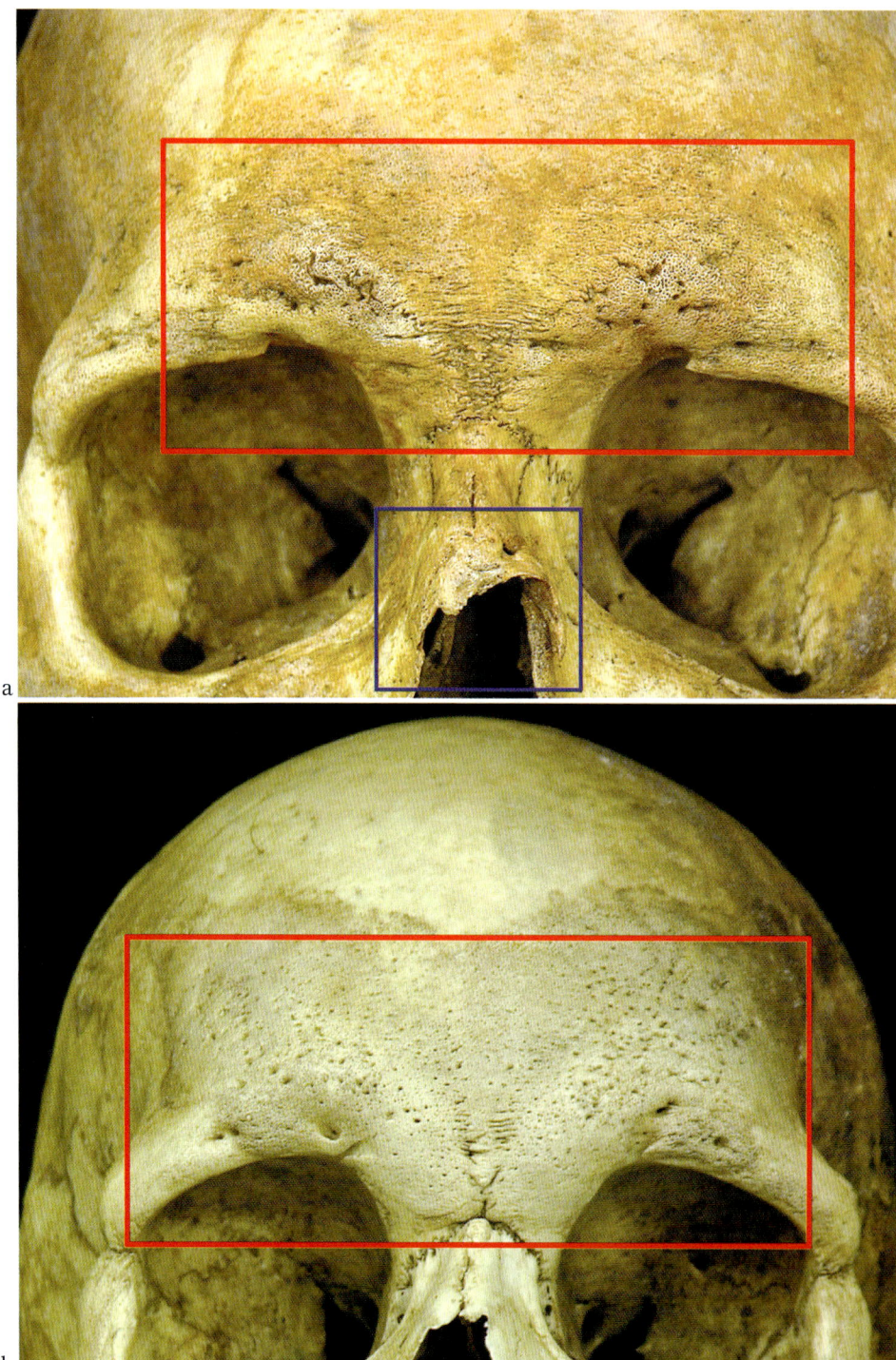

Figure 11a-b. Male vermiculate pattern in two adults (UTK). (a) Note the small pits in the frontal bone (rectangle), some of which coalesce, and tiny lines that resemble "knicks" giving the frontal bone a rough appearance and a healed broken nose (blue square). This pattern is usually restricted to the region above the orbits and along the brow ridges and is likely the result of osteoporosis. (b) Example of the male vermiculate pattern (rectangle) in another adult. Both individuals exhibit remnants of a supranasal suture. Common to uncommon findings.

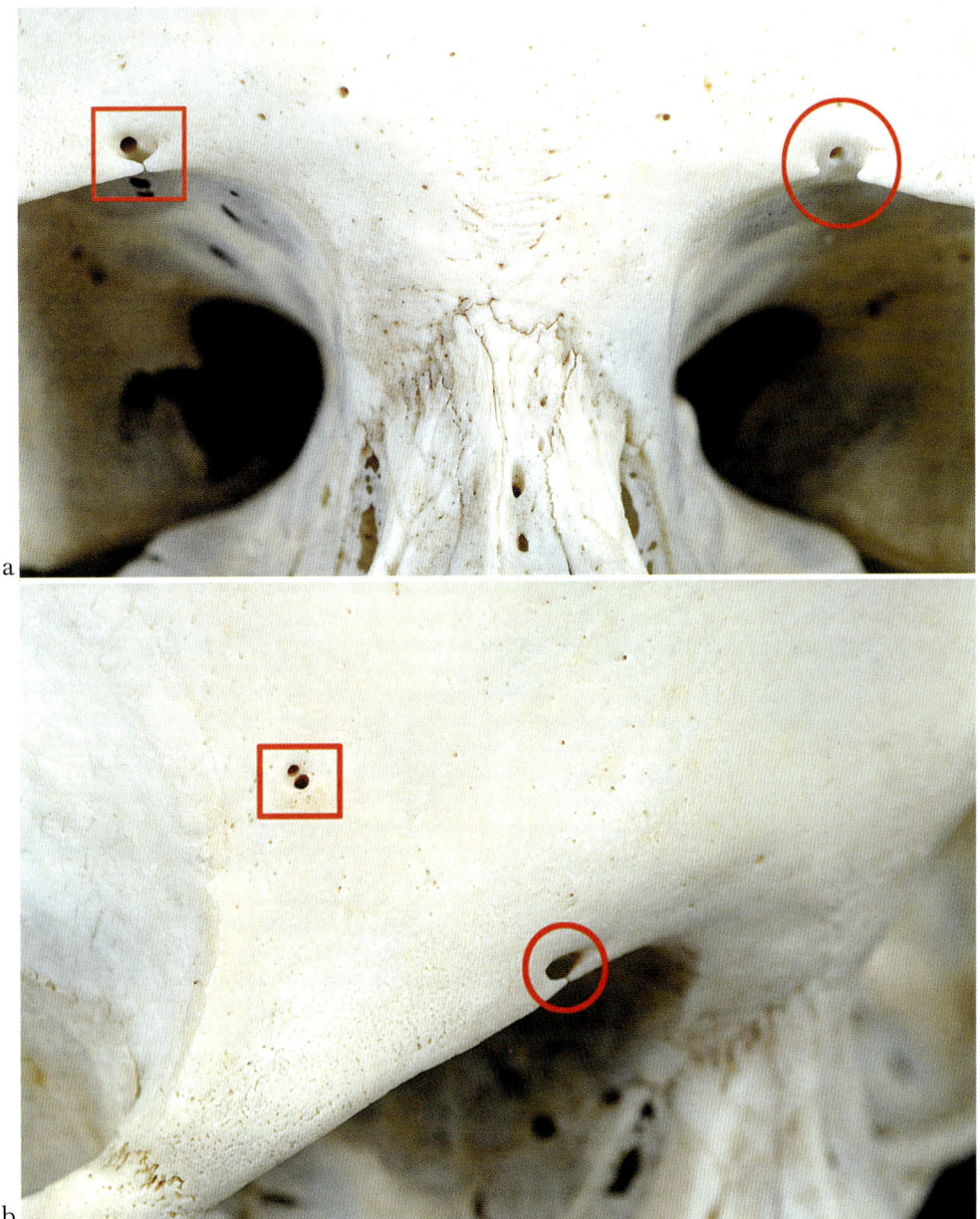

Figure 12a-b. Variants of supraorbital canals and foramina and double/divided frontal foramen in two adult Thai skull (KKU). (a) Frontal view illustrating supraorbital canals (square and circle), foramina and a double frontal foramen. Note that a notch and foramen (circle) may co-exist at the same location. (b) Right oblique view of the foramina (square and circle). Common findings. Cf. Hanihara and Ishida (2001b); Hauser and DeStefano (1989); Liu et al. (2011); Trivedi et al. (2010).

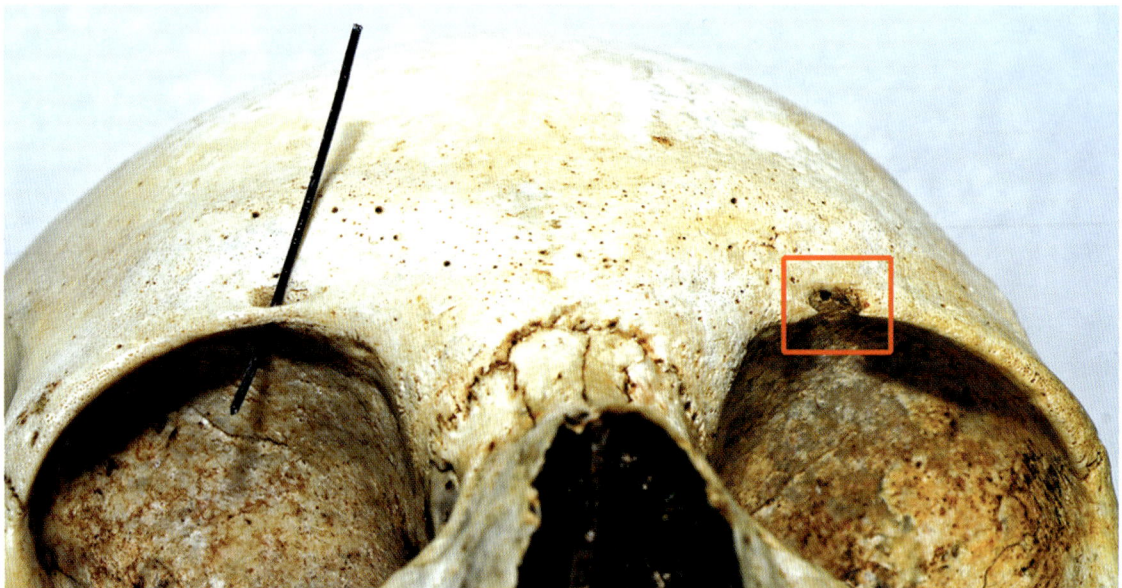

Figure 13. Supraorbital foramen (wire probe) above the right orbit and supraorbital notch (square) above the left orbit in an adult Thai female (KKU). Normal anatomy and common findings. Cf. Hauser and DeStefano (1989).

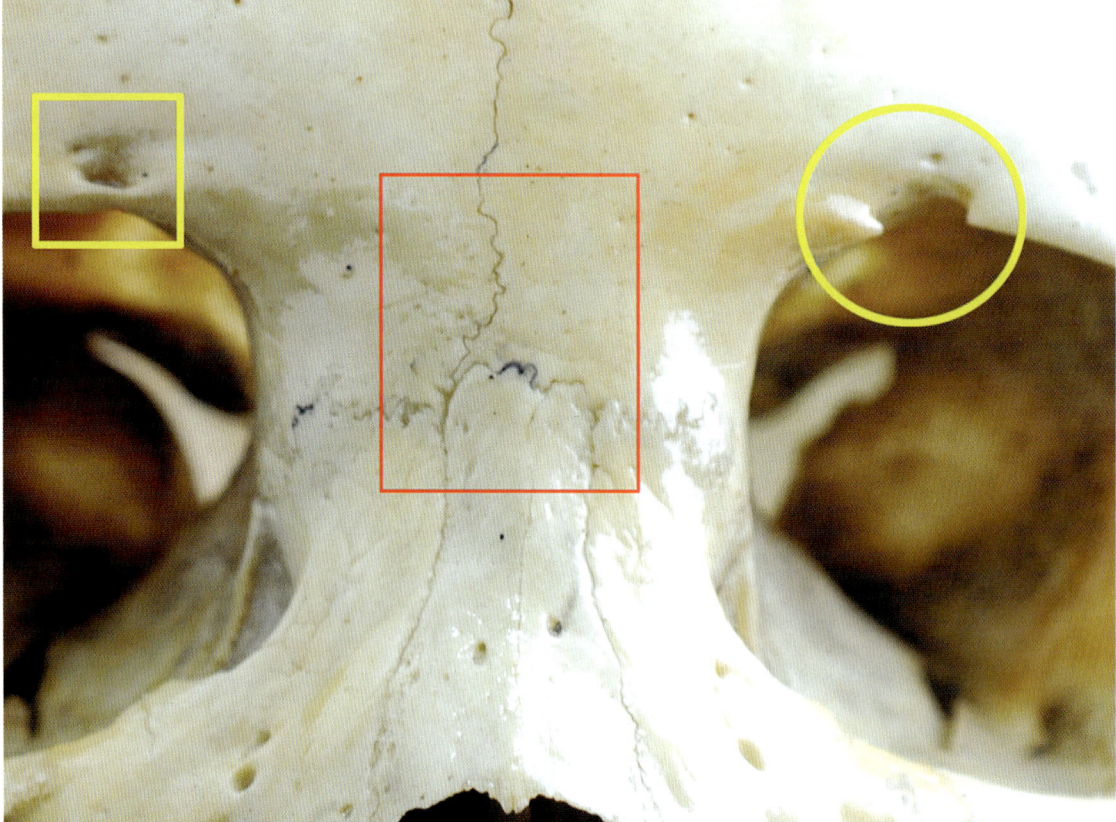

Figure 14. Right supraorbital bridge (yellow square), left supraorbital notch (yellow circle) and metopic suture that does not align with the internasal suture of the nasal bones in an adult Thai (KKU 053).

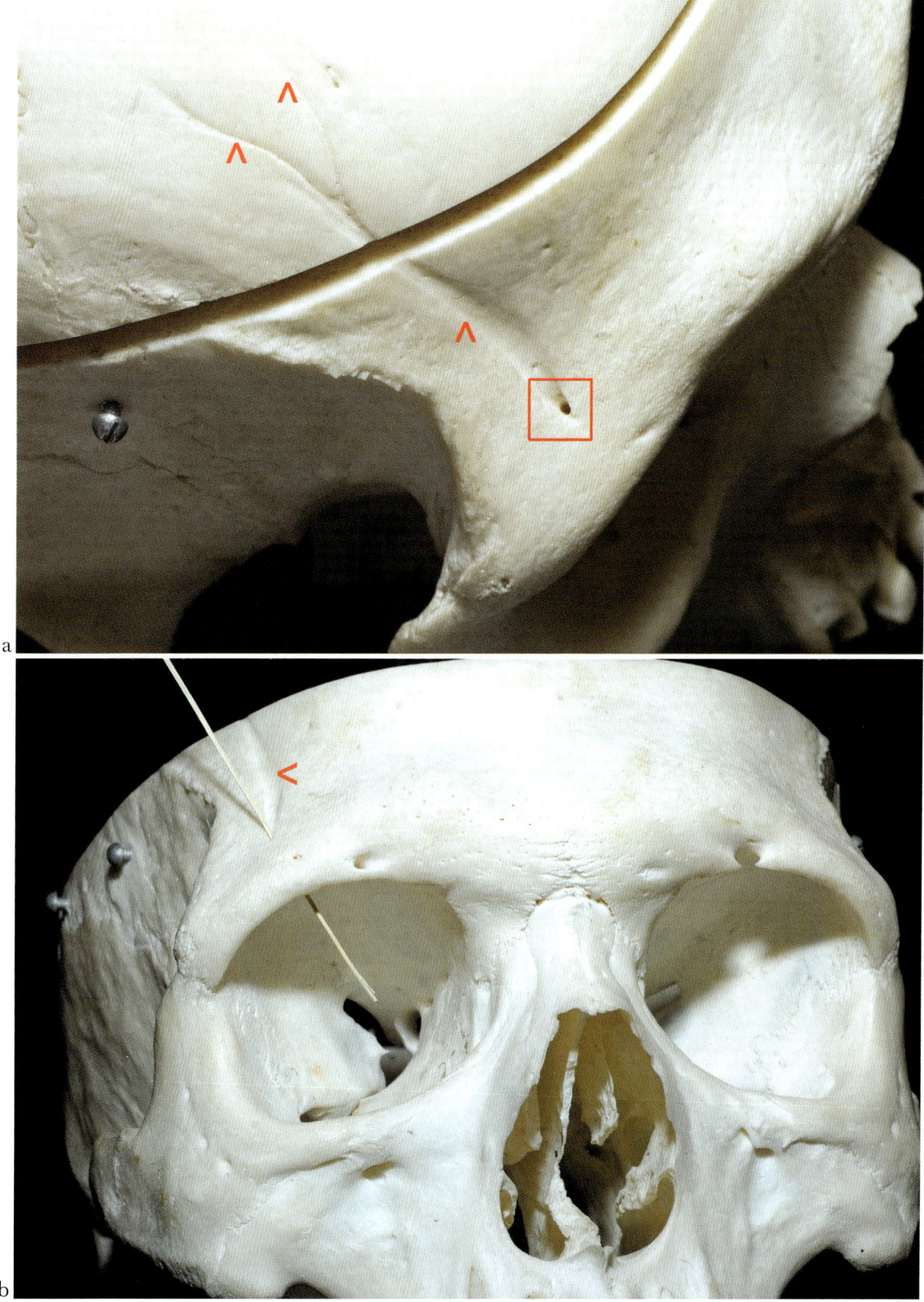

Figure 15a-b. Accessory frontal grooves (∧ and <) and foramen (probe and rectangle) piercing the right orbit of an adult Asian (JABSOM). (a) Right lateral view of these features and (b) frontal view.

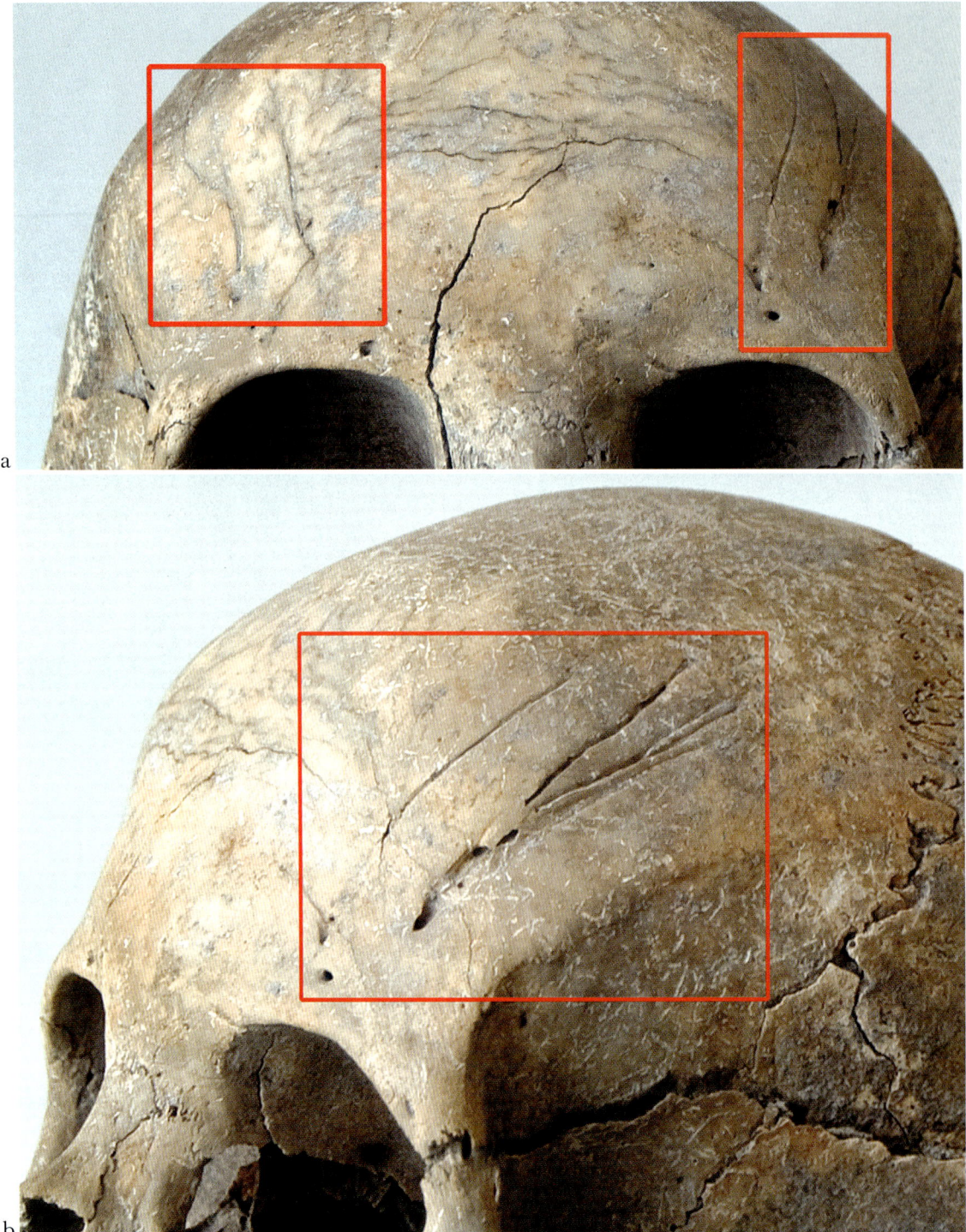

Figure 16a-b. Unusually complex frontal grooves/sulci and foramina transmitting vessels in an adult from Hungary (NHMH 65.6.9 Gyor. Szich). (a) Frontal view of the vertical fracture/breakage in the frontal bone, medial to the right orbit occurred postmortem. (b) Left oblique view showing the morphology of the multiple vessel grooves. Cf. Dixon (1937).

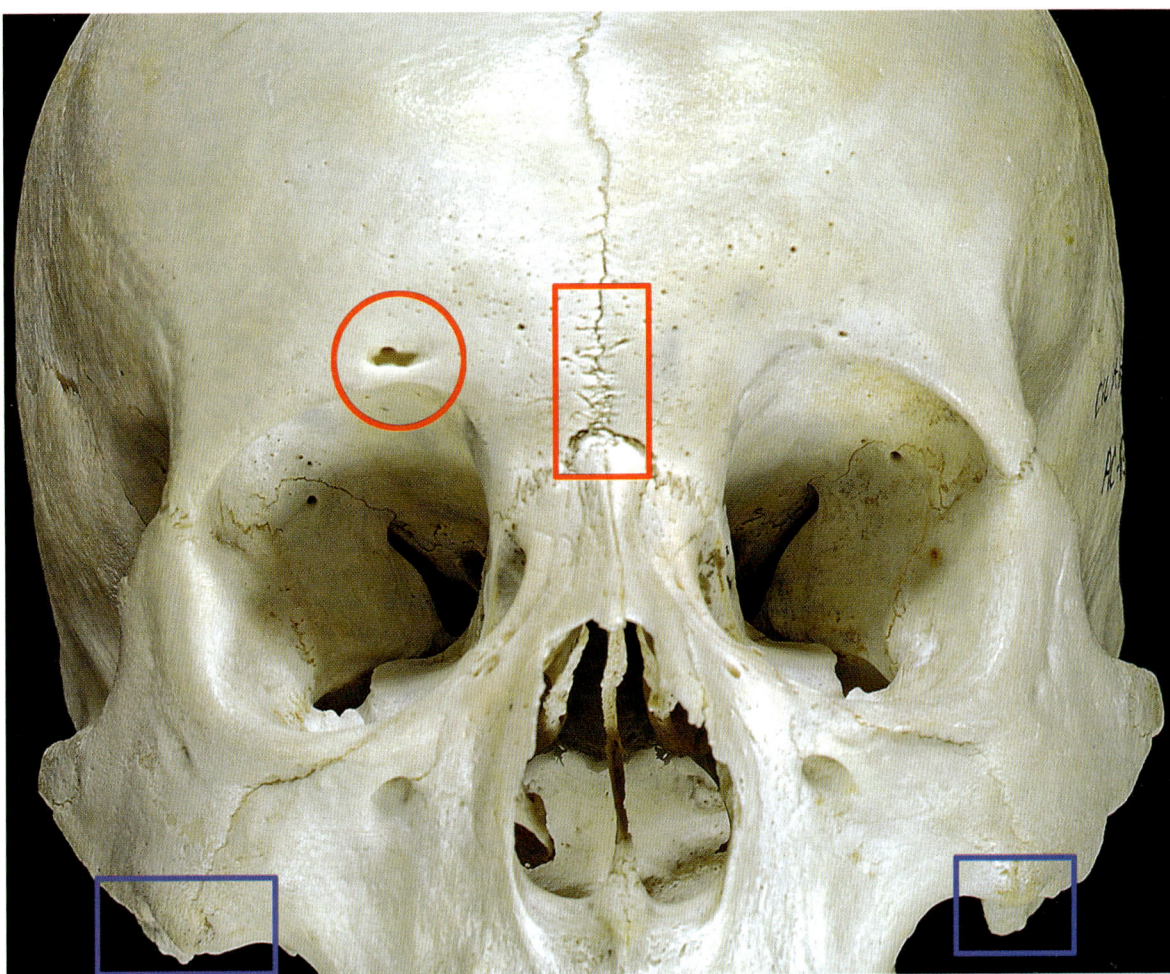

Figure 17. Metopism, supranasal suture and prominent zygomaxillary tubercles (blue) in an adult Thai (KKU). Note the large right supraorbital foramen (circle), glabellar porosity and supranasal suture restricted to a 1 to 2 cm area above Nasion (red rectangle). A radiographic study of 325 healthy patients revealed nine individuals (0.025%) with metopism (Tetradis and Kantor 1999). Common findings. See Dutton (2011) for anatomy of the orbit. Cf. Weinzweig et al. (2003) for discussion of the timing of metopic synostosis. See Yadav et al. (2010) for examples of metopism (frontal suture) in skulls of North India; Vu et al. (2001).

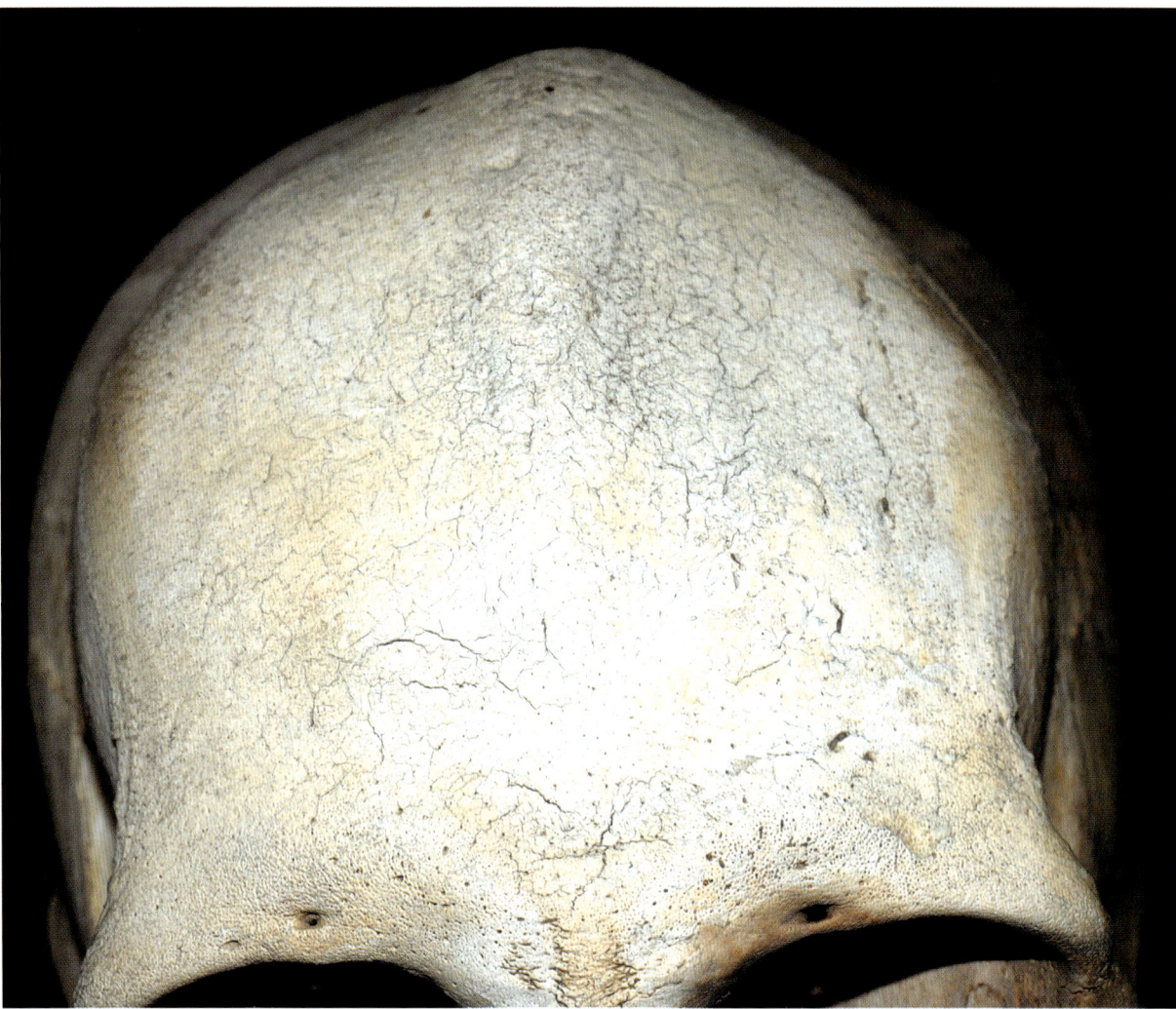

Figure 18. Keeled/steepled frontal bone along the metopic suture in an ancient adult ancient Peruvian male (SI). Frontal or sagittal keeling/steepling, as in this individual, is not necessarily the result of premature or rapid closure of the metopic or sagittal sutures. Keeling may be found in individuals in patent (open) sutures. Uncommon to common finding.

Frontal View of the Skull

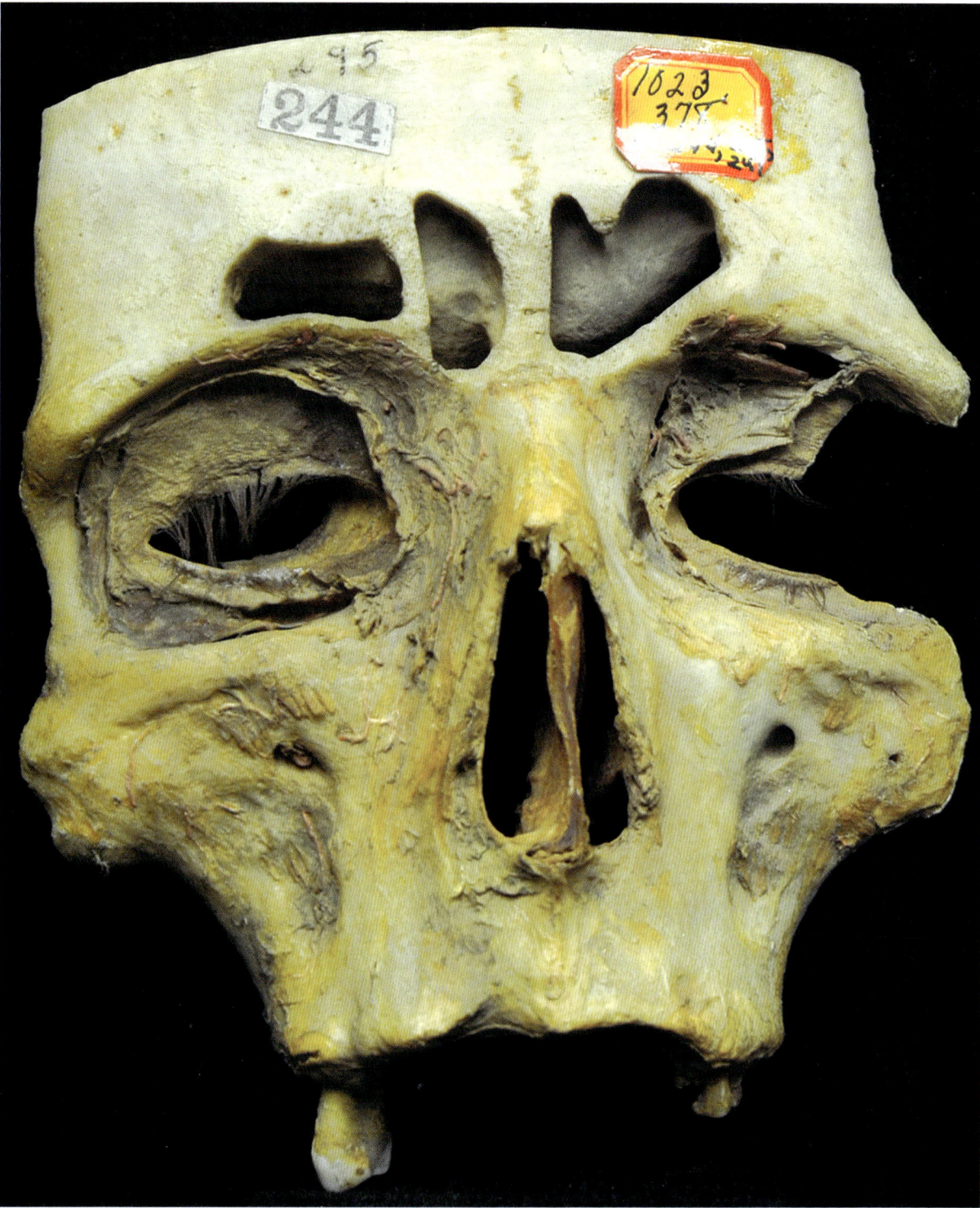

Figure 19. Frontal (external) view of the facial region of an adult showing soft-tissue attachment of the orbits, exposed frontal sinuses, mild deviated nasal septum and an extremely narrow nasal aperture (Mütter Museum 1023.378). See Nambiar et al. (1999) for information on frontal sinus variability.

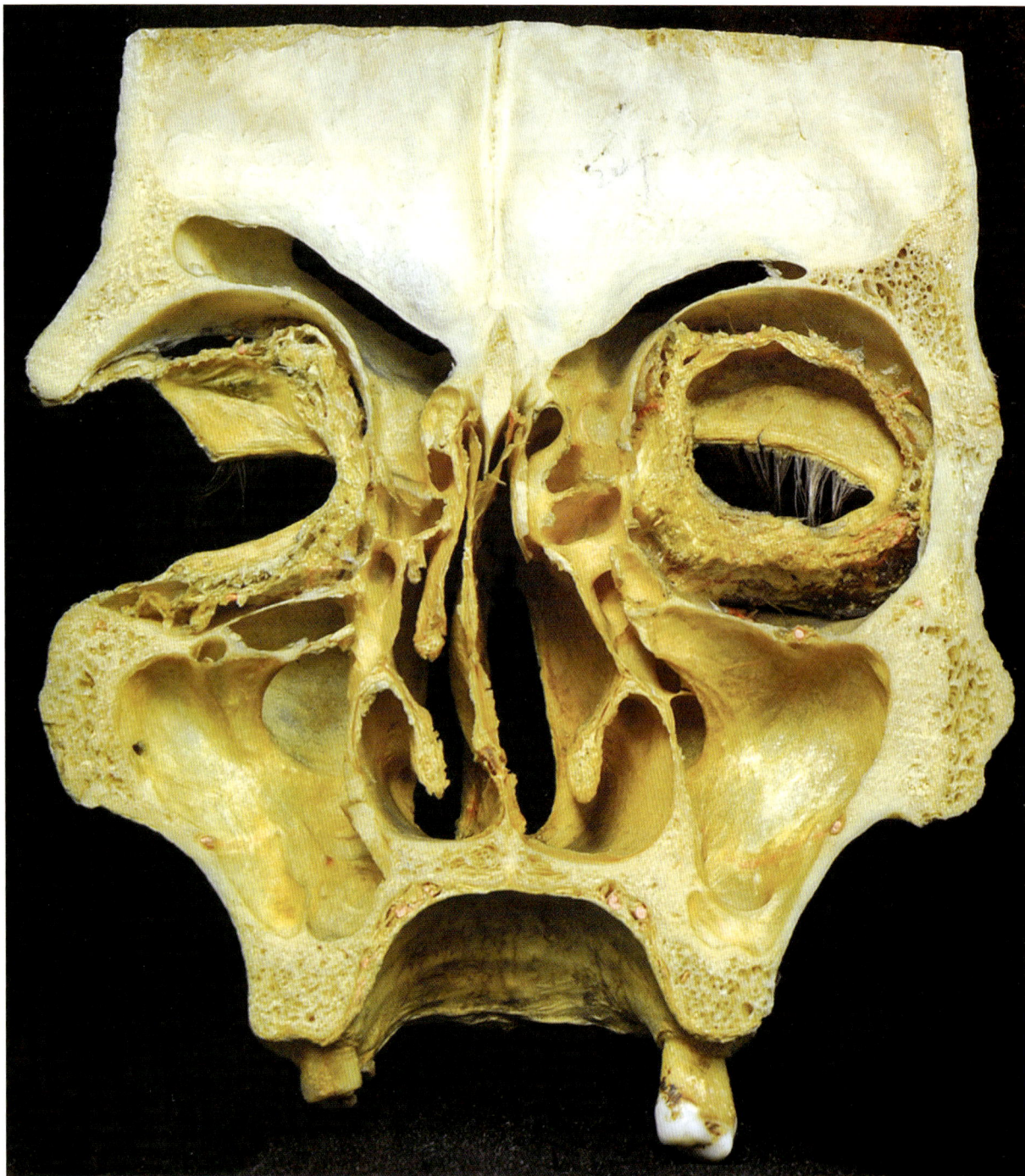

Figure 20. Internal view of the facial region of an adult, showing soft-tissue attachment of the orbits, and exposed frontal, ethmoidal and maxillary sinuses (Mütter Museum 1023.378). Note the yellowish, translucent soft tissue covering the maxillary antrums and the mildly deviated nasal septum, the latter of which is found in 8% of 325 healthy patients (Tetradis and Kantor 1999). See also Ozcan et al. (2008) for variation in turbinates.

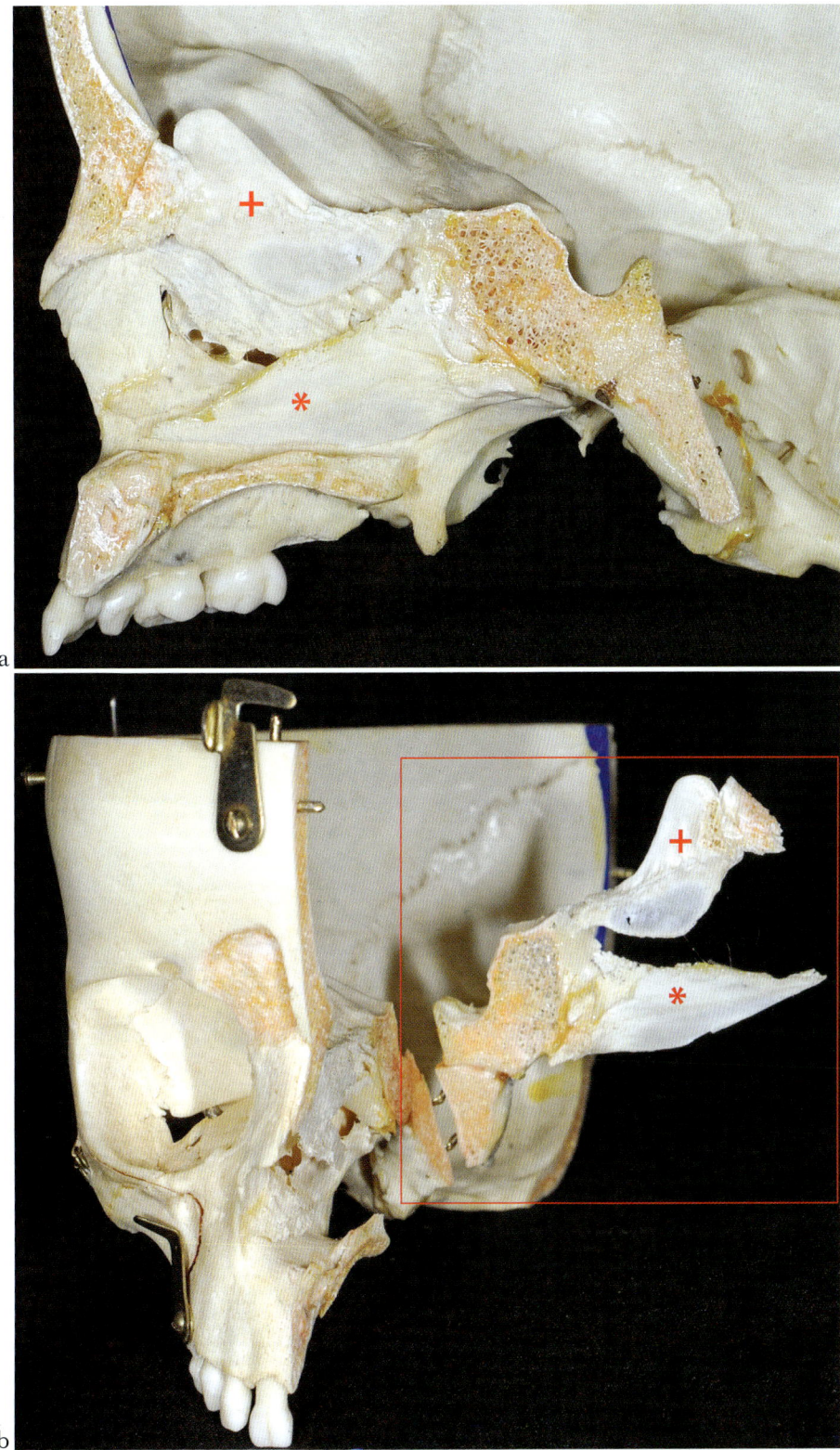

Figure 21a-b. Kilgore International demonstration skull showing the ethmoid bone and vomer in an approximately 5-year-old child (JABSOM). (a) Hinged sagittal section and left oblique view showing the perpendicular plate of the ethmoid bone and crista galli (+) and vomer (*). (b) Left oblique view of the perpendicular plate of the ethmoid bone and crista galli (+) and vomer (*).

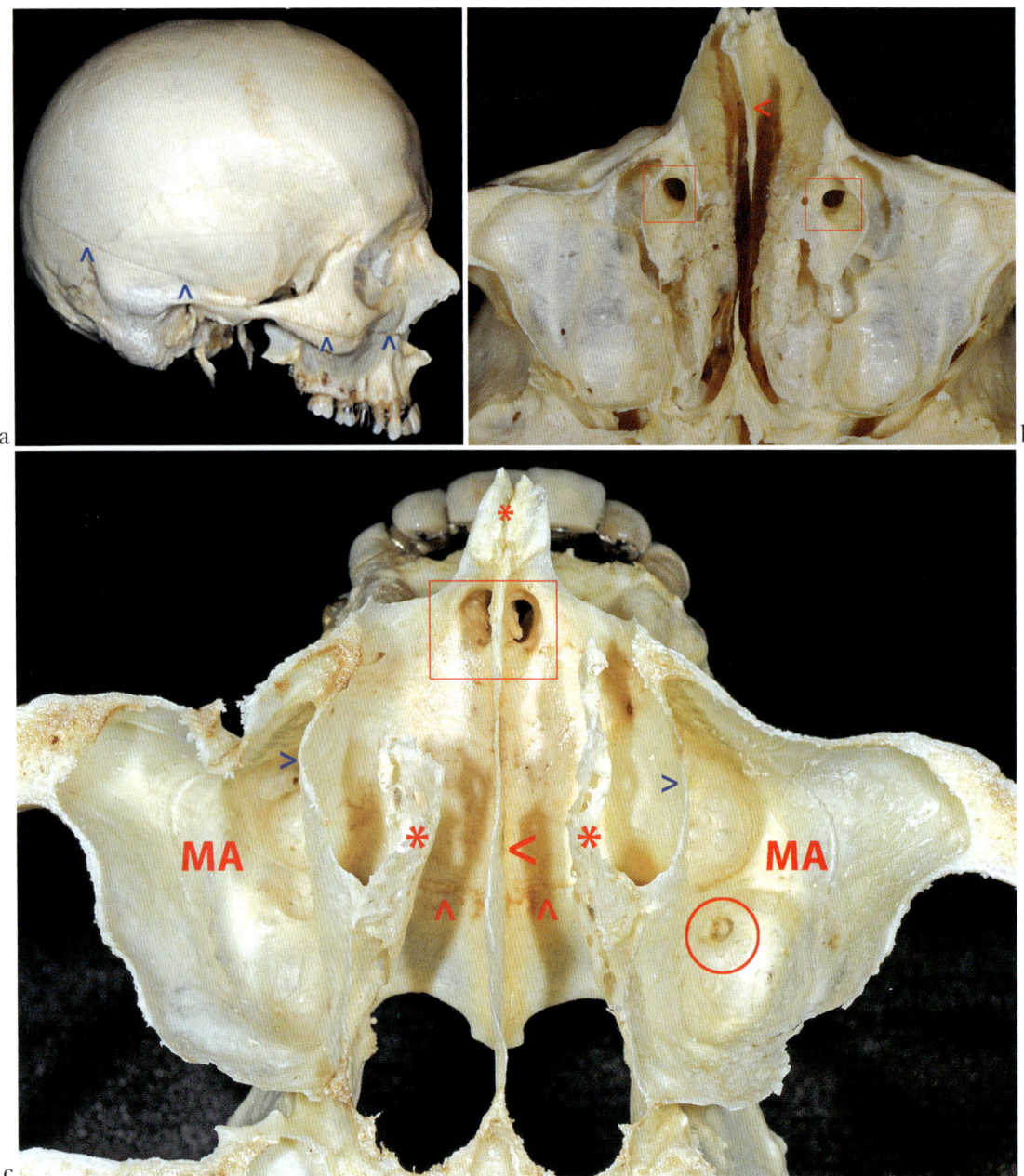

Figure 22a-c. Sectioned adult cranium through the occiptial bone and nasal aperture (934 JABSOM). (a) Right lateral view showing transection (∧). (b) Inferior-superior view through the facial region revealing the nasal septum (<) and nasolacrimal ducts (squares). (c) Superior-inferior view through the facial region showing the anterior nasal spine (*), incisive fossa (rectangle), maxillary antrum (MA), middle turbinate bones (*), transverse palatine suture (∧), the piriform aperture (blue >) and a molar root that has perforated into the right maxillary antrum/sinus (circle).

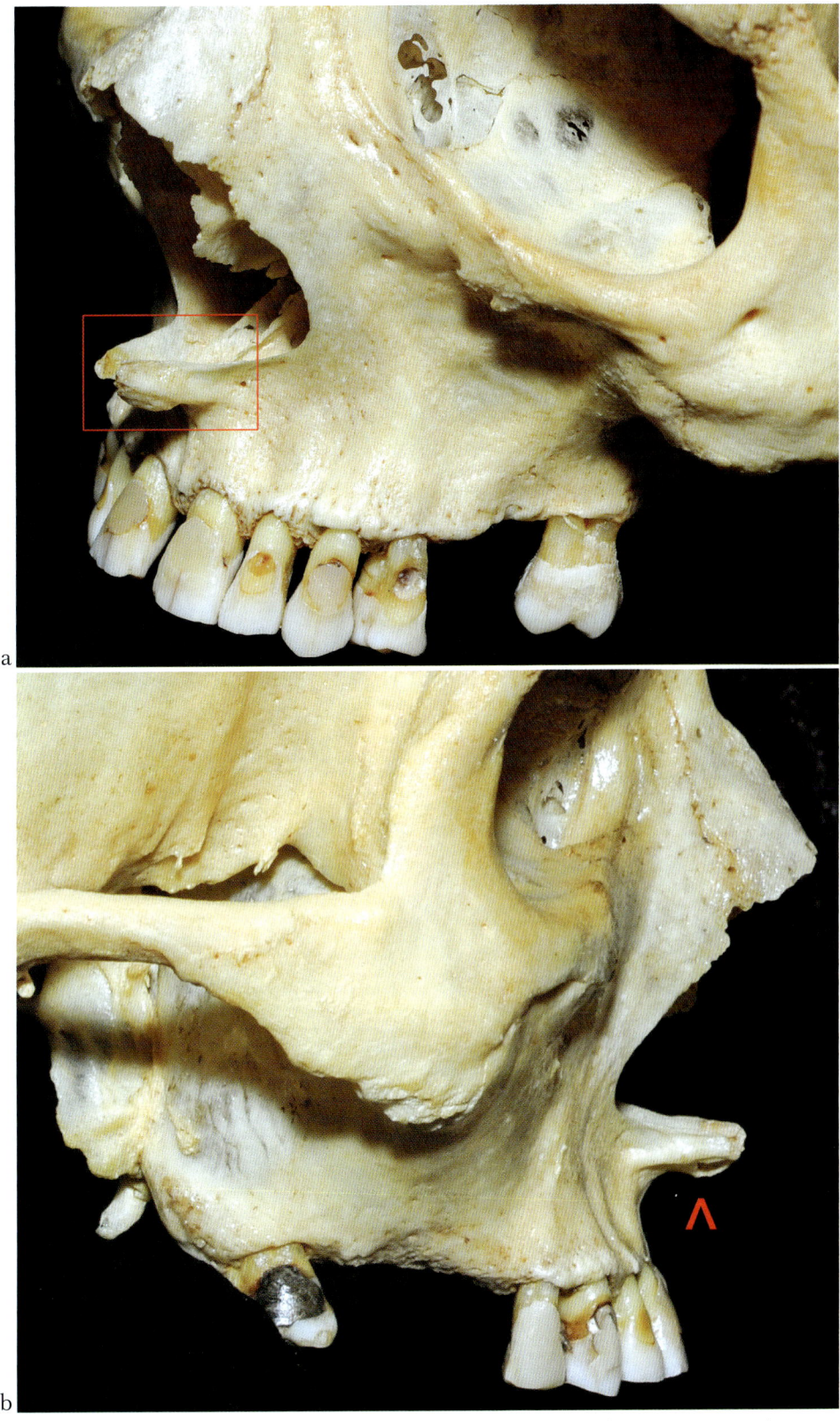

Figure 23a-b. Example of an unusually large anterior nasal spine. (a) Left oblique and (b) right lateral views of an unusually long anterior nasal spine (rectangle and ∧) in a Caucasoid adult (JABSOM).

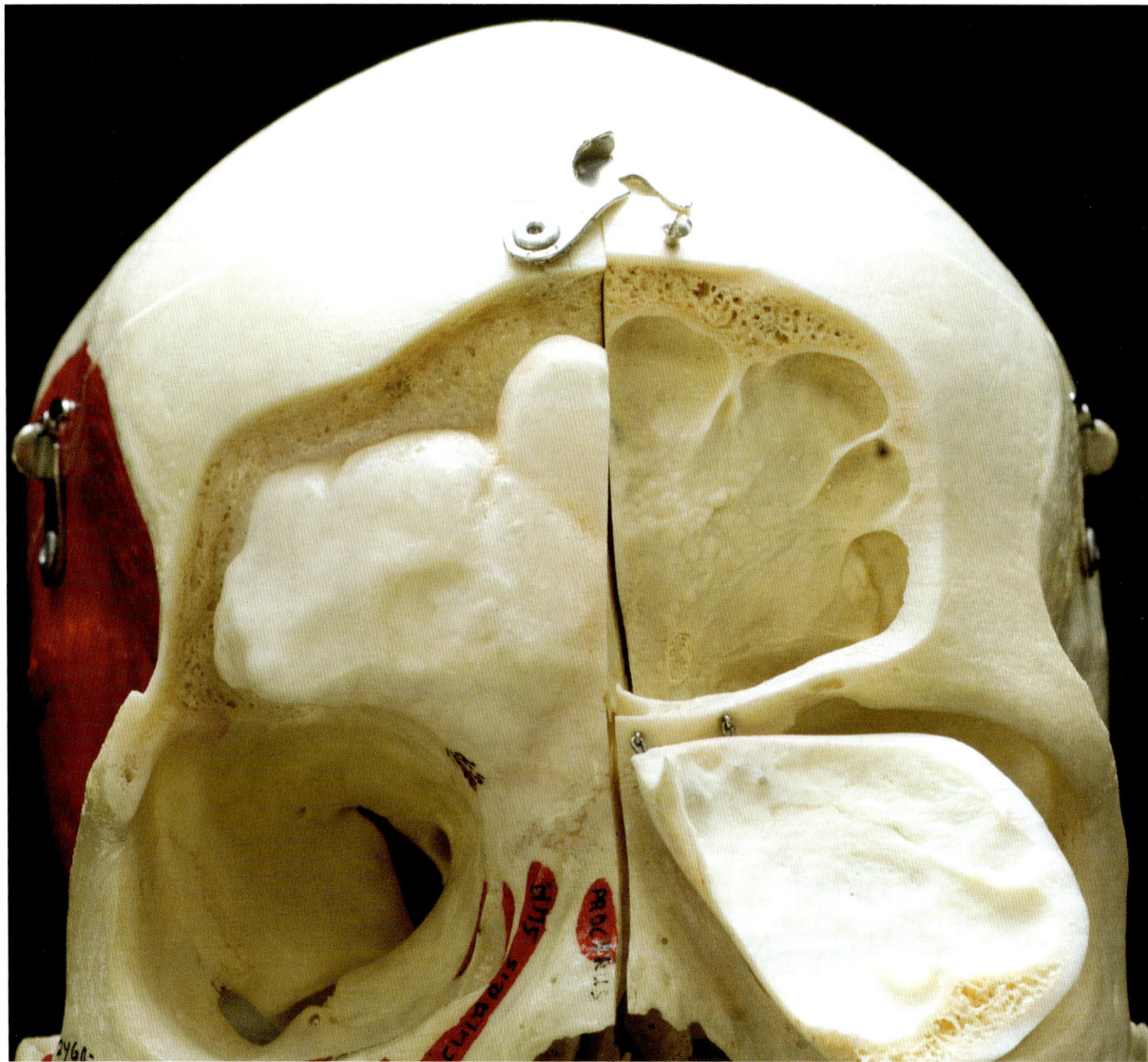

Figure 24. Normal anatomy of the frontal sinuses in an adult Asian (FSA AC049). The left half (anterior table) of the frontal bone has been cut away to expose the inside of the sinuses, while the right half has been removed/sanded to expose the sinuses and the posterior table in their entirety. The frontal sinuses are usually absent at birth and slowly develop, attaining their full size at about 15 years. Symmetry and asymmetry of the frontal sinuses was noted radiographically in 58% and 32%, respectively, of 50 Indian patients (David and Saxena 2010). Bilateral aplasia (absence) of the frontal sinuses were found in two individuals (4%) and unilateral aplasia in three (6%) individuals.

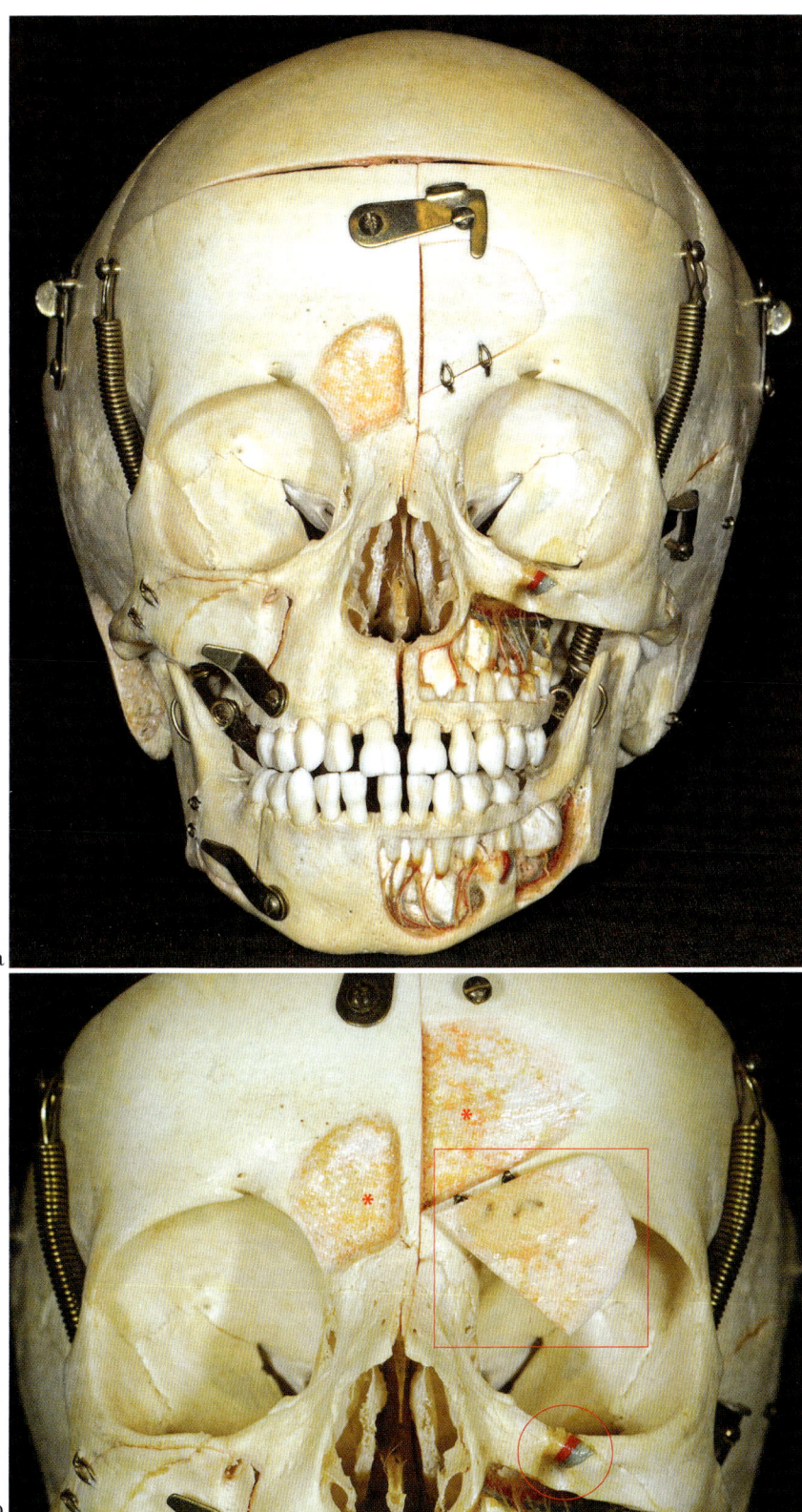

Figure 25a-b. Demonstration skull (Kilgore International) showing normal anatomy in a 5-year-old child (JABSOM). (a) Frontal view showing exposed right frontal sinus and developing teeth in the maxilla and mandible. (b) Close-up showing a bone flap (square) revealing the underlying bone and absence of frontal sinuses or compartments (*) and the neurovascular bundle (circle) through the left infraorbital foramen.

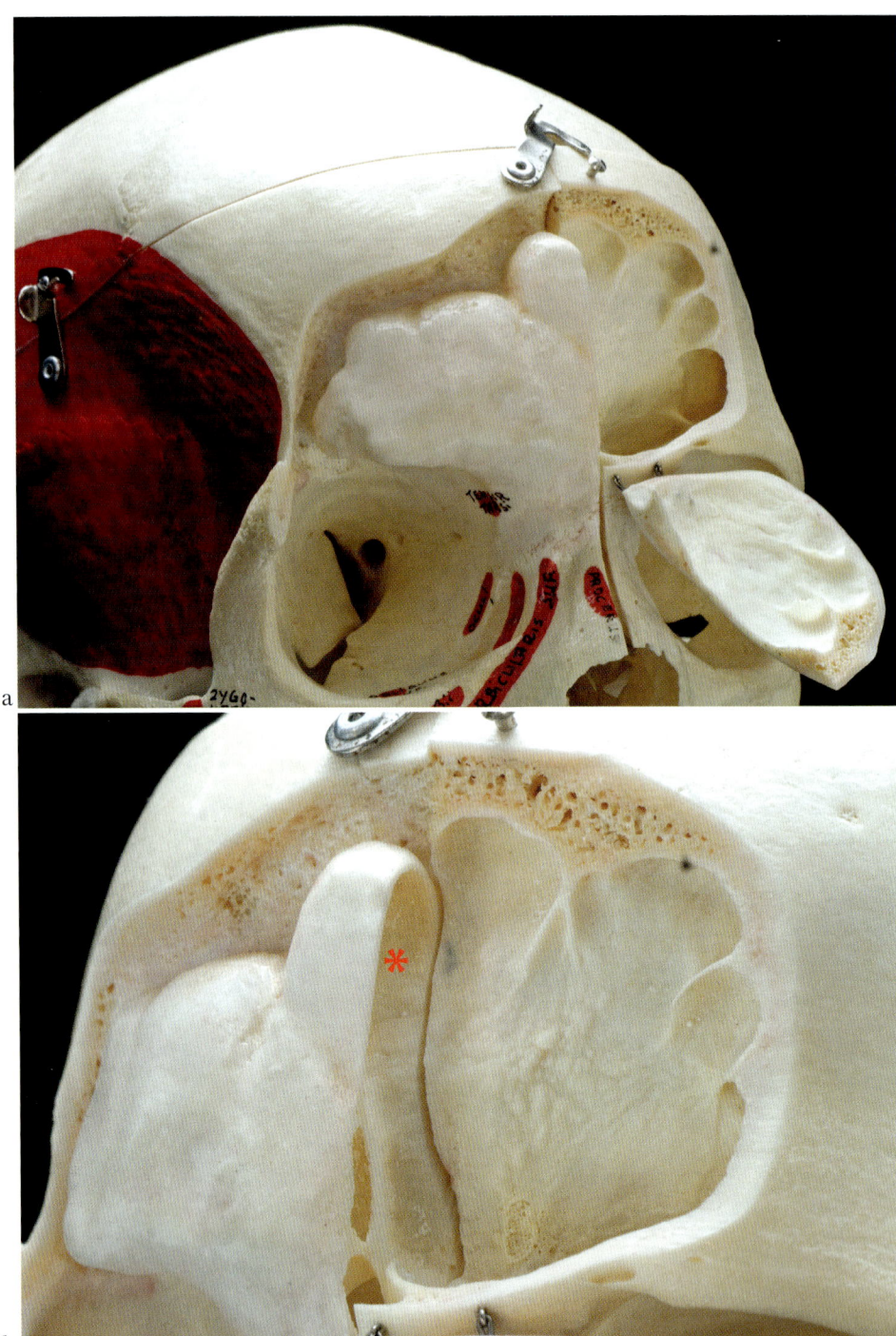

Figure 26a-b. Frontal sinus morphology in an adult Asian (FSA AC049). The left half of the frontal bone has been cut away to expose the inside of the sinuses, while the right half has been removed to expose the sinuses in their entirety. Note that the right sinus is hollow and cavernous (*). (The cranium is sagitally sectioned.) Cf. Aydinhigou et al. (2003) Kondrat (1995); Nambiar et al. (1999); Shankar et al. (1993); and Stilianos et al. (2005).

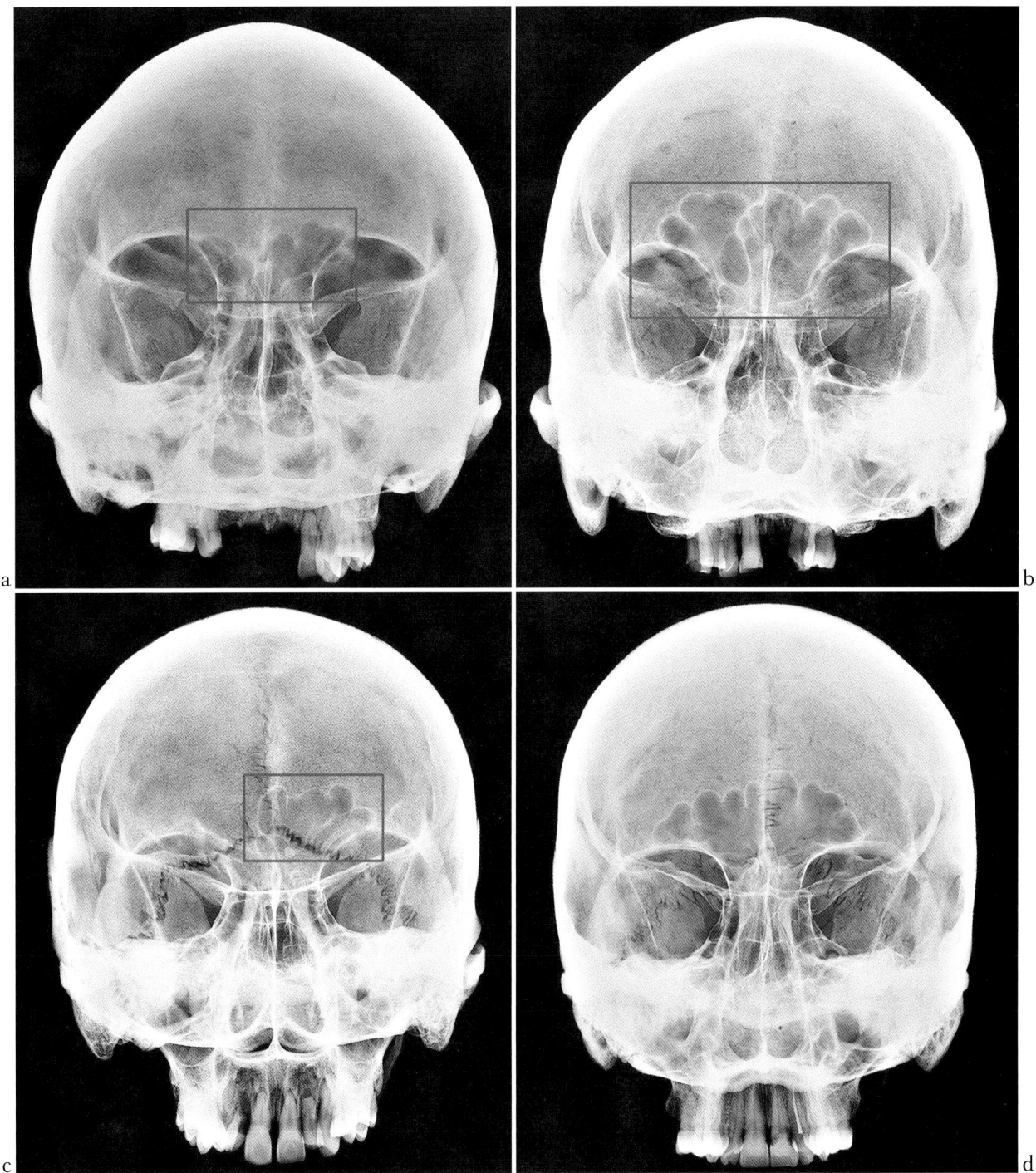

Figure 27a-d. Anterior-posterior X-rays showing variation in adult frontal sinus patterns in four teaching skulls (FSA, by Cortland Sciotto). (a) AC023. (b) AC019. (c) DS008. (d) AC055. See Patil et al. (2012) and Quatrehomme et al. (1996) for discussion on using frontal sinuses for personal identification, and Christensen (2004) on the impact of use by Daubert standards.

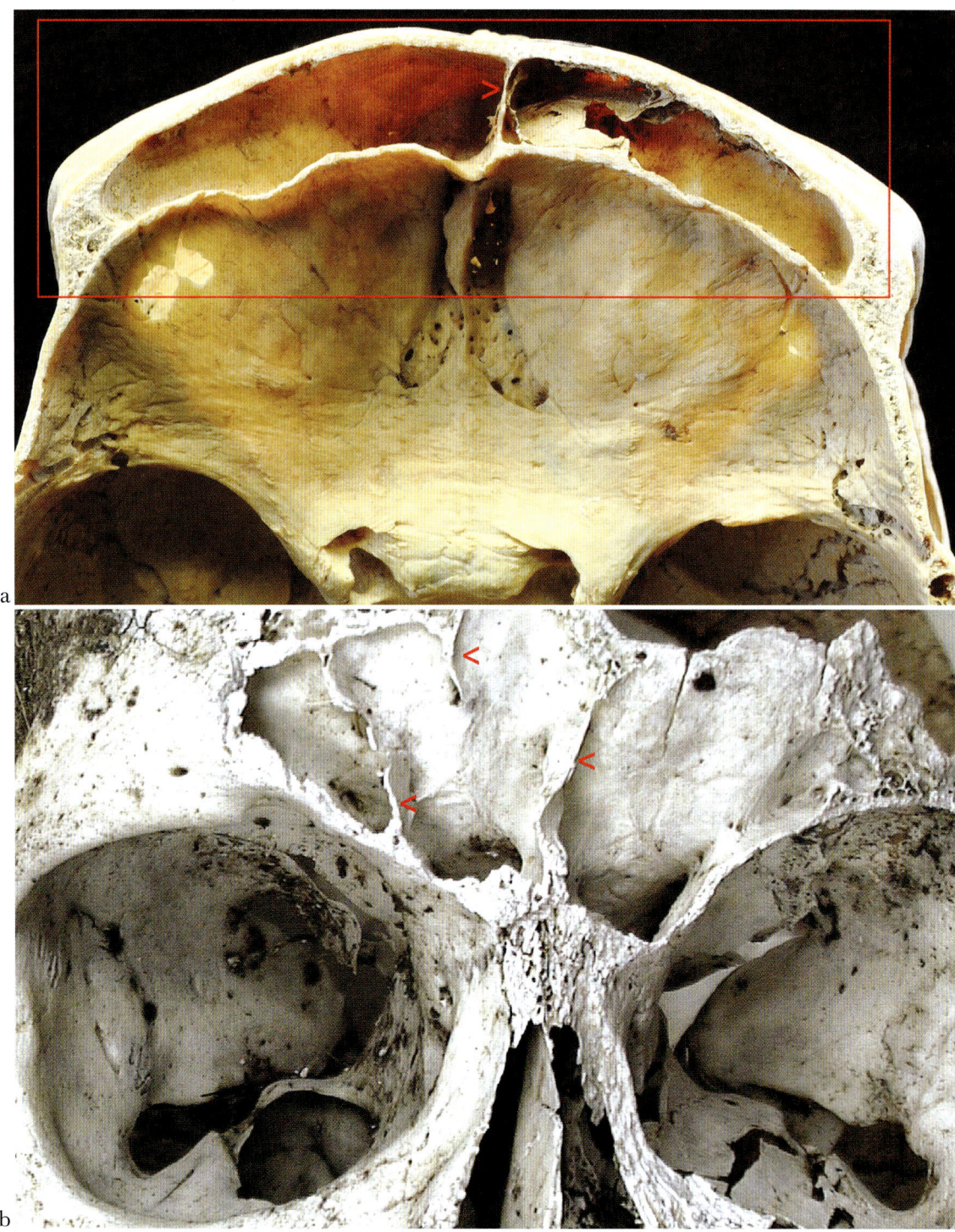

Figure 28a-b. Frontal sinus paterns in two adults. (a) Large frontal sinuses (rectangle), adhering soft tissue and a single bar of bone (>) spanning the outer and inner tables in an adult African (University of Pretoria). (b) Exposed frontal sinuses showing the vertical partitions (<) that separate the sinuses in an adult.

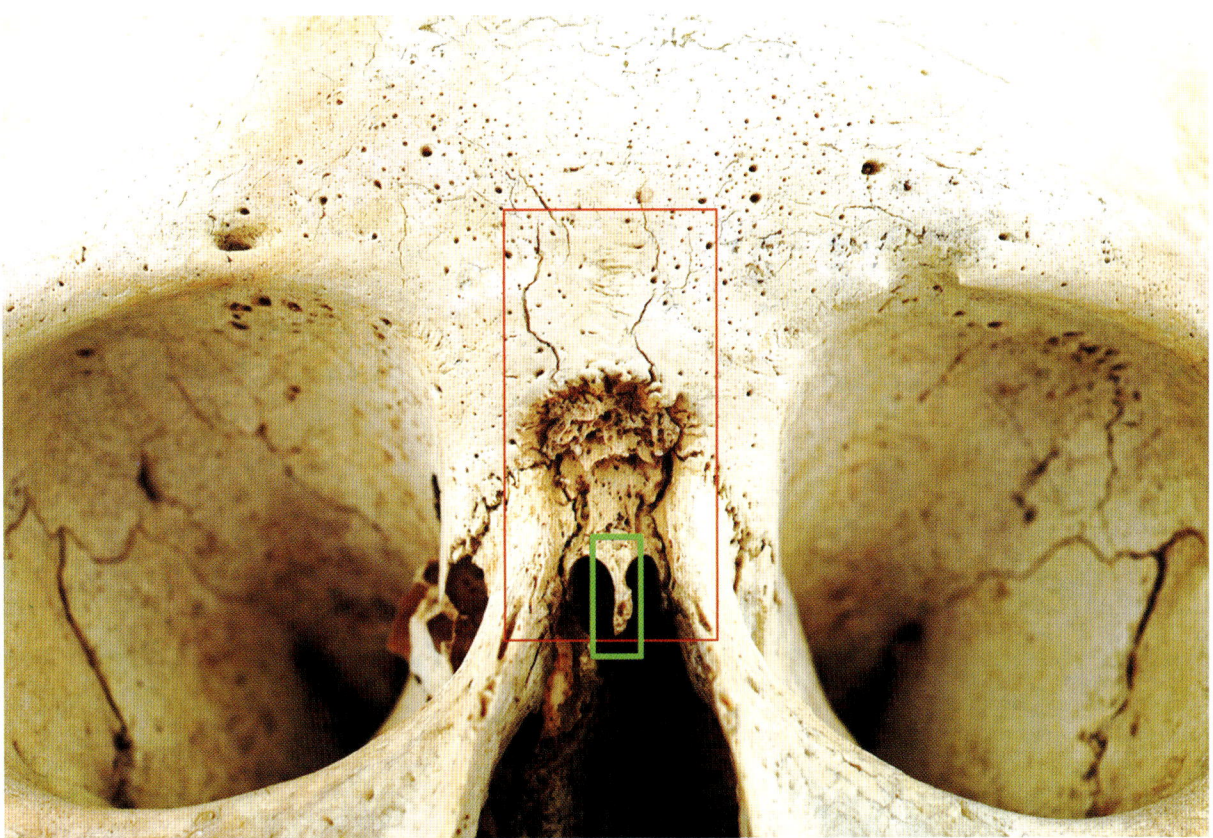

Figure 29. Postmortem breakage resembling downhill skier's tracks (red rectangle) which could be mistaken for the supranasal suture (none present), bilateral cribra orbitalia (pitting) in the upper orbital postmortem loss of the nasal bones resulting in exposure of the frontonasal suture (showing its normal anatomy) with its complex "woody" appearance and portion of the normal nasal spine/nasal spinalis (green rectangle) of the frontal bone in a subadult Thai (KKU). The pitting in the frontal bone is likely the result of osteoporosis rather than vascular impressions.

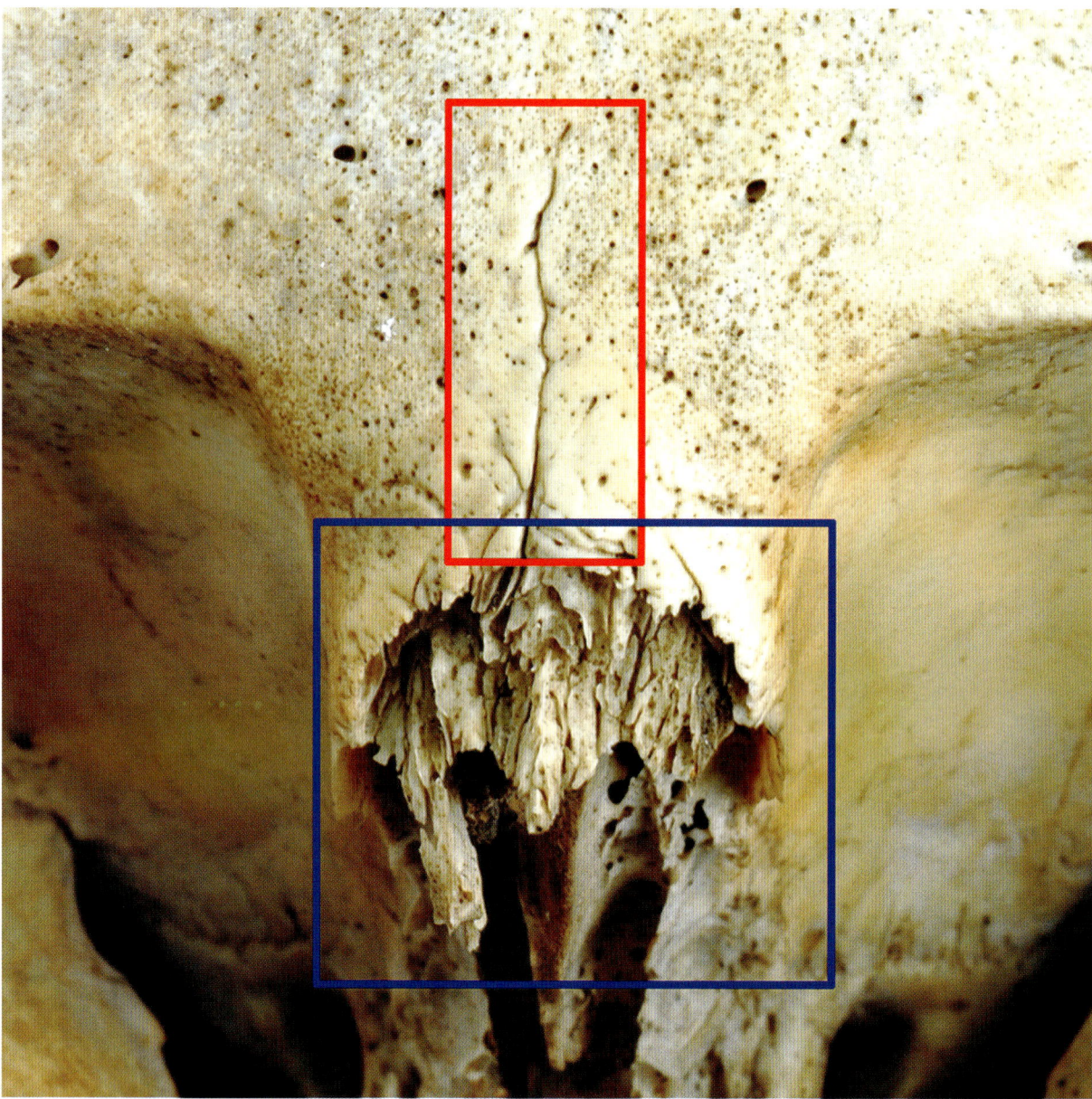

Figure 30. Trace of the metopic/frontal/interfrontal/median frontal suture (red rectangle) in a child, pinpoint porosities (osteoporosis) above and medial to the orbits, and the normal "woody" morphology of the frontonasal suture (margo nasalis) of the frontal bone resembling stalagtites (blue square) (KKU). Common findings.

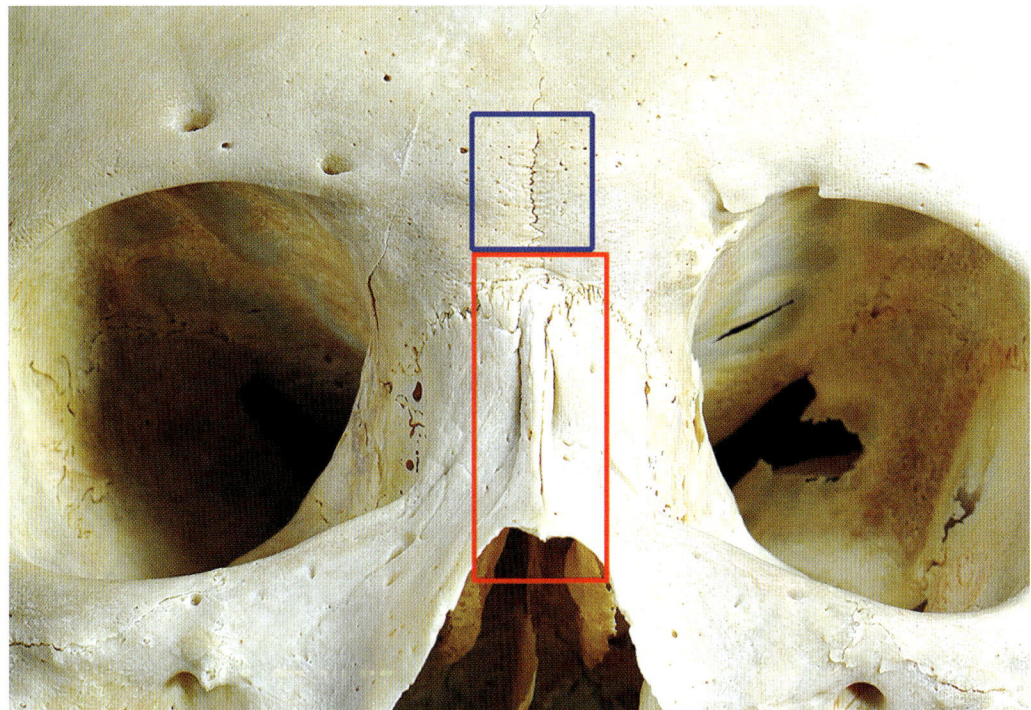

Figure 31. Hypoplastic nasal bones (red) and trace of a metopic suture (blue) (KKU). Hypoplastic nasal bones is an uncommon to rare finding, but common in trisomy 21. Cf. Manning and Singh (1977); Wahby (1903).

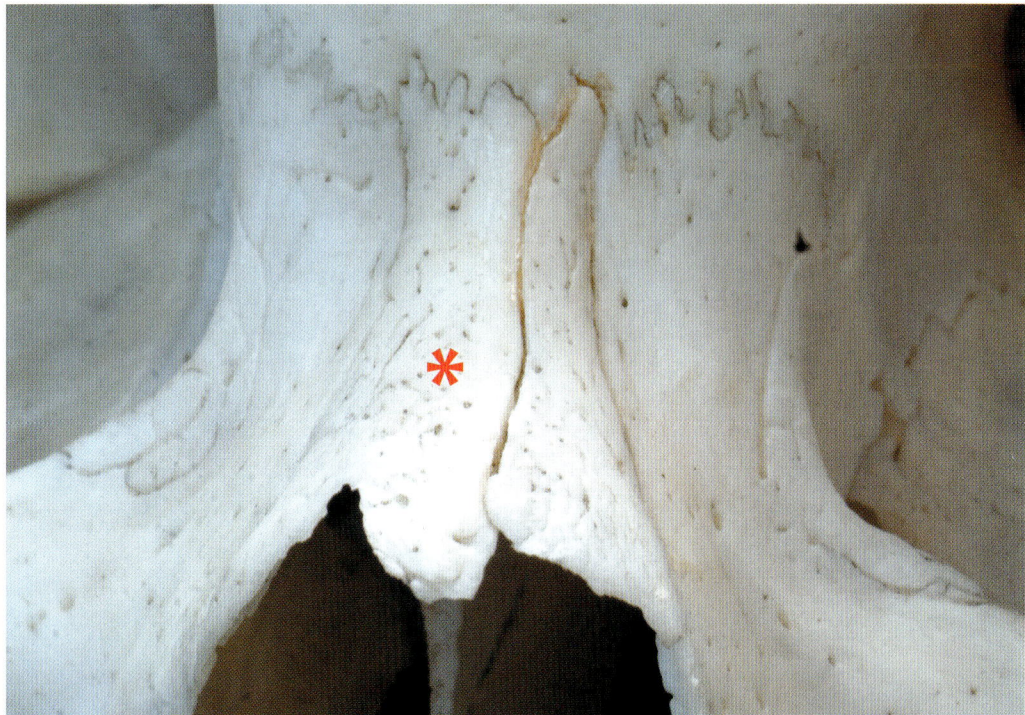

Figure 32. Asymmetrically sized nasal bones in an adult Asian (FSA AC043). Note that the right nasal bone (*) is wider and longer than the left nasal bone. Common finding.

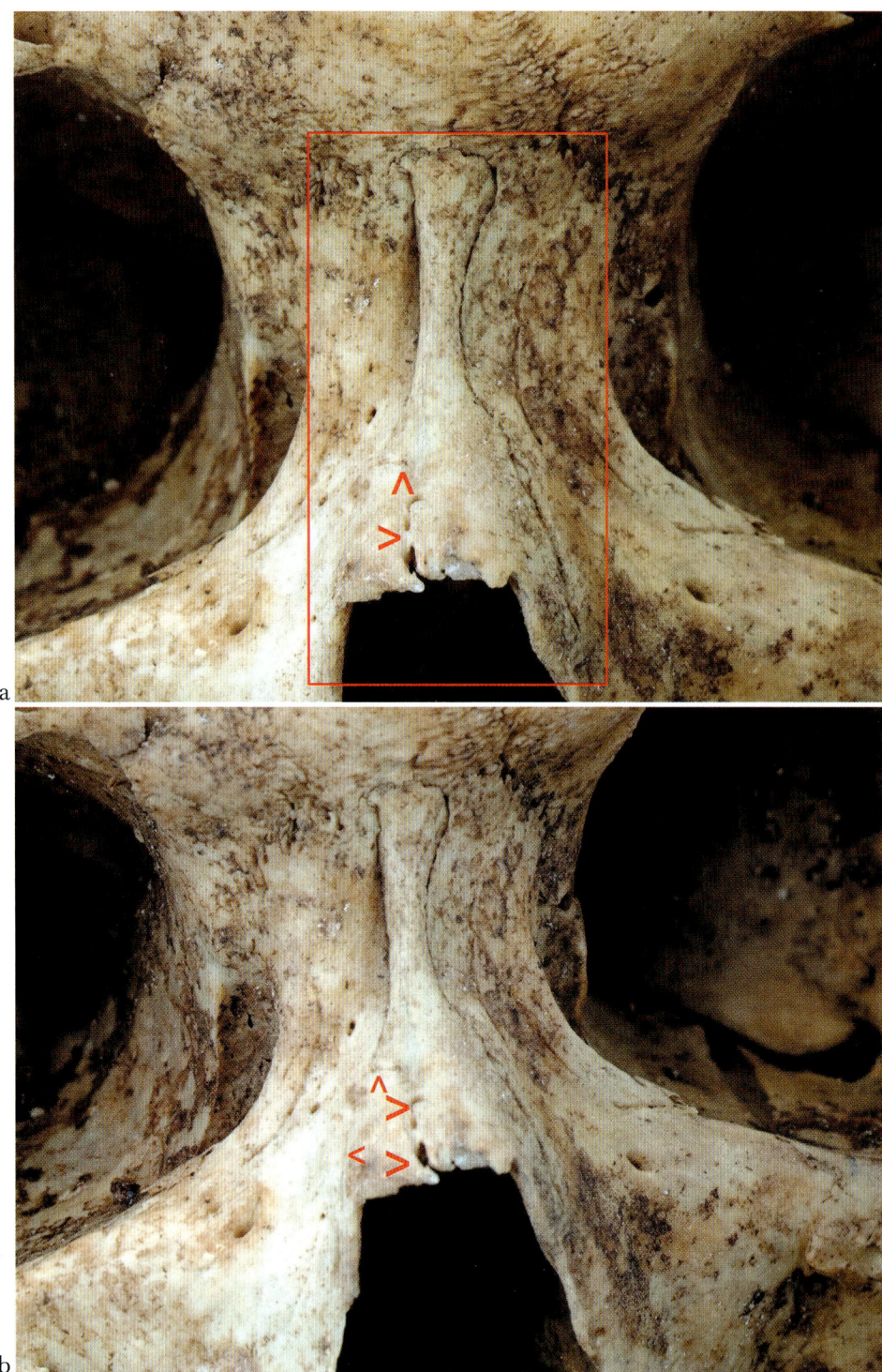

Figure 33a-b. Possible agenesis of the right nasal bone. (a) Fractured and healed nasal bones and possible agenesis of the right nasal bone. Single left nasal bone with probable fracture (∧ and >) in a 60-year-old Thai male (CMU 23 53). A portion of the right margin of the left nasal bone has obliterated (<) but is faintly visible. The right nasal bone appears to be congenitally absent (agenesis/aplasia), an uncommon to rare condition. (b) Right oblique view showing fracture (>) and right margin of the left nasal bone (<).

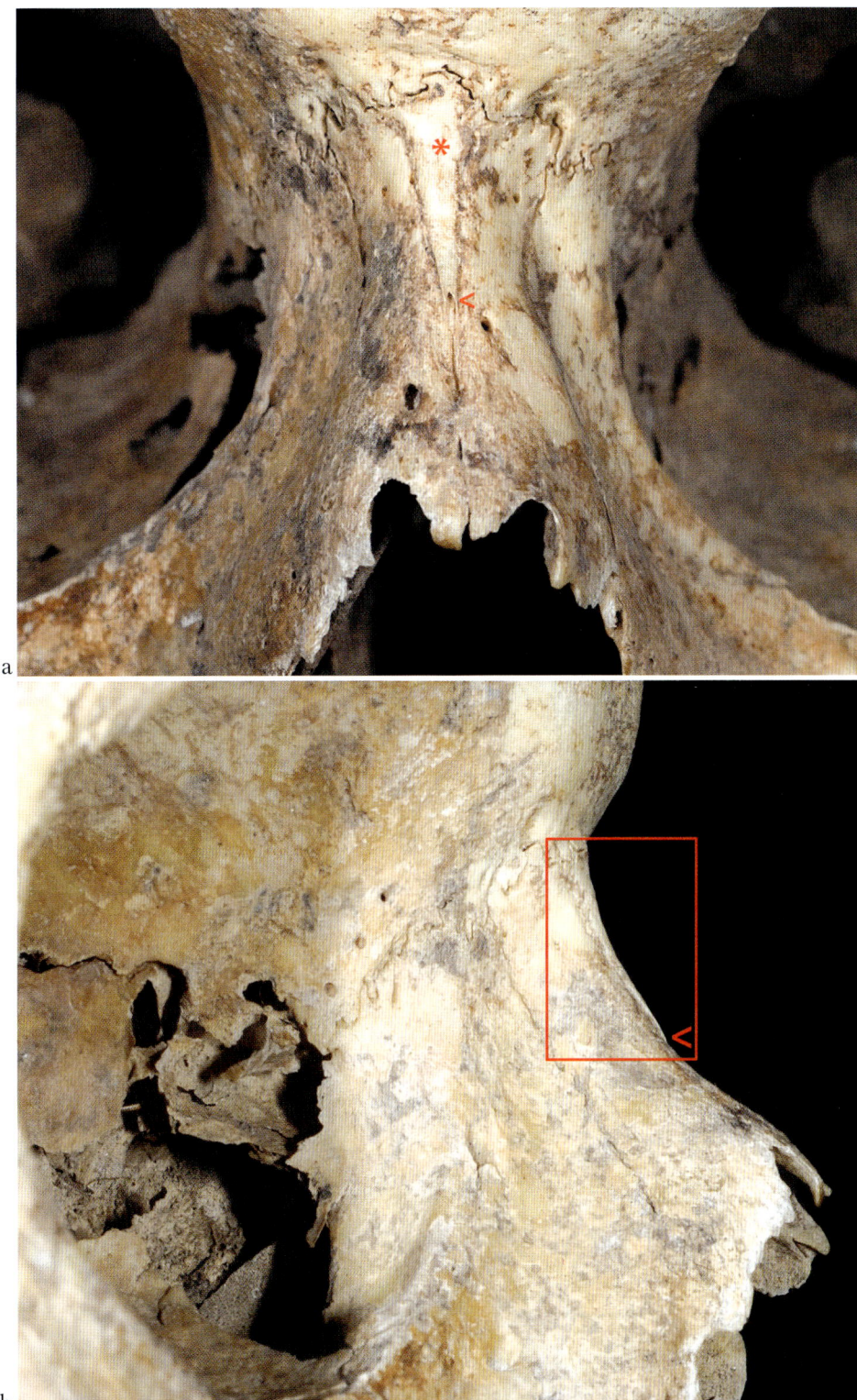

Figure 34a-b. Possible tripartite nasal bone (CIL). (a) Frontal view of possible V-shaped internasal bone (*), sometimes called tripartite nasal bones, in a young adult male. Note the small tunnel (<) formed by the internasal suture running beneath this accessory bone. (b) Right lateral view illustrating that the possible internasal bone (rectangle) is raised (<) above the nasal bones. Uncommon to rare trait.

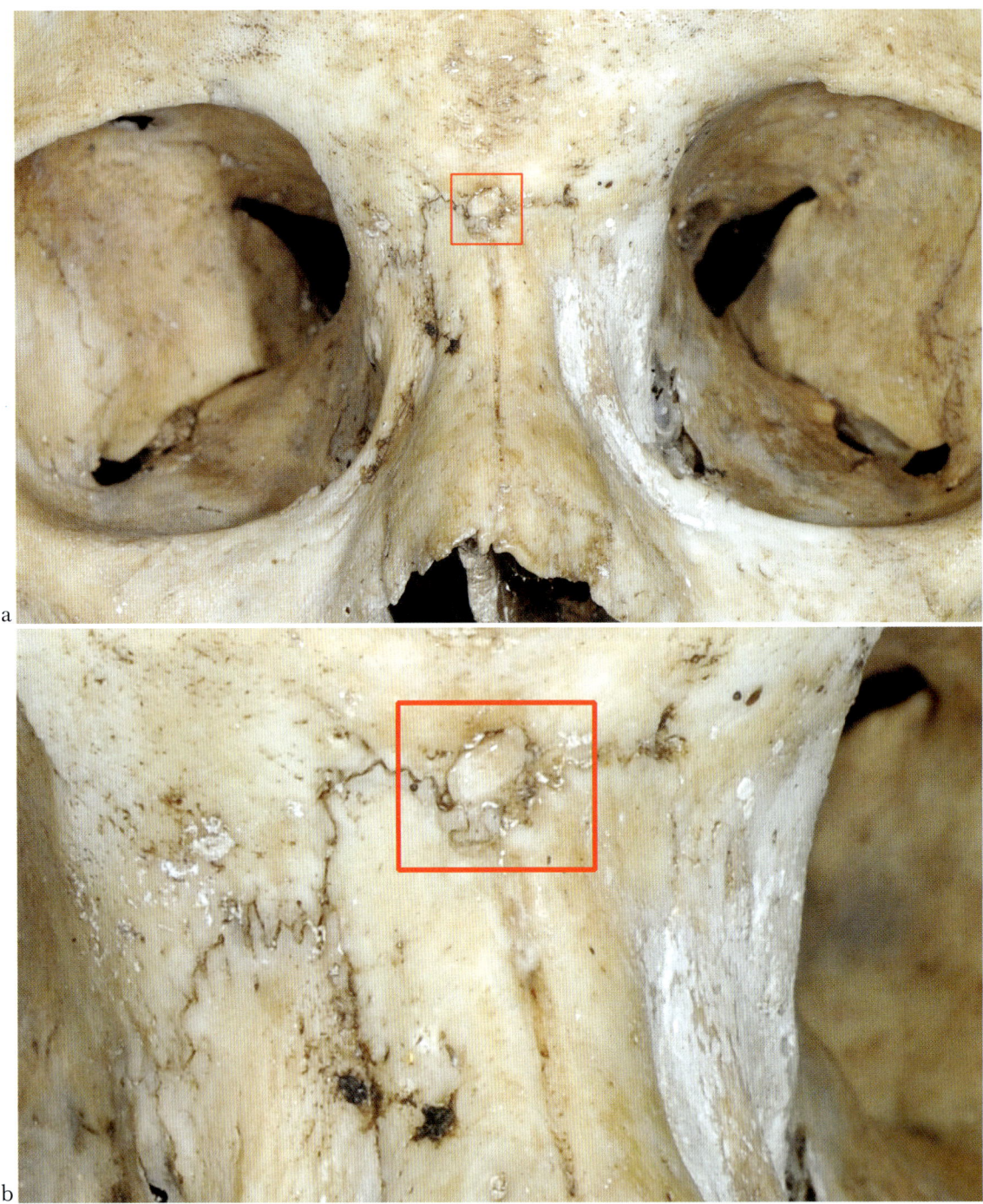

Figure 35a-b. Nasofrontal or metopic ossicle. (a) Frontal view of a small nasofrontal or metopic ossicle (square) situated above Nasion in an adult Thai (KKU A4 106). (b) Close-up of the ossicle showing that it forms a separate island of bone. Uncommon to rare trait.

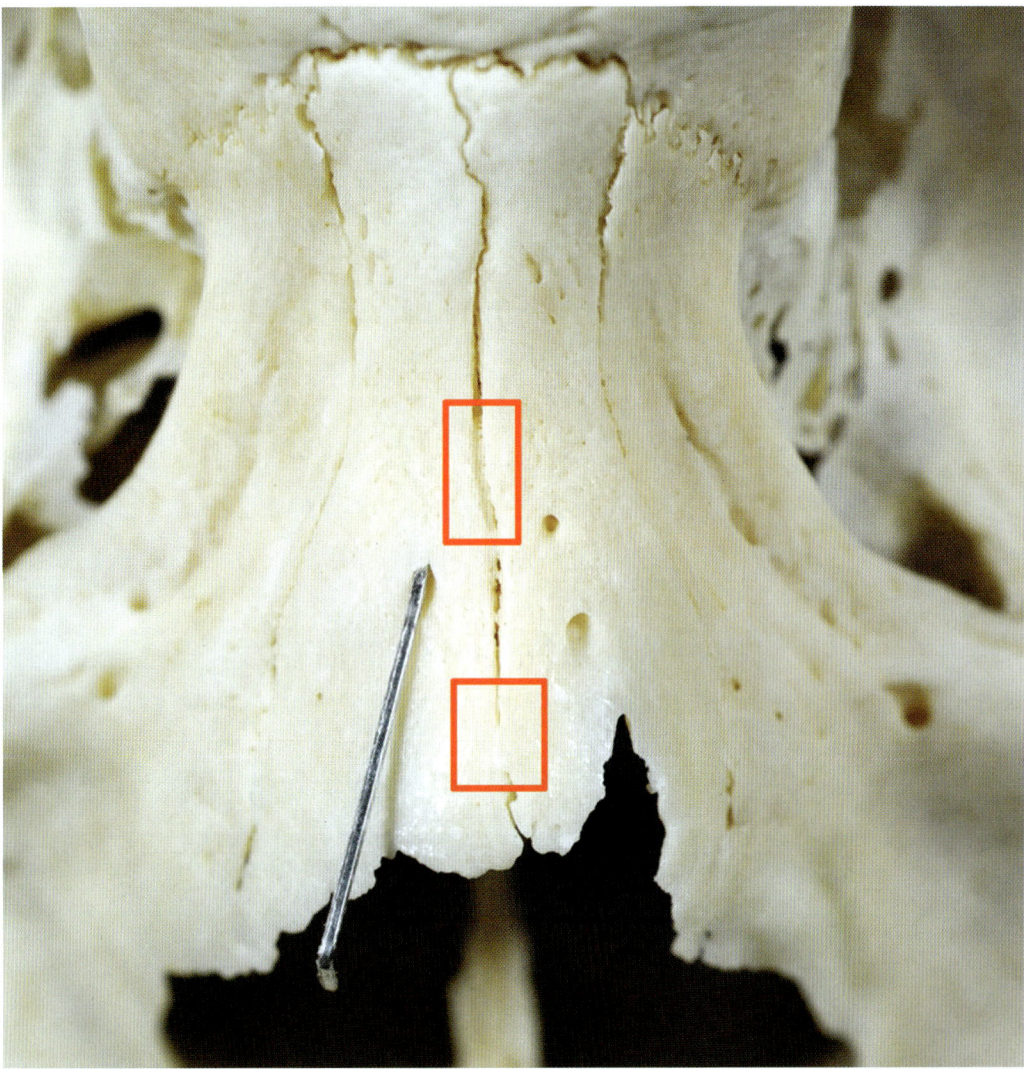

Figure 36. Double foramina in the left nasal bone and a single foramen in the right nasal bone of an adult Thai male (KKU). The wire inserted into the right foramen reflects the steep orientation of the foramen as it courses upward through the right nasal bone. Note the jagged and scalloped, but normal, non-articular edges of the nasal bones and obliteration and bridging of portions of the internasal suture (red square). Preliminary analysis suggests that the amount or pattern of obliteration of the nasal bone sutures may reflect age at death. Common findings. Cf. Hauser and DeStefano (1989).

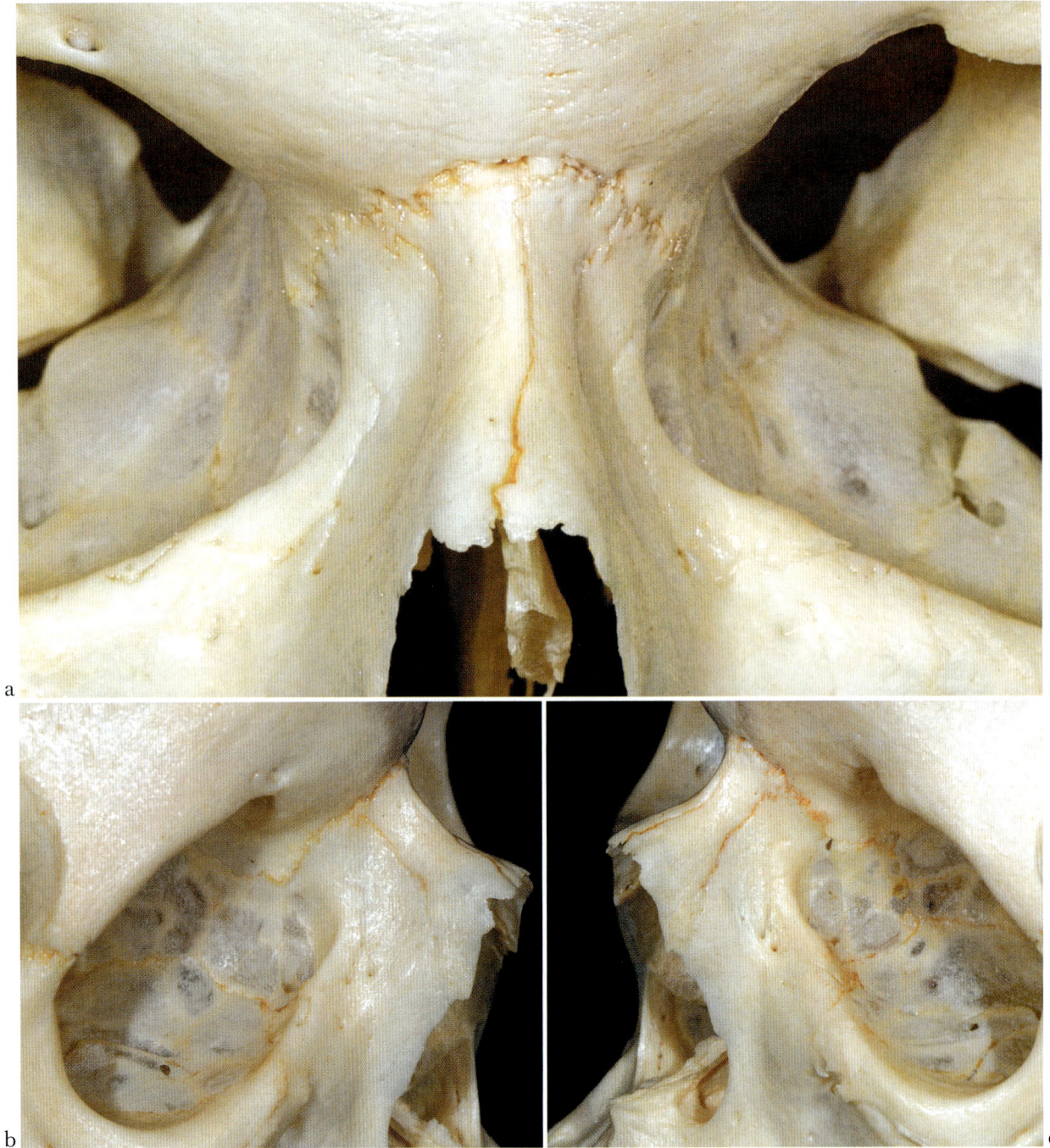

Figure 37a-c. Absence of nasal bone foramina in Thai adult (1134 JABSOM). (a) Frontal view showing absence of foramina in the nasal bones. (b) Right oblique and (c) left oblique views showing absence of foramina in the nasal bones. Note that the bones of the orbits are extremely thin/translucent.

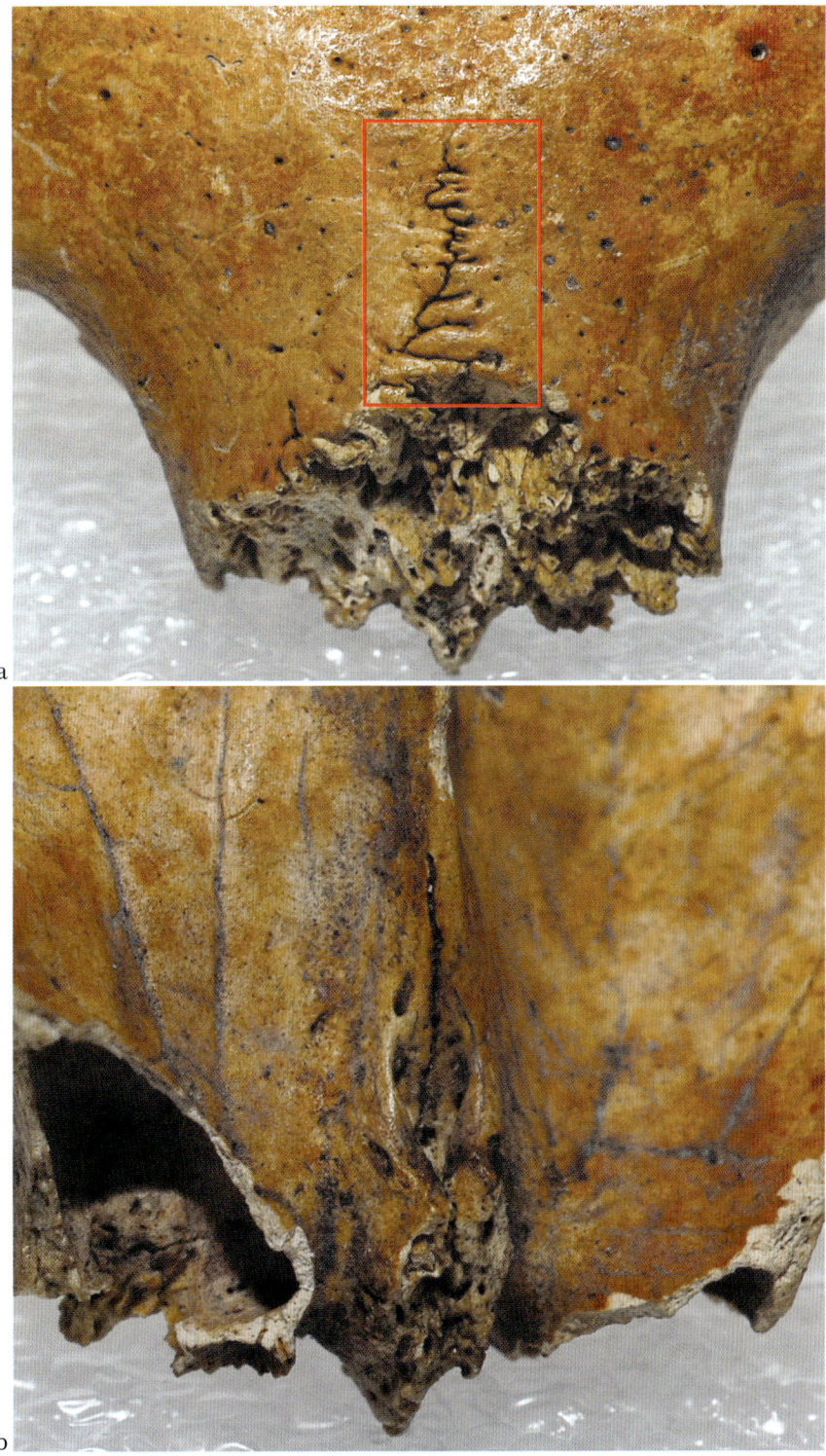

Figure 38a-b. Supranasal suture (SNS) in a teenager. (a) Ectocranial and (b) endocranial views of the supranasal suture. The jagged and horizontal nature of the suture ectocranially is represented by a more simple and straight articulation endocranially. The hollow cavernous areas are the frontal sinuses and the metopic suture superior to the SNS has fully obliterated. Normal anatomy.

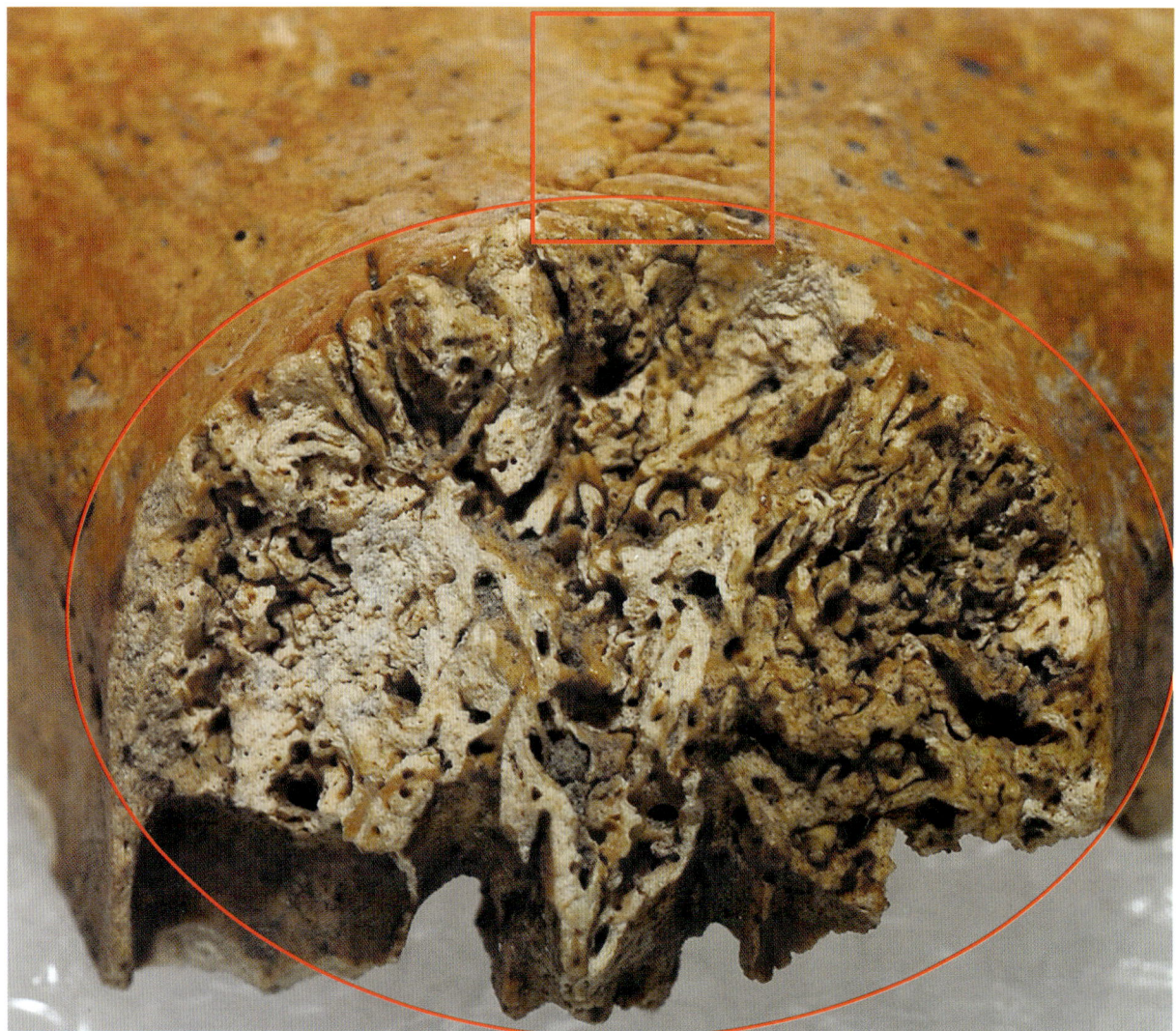

Figure 39. Inferior close-up view of the supranasal suture (square) and nasofrontal suture (oval) in a teenager. Note the width and depth of the nasofrontal suture as well as its tortuous morphology for distributing biomechanical stresses from the maxilla to the frontal bone. Normal anatomy in subadults.

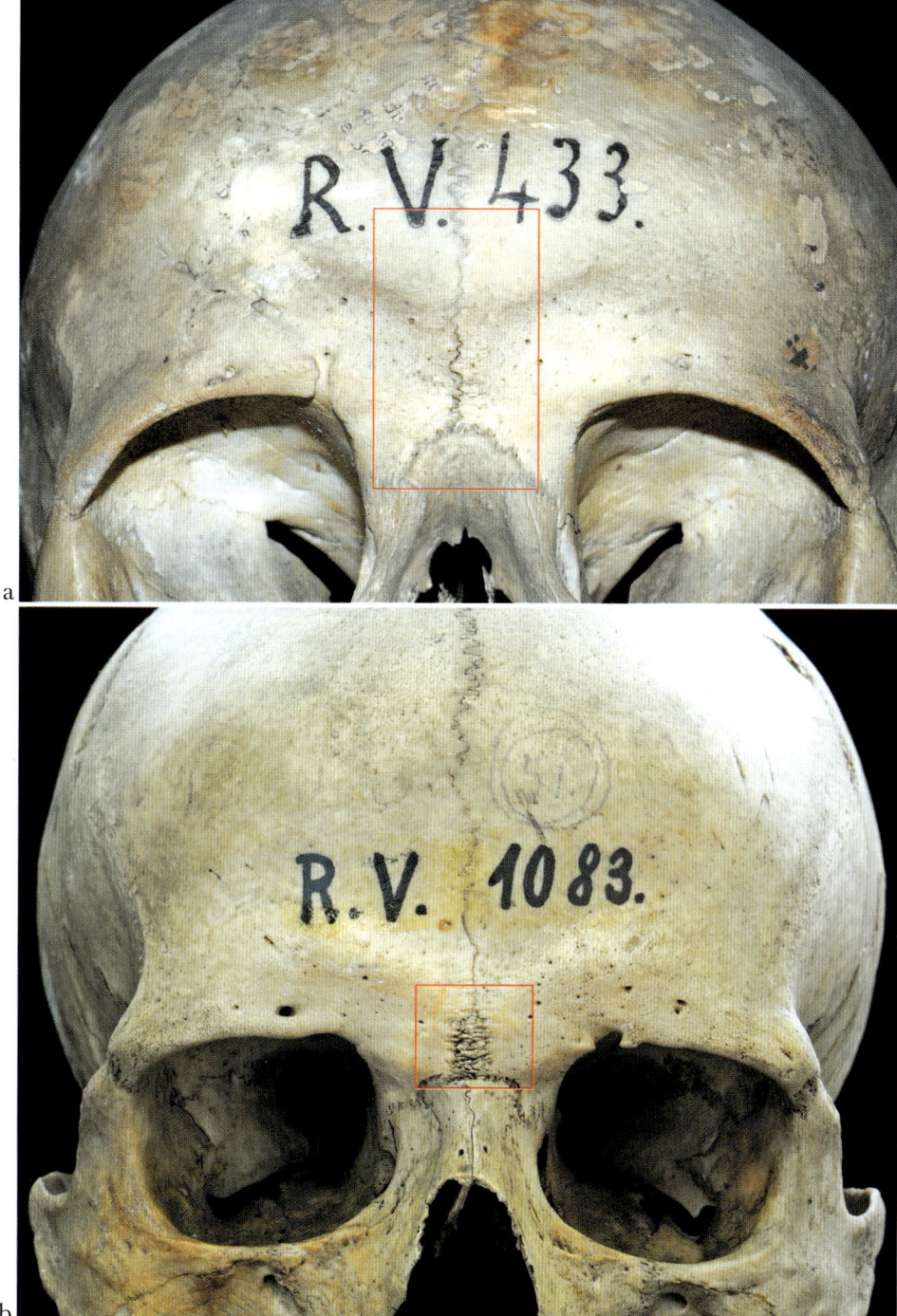

Figure 40a-b. Metopic suture and a supranasal suture (SNS) in two adults. (a) Relatively simple metopic suture (rectangle; RV433) without a SNS, compared to (b) an open metopic suture and complex supranasal suture (square) situated immediately superior to Nasion (RV1083). The metopic and supranasal sutures have been reported as two separate sutures (Hauser and DeStefano 1989) that form at different times in subadults and obliterate at different ages. Remnants of the SNS are often misidentified as a "trace" of the metopic suture. The metopic suture typically obliterates by about age 8 months, but as late as 2 years or older, while the SNS often does not obliterate until adulthood. Wood (2012) found a correlation between the presence of the SNS, maturation of the frontal bone in males and the size of the superciliary arch (browridge). Cf. Vu et al. (2001).

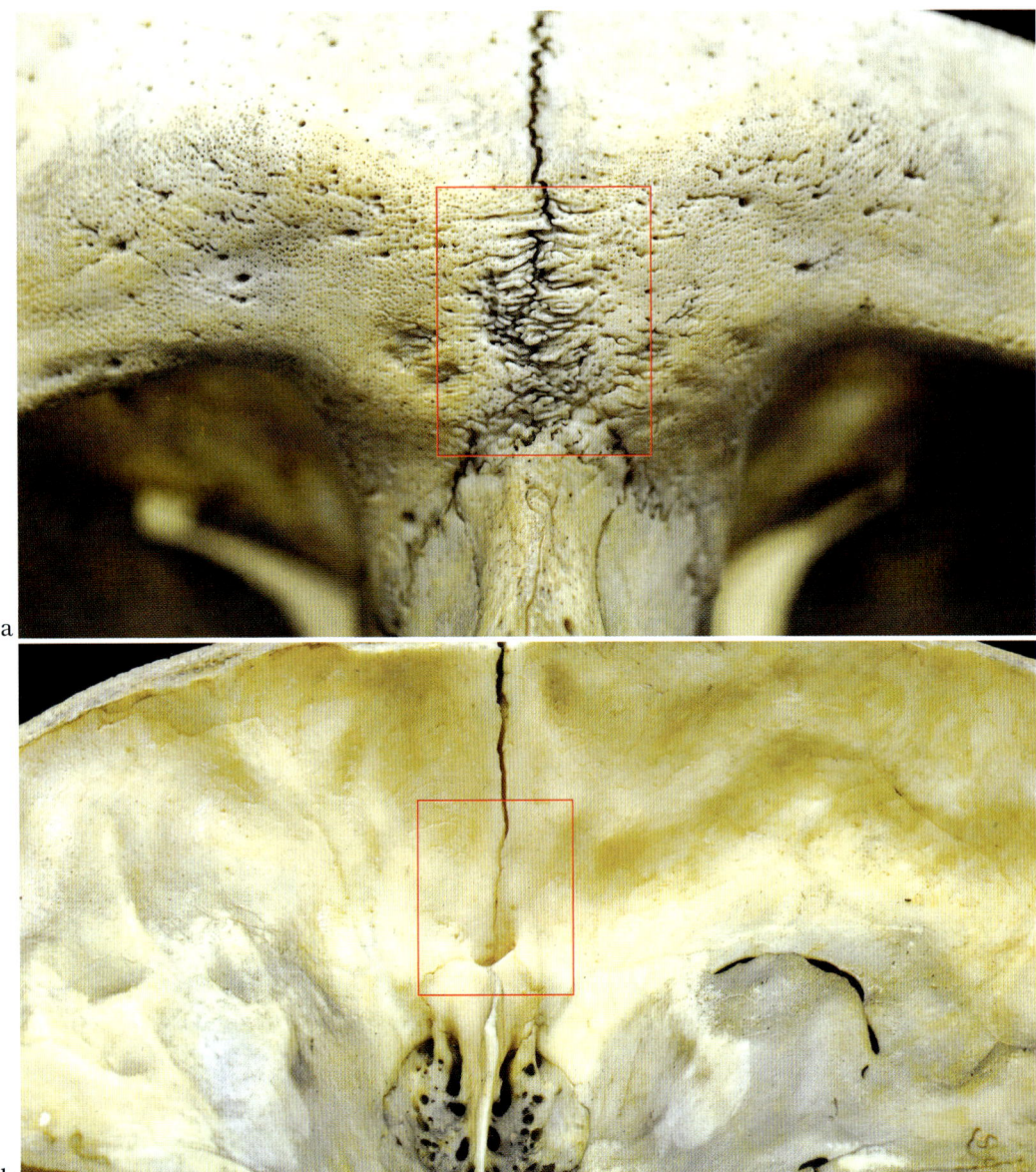

Figure 41a-b. Example of a metopic and supranasal suture. (a) Ectocranial and (b) endocranial views of the metopic and supranasal sutures and the foramen cecum (red square, that transmits a vein) in an adult White male (Mütter Museum 1008.48). Note the normal numerous perforations in the cribriform plate, to either side of the vertically-oriented crista galli that divides the cribriform down the midline. The supranasal suture forms superior and subsequent to metopic suture closure. This individual exhibits numerous pits and horizontally-oriented striations/grooves in the supraorbital region consistent with the male vermiculate pattern (cf. Tappen 1983). While the etiology of the vermiculate pattern is not well understood, it is often present in males (cf. Schiwy-Bochat 2001; Tappen 1983). See Hauser and DeStefano (1989) for examples of the supranasal suture. Common findings. Cf. Vu et al. (2001).

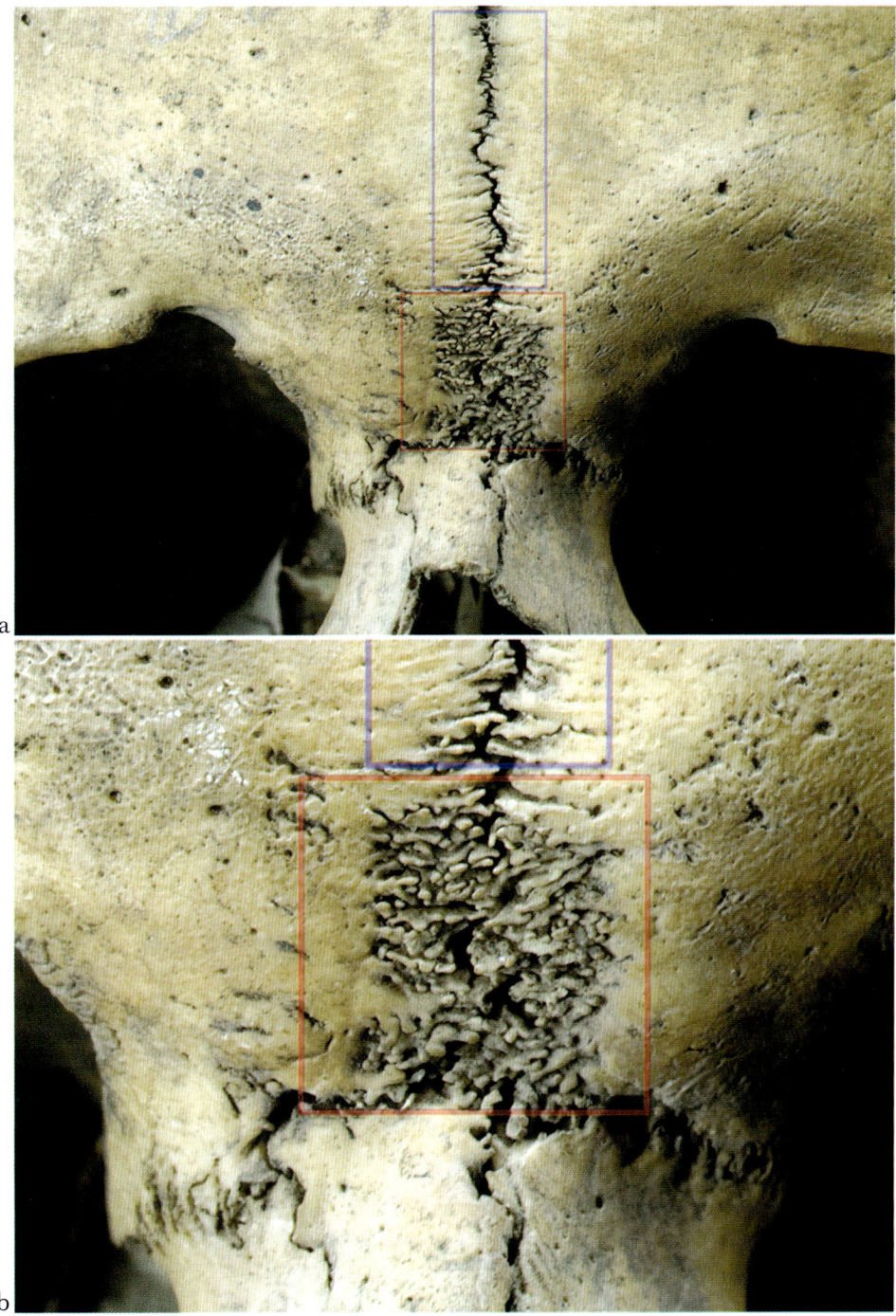

Figure 42a-b. Metopic suture (purple) and unusually complex supranasal (SNS) suture in an adult male from the catacombs of Paris (UPenn 664 L606). (a) Morphology of a relatively simple metopic suture (purple rectangle) leading into a much more complex supranasal suture (red square). (b) Close-up of the horizontally oriented (zigzag) supranasal suture (red square). The complexity of the metopic and SNS likely reflects biomechanical stresses related to mastication and stresses transmitted from the teeth and palate up through the maxilla and to the frontal bone. More research is needed to better understand how, when and why the SNS forms.

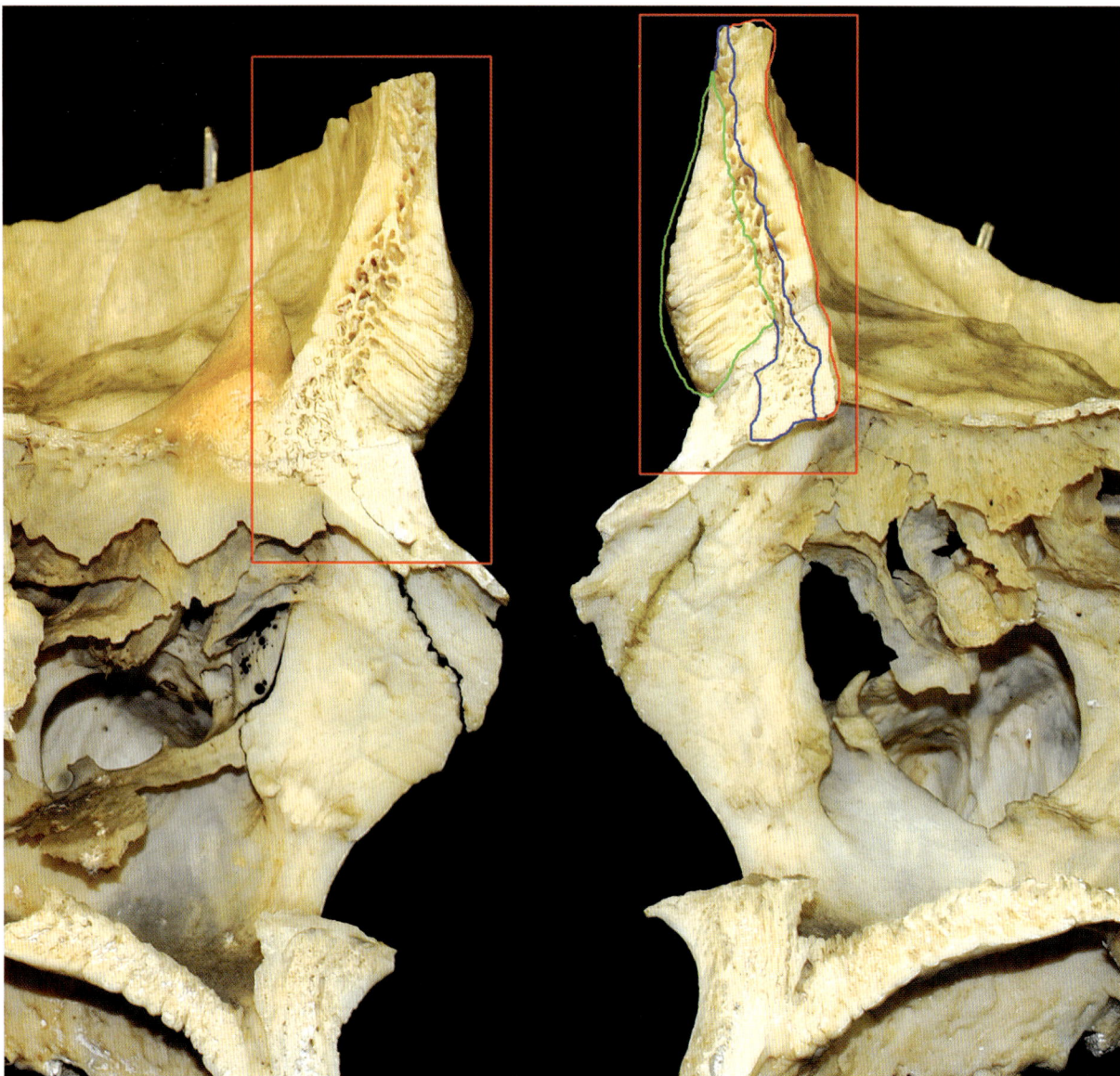

Figure 43. Sagittal section through the skull of a 45-year-old White male who died in 1881 or 1882 and showing the morphology of the supranasal (SNS) suture (rectangles) (Tübingen University, 794). This figure reveals that the SNS in the glabellar region is not superficial and involving only the outer table (the so-called "zigzag" pattern of striations), but appears to consist of three components or "zones" (roughly outlined in green, blue and red): 1) a complex anterior-posteriorly orientated outer table (green); 2) a medial-lateral horizontal morphology in the middle (blue); 3) a thick inner table (red) without interdigitations or horizontal striations. Note that the SNS involves only the glabellar region (approximately 1–2 cm above Nasion). Preliminary research reveals that the morphology, development and interrelated nature of the metopic and supranasal sutures are complex and require further research to better understand their anatomy and function. Normal anatomy.

Frontal View of the Skull

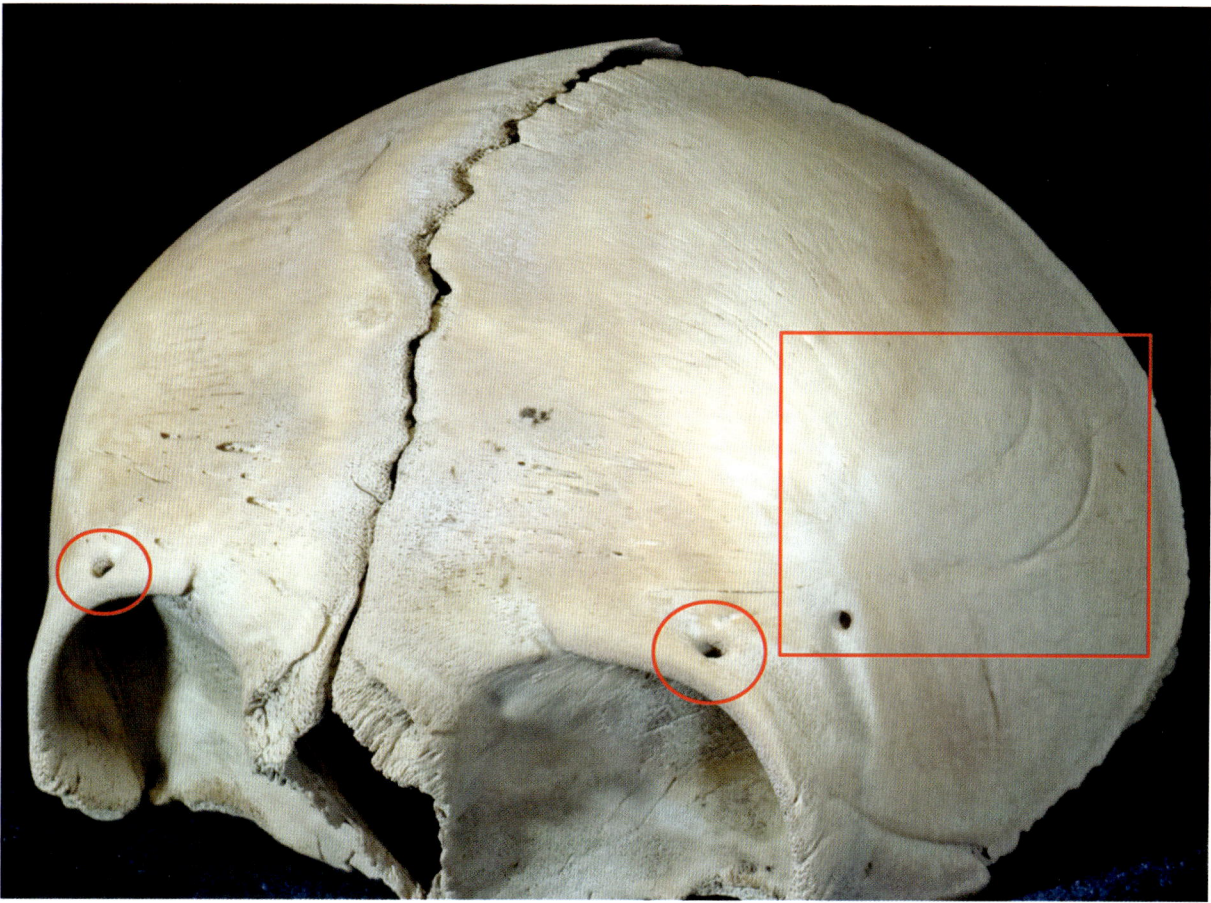

Figure 44. Open metopic suture, lateral supraorbital foramina (circles) and a lateral frontal foramen and grooves (rectangle) in a newborn (SI 228803 white female). Common findings.

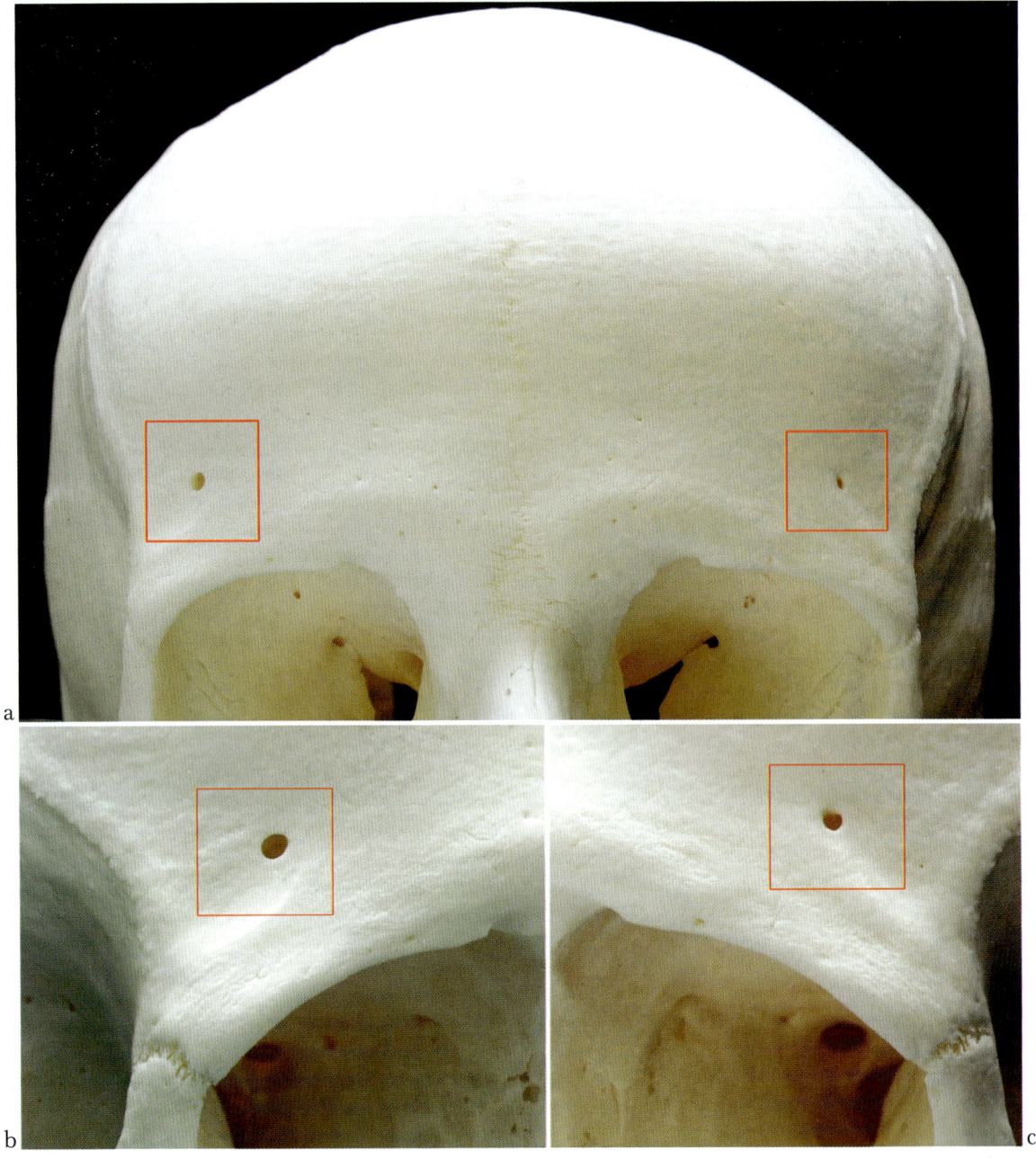

Figure 45a-c. Laterally positioned, but normal, supraorbital or frontal foramina in an elderly individual (FSA AC052). (a) Frontal view showing the position of the frontal foramina. (b) Oblique view of a large right foramen. (b) Oblique view of the smaller left foramen. Unusual positions and uncommon to common findings.

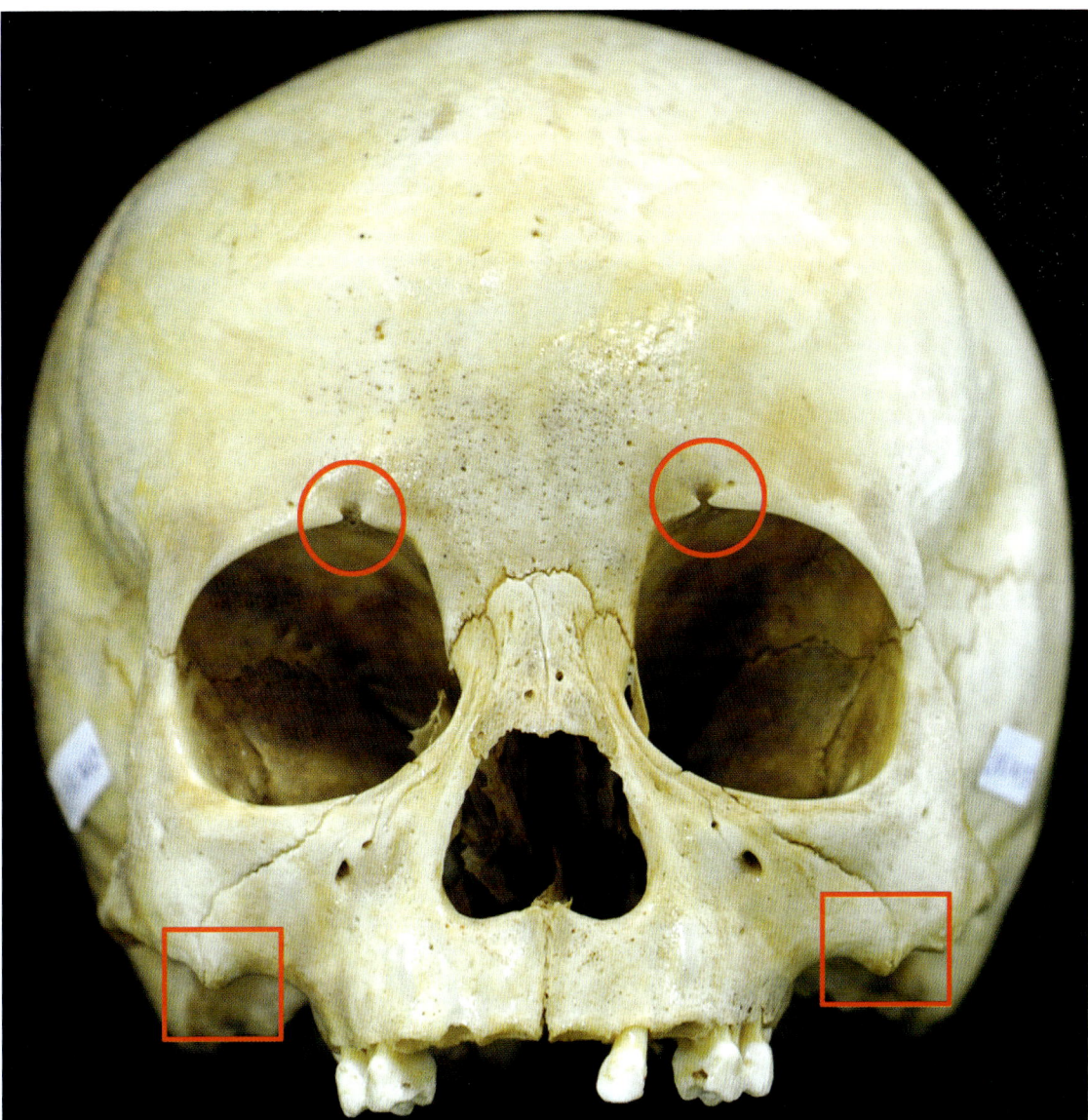

Figure 46. Normal morphology of a 4- to 6-year-old Thai child (KKU). Note the supraorbital notches (circles), mildly deviated septum inside the nasal opening, porosity above and medial to the orbits (glabella region), and prominent zygomaticomaxillary tubercles (squares) often seen in Asian individuals. These tubercles may form at the inferior margin and junction of the zygomaticomaxillary sutures, or medial, or lateral to them. Common findings. Cf. Hauser and DeStefano (1989). The contour of the zygomaticomaxillary sutures, although subject to much variation, is often used as an indicator of ancestry. Cf. Chung et al. (1995); Sholts and Wärmländer (2012). Note that in some of the older literature, the zygomatic bone/zygoma was known as the jugal bone and the "L-shaped" junction where the vertical and horizontal portions join as the "jugal point."

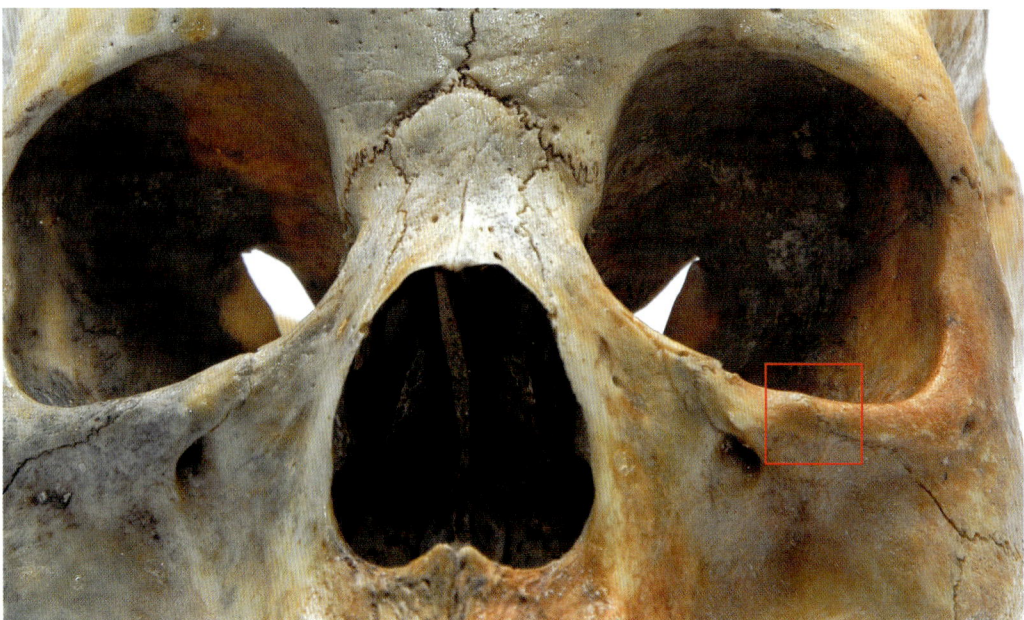

Figure 47. Small left tubercle (square) of the zygomaticomaxillary suture and absence of the tubercle on the right side in an adult Thai (KKU). The left tubercle in this specimen can be observed and palpated. Common finding and of unknown significance.

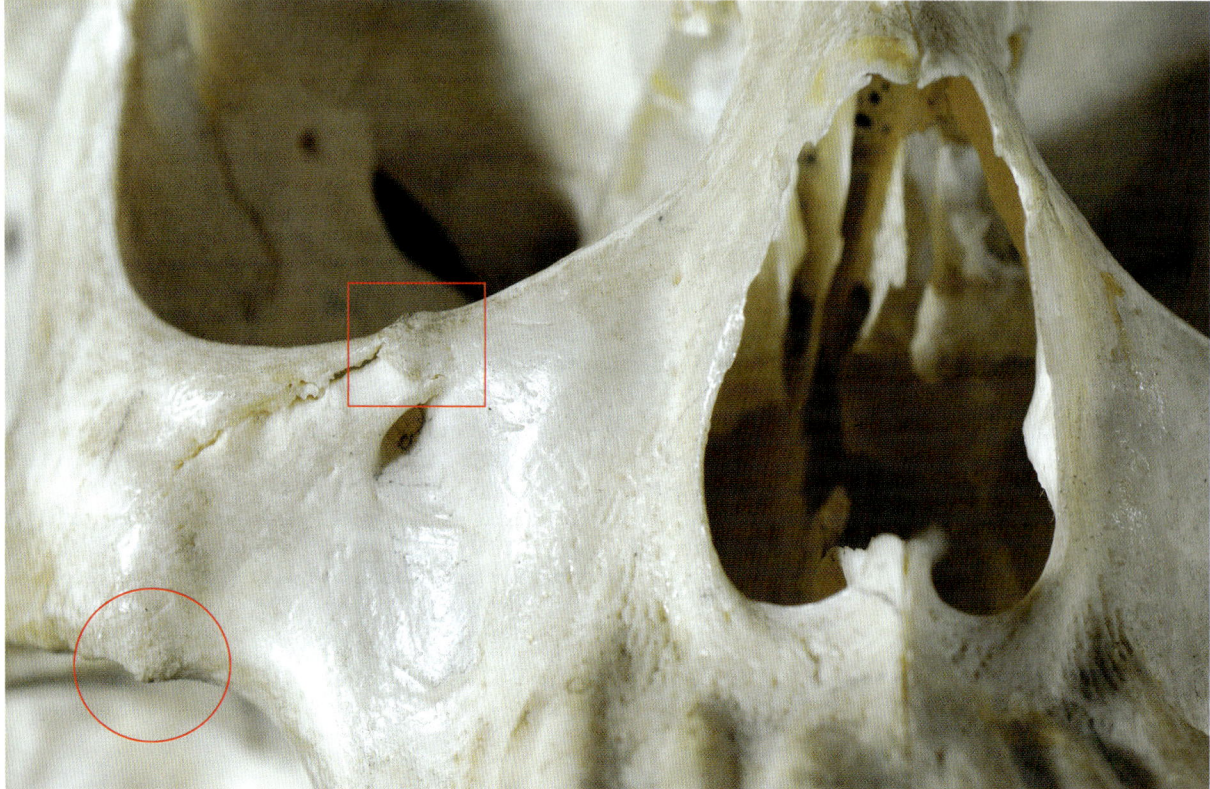

Figure 48. Small right tubercle (square) of the zygomaticomaxillary suture and zygomaxillary/malar tubercle (circle) in an Asian female (CSC AC007). These tubercles do not necessarily form on, at the apex, or along the zygomaticomaxillary suture. Common findings.

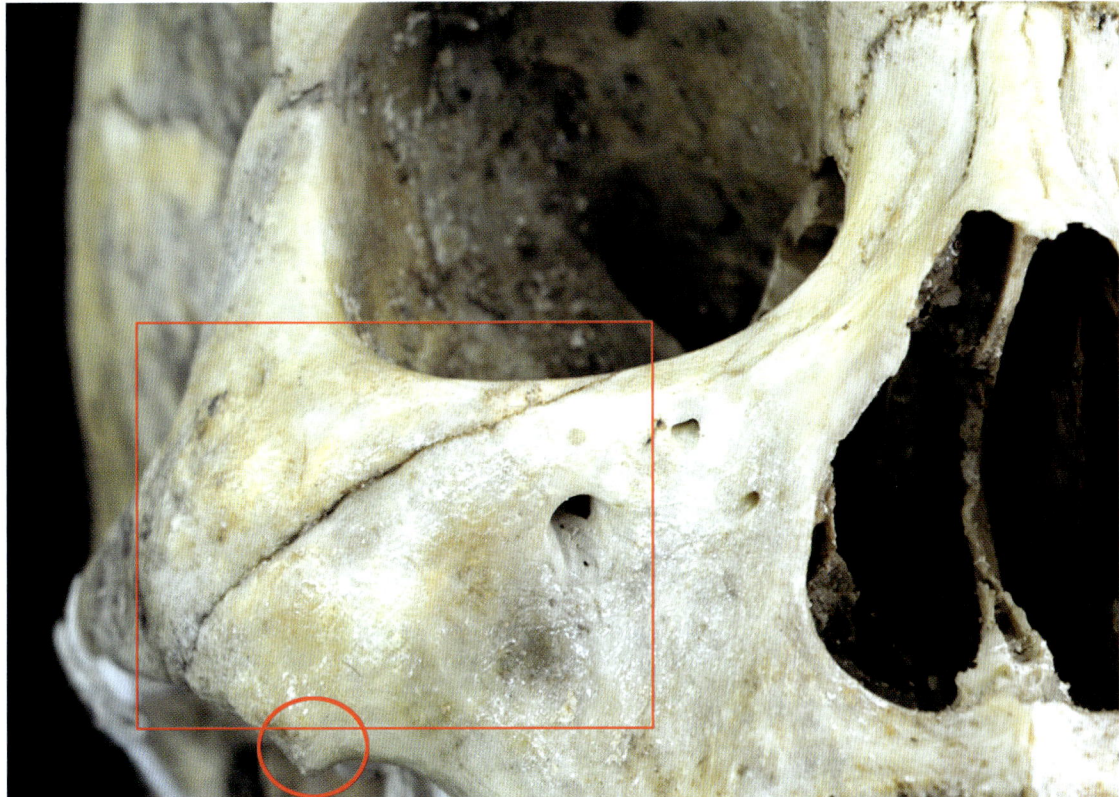

Figure 49. Unusually straight and diagonally-oriented zygomaticomaxillary suture in a Thai (KKU). Note the small malar tubercle (circle) far medial to the zygomaticomaxillary (ZM) suture. This tubercle can form distal to the ZM suture, not necessarily along it. Common findings.

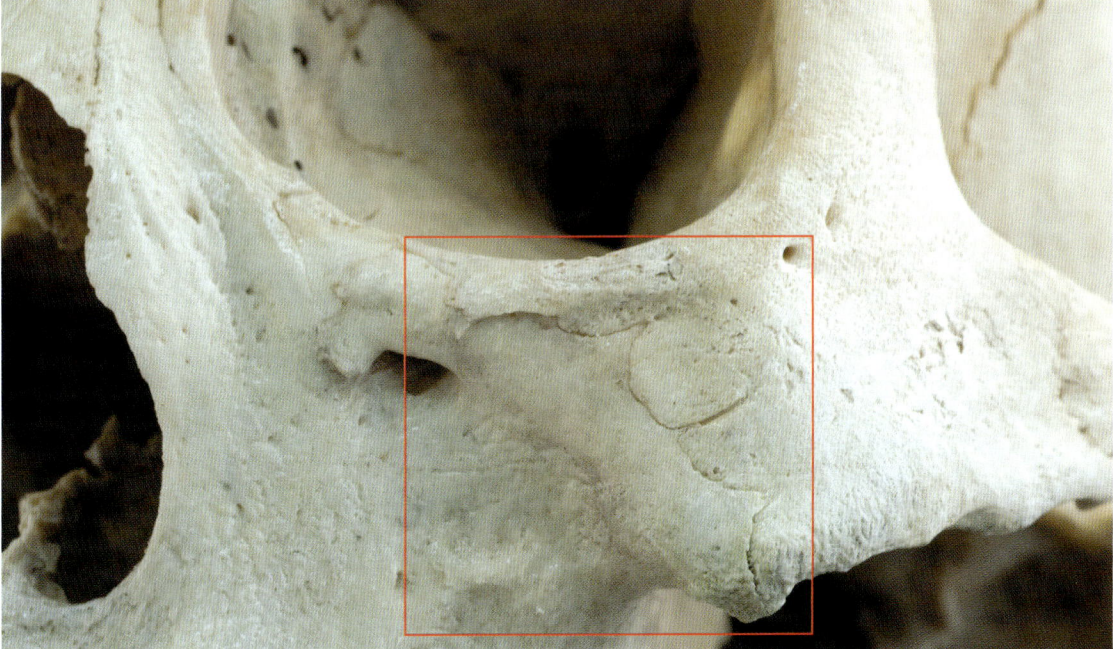

Figure 50. Bilateral zygomaticomaxillary suture (square) with unusually long, but normal extensions (CSC).

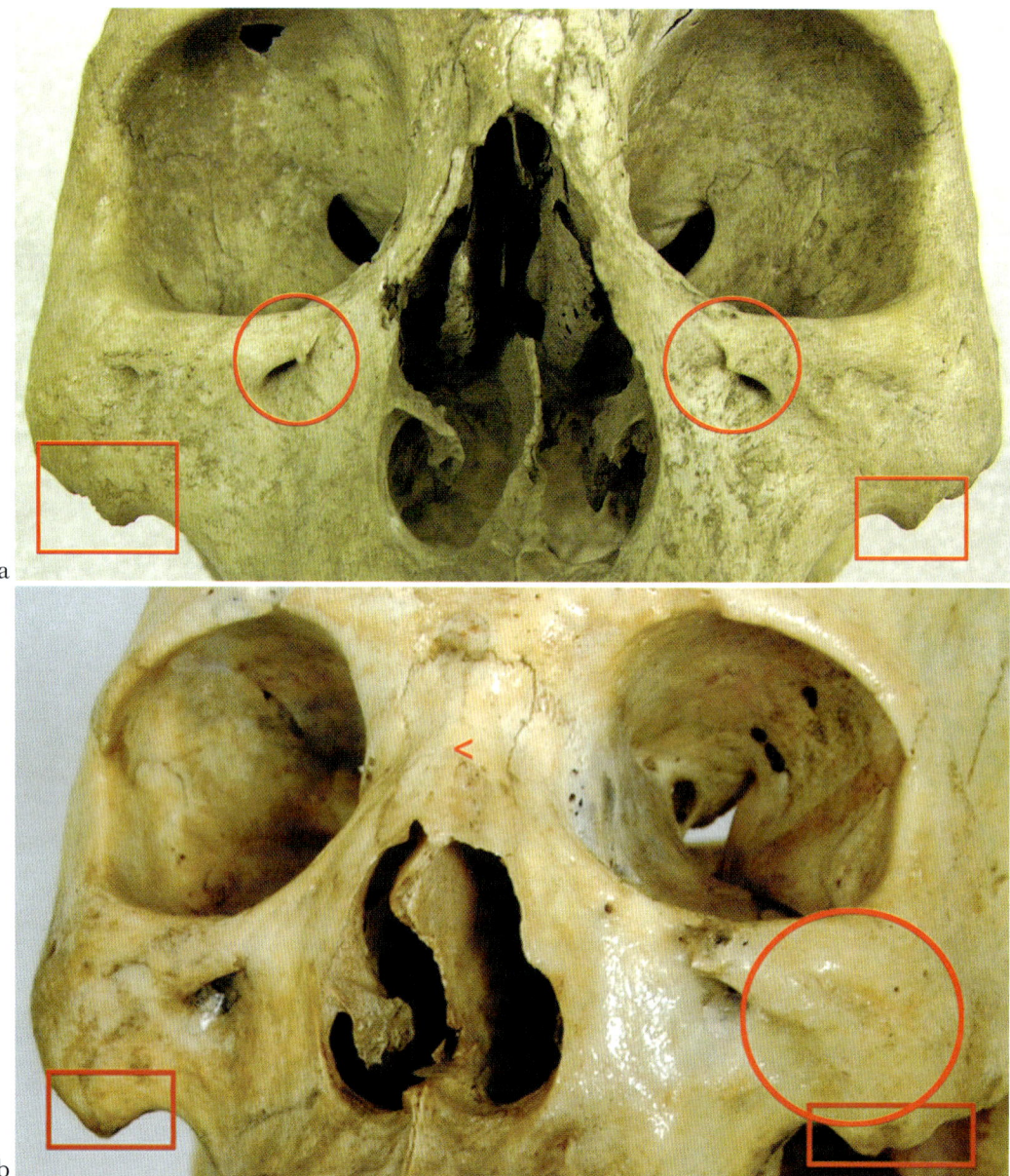

Figure 51a-b. "Folded" or overhanging of the infraorbital suture and prominent zygomaticomaxillary tubercles in two Thai adults (KKU). (a) Frontal view showing bone overhanging the infraorbital sutures (circles) and malar tubercles (rectangles) forming where the zygomaticomaxillary suture comes to an inverted cone at its apex, medial, or lateral to it. (b) Left oblique view showing the malar tubercles (rectangles), left zygomaticomaxillary suture (circle) and the internasal suture (<) that have completely obliterated, a situation not often present at any age. "Folded" sutures are uncommon findings and tubercles are common findings in some groups. Cf. Hauser and DeStefano (1989).

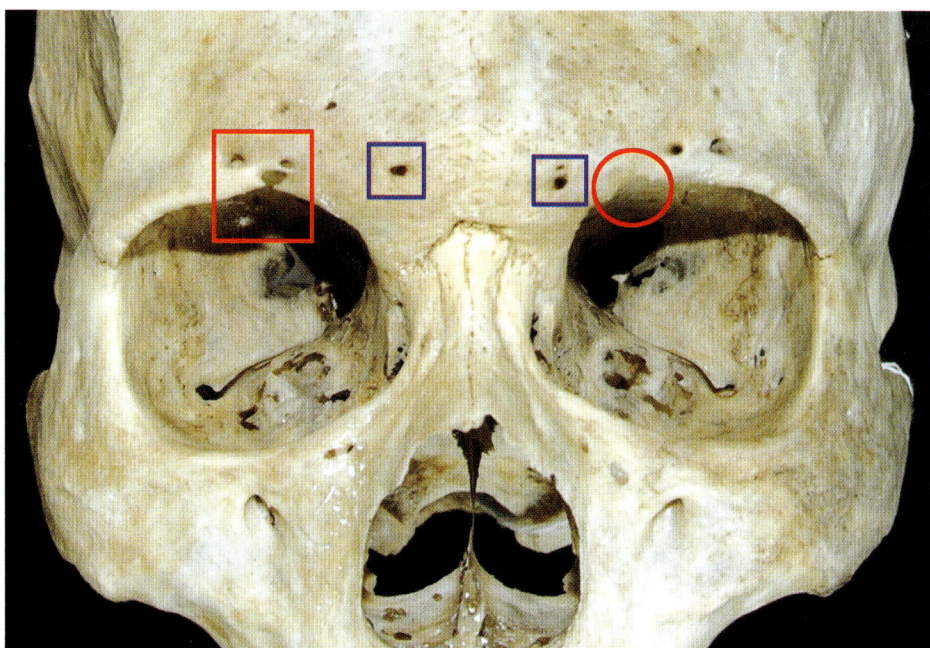

Figure 52. Right medial supraorbital notch and foramina (red square), left medial supraorbital notch (circle), supratrochlear foramina (blue squares) and numerous large supraorbital foramina in an adult Thai male (KKU). Multiple foramina such as this are an uncommon finding. Cf. Dutton (2011) for anatomy of the orbit; Chung et al. (1995) and Hauser and DeStefano (1989) for frequencies of supraorbital foramina and notches.

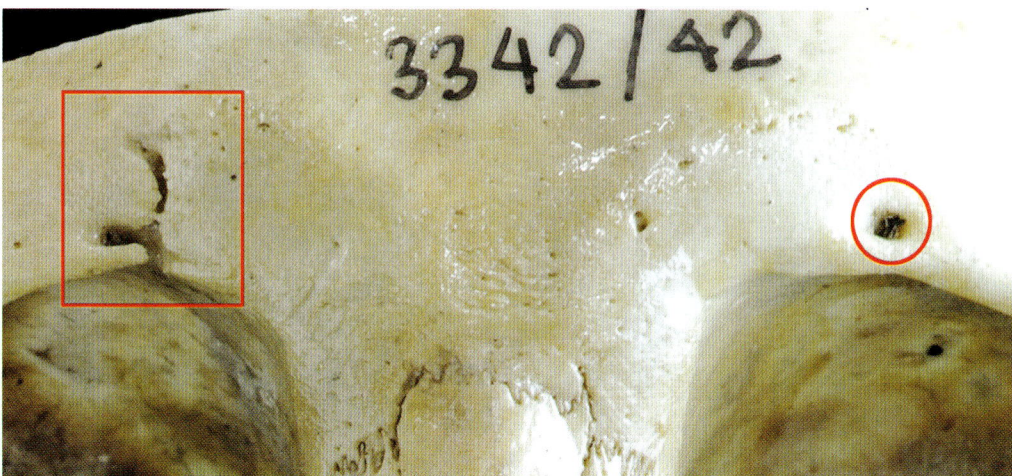

Figure 53. Left supraorbital foramen (circle) and a notched right supraorbital foramen and groove (square) in an adult Thai (KKU). Cf. Ashwini et al. (2012); Hauser and DeStefano (1989).

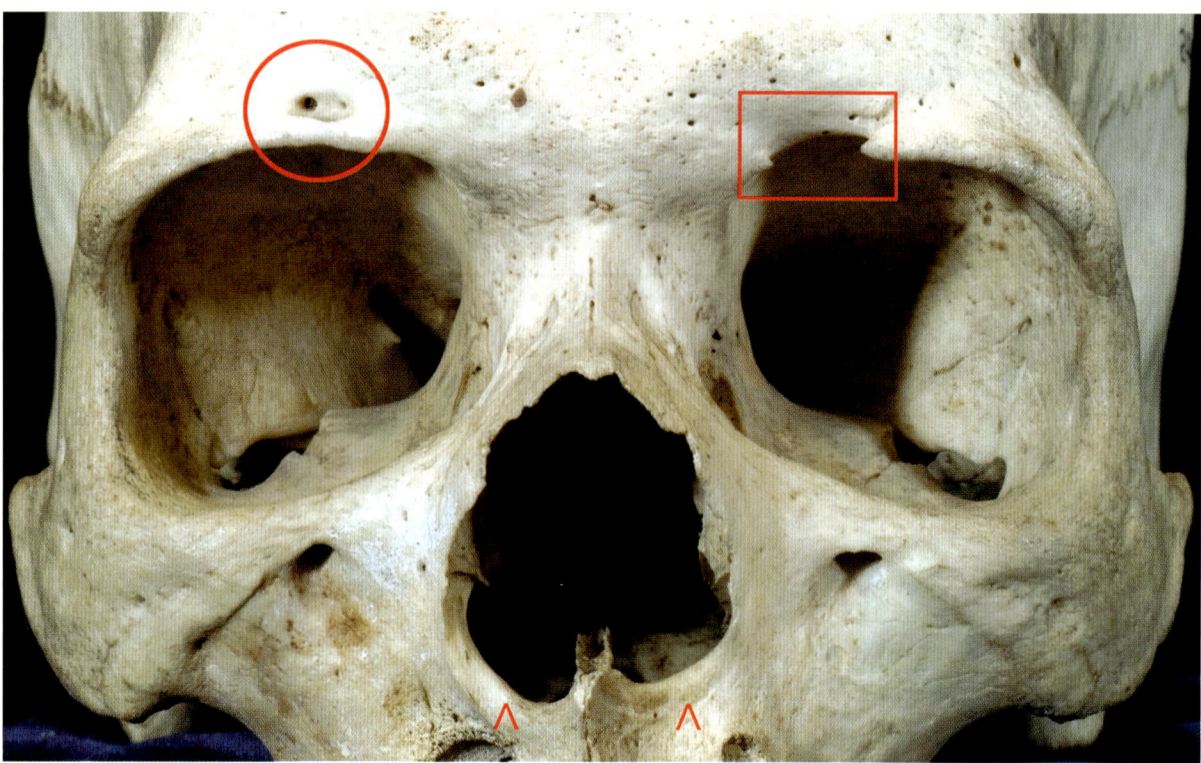

Figure 54. Supraorbital foramen (circle), unusually wide left supraorbital notch (rectangle) and nasal guttering resembling crescents (∧) in an adult Black (SI 244088). Although nasal guttering is often viewed as a Black/Negroid trait, it is commonly found in Asians and other groups. Cf. Ashwini et al. (2012) for supraorbital foramen and supraorbital notch.

Frontal View of the Skull

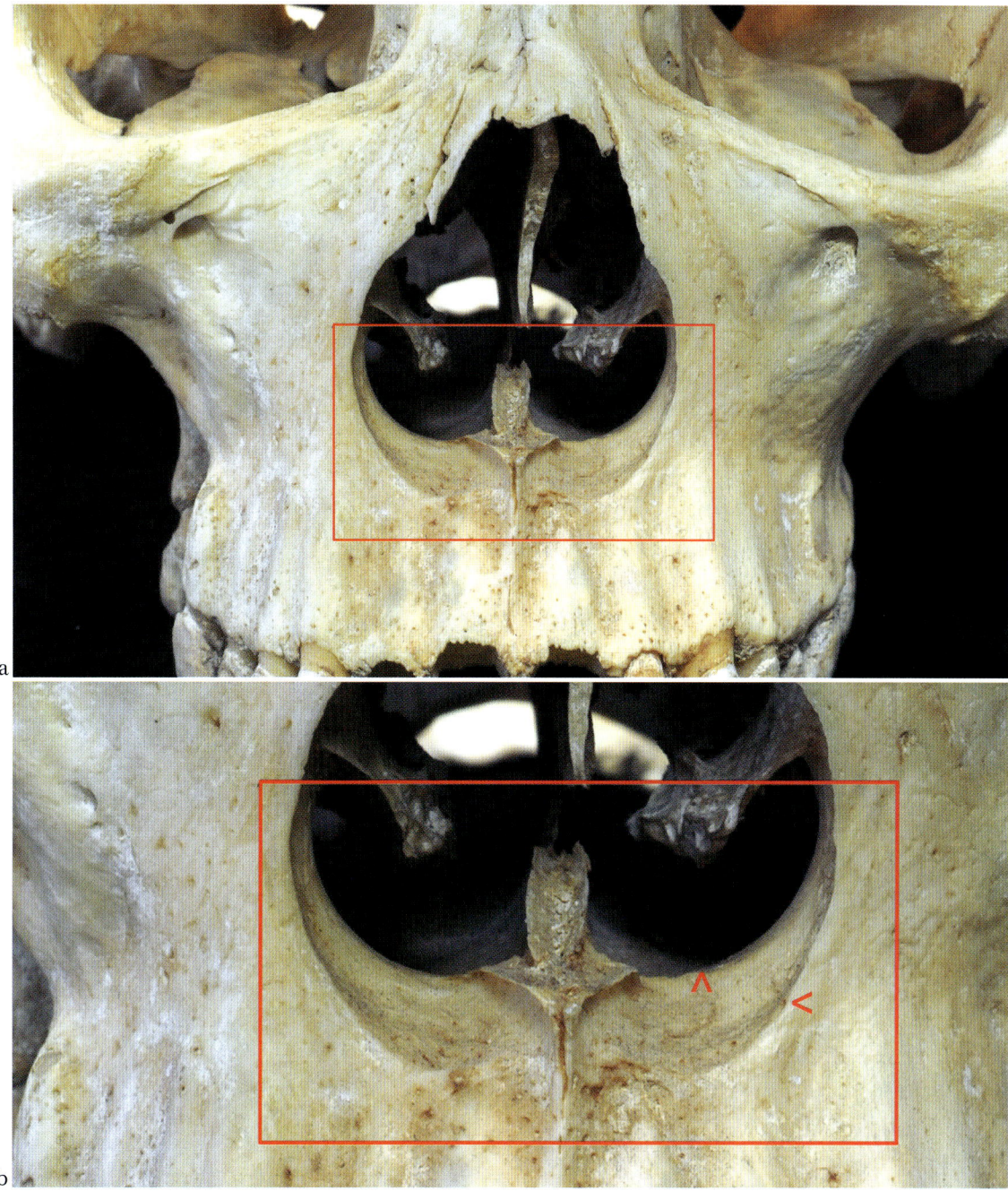

Figure 55a-b. Prominent nasal guttering in an adult African (University of Pretoria). (a) Note the wide and rounded shape of the nasal aperture and presence of "nasal guttering" (rectangle). (b) Close-up of nasal guttering showing inner (∧) and outer (<) ridges forming the anteriorly-sloping area known as "nasal guttering" along the inferior half of the nasal aperture.

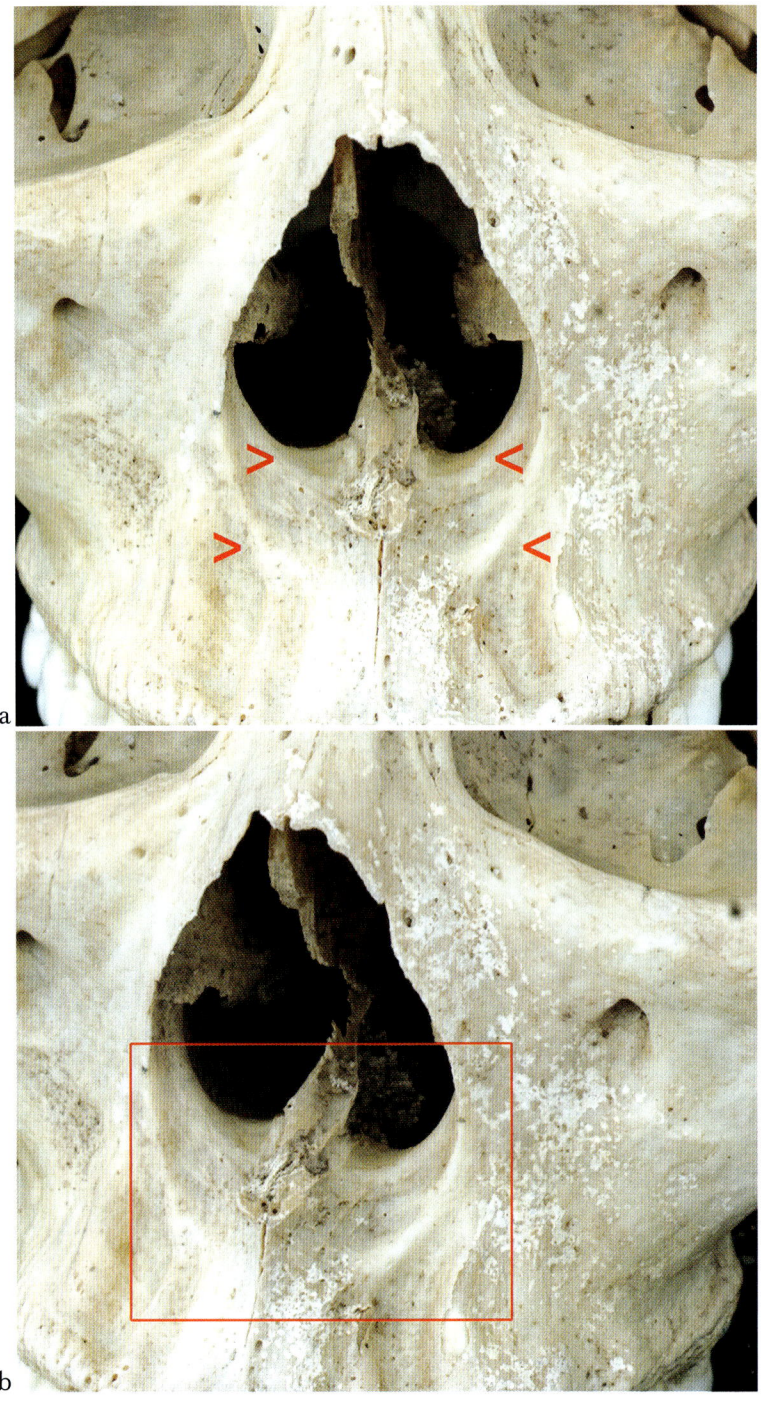

Figure 56a-b. Nasal guttering in a 57-year-old Thai male (CMU 190 52). (a) Frontal view showing the internal and external ridges (> and <) forming an inverted "V" (nasal guttering) along either side of the nasal opening. (b) Left oblique view of the nasal aperture and guttering (rectangle).

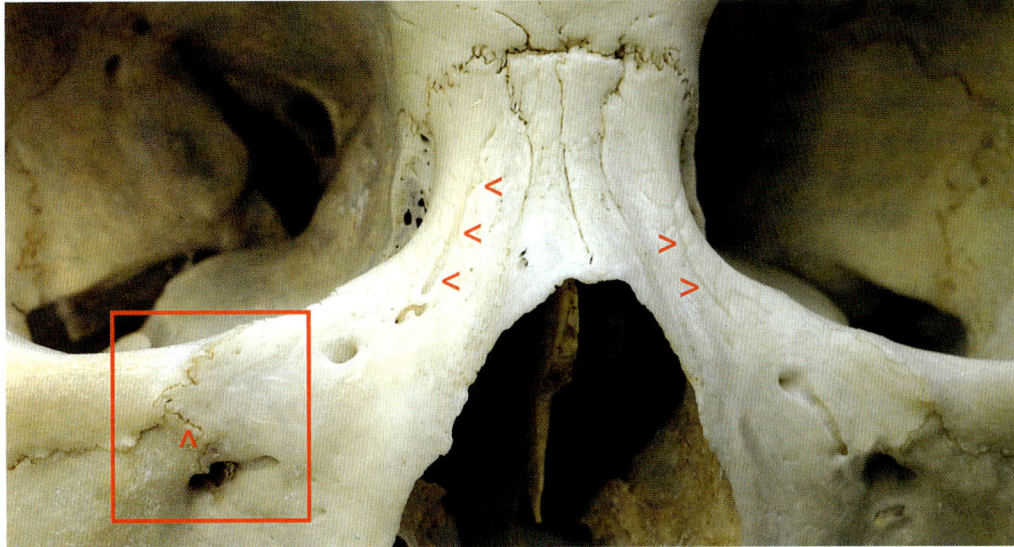

Figure 57. Bilateral infraorbital sutures into the infraorbital foramen (square and ∧) and sutura notha (< >) in a Thai (KKU). The sutura notha ("false suture") is situated approximately 3–5 mm from the anterior lacrimal crest and has been described either as a shallow groove that holds a small vein and was once believed to be an articulation that penetrated the full thickness of the bone (Flecker 1913), as a groove that separates the frontal process of the maxilla and the lacrimal bone (Isloor 2014), or as an embryonic facial fissure (Wobig and Dailey 2004), among others. Common findings. Cf. Boopathi et al. (2010); Hauser and DeStefano (1989); Last (1966); Turner (1885) for more on these foramina.

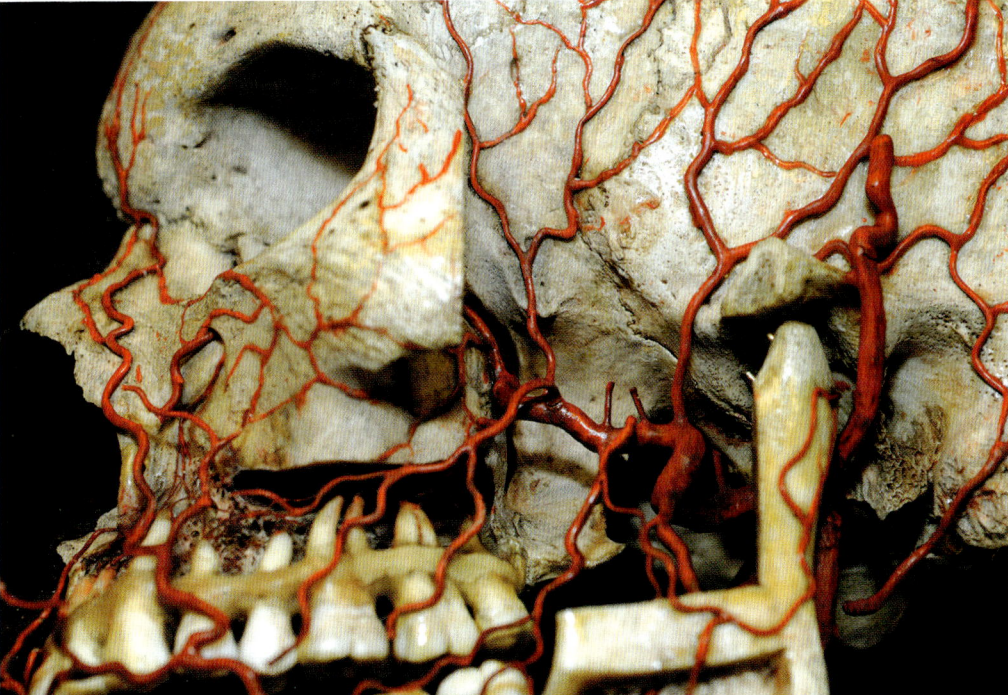

Figure 58. Arteries of the left side of the face and temporal region showing their position as they pass along the surface of the bones (produced by the corrosion method; Mütter Museum 6337). Normal anatomy. Cf. Dutton (2011) for vascular anatomy of the orbit and any version of Gray's Anatomy for arterial and venous anatomy of the face and head.

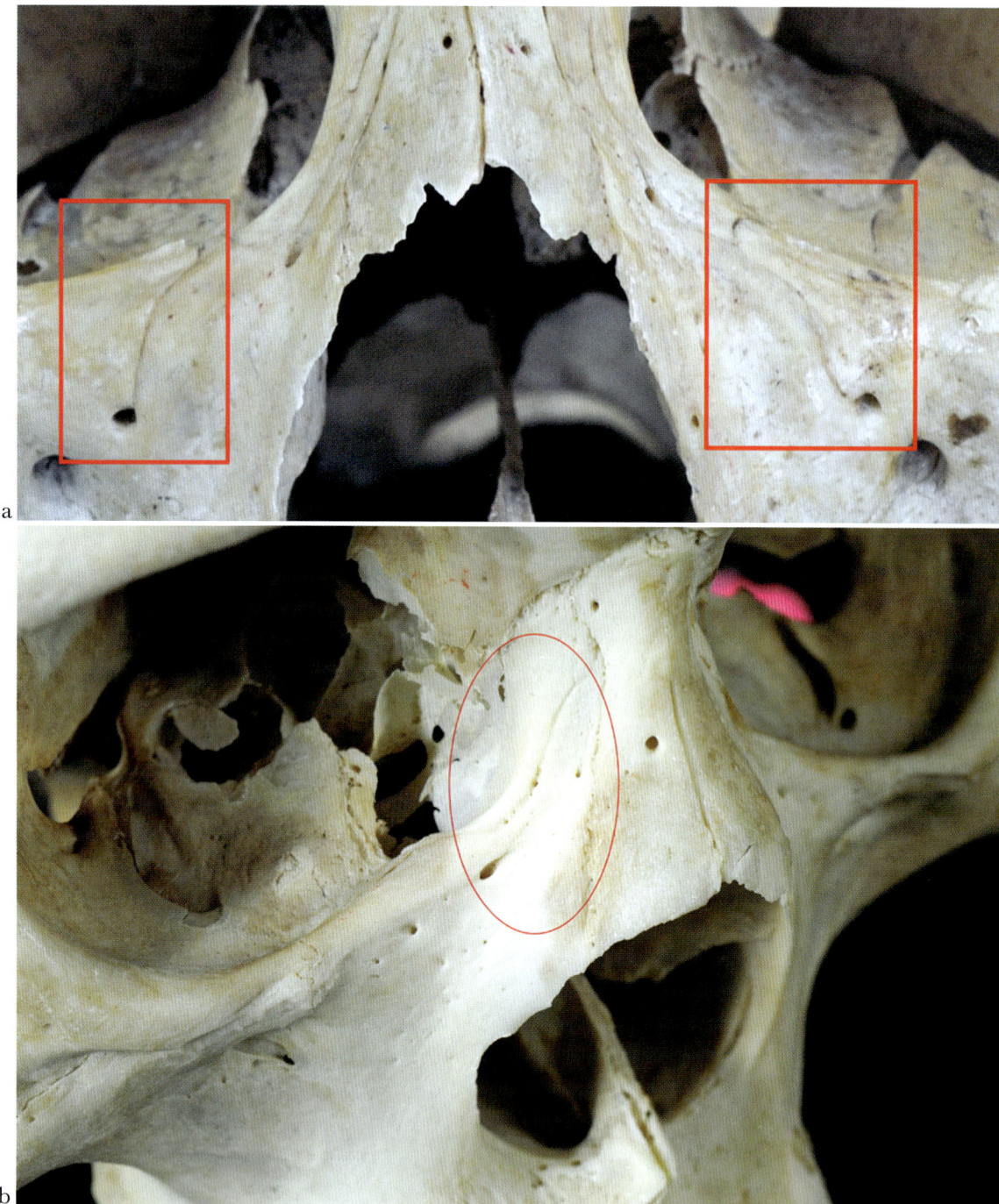

Figure 59a-b. Possible sutura notha ("false suture") (rectangles) in a Thai adult (KKU). (a) Frontal view showing narrow, shallow grooves (sutura notha) anterior to the lacrimal crest; note that these grooves are not serrated like typical infraorbital sutures. (b) Oblique view showing the right sutura notha; these shallow grooves contain small vessels "twigs" (Whitnall 1921) of the infraorbital artery lying beneath the periosteum (Werb 1974; Caesar and McNab 2004). Common finding. Cf. Flecker (1913); Hanihara and Ishida (2001b); Last (1966); Warwick (1976).

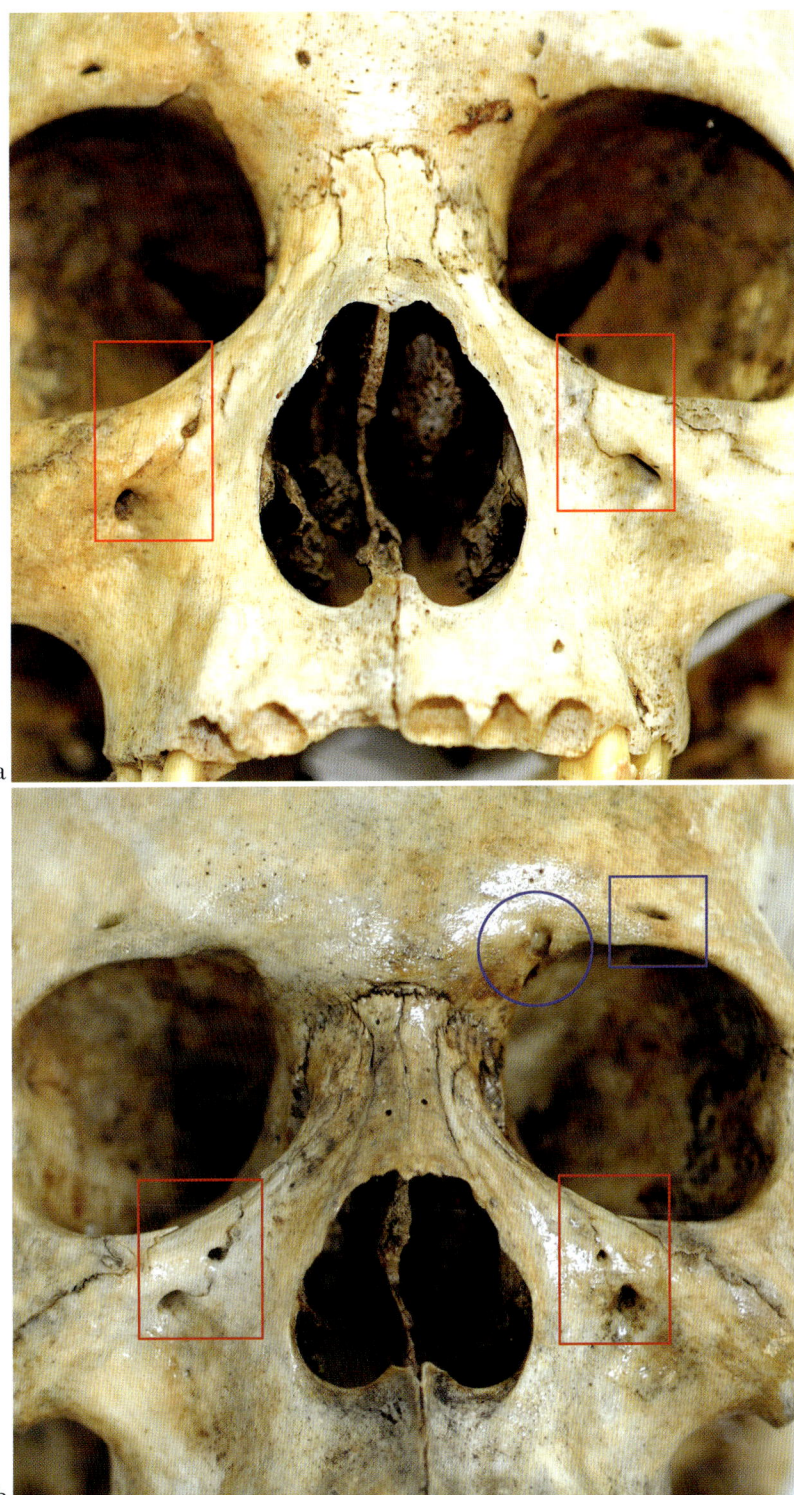

Figure 60a-b. Variants of the infraorbital suture extending into the infraorbital foramen. (Top) Double right foramina and single left foramen. (Bottom) Bilateral double foramina (red rectangles). Note the supraorbital notch (blue circle) and foramen (blue square) above the left orbit. Common findings. Cf. Bressan et al. (2004); Hanihara and Ishida (2001b) and Hauser and DeStefano (1989) for accessory infraorbital foramina.

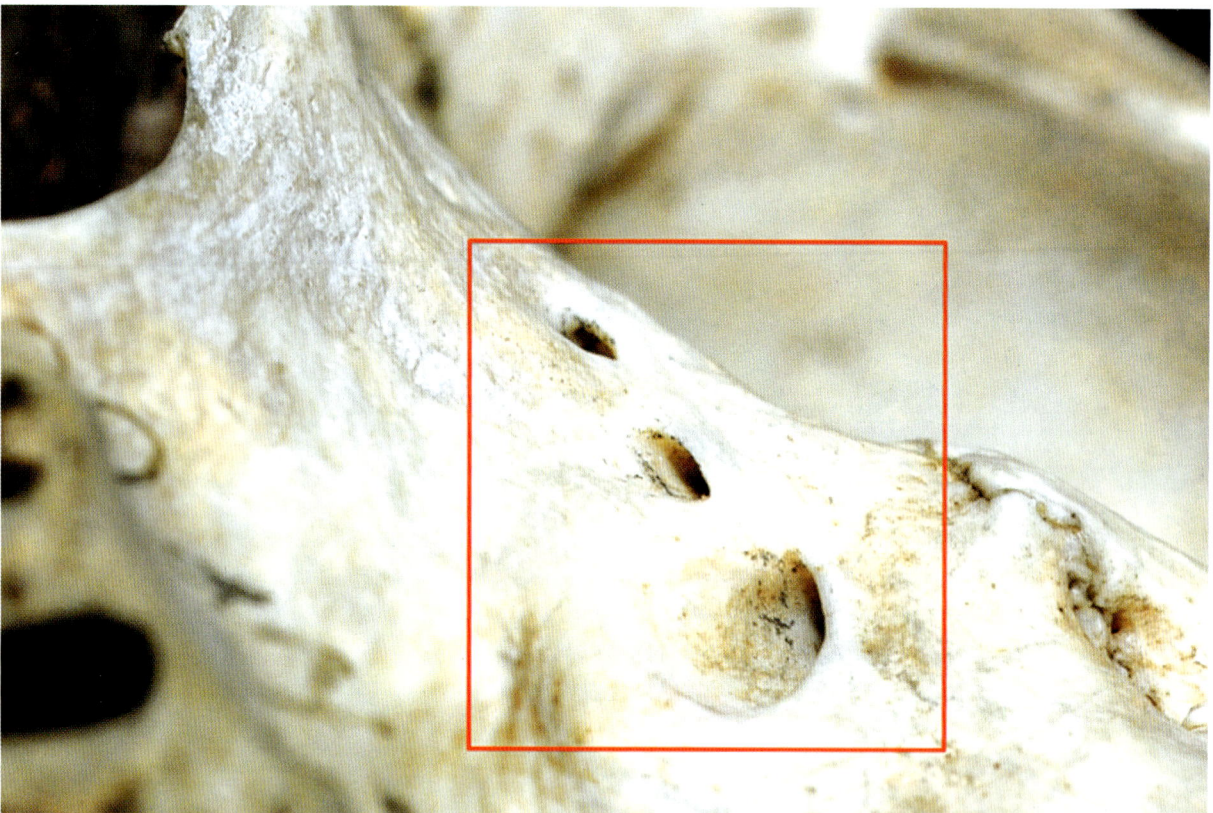

Figure 61. Uncommon triple left infraorbital foramina in an adult male (Mütter Museum 1008.80). A study of 80 South Indian skulls (Boopathi et al. 2010) revealed 13 skulls (16%) with accessory infraorbital foramina, the greatest number being three in an individual. Canan et al. (1999) reported 1.2% of 348 crania and maxillae with two or more infraorbital foramina. Numerous studies have been conducted on the direction, position and size of infraorbital foramina for anesthesia and surgery. Cf. Bressan et al. (2004); Hanihara and Ishida (2001b); Hauser and DeStefano (1989).

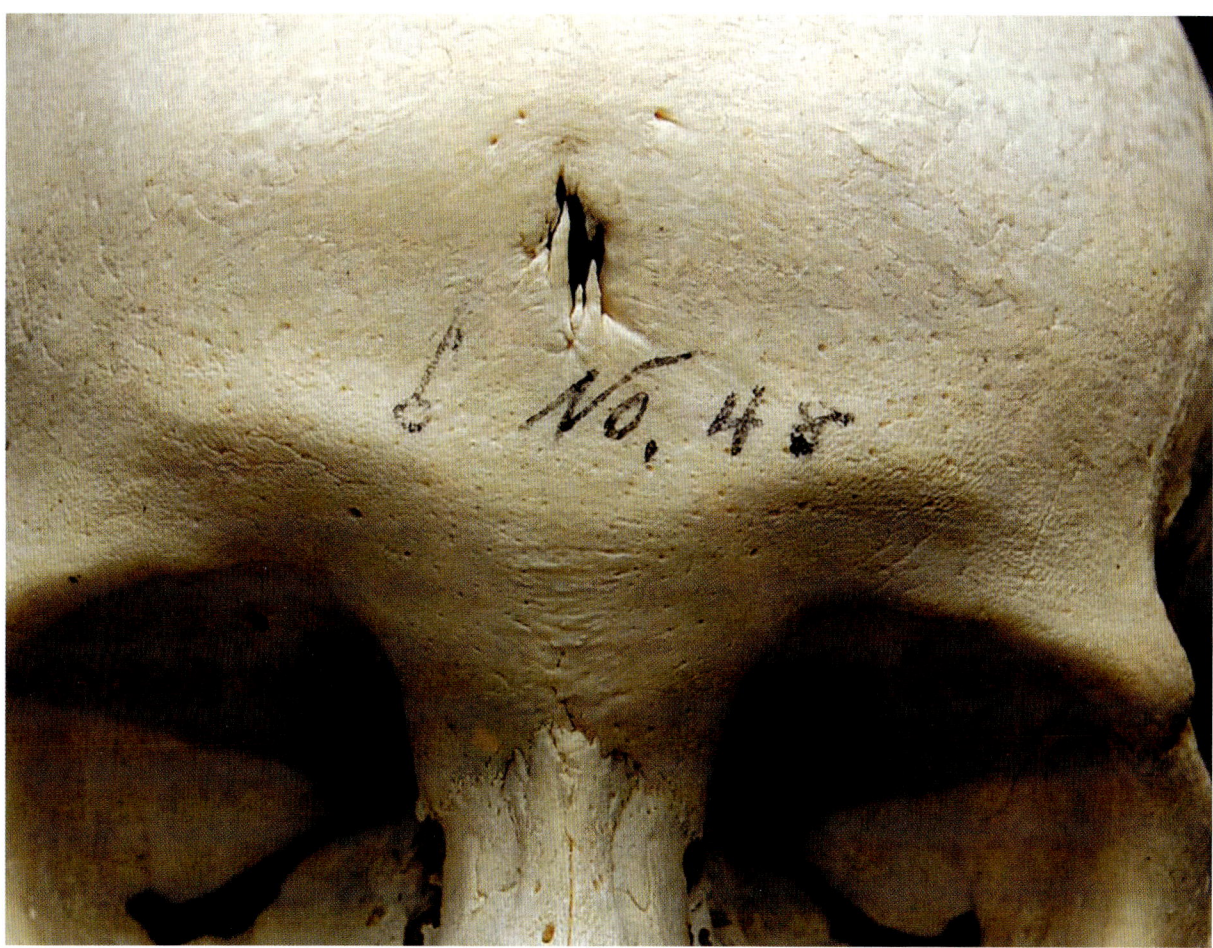

Figure 62. Vertically-oriented metopic fissure likely the result of incomplete ossification of the interfrontal/frontal/metopic suture that perforated the endocranium in a Japanese adult male (CU, Tuller). Note that the fissure is an isolated remnant of the metopic suture. Uncommon to rare finding, present in approximately 2% of adults and with a ratio of nearly 2:1 male:female (Hauser and DeStefano 1989; Schwalbe 1901). Cf. Schultz (1918, 1929); Woo (1949).

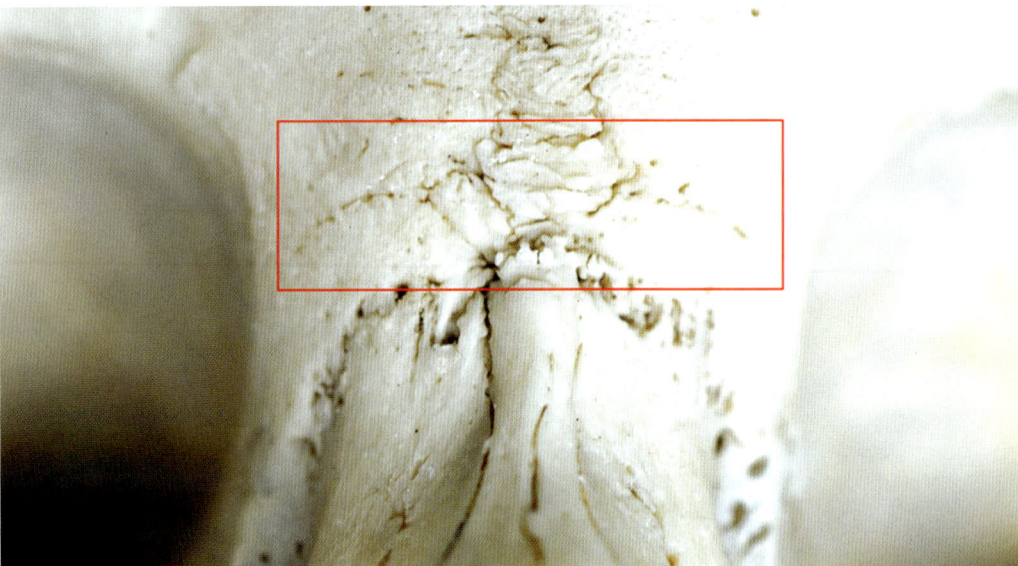

Figure 63. Supranasal triangle with lateral extensions (red rectangle) in an adult Thai (KKU). The region superior to Nasion varies greatly in the complexity of the metopic and supranasal sutures (two different sutures that form at different ages). Distinguishing the supranasal suture from the metopic suture (if indeed they are separate sutures) can be challenging for two reasons. First, some researchers identify the supranasal suture as ". . . that part of the metopic suture situated 1–2 cm above Nasion" (quotation marks added) (see Tavassoli 2001). Second, the general region superior to Nasion is commonly and accurately referred to as the "supranasal" or glabellar region, even when not referring to the metopic or supranasal sutures. While some researchers consider the supranasal suture as independent of the *metopic* suture (see Hauser and DeStefano 1989), others consider both sutures as one (metopic) (see Scheurer and Black 2000). Hauser and DeStefano (1989) reported the supranasal suture as present in 89% of 100 European adult males. There appears to be an association between the size and morphology of the supraciliary arches, sometimes called "superciliary arches" and the complexity and form of the supranasal suture (Brash 1953). The supranasal suture warrants further research to ascertain its etiology, development and timing of closure and obliteration. Cf. Pietrusewsky and Douglas (2002).

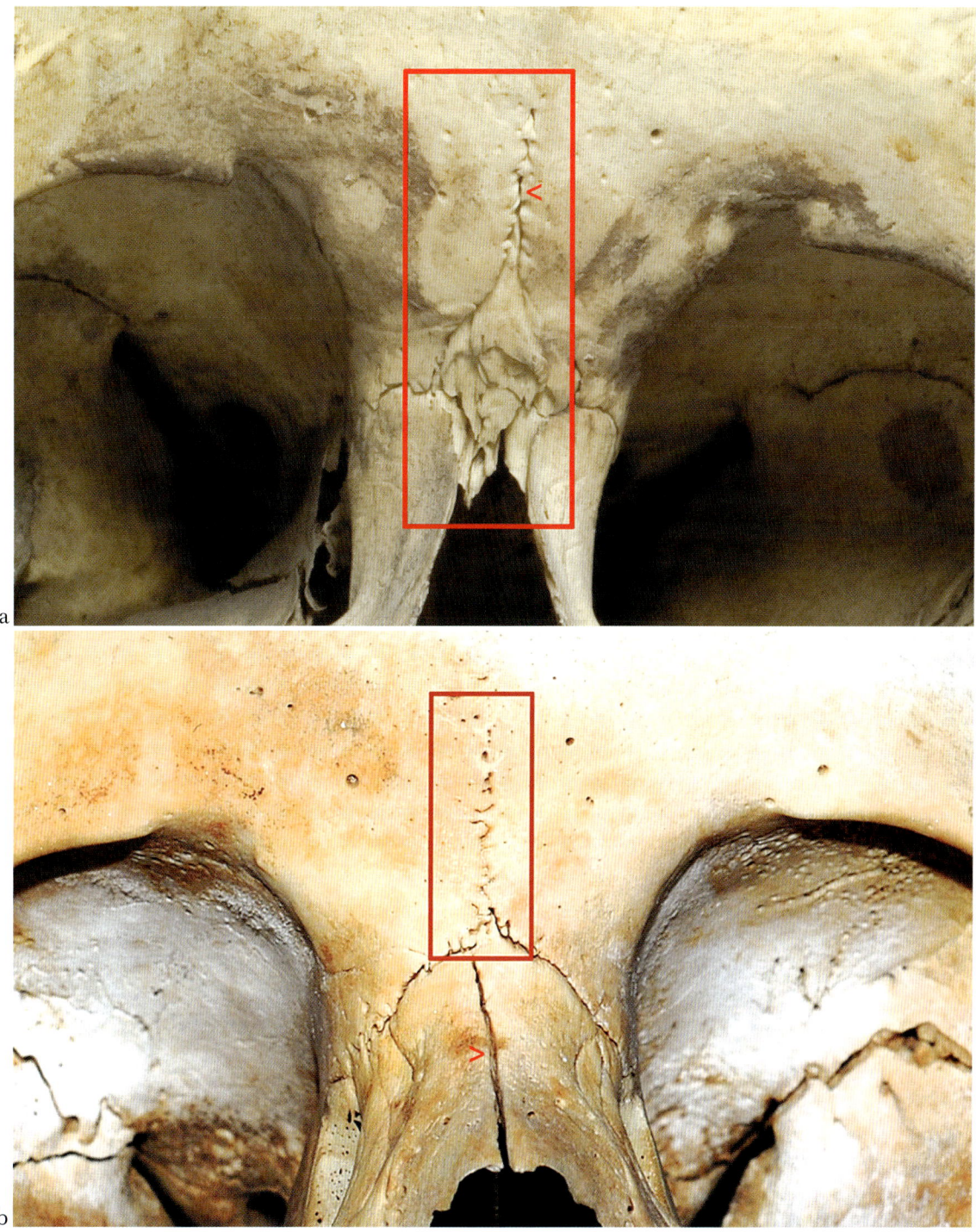

Figure 64a-b. Remnant of metopic suture. (a) Metopic/interfrontal suture (rectangle and <) leading into an unusually complex and diamond-shaped nasofrontal suture, possibly a frontonasal or metopic ossicle, in a 3- to 4-year-old child (UPenn L606 29). (b) Remnant/trace of the metopic/interfrontal suture (rectangle) in another child; note that the trace metopic does not align with the internasal suture (>).

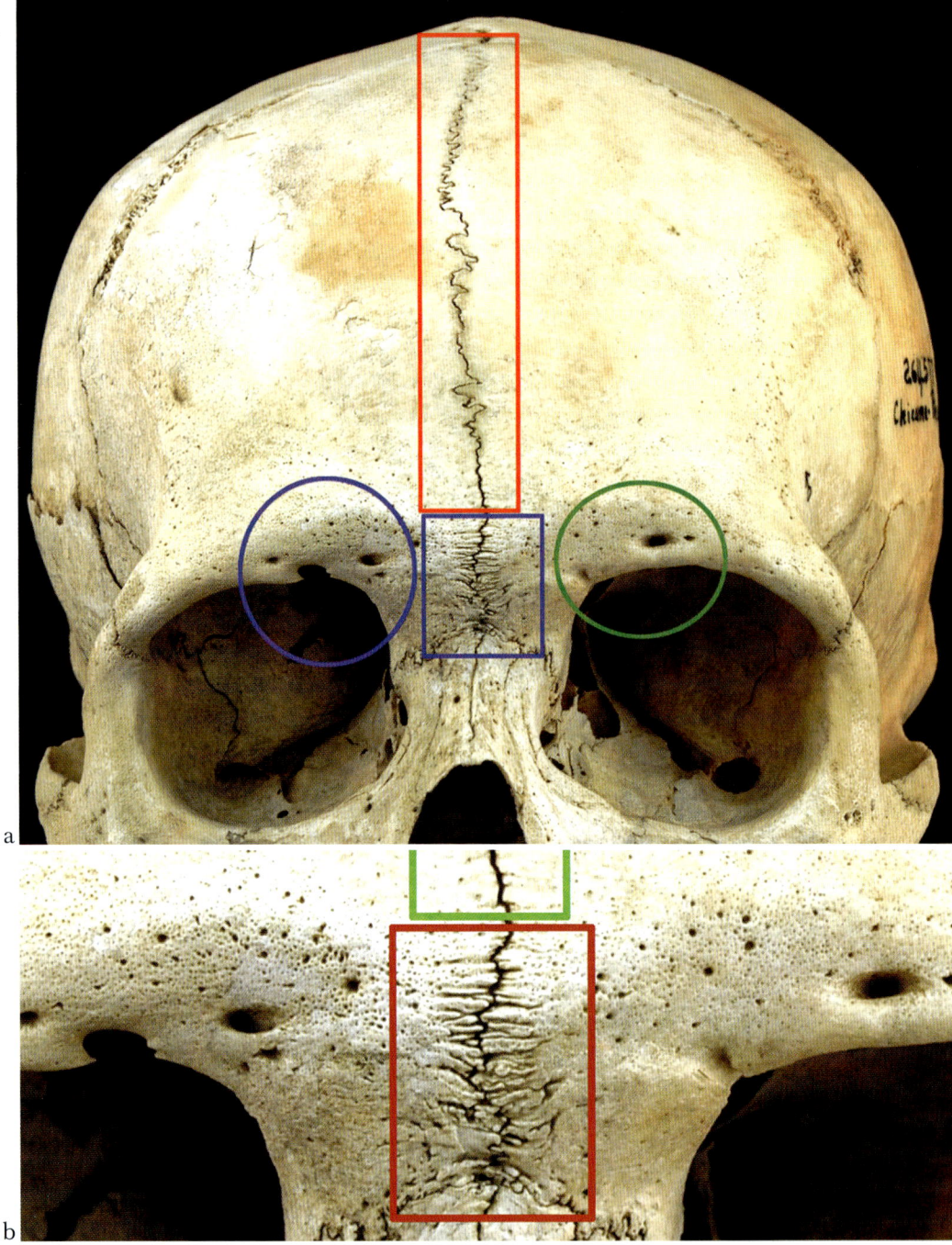

Figure 65a-b. Metopic and supranasal sutures, supraorbital foramina and notches. (a) Right supraorbital notch and foramina (blue circle), small left supraorbital notch and foramen (green circle), supranasal suture (blue square) and metopism (red rectangle) in an adult ancient Peruvian male (SI). (b) Close-up of the supranasal suture (red rectangle) and frontal porosity (porotic hyperostosis) above the orbits. Common findings. Cf. Dutton (2011); Hanihara and Ishida (2001b); Hauser and DeStefano (1989); Sant'Ana Castilho et al. (2006).

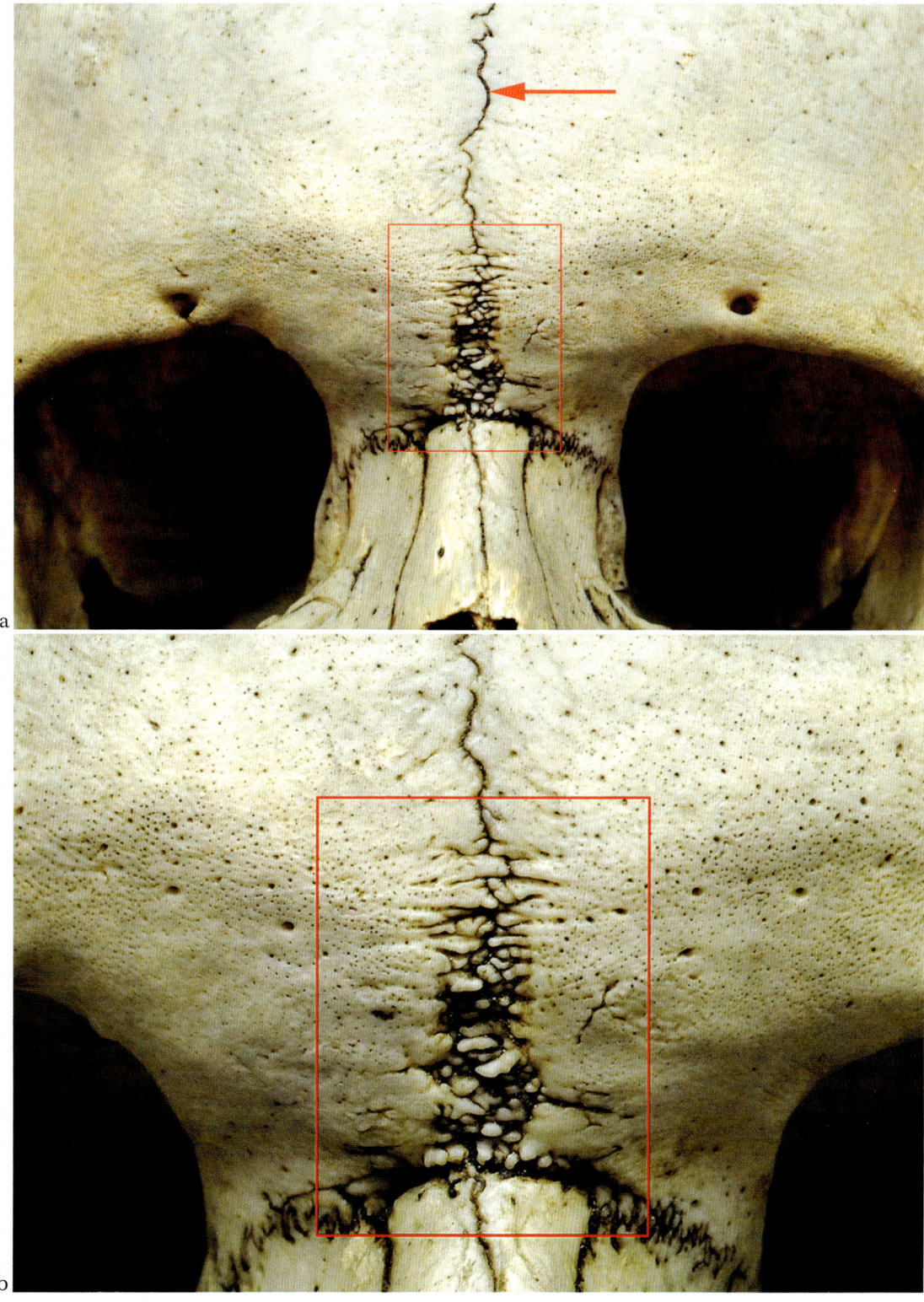

Figure 66a-b. Metopic and supranasal sutures in an adult skull (Mütter Museum 1997 1007 04). (a) Frontal view of a relatively simple metopic suture (arrow) superior to the much more complex and horizontally-oriented ("zigzag") supranasal suture (SNS) (red rectangle). (b) Morphology of an unusually complex SNS resembling grains of sand – these "grains" are horizontal projections within the SNS that likely dissipate biomechanical stresses associated with chewing.

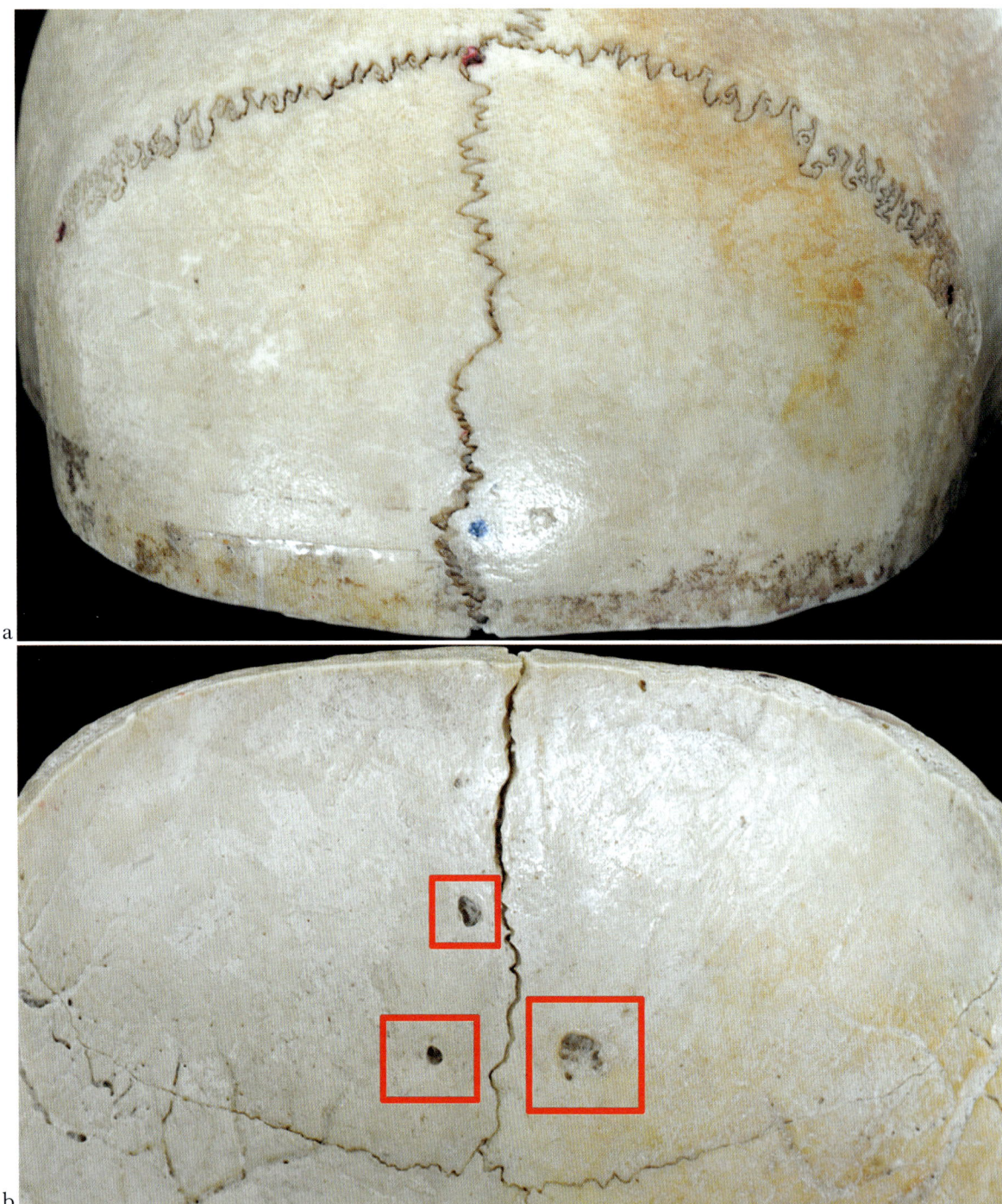

Figure 67a-b. Example of an open/patent metopic suture and Pacchionian pits. (a) Ectocranial and (b) endocranial views of patent/open metopic suture (sutura frontalis persistens) and Pacchionian pits (squares) in an adult Thai (KKU). Note that the metopic and coronal sutures are more complex ectocranially than endocranially, a pattern seen in nearly all humans. Some early researchers believed that narrow (dolicocephalic) skulls were less likely to exhibit metopism than wide (brachycephalic) skulls (Holden and Langton 1879), although other researchers disagree (Bolk 1917; Scheuer et al. 2000). Freyschmidt et al. (2002) report metopism as present in 5%–8% of adults. Cf. Yadav et al. (2010) for metopism.

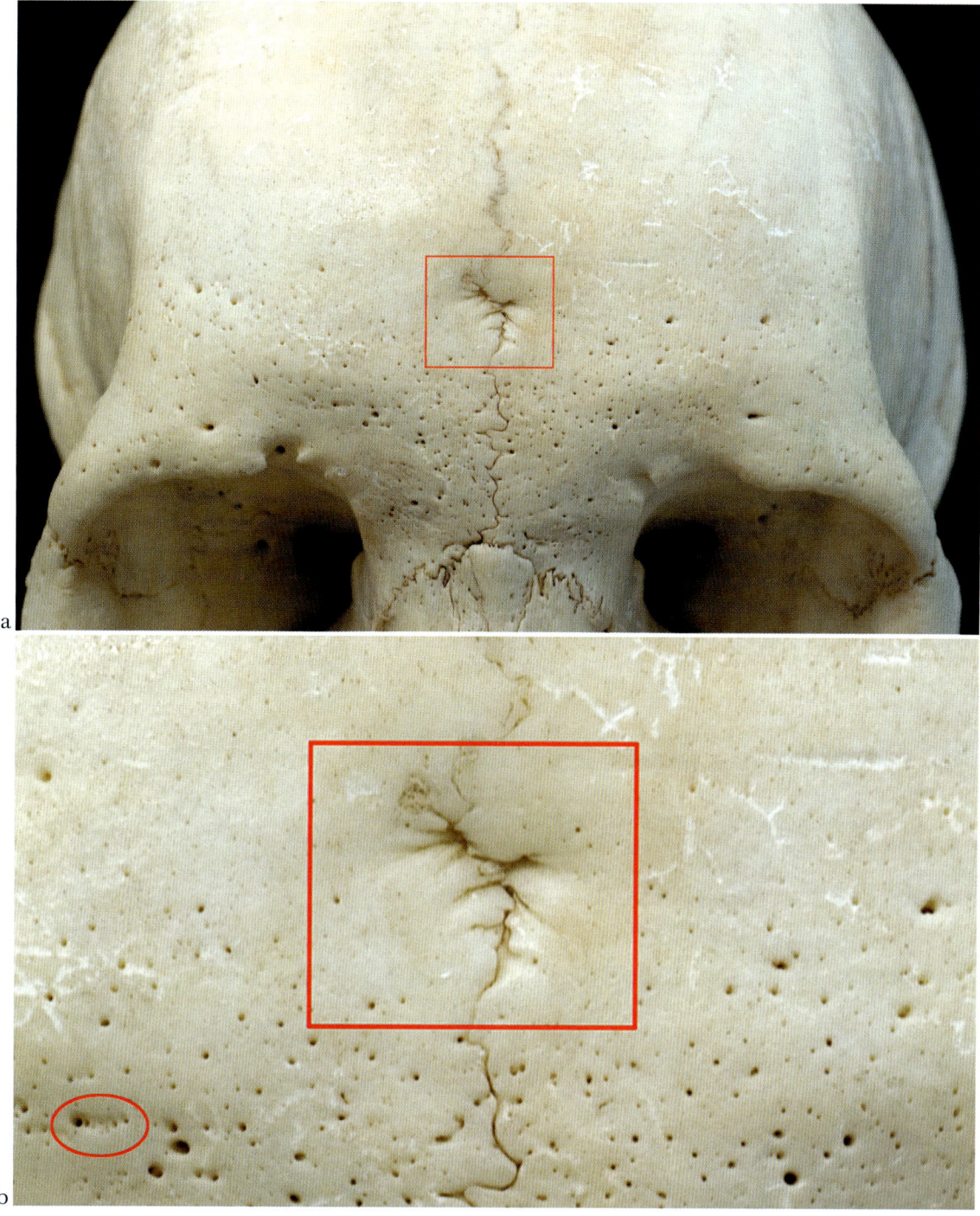

Figure 68a-b. Metopism and a metopic/frontal/interfrontal fissure in an adult Asian male (CSC AS022). (a) Frontal view of a persistent (open) metopic suture, sometimes referred to a remnant of the metopic suture (Yadav et al. 2010) and a metopic fissure (square). (b) Close-up of the fissure (square) showing that, when present, it may be visible endocranially along the frontal crest. Some of the pitting/foramina formed along a groove (circle) may have transmitted vessels, while others are likely due to porotic hyperostosis or attachment of the periosteum. Metopic fissure is an uncommon finding. Cf. Hauser and DeStefano (1989); Schultz (1918, 1929).

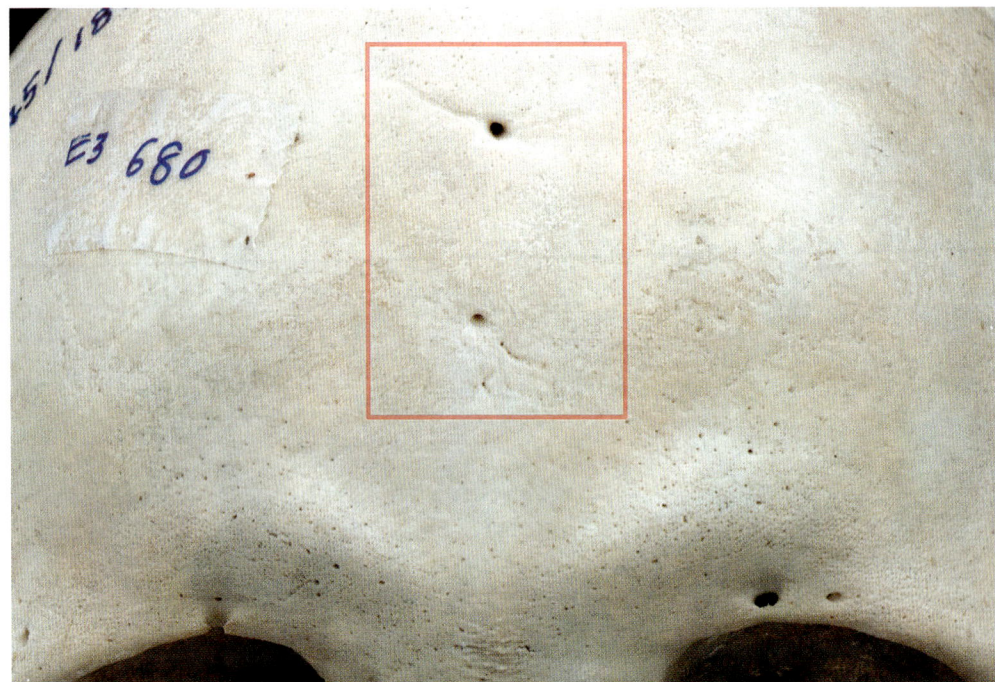

Figure 69. Two foramina along what is now an obliterated interfrontal/metopic suture (rectangle) – note that both foramina are associated with shallow grooves suggesting that the foramina are for extracranial vessels (KKU 45-188). Frontal foramina, while uncommon, are typical variants.

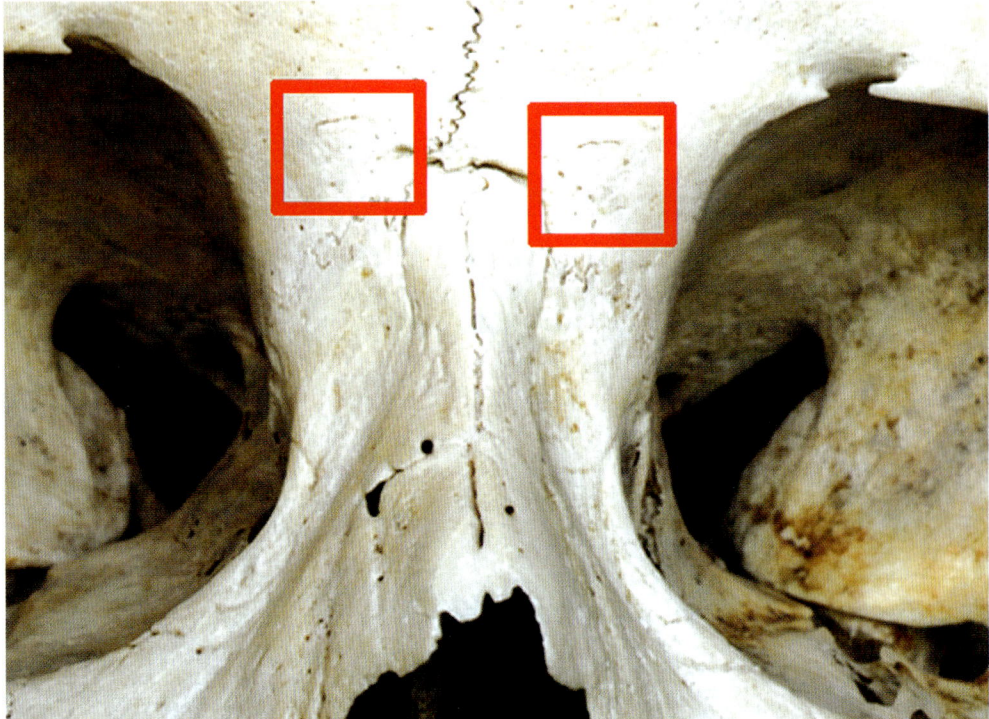

Figure 70. Small depressions likely serve as attachments for the procerus muscles (squares) in a Thai adult (KKU). Note the fractured and healed nasal bones resulting in deviation of the internasal suture (misalignment of the metopic and internasal sutures was developmental).

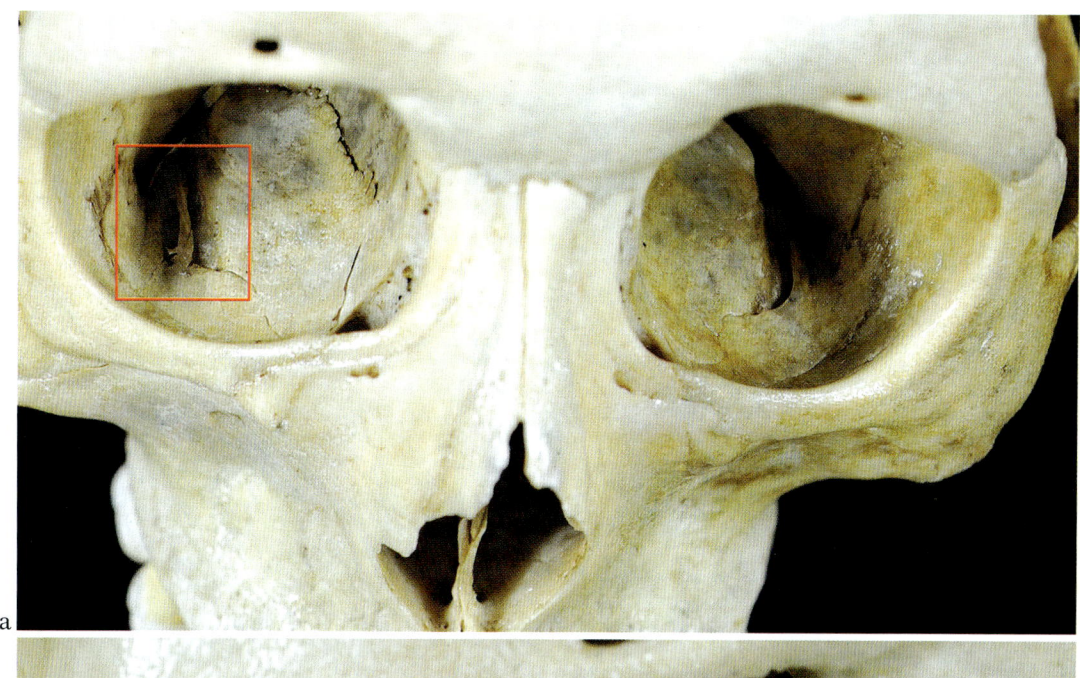

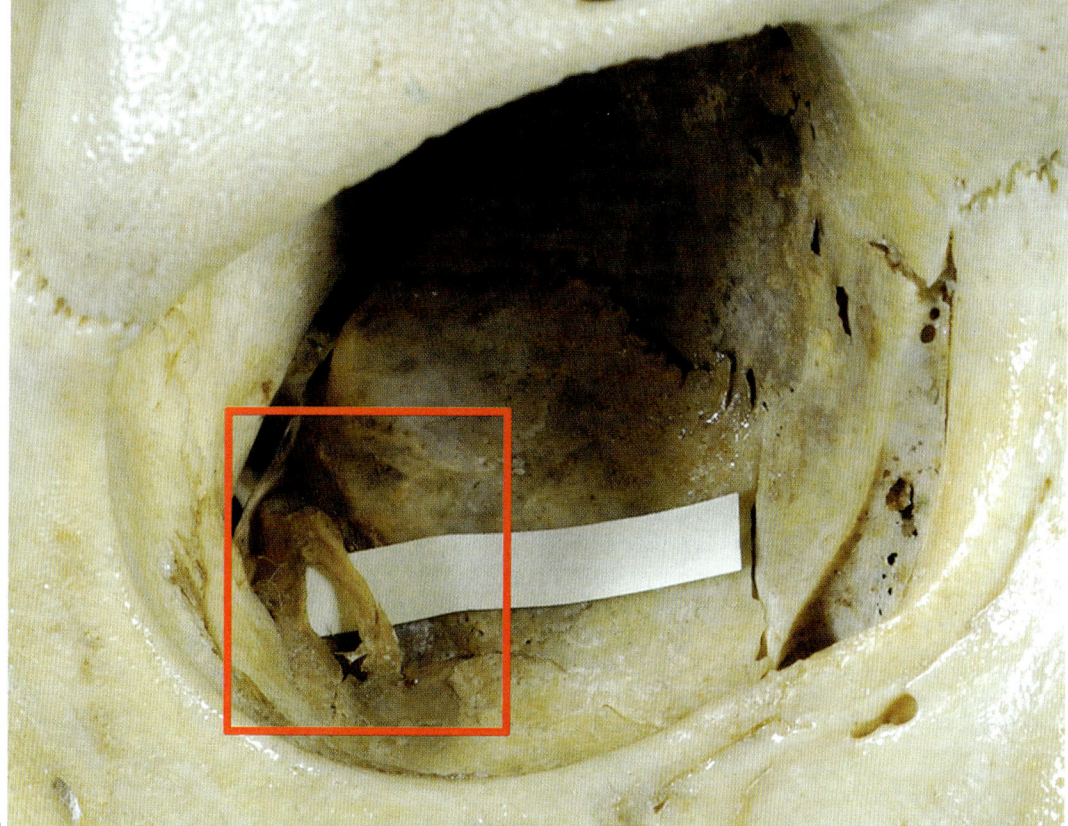

Figure 71a-b. Raised, overhanging medial "shelf" in the right orbit in an adult Asian (CSC AC011). (a) Frontal view of an overhanging "shelf" of bone and an elongated opening/aperture (rectangle) formed from the right zygoma that may transmit vessels and nerves. This shelf of bone may represent periorbital calcification of the soft tissues or localized resorption of the bone and is only the second example of its kind that the authors have encountered. (b) Detail of the bony "shelf" (square) and opening in the right orbit highlighted from beneath with a piece of white paper. Rare finding. Cf. Ozer et al. (2009) for an anatomical study of the orbital fissure.

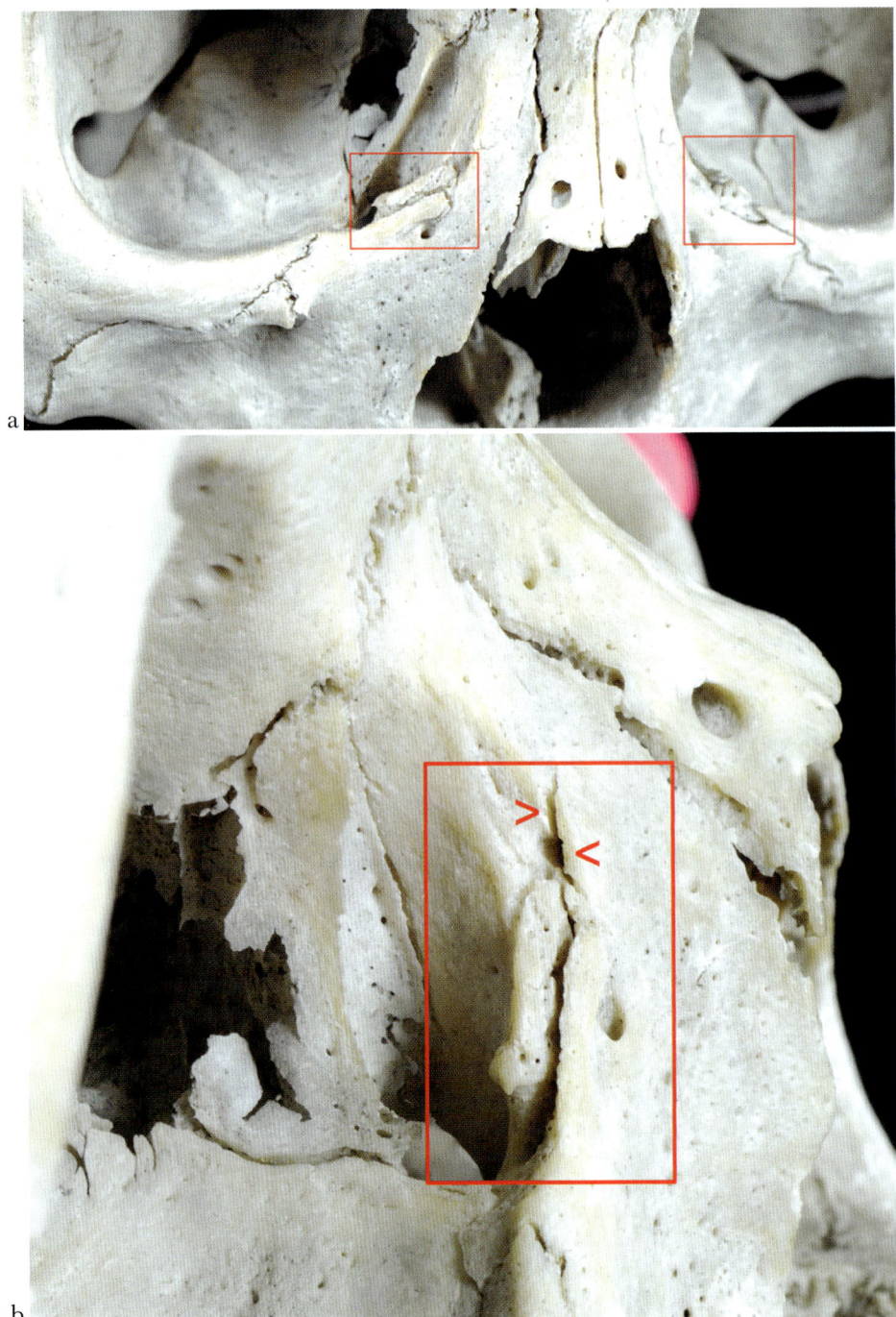

Figure 72a-b. Lacrimal or perilacrimal ossicles in an adult Thai (KKU). (a) Oblique view of small islands/ossicles of bone in the lacrimal region along the anterior lacrimal crest (possibly what Flecker (1913) called the Ossicle of Infraorbital Margin, or Ossicle of Lacrimal Groove). Note the lacrimal ossicle in the left orbit is situated at the origin of the zygomaticomaxillary suture. The lacrimal canal houses the lacrimal sac in the living. (b) Close-up of the right perilacrimal ossicle (rectangle), foramen (<) and small suture (>) medial to the ossicle. The etiology of these islands, many of which are loosely attached and mobile, may reflect a genetic component. The lacrimal bone ossifies from more than one intra-membranous center. Perilacrimal ossicles are uncommon finding. Cf. Flecker (1913) and Macalister (1884) for six types of lacrimal ("lachrymal") ossicles.

Frontal View of the Skull

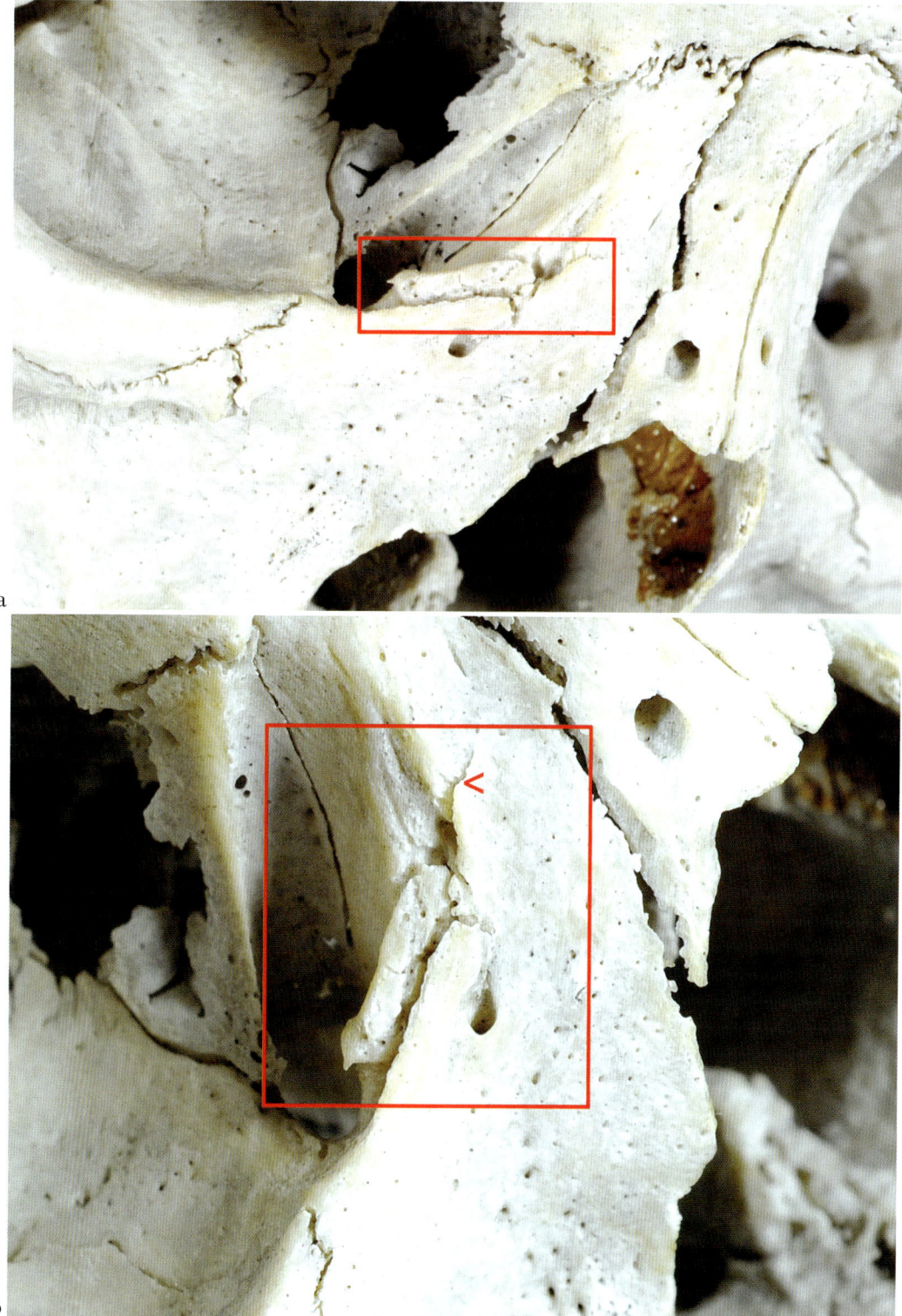

Figure 73a-b. Lacrimal ossicle along the right orbit. (a) Close-up of the movable, but attached, lacrimal ossicle (rectangle) along the right anterior lacrimal crest and large but normal nasal foramina in a Thai adult (KKU). (b) Close-up of the ossicle and small suture (square and <) medial to the ossicle. Uncommon finding. Cf. Flecker (1913); Macalister (1884).

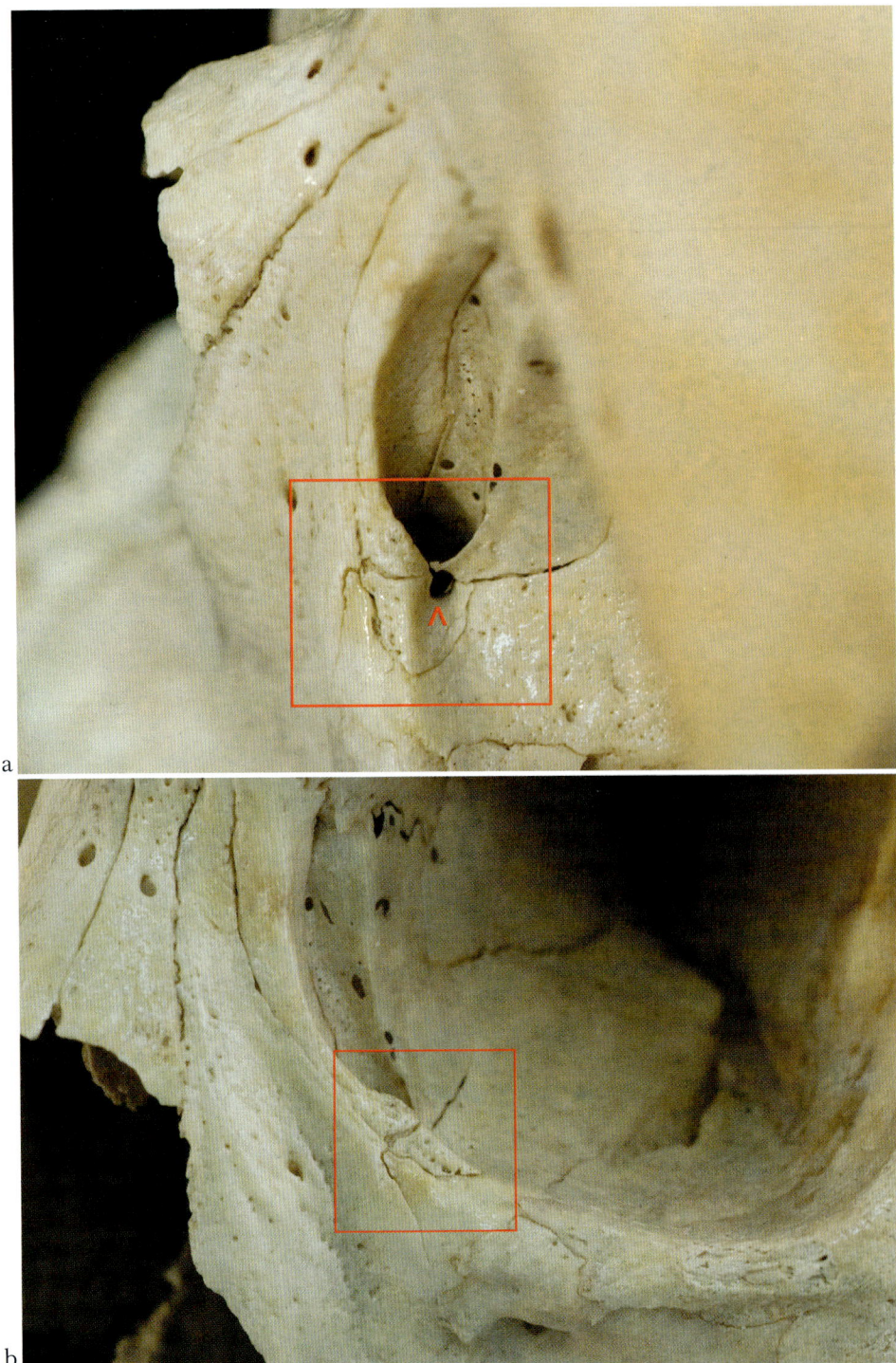

Figure 74a-b. Lacrimal ossicle and foramen in an adult Asian skull. (a) Superior view showing a lacrimal ossicle (square) and small inconstant foramen (∧) that communicates with the lacrimal canal in the left orbit (the lacrimal canal houses the lacrimal sac). (b) Oblique view of the ossicle (square) and its position along the orbital rim. This lacrimal bone variant, one of six identified by Macalister (1884) as ossiculum canalis naso-lachrymalis, is part of the maxilla, not the lacrimal bone. This trait is bilateral in this individual and the ossicle is attached and stationary, not mobile. Cf. Flecker (1913). It is sometimes necessary to use a magnifying glass or stereoscopic microscope to identify the smaller ossicles. Uncommon trait.

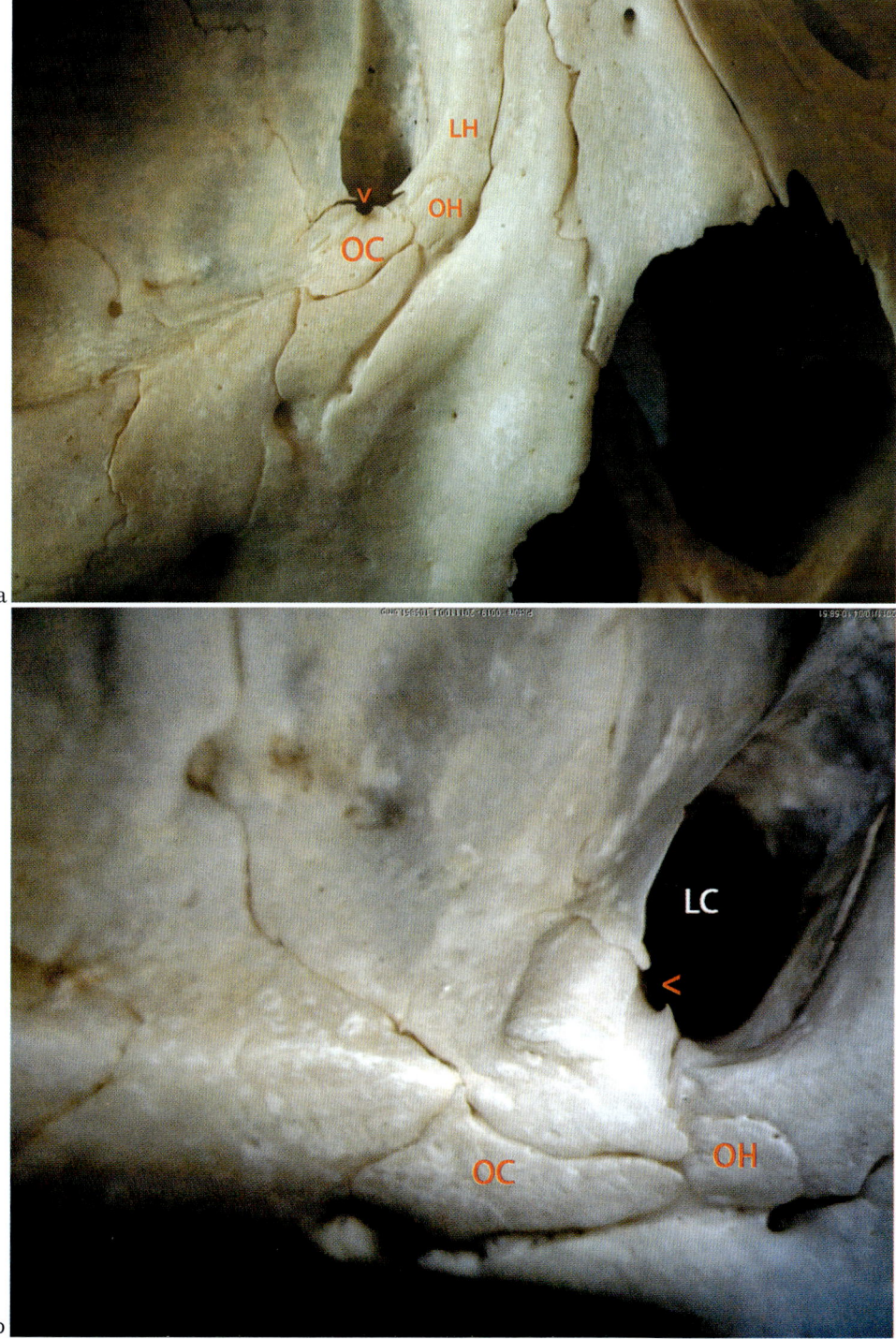

Figure 75a-b. Bilateral lacrimal ossicles in a young adult Asian female (CSC AC026). (a) Magnified view illustrating the morphology of the lacrimal canal and incomplete foramen (∨), the ossiculus canalis (OC) and ossiculus hamuli (OH) in the right orbit. "LH" is the lacrimal hamulus that, near its inferior tip, has a small ossicle (OH). (b) Superior view of the lacrimal canal (LC), ossiculus canalis (OC), ossiculus hamuli (OH) and an osseous notch communicating with the lacrimal canal in the right orbit. The frequency of this foramen and its function are unknown. While the ossicles in this individual appear to be separate, they are anchored and immobile. Cf. Macalister (1884).

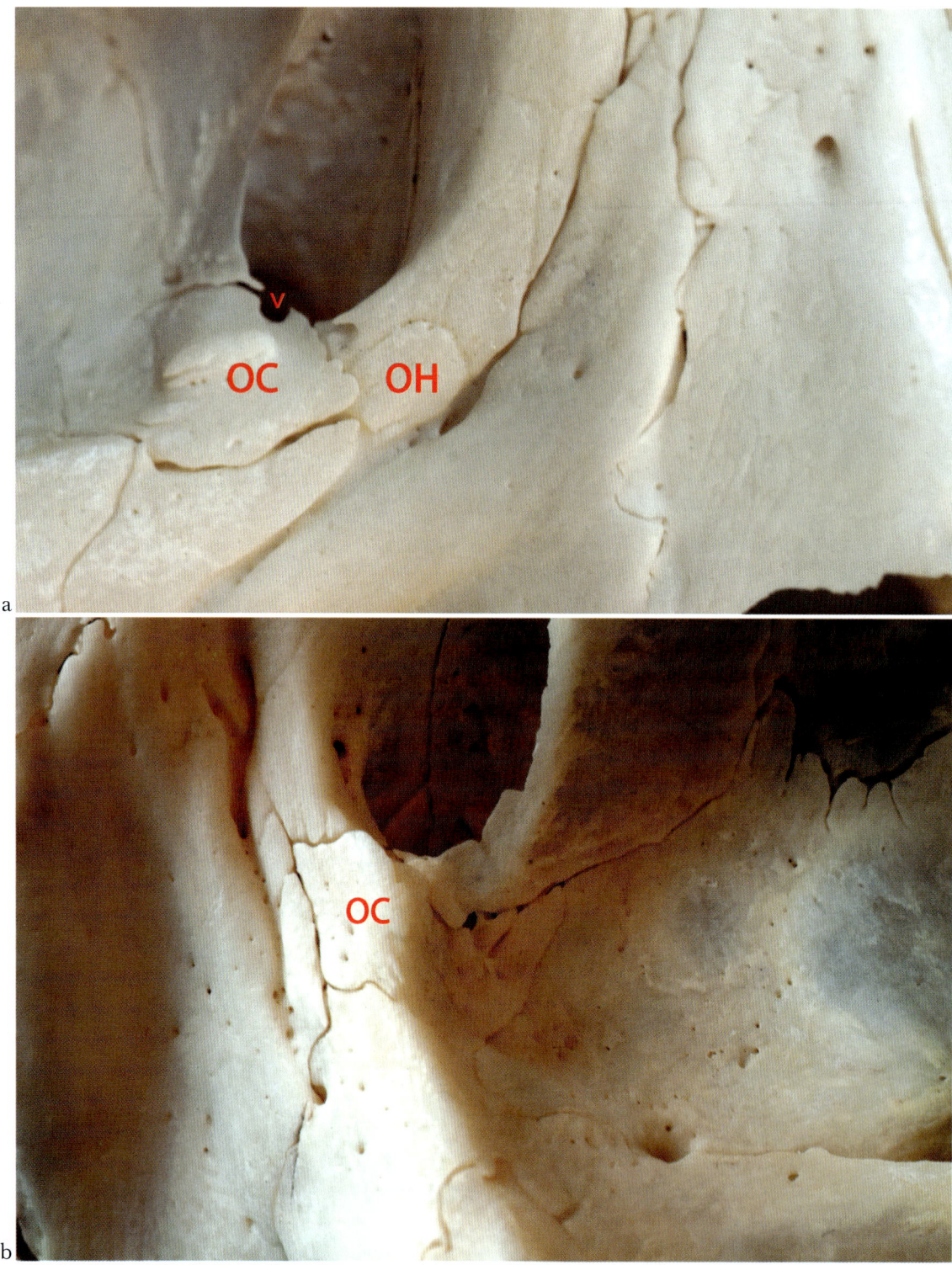

Figure 76a-b. Orbital ossicles and lacrimal foramen. (a) Close-up of ossiculus canalis (OC), ossiculus hamuli (OH) and an inconstant foramen (∨) of unknown etiology in the right orbit. (b) A single ossiculus canalis (OC) in the left orbit. See Macalister (1884) for more on the foramen.

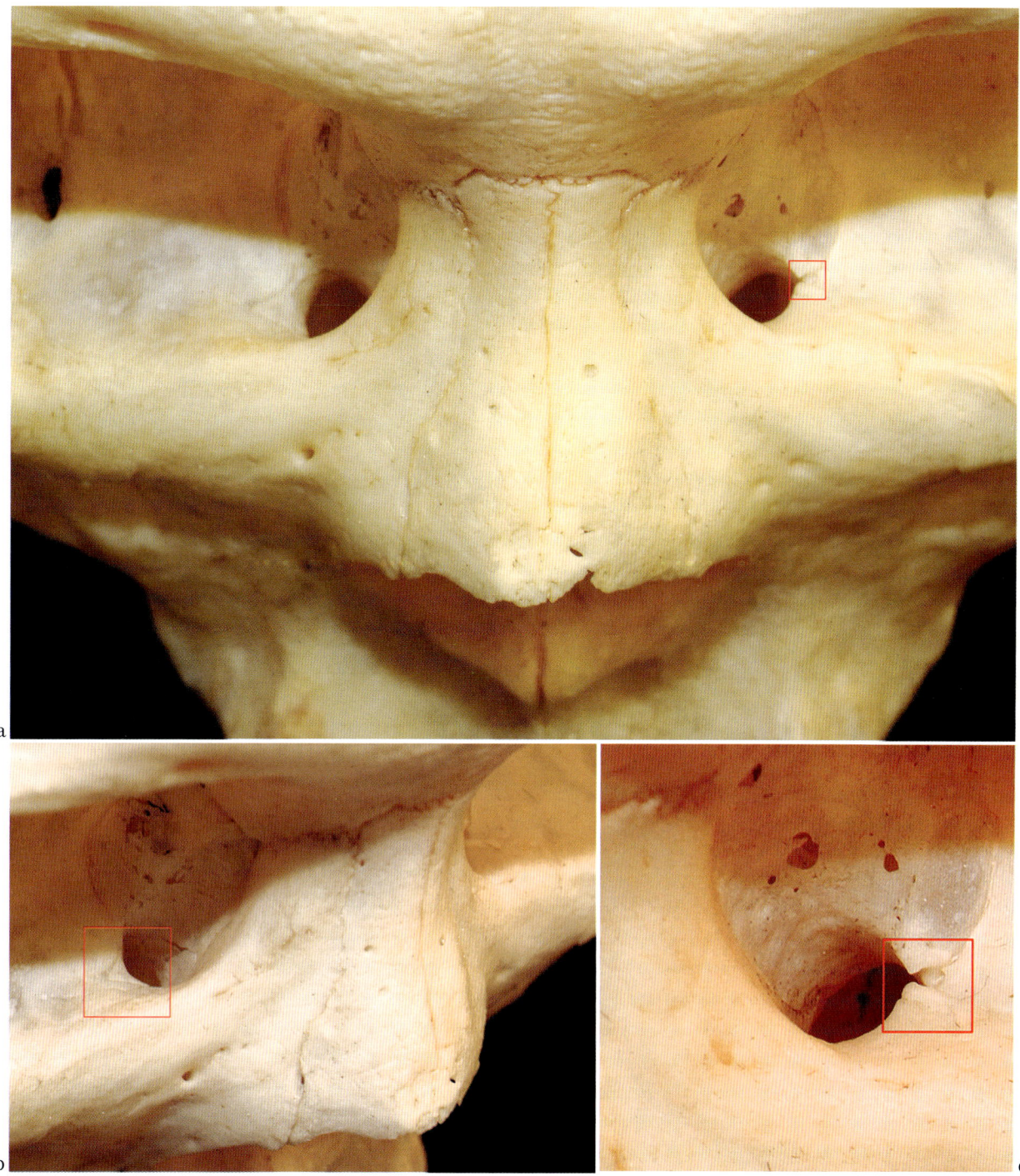

Figure 77a-c. Partial bridging of the left lacrimal foramen in a 91-year-old Asian female (JABSOM 1367). (a) Incomplete bridging of the lacrimal foramen (square) in the left orbit and absence in the right orbit. (b) Close-up showing absence of a foramen (square) in the right orbit. (c) Close-up of the incomplete formation/partial bridging of a foramen in the left orbit (square). The lateral margin of the lacrimal canal may exhibit a complete or partially-formed foramen that communicates with the lacrimal canal and may transmit a vessel. A small pilot study (N=25) consisting primarily of Asian skulls revealed a foramen in 20% of the crania. Three possible features were noted: a foramen, a partial foramen or an absence of both. Macalister (1884) refers to this feature simply as a "vascular foramen."

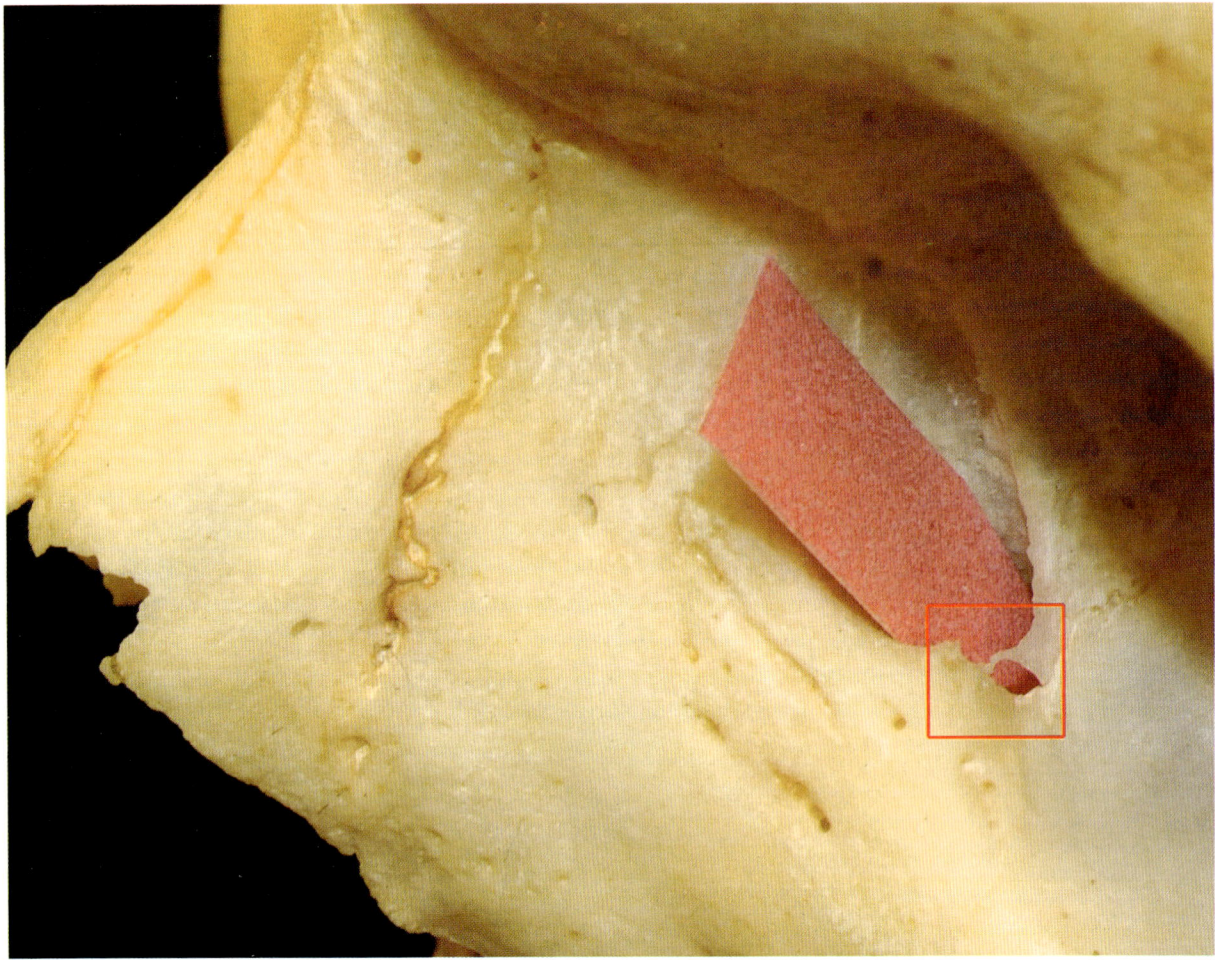

Figure 78. Left lacrimal foramen (square) in a 70-year-old Caucasoid male (JABSOM 1353). Note in this individual that the foramen is formed by a thin, delicate bridge of bone. There was no evidence of a foramen in the right orbit. Cf. Macalister (1884).

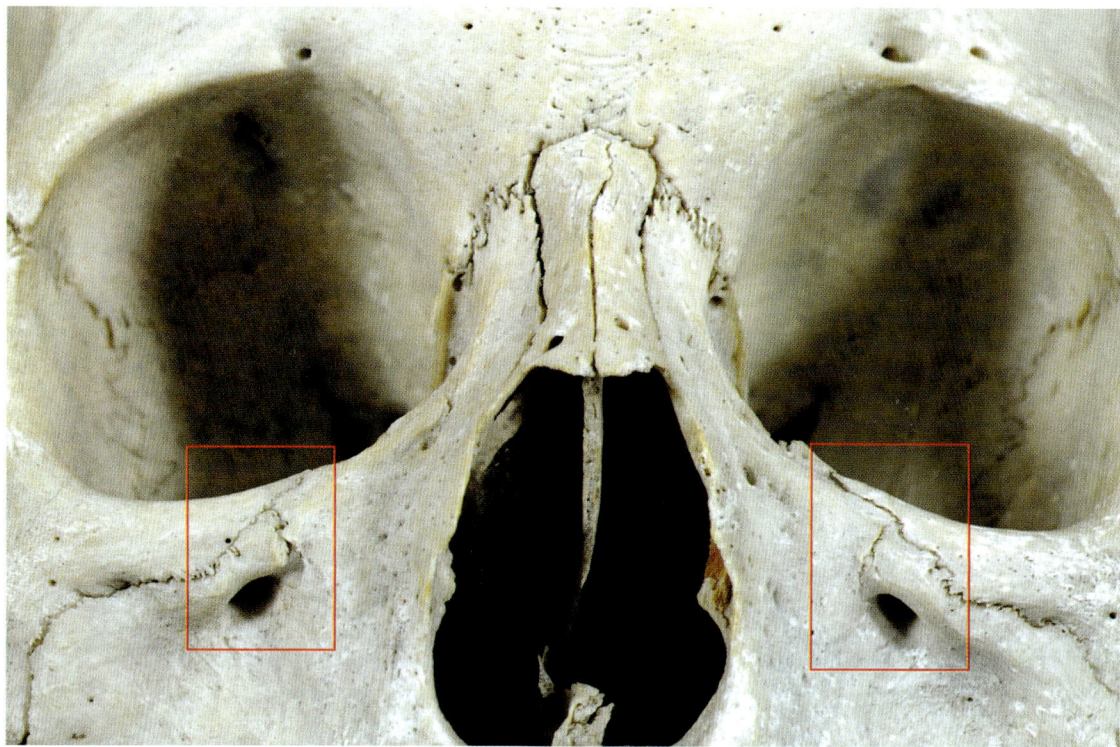

Figure 79. Bilateral infraorbital sutures (rectangles) into the infraorbital foramina in a Thai adult skull (KKU). While there is variation in the origin of these short and inconstant sutures (rectangles), most extend from the zygomaticomaxillary suture into the infraorbital foramina. Common finding. Cf. Boopathi et al. (2010); Hauser and DeStefano (1989); Pietrusewsky and Douglas (2002); Turner (1885).

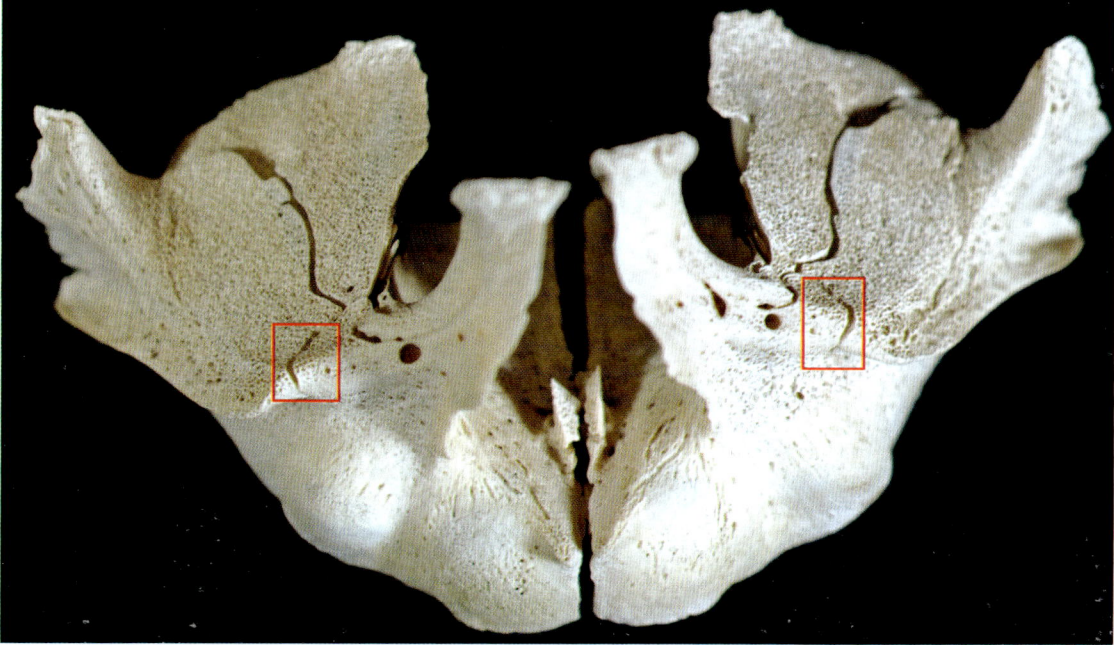

Figure 80. The path of the infraorbital suture (squares) along the floor of the orbits of a fetus (SI 249551). Note the porous nature of much of the bone, particularly in the orbits. Normal anatomy and common finding.

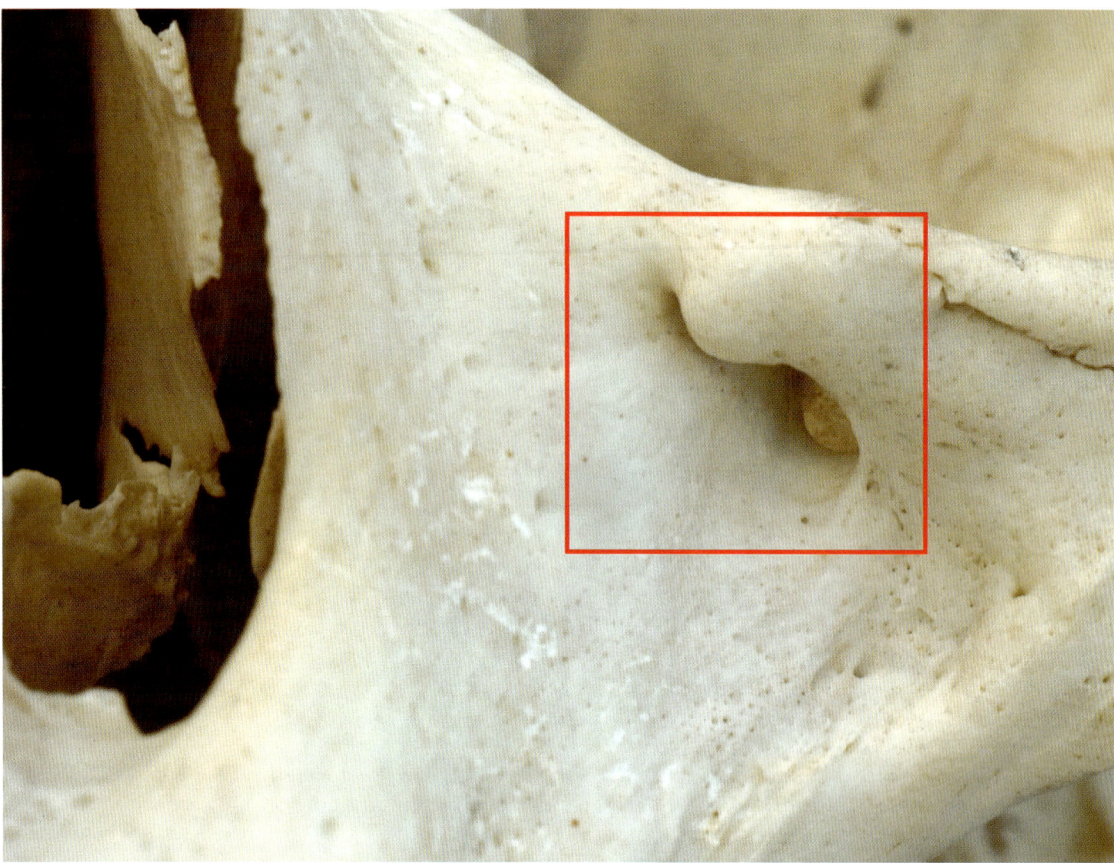

Figure 81. "Folded" or overhanging margin of the left infraorbital foramen (bilateral) in a robust adult Asian male (CSC AS022). Cf. Leo et al. (1995) for more on infraorbital foramen.

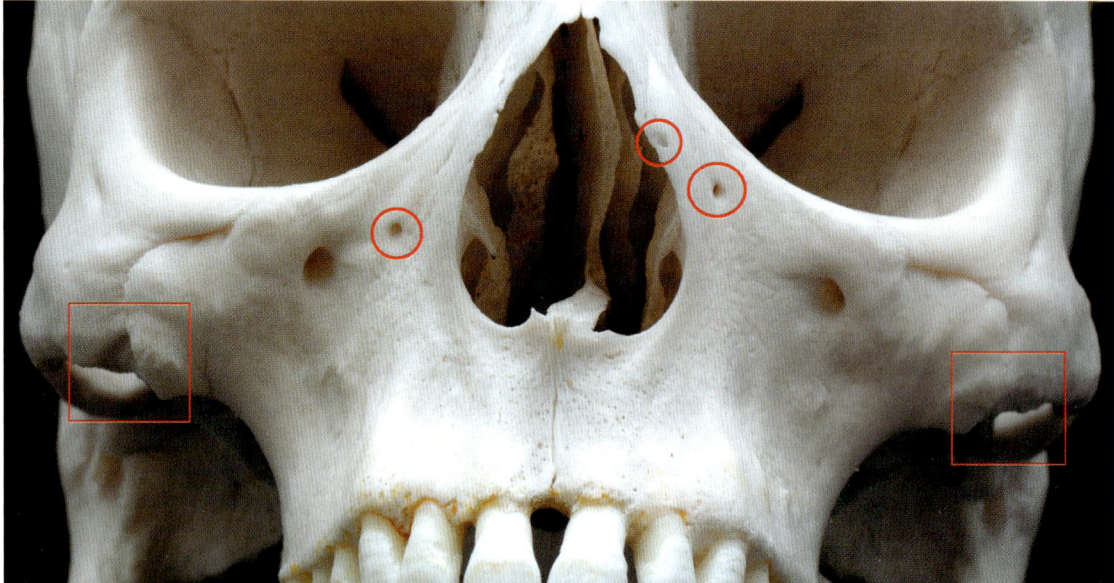

Figure 82. Accessory maxillary/infraorbital foramina (circles) and unusual morphology (squares) of the zygomaxillary tubercles for attachment of the masseter muscle in an adult male (FSA AC051). The foramina are common typical variants. Cf. Hauser and DeStefano (1989).

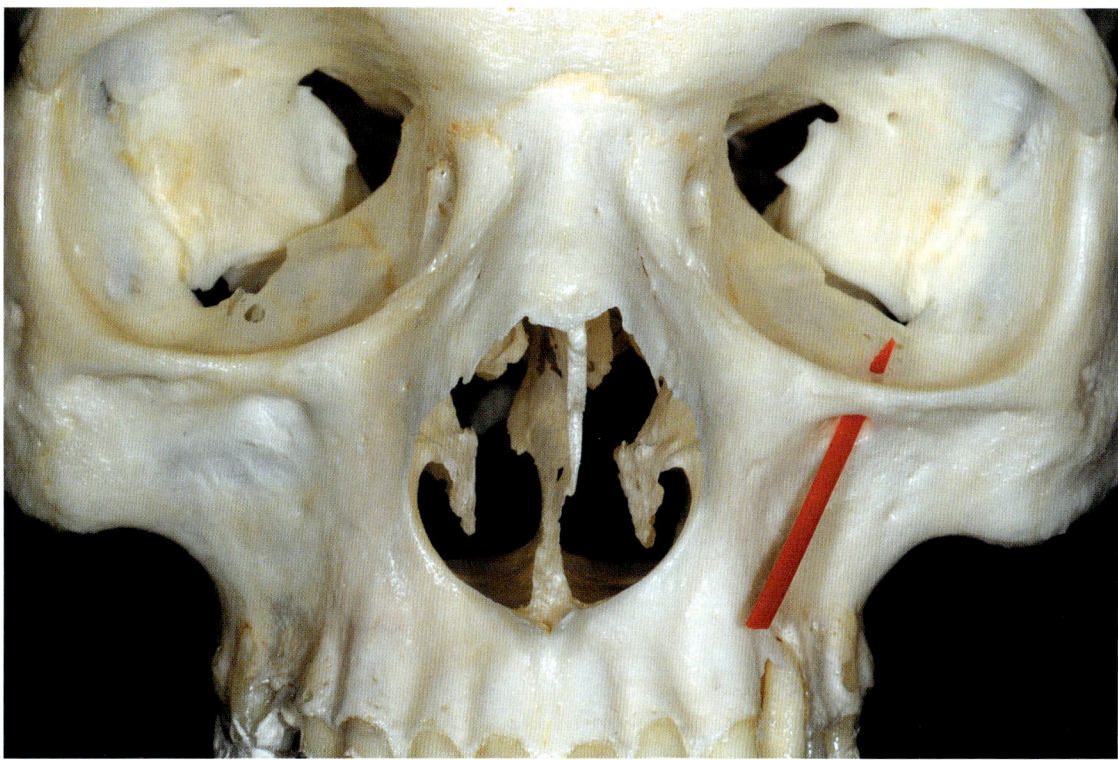

Figure 83. The path of one of the lesser infraorbital foramina (probe) into the lower orbital border in an adult (JABSOM). This foramen transmits the infraorbital vein, artery and nerve. See Macedo et al. (2009) for more on the position of this foramen.

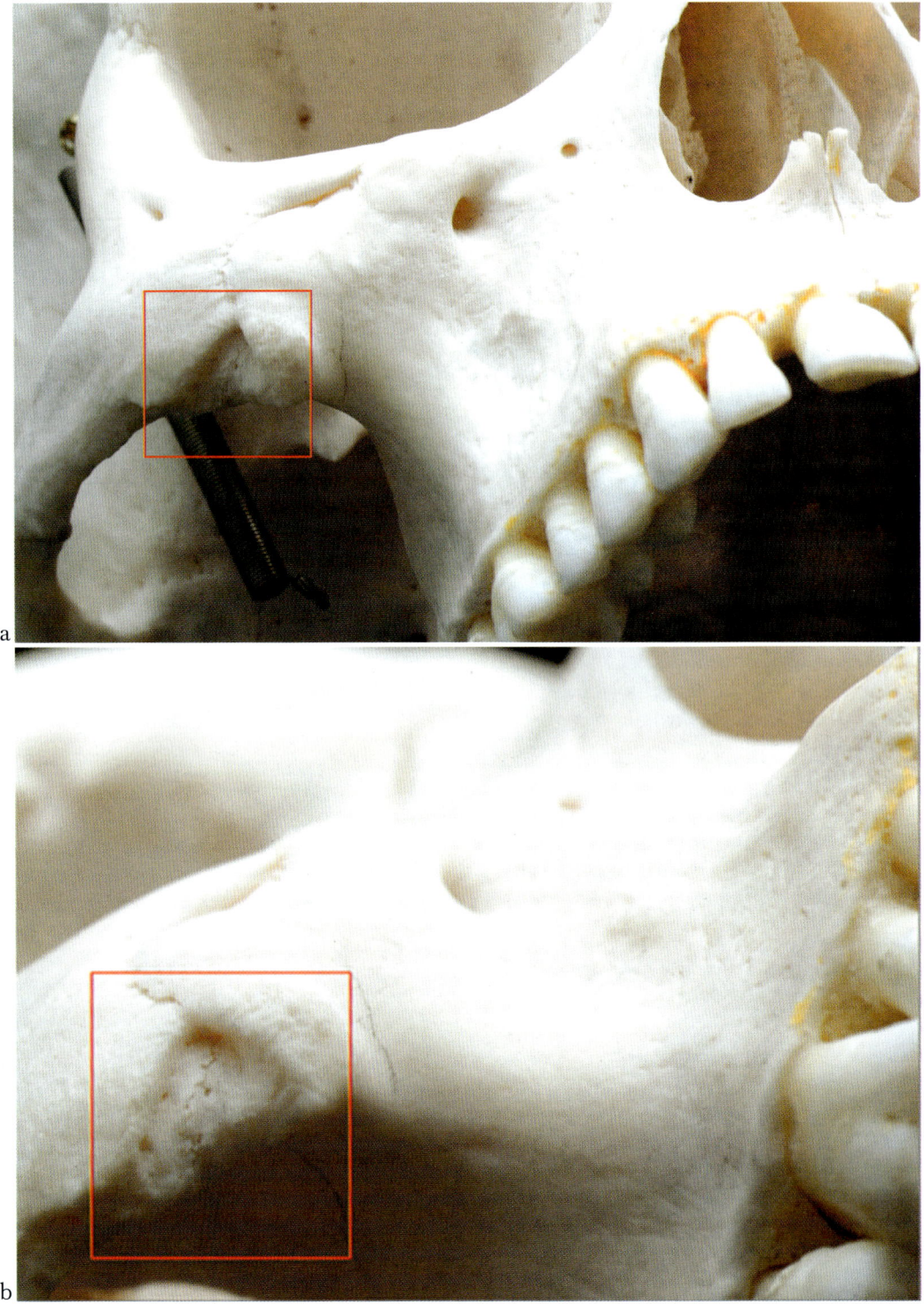

Figure 84a-b. Unusually deep right inferior malar tubercle in an adult male (FSA AC051). (a) Unusually deep depression (square) in the right zygomatic bone with the zygomaticomaxillary suture dividing and running along the floor of this depression; this is not an os Japonicum (the depression in the left tubercle of this individual is not as pronounced as in the right tubercle). (b) Close-up of the depression and zygomaticomaxillary suture (square). Cf. Hauser and DeStefano (1989).

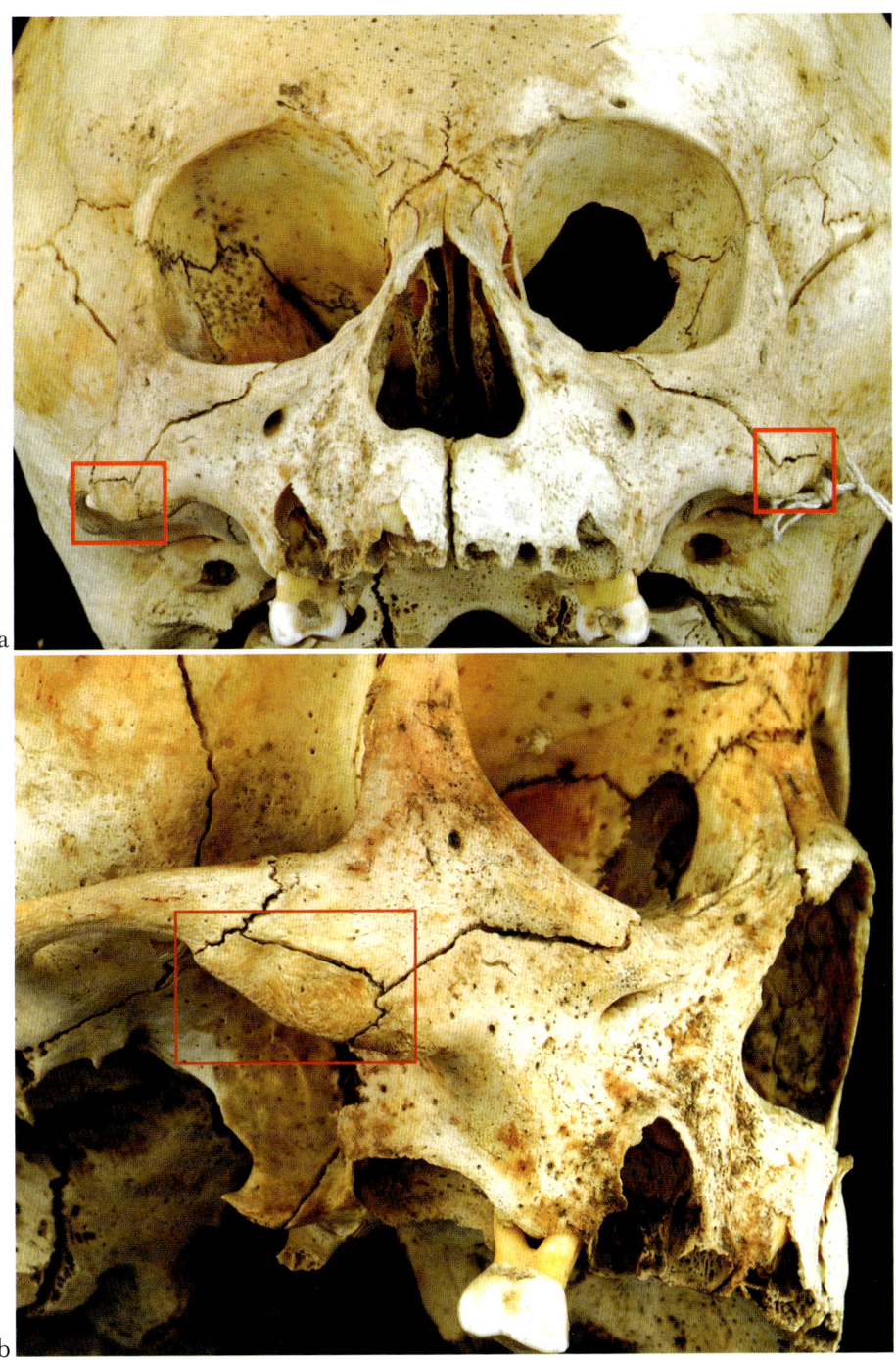

Figure 85a-b. Bilateral os Japonicum in an ancient Peruvian child (SI). (a) Bilateral os Japonicum (squares) showing the transversozygomatic suture dividing the zygomas. (b) Right oblique view and close-up of the right os Japonicum (rectangle). Common to uncommon finding depending on the group examined. Cf. Hanihara et al. (1998) for extensive research on this feature in many human groups.

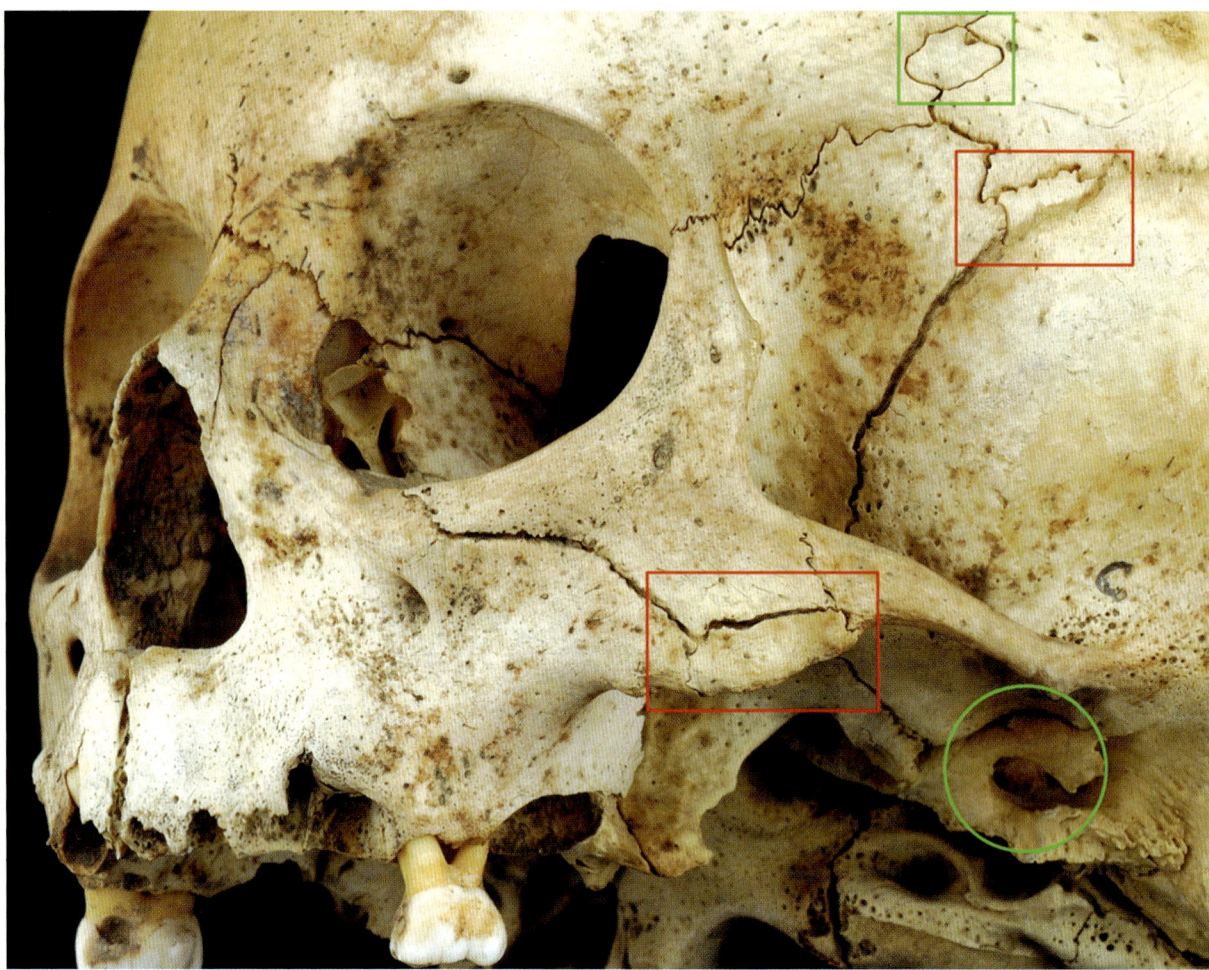

Figure 86. Coronal ossicle (green square), small squamosal ossicle (upper red rectangle), os Japonicum, also known as the os zygomaticum bipartitum (lower red rectangle) and a large tympanic dehiscence (green circle) in an archaeological Peruvian child (SI). os Japonicum, a term first used in 1879 to refer to bipartite/divided zygomatic bones in Japanese crania, are present in many groups around the world. Frequent finding in some groups. Cf. Hanihara et al. (1998) for diverse frequencies of the os zygomaticum bipartitum; see Hauser and DeStefano (1989) for information on all four traits.

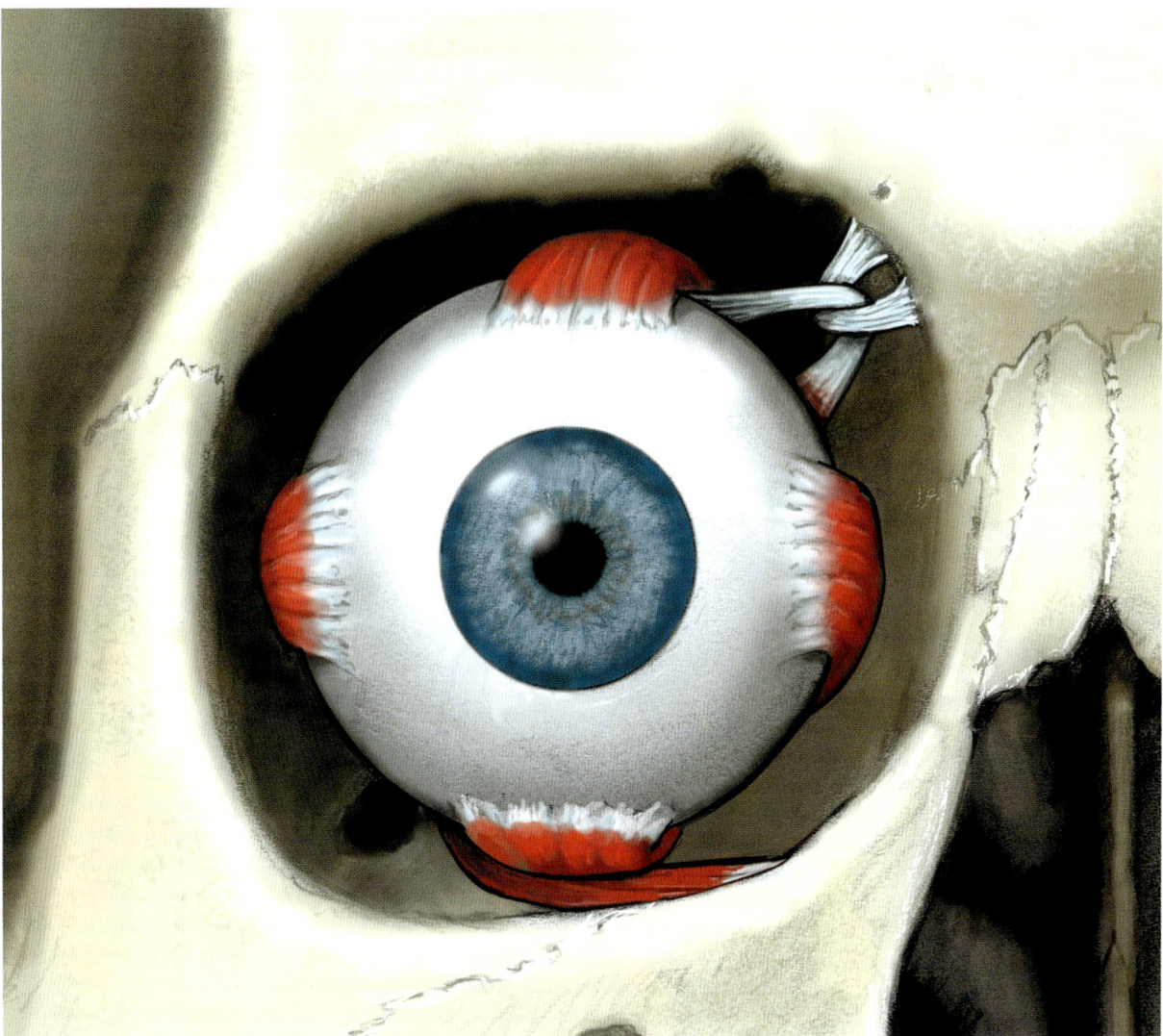

Figure 87. Anatomy of the right orbit showing the U-shaped trochlear apparatus (pulley) and superior oblique muscle running through it (illustration by Beth Lozanoff). An ossified/calcified trochlear pulley was found in 35 of 216 Korean patients and believed to be benign, showed a significant sex difference, may not represent a degenerative process, and appears to occur regardless of chronic disease (Ko and Kim 2010). Occasionally there is a shallow trochlear fossa or indentation where the pulley attaches to the medial orbit. Note where the inferior oblique muscle attaches along the inferior margin of the orbit. See Dutton (2011) for detailed information on the orbit and its structures.

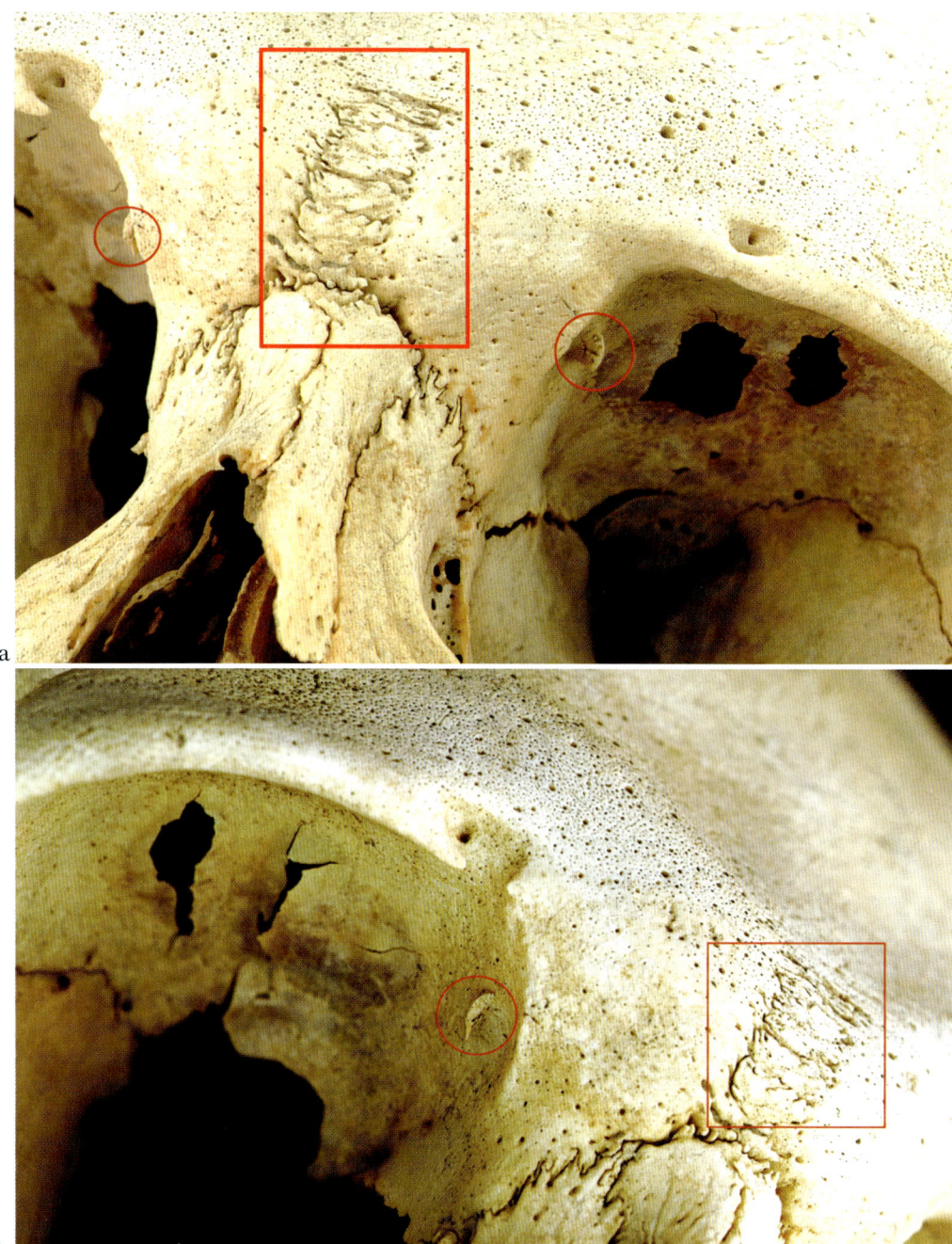

Figure 88a-b. Bilateral calcified/ossified trochlear apparatus in an adult Thai skull (KKU). (a) Trochlear apparatus (circles), sometimes known as spina trochlearis, trochlear spine and trochlear spur, a supranasal suture (rectangle) and male vermiculate pattern (pitting and irregular grooves above the orbits). While the trochlea/trochlear pulley (hyaline cartilage) is often attributed to calcification accompanying middle and old age, it is often present in the shape of a small hook or spike in adolescents or younger. (b) Inferior view of the right trochlear spur (circle) and the supranasal suture (square). A completely calcified U or ring of bone is an extremely rare occurrence (the authors have never seen one). The trochlea serves for passage of the superior oblique. Growth and calcification of the pulley usually begin superiorly and progress inferiorly. Cf. Dutton (2011); Hart et al. (1992); Hauser and DeStefano (1989); Ko and Kim (2010); Ossenberg (1970); Tappen (1983); Toldt (1928). Common findings.

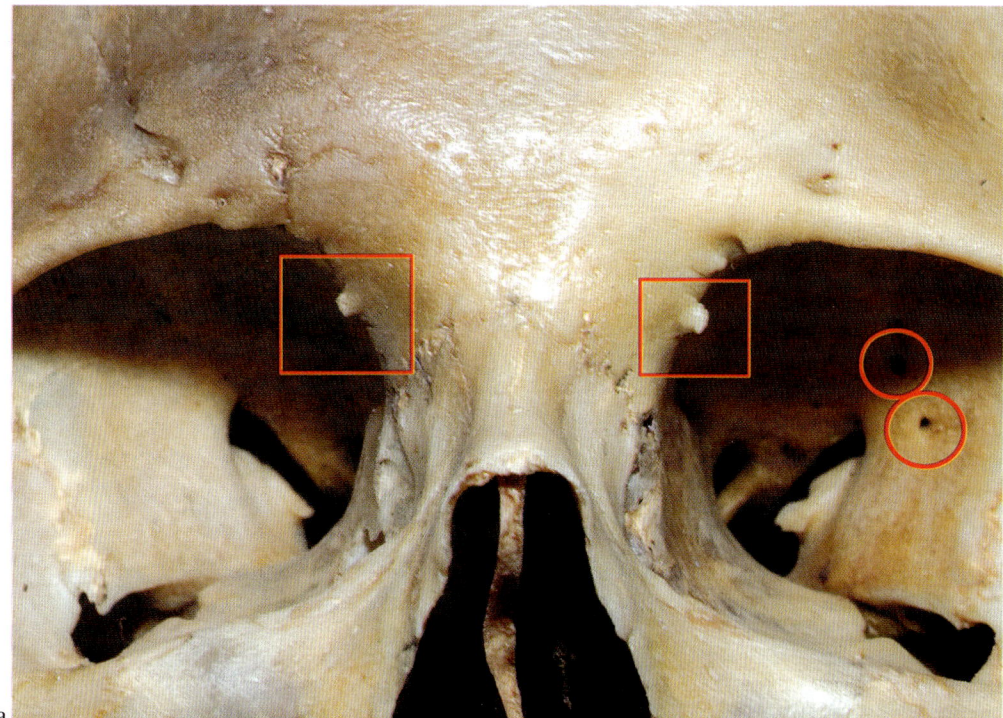
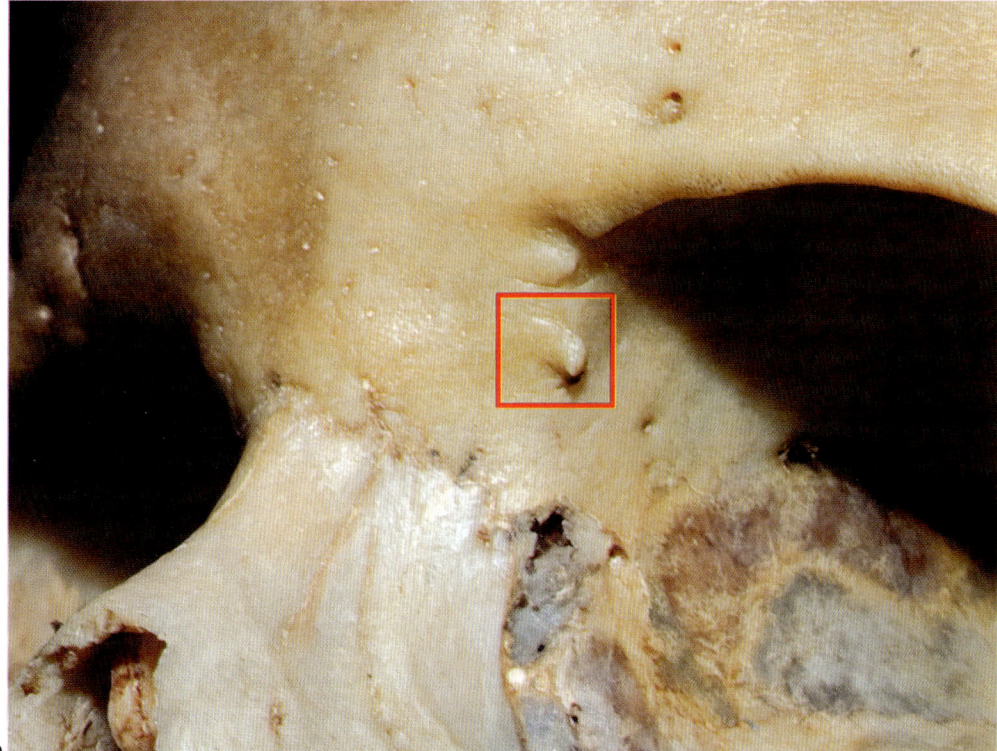

Figure 89a-b. Osseous projections and orbital foramina in an elderly White female (SI Terry 293R). (a) Small, bilateral bony projections (squares) of unknown etiology and frequency and foramina in the orbits (circles). Based on the anterior position and blunt shape of the bony projections, they may be calcified trochlear spurs that deflect anteriorly. The left orbit has three meningo-orbital foramen (circles), also known as foramen of Hyrtl and lacrimal foramen, among others (common finding). (b) Inferior view of the bony projection (square) in the left orbit. Cf. Jovanovic et al. (2003); Krishnamurthy et al. (2008); Neto et al. (1984); O'Brien and McDonald (2007); Vázquez et al. (2001).

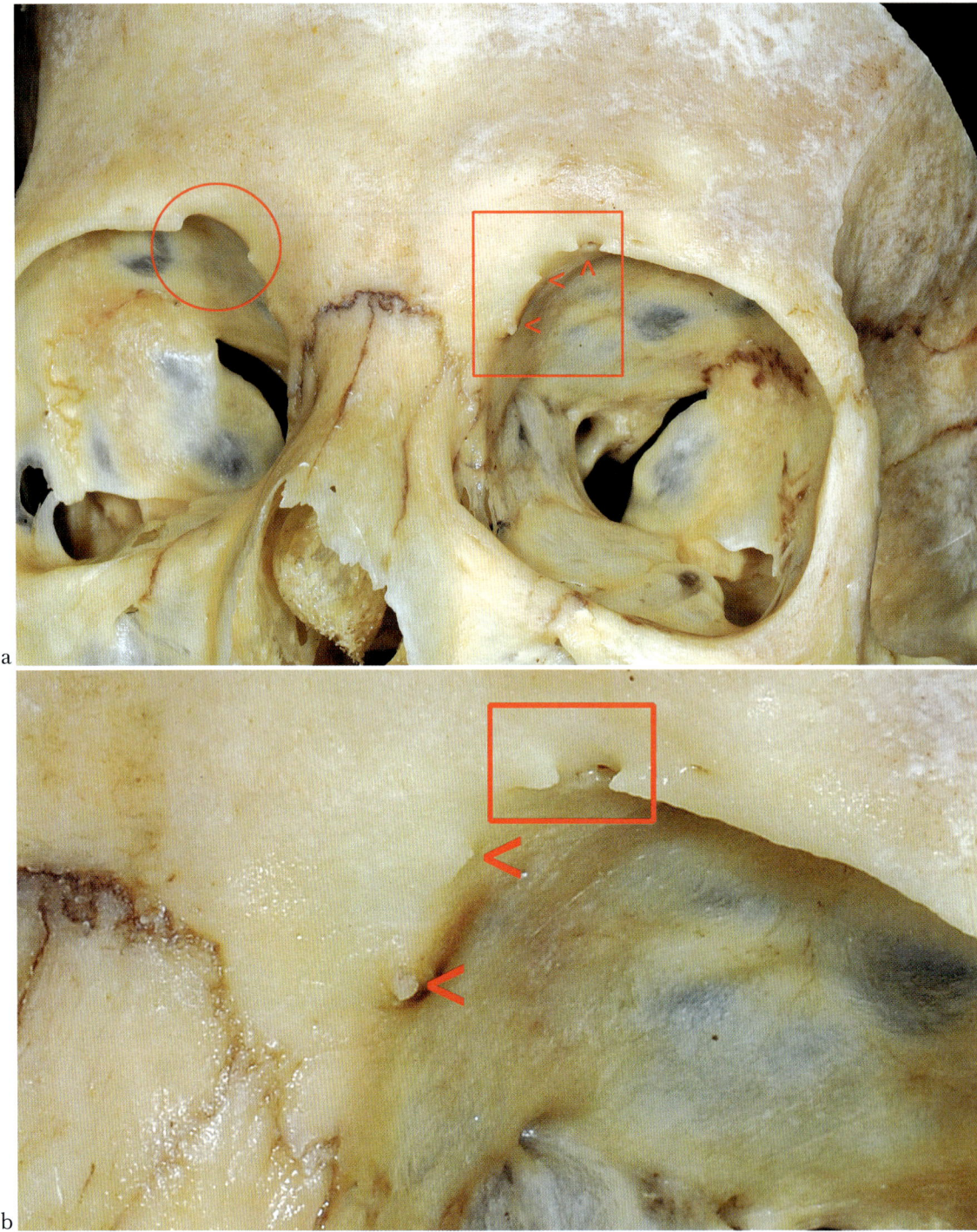

Figure 90a-b. Supraorbital notches and orbital rim spurs in a 54-year-old Asian male skull (JABSOM 1198). (a) Note the unusually large, but typical right supraorbital notch (circle) and small left supraorbital notch (∧), but two small osseous projections (<) along the medial border of the orbit. (b) The supraorbital notch (rectangle) has a small supraorbital foramen (normal variant). The location of the orbital rim spurs (<) appears to be positioned too far anteriorly to be trochlear spurs, although they may be a variant of trochlear spur. The notches are common variants. The function of the orbital rim spurs is unknown, but appear to be uncommon to rare.

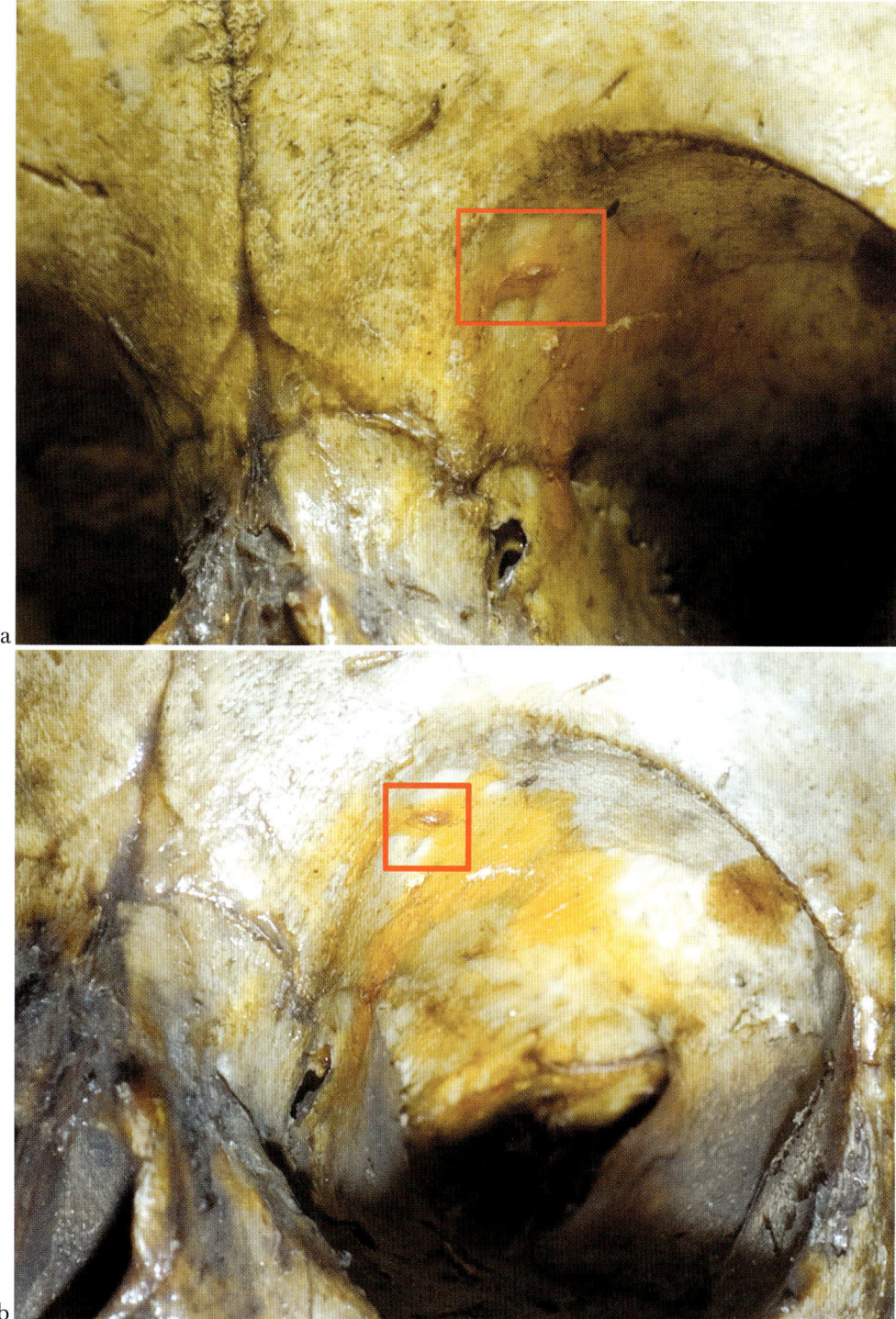

Figure 91a-b. Small trochlear spur in a 6-month-old child (UPenn L-606 66). (a) Frontal view of a small trochlear spur (square) in the left orbit. Although much of the facial region is covered in varnish or shellac that has yellowed over the years, the whitish trochlear spur in the left orbit is still clearly visible and palpable in the center of the square. The trochlea may be represented by a small spine, a shallow fossa, or both. (b) Close-up of the left trochlear spur (square). Common finding in adults, but with an unknown frequency in children. While the size and frequency of trochlear spurs may be correlated with age and some may view them an indicator of age, these osseous spurs may be found in very young children.

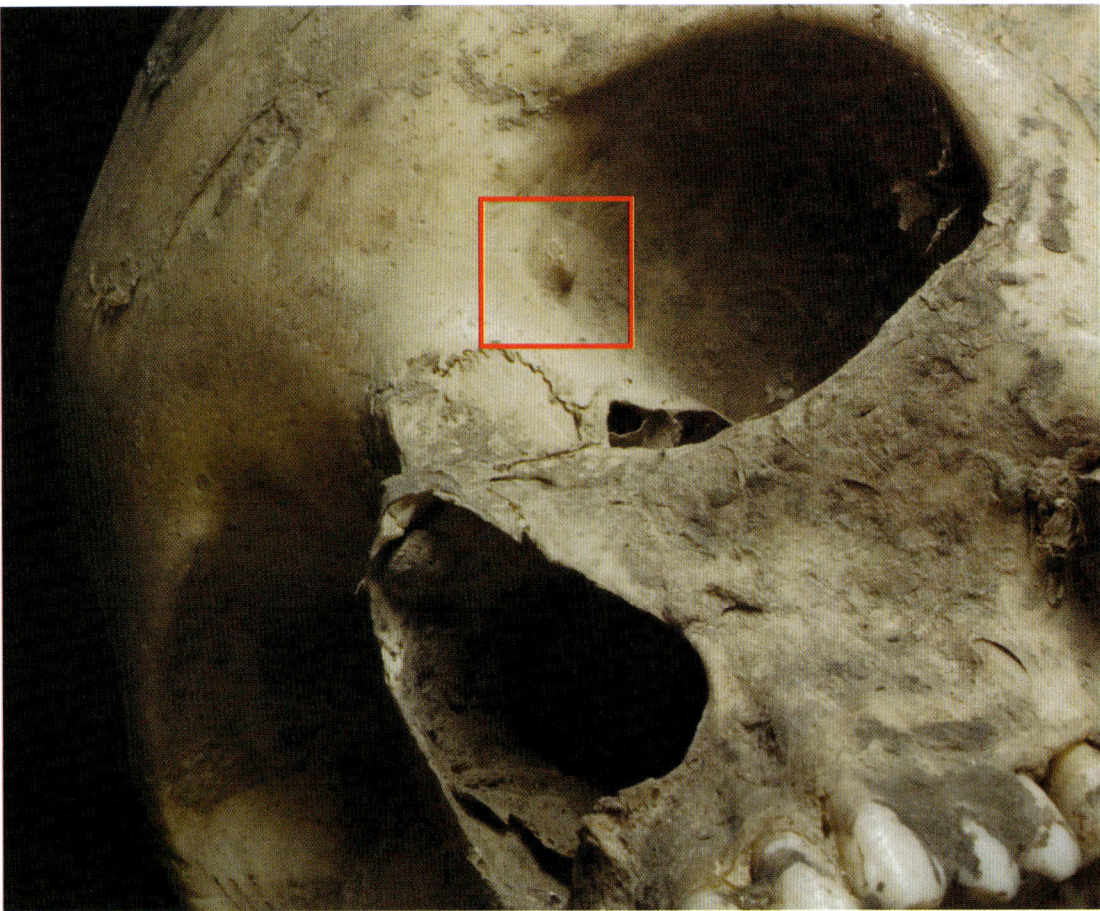

Figure 92. Left trochlear spur (square) in an approximately 6-year-old child from Peru (UPenn L-606 88).

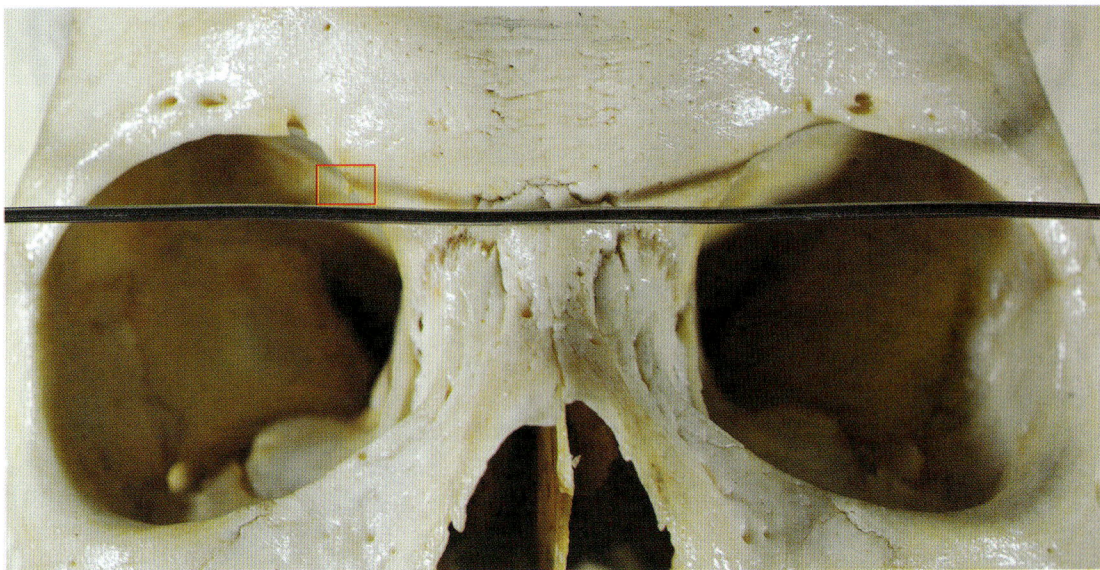

Figure 93. Location of unilateral trochlear spur (rectangle) above a straight line (probe) approximately across Nasion (KKU). Trochlear spurs and fossa are located above this line. Common finding.

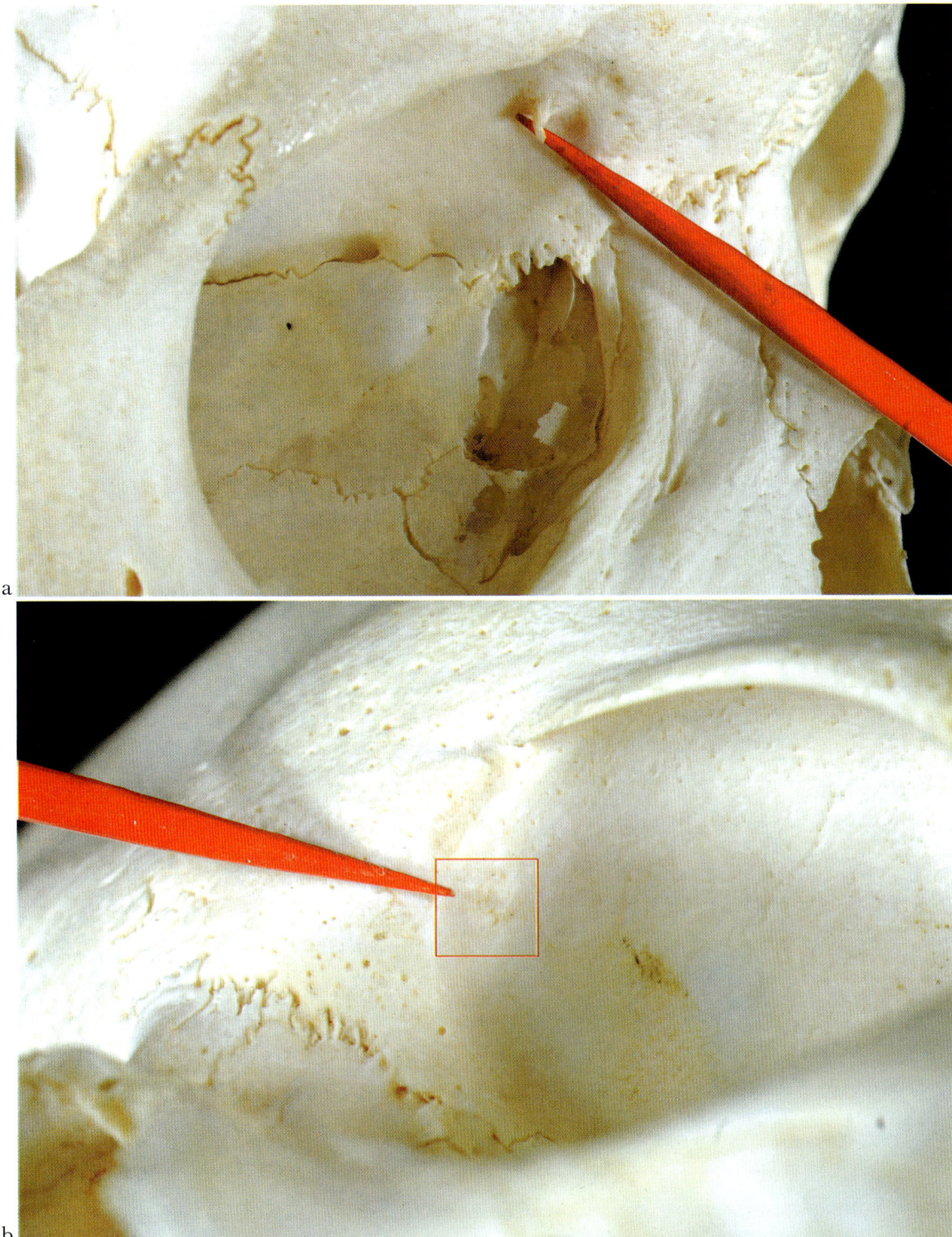

Figure 94a-b. Trochlear spur and fossa in an adolescent male skull (CSC AS 005). (a) Typical hook-shaped trochlear spur (probe) in the right orbit. (b) Trochlear fossa (square and probe) with absence of a trochlear spur in the left orbit. The trochlear fossa in the left orbit of this individual is represented by a small, shallow and roughened depression, but no spur or bony projection. These spurs may be present in subadults and are not necessarily a result of aging. Common findings.

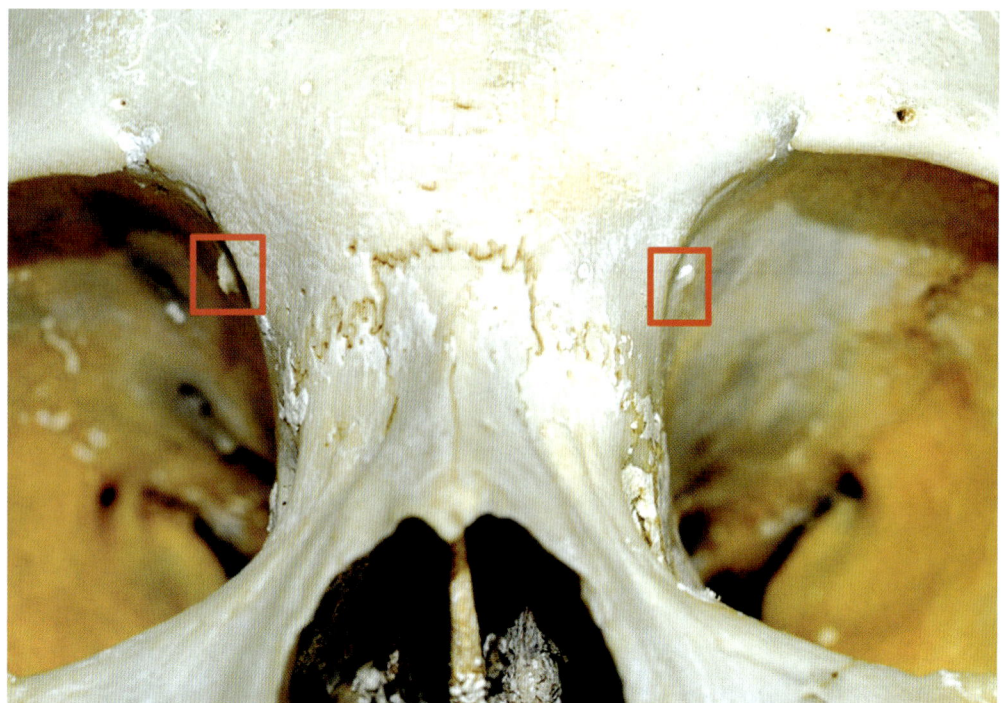

Figure 95. Bilateral trochlear spurs in a Thai adult (KKU). Common finding.

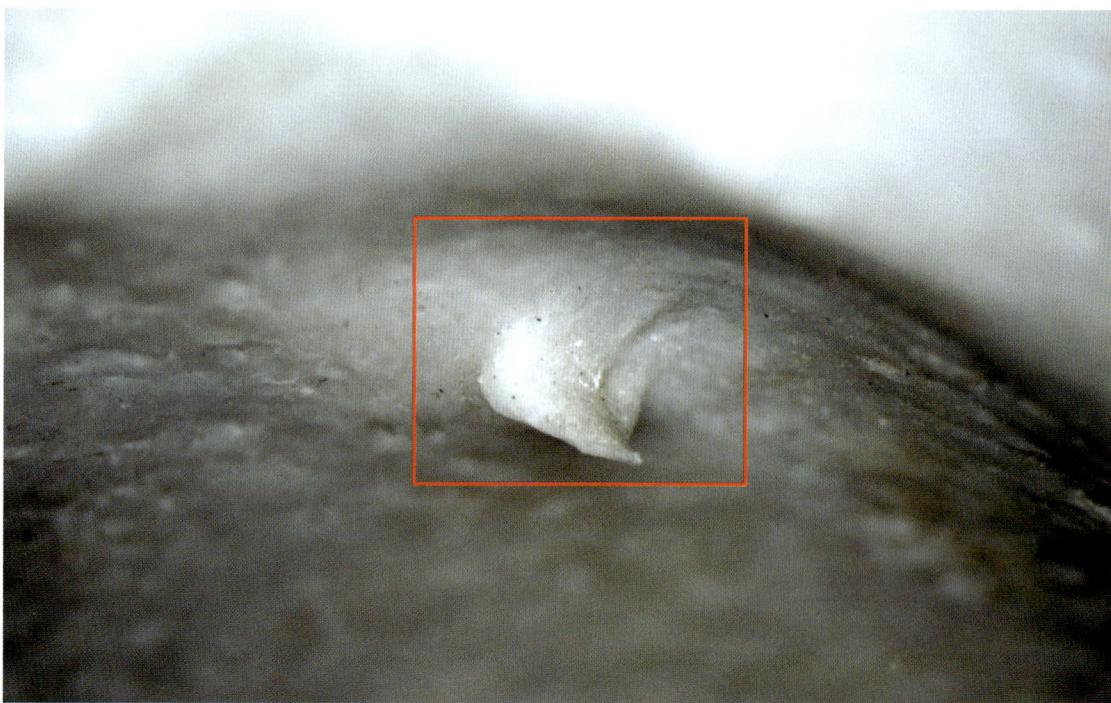

Figure 96. Low-power microscopy of trochlear pulley/spur in the right orbit of an adult Asian skull (CSC AC026). The spur is pointing towards the midline.

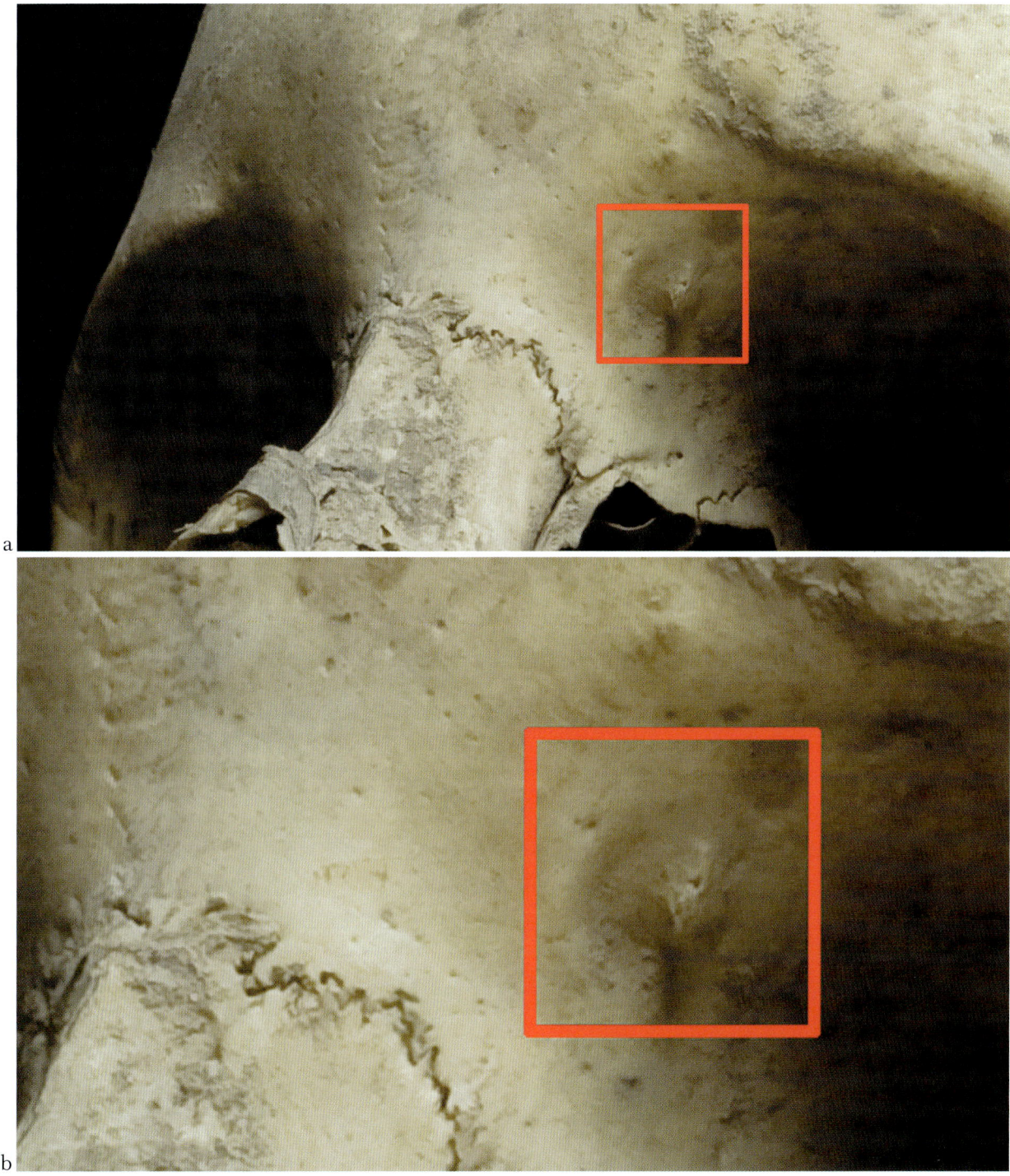

Figure 97a-b. Small trochlear mound and spur in a child (UPenn L606 88). (a) Small hook-shaped trochlear spur atop a bony mound in an approximately 4-year-old child (UPenn L606 88). (b) Close-up of the left trochlear spur and mound (square). Normal findings.

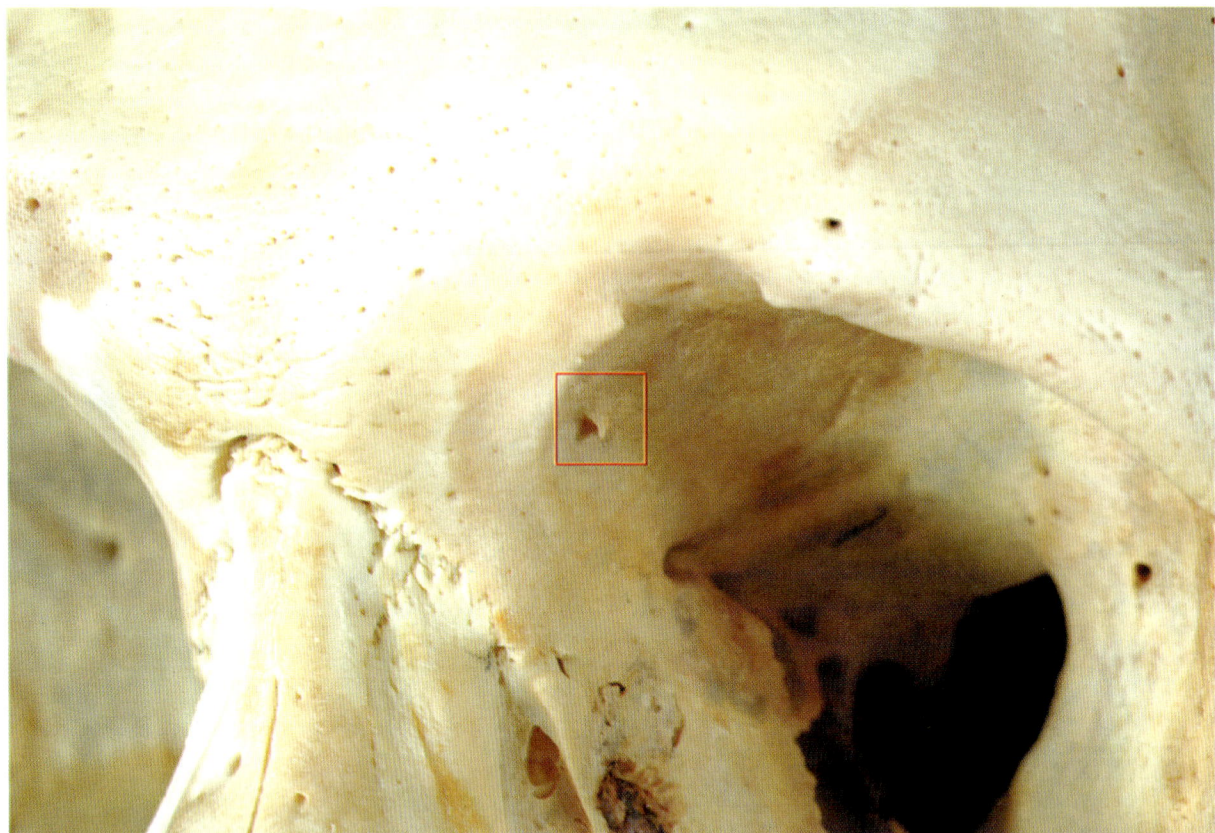

Figure 98. Calcified trochlear spur (square) in the left orbit. This spur, which is part of the U-shaped trochlear apparatus, may be unilateral or bilateral. A spur such as this is a common finding, while ossification of the entire U-shaped ligament is rare.

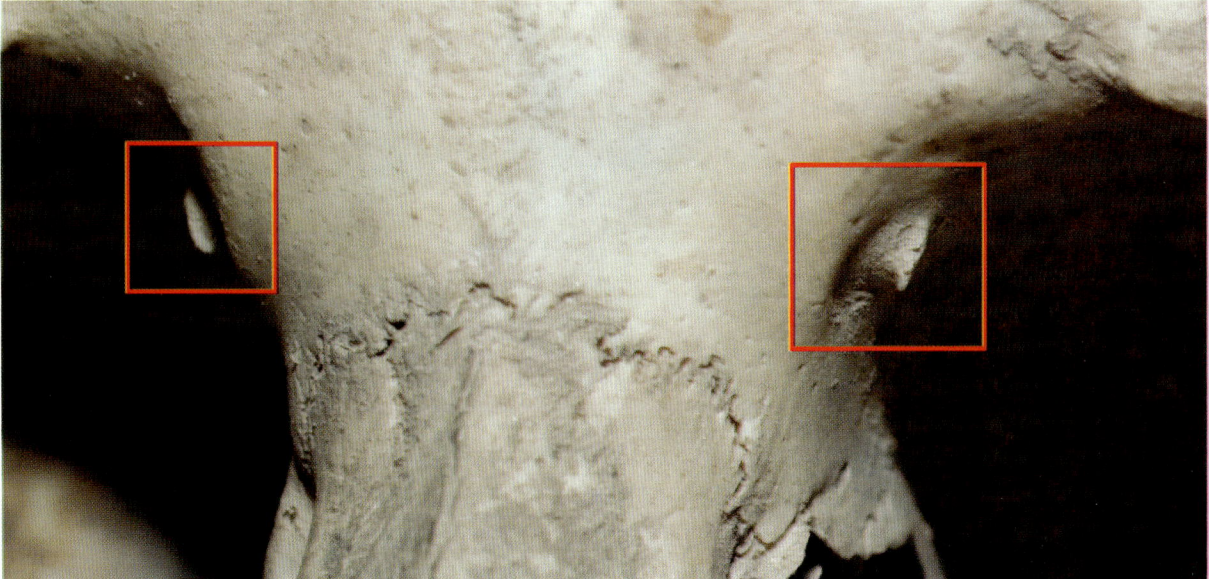

Figure 99. Bilateral trochlear spurs (squares) in a 12–16-year-old probable female (UPenn 83-67-668).

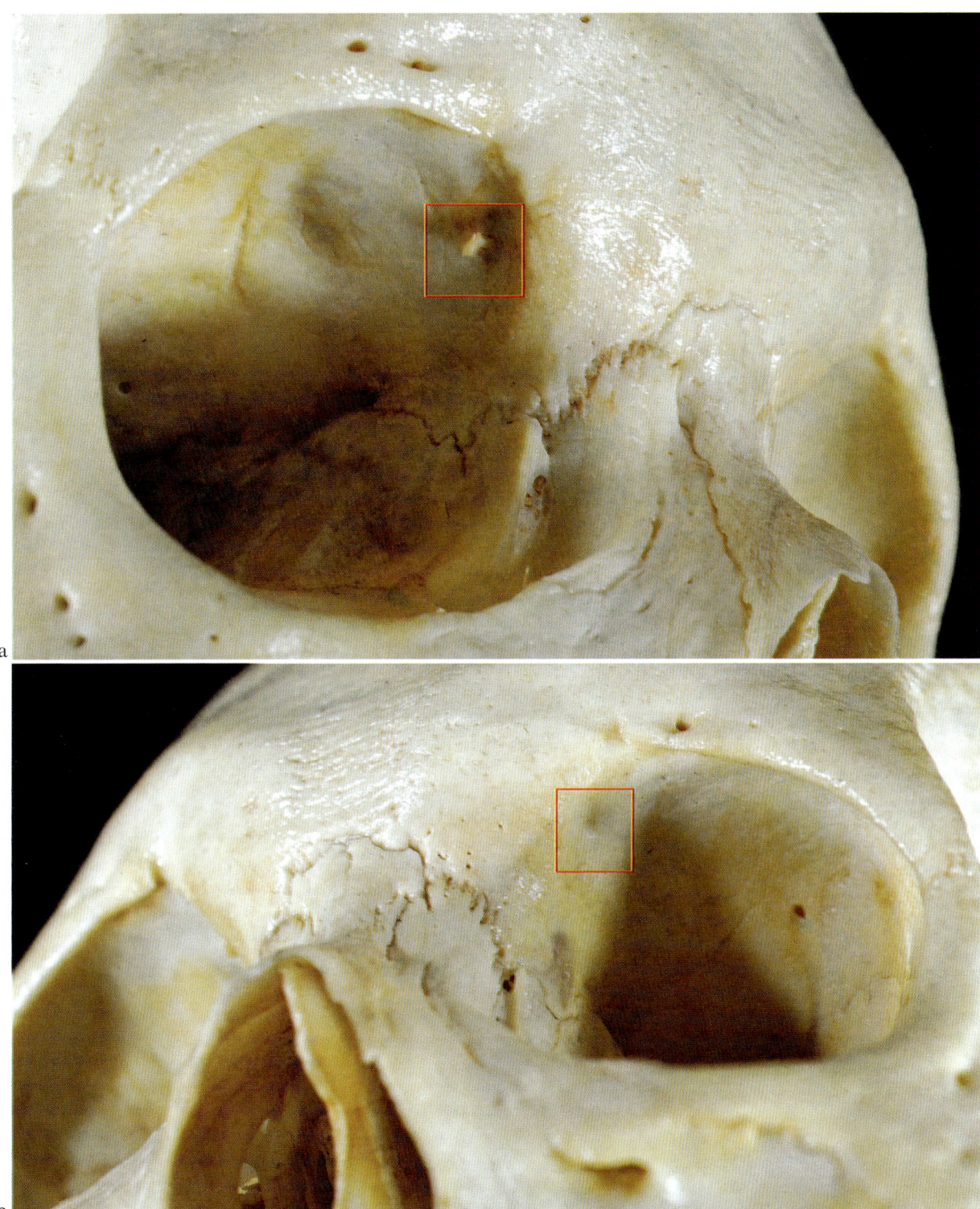

Figure 100a-b. Trochlear spur and fossa. (a) Trochlear spur (square) in the left orbit of an adult Asian skull (CSC DS005). (b) Trochlear fossa (square) with no evidence of a trochlear spur in the left orbit of the same individual. Both are commonly encountered typical variants.

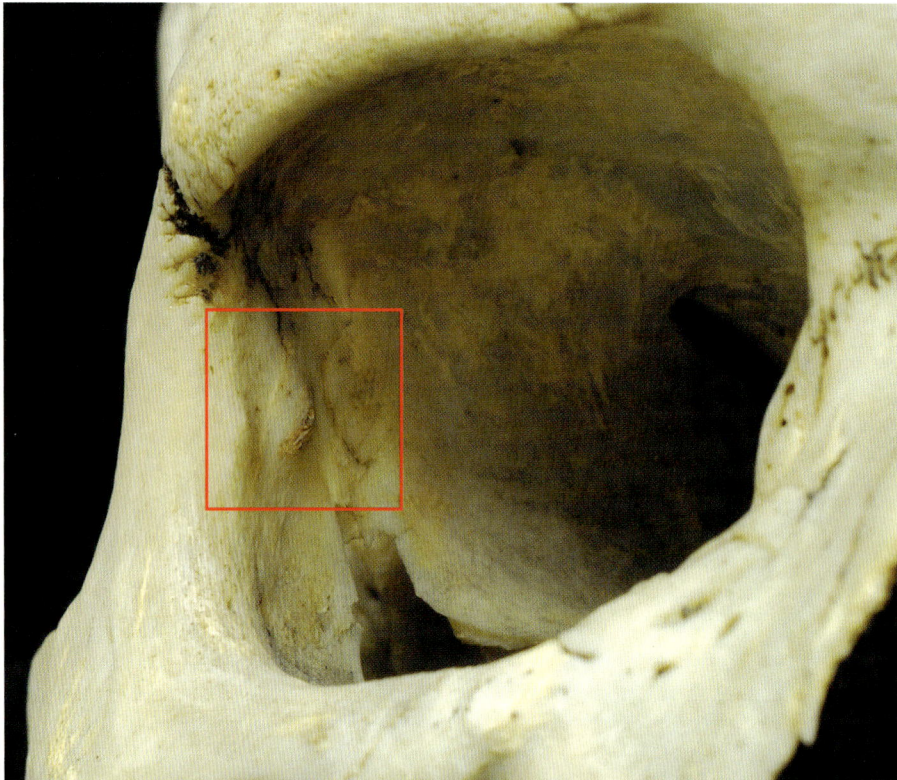

Figure 101. Prominent lateral tubercle (square), sometimes referred to as the orbital tubercle of the malar bone (Whitnall's tubercle), for attachment of the lateral rectus muscle of the right orbit (Mütter Museum 107.04). Examination of 2,000 skulls from around the world revealed tubercles in more than 95% of skulls (Whitnall 1911, 1921). Common finding.

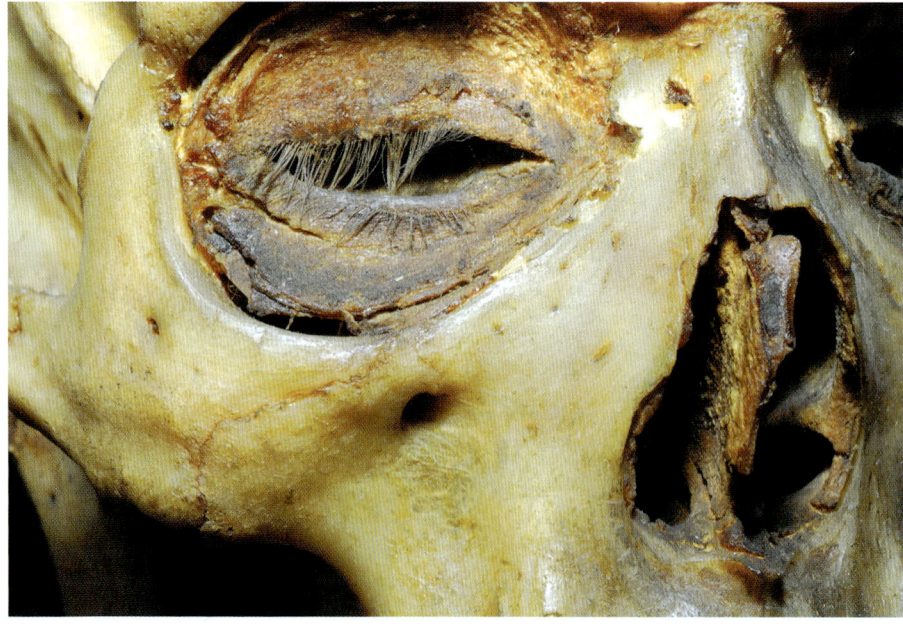

Figure 102. The right orbit showing attachment of the tarsal component of the orbicularis oculi (Mütter Museum 1007.72). Normal anatomy.

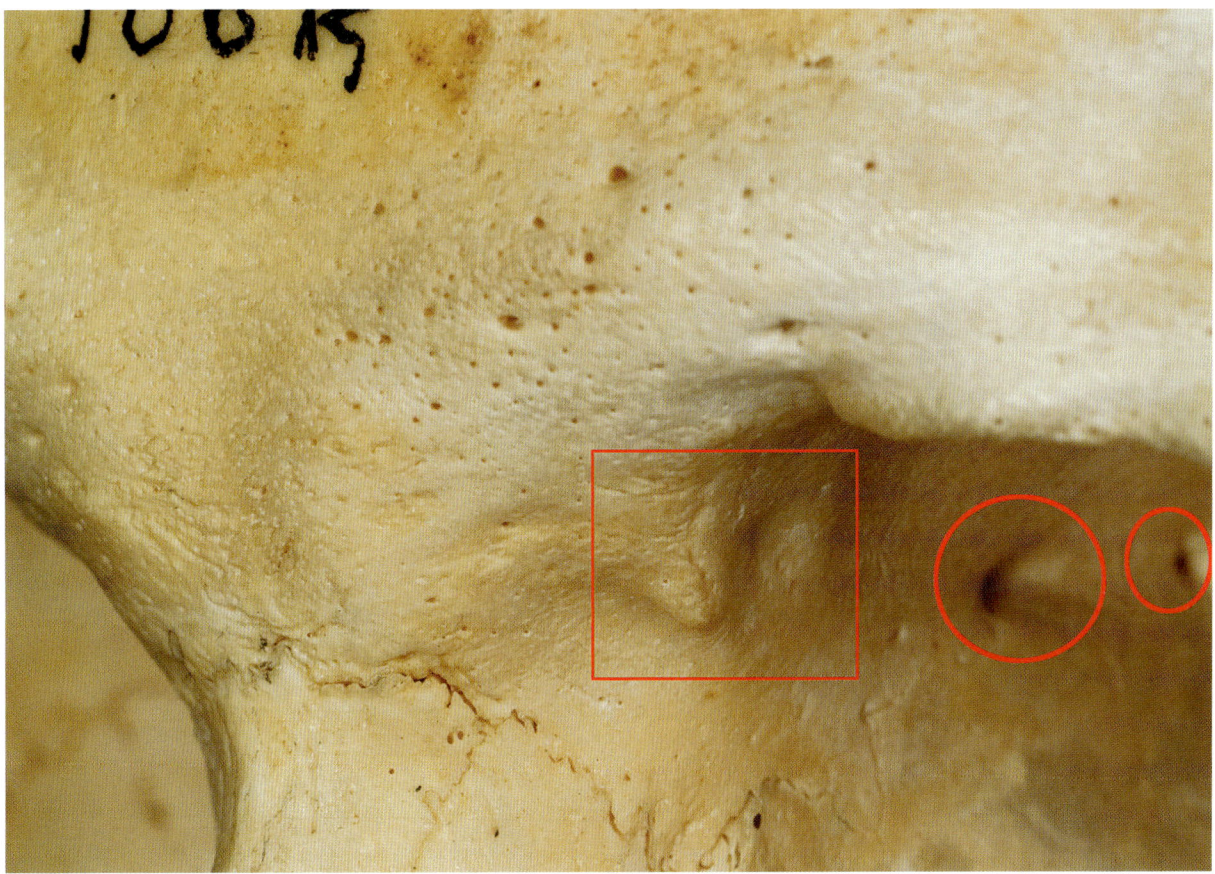

Figure 103. Small left trochlear projection (red square) with a shallow posterior depression (SI Terry106R (adult Black) – this feature was bilateral (common to uncommon finding). Anterior ethmoidal foramen (large circle) and posterior ethmoidal foramen (small circle) along the suture. A study of 100 India crania (Mutalik et al. 2011) revealed the anterior ethmoidal foramen present in all 100 skulls and posterior ethmoidal foramen in 98 skulls. The authors found 20 right and 22 left accessory foramina, all exsutural, located inferior to the optic canal. Each orbit typically has an anterior and posterior foramina, but may have as many as five (Abed et al. 2011). While most (85%) ethmoidal foramina lie on the frontoethmoidal suture, they may be above or below it (Abed et al. 2011; Huanmanop et al. 2007). Cf. Dutton (2011) for anatomy of the ethmoidal foramen.

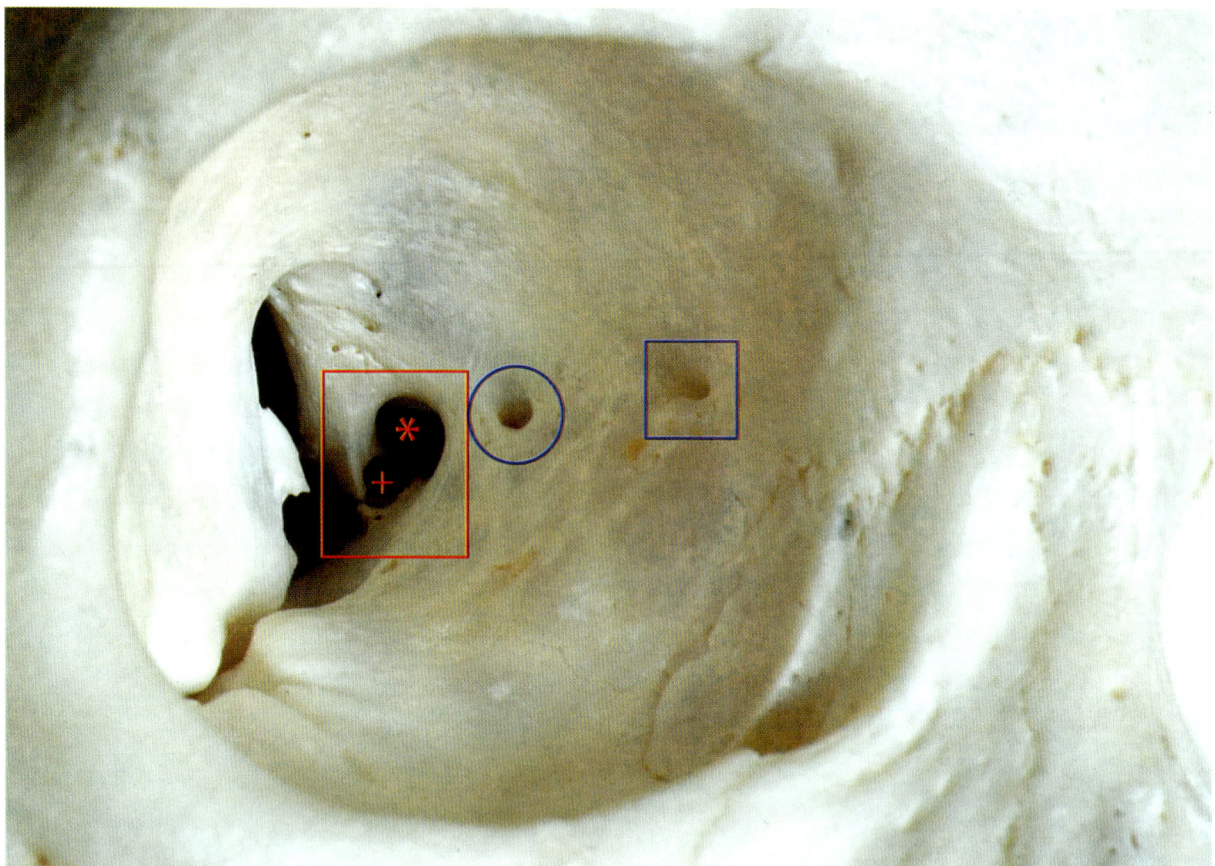

Figure 104. Incomplete right optic foramen (red square), anterior ethmoidal foramen (blue square) and posterior ethmoidal foramen (blue circle) in an adult Asian male (CSC DS034). The small bony projection between the * and + in the left orbit is the posterior strut that, when ossified, separates the main and lesser canals. Unilateral double optic foramen is a rare trait (2.75% or 11 of 400 skulls) and bilaterally (1.66% or 7 of 400 skulls) (Patil et al. 2011) is extremely rare. The large canal (asterisk) carries the optic nerve and meninges and the smaller canal (+) the opthalmic artery. Cf. Choudhry et al. (1988, 1999, 2005); Clegg (1936); Freyschmidt et al. (2002); Ghai et al. (2012); Keyes (1935); Singh (2005); Vázquez et al. (2001); Warwick (1951).

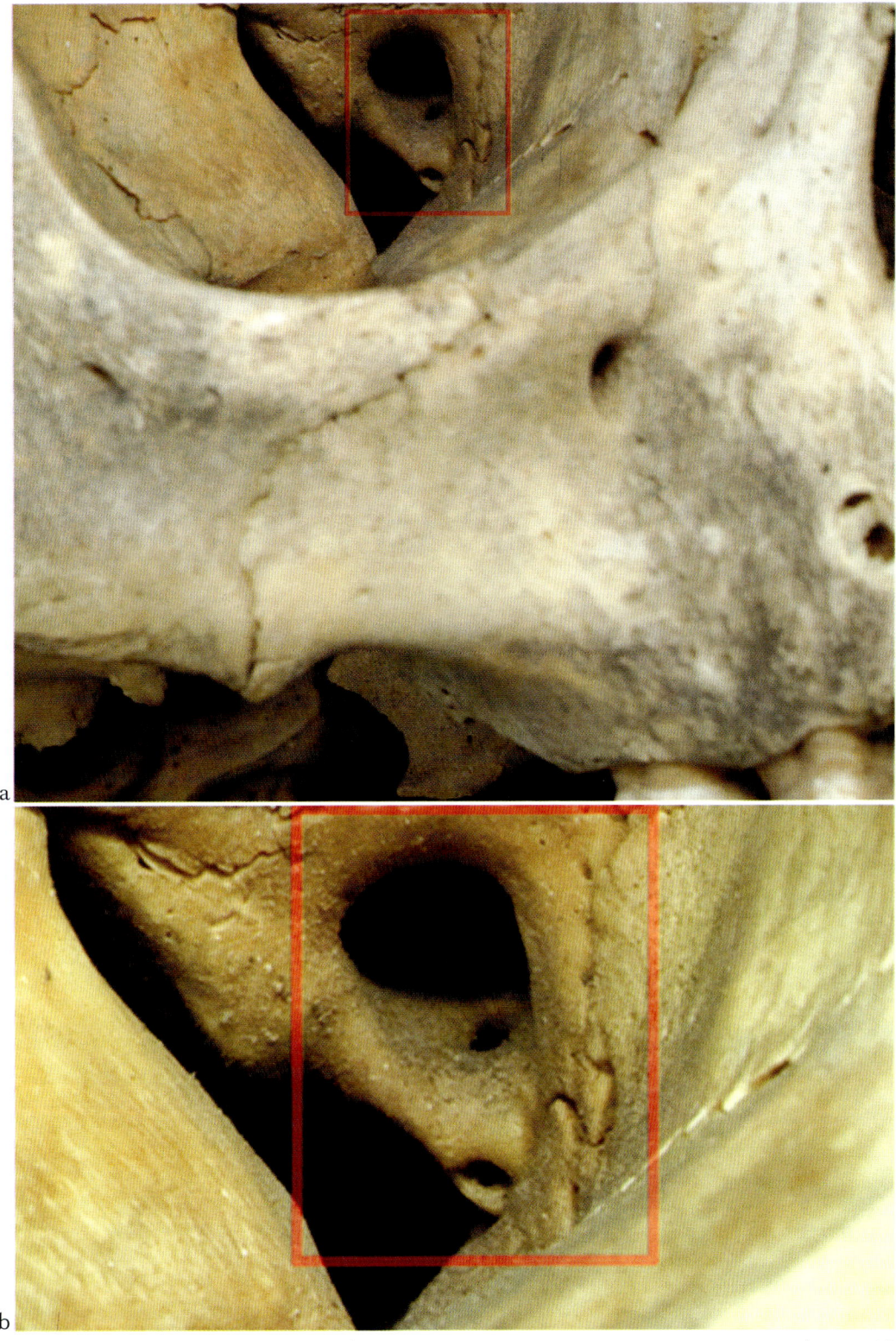

Figure 105a-b. Triple optic foramina. (a) Uncommon to rare triple foramina in the left orbit (rectangle) of a 6- to 8-year-old child (UPenn 1492 L606). (b) Close-up of the three foramina consisting of the typical large optic foramen above two smaller foramina.

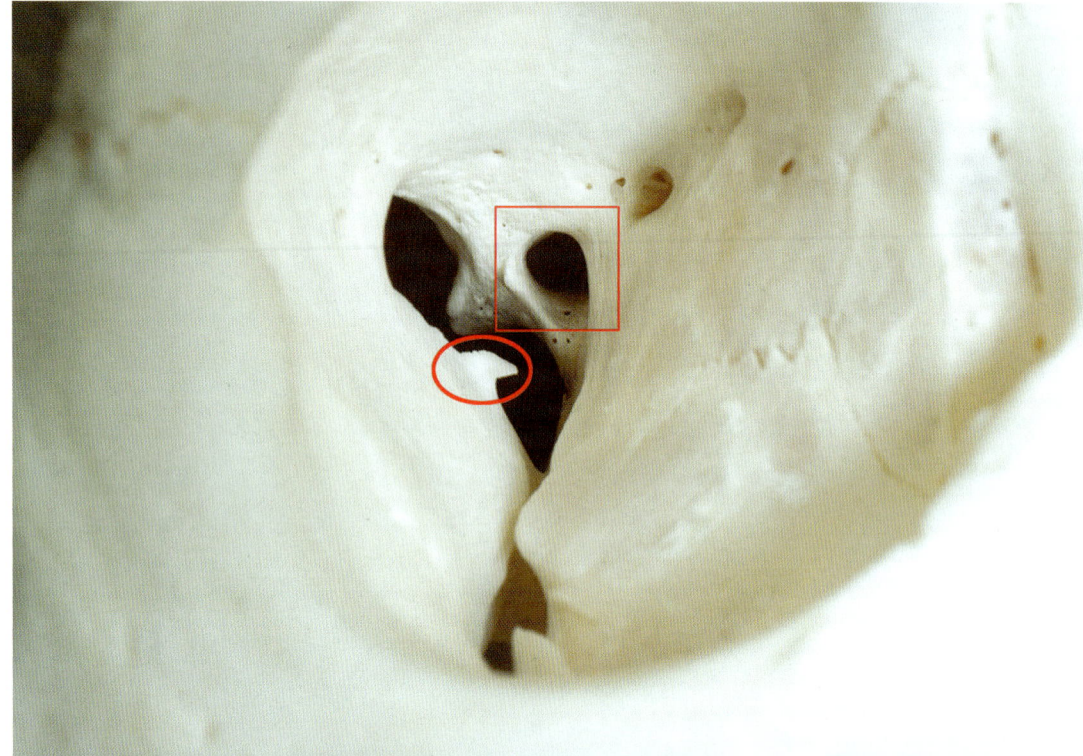

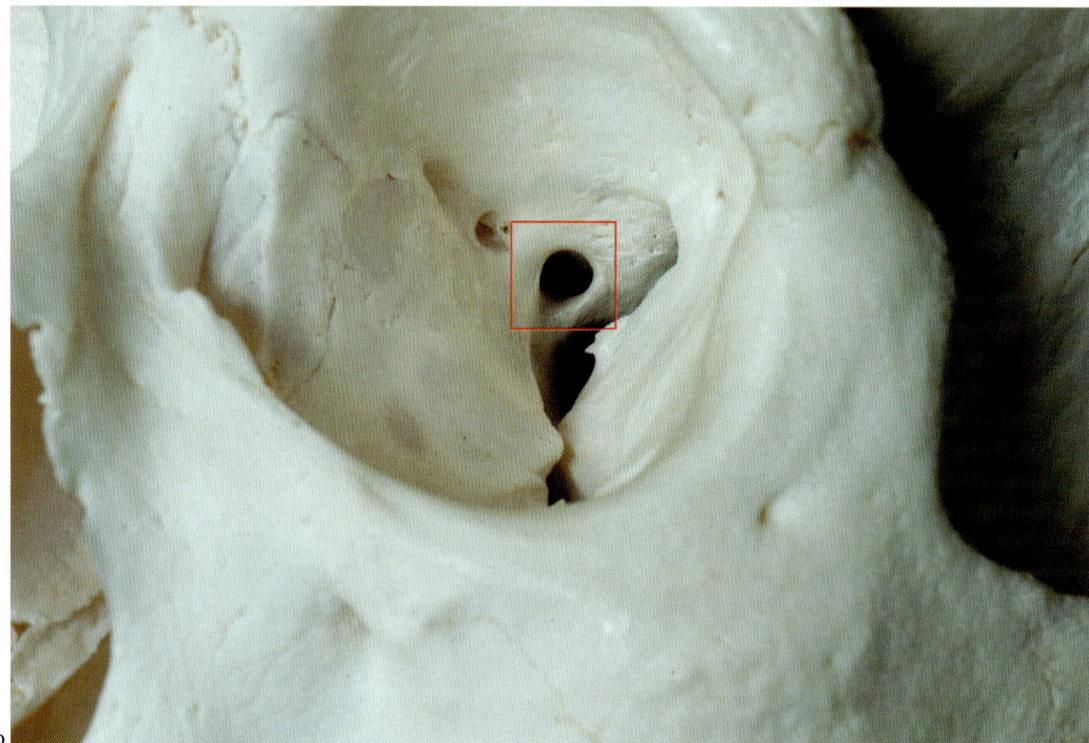

Figure 106a-b. Single optic foramen. (a) Single right (square) and (b) left (square) optic foramen in a robust adult Asian male skull (CSC DS035). Note the small bony spine (top; oval) known as the spina recti lateralis for attachment of the rectus lateralis muscle.

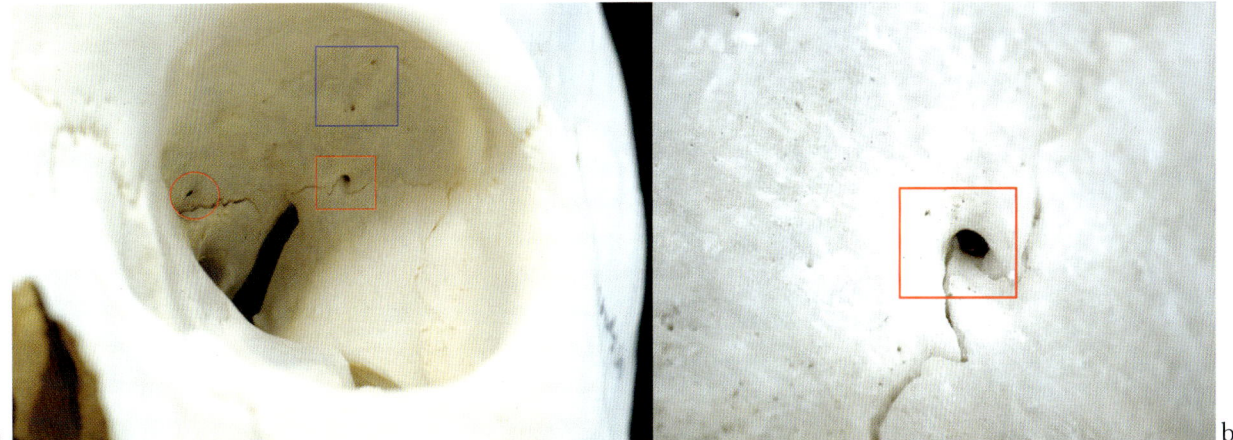

Figure 107a-b. Depiction of meningo-orbital foramen. (a) A meningo-orbital foramen (red square), also known as foramen meningo-orbitale, foramen of Hyrtl and lacrimal foramen, among others, in the sphenofrontal suture, posterior ethmoidal foramen (red circle) and two tiny meningo-orbital foramina (blue square) in the left orbit of an adult Asian skull (CSC AC026). (b) Close-up of the meningo-orbital foramen (square). Frequency of the meningo-orbital foramen varies from 6% (Neto 1984) to 83% of skulls (Erturk et al. 2005). See Babu et al. (2011); Jovanovic et al. (2003); Krishnamurthy et al. (2008); Kwiatowski et al. (2003); O'Brien and McDonald (2007).

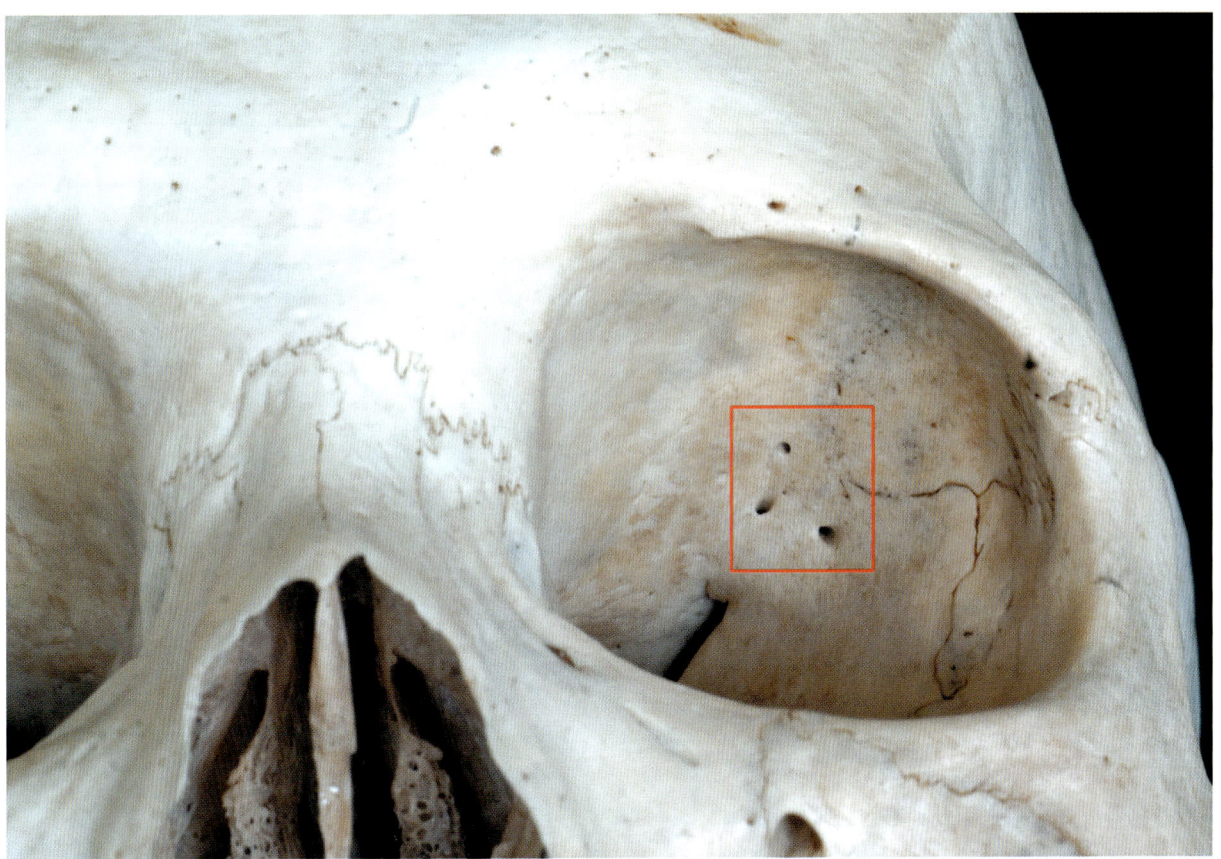

Figure 108. Three left meningo-orbital foramina (square) in an adult Thai female (KKU 4778 43).

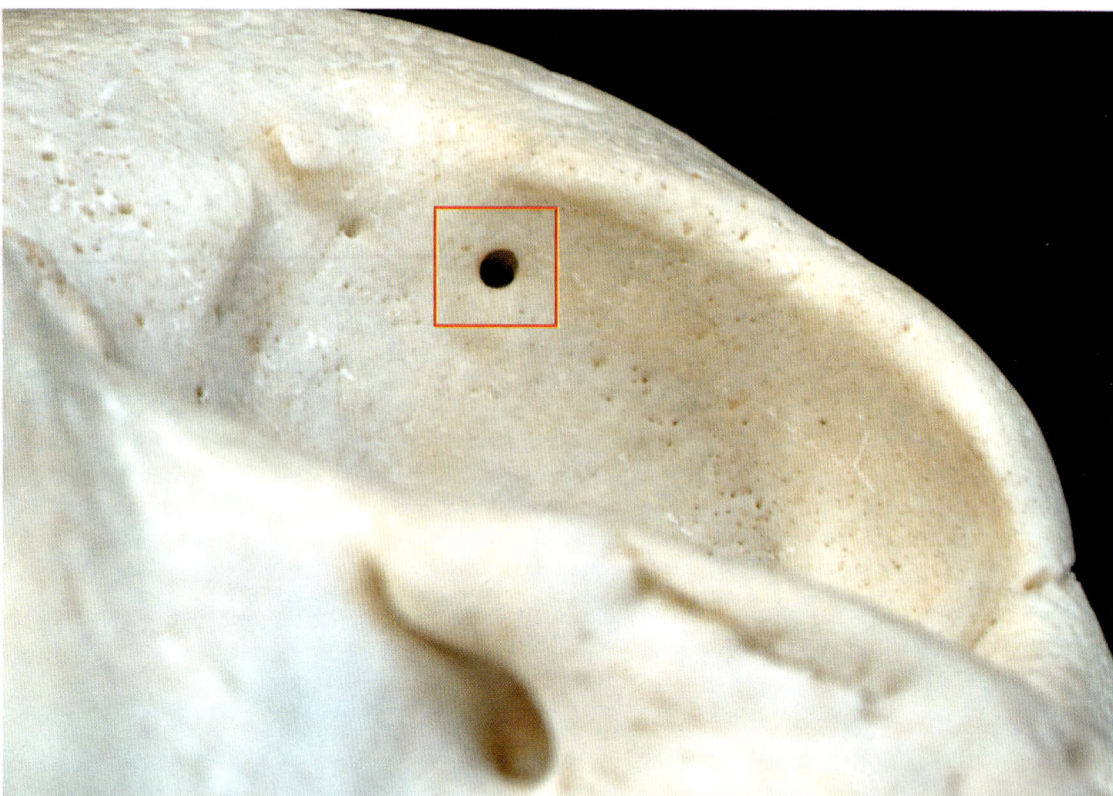

Figure 109. Unusually large foramen (square) in the left upper orbital plate in an adult Asian male (CSC AS022). This foramen and others like it usually communicate with a foramen and/or groove in the frontal bone.

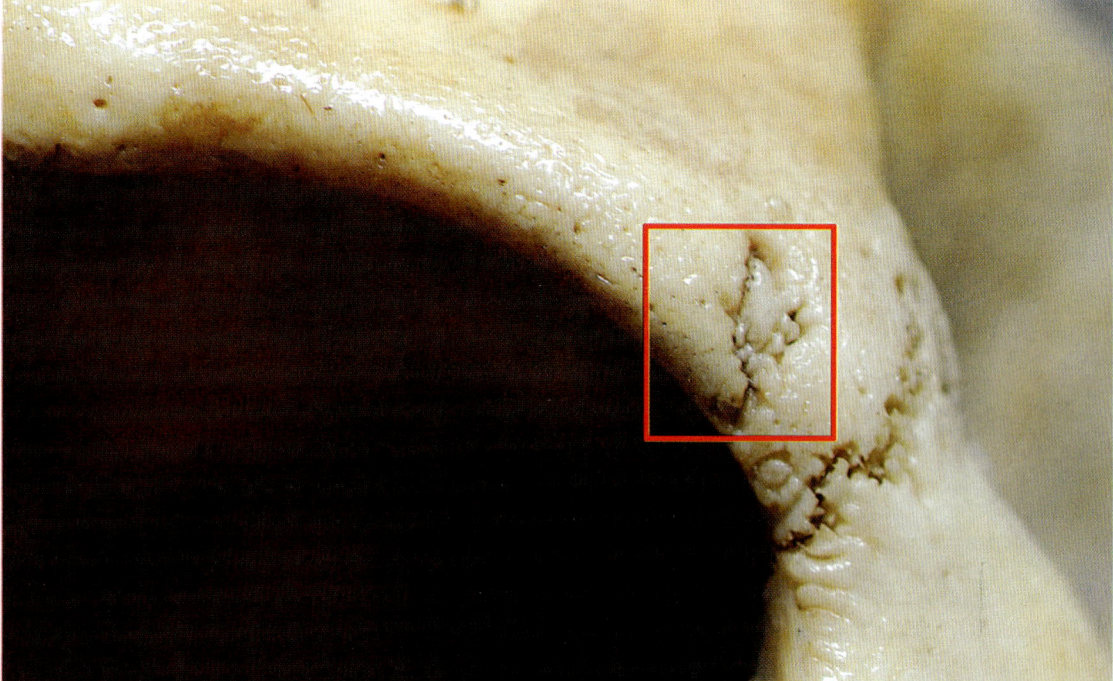

Figure 110. Accessory zygomaticofrontal suture (square) in the left orbit of an adult, probable Asian (CSC). Uncommon to rare.

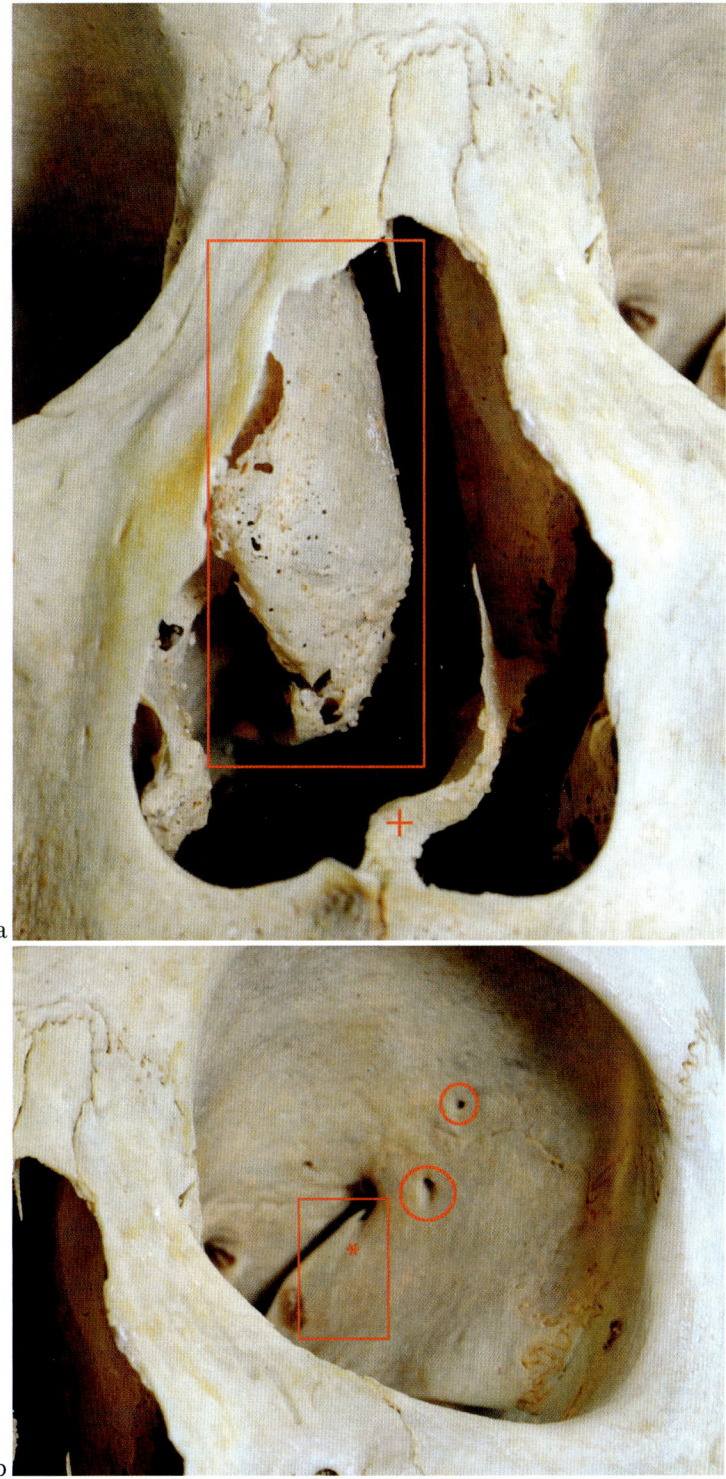

Figure 111a-b. Unilateral concha bullosa, deviated septum and multiple foramina in the orbits. (a) a deviated nasal septum (AC), anolateral concha bullosa (CB) and accessory left infraorbital foramen (red circle). (b) Partial foramen at the lateral end of the superior orbital fissure and a shallow groove/depression (rectangle and *) extending inferiorly (KKU). Cf. Babu et al. (2011); Cukurova et al. (2012); Jovanovic et al. (2003); Krishnamurthy et al. (2008); Kwiatowski et al. (2003); O'Brien and McDonald (2007) for Meningo-orbital foramen and foramen of Hyrtl; Kwiatkowska et al. (2009) for concha bullosa.

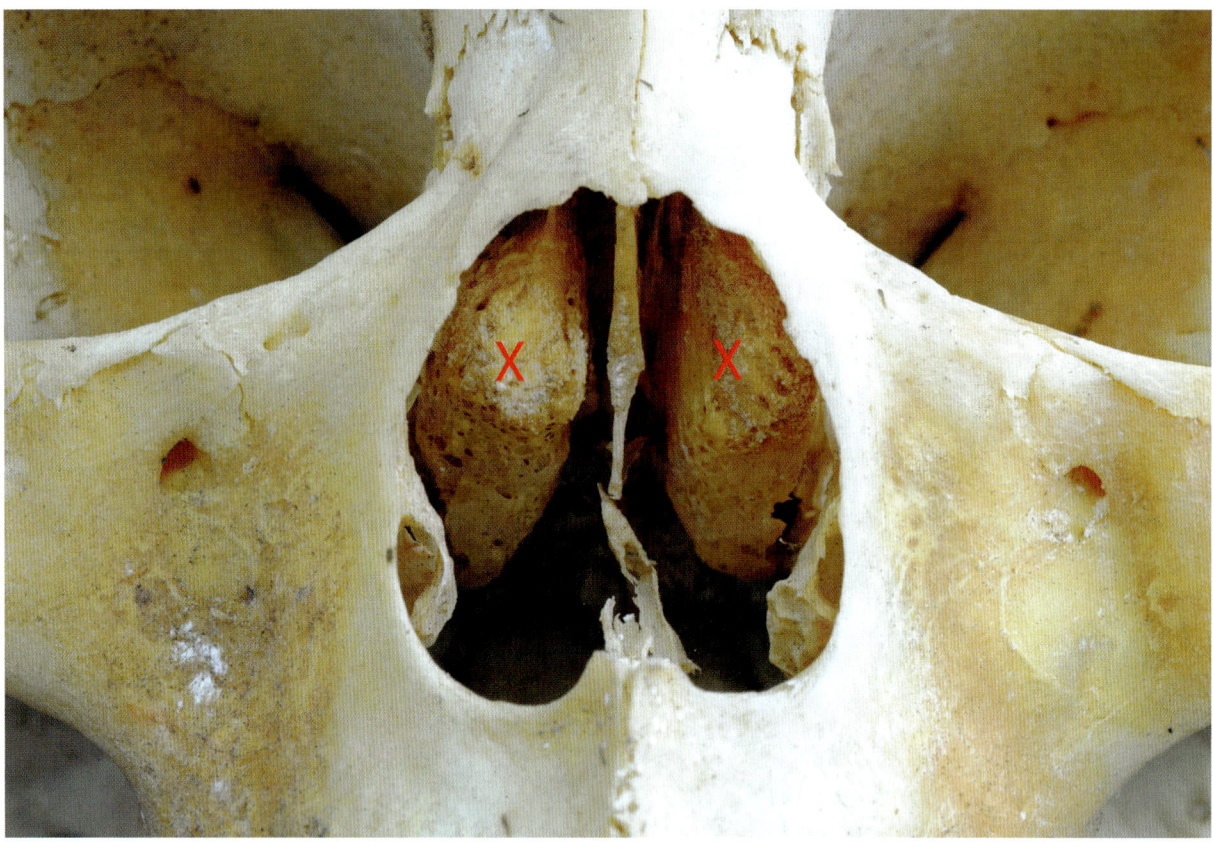

Figure 112. Bilateral concha bullosa (X) in a Thai adult (KKU 199). Cf. Kwiatkowska et al. (2009) for concha bullosa.

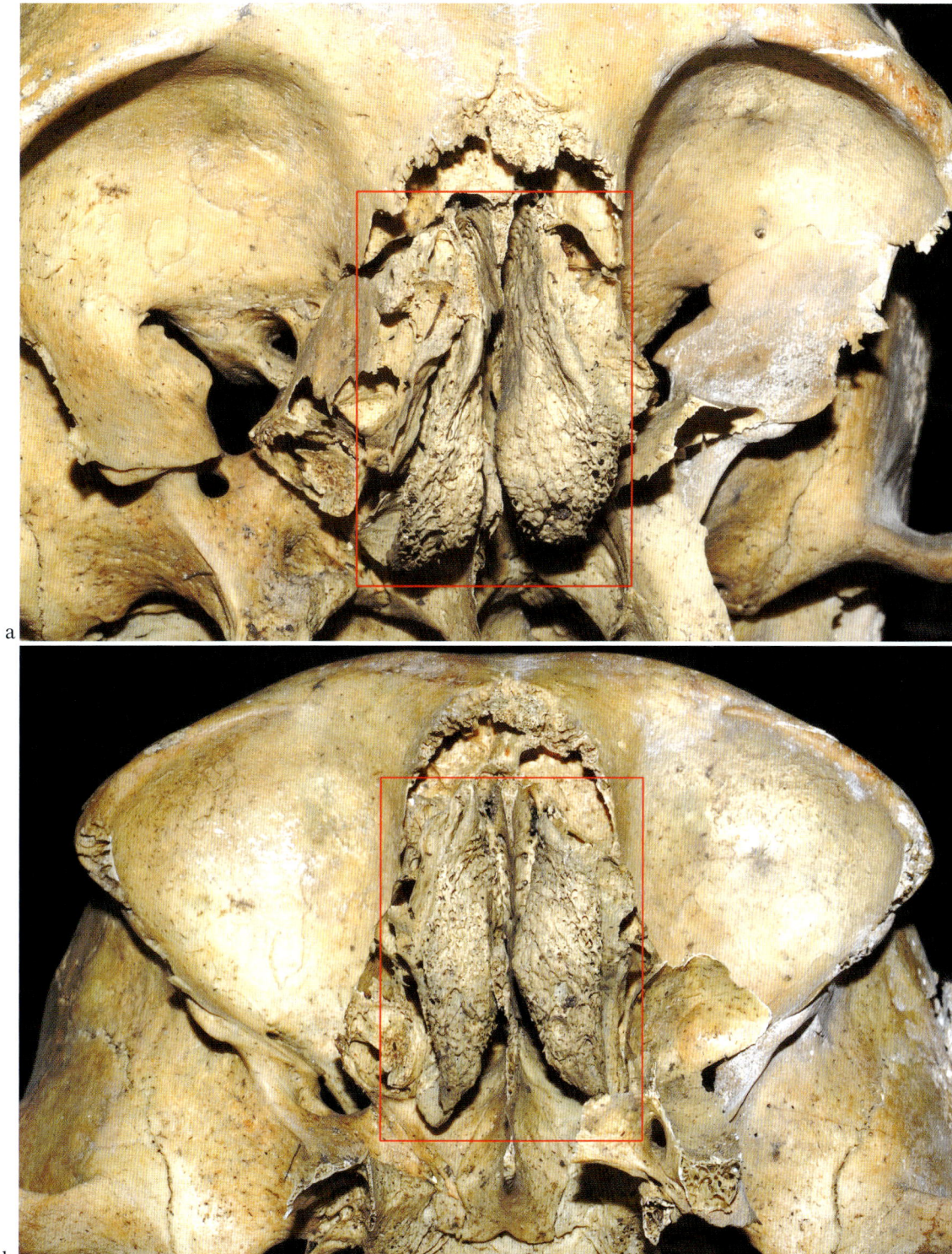

Figure 113a-b. Bilateral concha bullosa in an adult (RV778). (a) Oblique view showing perimortem trauma or postmortem breakage of the facial region revealing enlarged/hypertrophied/pneumatized middle turbinates (rectangle), also known as concha bullosa. Concha bullosa is one of the most common anomalies in the paranasal sinuses. (b) Inferior view and close-up of concha bullosa. Unilateral or bilateral hypertrophied turbinates and a deviated nasal septum are often present together. Cf. Cukurova et al. 2012.

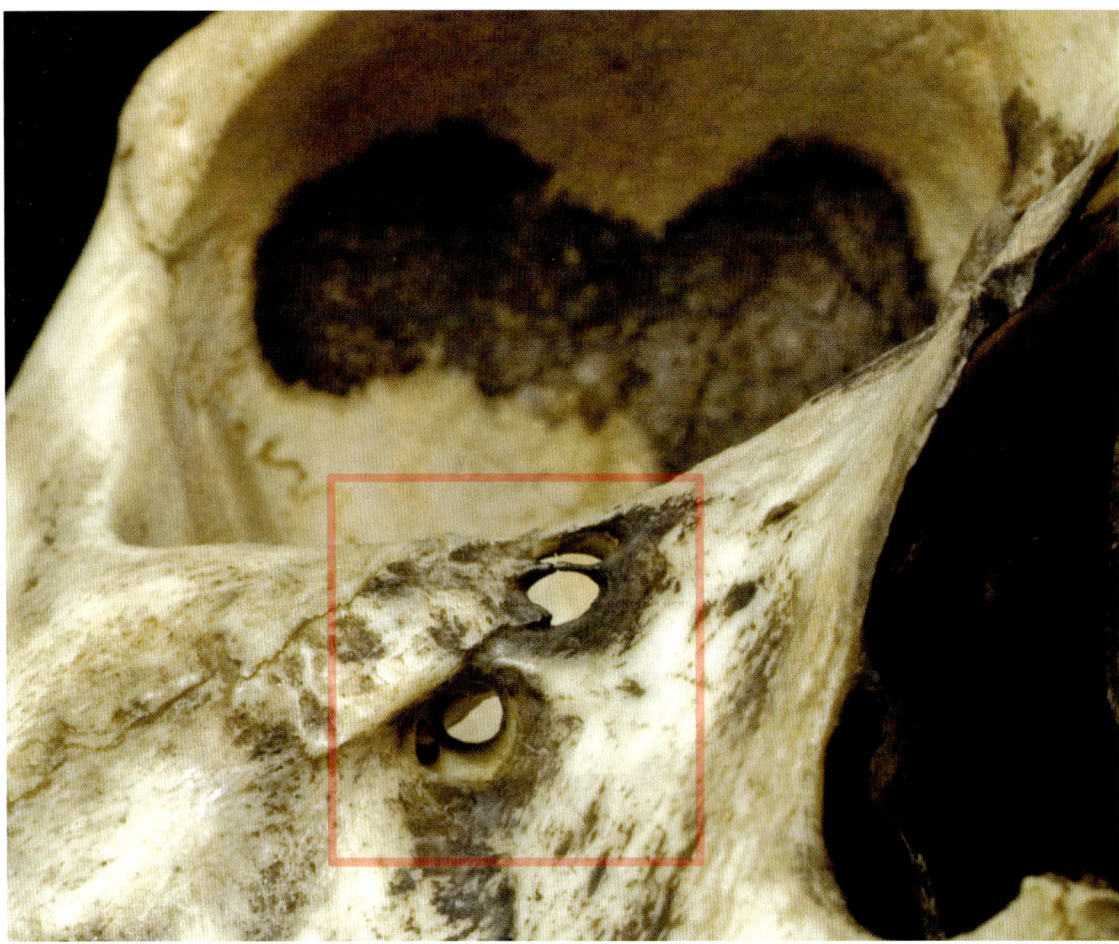

Figure 114. Four right infraorbital foramina (square) in a 60-year-old individual (Mütter Museum 1006-111). Some researchers might classify this as two or double foramina, each of which is divided into two foramina consisting of one major and one minor foramina. Cf. Boopathi et al. (2010); Leo et al. (1995); Vázquez et al. (2001). See Riesenfeld (1956) for more on multiple infraorbital foramina. Unusual to rare finding.

Frontal View of the Skull

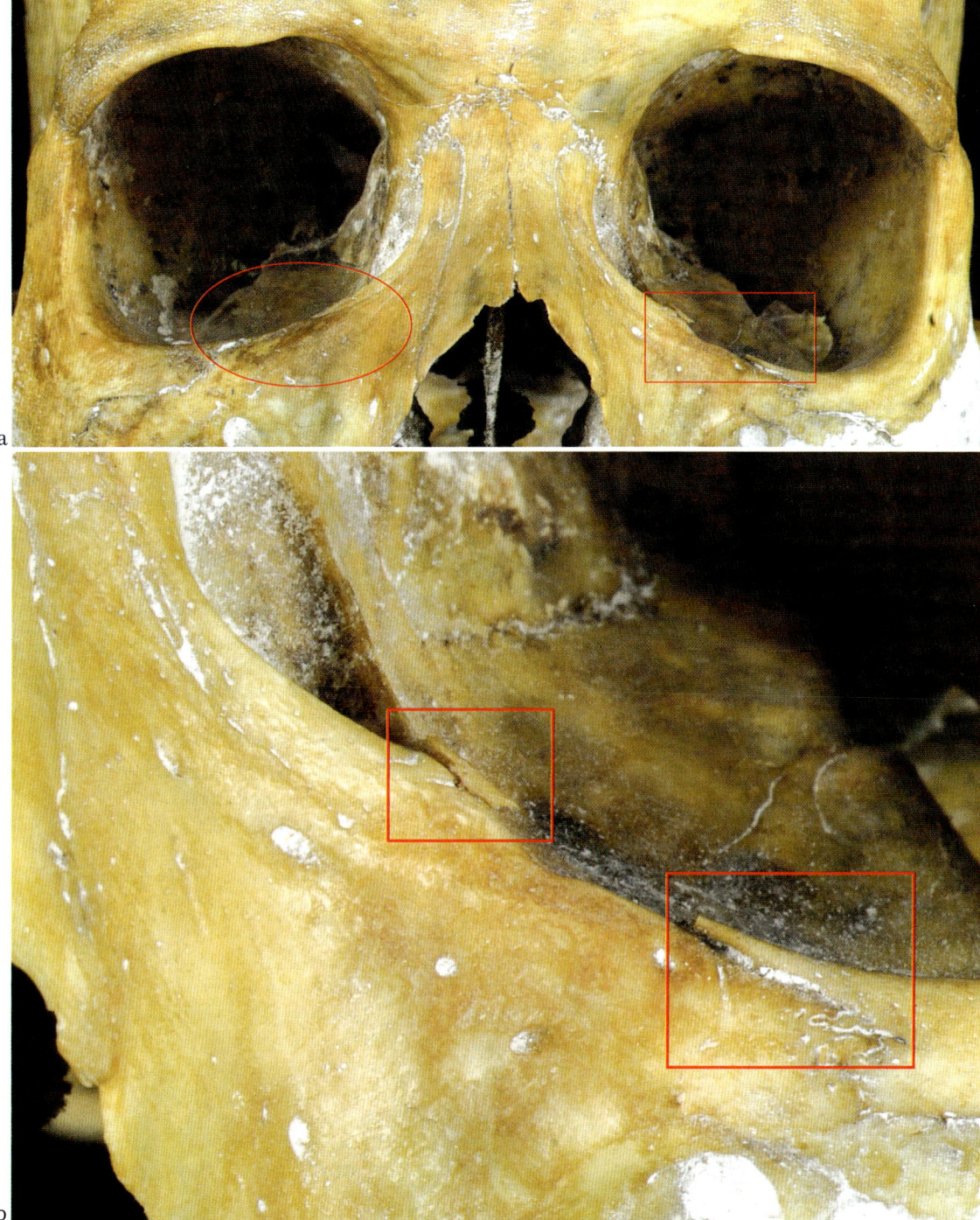

Figure 115a-b. Calcification along the inferior border of the left orbit in an adult Thai (KKU). (a) Calcification (rectangle) and absence (oval) of bony projections in the right orbit. Note that the lateral "finger-like" bony extension in the left orbit is an extension of the zygomatic bone along the zygomaticomaxillary suture and attachment of the inferior oblique muscle and small lacrimal bone (ossiculum canlis; small square). (b) Magnified view of the finger-like projection (rectangle) along the left orbit. Uncommon finding.

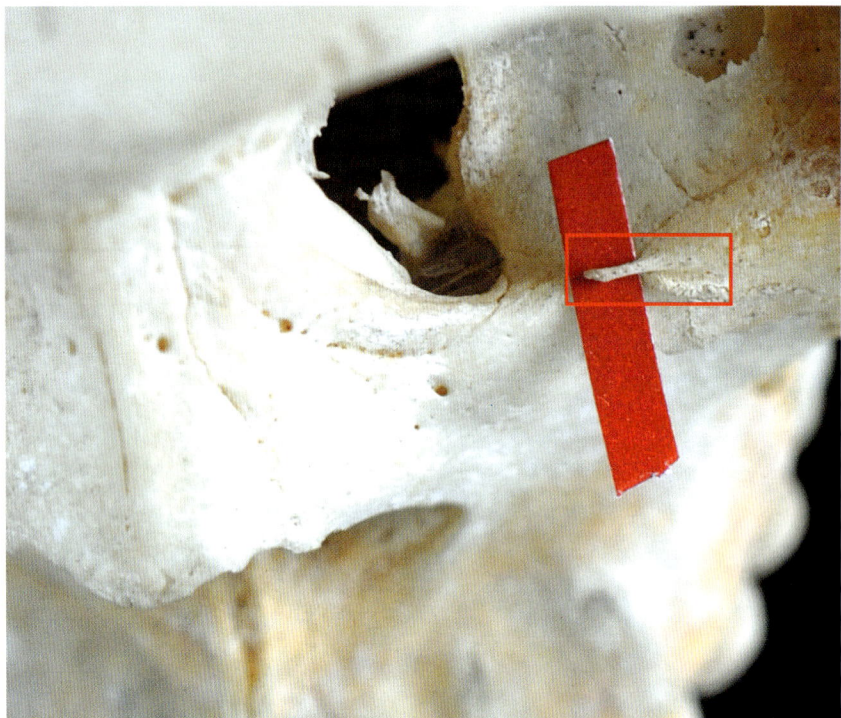

Figure 116. Calcification (red rectangle) in the general area of attachment of the inferior oblique muscle in an adult Thai (KKU). This finger-like spur is an uncommon finding.

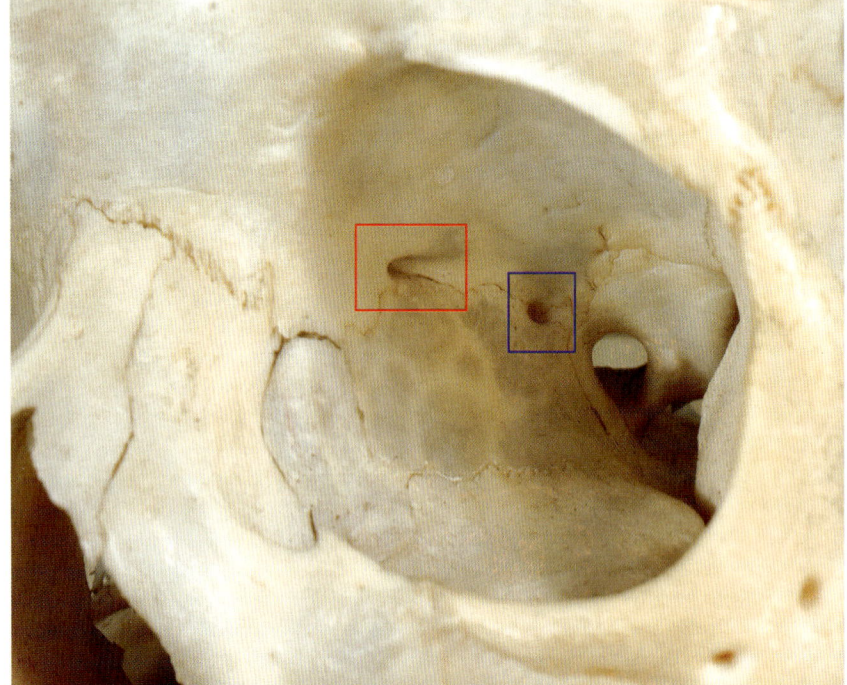

Figure 117. Anterior (red) and posterior (blue) ethmoidal foramina (CSC AS007) along the fronto-ethmoidal suture. Normal anatomy.

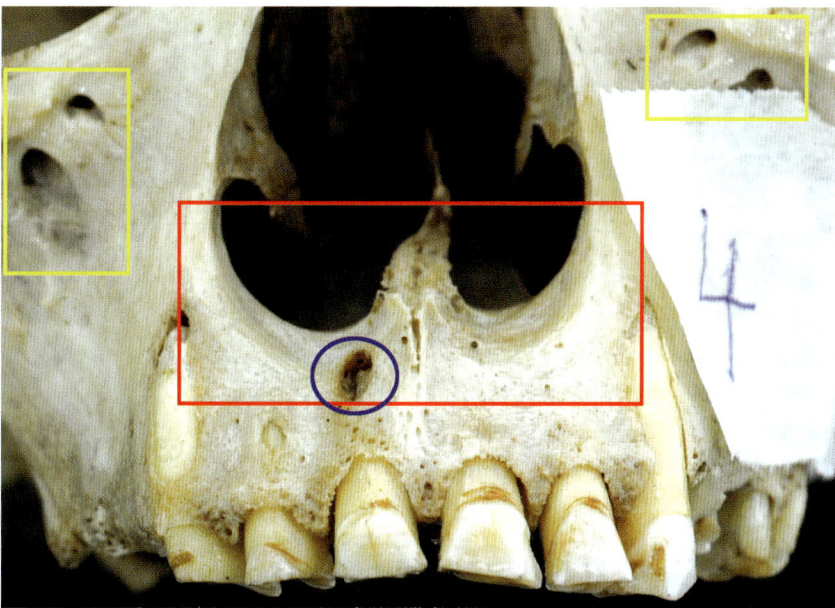

Figure 118. Guttered inferior nasal margin (rectangle) in a Thai adult; this is a common feature in most Negroid and many Asian individuals (KKU). Note the marked dental attrition of the occlusal surfaces of the teeth. Also note the periapical lesion/abscess at the base of the right central incisor (circle), mild left deviation of the nasal septum and double infraorbital foramina (yellow rectangles). Cf. Hauser and DeStefano (1989) and Vázquez et al. (2001) for double infraorbital foramina.

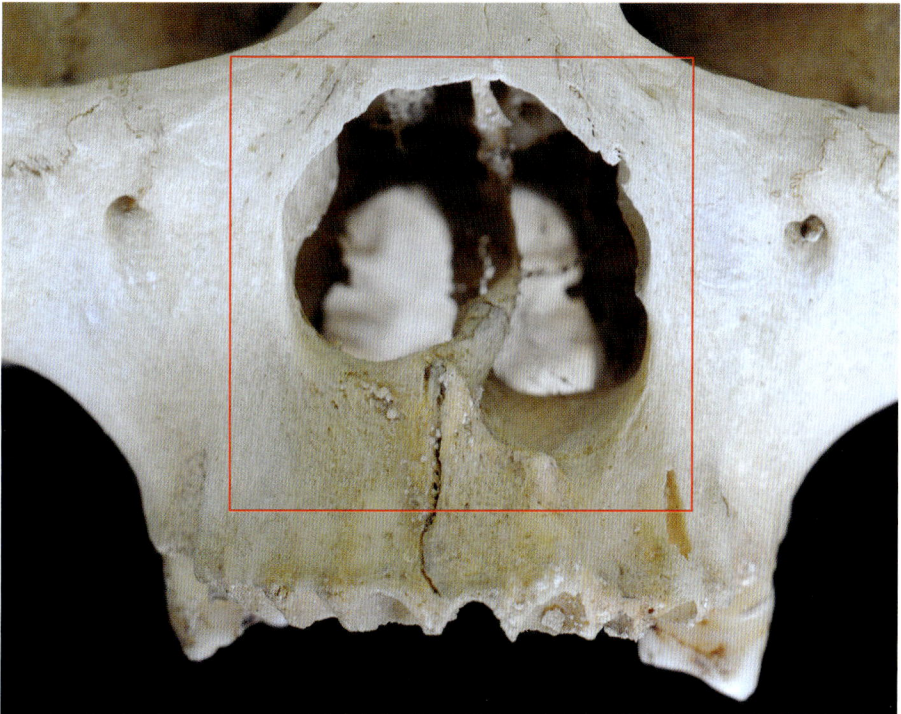

Figure 119. Asymmetrically shaped and guttered nasal aperture (square) in an adult Thai (KKU) – note the septum is deviated to the individual's left. Guttering is common, but such asymmetry is rare.

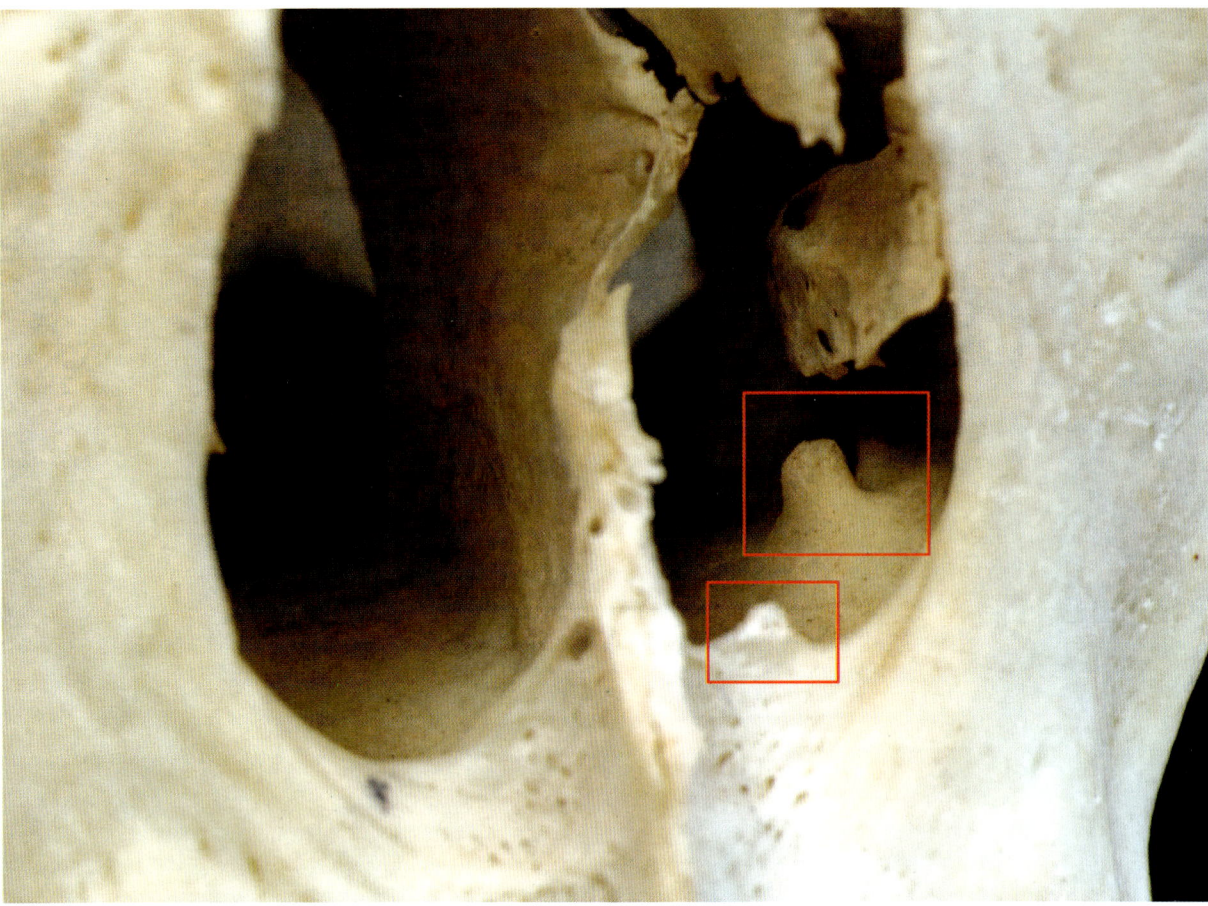

Figure 120. Three bony tumor-like projections on the floor of the left nasal cavity in an adult Asian male (CSC AS022). Note that the anterior projection is along the innermost portion of the nasal margin and the other two projections lie deeper within the cavity. The right nasal cavity is free of these projections and those in the left do not appear in any way to be connected or communicate with the tooth roots. This is the first example of its kind that the authors have seen.

Frontal View of the Skull

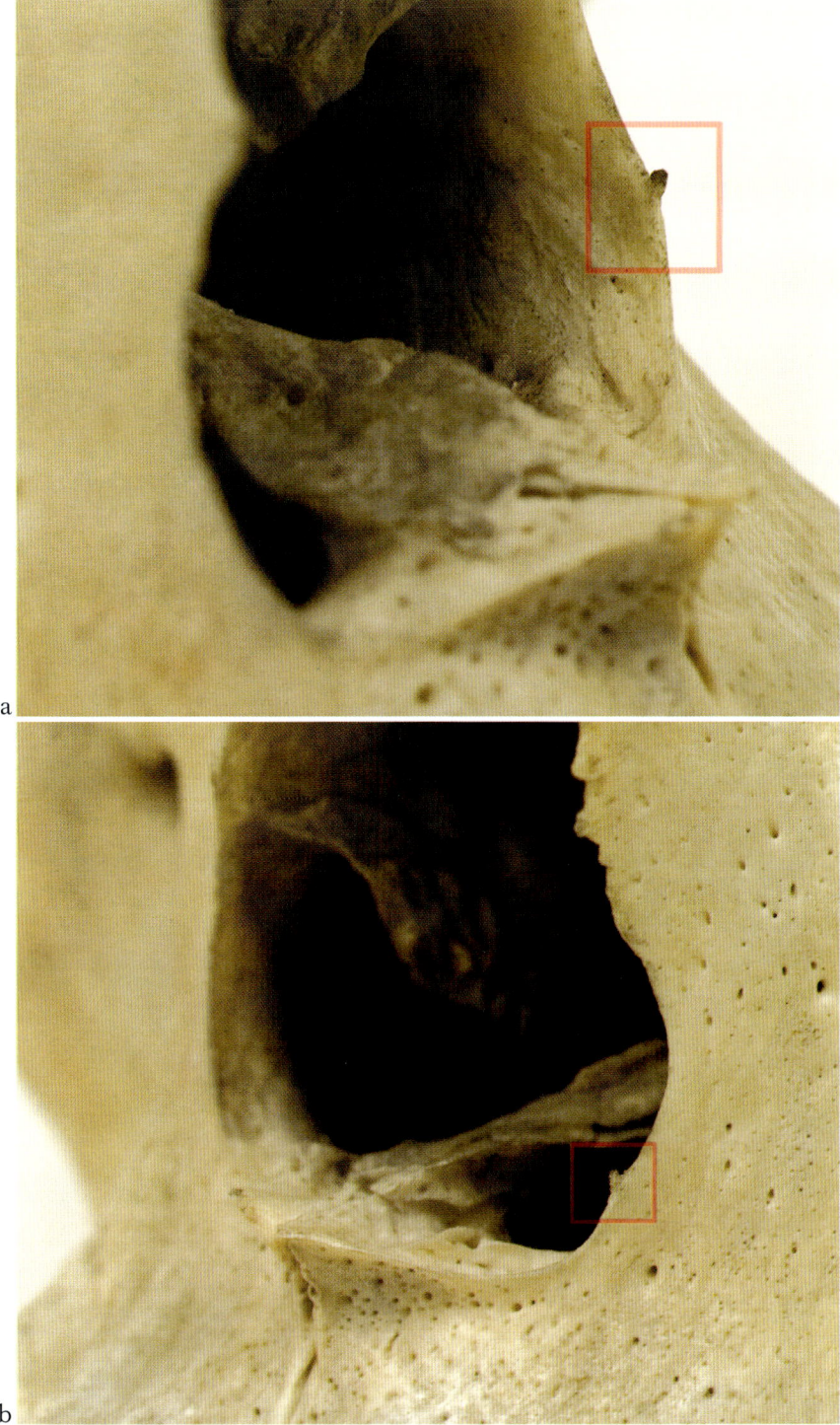

Figure 121a-b. Nasal rim spine in a 24-year-old male (Mütter Museum 1006.076). (a) Right oblique showing a small bony projection/spine (square) along the left lateral rim of the nasal aperture resulting in what the present authors call a "nasal rim spine". (b) Left oblique view of the left nasal rim spine (square). Duckworth (1906) first reported on these spines, which may be unilateral or bilateral, in three New Guinea skulls along with two other crania that had small elevated ridges in this area. What attaches to these spines and their function is unknown. Cf. Hauser and DeStefano (1989); Toldt et al. (1919). Uncommon to rare trait.

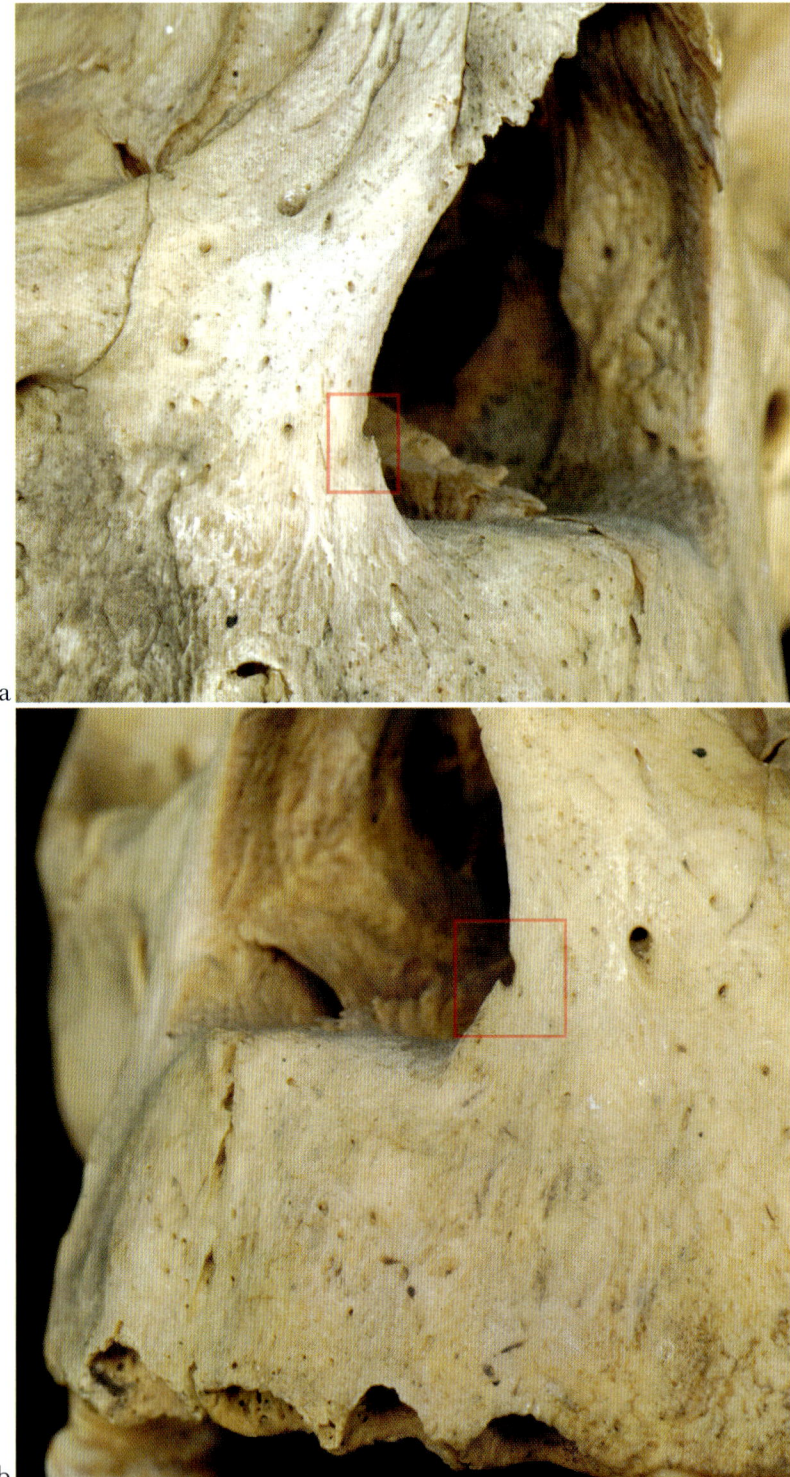

Figure 122a-b. Bilateral and symmetrical nasal rim spines and notches in a 6- to 8-year-old child (UPenn 1492 L606). (a) Right oblique view showing a small notch and spine (rectangle) along the inferior portion of the right nasal aperture. (b) Small notch and spine (square) along the left rim/margin of the nasal aperture. Although possible, these spines do not appear to result from ossification of soft tissues along the piriform aperture (nasal sill/rim), although they may somehow relate to the lesser alar cartilages.

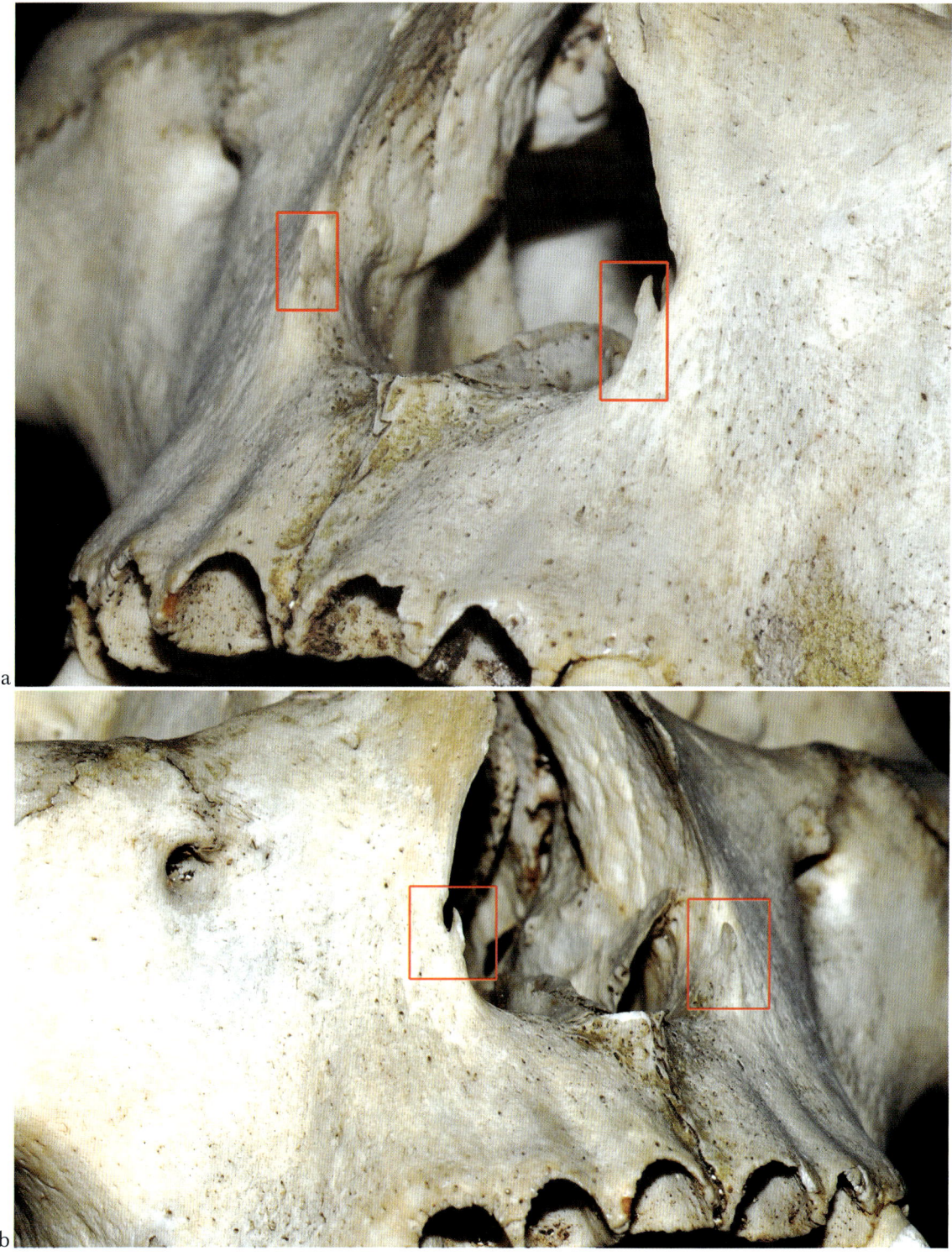

Figure 123a-b. Nasal rim spines that resemble horns in a young adult (RV1503). (a) Left oblique and (b) right oblique views of the upwardly-projecting spines. These tiny projections, first reported by Duckworth in 1906, are usually bilateral, form along the inferior portion of the nasal aperture and may have notches situated superior to them. Uncommon to rare trait of unknown frequency and function, but may possibly be connected to the lesser alar cartilages.

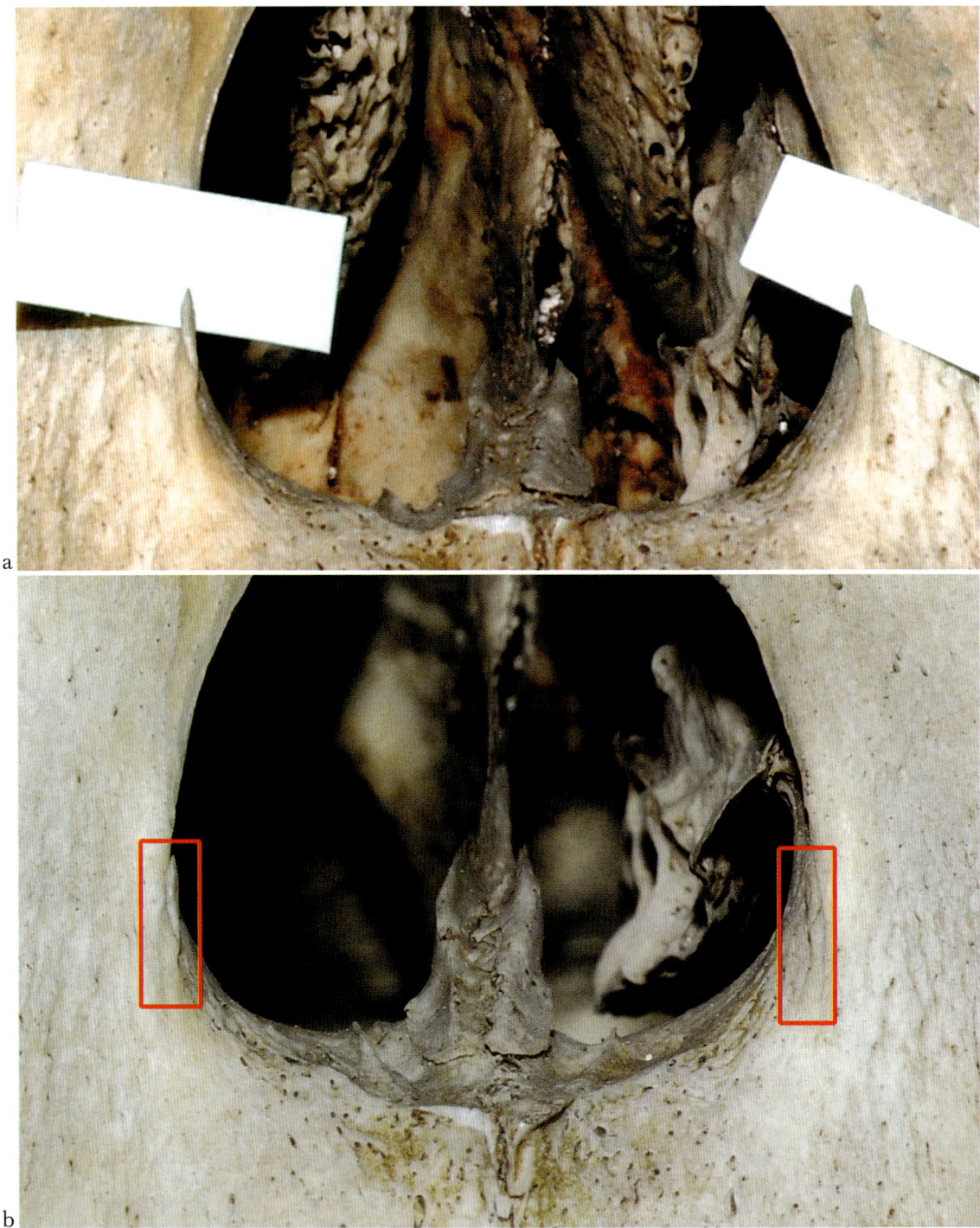

Figure 124a-b. Anterior view of "nasal rim spines" in a young adult (RV1503). (a) Close-up of the spines showing that they follow the curvature of the nasal sill and are not perfectly straight, curving most at their bases. (b) Note that the bases of the slender and upwardly projecting spines (rectangles) in this specimen originate slightly lateral to the nasal sill. The function and etiology of these spines are unknown.

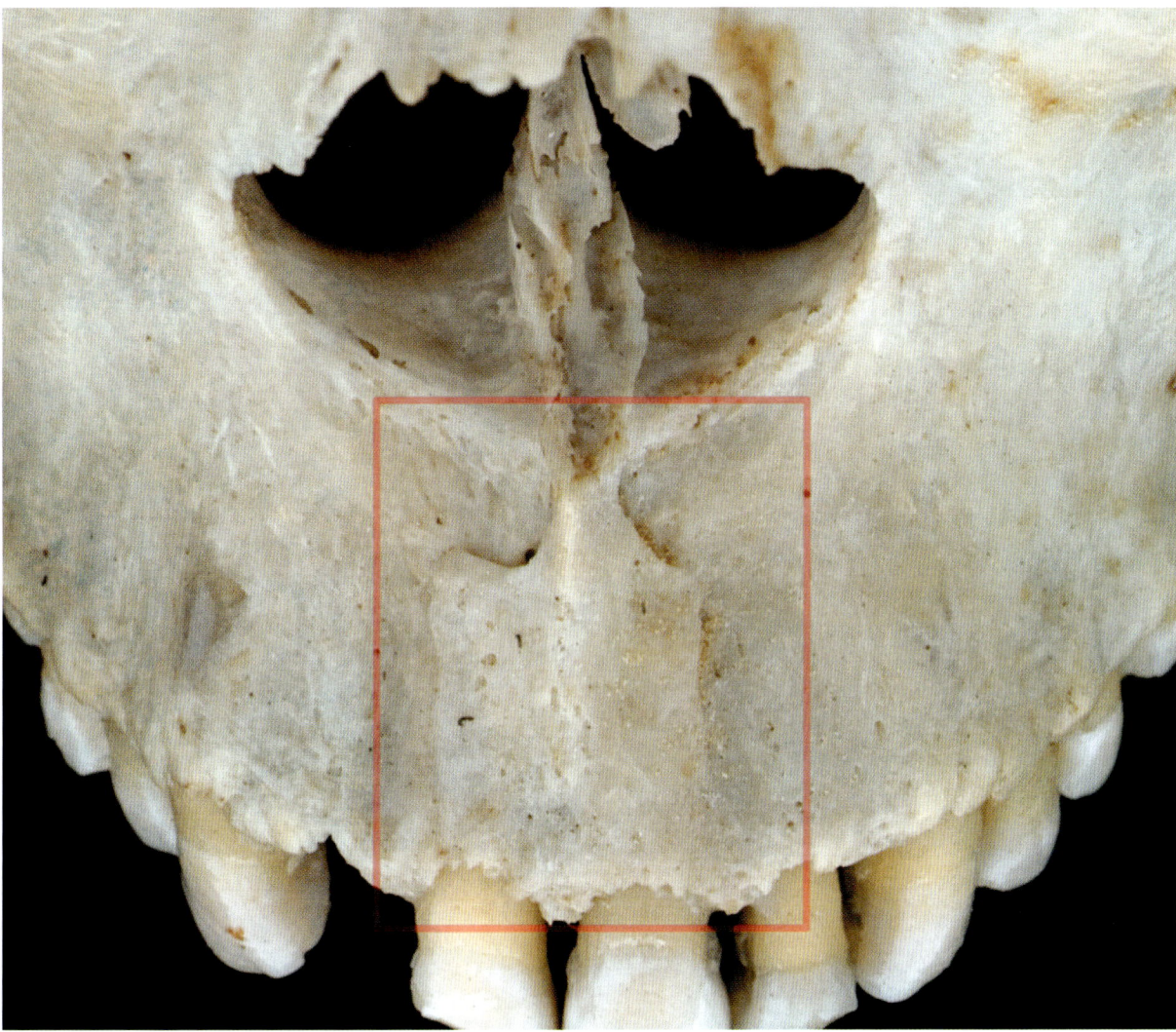

Figure 125. A rare, shield-shaped area of bone extending inferiorly from the anterior nasal spine to the alveoli of the central incisors in an elderly Thai female skull (KKU 51-1859). This raised area of bone does not appear to be the result of trauma or disease and does not communicate with the hard palate or involve the teeth.

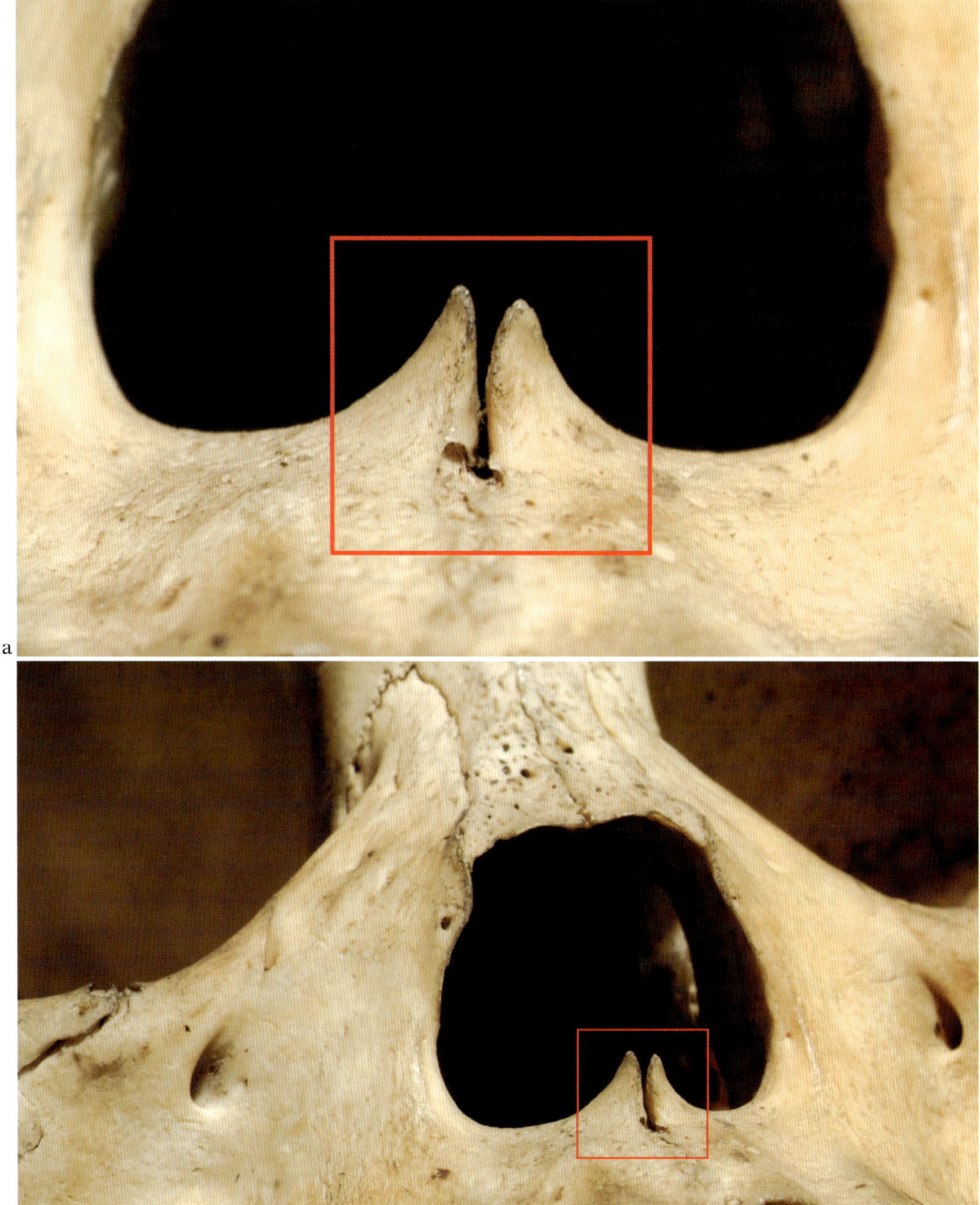

Figure 126a-b. Normal divided anterior nasal spine (square) in a 12- to 16-year-old African, probable female (TM 107, Ditsong Museum). (a) Frontal and (b) right oblique views showing that the nasal spine (squares) is separated along its superior portion. Although the nasal spine may remain divided along the midline, the two projections often join and their line of union obliterates in childhood.

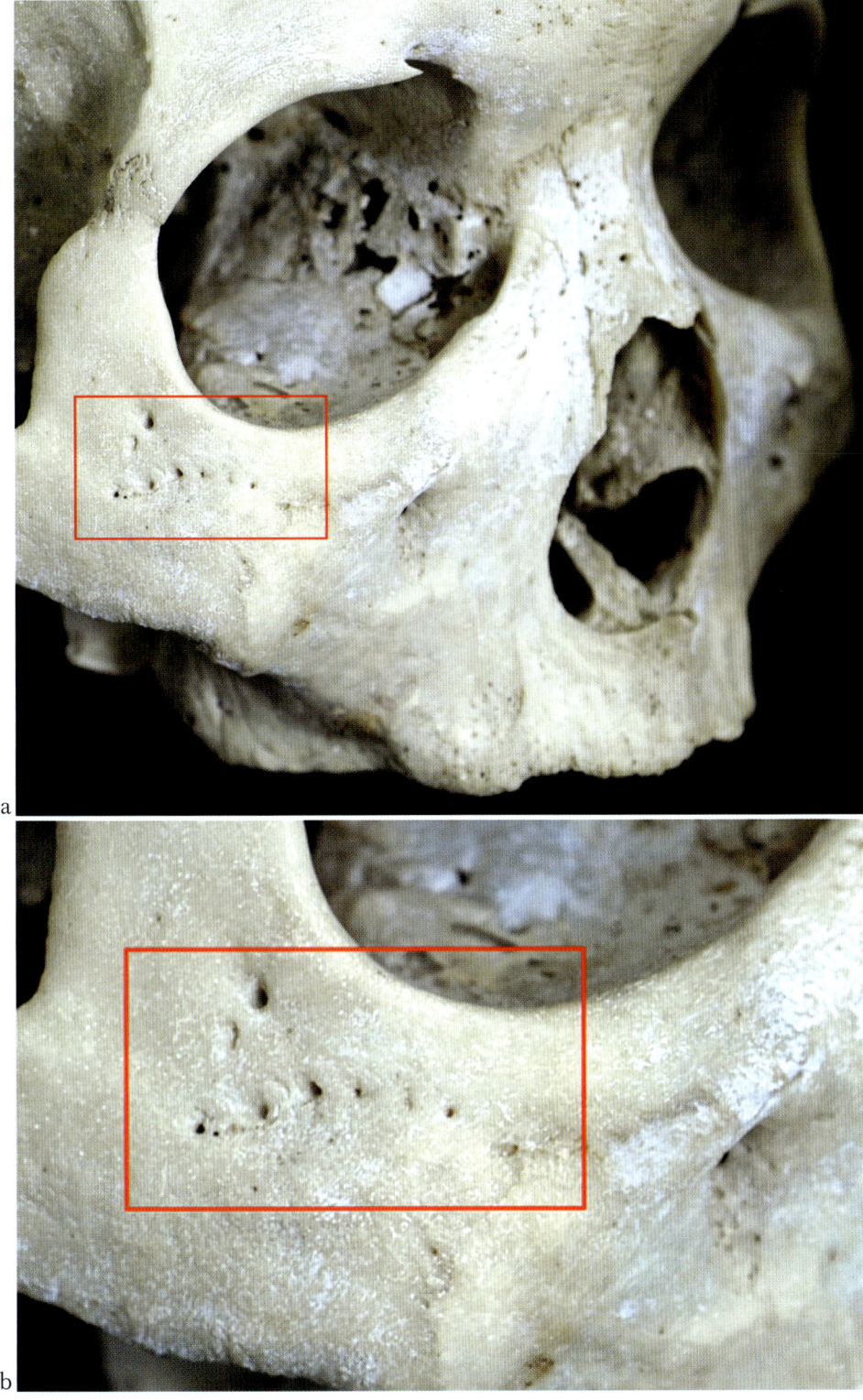

Figure 127a-b. Multiple zygomatic foramina for vessels in an adult Thai skull (KKU). (a) Position of the foramina (rectangle) in the right zygoma. (b) Close-up of the foramina (rectangle) forming a groove in the right zygoma. Note that the two largest foramina are oriented vertically, while the smaller foramina form a horizontally groove, likely for passage of one or more vessels, in the zygoma. Uncommon to common finding.

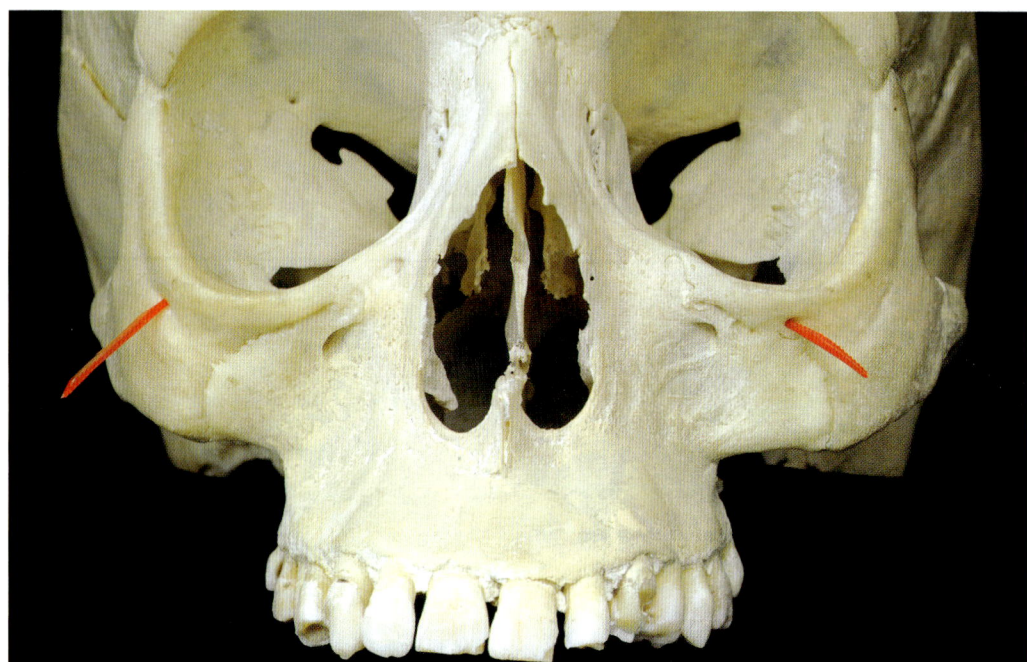

Figure 128. Medially positioned zygomaticomaxillary foramina (red probes) (FSA DS041). Note the asymmetry in the position of the foramina such that the left foramen lies close to the zygomaticomaxillary suture.

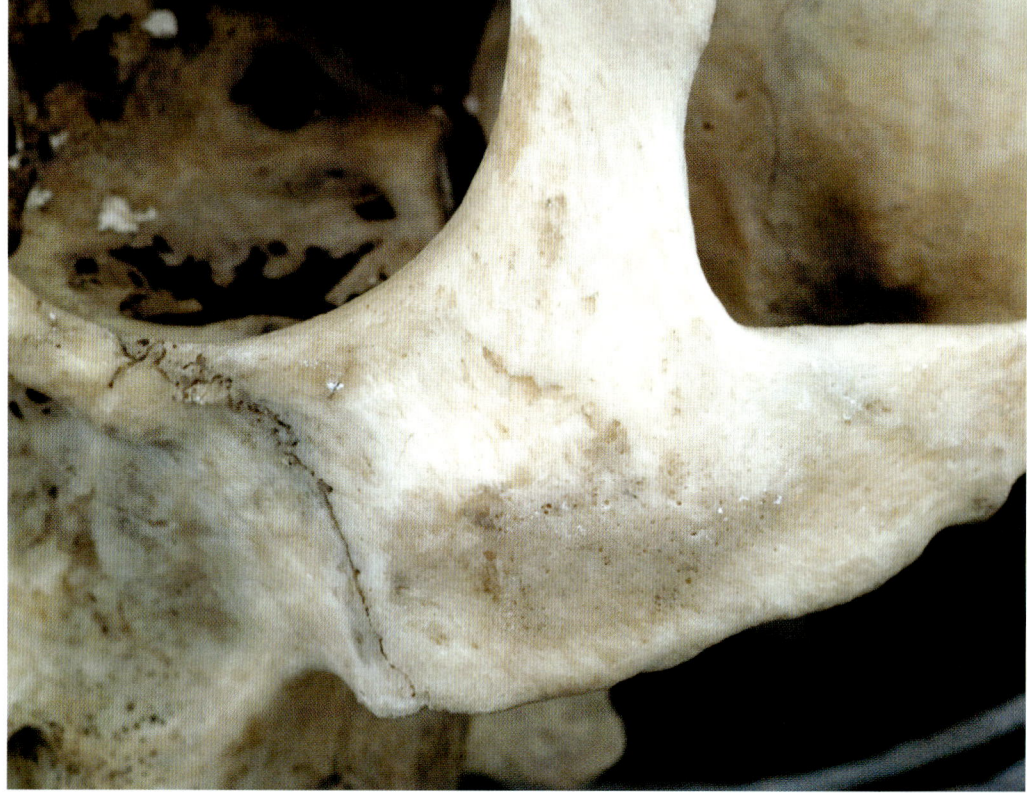

Figure 129. Left zygoma without a zygomaticomaxillary foramen (KKU 2557-42).

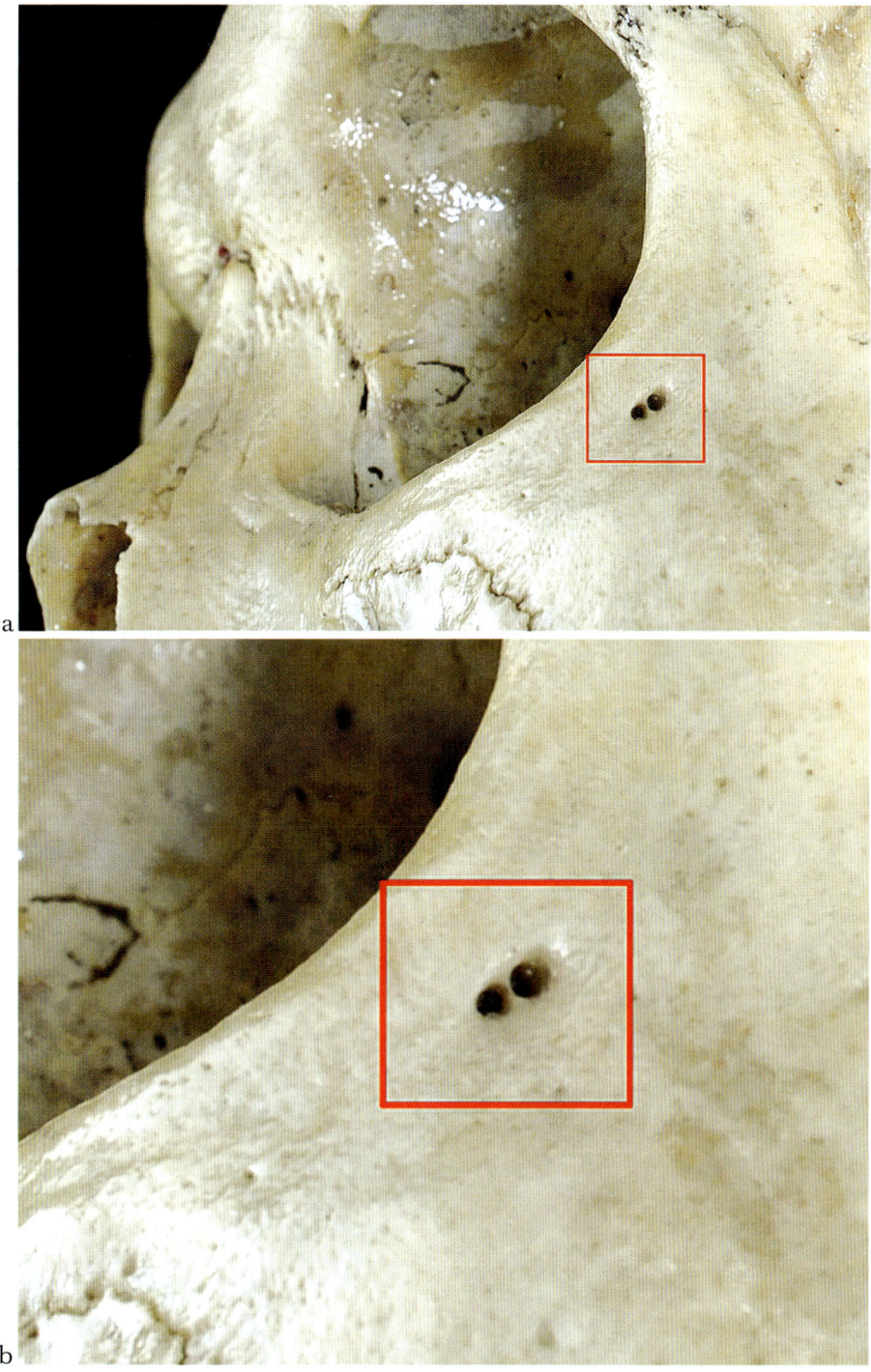

Figure 130a-b. Type II left zygomaticofacial foramen (see Loukas et al. 2008). (a) Divided or double zygomaticofacial foramen (square) in an adult (KKU). This trait may appear as two external and internal foramina, or a single internal foramen that is externally divided/bridged (raising the question whether this is two completely separate foramina, or one foramen that is divided, both conditions of which may transmit separate vessels). These foramina may be internally or externally divided. (b) Note that both foramina have rounded entrances, indicating something passed through each of them. Common finding. Cf. Aksu et al. 2009 for a study of zygomaticofacial foramen; Mangal et al. (2004); Wartmann and Loukas (2009).

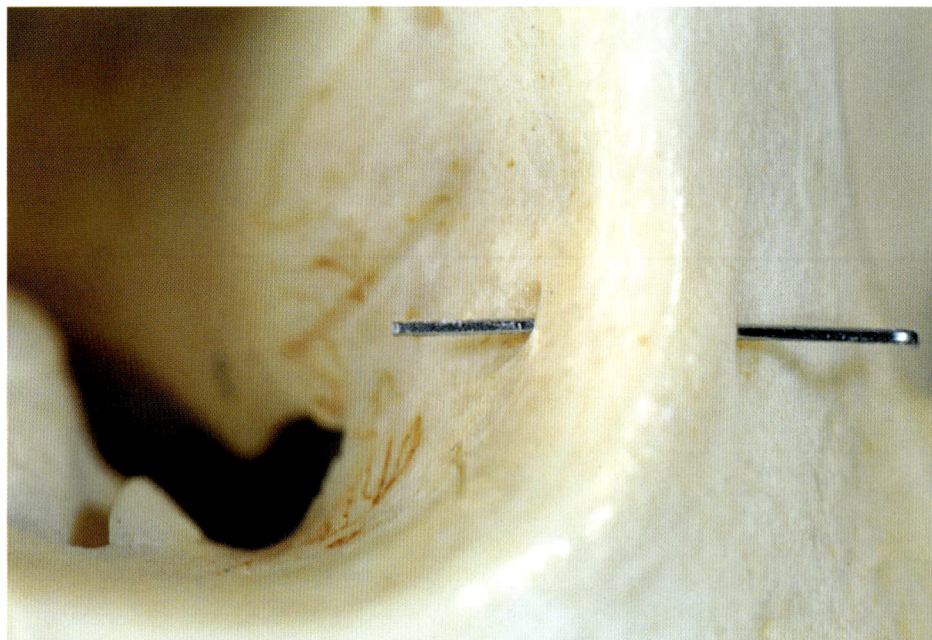

Figure 131. Type I zygomaticofacial foramen (wire) in the lateral border of the left orbit of a Thai adult skull for transmission of the zygomaticofacial nerve (KKU). Typical anatomy and variant. Cf. Aksu et al. (2009); Mangal et al. (2004).

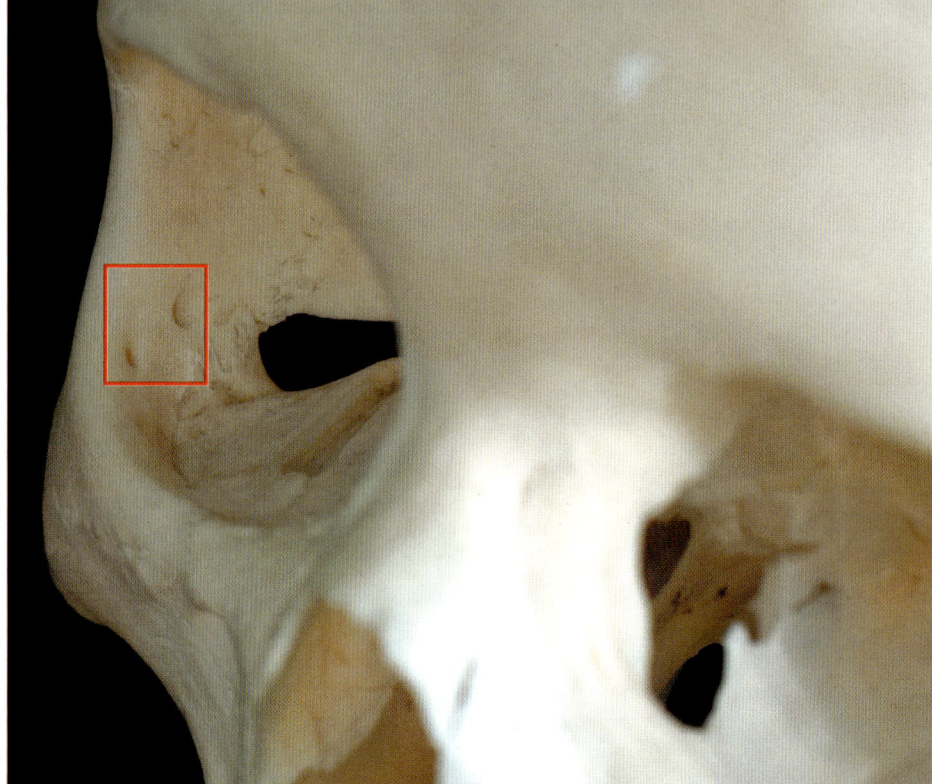

Figure 132. Two zygomaticofacial foramina, often referred to as zygomatico-orbital foramina (square), that transmits the zygomaticofacial nerves (CSC AC 027). Cf. Aksu et al. (2009).

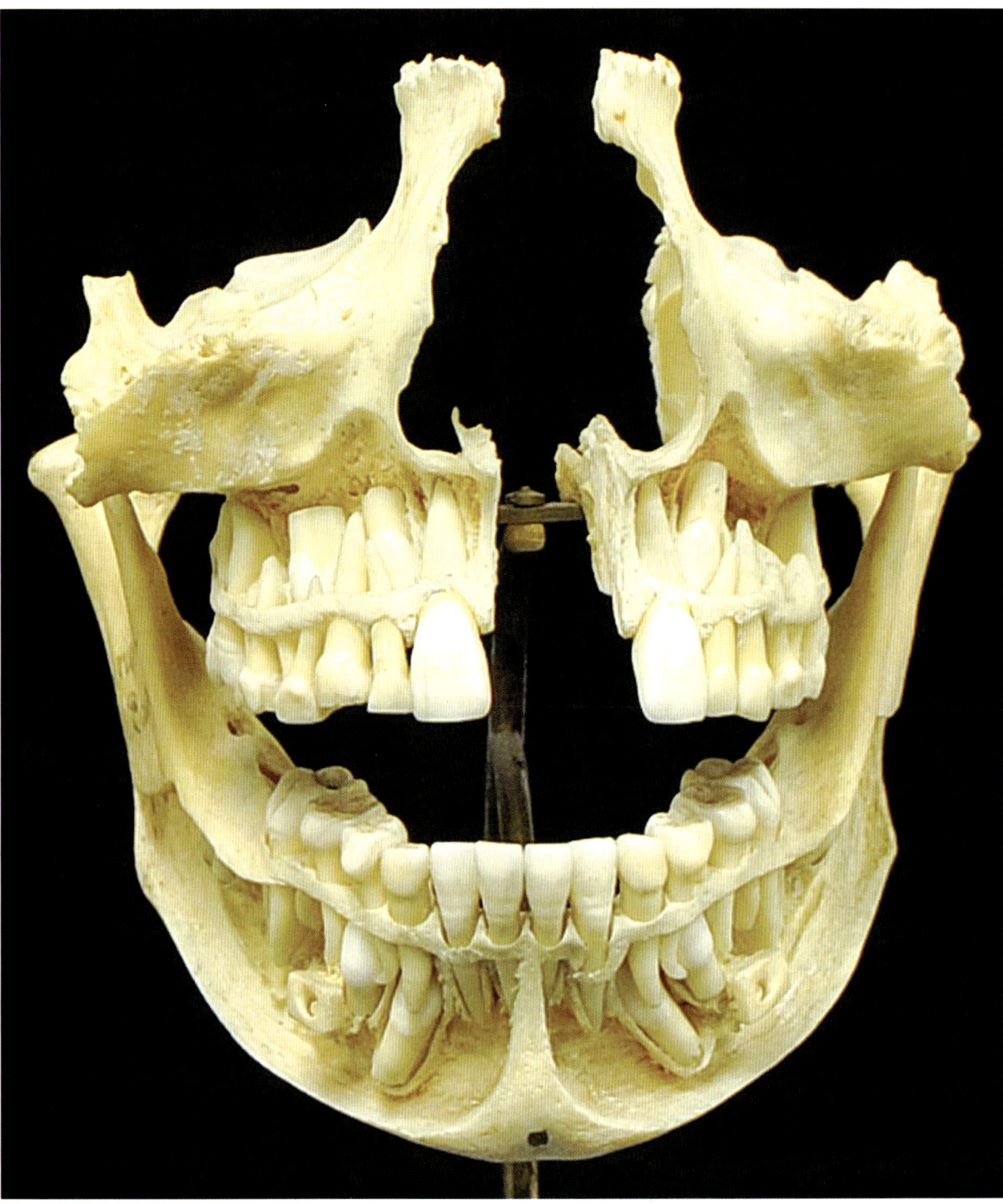

Figure 133. Normal developmental anatomy of the jaws and teeth in an 8- to 10-year-old child (Mütter Museum 1919.1098.10). Note the position of the deciduous teeth within their bony crypts and the linear hypoplastic lines near the cementoenamel junction of the mandibular incisors.

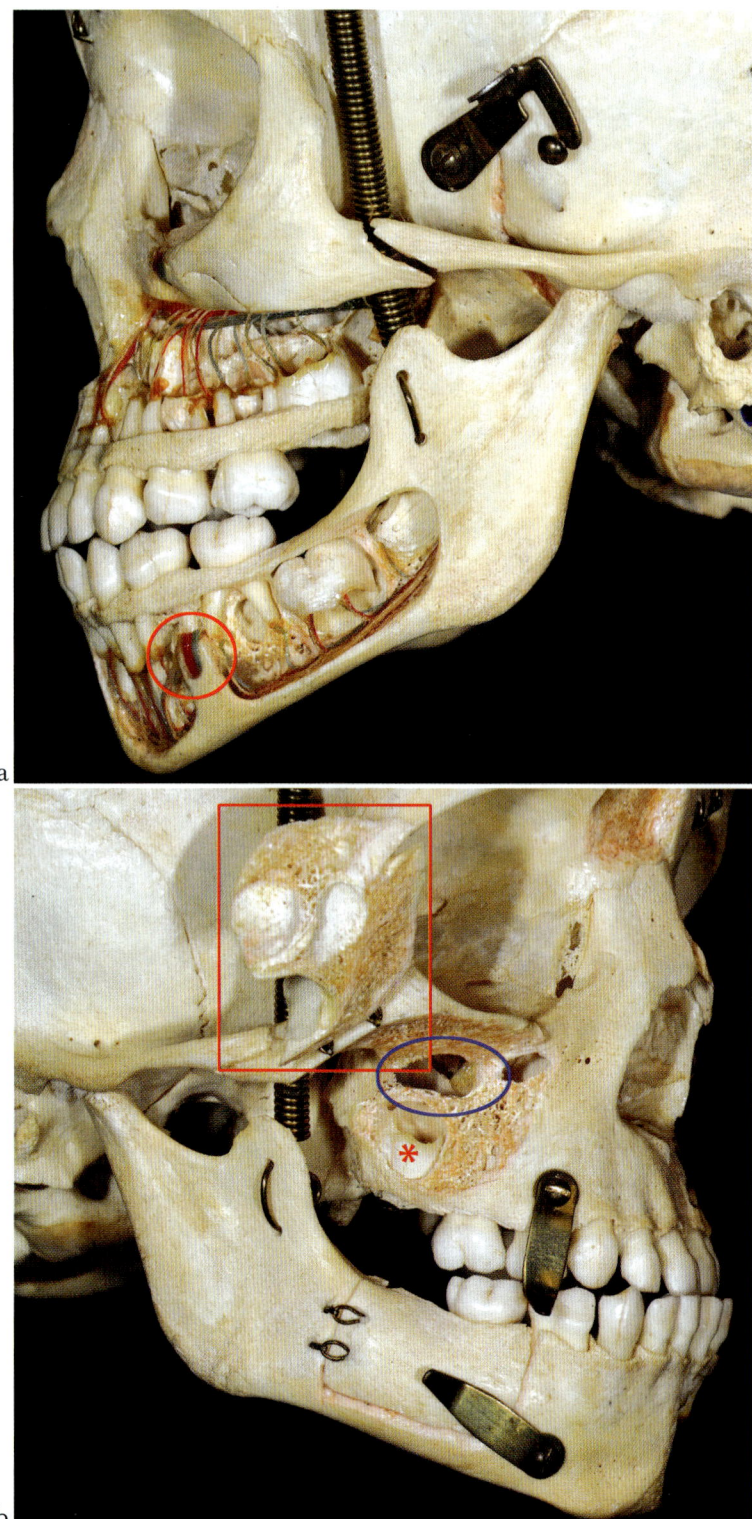

Figure 134a-b. Typical anatomy of the maxilla and mandible in a child (Kilgore International; JABSOM). (a) Normal anatomy of the maxilla and mandible in an approximately 5-year-old child showing the veins, arteries and nerves supplying and innervating the teeth and exiting the left mental foramen (circle). (b) A sectioned bone flap (rectangle) exposes the right maxillary antrum (blue oval) and right first (6 year) permanent molar (*).

Frontal View of the Skull

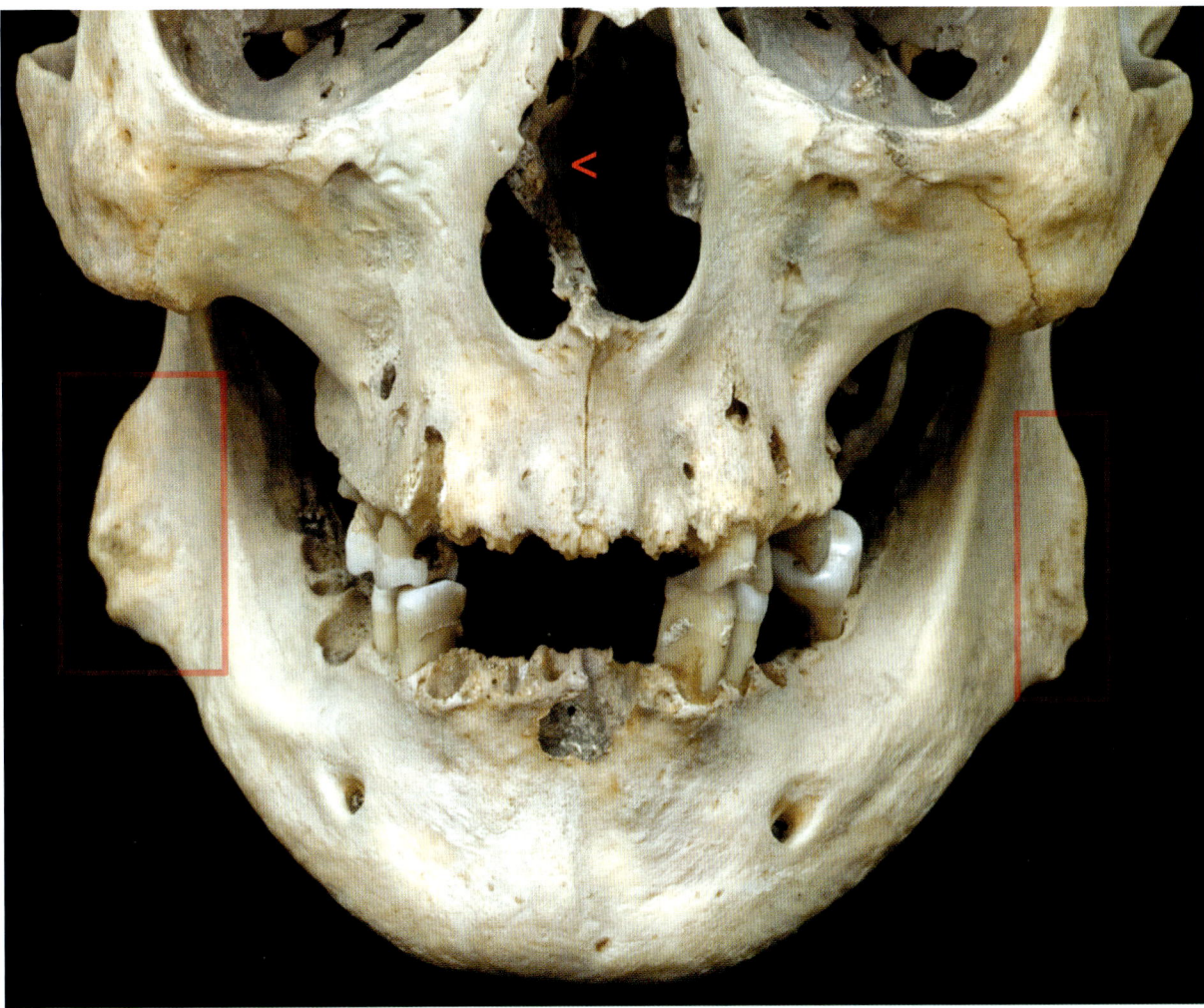

Figure 135. Significantly flared/everted gonial angle (rectangles) and right deviated nasal septum (<) in an adult male skull (Mütter Museum 1006-107). Gonial flaring is a common male trait, although it is present in some females.

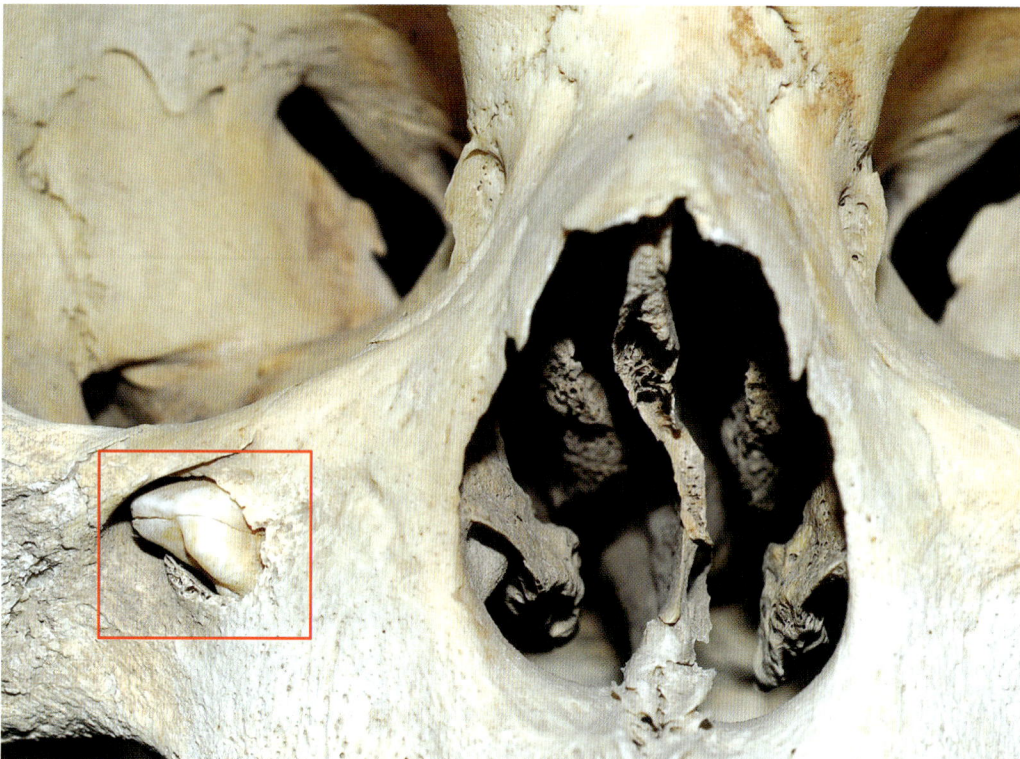

Figure 136. Displaced/malpositioned/ectopic right canine tooth (square) through the right infraorbital foramen due to development of a tooth bud in the maxillary antrum (KKU). Uncommon finding.

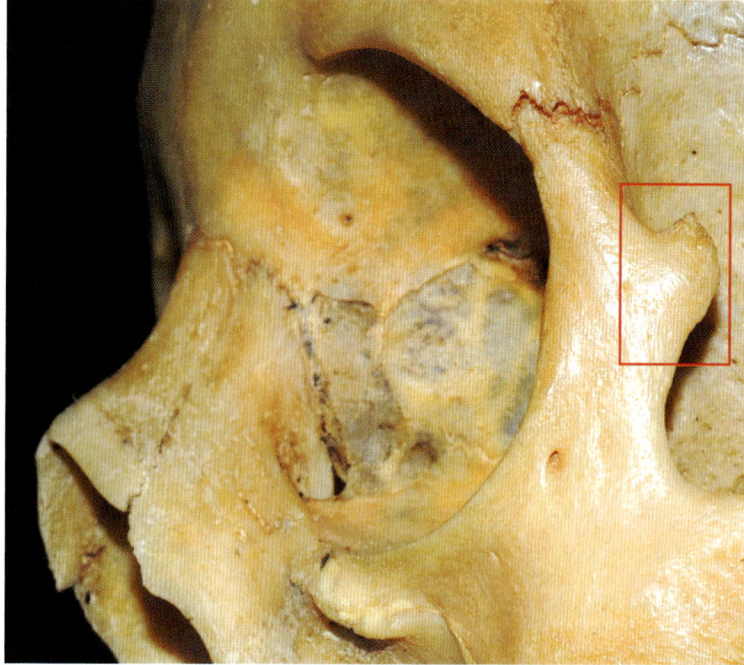

Figure 137. Prominent marginal tubercle (rectangle), also known as tuberculum marginale, processus marginalis of Sömmering, spina zygomatica, in an adult Thai male skull (KKU). This trait is often bilateral, but not necessarily symmetrical. Common to uncommon finding. Cf. Hauser and DeStefano (1989).

Chapter 2

RIGHT LATERAL VIEW OF THE SKULL

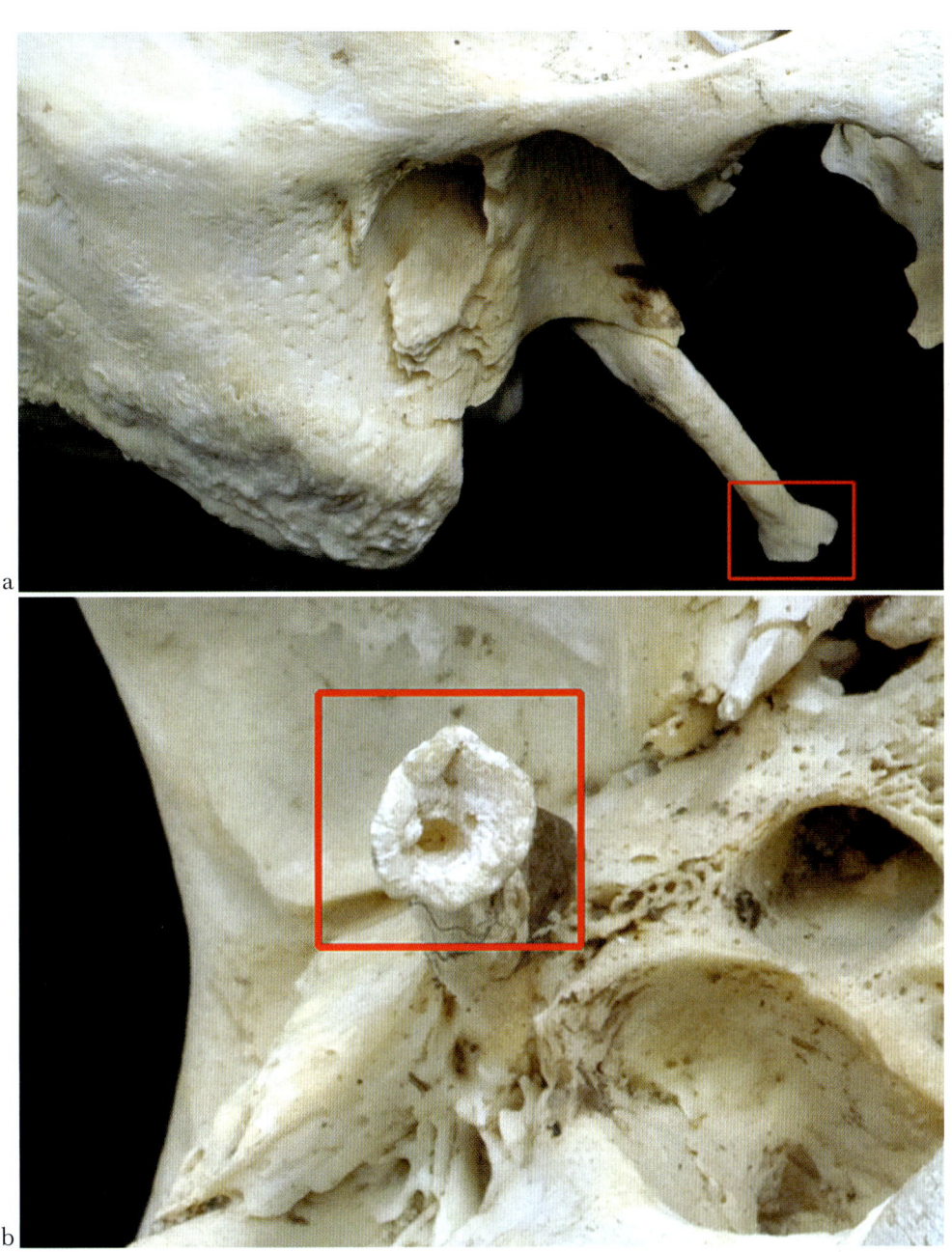

Figure 138a-b. Variant of elongated styloid process of the temporal bone. (a) Right lateral view of a segmented (red square) right styloid process resulting in partial or non-union of the styloid process to the ossified stylohyoid portion of the styloid chain in an elderly Thai male (CMU 128 50). (b) Inferior view of the internal morphology of the temporal styloid process in this individual. See Langlais et al. (1986) for classification of styloid processes. Styloid processes can increase in length during aging, are typically longer in males, may vary in length from side to side in the same individual, may be symptomatic, and a radiographic frequency of 2 to 28% of adults (More and Asrani 2010). Cf. Yaczi et al. (2008).

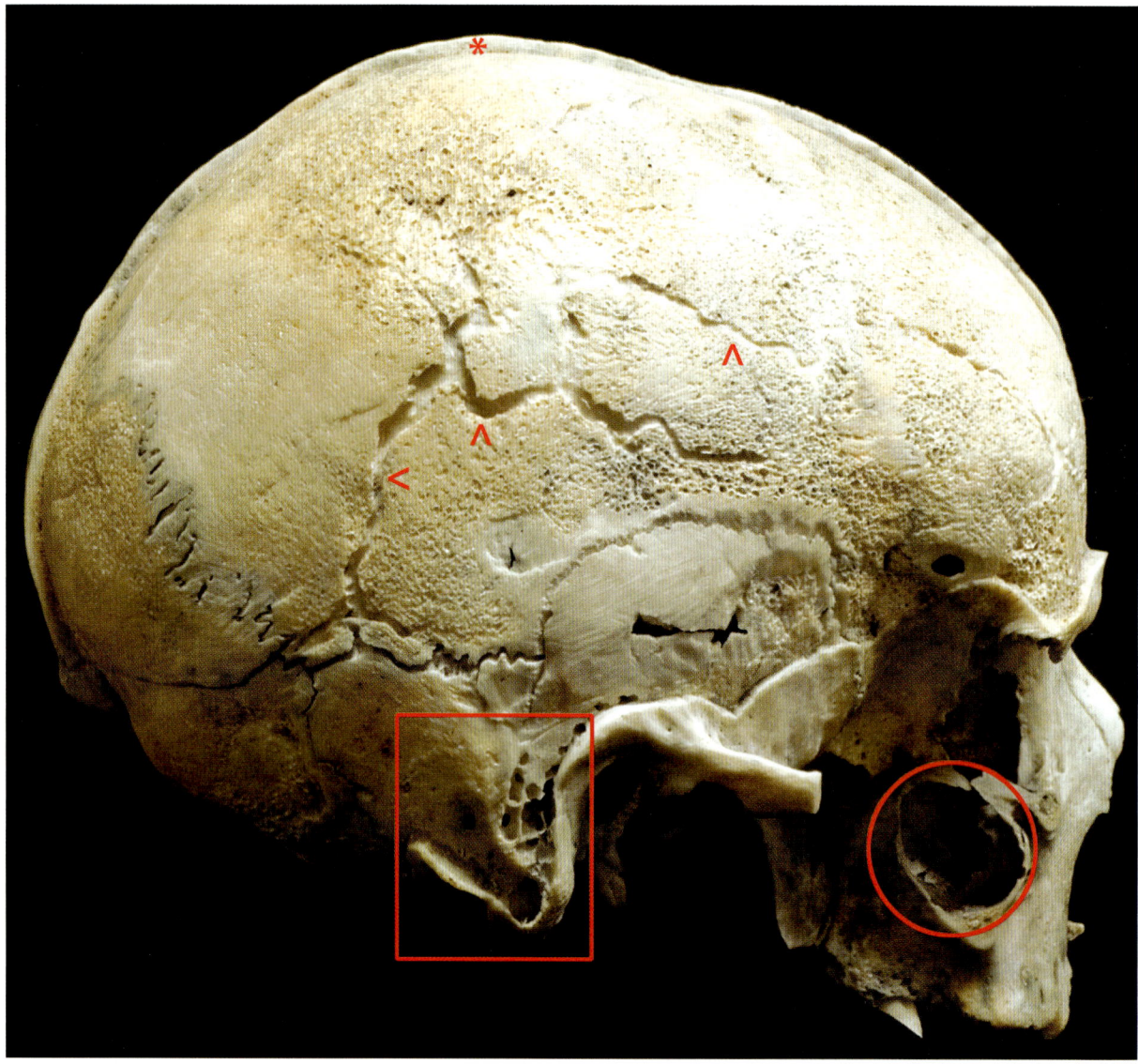

Figure 139. Removal of the outer lamina/table (*) of the cranium revealing the diploic veins (< and ∧), mastoid air cells (rectangle) and right maxillary antrum (circle) in an adult (UPenn). Typical anatomy.

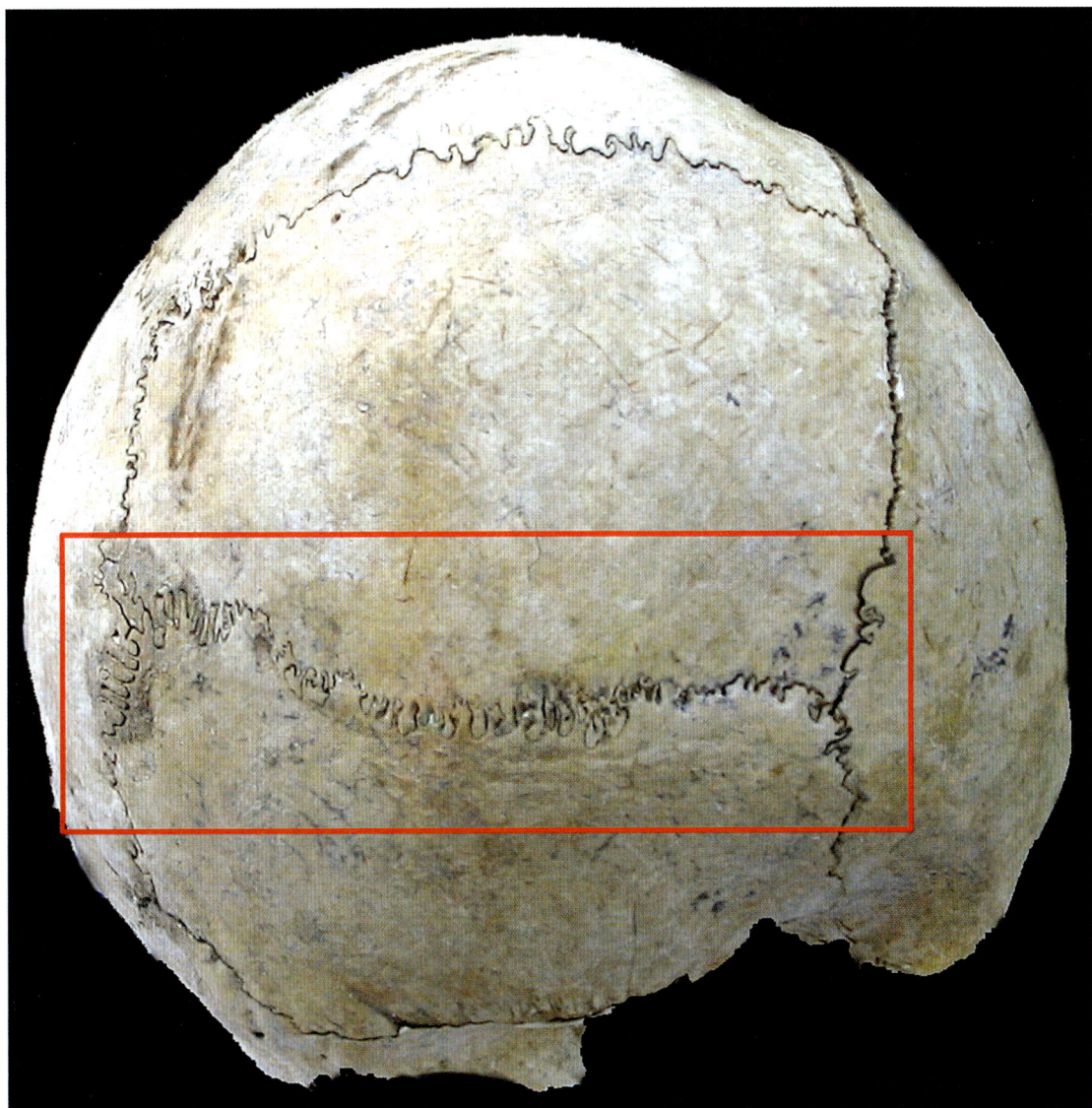

Figure 140. Extremely rare bipartite right parietal bone (red square) from Hungary (Ivett Kövári, Herman Otto Museum, Hungary), also known as os bipartite divisum (Hauser and DeStefano (1989), os parietale bipartitum (Berry 1910), os parietale divisum (Becker et al. 2005), parietal sagittal suture (Nickel 1971), and bifid parietal (intraparietal suture). Note this accessory suture (subsagittal suture), which is present only on the right side in this individual, is more complex than the sagittal suture, divides the right parietal bone into two portions, runs parallel to the sagittal suture, forms a "Bregma-like" junction where it joins the lambdoidal suture, and does not have an "Obelion." Shapiro (1972), in examining 25,000 radiographs, found only three examples (0.00012%) of complete bipartite parietal bones. Bipartite parietal bones are believed to form as a result of the two centers of ossification that fail to unite Cf. Becker (2005); Gray (1901); Hrdlička (1903); Shapiro (1972); Tharp and Jason (2009); Toldt (1883). Accessory sutures such as this may be mistaken as fractures. There is considerable anatomic variation of bipartite parietal bones such that there may be complete or incomplete separation and oriented vertically, diagonally or horizontally. See Turner (1891, 1901) for brief descriptions of a double right and left parietal bones, respectively.

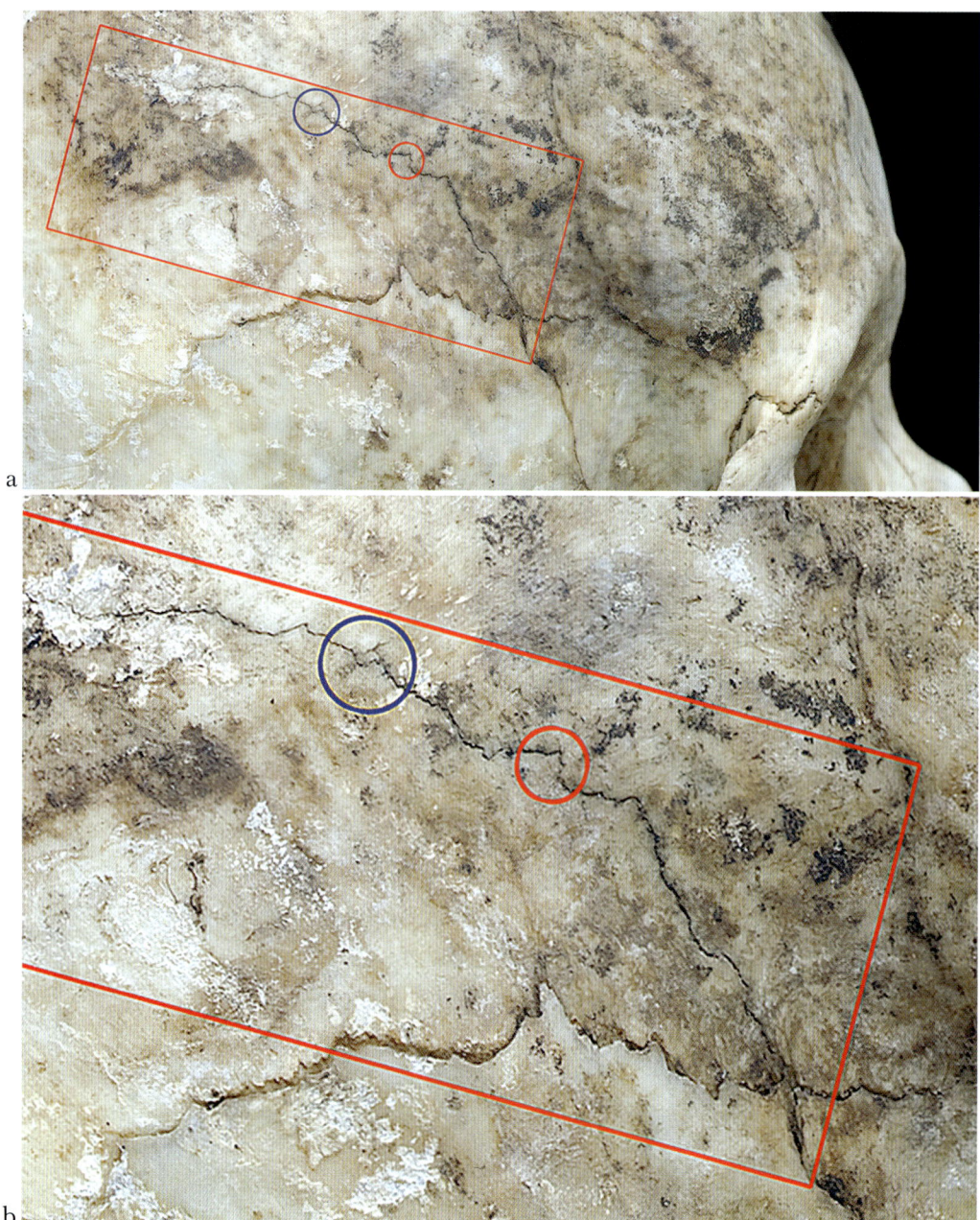

Figure 141a-b. Possible accessory (bipartite) right parietal or squamosal suture in a 55-year-old Thai male (CMU 35 52). (a) Right lateral view depicting the morphology of this possible suture, which shares some features with postmortem breakage. (b) Note that this feature continues its course as an extension of the squamosal suture and exhibits suture-like morphology with interdigitations, deviations (red circle) and a small bone island (blue circle). This feature may not be a suture since it does not communicate with the sagittal or lambdoidal suture and postmortem breakage occurs inside the left orbit. Regardless of the etiology, this example highlights the difficulty of distinguishing some antemortem and postmortem features.

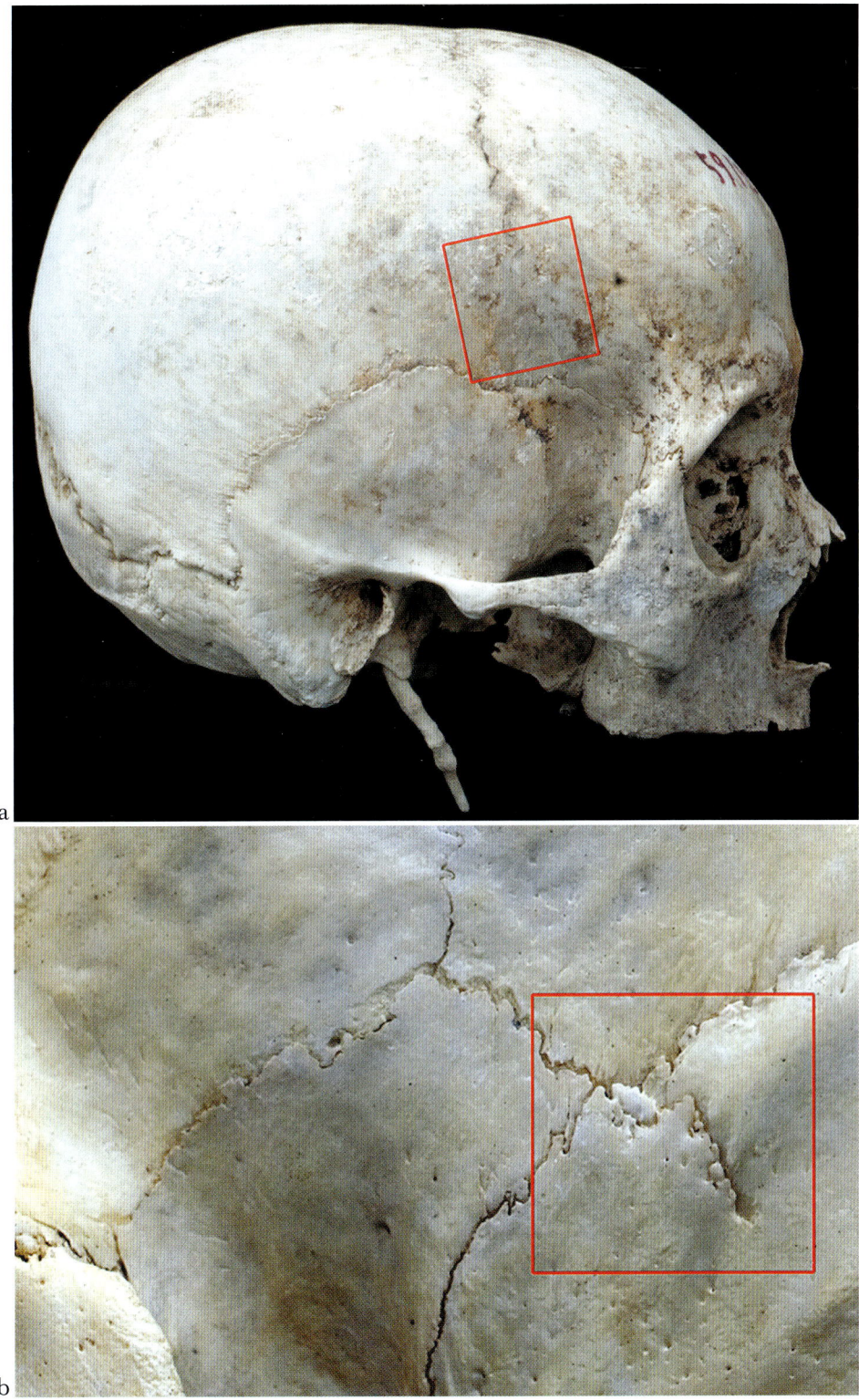

Figure 142a-b. Bilateral partial division (transverse suture/bipartite temporal bone) in the right and left temporal squama of a 36-year-old Thai female skull (CMU 122 50) resulting in bilateral extension of the sphenofrontal sutures. (a) Right lateral view showing the location of the accessory suture (square). (b) Close-up of the left accessory suture (square). Transverse accessory suture (square) in the left temporal squama. Uncommon to rare variant. Cf. Hauser and DeStefano (1989).

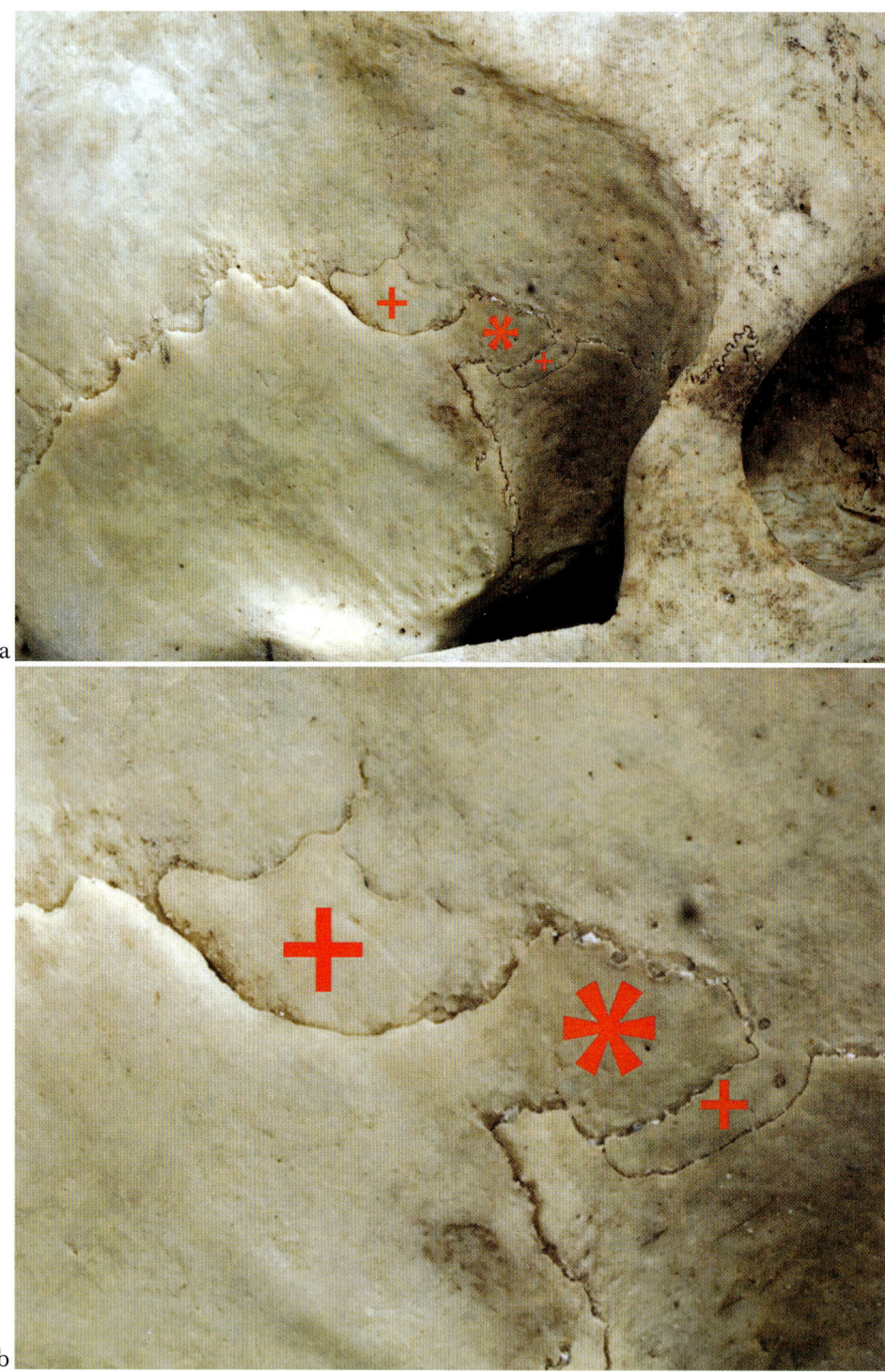

Figure 143a-b. Temporal extension and epipteric bones (CMU 193 52). (a) Two right epipteric bones (+) and a temporal extension (*) in a 65-year-old Thai female. The suture between the frontal bone and the smaller epipteric bone (+) is obliterated, making it appear as though it is a bony extension and not an ossicle, which it is. However, there is no endocranial or ectocranial separation of the temporal extension (*). (b) Magnified view of the temporal extension (*) and epipteric ossicles (+).

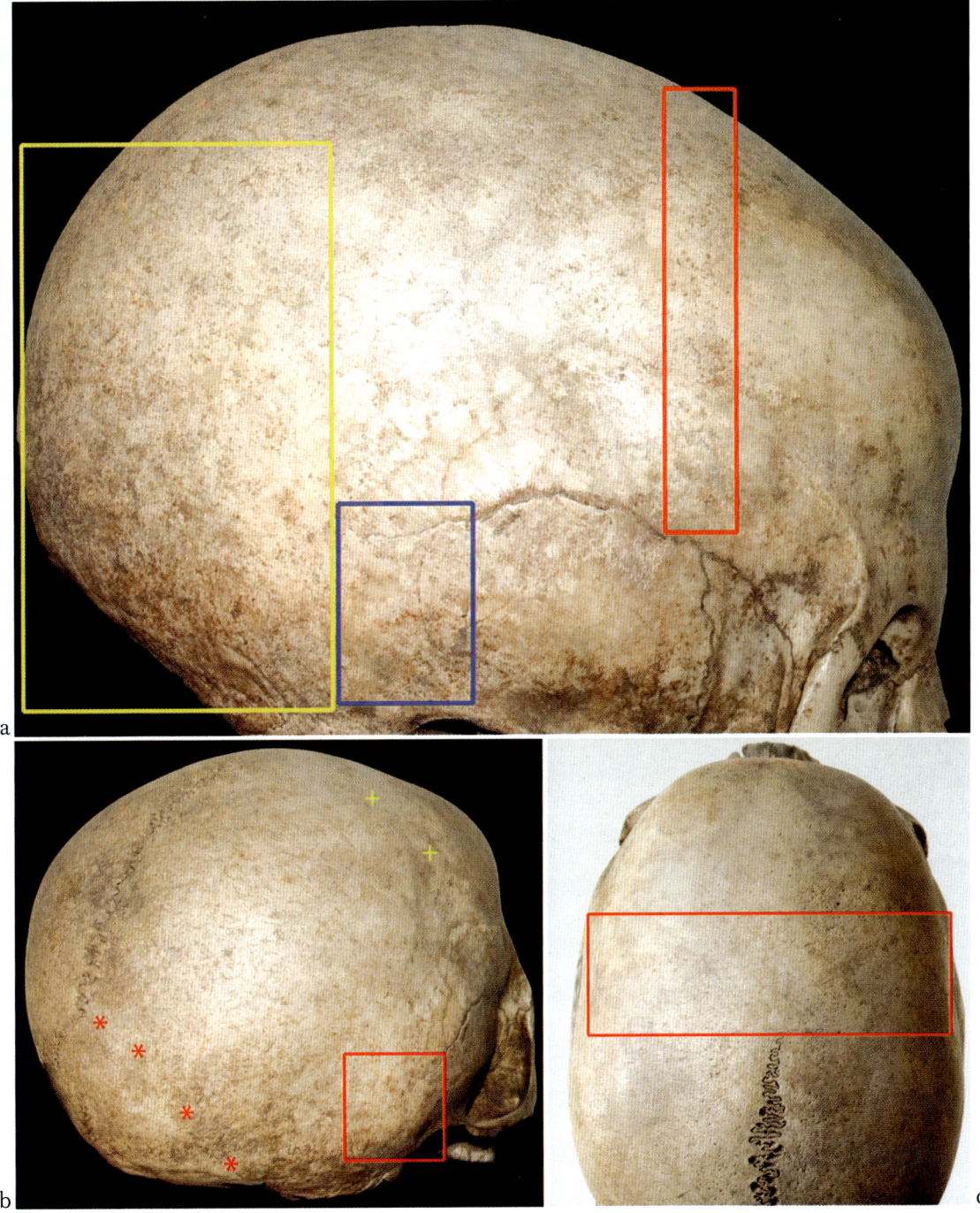

Figure 144a-c. Premature craniosynostosis in an adult (Budapest, Hungary). (a) closure of the coronal (red square), lambdoidal (yellow square) and squamosal sutures (blue square). (b) Obliteration of the right lambdoidal (*), squamosal (red square) and coronal sutures (+). (c) Complete craniosynostosis of the coronal suture (red square). The combination of synostoses in what appears to be a young adult is unusual and possibly pathological. However, scaphocephalic and plagiocephalic features were not present.

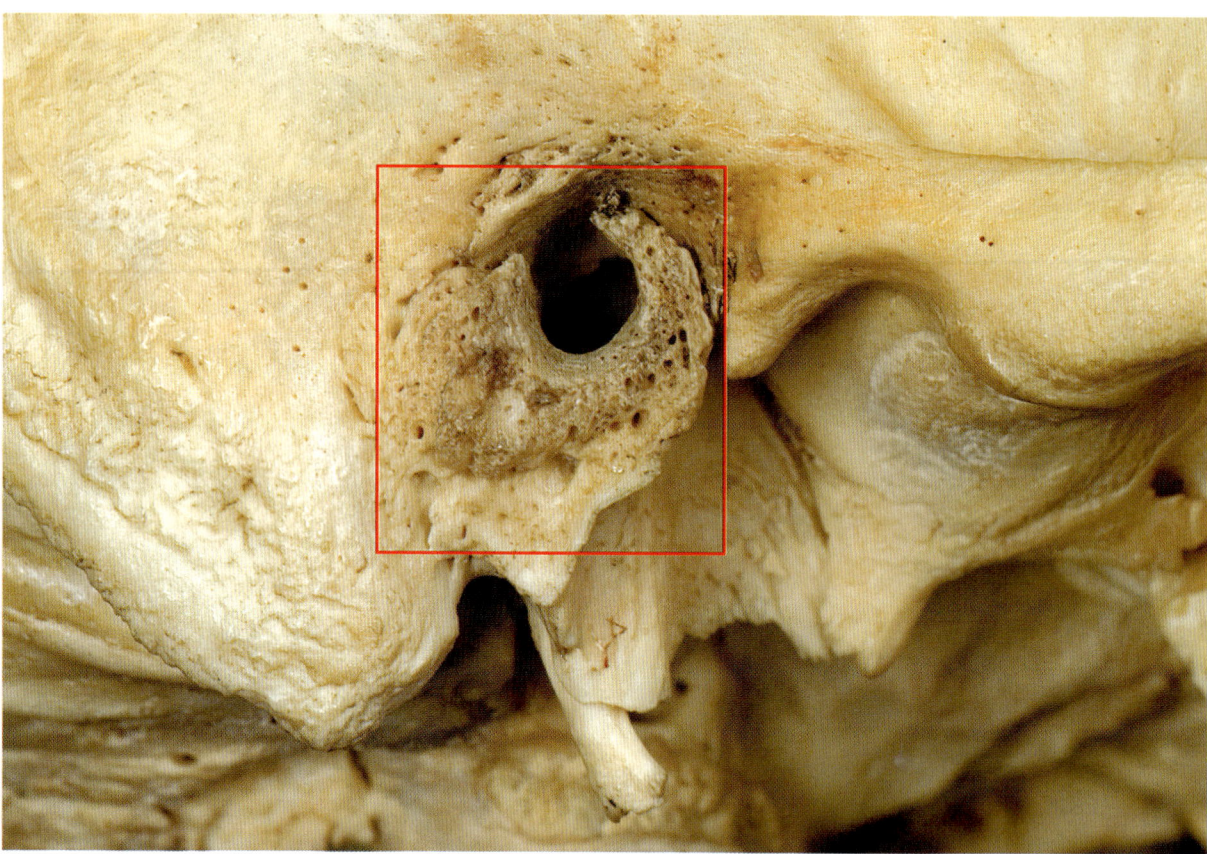

Figure 145. Thickened pars tympanica (bilateral) of unknown etiology in an adult Black male skull (SI Terry106R) (compare with Figure 134). Tympanic thickening, also known as os tympanicum hyperostosis, is more common in males and does not appear to be a result of infection. Oetteking (1930) found this feature in 98% of Pacific Northwest aboriginal crania. Uncommon to common finding depending on the group being examined. Cf. DeVilliers (1968); Halpern (1973); Stewart (1933); Wood-Jones (1931).

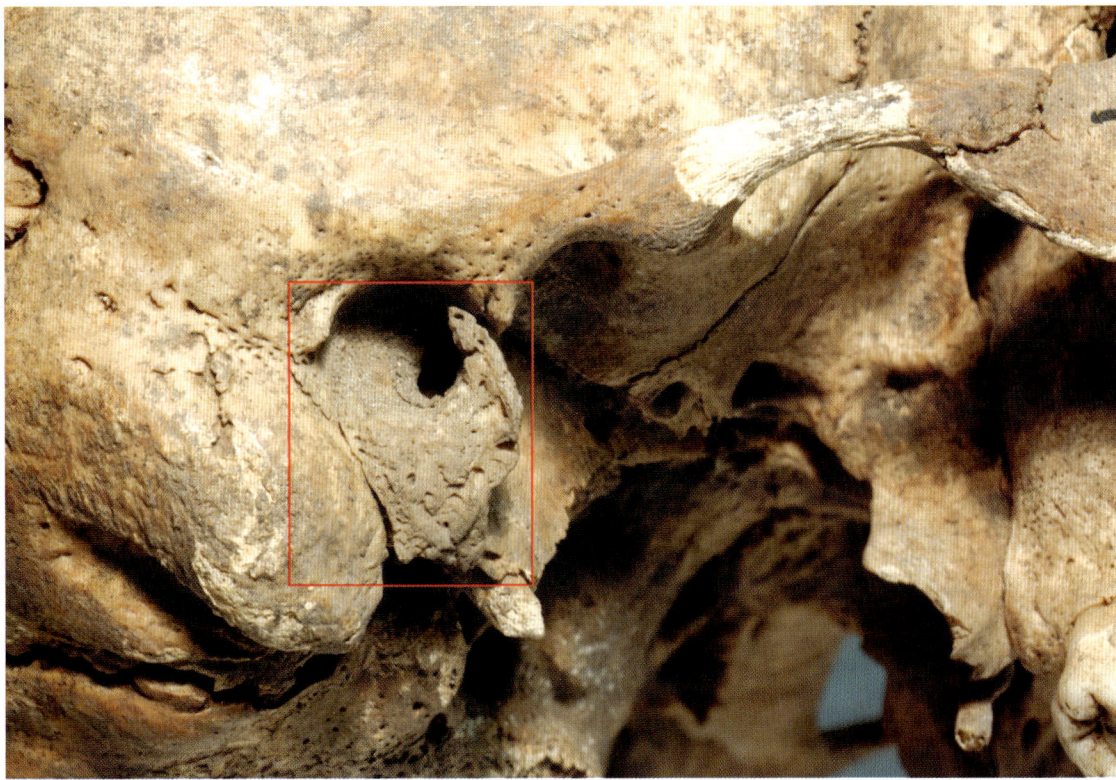

Figure 146. Greatly thickened pars tympanica (rectangle) in an adult African – note that the external auditory meatus has narrowed (TM 91, Ditsong Museum).

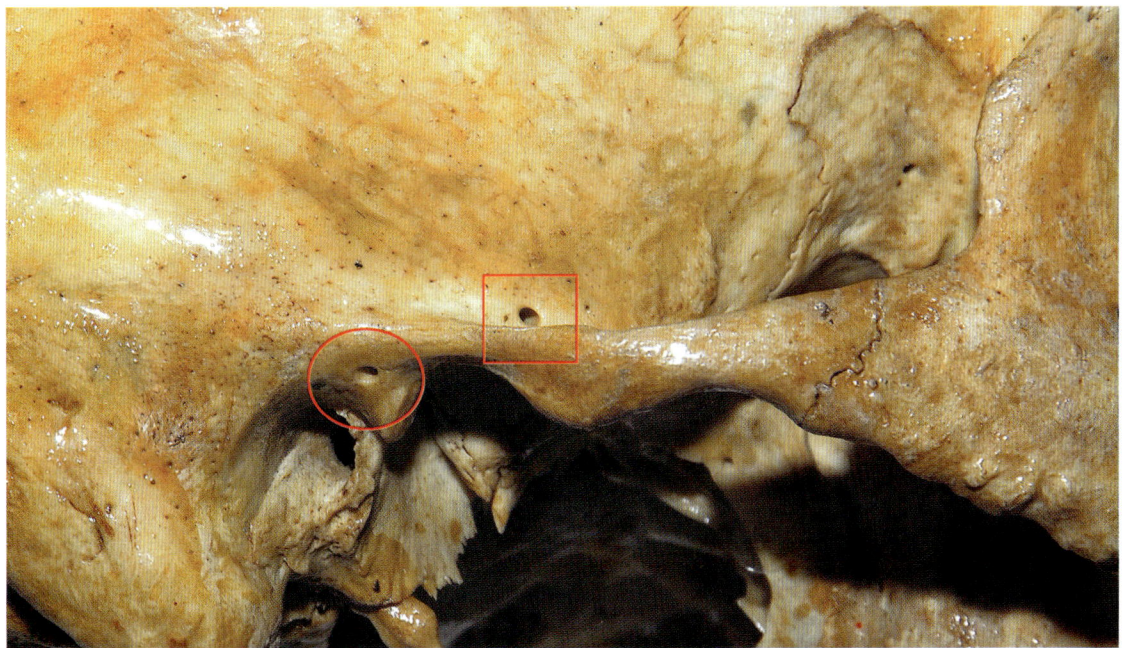

Figure 147. Inferior squamosal foramen (square) typically transmitting an emissary vein (Boyd 1930; Butler 1957, 1967; Hauser and DeStefano (1989) and postglenoid/supraglenoid foramen (circle), sometimes referred to as an inferior squamosal foramen (reported incidence of 0.9%; Vázquez et al. 2001) in an adult Thai (KKU). Uncommon findings warranting further research. Cf. Chauhan et al. (2011).

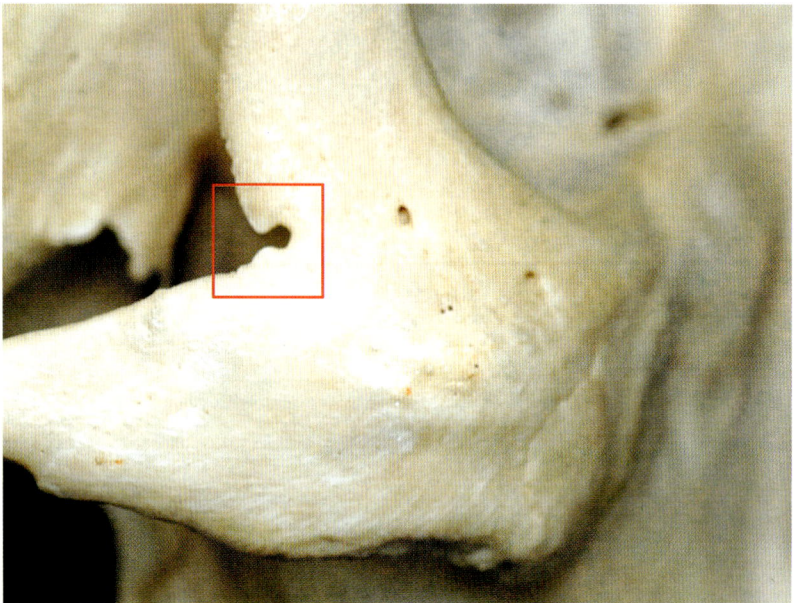

Figure 148. Notch or partial foramen (square) along the lateral margin of the right malar in an adult Thai skull (KKU). While the origin and purpose of this trait (possibly a zygomaticotemporal foramen) is unknown, it is an uncommon to rare finding at this location, sometimes referred to as the jugal point in the earlier literature (see Brash 1953).

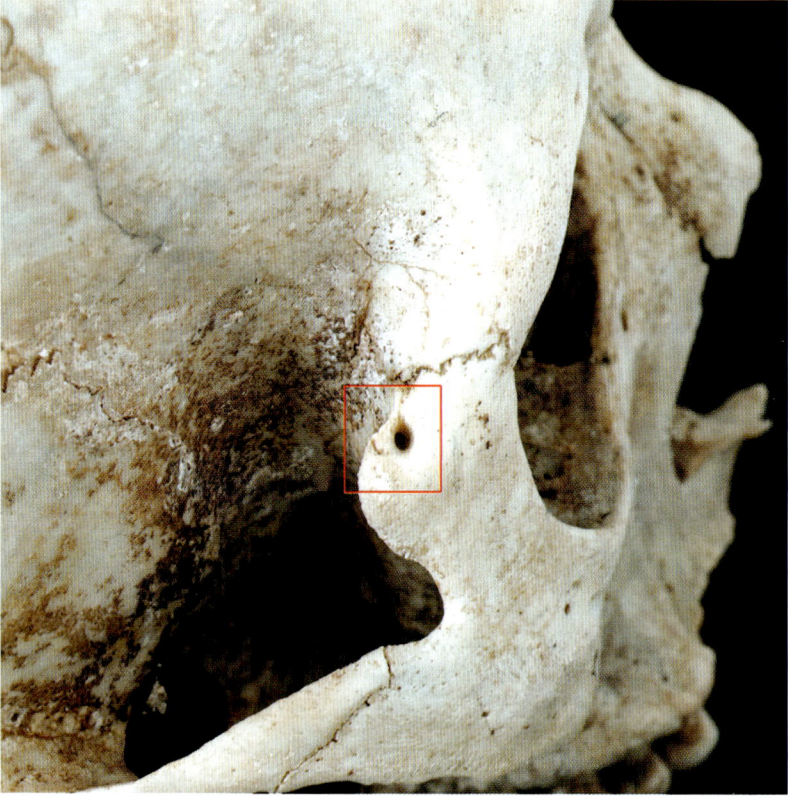

Figure 149. Foramen (square) high in the lateral margin of the right malar tubercle in a 64-year-old Thai male skull (CMU 101 52). This foramen perforated the lateral wall of the right orbit. Uncommon to common normal variant.

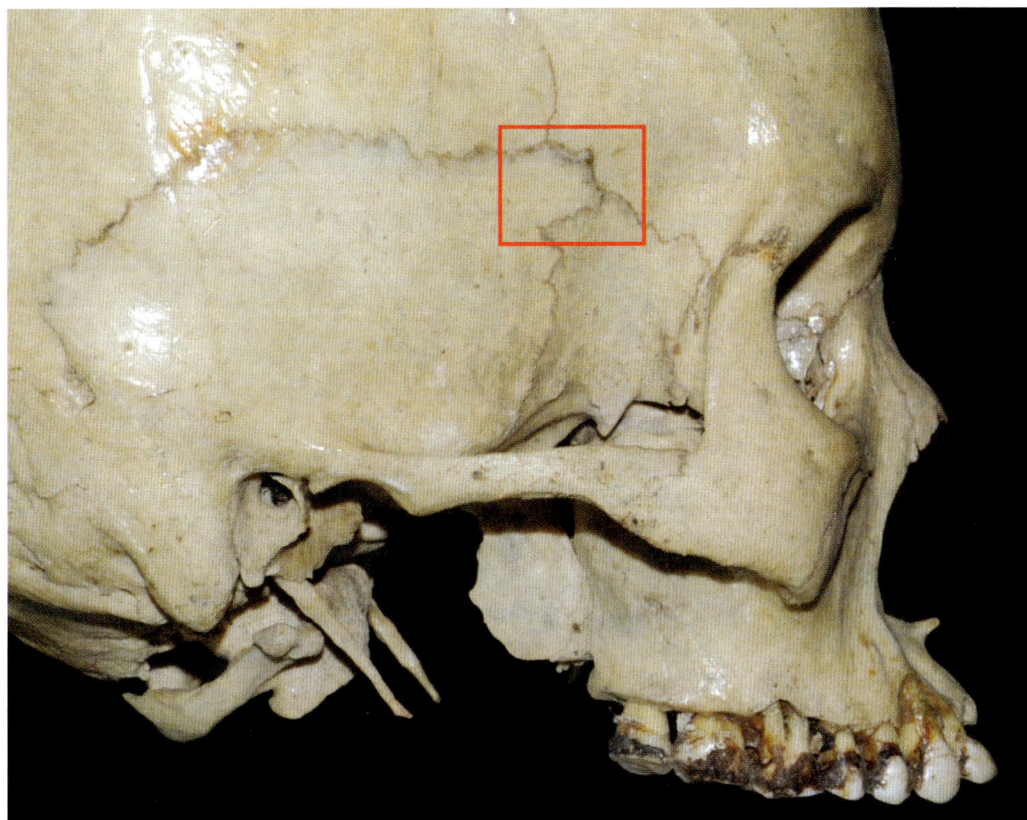

Figure 150. Bilateral fronto-temporal articulation (rectangle) in an adult Thai female skull, an uncommon finding in most groups (KKU). Note atlanto-occipitalization at the base of the skull, bilateral elongated styloid processes, and blackened teeth (betel nut chewing). Cf. Asala and Mbajiorgu (1996) and Bauer (1915) for Pterion; Gladstone and Erichsen-Powell (1915), Gladstone and Wakeley (1925) and Green (1930) for occipitalization; Collins (1926) and Vázquez et al. (2001) for fronto-temporal articulation and Hauser and DeStefano (1989) for all traits; Yaczi et al. (2008).

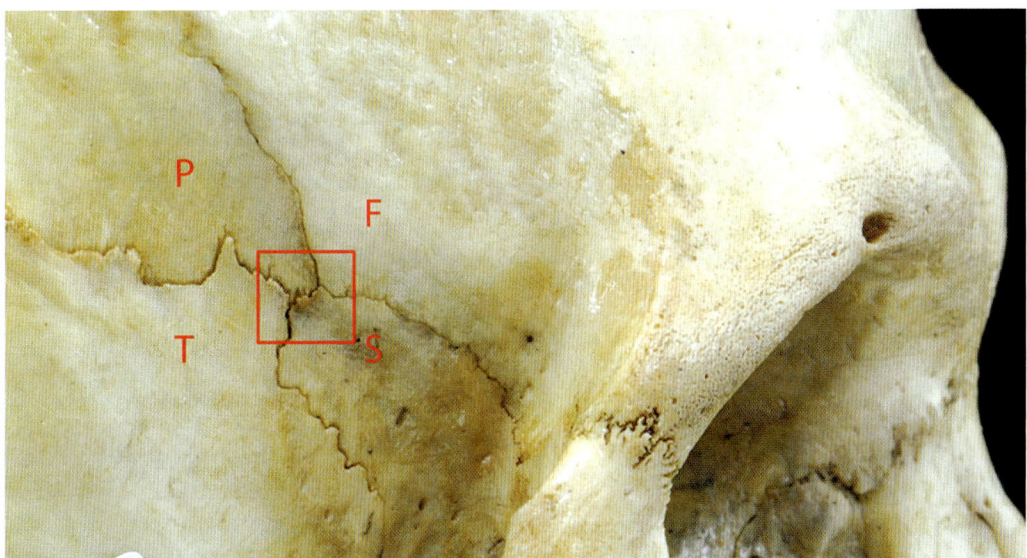

Figure 151. H-shaped pterion (square) at the junction of the frontal (F), sphenoidal (S), temporal (T) and parietal (P) bones in an adult Asian male (KKU). Cf. Hauser and DeStefano (1989).

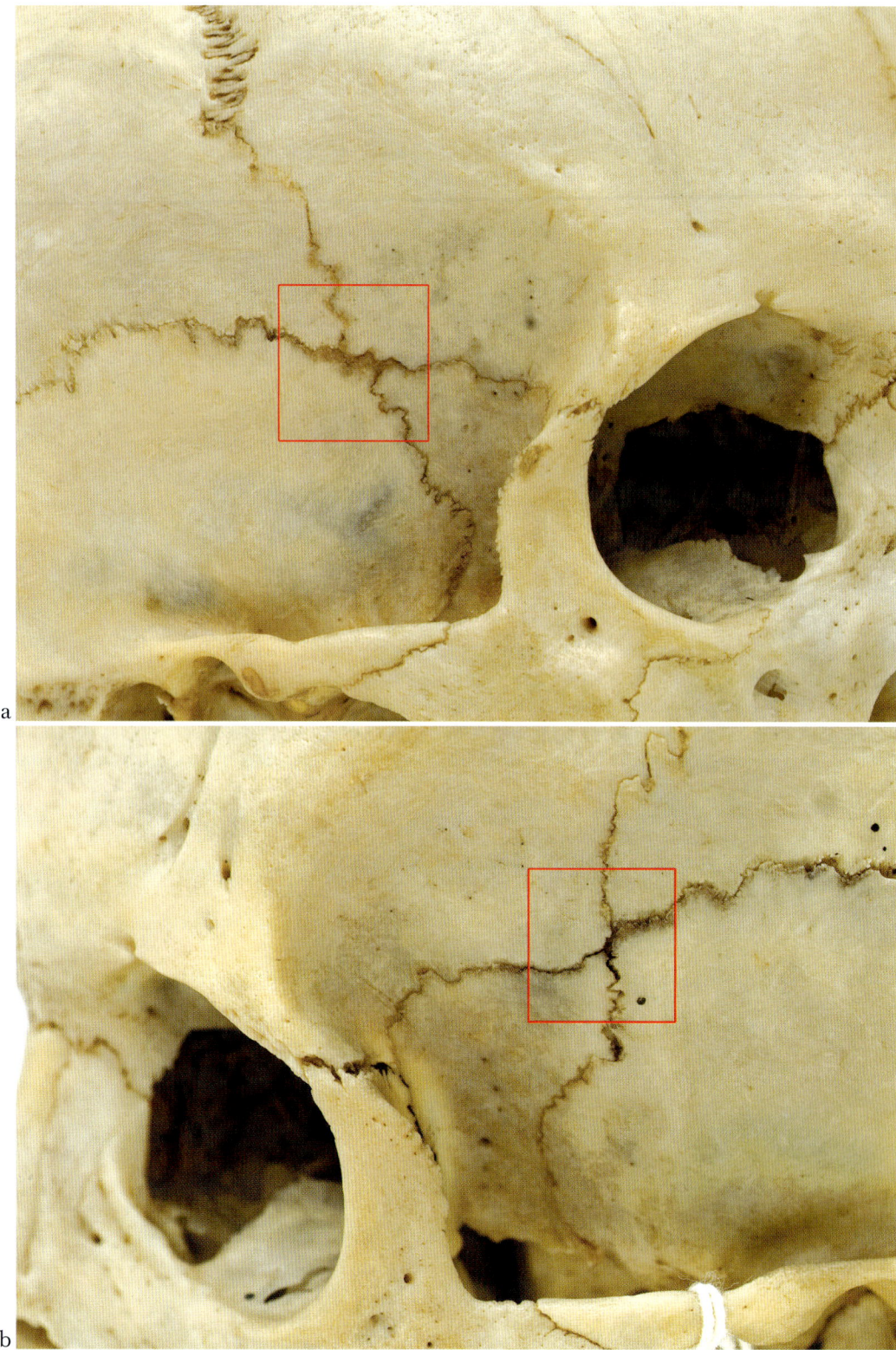

Figure 152a-b. Asymmetry in the shape of pterion in an adult male (Mütter Museum). (a) Right pterion appears as an "x" and (b) while the left assumes a "+" form. Typical variation.

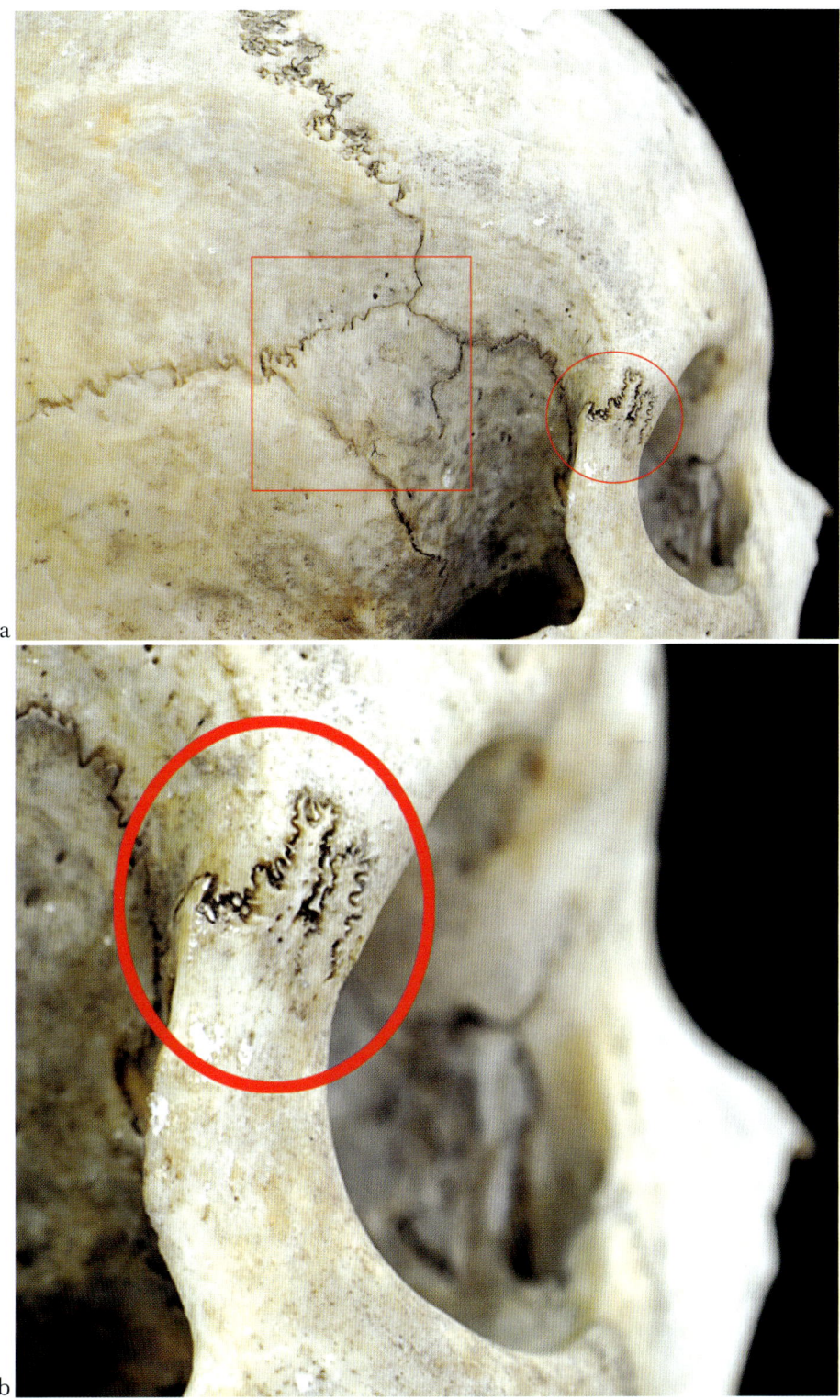

Figure 153a-b. Right epipteric (epiteric) bone and an unusually-shaped and double-looped frontomalar suture (KKU). (a) Large right epiteric/epipteric bone (square) and accessory or sutural extensions of the frontomalar suture (circle). (b) Higher magnification of the accessory sutural extensions in the right frontomalar suture. Both are common findings. Cf. Hauser and DeStefano (1989).

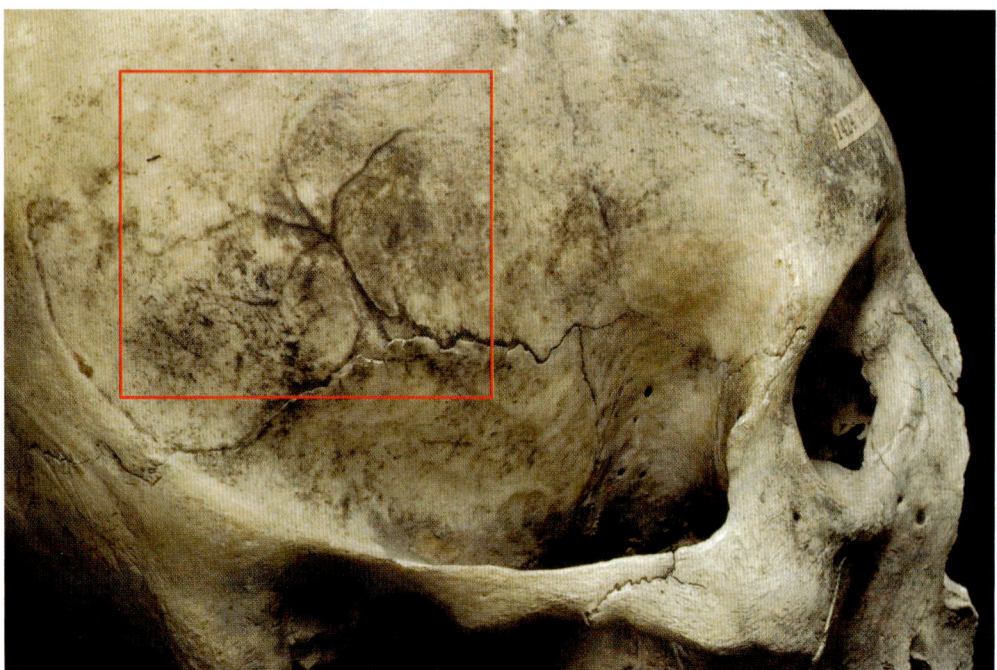

Figure 154. Unilateral small ossicle (red square) along the upper portion of the right sphenoidal bone (not at pterion) and grooves in the parietal bone for transmission of the superficial temporal artery in an Asian child (CSC AC 003). Uncommon finding. Cf. Hauser and DeStefano (1989).

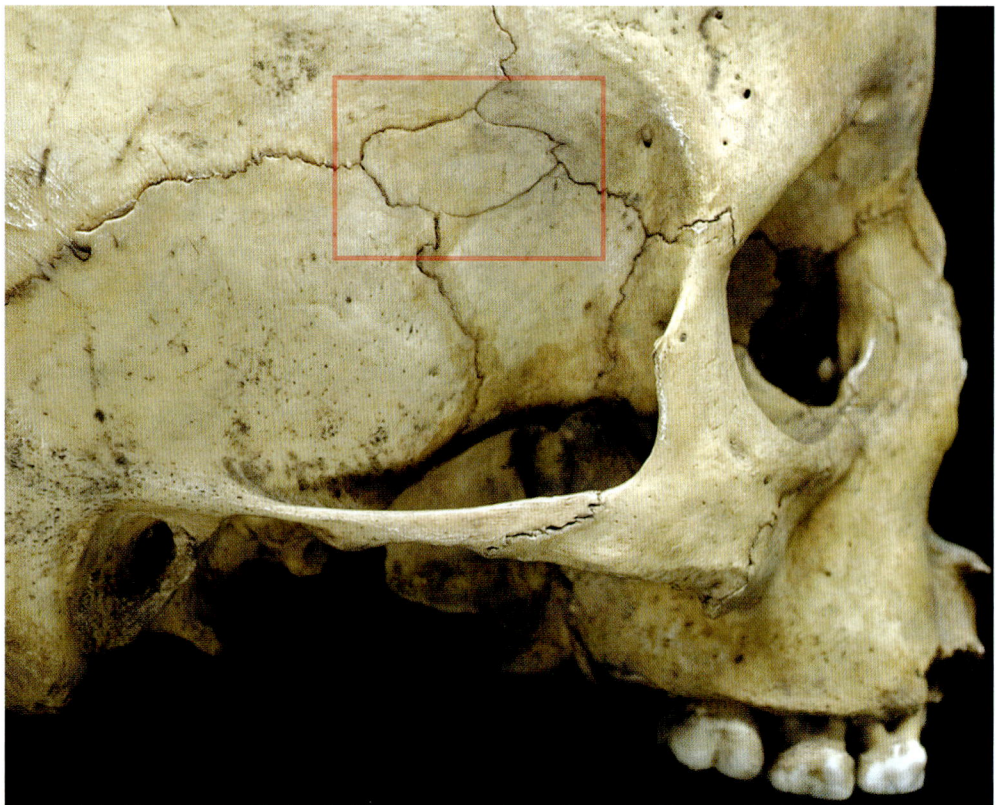

Figure 155. Large right epipteric (epiteric, Wormian os Ptericum) bone connecting the frontal, sphenoidal, temporal and parietal bones in a 6- to 8-year-old Peruvian child (UPenn 1933 L606). Common finding.

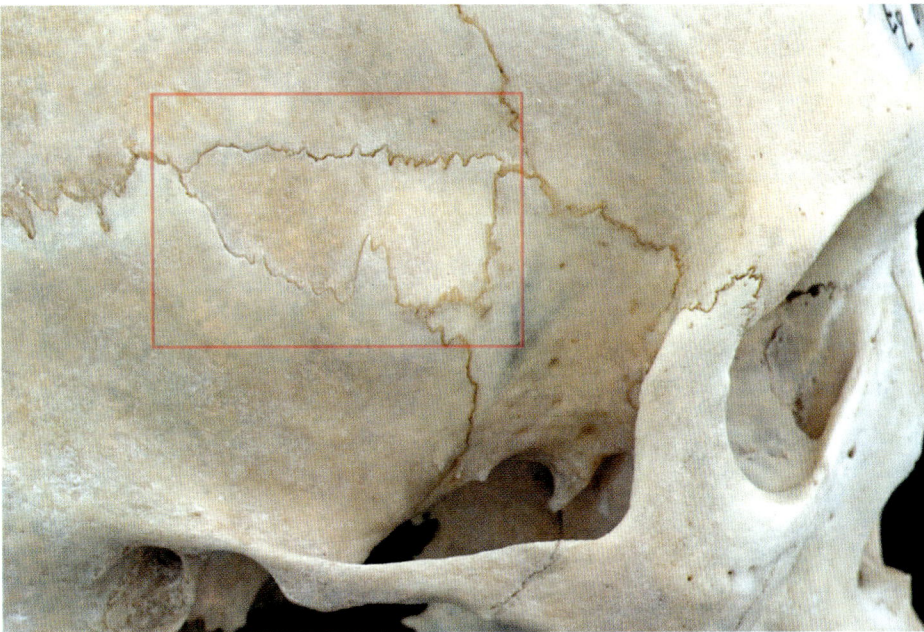

Figure 156. Unusually large, elongated right epipteric bone (rectangle) that joins with the sphenoid bone in an adult Thai male (KKU 3969-42). Uncommon finding.

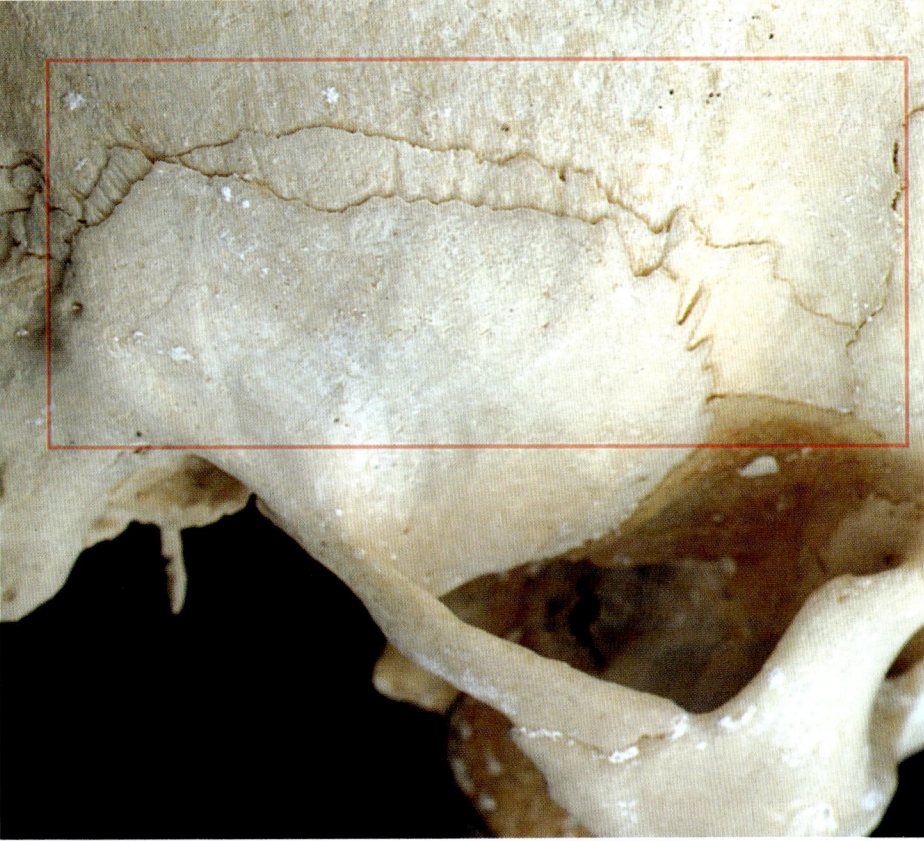

Figure 157. Uncommon to rare example of an epipteric/epiteric bone (rectangle) that spans the length of the right temporal squama in an adult Thai (KKU 1441-39).

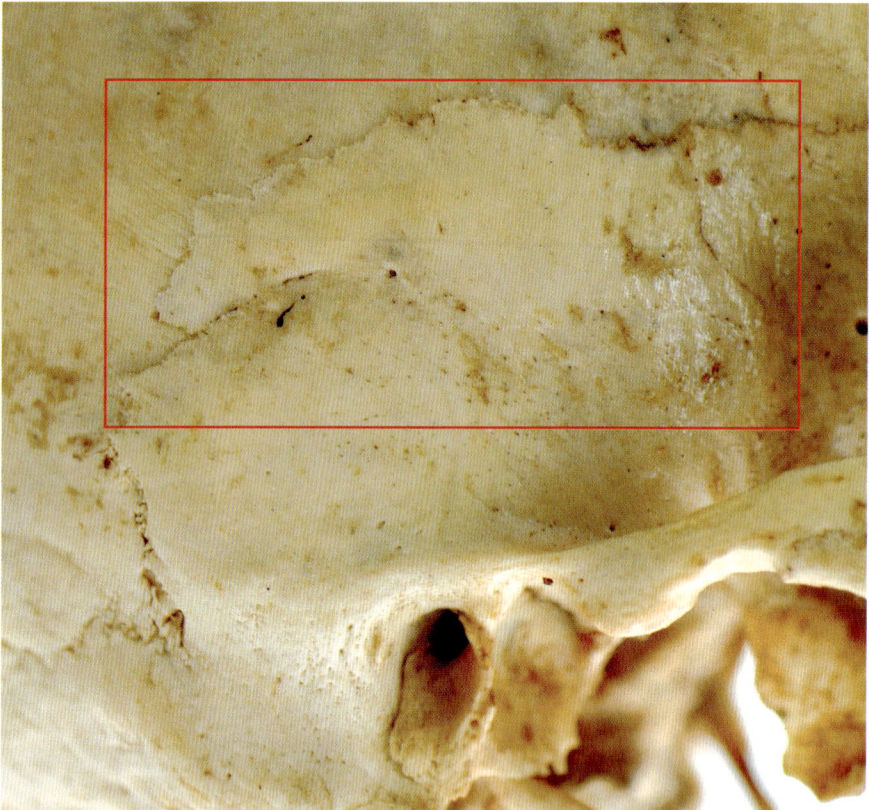

Figure 158. Possible bipartite right temoral bone (rectangle) or an unusually large squamosal ossicle or epipteric bone in an adult Thai male skull (KKU). Note the difficulty in differentiating a bipartite bone from an accessory ossicle, both representing a similar process (hyperostotic traits). Uncommon finding.

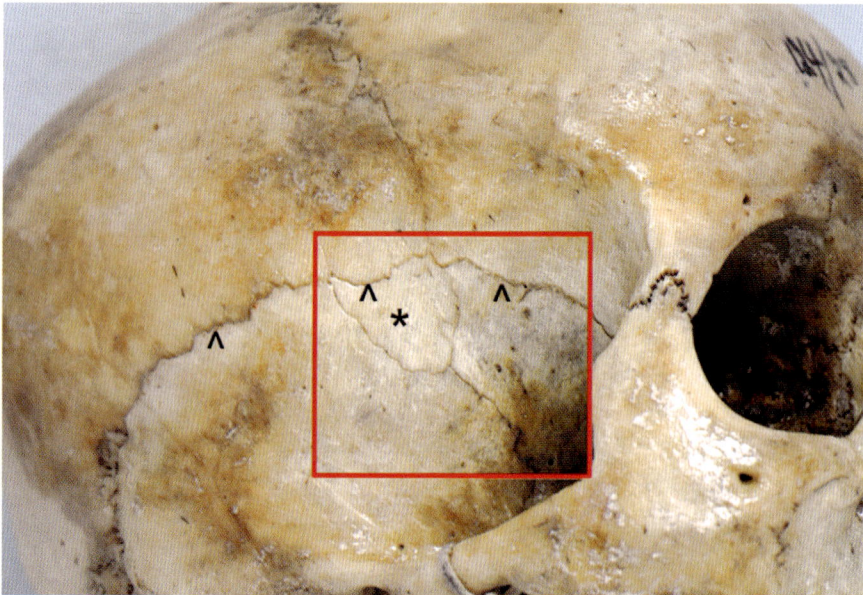

Figure 159. Epipteric bone in an adult Thai male skull (KKU). Note that the squamosal suture of the epipteric bone (middle ∧) is an extension of and at the same level as the superior margin of the temporal (left ∧) and sphenoidal bones (right ∧). Common finding. Cf. Sutton (1884); Hauser and DeStefano (1989).

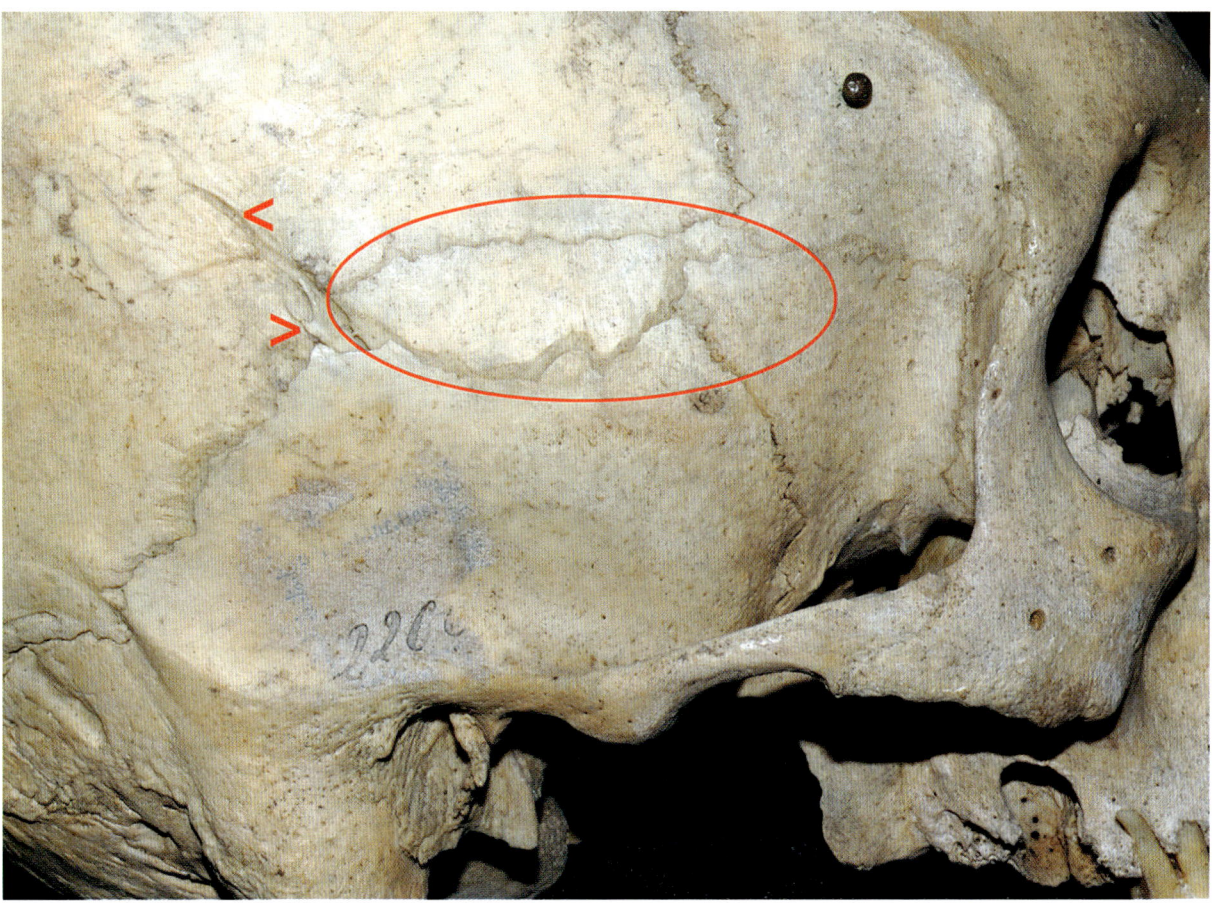

Figure 160. Parietal extension (<) with a small ossicle (>) and a large epipteric bone/squamosal ossicle (oval) in an adult Peruvian male (RV1365).

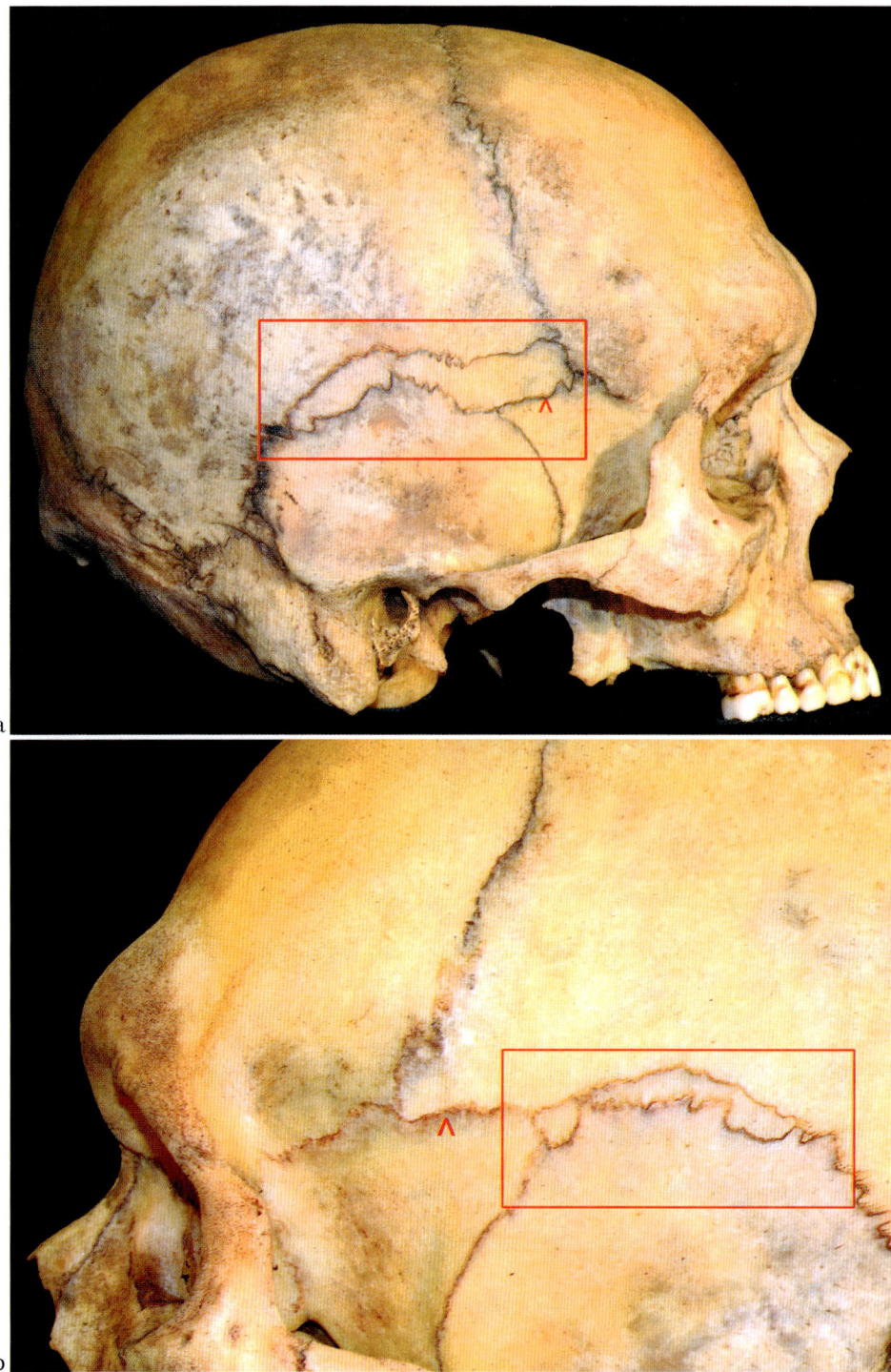

Figure 161a-b. Variants of squamosal ossicles and epipteric bone. (a) A large crescent-shaped epipteric (epiteric) bone (rectangle) along much of the right temporal bone and that terminates into the coronal suture (uncommon, but typical variant). The (∧) indicates the sphenoparietal suture that forms the inferior margin of the epipteric bone. (b) Commonly found squamosal ossicles (rectangle) and the sphenoparietal suture (∧) (typical anatomy) on the left side of the same 43-year-old White male (JABSOM 1451).

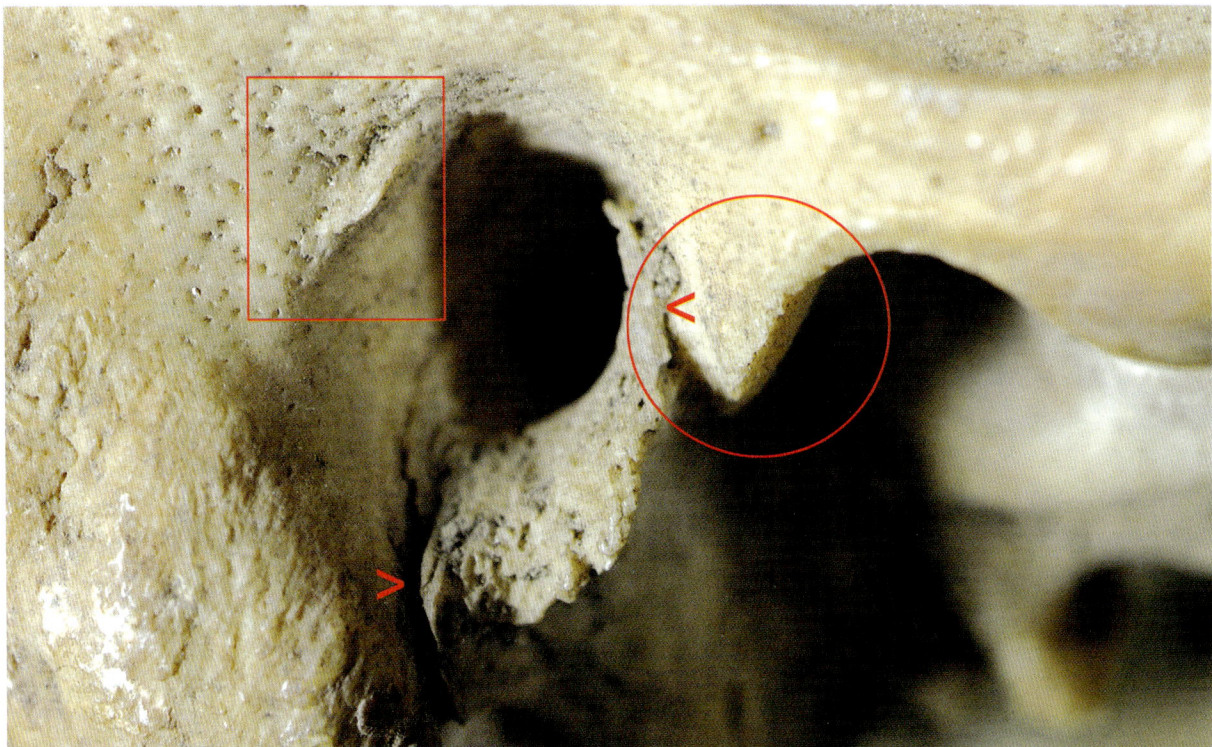

Figure 162. Small right suprameatal pit and prominent Spine of Henle (square) and a large, thick postglenoid tubercle/process (circle) in an adult Thai skull (KKU). Uncommon to common findings. Cf. Katsavrias and Dibbets (2002) for more on the postglenoid tubercle. Note the normally occurring tympanomastoid (>) and tympanosquamous (<) suture lines (partially dirt filled). These sutures may close with age or remodel and obliterate due to disease.

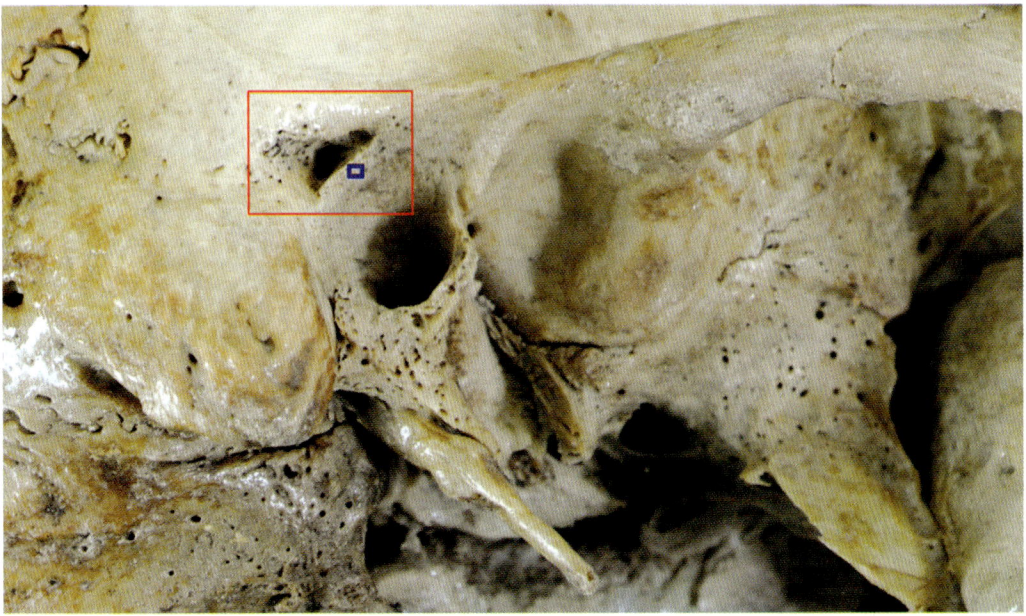

Figure 163. Deep suprameatal pit (rectangle) in the right temporal bone of an adult Thai skull (KKU). The small diagonal ridge of bone (blue) forming the inferior border of the pit is the Spine of Henle or suprameatal spine (of Henle), a surgical landmark representing the anterosuperior portion of the auditory meatus. Common to uncommon and typical variant. Hauser and DeStefano (1989).

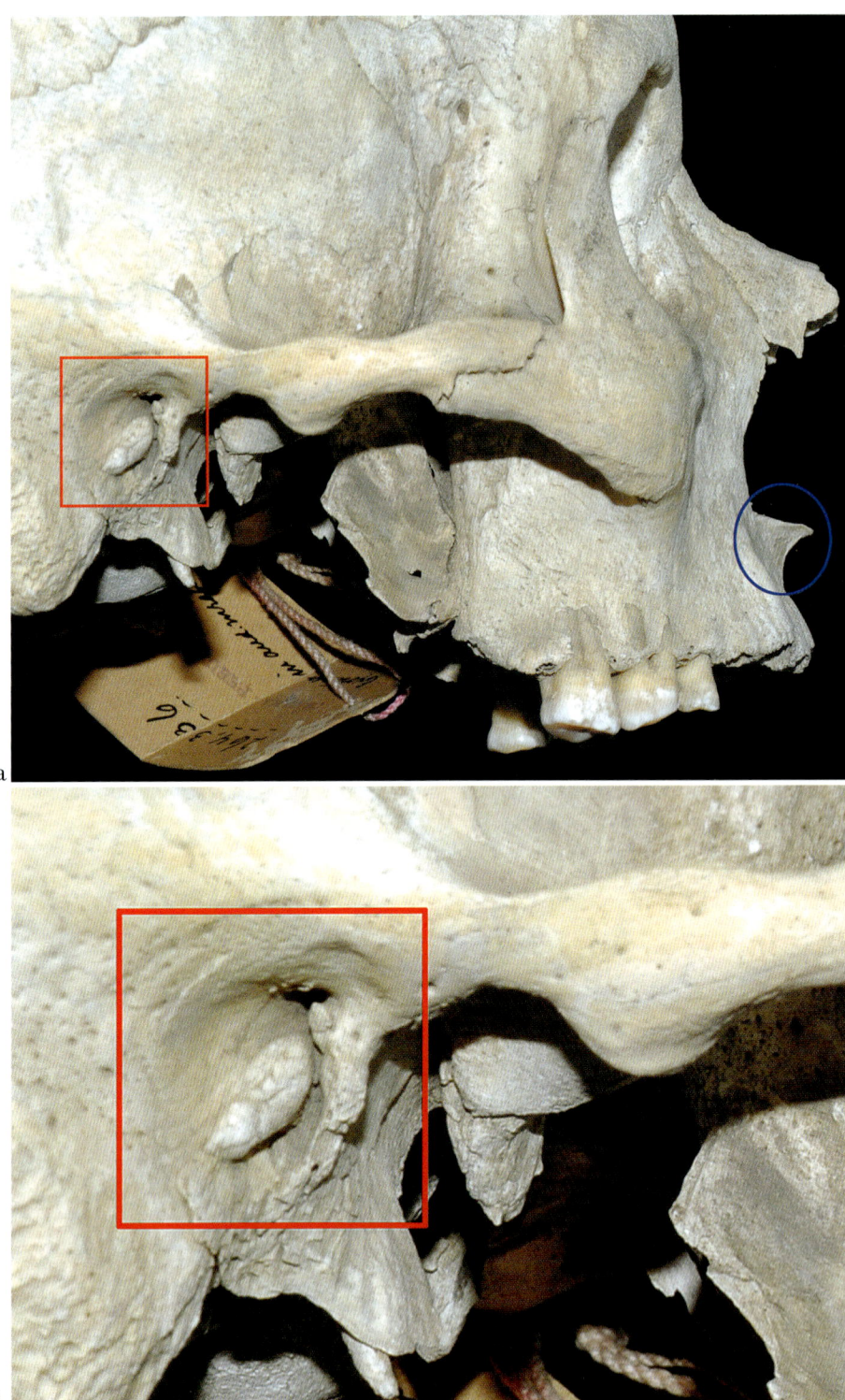

Figure 164a-b. Auditory exostoses, long nasal spine and nasal bone overhang in an adult Peruvian male skull (SI P264336). (a) Multiple exostoses in the right external auditory canal (square). (b) Higher magnification of the right auditory exostoses (square). Some researchers refer to an exostosis, also called an osteoma, hamartoma and "surfer's ear," as a pathological lesion/growth often associated with cold water, while others classify it as a non-metric trait. Uncommon to common findings depending on group. Cf. Kennedy (1986); Hauser and DeStefano (1989); Okumura et al. (2007); Sheehy (1982); Turner (1879).

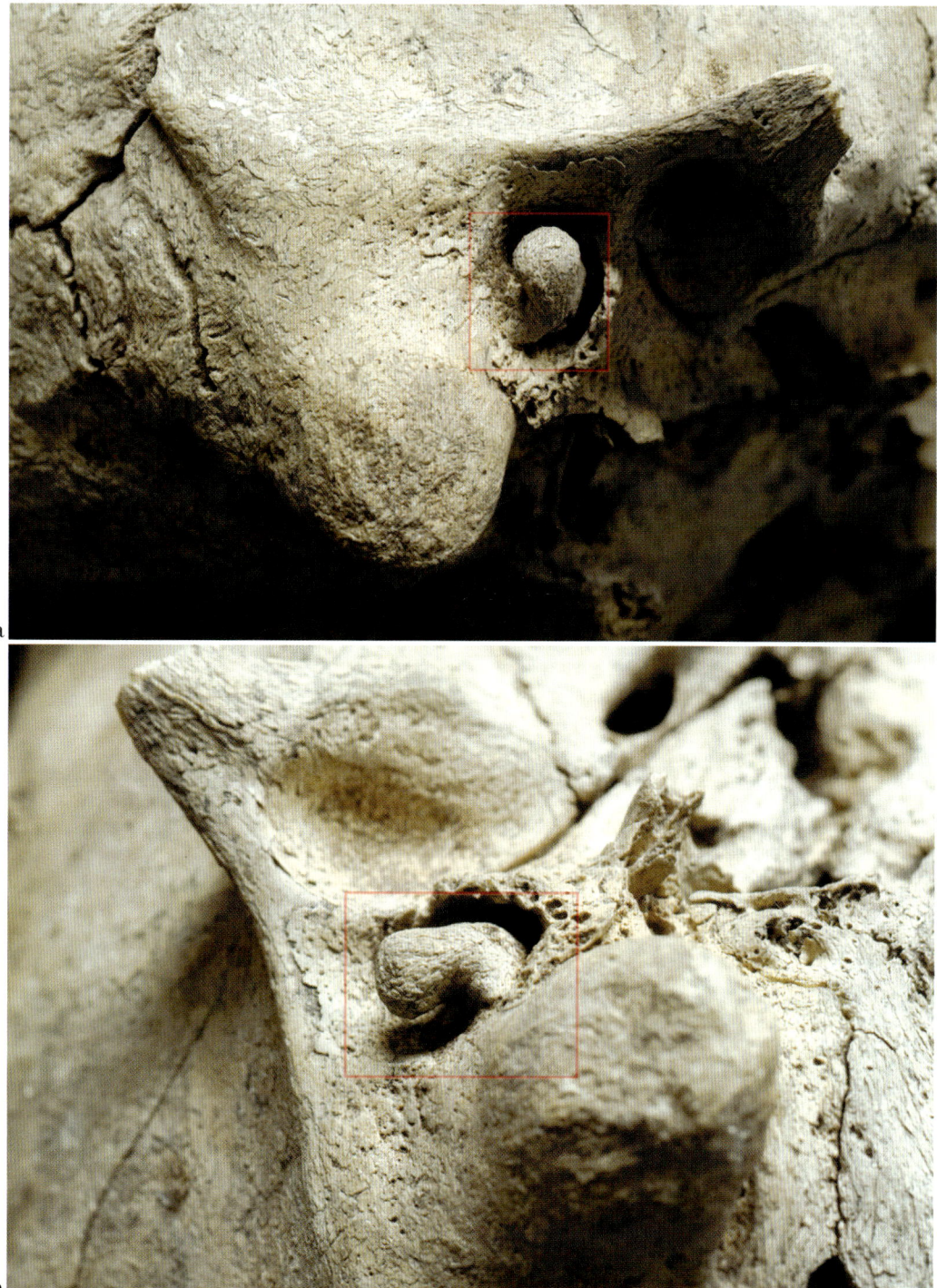

Figure 165a-b. Large, curved auditory exostosis extending from the posterior wall of the right auditory meatus in an adult Peruvian (UPenn). (a) Lateral view of a large, hook-shaped exostosis (rectangle) in the right auditory canal. (b) Higher magnification of the auditory exostosis (rectangle). Cf. Kennedy (1986); Hauser and DeStefano (1989); Okumura et al. (2007); Sheehy (1982); Turner (1879).

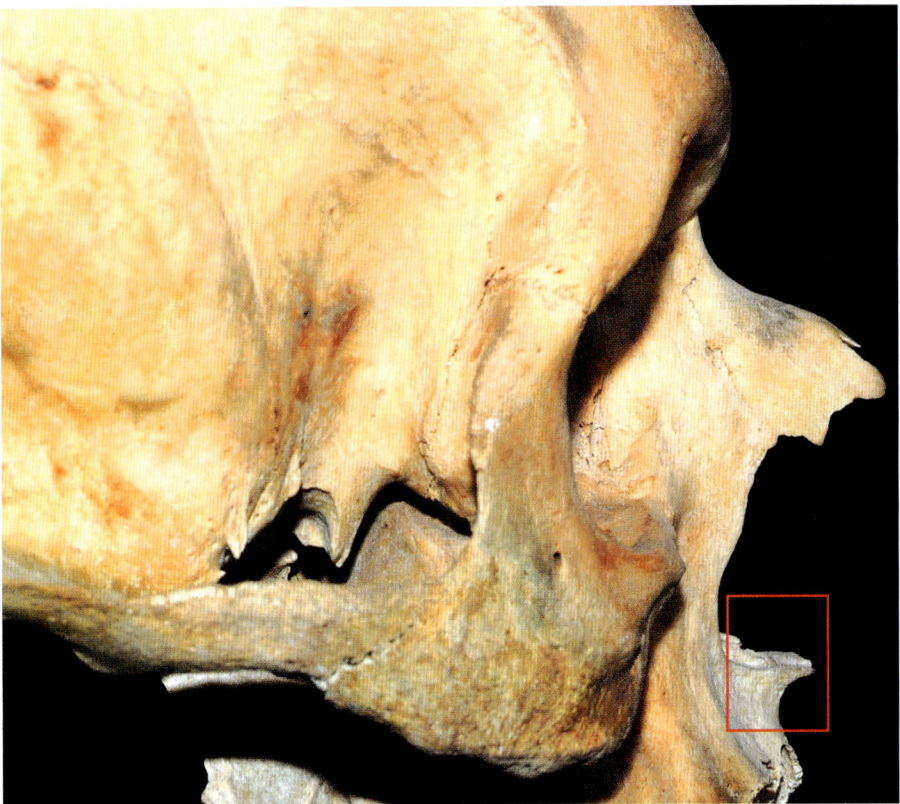

Figure 166. Prominent anterior nasal spine (square) and overhanging/projecting nasal bones in an adult Peruvian male (SI). Both are typical morphoscopic traits that are scored as non-metric traits. See Hefner (2015).

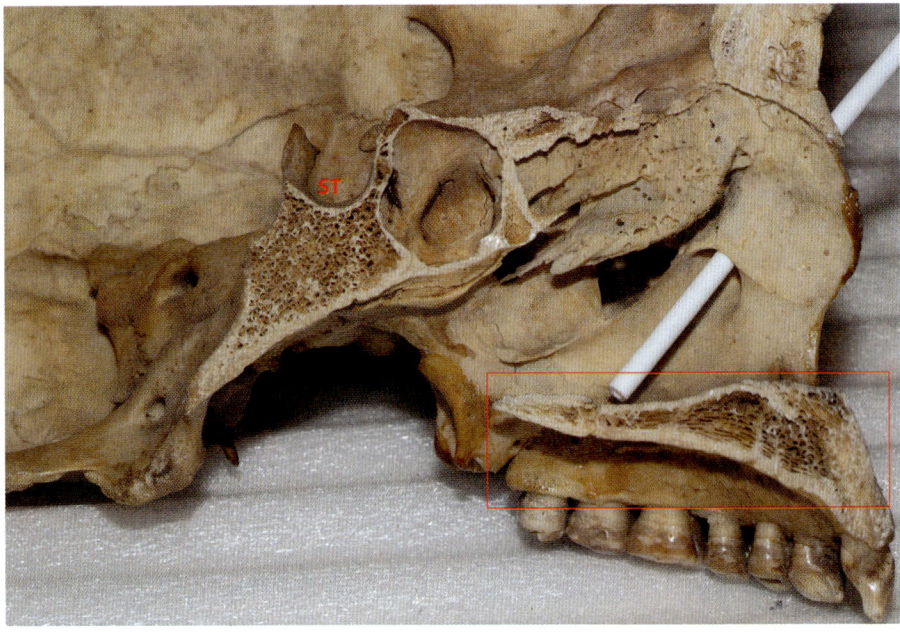

Figure 167. Typical internal morphology of the basilar bone (inferior to ST (sella turcica or "Turk's saddle" housing the hypophysis/pituitary gland)), the hard palate (rectangle) and angle and pathway of the nasolacrimal canal (probe) in an adult African (TM 38, Ditsong Museum).

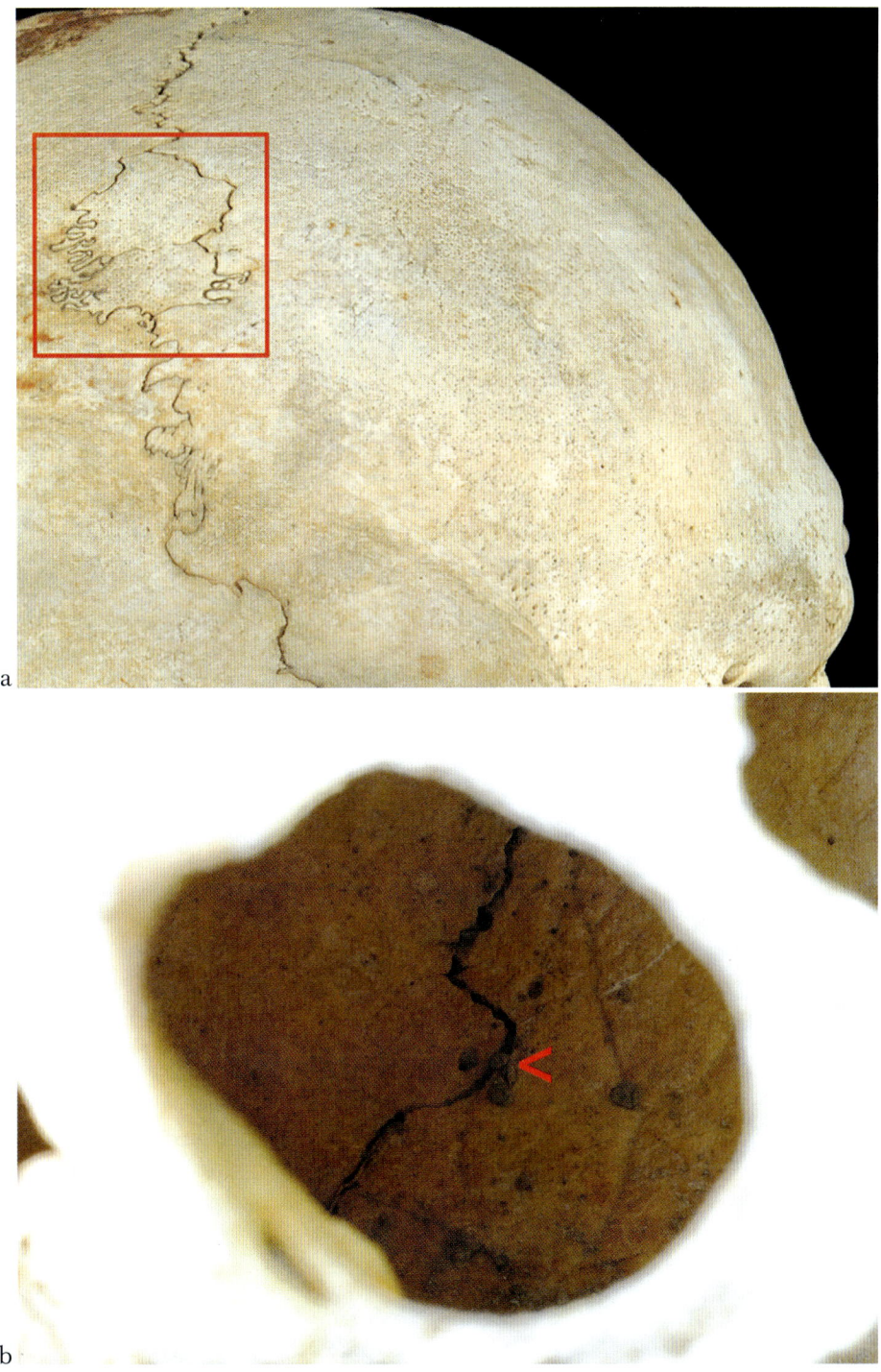

Figure 168a-b. Comparison of coronal suture morphology endocranially and ectocranially. (a) One small and two large coronal ossicles in an adult Thai skull (KKU). Note the complexity of the sutures ectocranially and the swirling "coastal" morphology of the coronal suture as it extends laterally. (b) Endocranial view showing that most of the sutures of the coronal ossicles have obliterated leaving only a portion in the parietal bone visible (<). Coronal ossicle uncommon to common finding. Cf. Hauser and DeStefano (1989); Saunders and Rainey (2008).

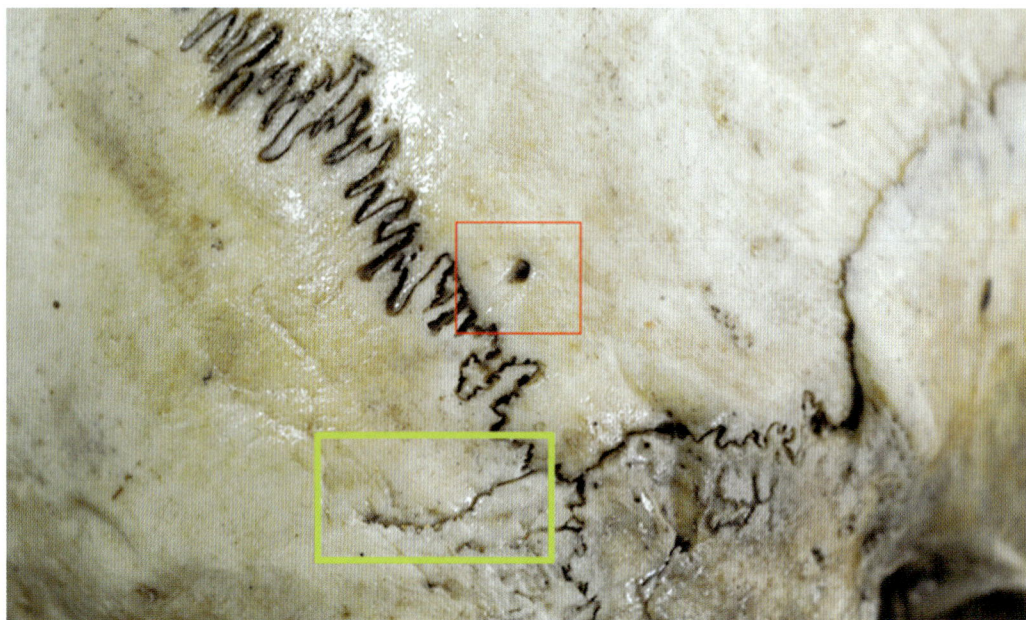

Figure 169. Foramen (red) superior to Asterion and trace right Mendosal suture (yellow) in an adult Thai skull (KKU). The Mendosal suture, also known as the biasterionic suture, may originate at, below, or above Asterion and may persist throughout a lifetime. Common findings. Cf. Gayretli et al. (2011); Hauser and DeStefano (1989); Tubbs et al. (2007).

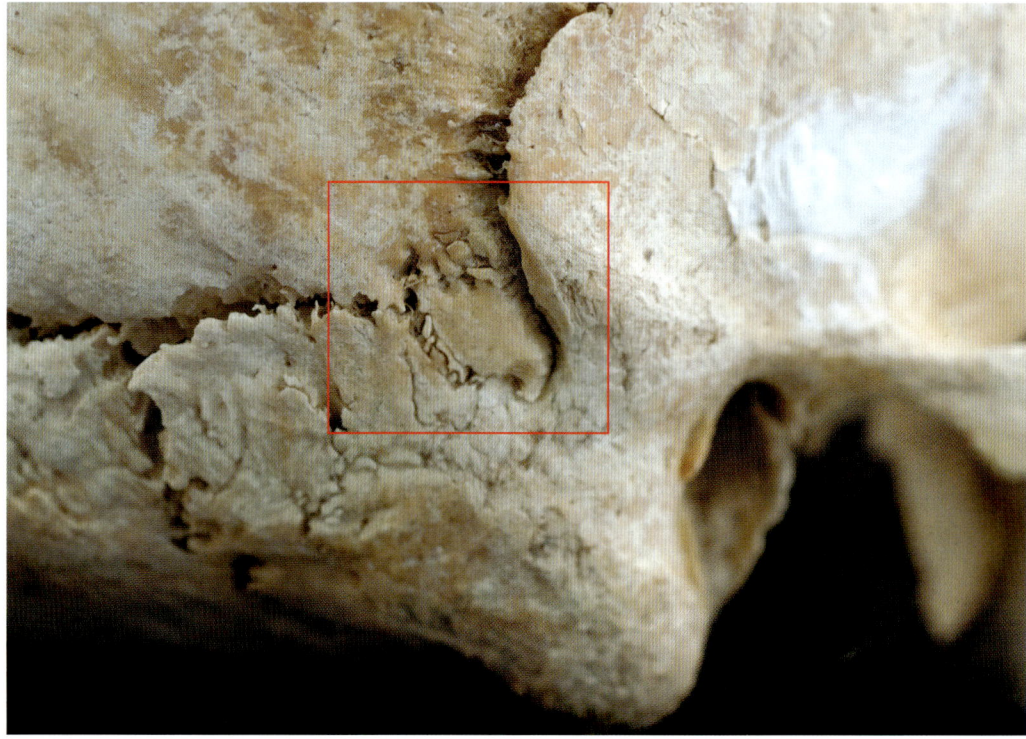

Figure 170. Small right mastoid notch bone (square) (CSC DS 008). Cf. Hauser and DeStefano (1989); Saunders and Rainey (2008).

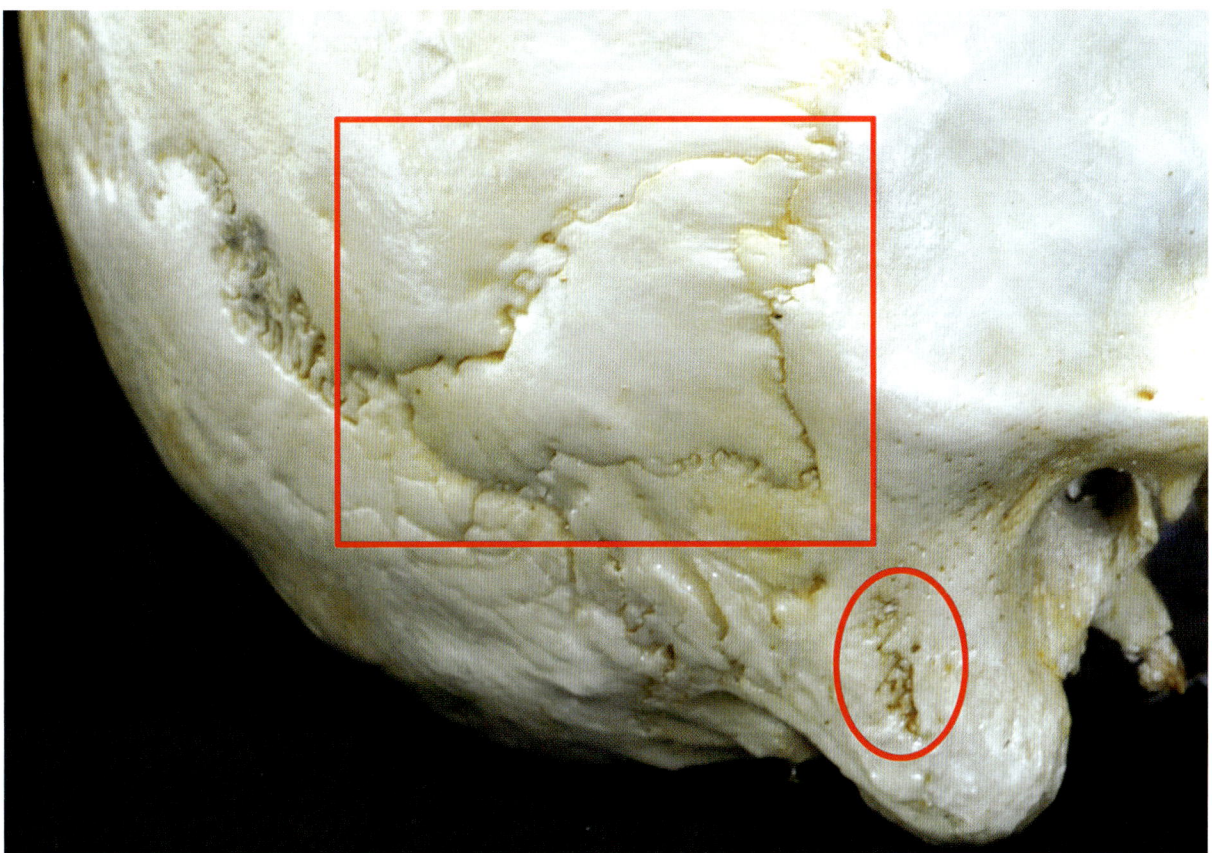

Figure 171. Large bone/ossicle (rectangle) spanning Asterion and the mastoid notch, and trace/remnant of the petro-squamous suture (oval; sometimes called the squamomastoid suture or sutura mastoideosquamosa) in an adult Thai skull (KKU). Uncommon to common findings. For Asterionic bone see Hanihara and Ishida (2001a); Hauser and DeStefano (1989); Konigsberg et al. (1993); Sternberg (1975); Wilson (2010).

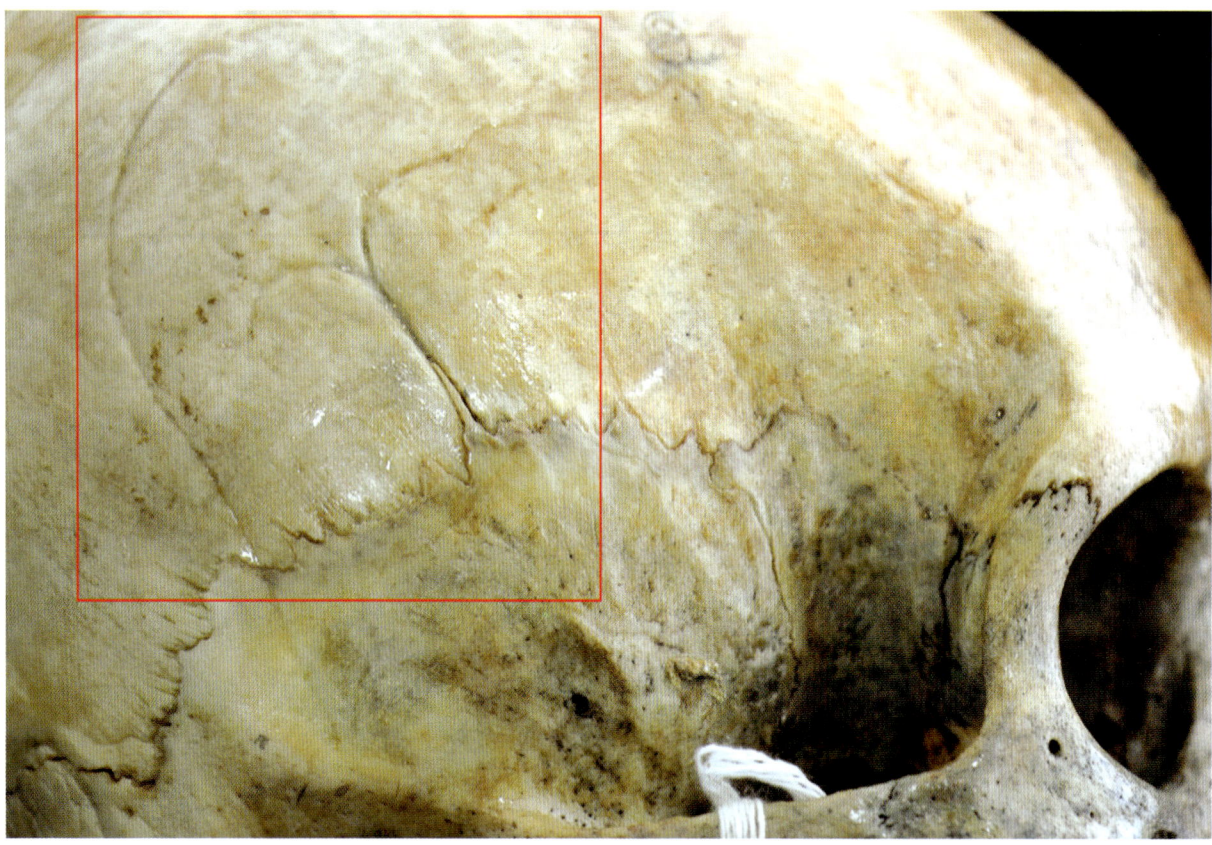

Figure 172. Unusually shaped parietal process of the temporal squama leading into a "fountain-like" groove. This bony extension in this adult Thai skull originates along/under the margin of the temporal squama and runs across the surface of the parietal bone where it bifurcates (KKU). These shallow grooves may serve as paths for branches of the superficial temporal artery. This is an unusual feature in the human skeleton, similar to frontal grooves, where a portion of one groove coursing across the parietal bone is filled with a bony projection while the remainder may hold a vein or artery. Perhaps some of these extensions and grooves are exaggerated variants of parietal striae of the squamosal suture. Uncommon to common finding. Cf. Hauser and DeStefano (1989). This serrate suture has a thin layer of fibrous tissue separating the squama and parietal bone (Lockhart et al. 1965).

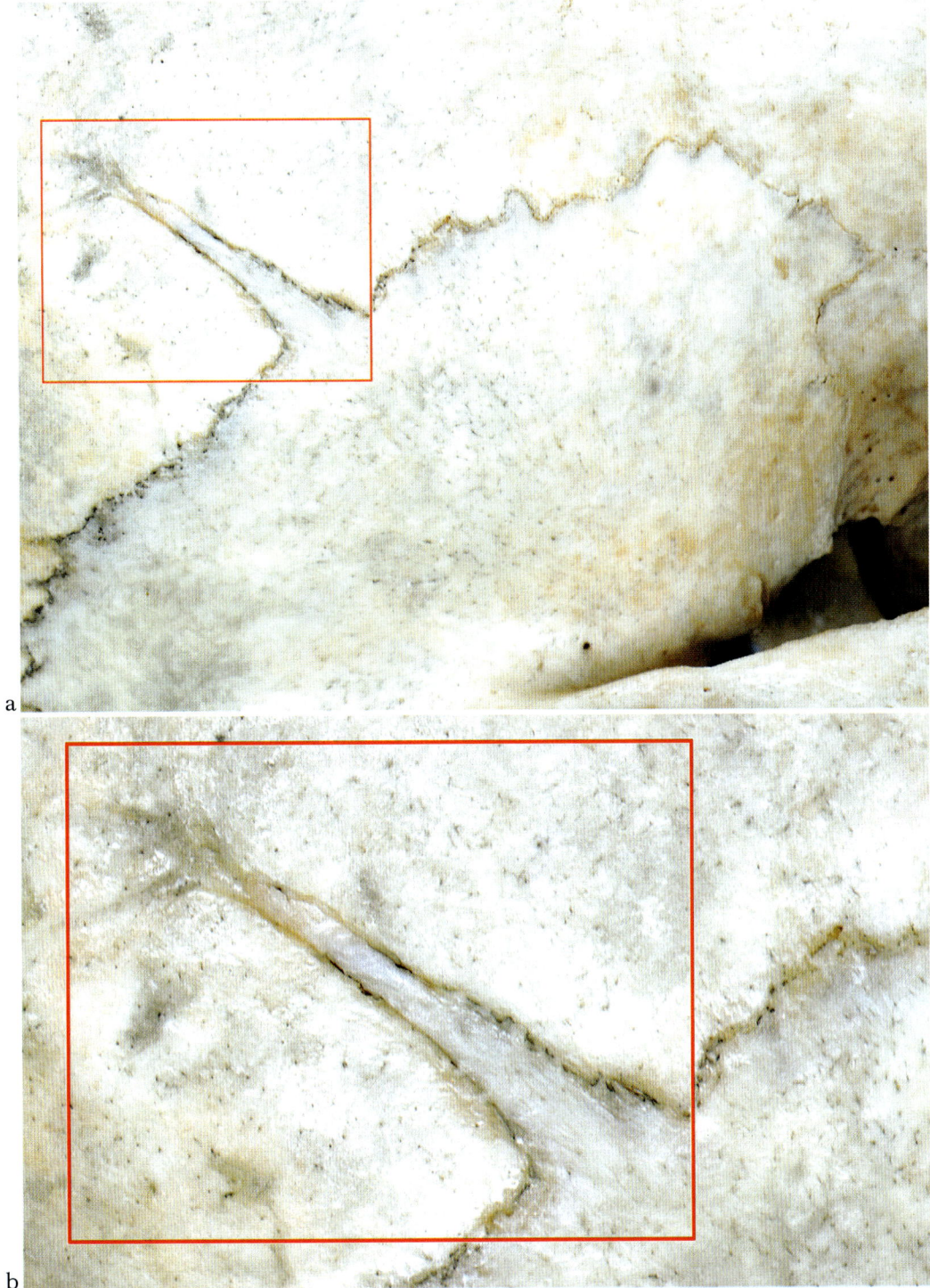

Figure 173a-b. Variant of the parietal process of the temporal squama. (a) Low and (b) high magnification of the "tree-like" appearance of the parietal process of the right temporal squama in an adult Asian skull (KKU). The bony extension originating along the margin of the temporal squama fills a correspondingly-shaped groove in the parietal bone. In this individual, the process and groove does not appear to serve for passage of a vein or artery across the parietal bone (that may be suggested if, as in this case, the bony extension separates, leaving only a groove in the parietal bone). A similar groove in the parietal bone, with or without a bony extension, may be found originating from beneath the temporal squama and carrying a vessel. Uncommon to common finding.

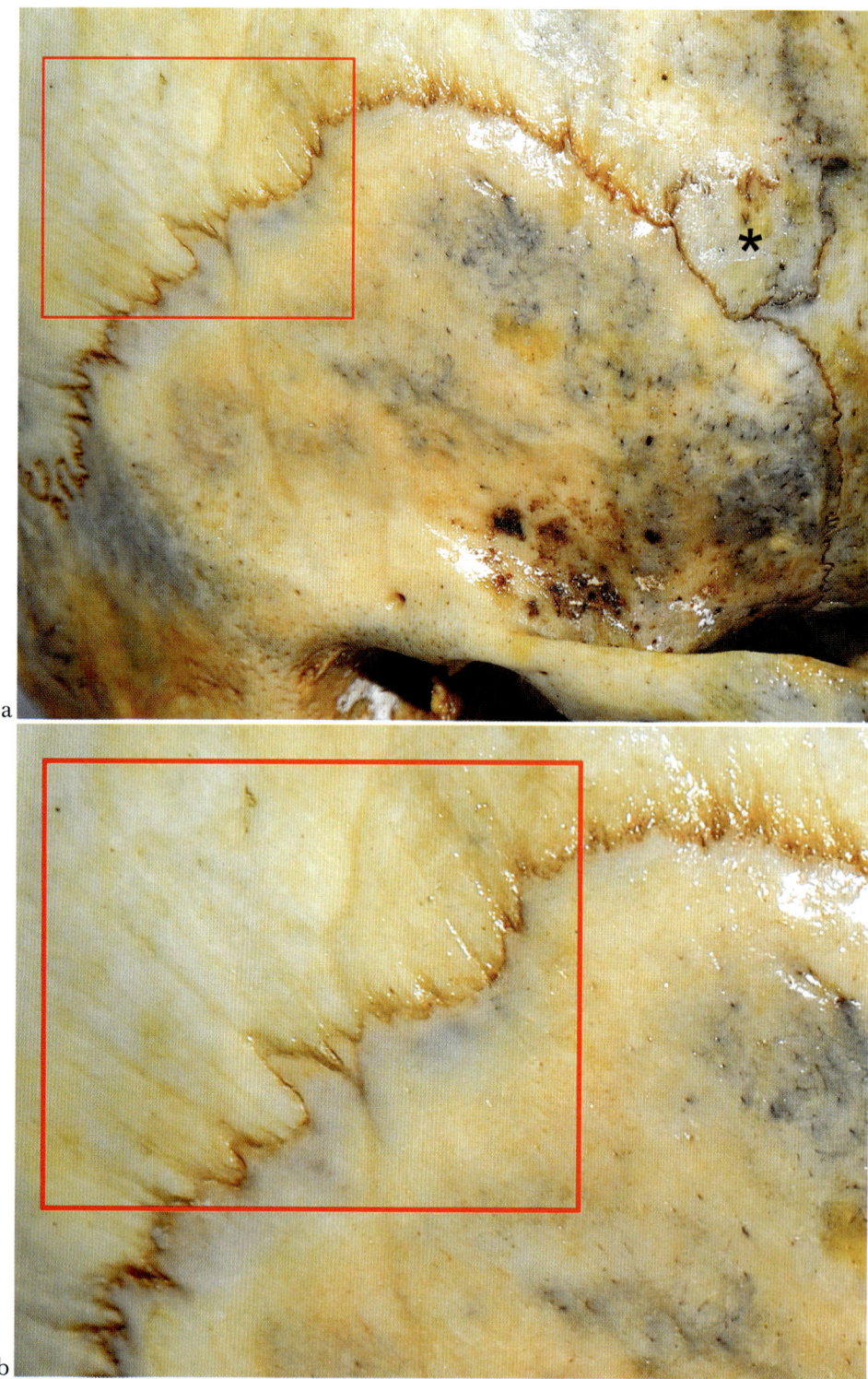

Figure 174a-b. Parietal striae ("rays") and epipteric bone in the right side of the skull. (a) Shallow grooves (rectangle) associated with finger-like interdigitations and extensions of the squamosal suture of the temporal bone and an epipteric bone (*). (b) Note that each groove (rectangle) is met with a bony extension from the temporal bone along the squamosal suture. It is likely that these grooves indicate the directionality of simultaneous growth of the temporal and parietal bones in subadults. Cf. White and Folkens (2005). Common findings.

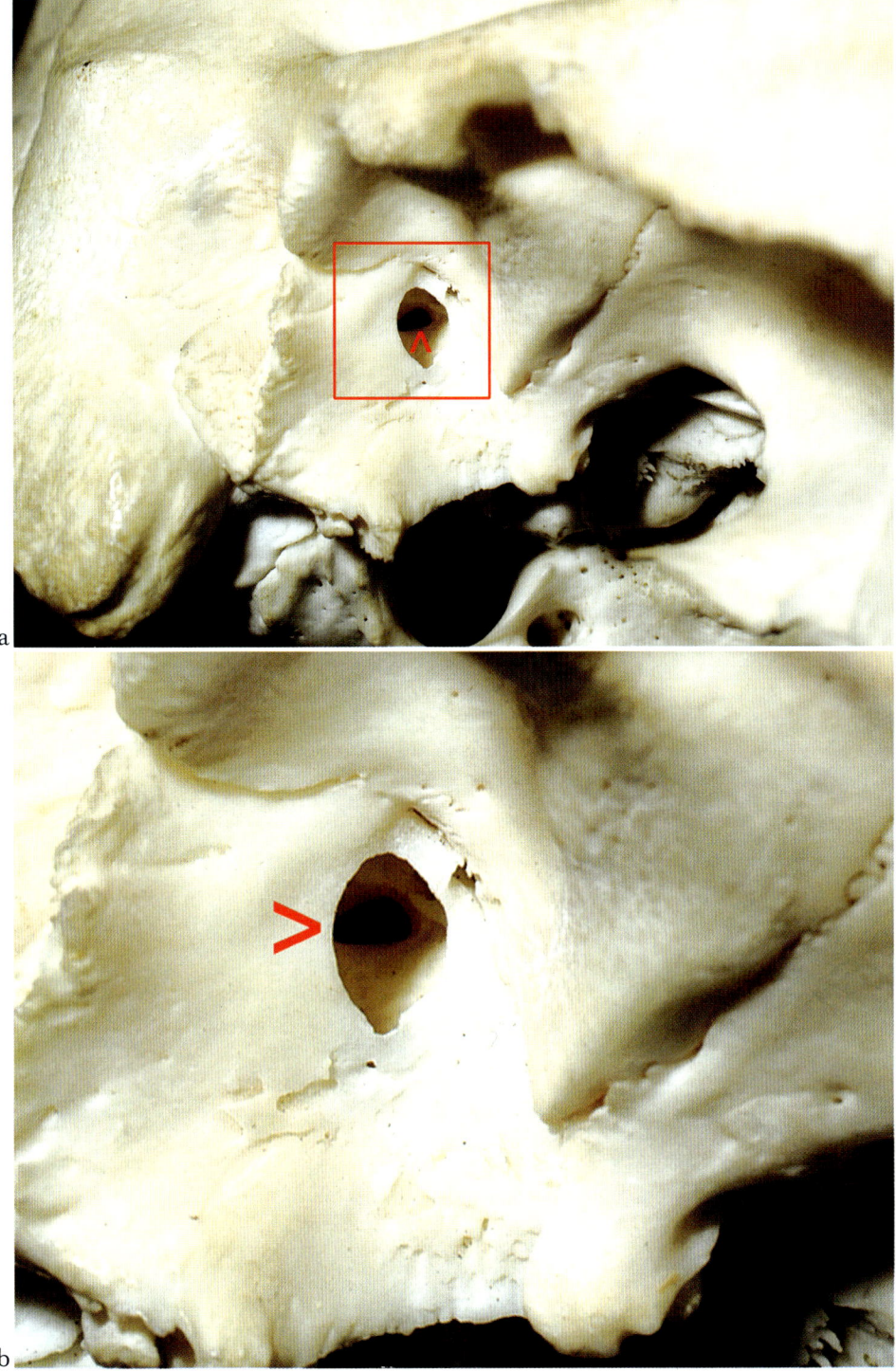

Figure 175a-b. Tympanic dehiscence revealing the right oval window in an adult (JABSOM). (a) Tympanic dehiscence (square), also known as the foramen of Huschke and foramen tympanicum, revealing the oval window (∧) that houses the base or foot of the stapes. The oval window, or fenestra of vestibule, opens into the middle ear. (b) Higher magnification of the oval window (>) as seen through the tympanic dehiscence. The oval window is a typical anatomical feature, as is the tympanic dehiscence in subadults. Persistence of this dehiscence into adulthood is an uncommon to common developmental defect. The oval window in this individual, because of the dehiscence, is visible by looking into both the tympanic dehiscence and the external auditory meatus.

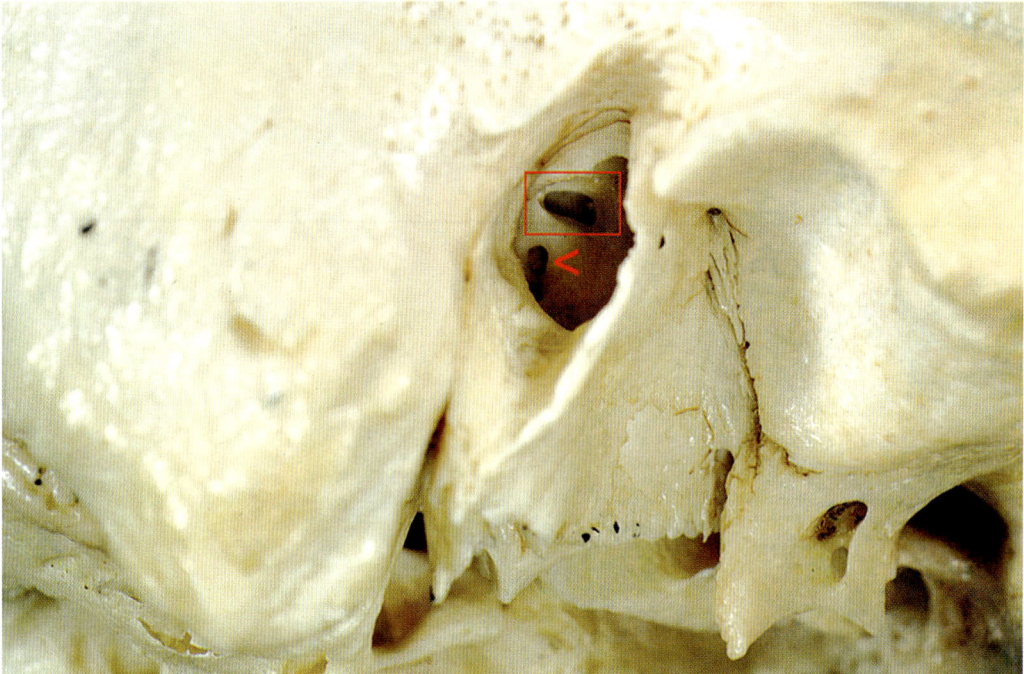

Figure 176. Oval window (fenestra vestibule; rectangle) that houses the base of the stapes in the right temporal bone of an adult Thai male skull. Note the round window/fenestra cochleae (<), which is covered by a membrane in the living below and to the left of the oval window (KKU) (rarely, the round window may be absent). Normal anatomical feature often used as an ancestry trait (Birkby et al. 2008; Gill and Rhine 1990; Napoli and Birkby 1990).

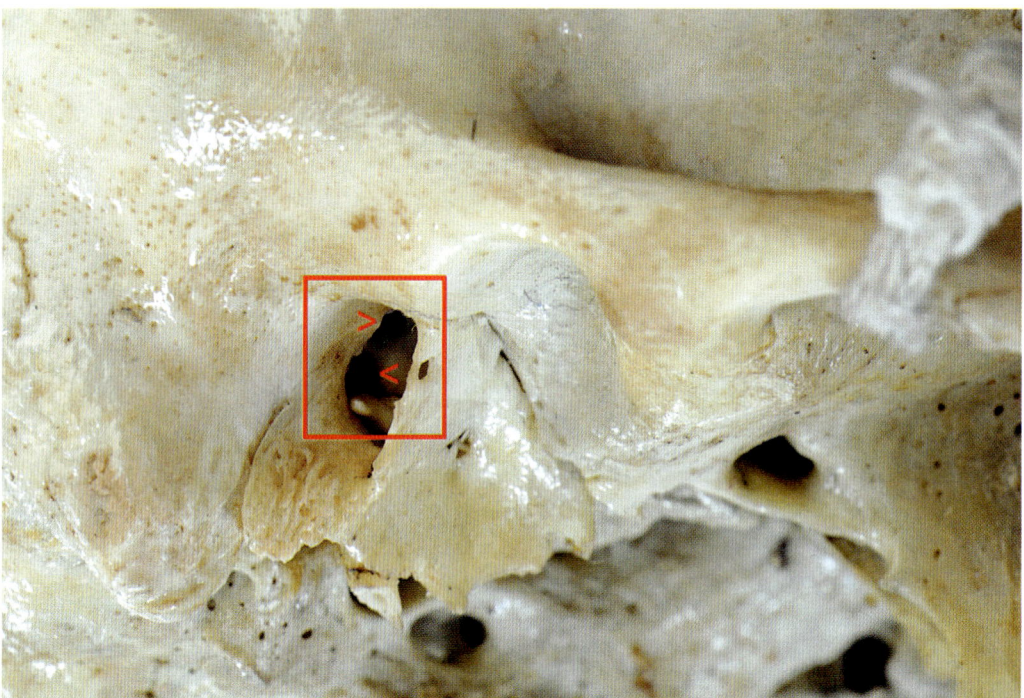

Figure 177. Oval window (square and >) and round window (square and <) in the right temporal bone of an adult Thai (KKU). Note that both windows are visible in this individual from a slightly antero-posterior view.

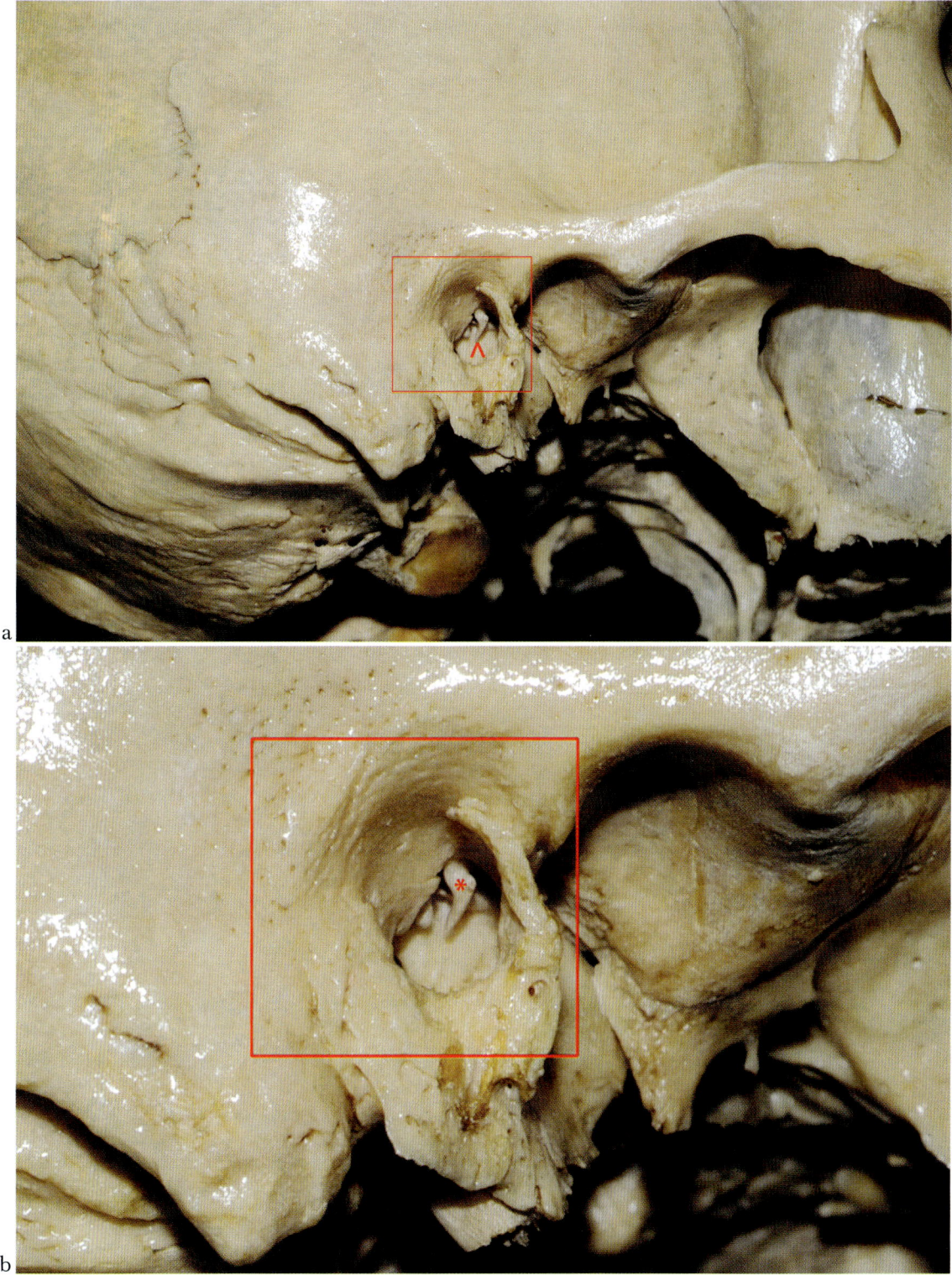

Figure 178a-b. Right auditory/ear ossicle in anatomical position. (a) The malleus (^) attaches to the incus and the incus to the stapes, the foot plate of which fills the oval window in the external auditory meatus (square) (JABSOM M04). (b) Higher magnification of the right malleus (square and *).

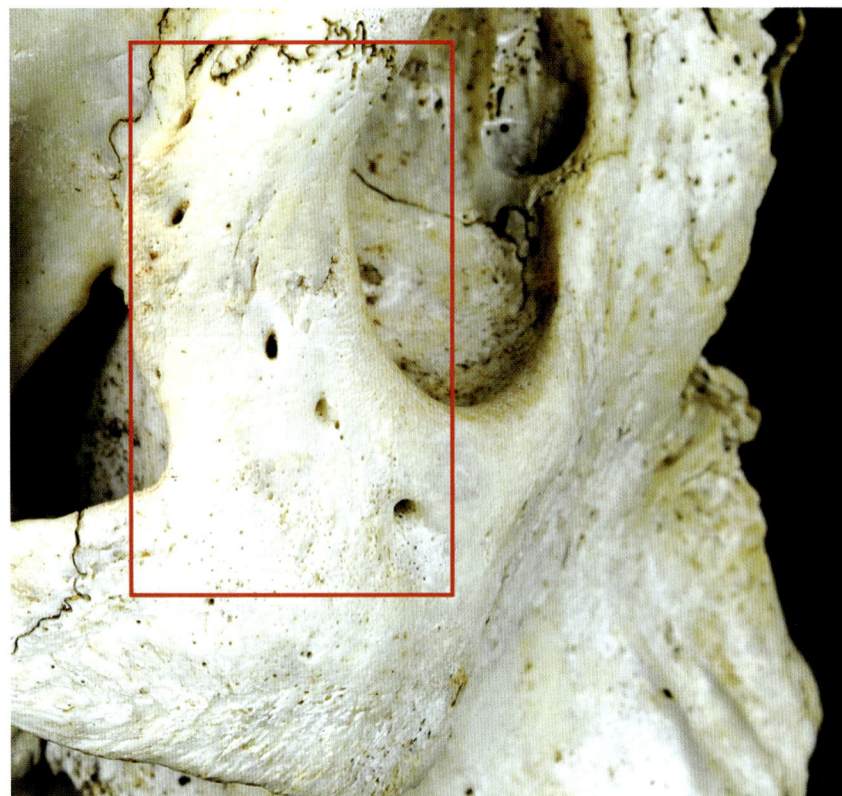

Figure 179. Five zygomaticofacial foramina (rectangle) in the right zygoma of an Asian adult skull (KKU). Mangal et al. (2004), found no foramen in 15.6%, one foramen in 44.4% (most common finding) and five foramina in 1.3% of 80 dry bone skulls. Five or more moderate to large foramina are a rare finding. See Hauser and DeStefano (1989).

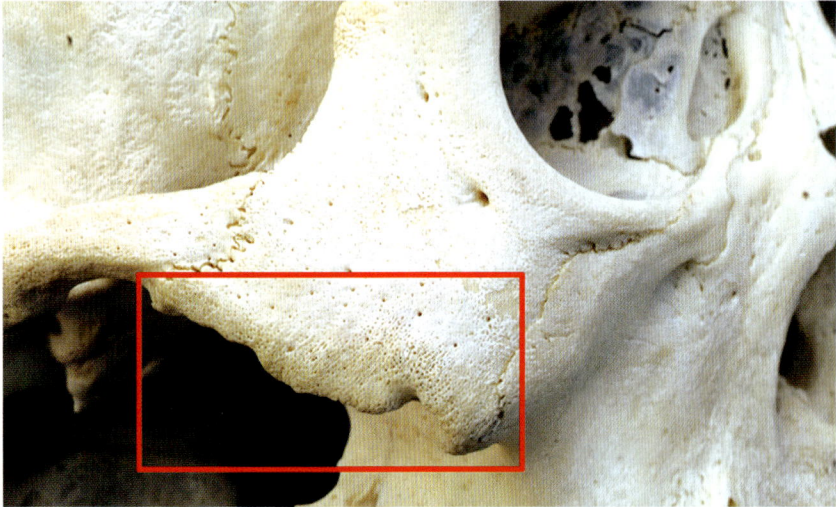

Figure 180. Undulating inferior border (rectangle) of the right zygomatic (malar) bone in an adult Asian skull (KKU). Development in this area is, to some extent, due to activity of the masseter muscle, but research is needed to determine whether there is a genetic component. Common finding.

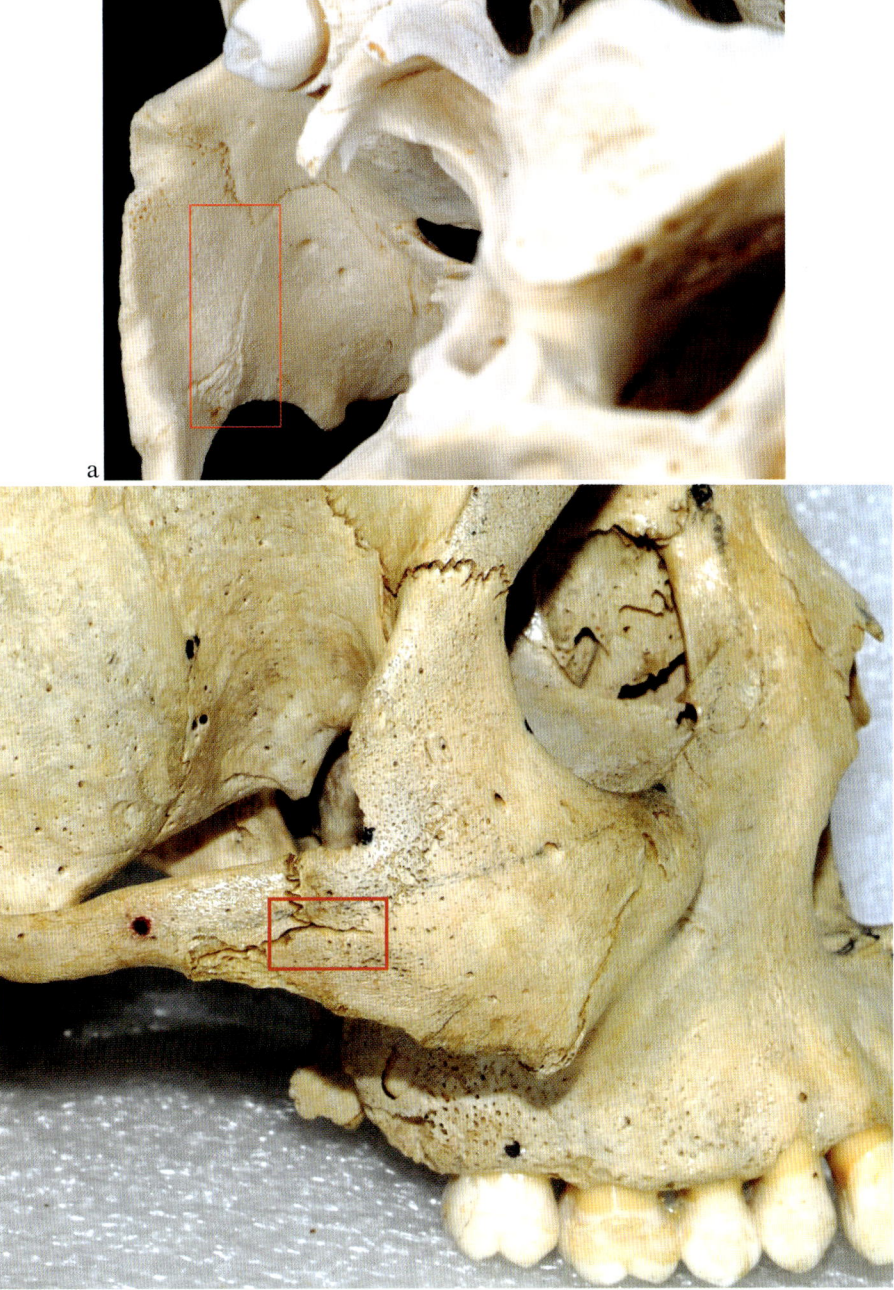

Figure 181a-b. Trace os Japonicum in a subadult. (a) Internal/temporal surface of a right zygomatic bone, from below, showing faintly visible trace of the os Japonicum/os zygomaticum bipartitum (rectangle). (b) Right lateral view demonstrating a trace of the os Japonicum (rectangle). Perhaps not surprisingly, the temporal trace is often visible in skulls that exhibit no evidence of ever having an os Japonicum on the lateral surface and it is not often mentioned in anatomy texts. That the lateral aspect of this suture may completely obliterate while the temporal surface does not, may be the result of muscular stresses associated with mastication and other activities. Many individuals exhibit what appears to be a trace os Japonicum (b; rectangle), although a similar "trace" may actually be a remnant of a "finger-like" extension of the zygomaticofacial suture. Common to uncommon findings. Cf. Hanihara and Ishida (2001b); Hauser and DeStefano (1989). MacCurdy (1914) refers to this as the os zygomaticum duplex.

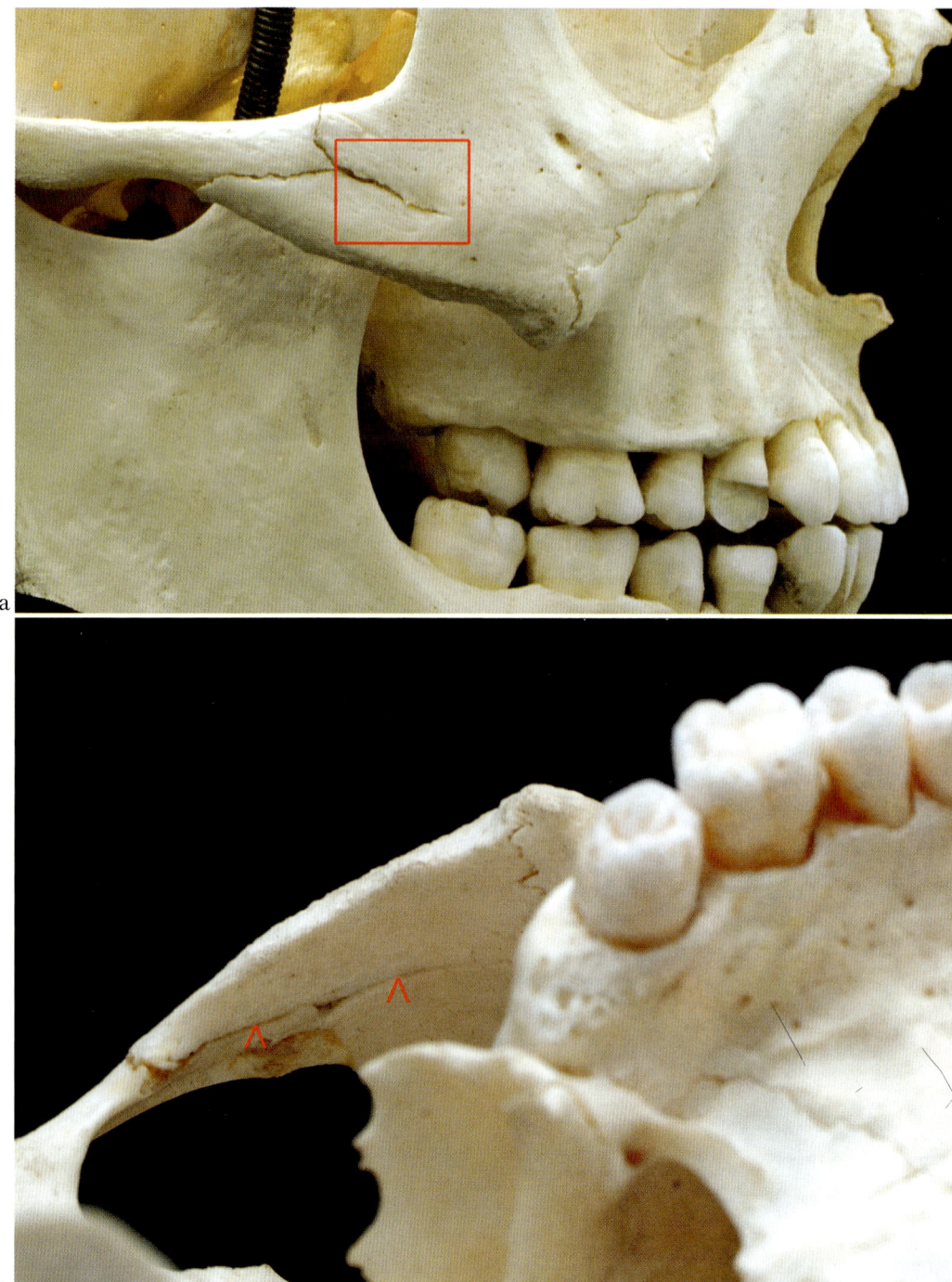

Figure 182a-b. Either a prominent trace/remnant of a right os Japonicum, or a vestige of the zygomatic suture in a young adult Asian male skull (FSA AS009). (a) Trace os Japonicum (rectangle) or a vestige of the right zygomatic suture (Hanihara and Ishida 2001a; Hanihara et al. 1998) resulting in what is commonly called a partially obliterated os Japonicum. (b) Internal surface of the right zygoma revealing a horizontal suture (∧) separating the zygoma into superior and inferior halves. Although this feature was present bilaterally and symmetrically on both the facial and inner/temporal surfaces of the zygomas, there was no unambiguous evidence that this represented a separate ossicle.

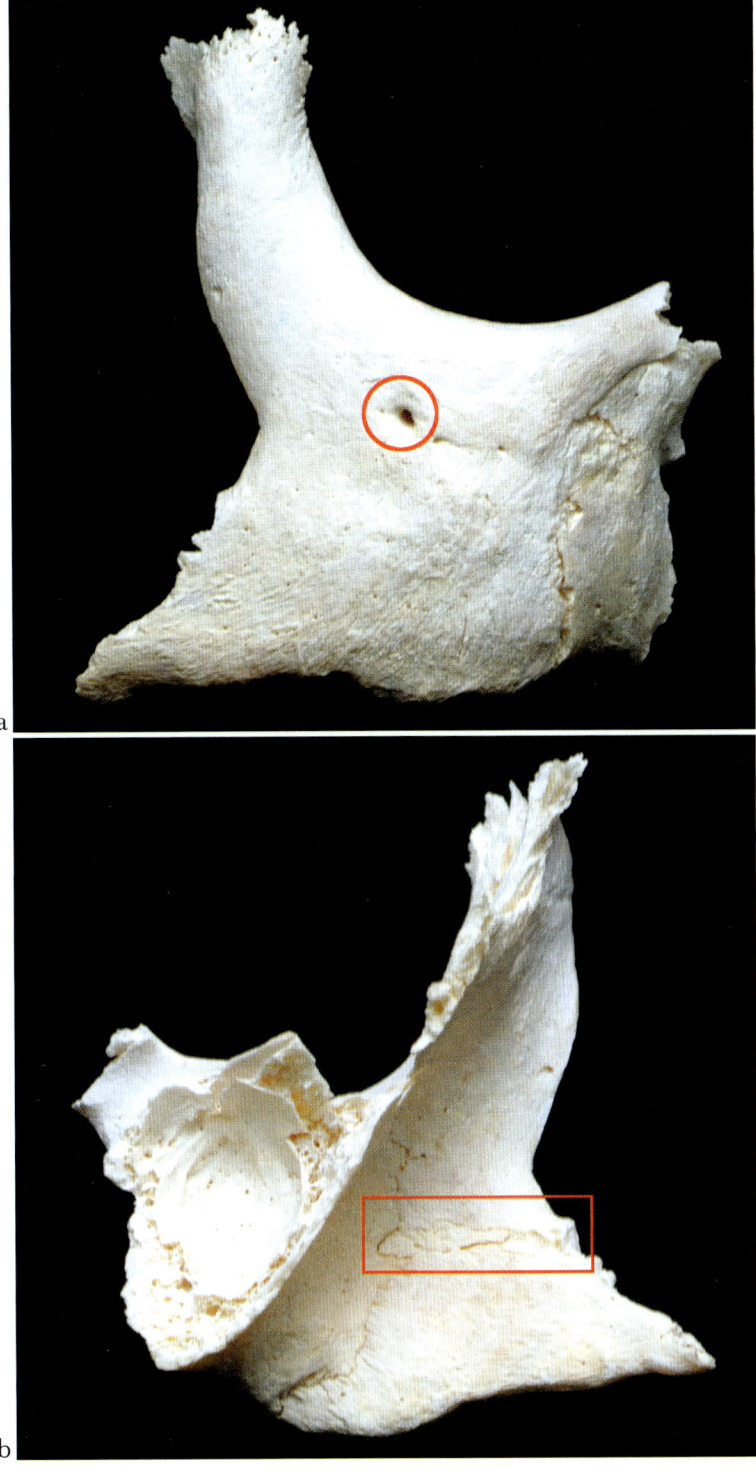

Figure 183a-b. Right zygoma showing no evidence of os Japonicum on the lateral surface, but a "trace os Japonicum" on the medial surface and a single zygomaticofacial foramen. (a) Lateral view of the right zygoma showing no visible trace of a suture associated with os Japonicum and a zygomaticofacial foramen (circle). (b) Sutural trace (rectangle) on the temporal/internal surface of the right zygoma suggestive of os Japonicum. Absence of a suture on the facial surface suggests this feature is not a trace os Japonicum. Cf. Aksu et al. (2009); Hanihara and Ishida (2001a); Hanihara et al. 1998; Mangal et al. (2004); Wartmann and Loukas (2009).

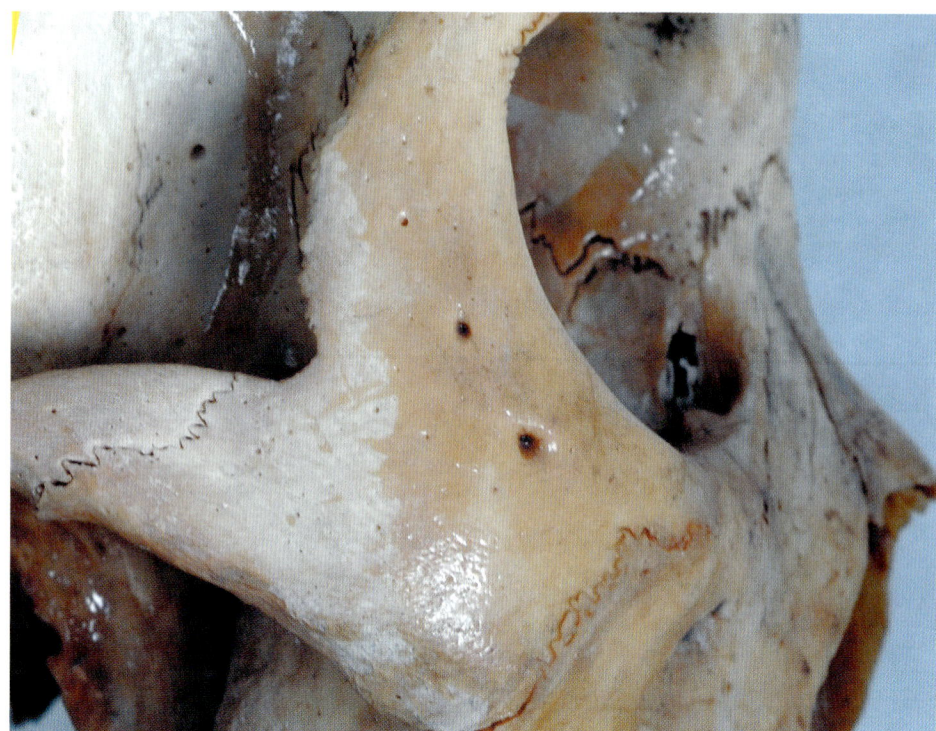

Figure 184. Right zygoma showing no evidence or trace of os Japonicum.

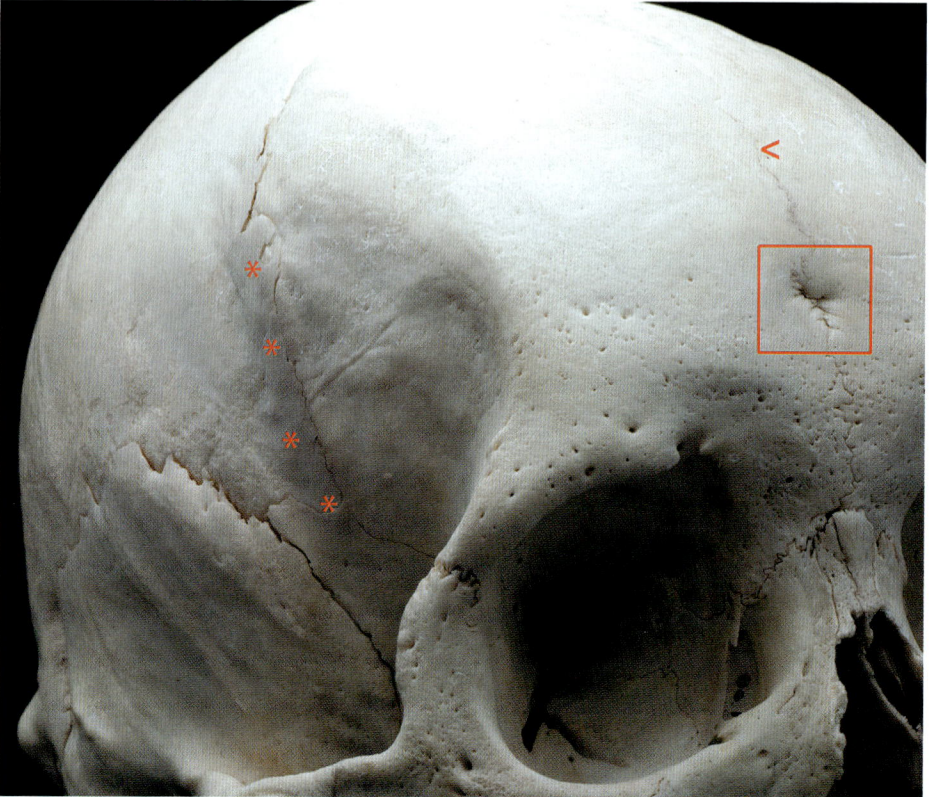

Figure 185. Metopic fissure (square), metopism (<) and sulcus of Gustav Schwalbe (*) in a probable adult Asian male (CSC018).

Chapter 3

LEFT LATERAL VIEW OF THE SKULL

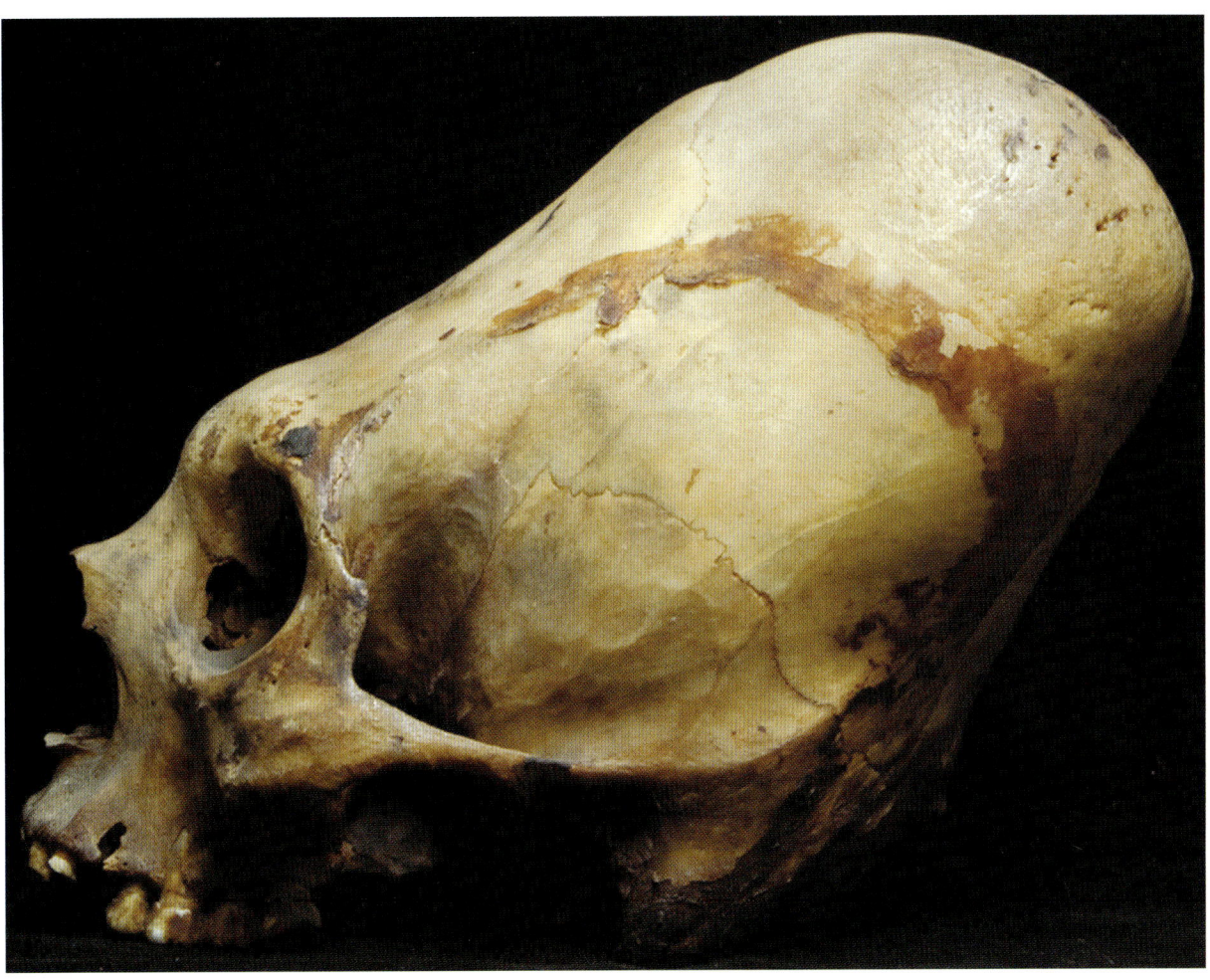

Figure 186. Artificial cranial modification due to wrapping or binding the head during early childhood in an ancient adult Peruvian (UPenn L-606). Artificial pressure exerted on a skull by binding or wrapping influences the complexity (serration) of the coronal suture and an increase in the number of ossicles/wormian bones; however it does not cause premature cranial synostosis. Cf. Dorsey (1897). Cranial modification such as this greatly alters the shape of the vault and can double its length.

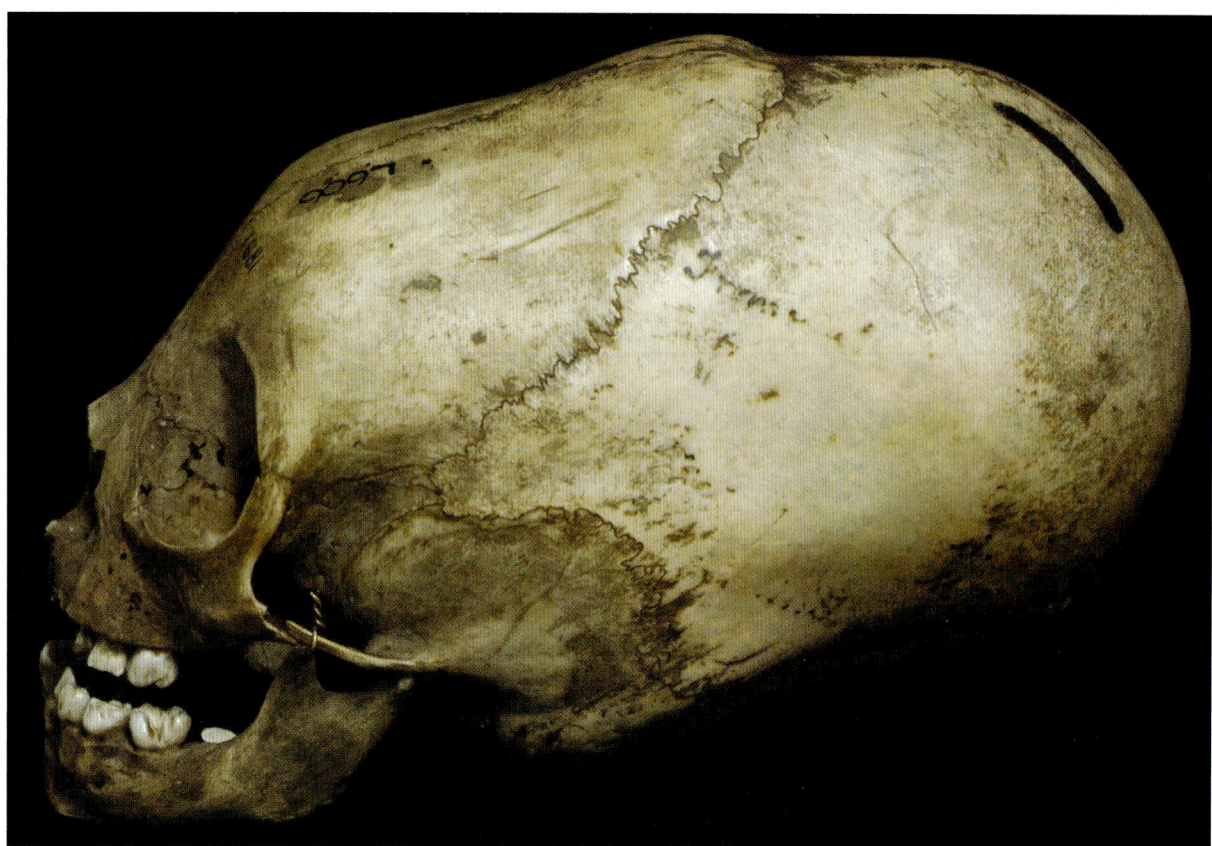

Figure 187. Extreme cranial modification in an ancient Peruvian child (3–5 years of age) (UPenn L-606).

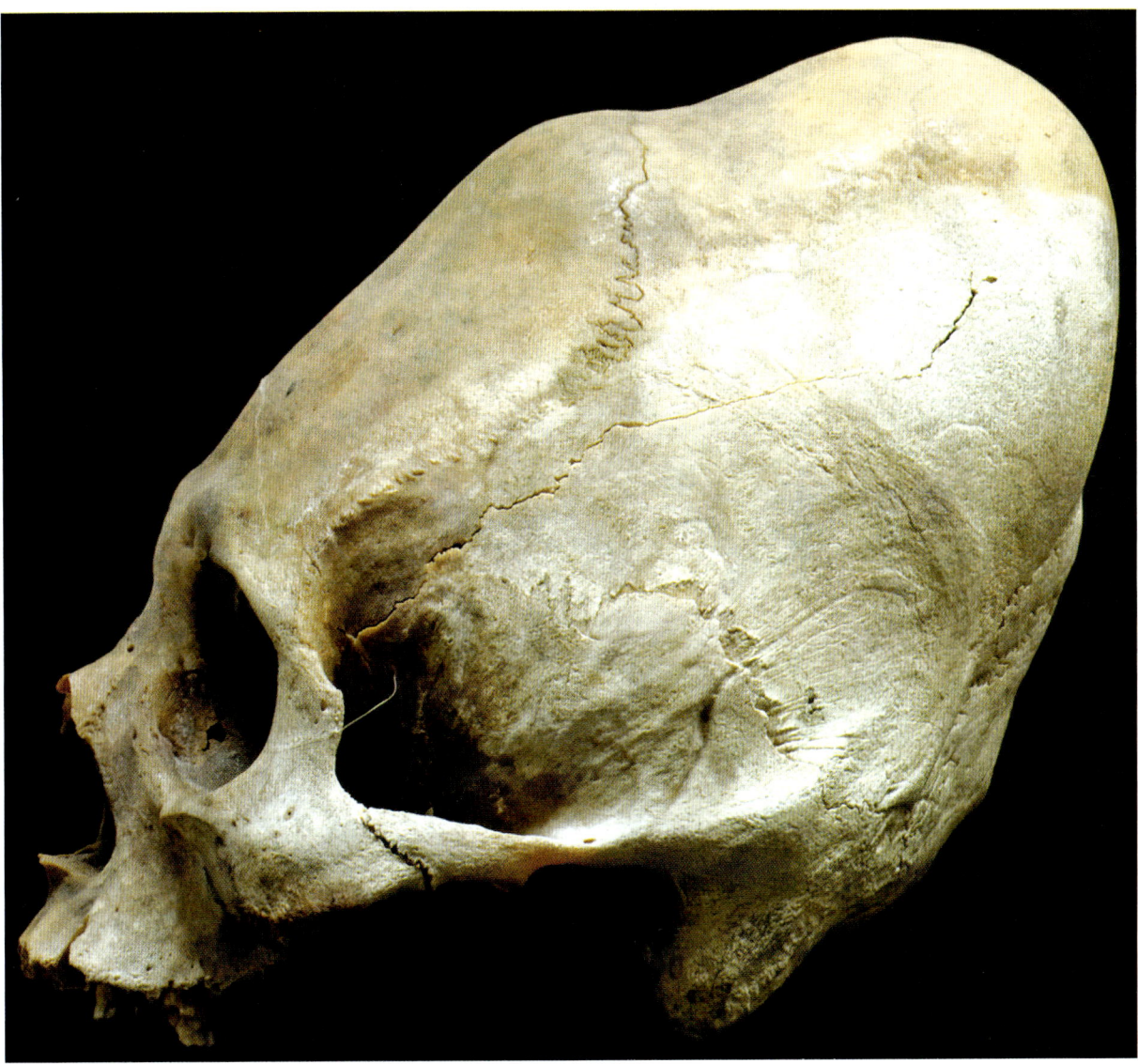

Figure 188. Artificial cranial deformation in an adult Peruvian (UPenn 29-144-13 L606). The left side of the skull exhibits postmortem breakage resembling a fracture.

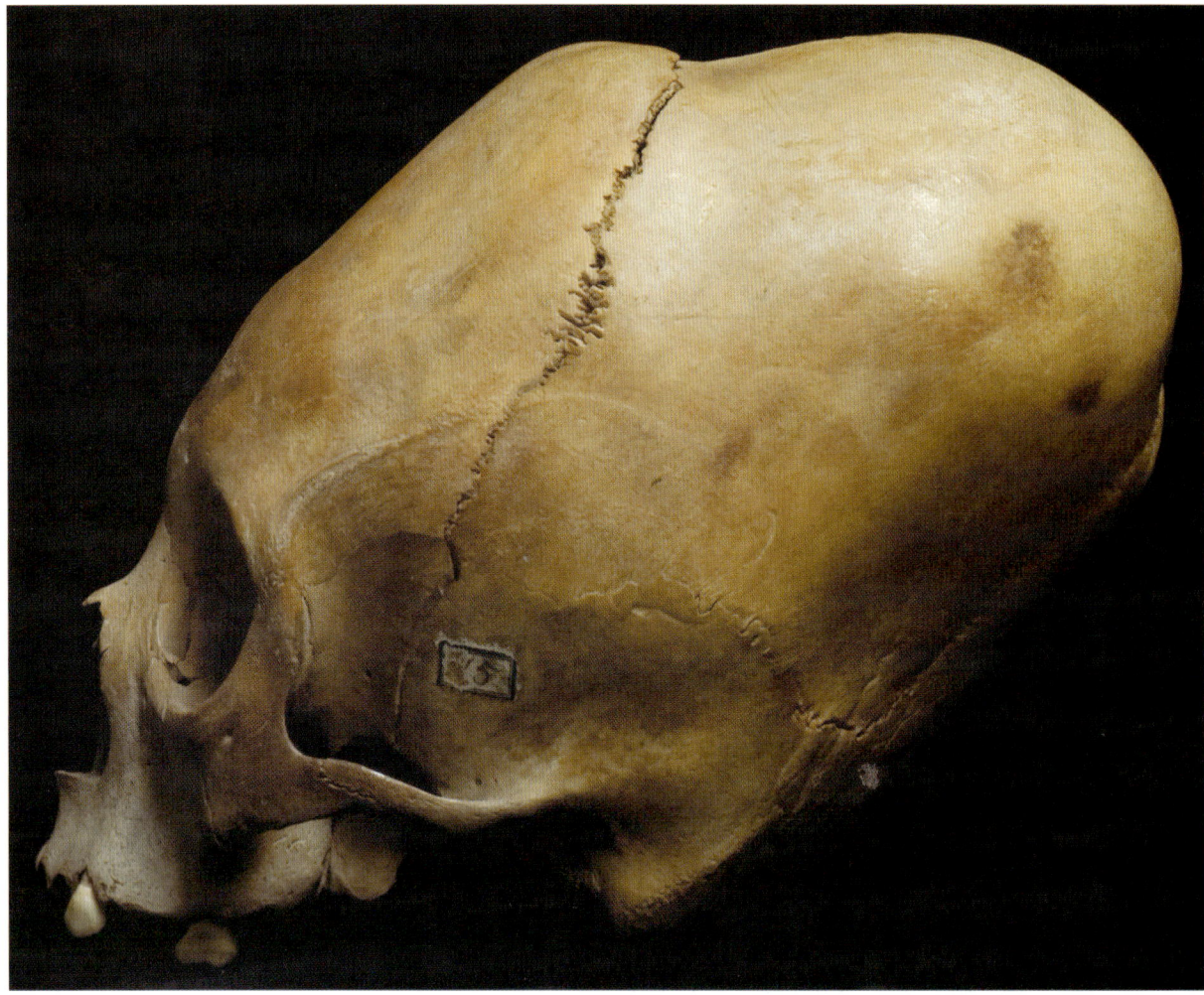

Figure 189. Artificial cranial deformation in a 12- to 15-year-old Peruvian subadult (UPenn 24-142-224). Note the vertically-oriented occipital region, sloping frontal bone and open coronal suture.

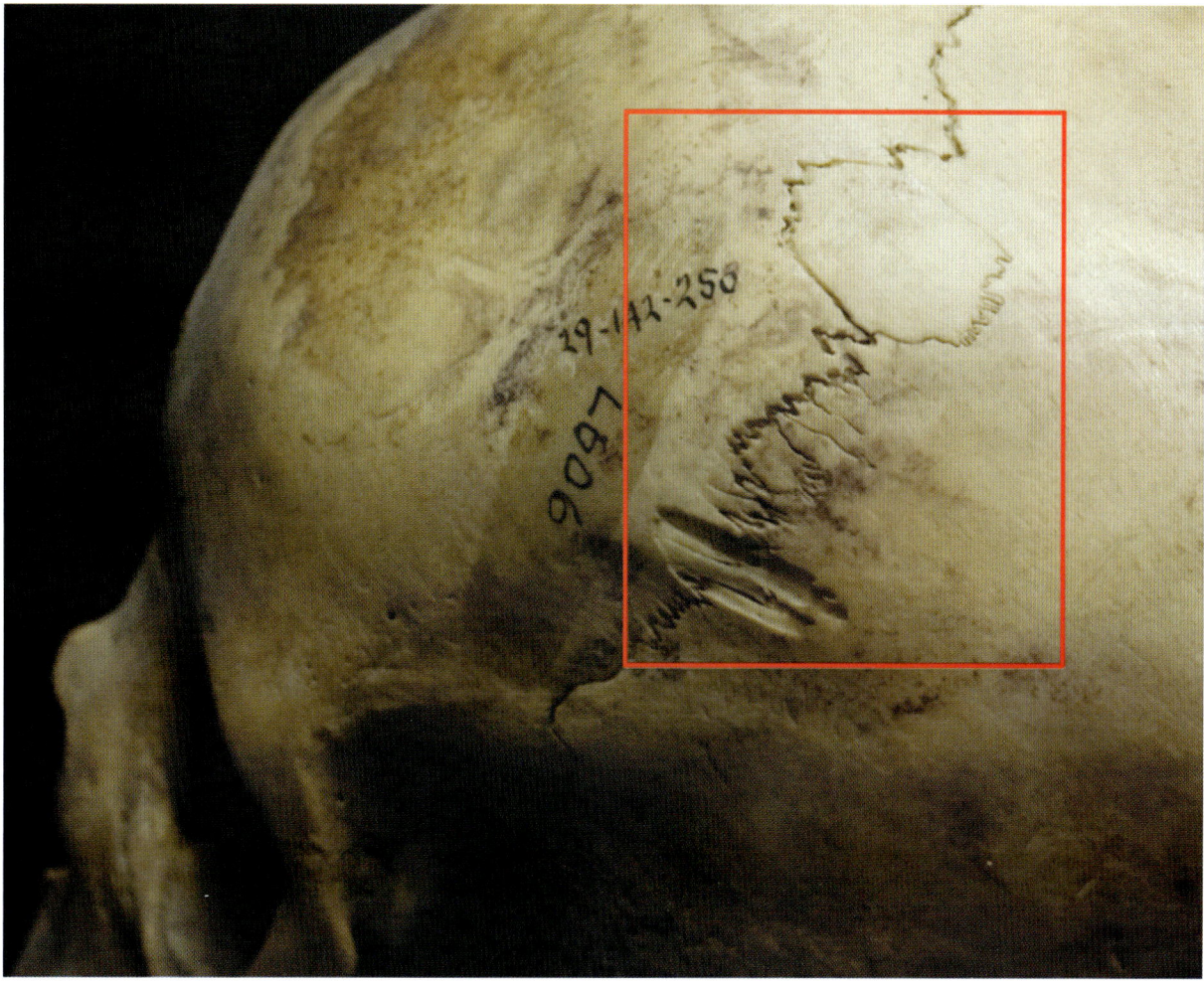

Figure 190. Numerous coronal ossicles (rectangle) in an ancient Peruvian child (Penn Museum L-606 29-142). Uncommon finding. See Dorsey (1897) for a discussion on increased sutural complexity and the formation of coronal ossicles associated with artificial cranial deformation. Multiple coronal ossicles such as in this individual are unusual, but not rare, depending on the group examined.

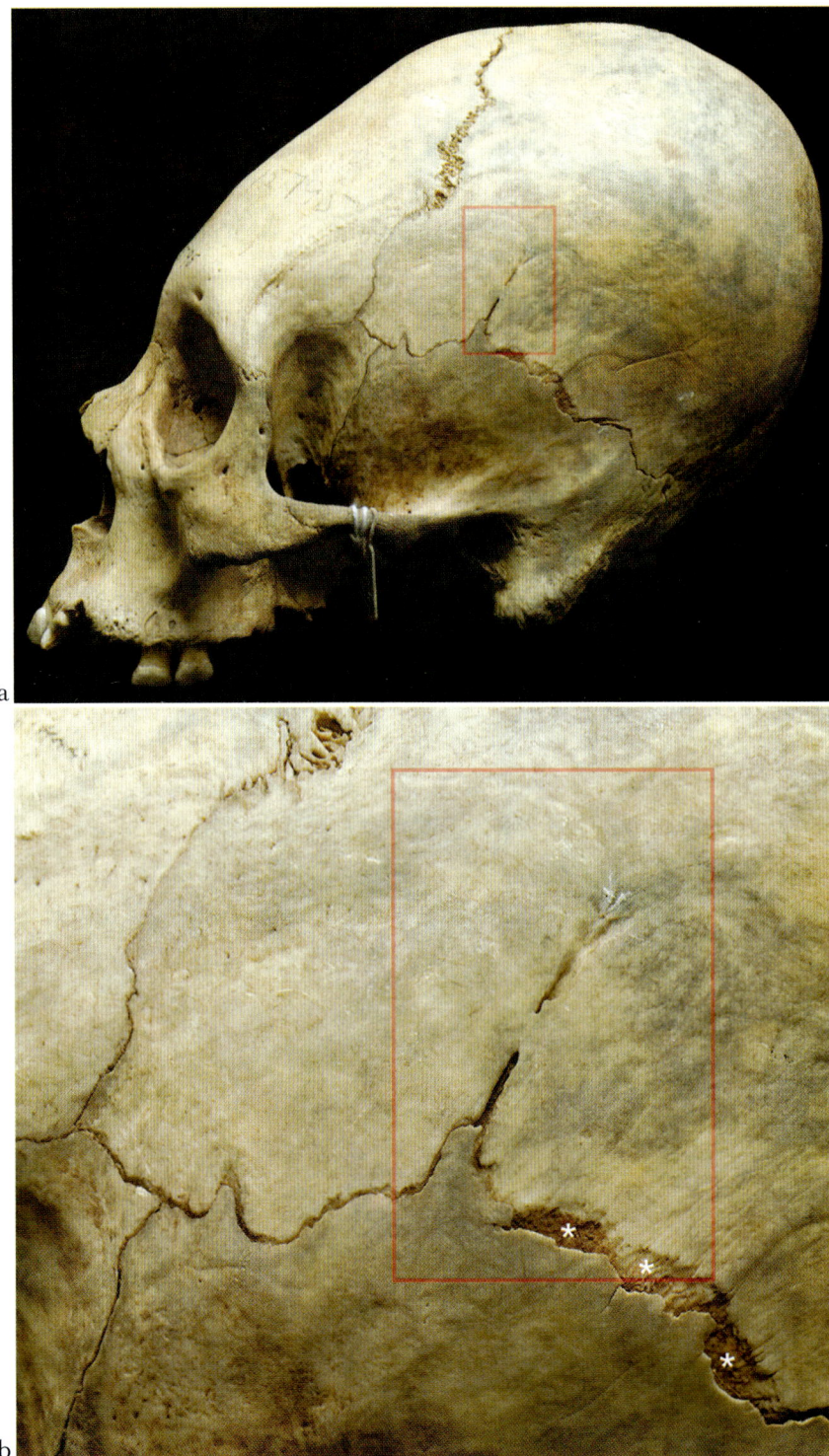

Figure 191a-b. Partially bridged left parietal process of the left temporal squamous portion in an adult. (a) Cranium of an ancient Peruvian with artificial cranial deformation, parietal process and groove (rectangle). (UPenn 15795). (b) Higher magnification of the parietal process groove and partial bridging (rectangle) that likely carried a vessel and remnant of a crescent-shaped squamosal ossicle(s) (*) that is missing postmortem.

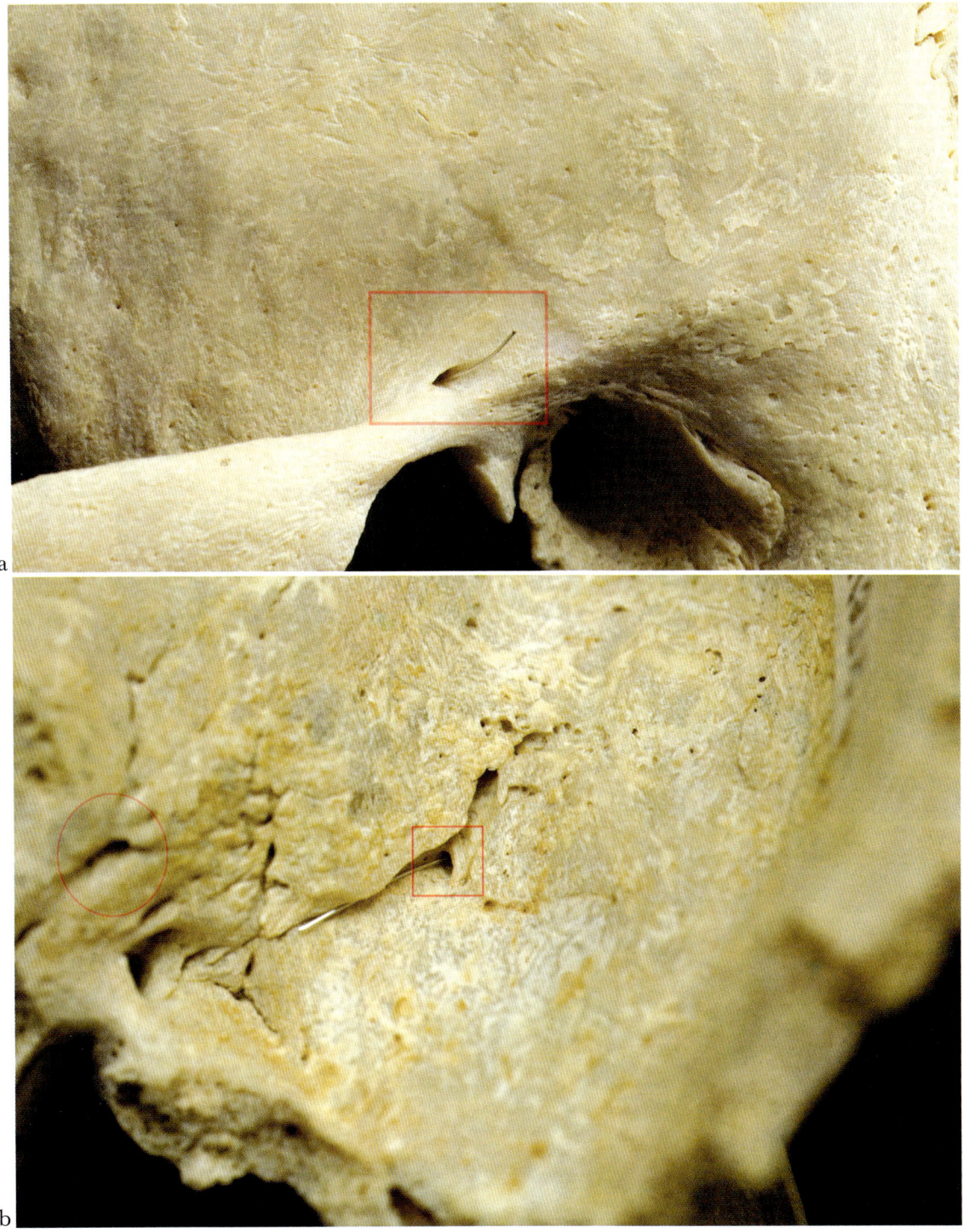

Figure 192a-b. Depiction of a left postglenoid foramen. (a) Left lateral view of a wire inserted into the squamosal foramen (rectangle). (b) Endocranial view of the foramen (square) as it enters posterior to the petrous and squamous bones (Mütter Museum F1993-123-5). This foramen is sometimes referred to as the squamosal (Boyd 1930), glenoid foramen (Alsherhri et al. 2011), inferior squamous foramen (Hauser and DeStefano 1989) or supraglenoid foramen.

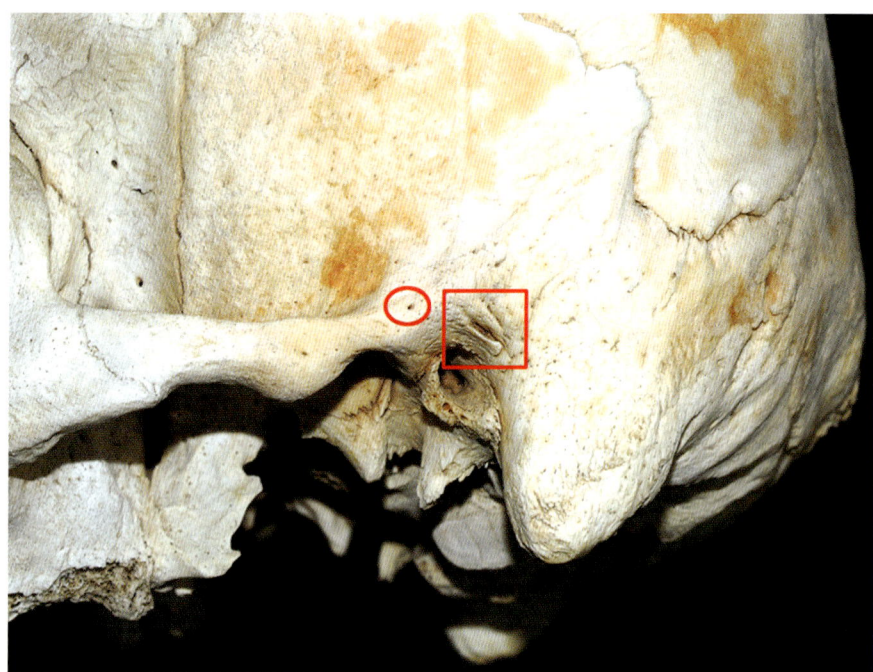

Figure 193. Suprameatal pit (square) and a tiny postglenoid or inferior squamosal foramen (circle) in an adult ancient Peruvian male (SI). Common findings. Cf. Boyd (1930) for more on the squamosal foramen.

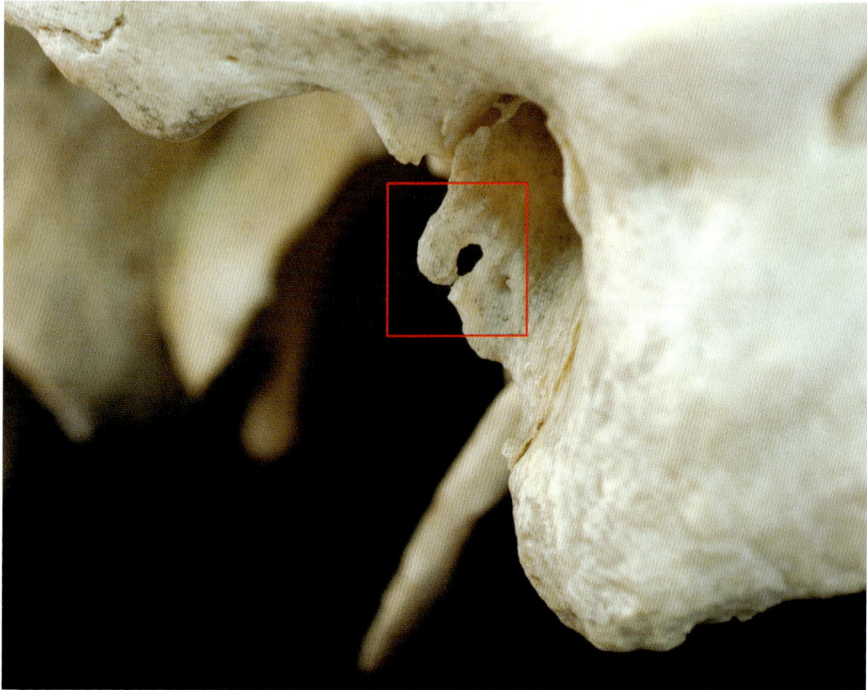

Figure 194. Partial foramen (square) of unknown etiology along the tympanic plate of the left temporal bone (CSC DS 008). Common finding.

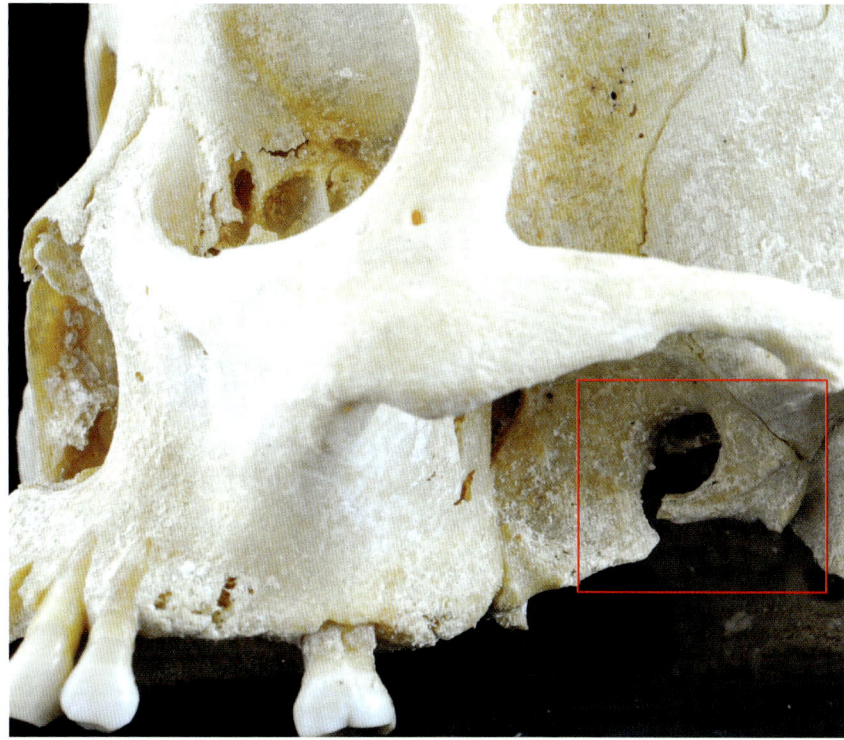

Figure 195. Incompletely formed pterygospinous bridge (rectangle) in an adult Thai skull (KKU). Common finding. Cf. Antonopoulou et al. (2008); Chouke (1946, 1947); Galdames et al. (2010); Nayak et al. (2007); Peker et al. (2002); Rossi et al. (2010); Skrzat et al. (2005); Sternberg (1975).

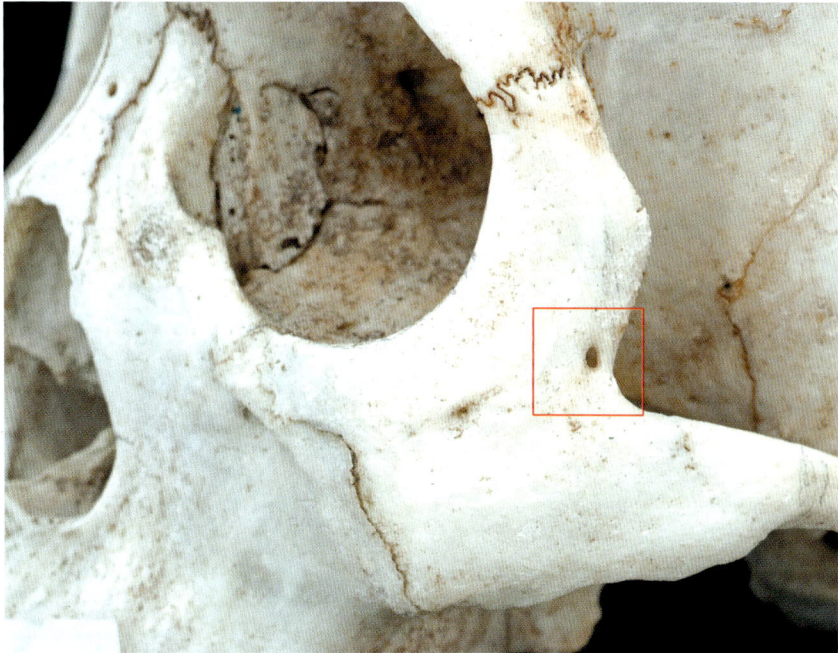

Figure 196. Foramen formed (square) along the margin (jugal) of the left malar bone (CMU 147 52). This may be a zygomaticofacial foramen.

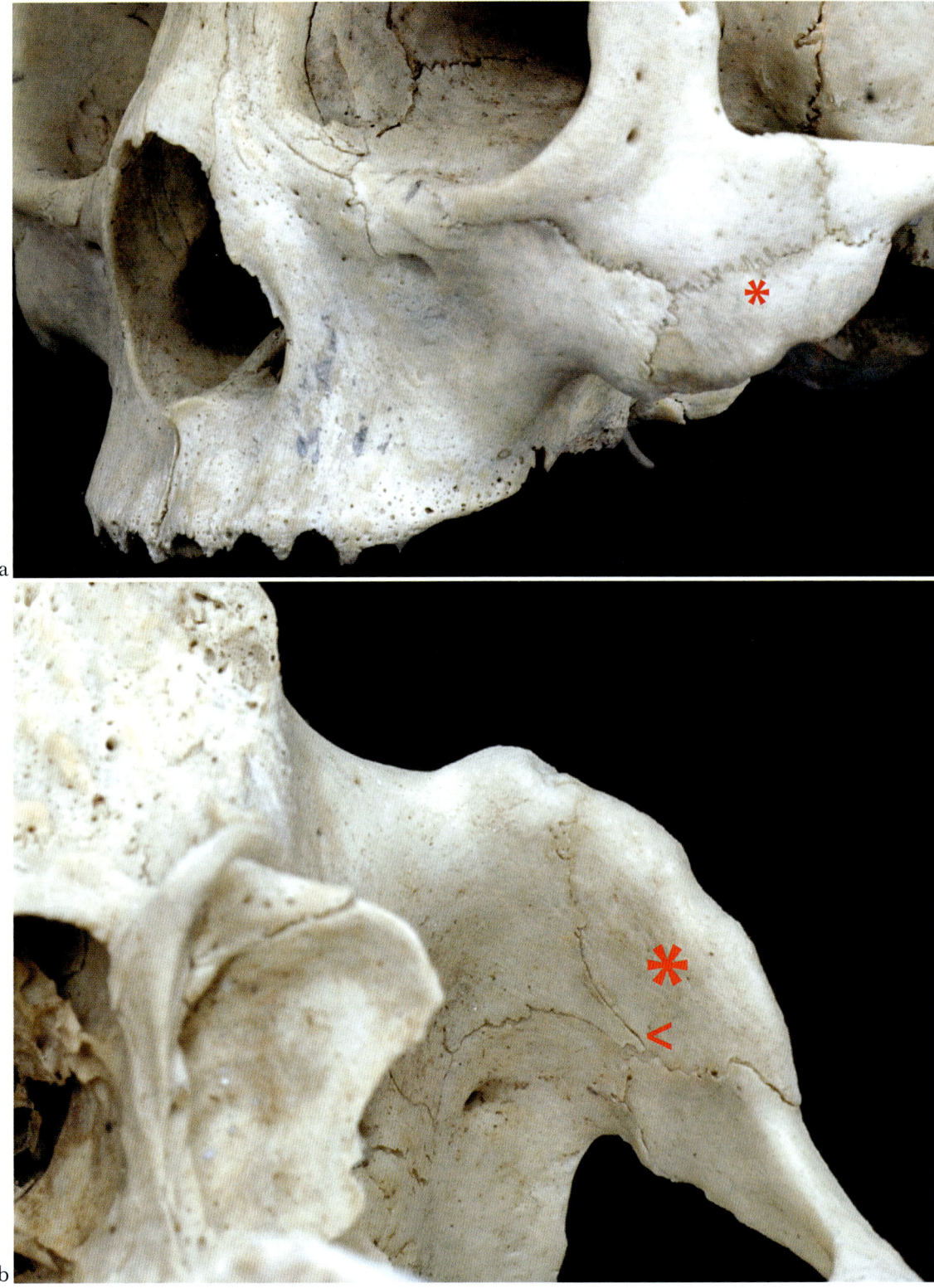

Figure 197a-b. Facial and internal views of left os Japonicum in a 65-year-old Thai female skull (CMU 53 52). (a) Facial view of os Japonicum (*). (b) The accessory suture (<) forming the os Japonicum (*) is visible internally and along its full length, even at this age. Cf. Hauser and DeStefano (1989).

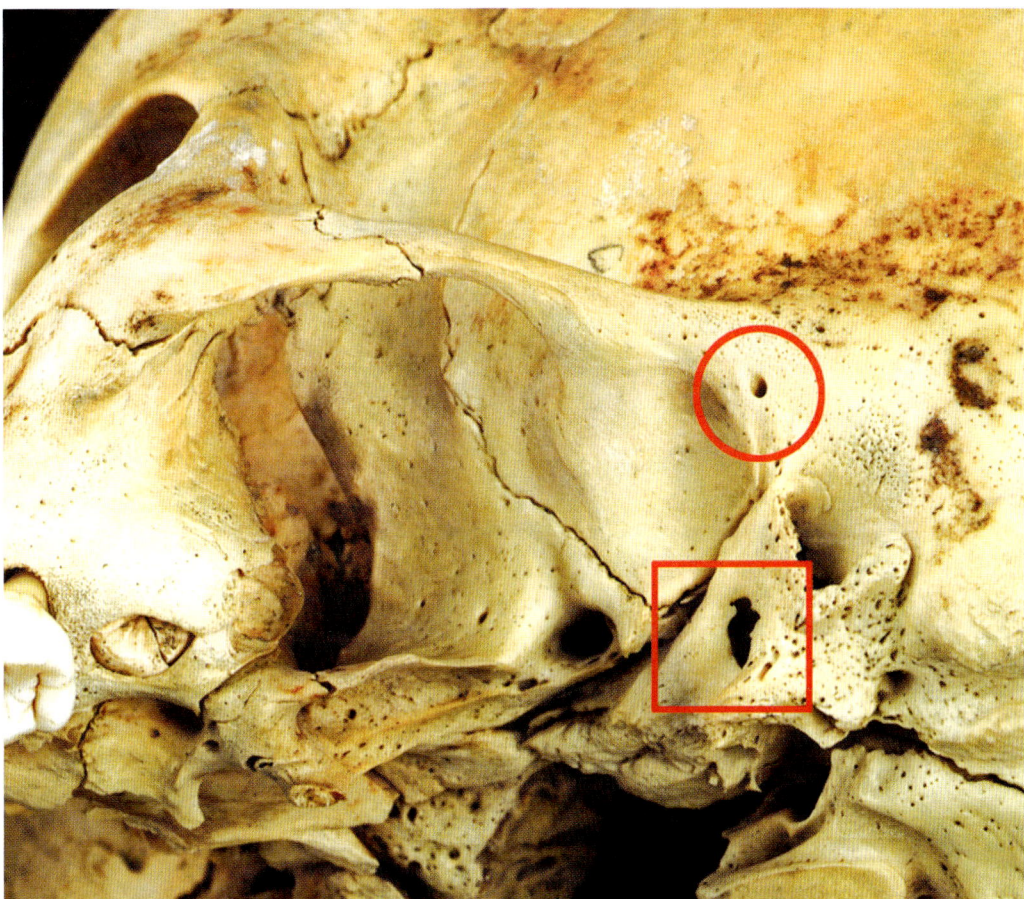

Figure 198. Inferior postglenoid foramen (circle) and tympanic dehiscence/foramen of Huschke/foramen tympanicum (square) in an ancient Peruvian subadult skull (SI). The postglenoid foramen, also known as squamosal foramen and foramen jugulare spurium of Luschka, appears in two locations either superior or inferior to the crest of the zygomatic arch, but most commonly at the root of the zygomatic process/arch. The postglenoid foramen, 1 to 5 mm in diameter, is present in fetuses but disappears, leaving a foramen in less than 1% of adults (Butler 1957). Wysocki (2002) found the postglenoid foramen in 2 of 50 adult male skulls and 5 of 50 adult female skulls (3.5% combined). The postglenoid foramen, sometimes referred to as the "false" jugular foramen/foramen jugulare spurium (Wysocki 2002) is an uncommon to rare finding. When scoring the tympanic dehiscence, also known as foramen tympanicum, the present author refers to this developmental defect as a foramen of Huschke only if it persists into adulthood. The foramen of Huschke/tympanicum is a normal entity present during embryonic development of the temporal bone and usually closes by five years of age. While the frequency of this foramen varies greatly, Wang and Colleagues (1991) found it in 7% of 377 adult dry skulls. See Hauser and DeStefano (1989); Humphrey and Scheuer (2005); Lacout et al. (2005); Vázquez et al. (2001) for more on the foramen of Huschke. See Boyd (1930); Butler (1957, 1967); LeDouble (1903); Wysocki (2002) for more on the postglenoid foramen and inferior squamous foramen (petrosquamous emissary). Note that the squamosopetrous foramen (and sinus) is located in this same general area, but it is usually situated medial to the sinus, not lateral to it, as in this example.

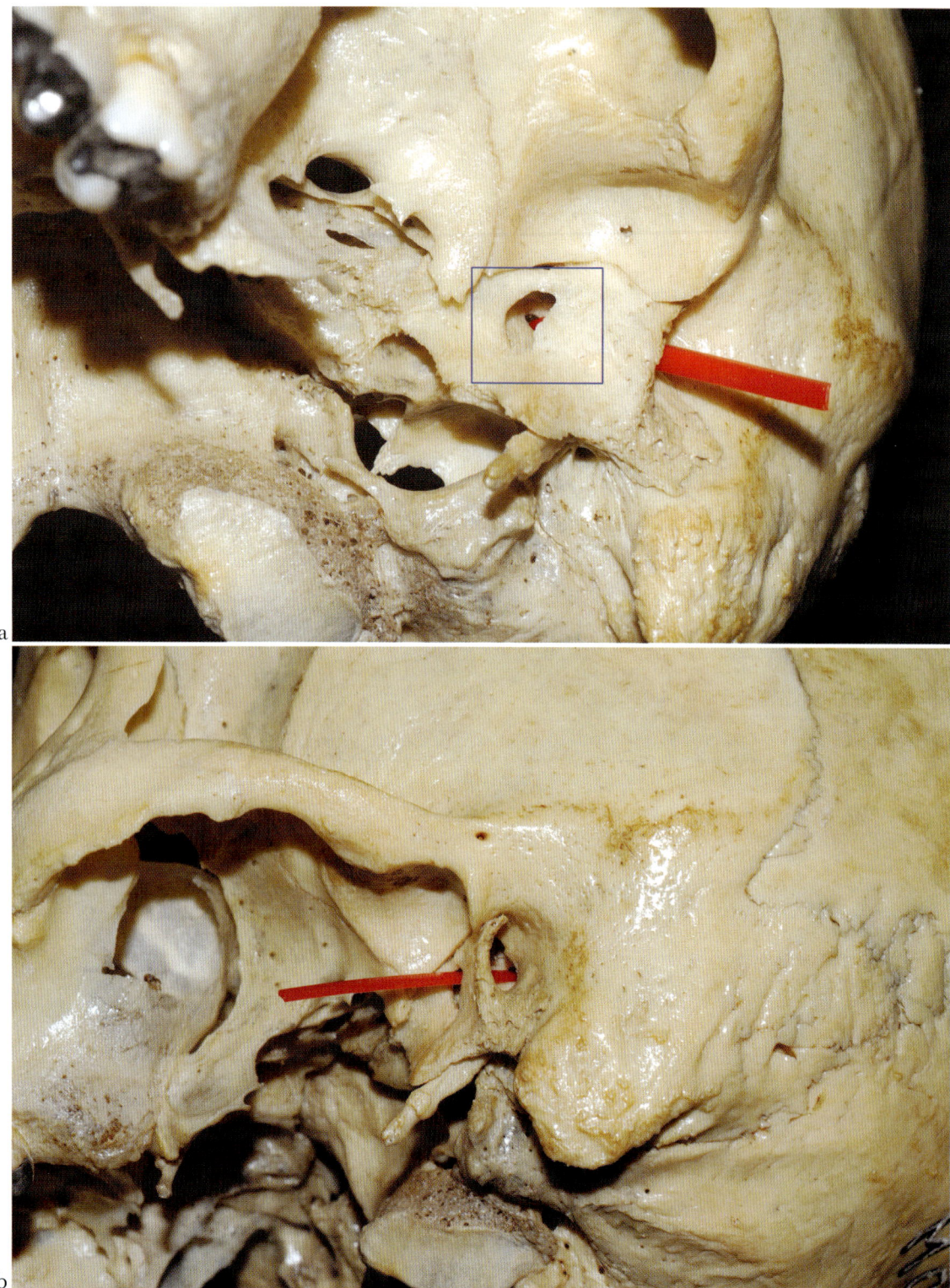

Figure 199a-b. Demonstration of a tympanic dehiscence and oval window. (a) Red probe inserted into the left external auditory meatus and pointing to the oval window through a small tympanic dehiscence (square), also known as a foramen of Huschke. (b) Left lateral view showing a red probe inserted through a dehiscence in the left tympanic plate and entering the oval window (JABSOM M02).

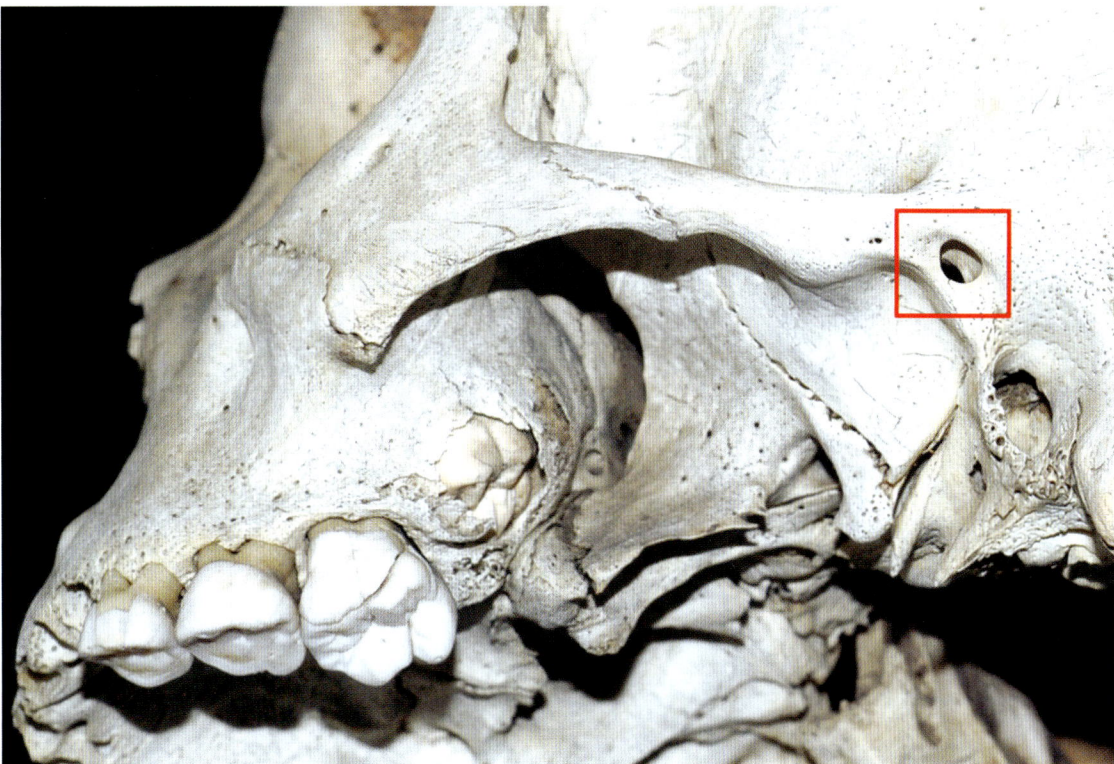

Figure 200. An unusually large postglenoid/supraglenoid/inferior squamous foramen (square) at the root of the zygomatic process in a Thai child (KKU); note that this foramen is below the supramastoid crest and far from the Glaserian or petrotympanic fissure. This is the largest foramen of its kind that the authors have noted. Foramina of this size are uncommon to rare and may reflect a pathological condition. While the size of foramen, which transmits an emissary vein, is usually largest in newborns and its incidence is higher in children and adolescents, the authors have seen foramen of this size in only one other child. Cf. Boyd (1930); Chauhan et al. (2011); Hauser and DeStefano (1989); Vásquez et al. (2001).

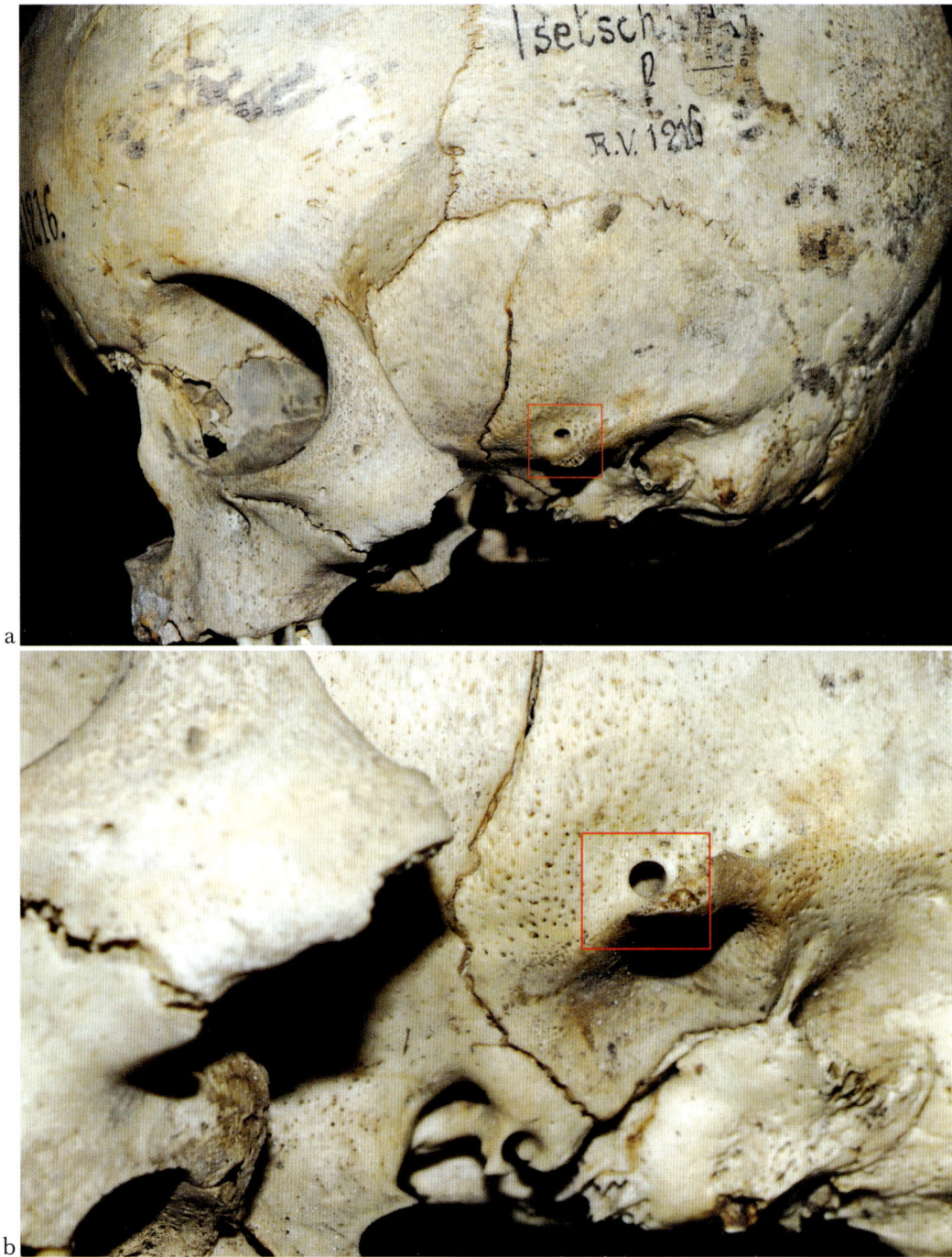

Figure 201a-b. Unusually large left inferior squamous foramen in a 3- to 5-year-old child (RV1216). (a) Left lateral view of the skull and inferior squamous foramen (square). (b) Higher magnification showing the sharp border of this foramen (square) and its internal morphology. This foramen is believed to transmit the petrosquamous emissary vein. See Hauser and DeStefano (1989) for more on this foramen.

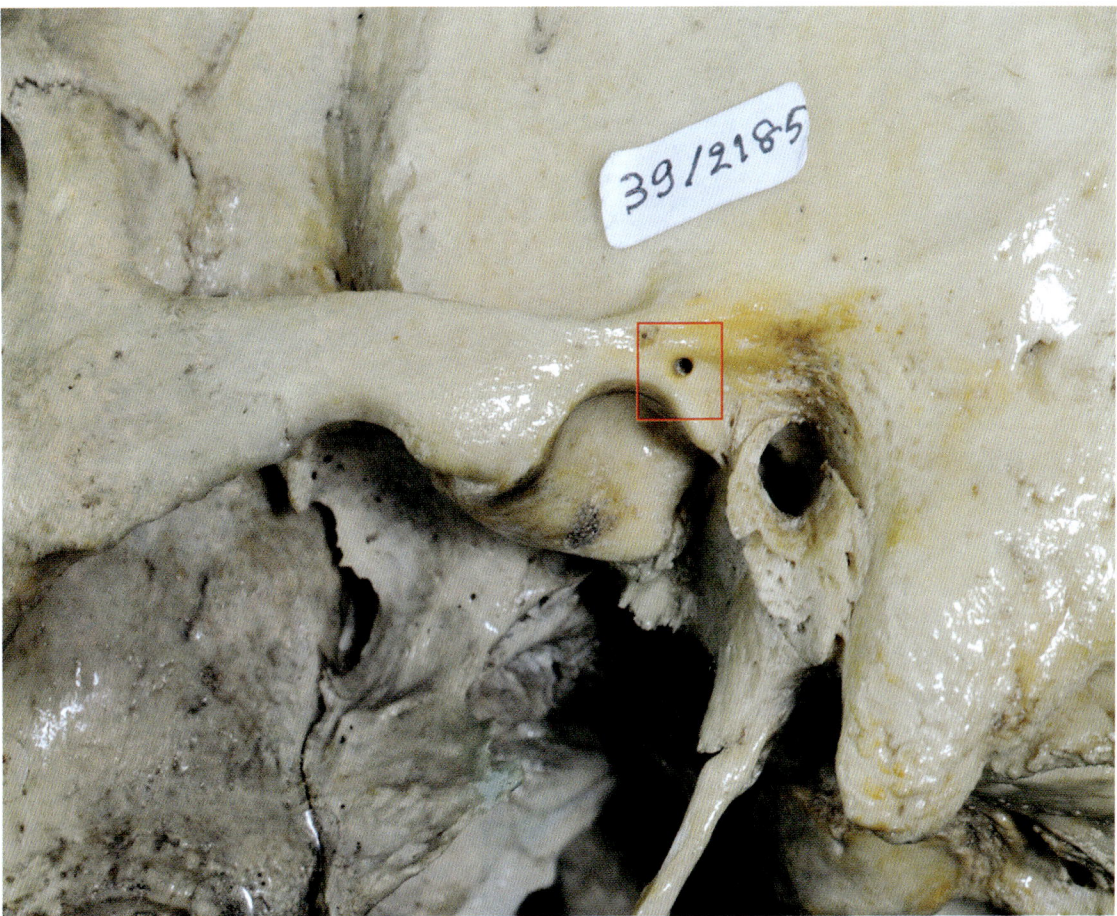

Figure 202. Small inferior squamosal or postglenoid foramen (square) in the left temporal bone in an adult Thai skull (KKU); this may be a variant of Figures 190, 192, 193, 198, 200, 201, 203, 228 and 229. There appears to be terminological confusion in the literature when referring to this foramen, since the squamosal foramen is above the root of the zygomatic arch and the postglenoid foramen is in the Glaserian fissure (Gray 1901). Uncommon finding. Cf. Boyd (1930); Brash (1953); Chauhan et al. (2011); Vázquez et al. (2001).

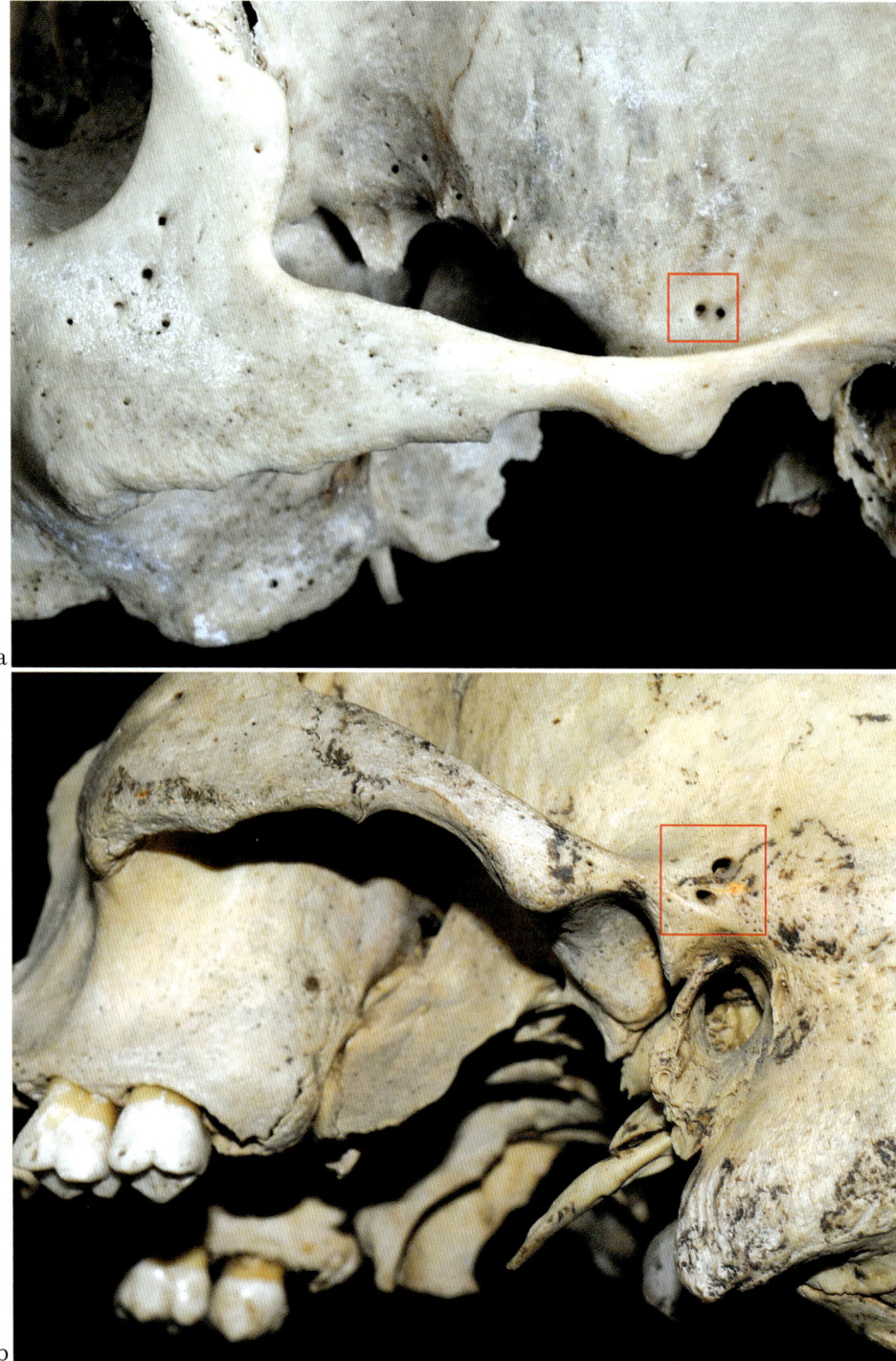

Figure 203a-b. Double or divided inferior squamous foramina situated next to one another and superior to the zygomatic arch (PAVN Forensic Institute). (a) Small squamous pits (square) superior to the zygomatic arch and that may house the petrosquamous emissary vessels. (b) Two large, double or divided squamous foramina situated at the root of the zygomatic arch (PAVN Forensic Institute). Double foramina such as these are uncommon findings. Cf. Boyd (1930); Hauser and DeStefano (1989).

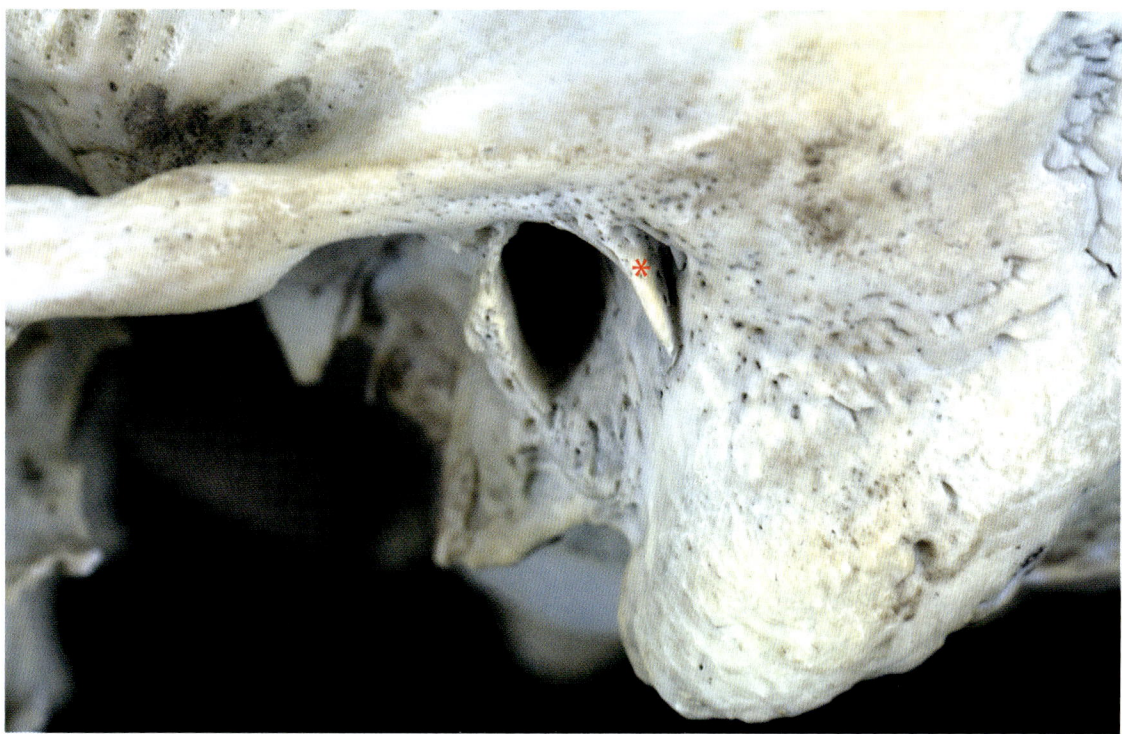

Figure 204. Prominent left spine of Henle (*), also known as the suprameatal spine of Henle, in a young adult White male (CIL).

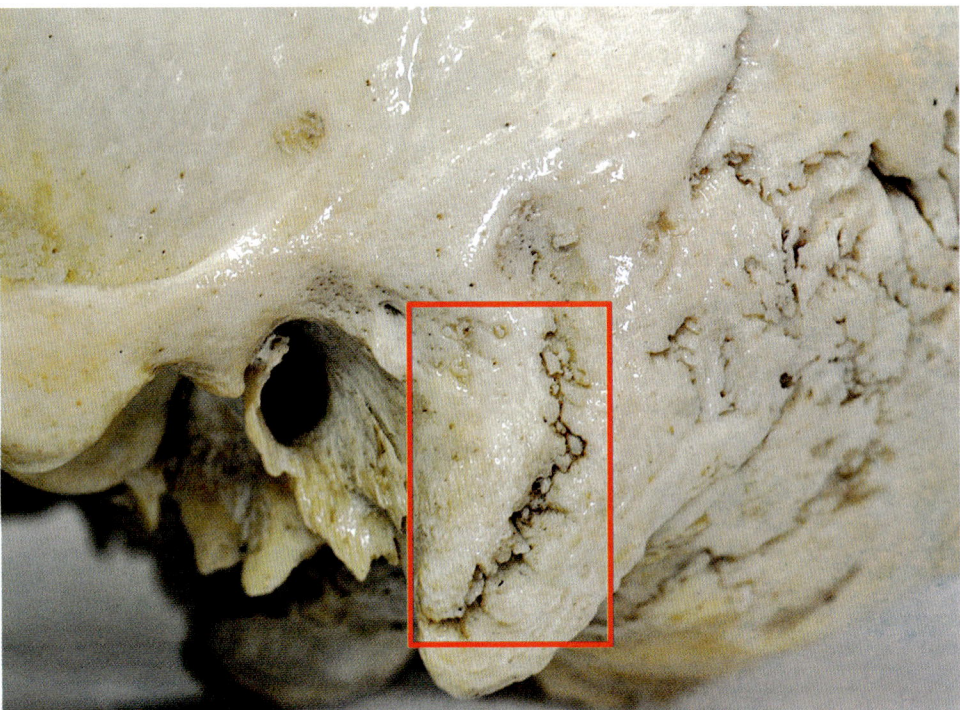

Figure 205. Remnant of the petrosquamous suture (rectangle), sometimes referred to as a "divided mastoid" (sutura mastoideosquamosa – Sternberg 1975), in the left mastoid process of an adult Thai male skull. A depression, as seen in this specimen, often forms at the superior termination of this suture (KKU). Common finding. Cf. Hauser and DeStefano (1989).

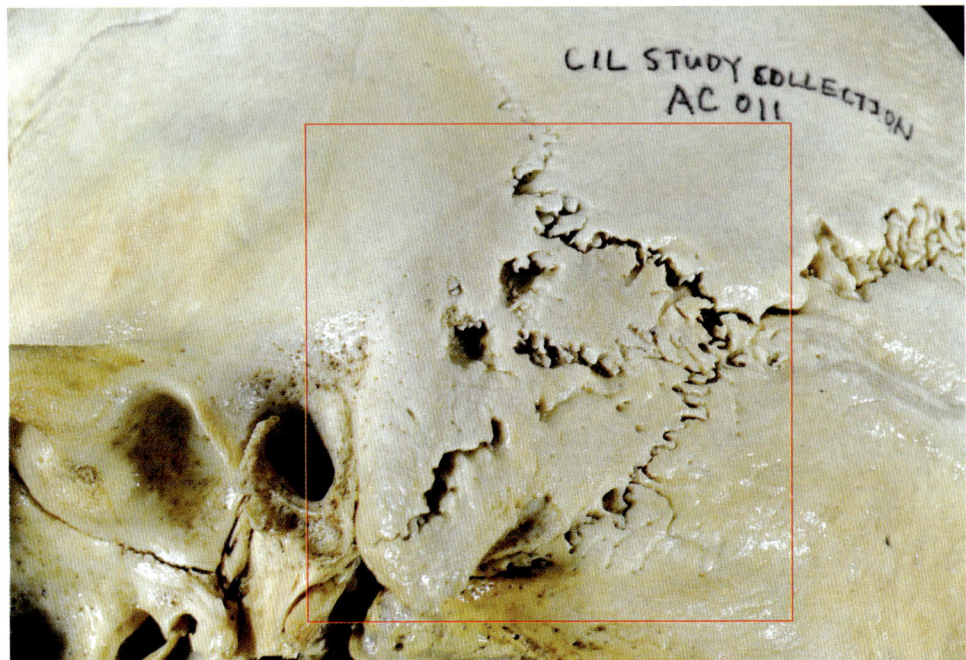

Figure 206. Unusually complex and jagged variant of the left parietal notch bone and petrosquamous suture (square) in an adult Asian skull (CSC AC 011). Note that the petrosquamous suture is wide and deep. Cf. Berry and Berry (1967); Sternberg (1975). Uncommon finding.

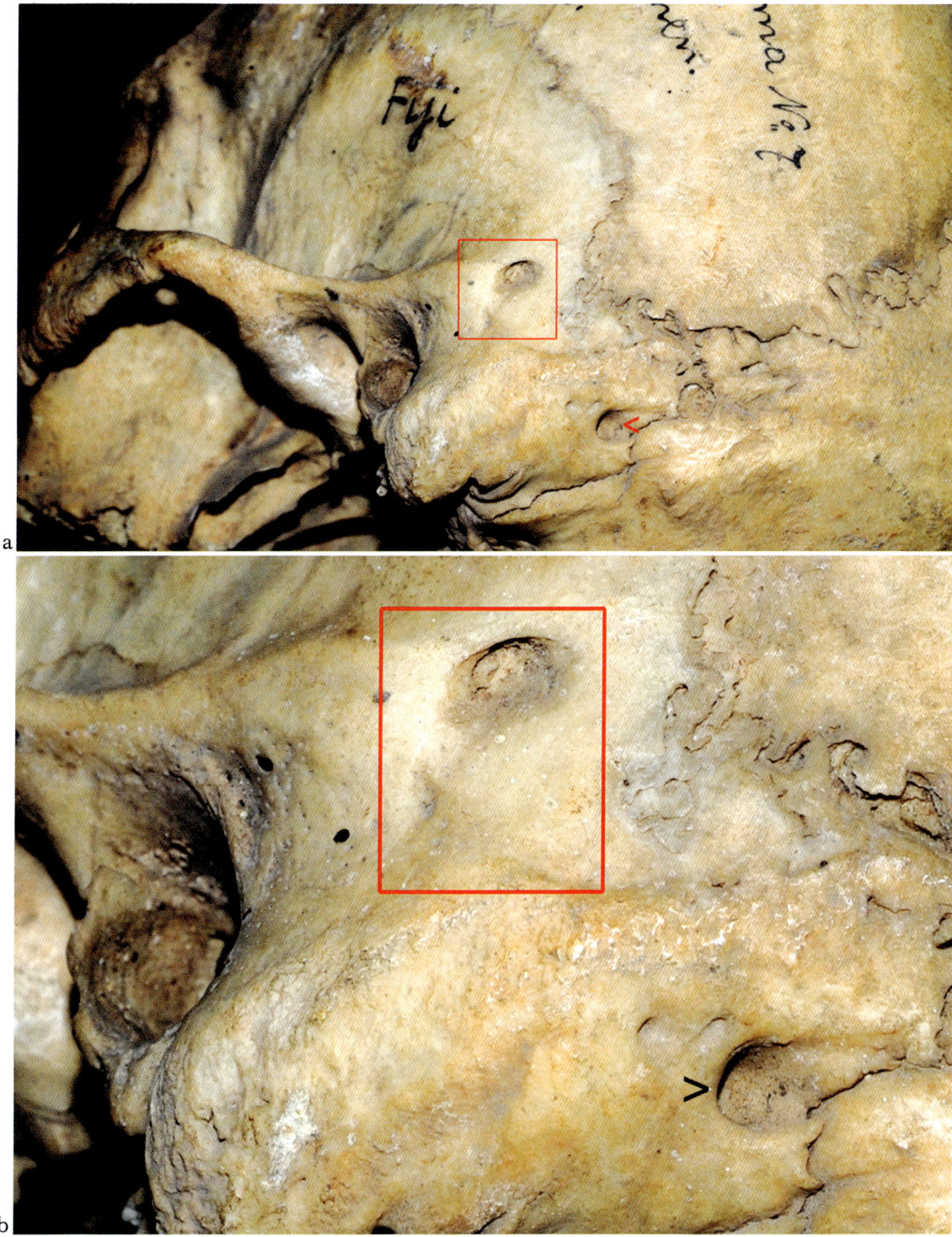

Figure 207a-b. Depression/pit at the superior portion of the left petrosquamosal suture and a mastoid foramen (RV794). (a) Left lateral view illustrating a depression (square) and normal mastoid foramen (<). (b) Close-up of the depression (square) and foramen (>). This uncommon trait was bilateral in this individual and is likely a trace, or faulty ossification and closure of the suture.

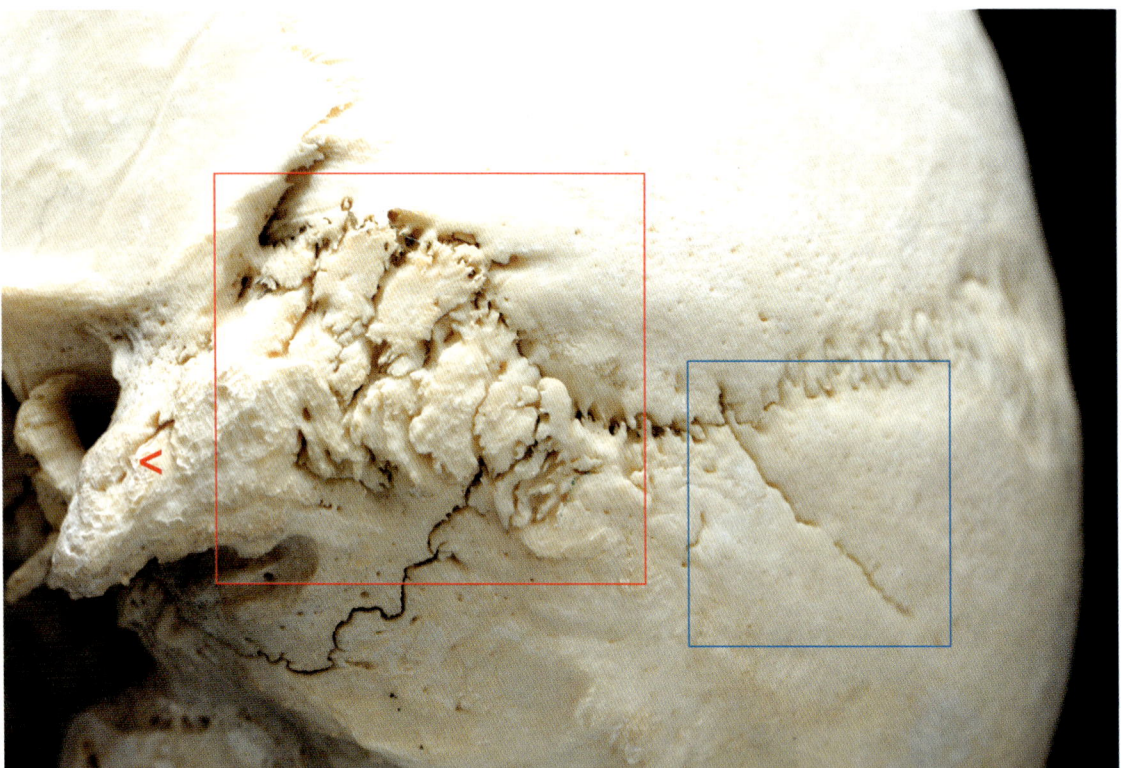

Figure 208. Exceptionally complex parietal notch bones (red square), trace Mendosal suture (blue square) and persistent petrosquamosal suture (<) in an adult male skull (FSA DS043).

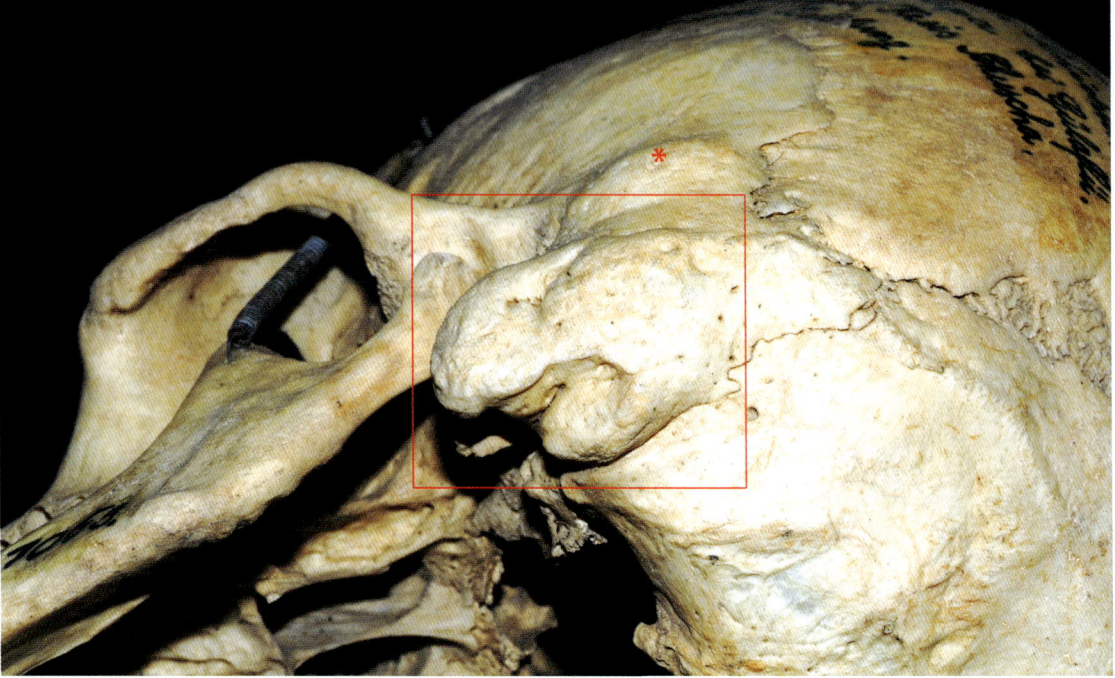

Figure 209. Unusually large, nearly duplicated, left mastoid process (square) and prominent suprameatal crest (*) in an adult male (RV1063). These features were present bilaterally.

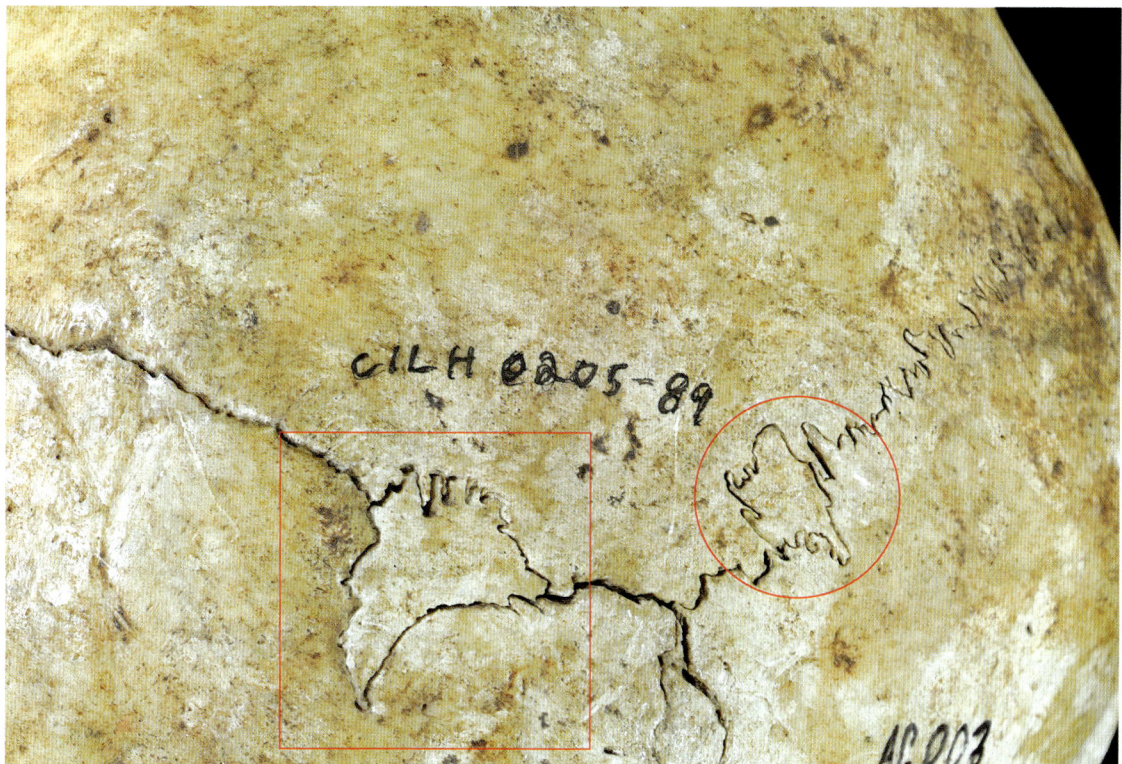

Figure 210. Left parietal notch bone/ossicle (square) and small lambdoidal ossicle (circle) in a 6- to 8-year-old Asian child (CSC AC 003). Common findings.

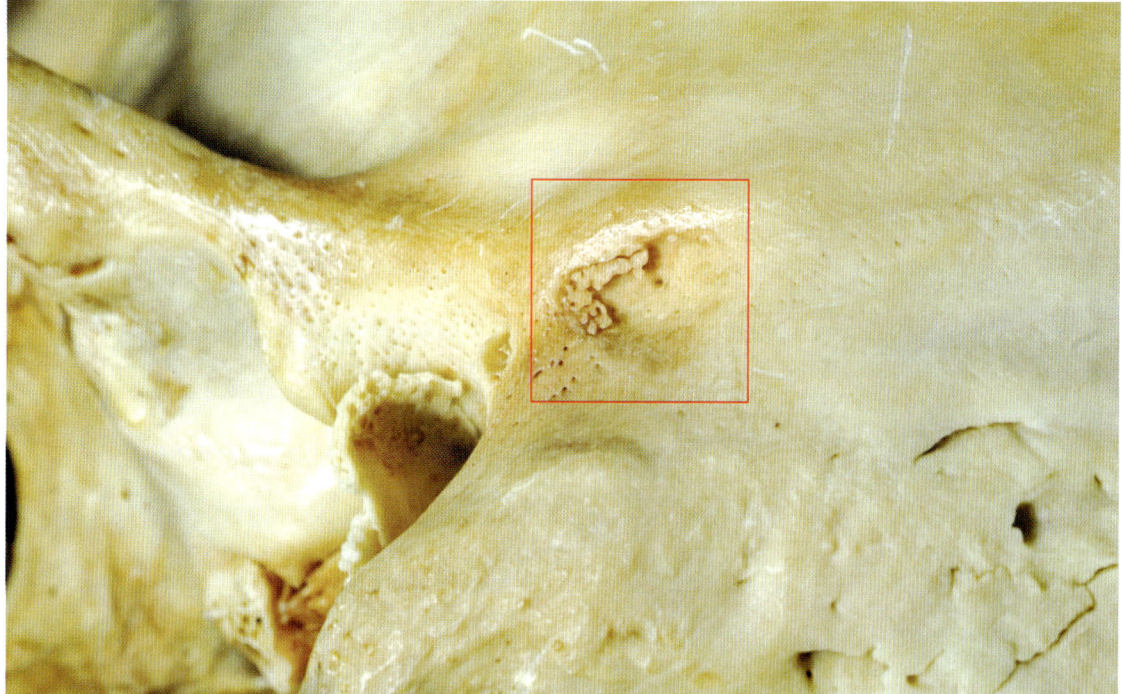

Figure 211. Depression partially filled with suture-like bone (square) in the left temporal bone of an adult Thai (KKU). This depression is an uncommon finding and pits filled with spicules are rare findings.

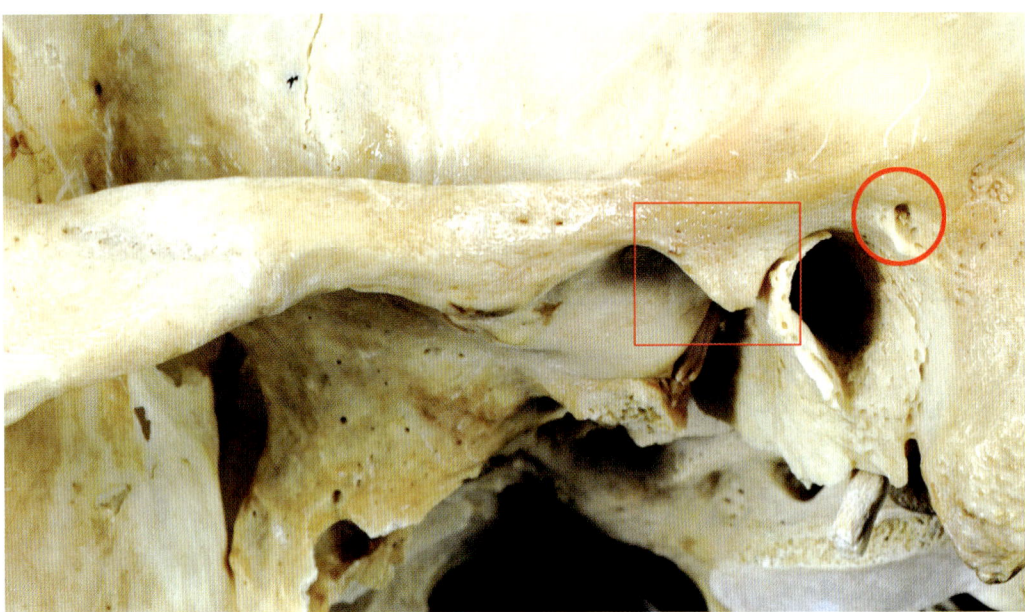

Figure 212. Small suprameatal pit or squamosal foramen (circle) and large postglenoid tubercle/process (rectangle) in an adult Thai skull (KKU). Cf. Boyd (1930); Chauhan et al. (2011); Hauser and DeStefano (1989). Uncommon findings.

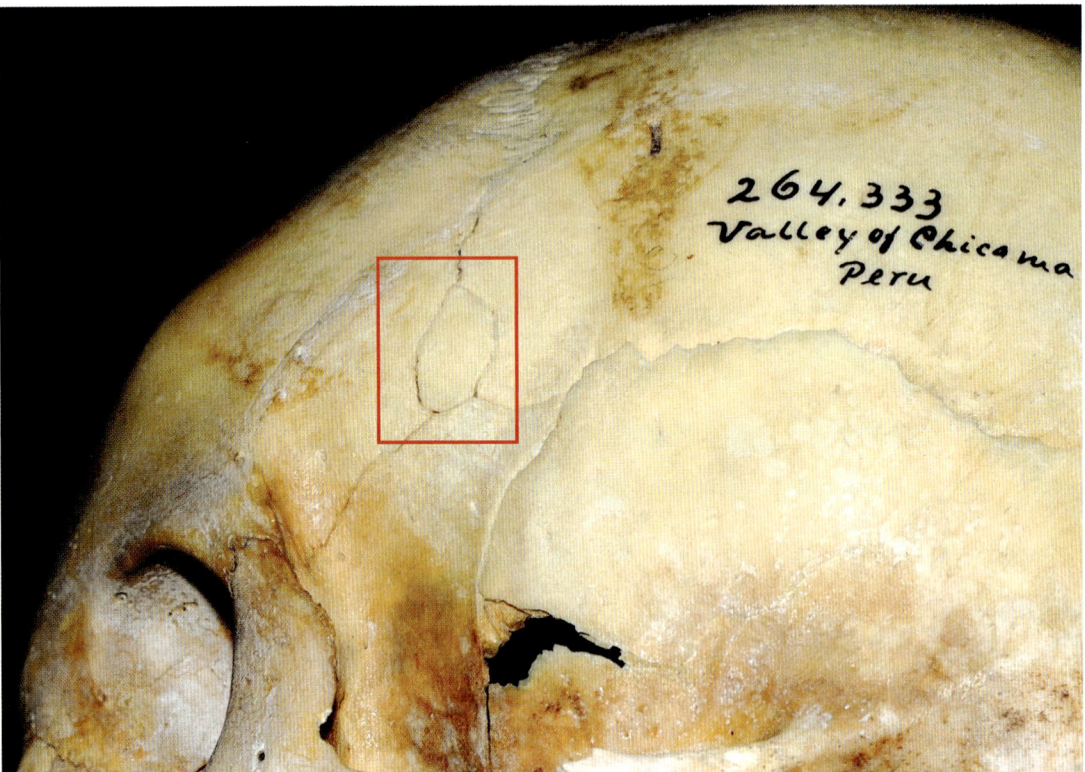

Figure 213. Coronal ossicle positioned low along the coronal suture (rectangle), immediately superior to the left sphenoid bone, in an adult ancient Peruvian skull (SI 264333). An epipteric bone would be positioned more posteriorly. Uncommon finding. Cf. Hauser and DeStefano (1989).

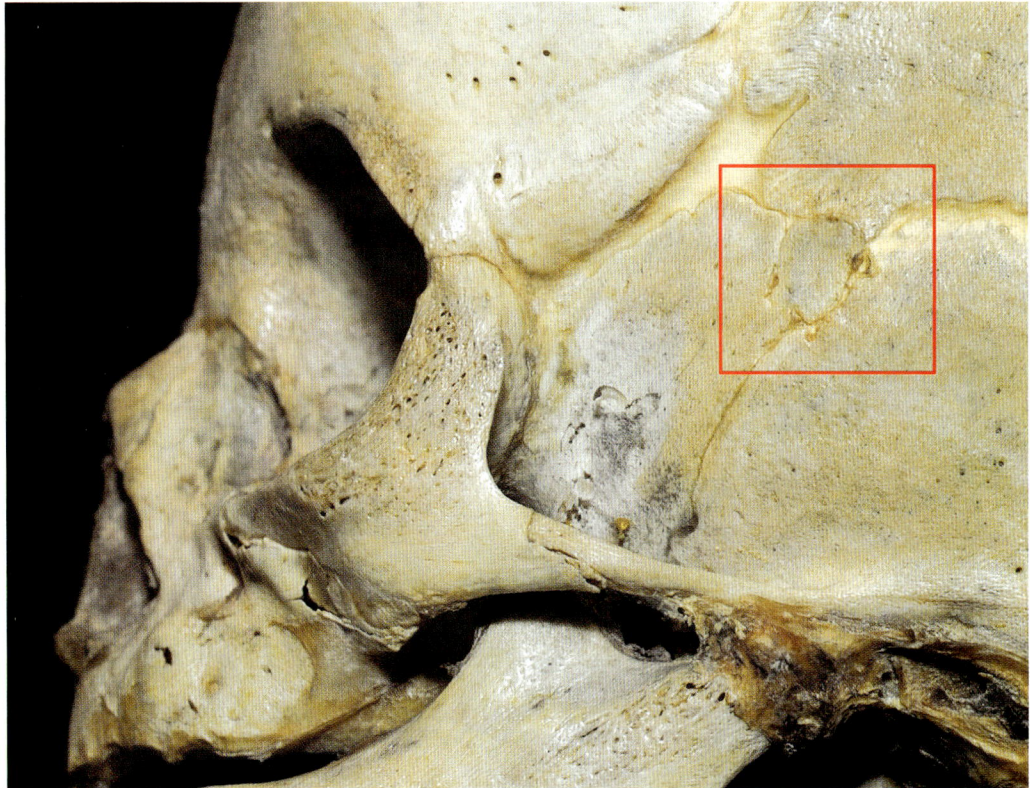

Figure 214. Small epipteric bone/ossicle (square) between the sphenoid, parietal and temporal bones in a child (Mütter Museum 17836.35). Common finding.

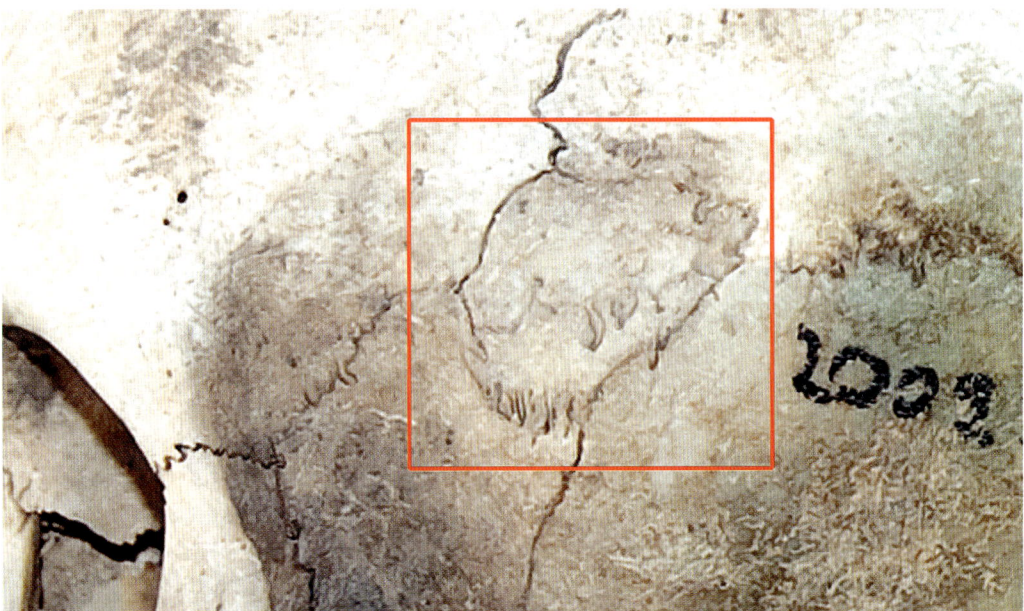

Figure 215. Horizontally divided left epipteric/epiteric bone (square) in a subadult skull (NHMH Soet-Tetelhegy 2003.32.B3). Uncommon finding.

178 *Photographic Regional Atlas of Non-metric Traits*

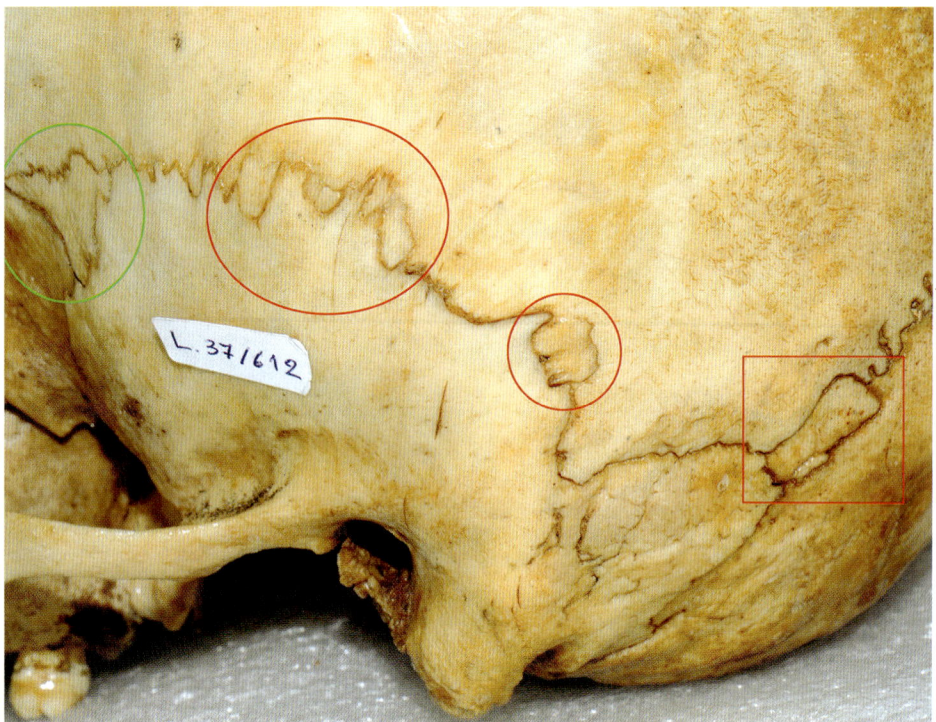

Figure 216. Multiple squamosal ossicles (red circles), asterionic ossicle (square) and an epipteric bone (green circle) in an adult Thai skull (KKU). Common findings. Cf. Sutton (1884); Hauser and DeStefano (1989).

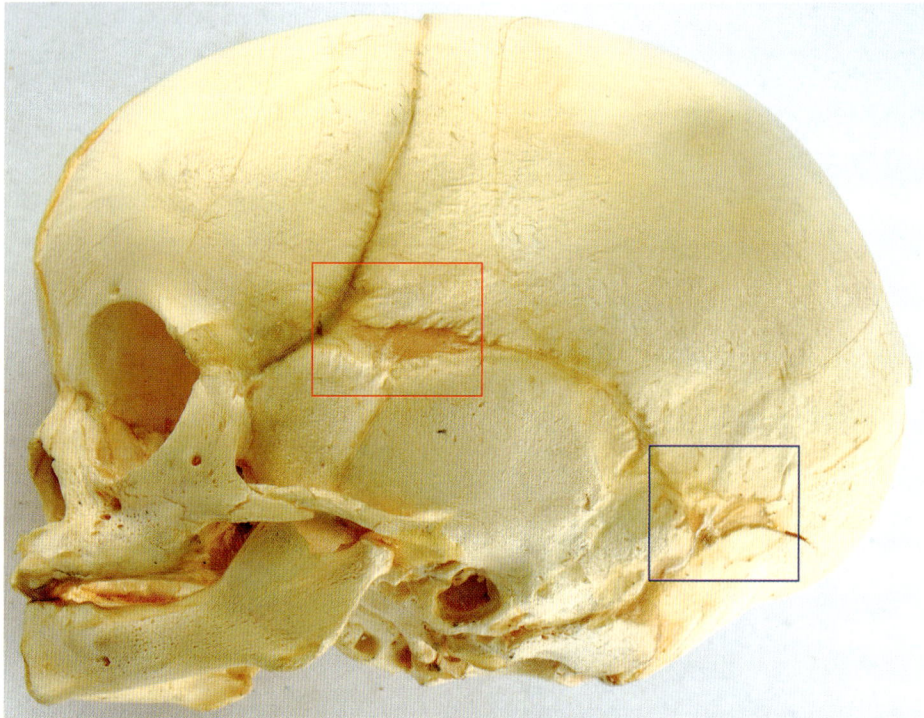

Figure 217. Typical anatomy of an Asian fetal cranium (KKU). Note the anterolateral (red rectangle) and posterolateral (blue rectangle) fontanelles.

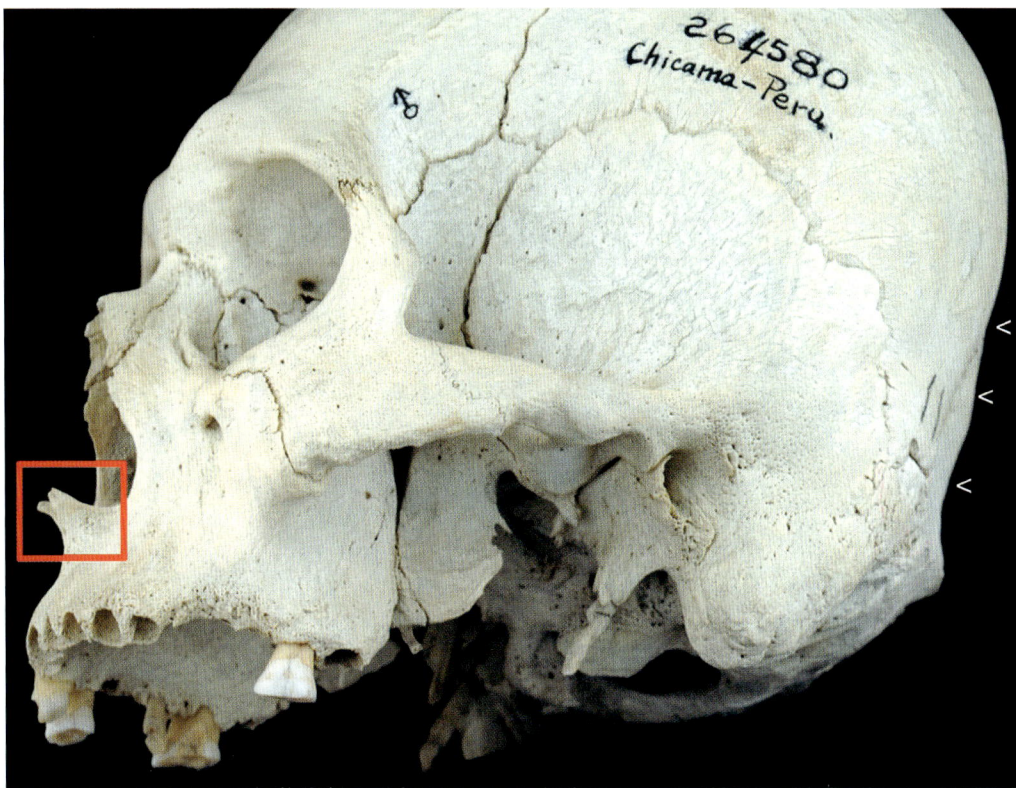

Figure 218. Artificial cranial modification or deformation (resulting in brachycephaly in this individual), prominent anterior nasal spine (square) and a flattened occipital region (<) in an adult ancient Peruvian male (SI 264580). The morphology and frequency of flattened occipital bones, which is often seen in Asian individuals, is worthy of research as a possible ancestry trait. Common findings.

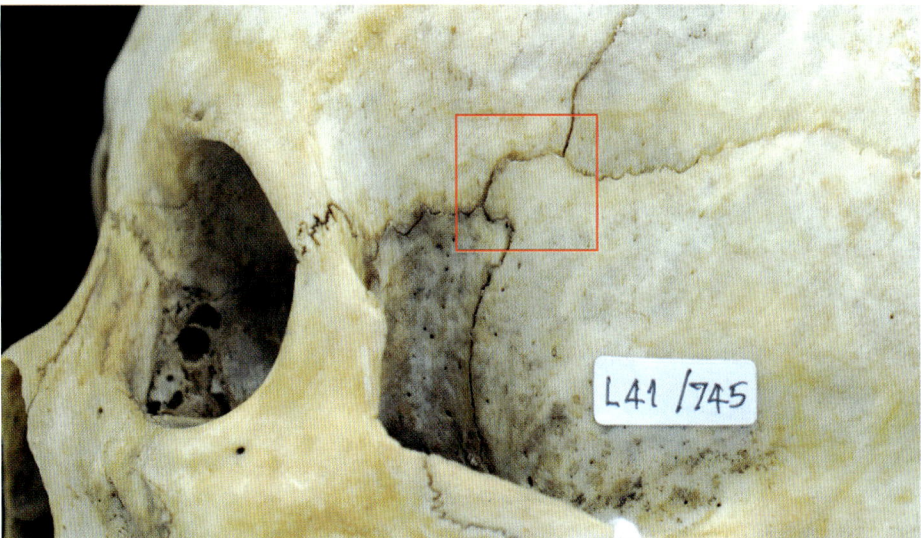

Figure 219. Frontotemporal articulation (square) in a Thai adult skull (KKU). This is an uncommon to common variant. The frontal bone usually articulates with the parietal and sphenoidal bones, not the temporal bone. Ilknur et al. (2009) found 2 of 44 skulls (4.5%) with frontotemporal articulation and Saheb et al. (2011) found this feature in 17.35% of adult Indian skulls. The frequency of this trait varies greatly by group examined. Cf. Bauer (1915); Hauser and DeStefano (1989).

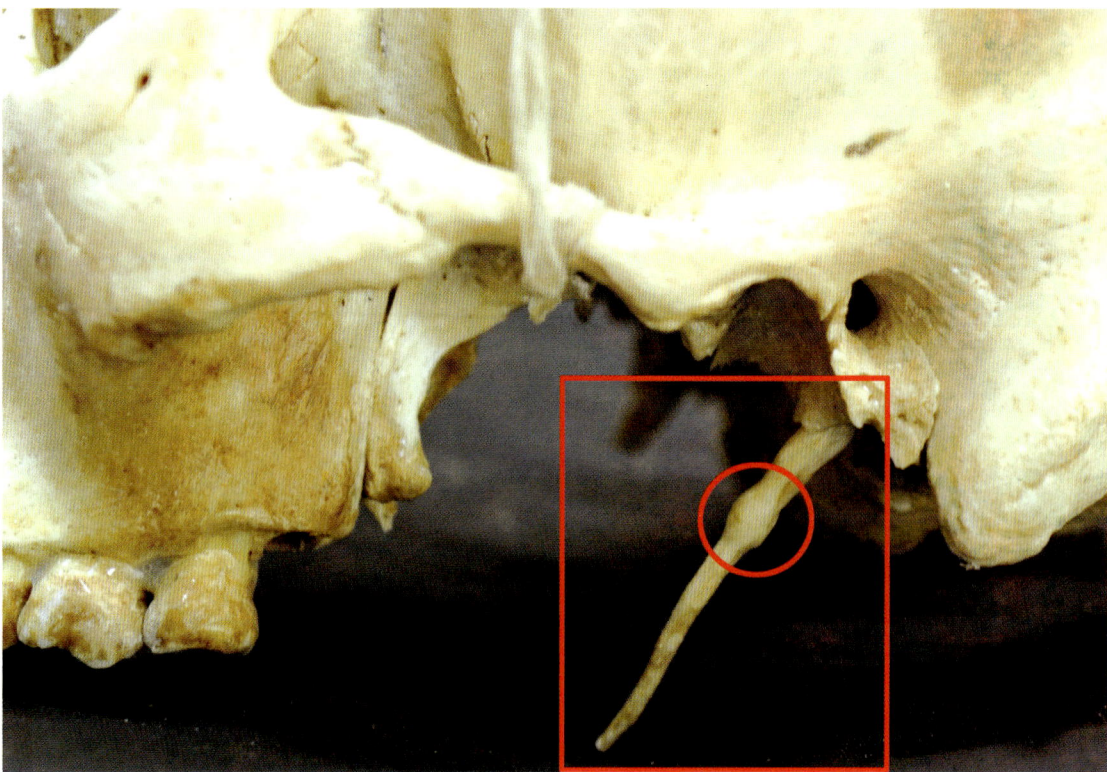

Figure 220. Elongated ossified styloid process (rectangle), often known as Eagle's syndrome (when longer than 30 mm) in an adult Thai male (KKU). Note the "knee joint" (circle) representing the connection of the styloid process (bone, the stylohyal portion) with the calcified stylohyoid ligament (Piagkou et al. 2009). Correll et al. (1979) conducted a large panoramic radiographic study of patients and found 18.2% of 1,771 individuals with an elongated styloid process. Asymptomatic elongated styloid processes have been reported to attain a length of 140 mm (Kubikova and Varga 2009) and develop as a result of increased calcium salts being deposited into the ligaments and processes (Unlu et al. 2008). Elongated processes tend to be more common in older individuals and women, may be bilateral or unilateral, vary greatly in length and shape, and often do not result in pain or discomfort. Thus, they do not develop into "Eagle syndrome," also known as "stylalgia." Uncommon to common finding. Cf. Eagle (1937, 1948); Kubikova and Varga (2009); Naik and Naik (2011); Prabhu et al. (2007); Ramadan et al. (2007); Gözil et al. (2001); Yaczi et al. (2008).

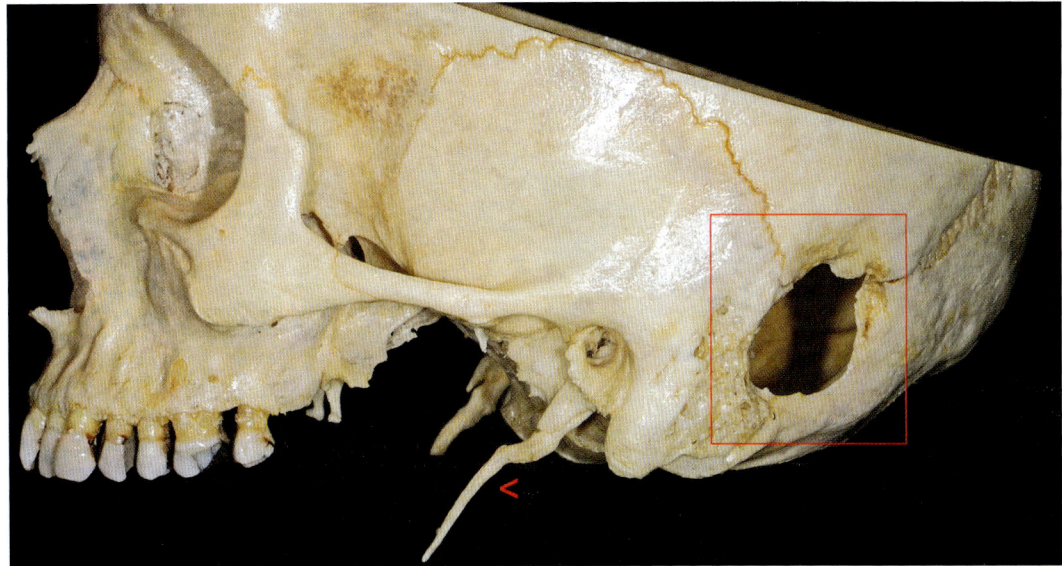

Figure 221. Segmented left styloid process (<) measuring 37 mm from the base of the process to its tip and healed craniotomy (square) in an elderly Japanese male (JABSOM 856). Cf. Yaczi et al. (2008).

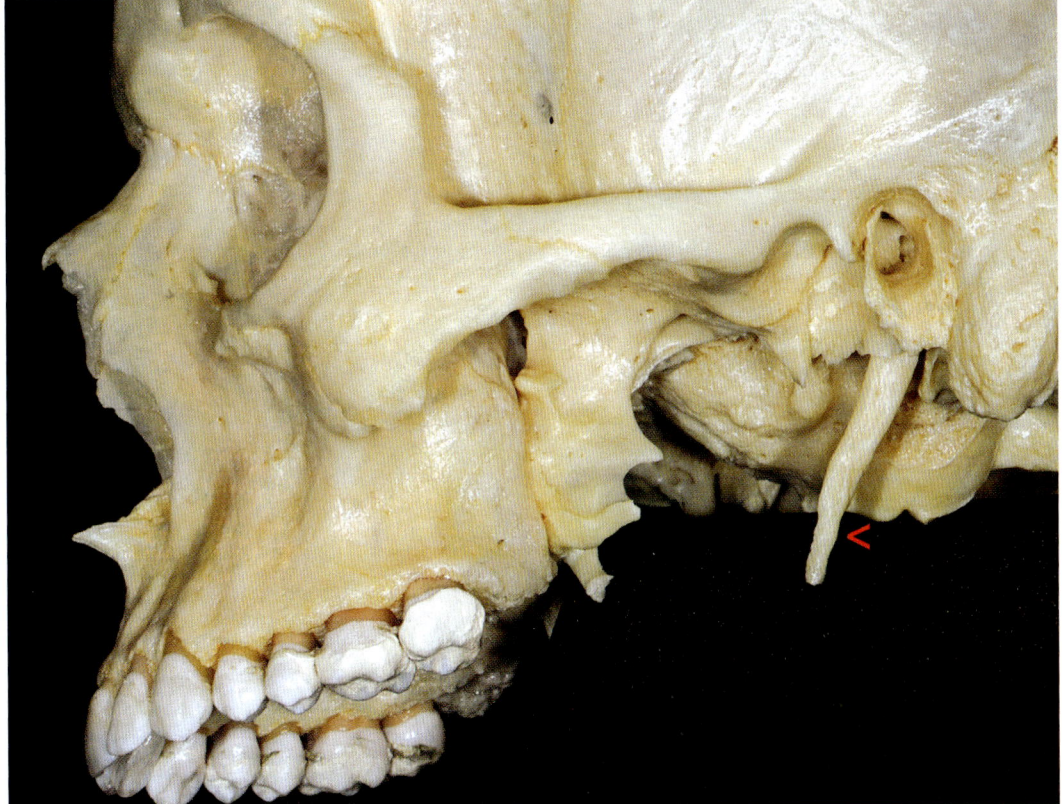

Figure 222. Typical non-segmented left styloid process (<) in a 35-year-old White male (JABSOM 1022).

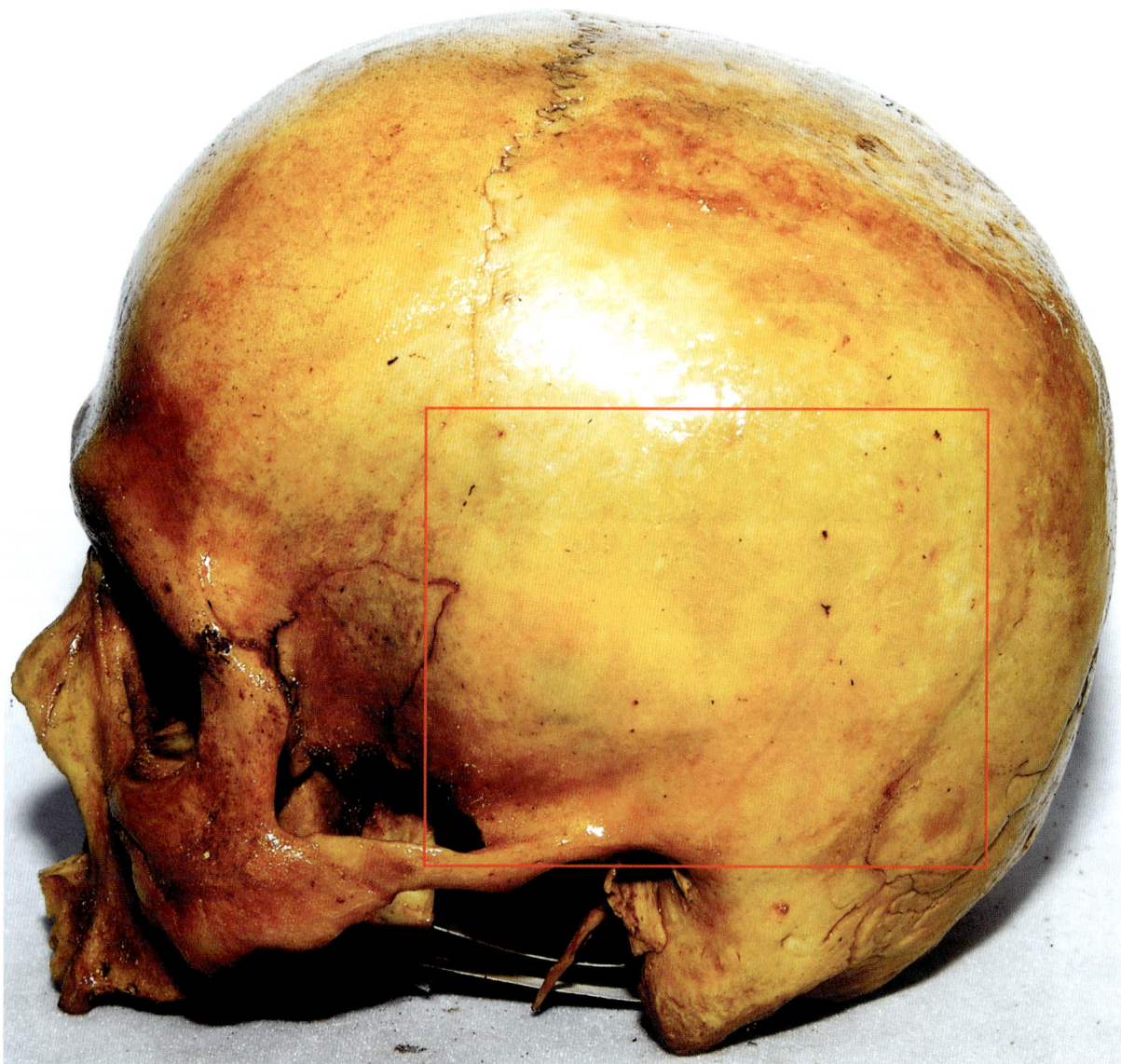

Figure 223. Complete obliteration of the squamosal suture (rectangle) in an adult Thai male skull (KKU). Note that the shape of the cranium is normocephaly, indicating that obliteration of the squamosal in this individual did not occur prematurely in the subadult years, but likely as a result of old age. Regardless of the person's age, complete obliteration of this suture as in this individual is unusual or rare. Lockhart et al. (1965) report this suture as obliterating at 80+ years of age.

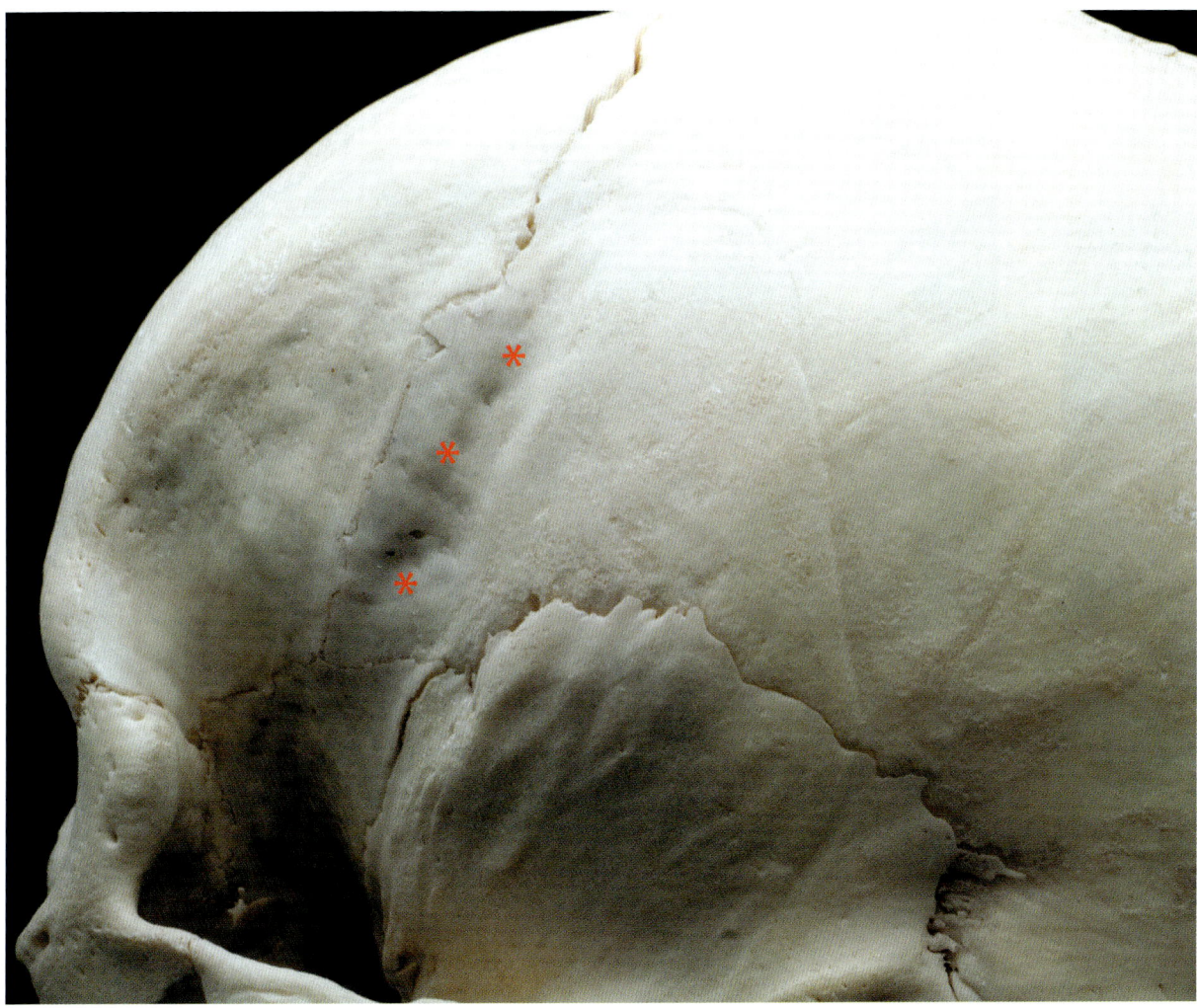

Figure 224. Sphenotemporal sulcus (*) of Gustav Schwalbe (CSC018), a feature reportedly present in about 50% of human skulls; Stibbe (1929) describes this sulcus as corresponding to the elevation along the posterior border of the lesser wing of the sphenoid bone.

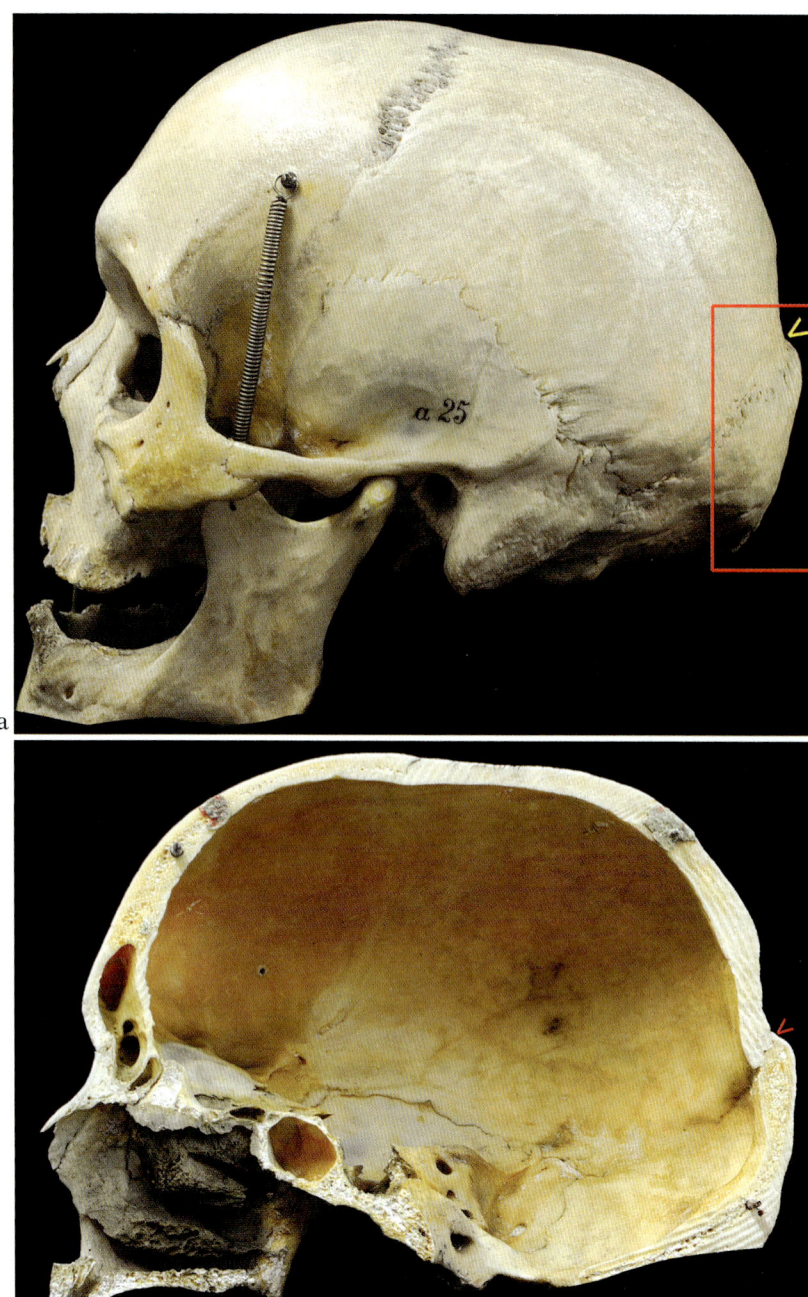

Figure 225a-b. Occipital bun in an adult male (Tübingen University OSUT 794) without artificial cranial deformation. (a) Lateral view showing an "occipital bun" (rectangle), sometimes referred to as bathrocephaly or "chignon" and a depression superior to the lambdoidal suture (<) in an adult from the 19th century in Germany. (b) Sagittally sectioned view of skull showing the occipital bun inferior to lambdoidal suture (<). Bathrocephaly, a protrusion or posterior bulging of the occipital bone inferior to the lambdoidal suture reportedly is not a result of premature craniosynostosis, but may result from a breech position in utero (Graham 2006), or a persistent Mendosal suture (Davanzo et al. 2014; Gallagher et al. 2013). Freyschmidt et al. (2002) attribute this normal variant to excessive growth of the lambdoidal suture. The authors have noted that some individuals with an occipital bun have an unusually high number of lambdoidal ossicles and postbregmatic depression. See Gunz and Harvati (2007 and 2011) for a discussion of "chignon" morphology and "hemibun" associated with the relative position of the cranial base.

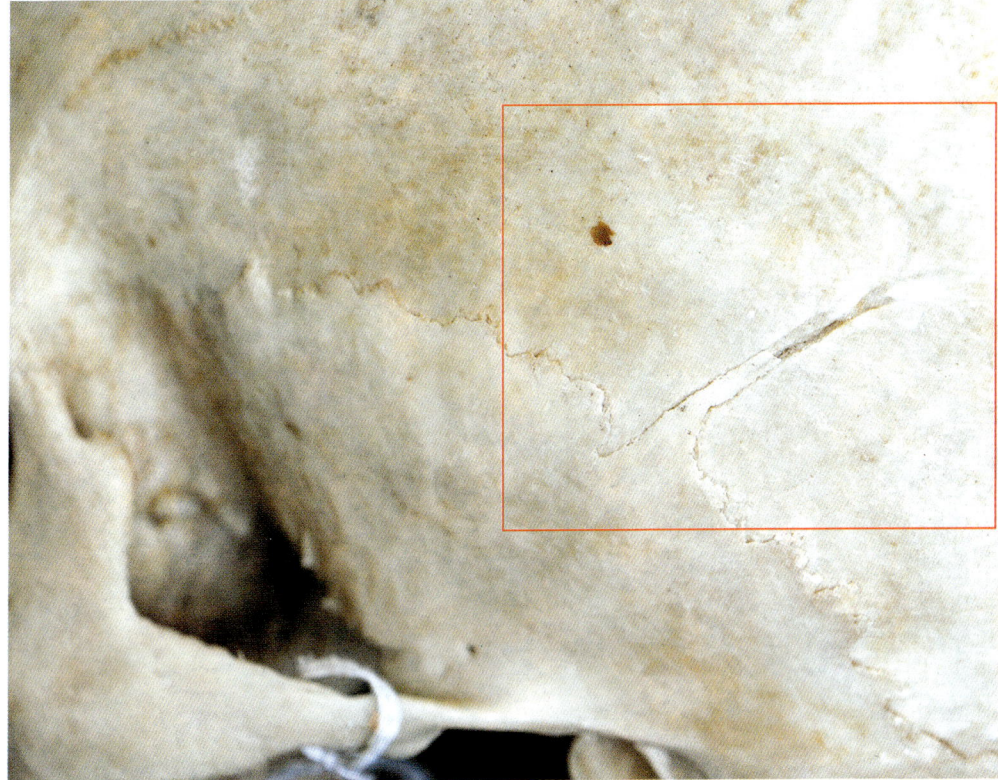

Figure 226. Parietal extension of the squamosal (square) that likely transmitted a vessel (KKU).

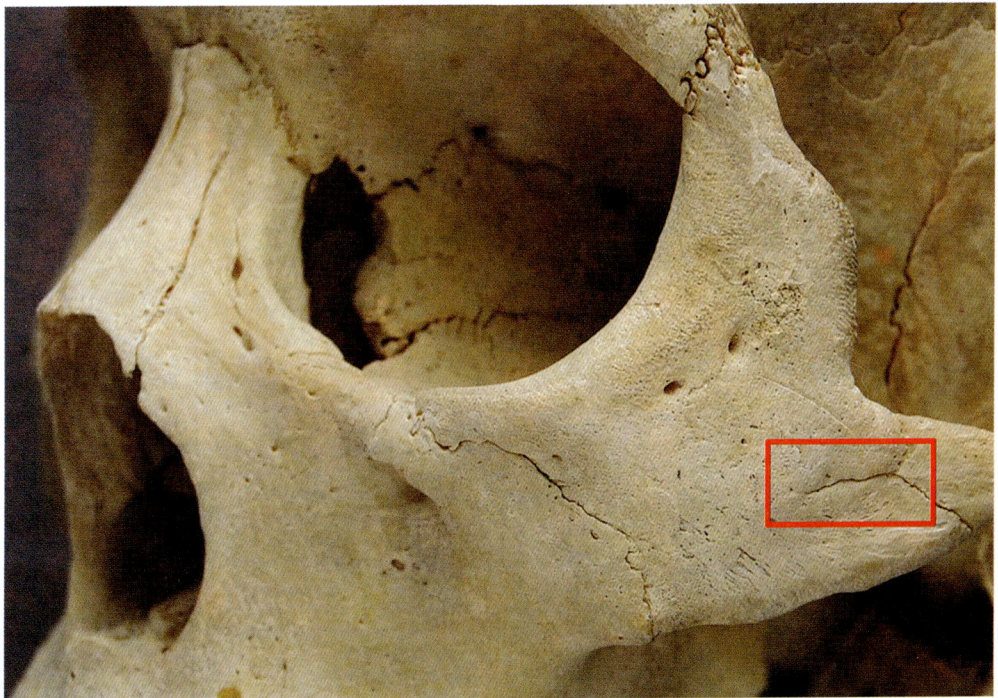

Figure 227. Trace left os Japonicum (rectangle).

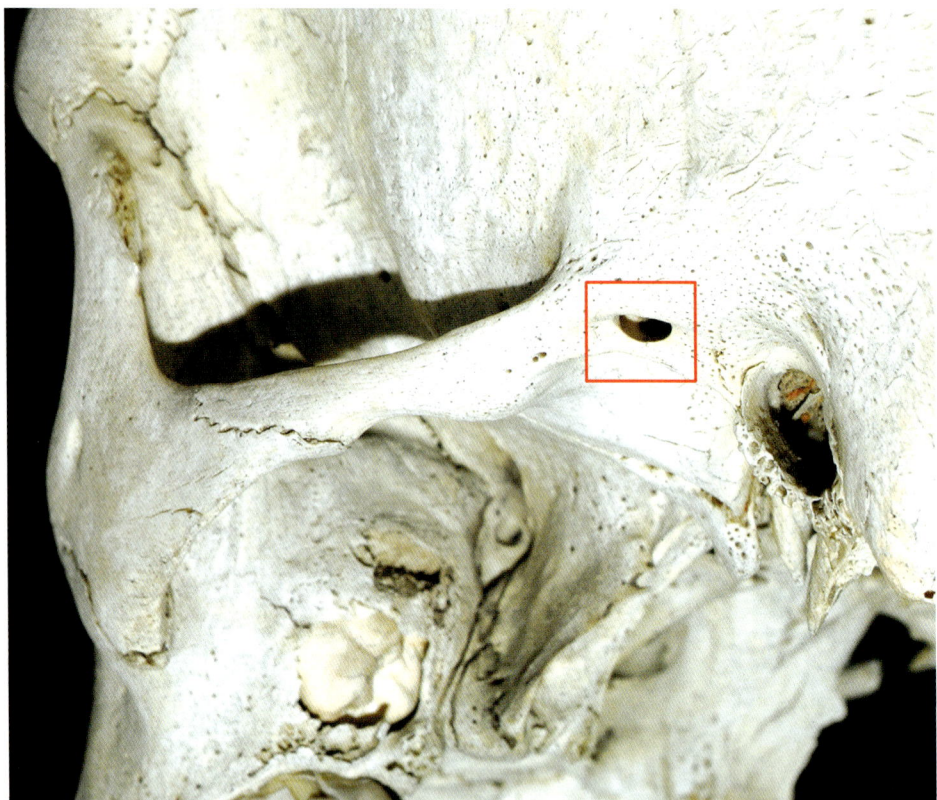

Figure 228. Unusually large postglenoid foramen in a child – this foramen does not appear to be pathological or the result of infection.

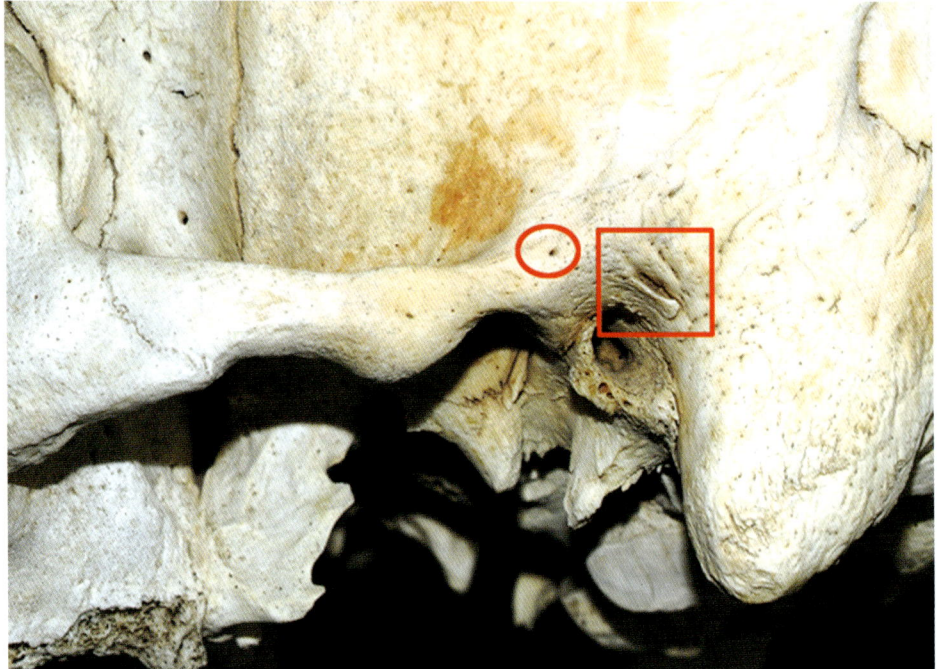

Figure 229. Small supraglenoid foramen (circle) and suprameatal pit (square) in an adult ancient Peruvian (SI).

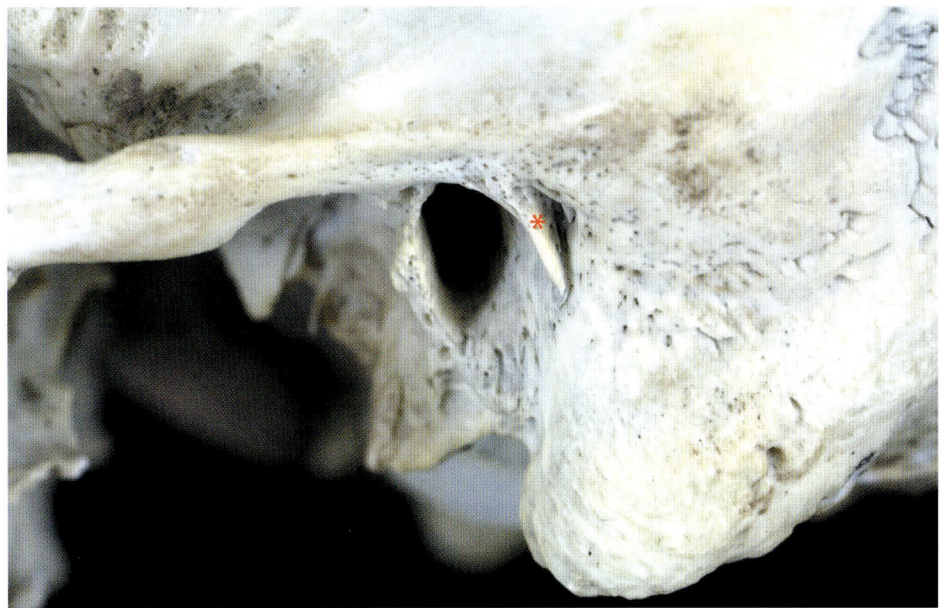

Figure 230. Large spine of Henle (*) (CIL).

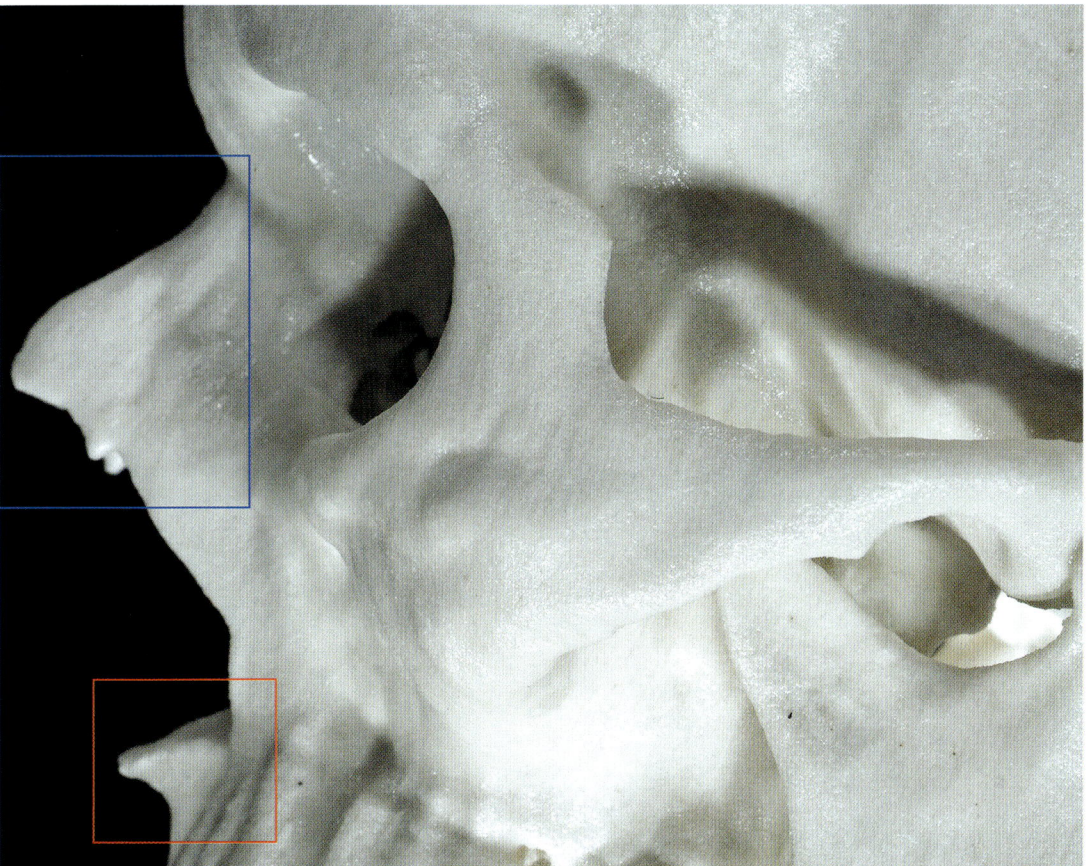

Figure 231. Large anterior nasal spine (red square) and overhanging nasal bones (blue rectangle) in a skull replica of an adult White male (RWM collection). See Hefner (2015) for more on morphoscopic traits representative of ancestry.

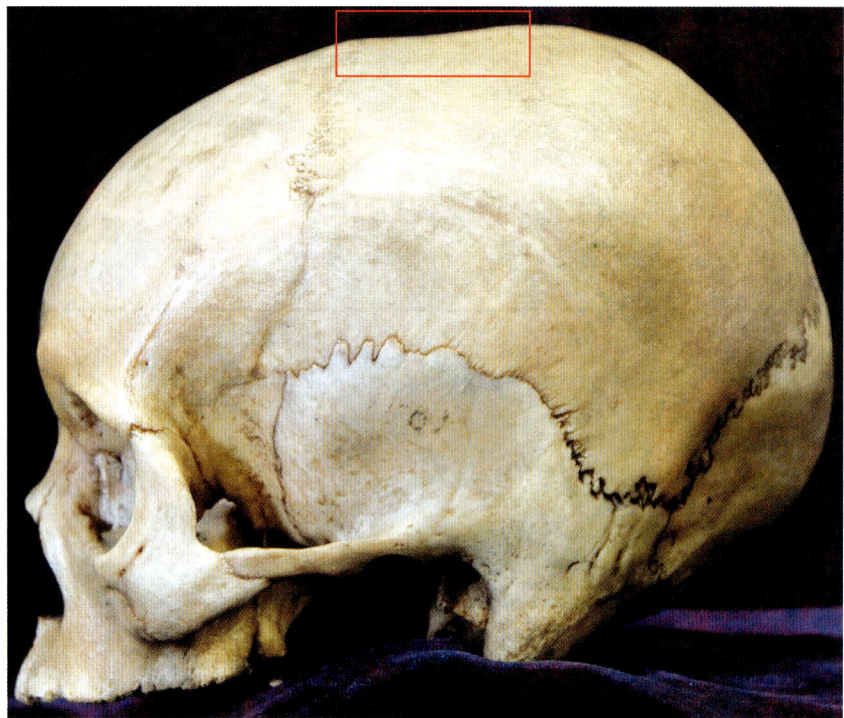

Figure 232. Post-bregmatic depression (rectangle) in a 78-year-old Black female (SI Terry1501). This morphoscopic trait (common finding) is usually considered a racial feature of individuals of Black/African American ancestry, but is sometimes found in Asians. Note the "wavy" squamosal suture (uncommon finding).

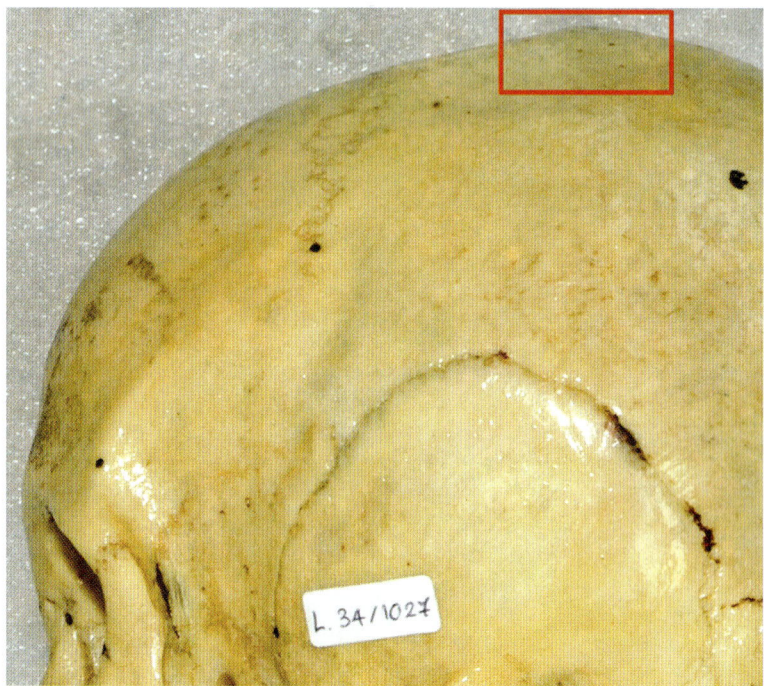

Figure 233. Subtle protrusion of the ectocranium (rectangle) in an elderly Thai due to erosion by arachnoid granulations (KKU L 34/1027).

Chapter 4

SUPERIOR VIEW OF THE SKULL

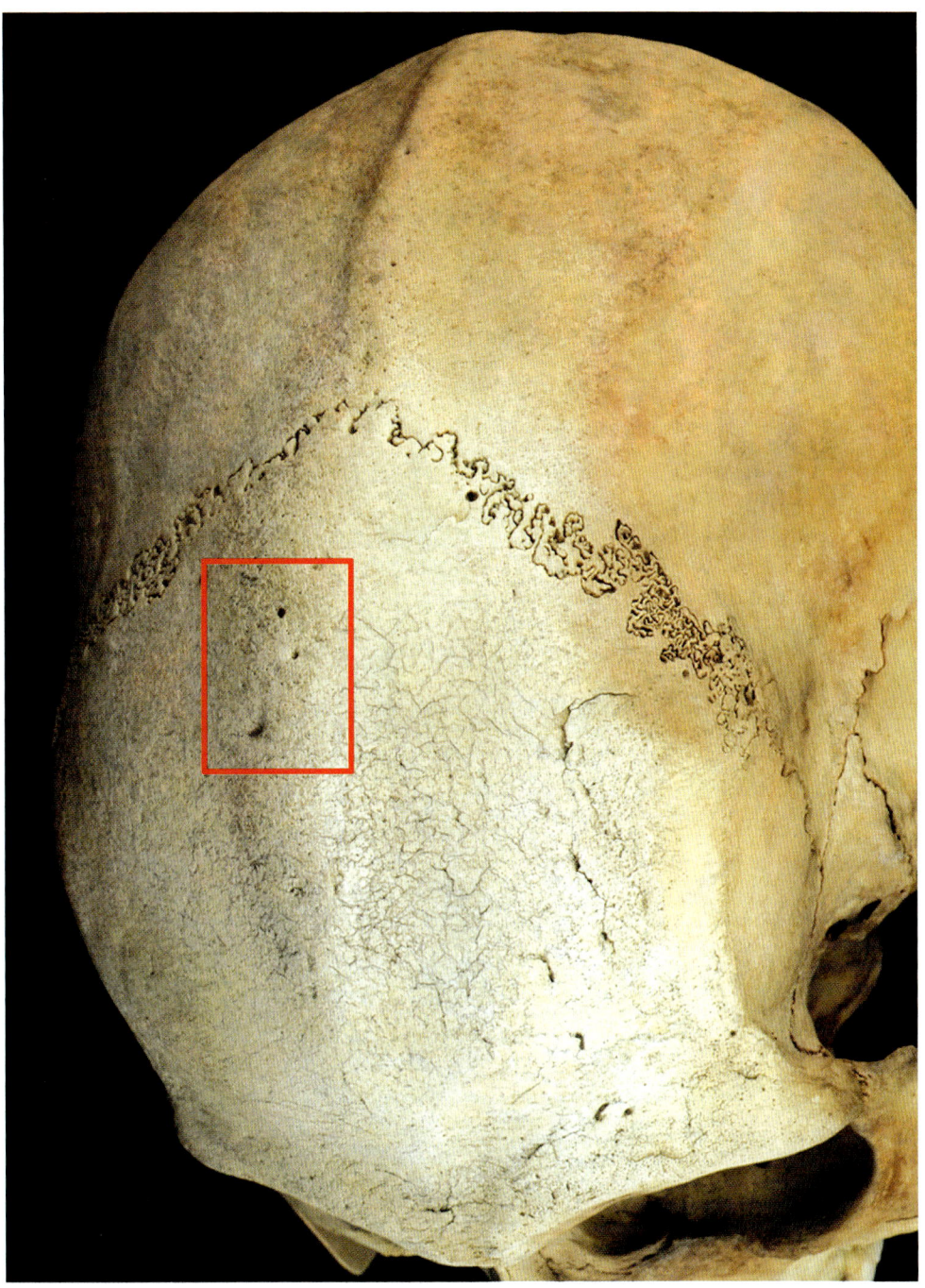

Figure 234. Keeling (and multiple foramina, rectangle) along the metopic (reliqua suturae frontalis) and sagittal sutures in a Peruvian male (SI). Both are uncommon to rare findings. The authors have seen frontal and sagittal keeling in individuals with completely open, unfused sutures, but this condition does not always accompany or reflect premature craniosynostosis.

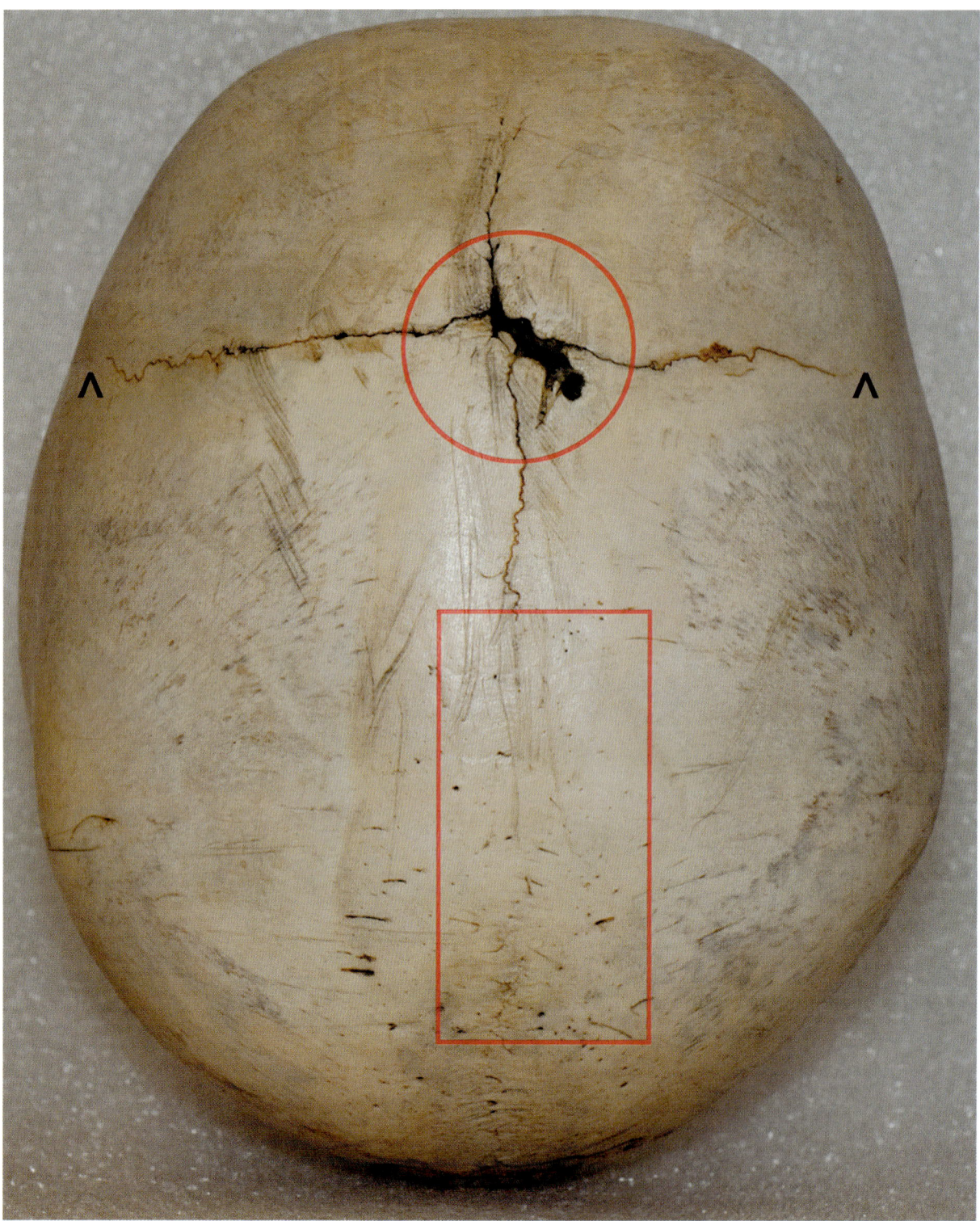

Figure 235. Premature craniosynostosis of the coronal suture (∧), sagittal suture (rectangle) and a remnant of the bregmatic fontanelle in a 2–3-year-old child (Mütter Museum 1006-86). Cf. Schultz (1929); Barclay-Smith (1910) for accessory ossicles in the bregmatic fontanelle.

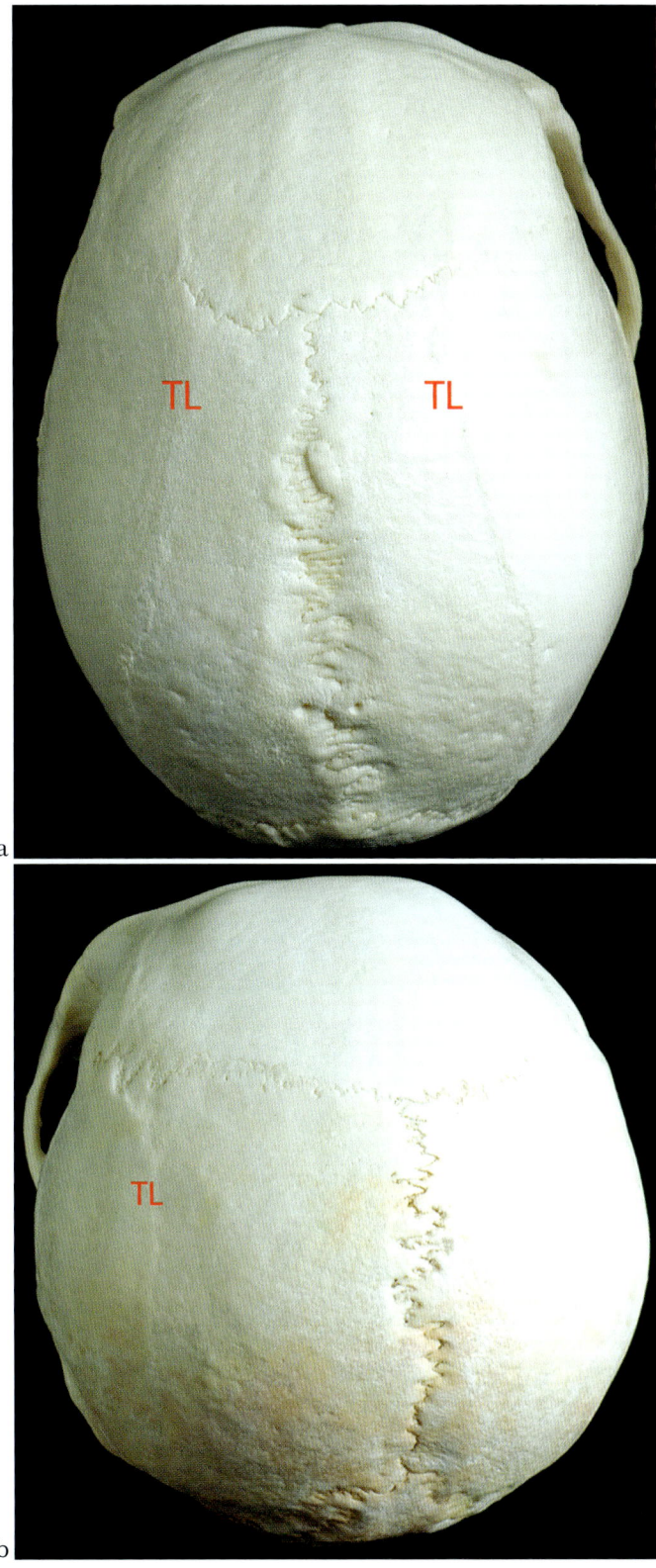

Figure 236a-b. Position of the superior temporal lines (TL) for attachment of the temporalis muscle. (a) Temporalis line positioned near the sagittal suture in a robust adult Asian male skull (CSC DS035). (b) Temporalis line positioned lower in a less robust adult Asian male.

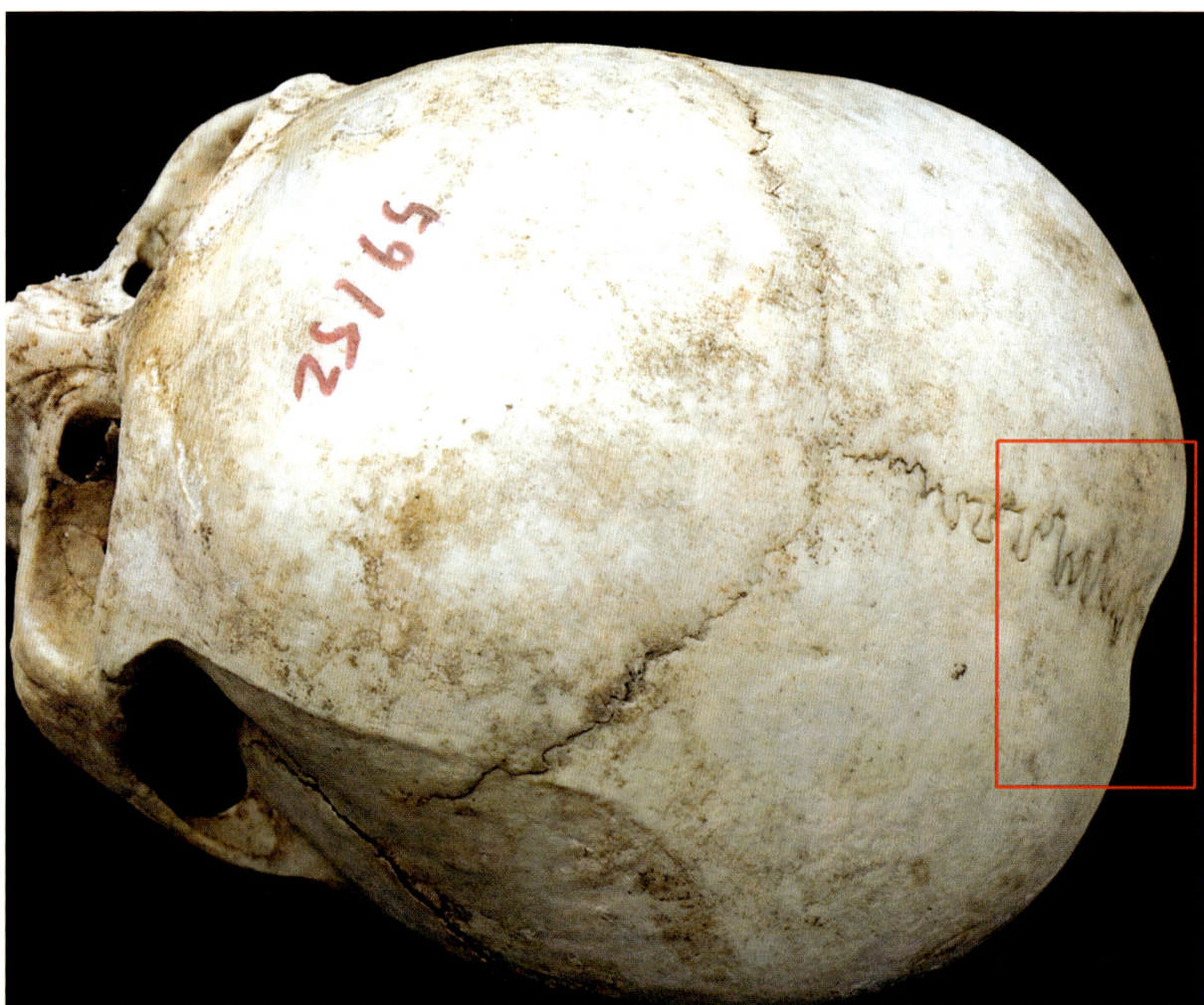

Figure 237. Sagittal/parietal groove (rectangle), usually in the region of Obelion, in an elderly female skull (CMU 60 52). Common finding in some groups, especially elderly individuals and those who have undergone artificial cranial deformation, or premature cranial synostosis.

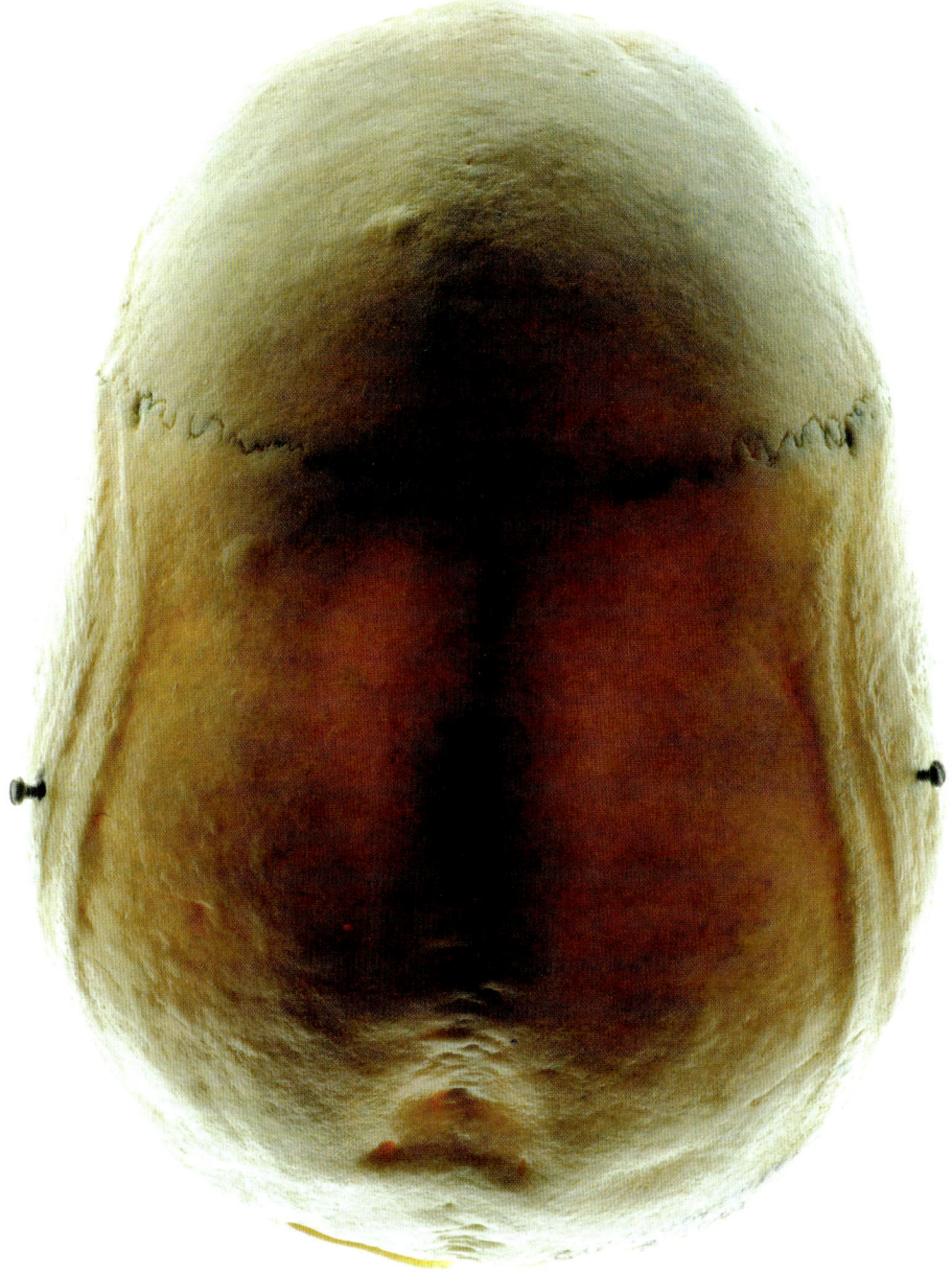

Figure 238. Backlighting of the cranial vault showing thin areas in the frontal and parietal bones, thickened bone along the coronal and sagittal sutures, pronounced temporal bone markings (wavy lines) for attachment of the temporalis muscles and a depression at the Inion in an adult Asian male skull (CSC AC001). Any or all of these features may be found in middle-aged and older individuals. Note the circular depression at Obelion and bilateral parietal foramina.

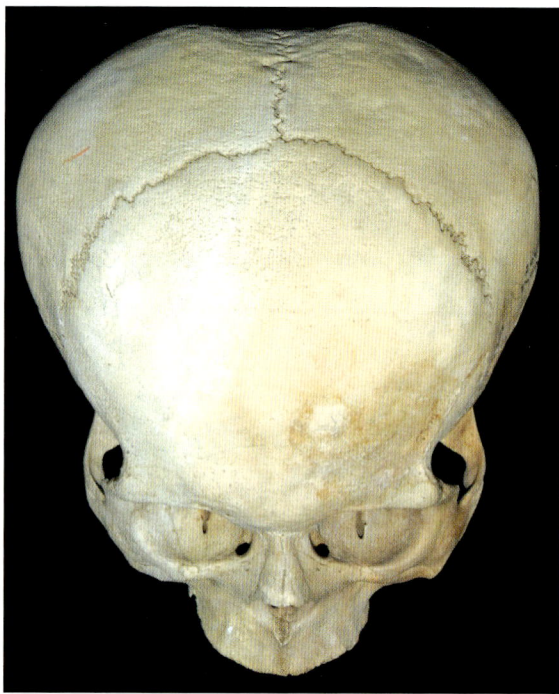

Figure 239. Artificial cranial deformation (fabric wrapping/binding) in an adult ancient Peruvian cranium (SI). Cf. Anton (1989); Dorsey (1897); Ossenberg (1970). Cf. Gottlieb (1978, Van Arsdale and Clark (2012) and Wilczak and Ousley (2009) for discussions of cranial deformation and ossicles.

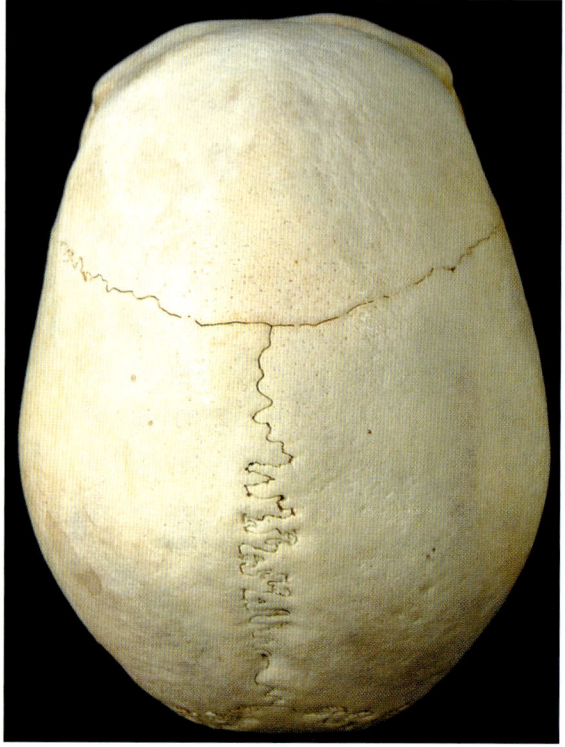

Figure 240. Simple coronal suture and moderately complex sagittal suture (CIL CSC AC021) both of which are typical morphoscopic variants. Cf. Mann et al. (2009); Skrzat and Walocha (2003a, b).

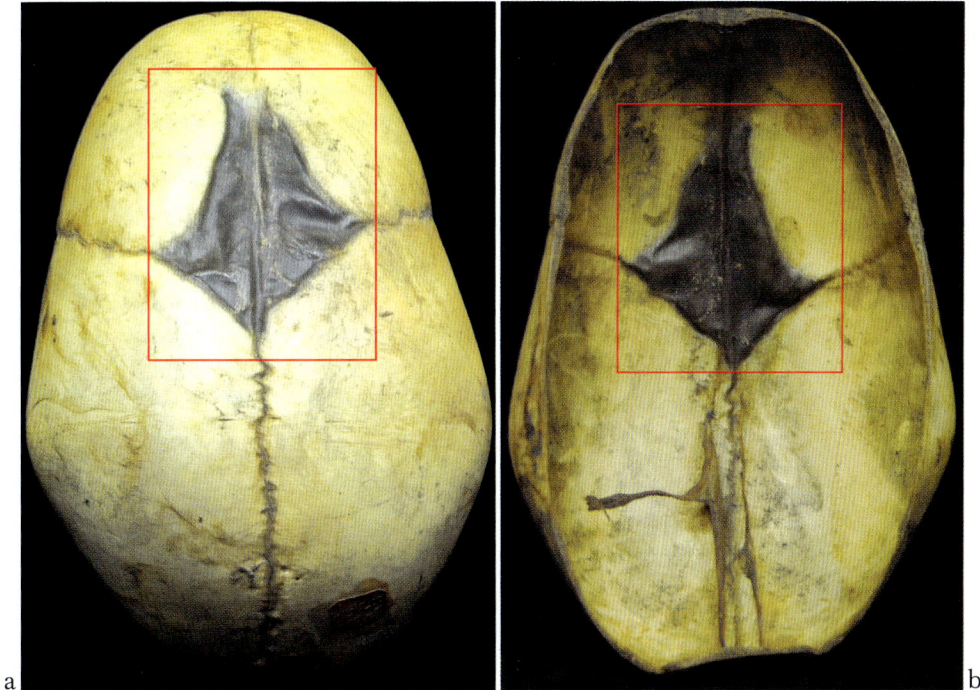

Figure 241a-b. Persistent anterior fontanelle in an adolescent (Mütter Museum 17830.54). (a) Ectocranial and (b) endocranial views showing the fibrous membrane (dura mater) that covers the diamond-shaped fontanelle (rectangle) and protects the brain.

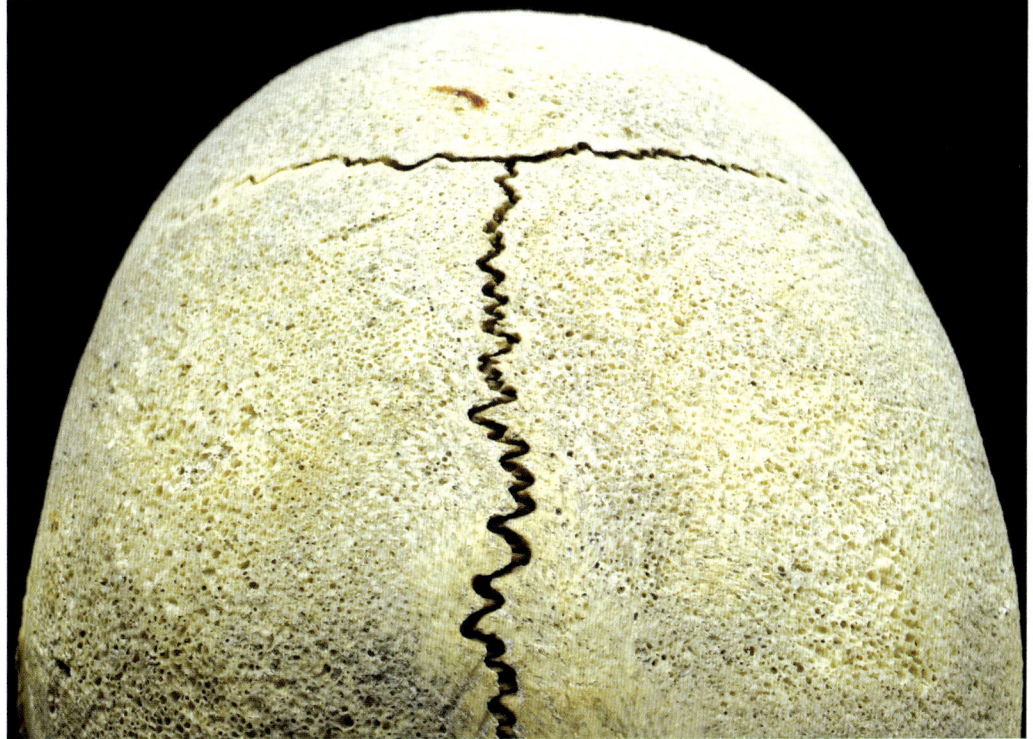

Figure 242. Postmortem removal (cutting) of the external lamina exposing the highly porous diploë that resembles a sponge or pumice (Mütter Museum 1007.06). Normal anatomy.

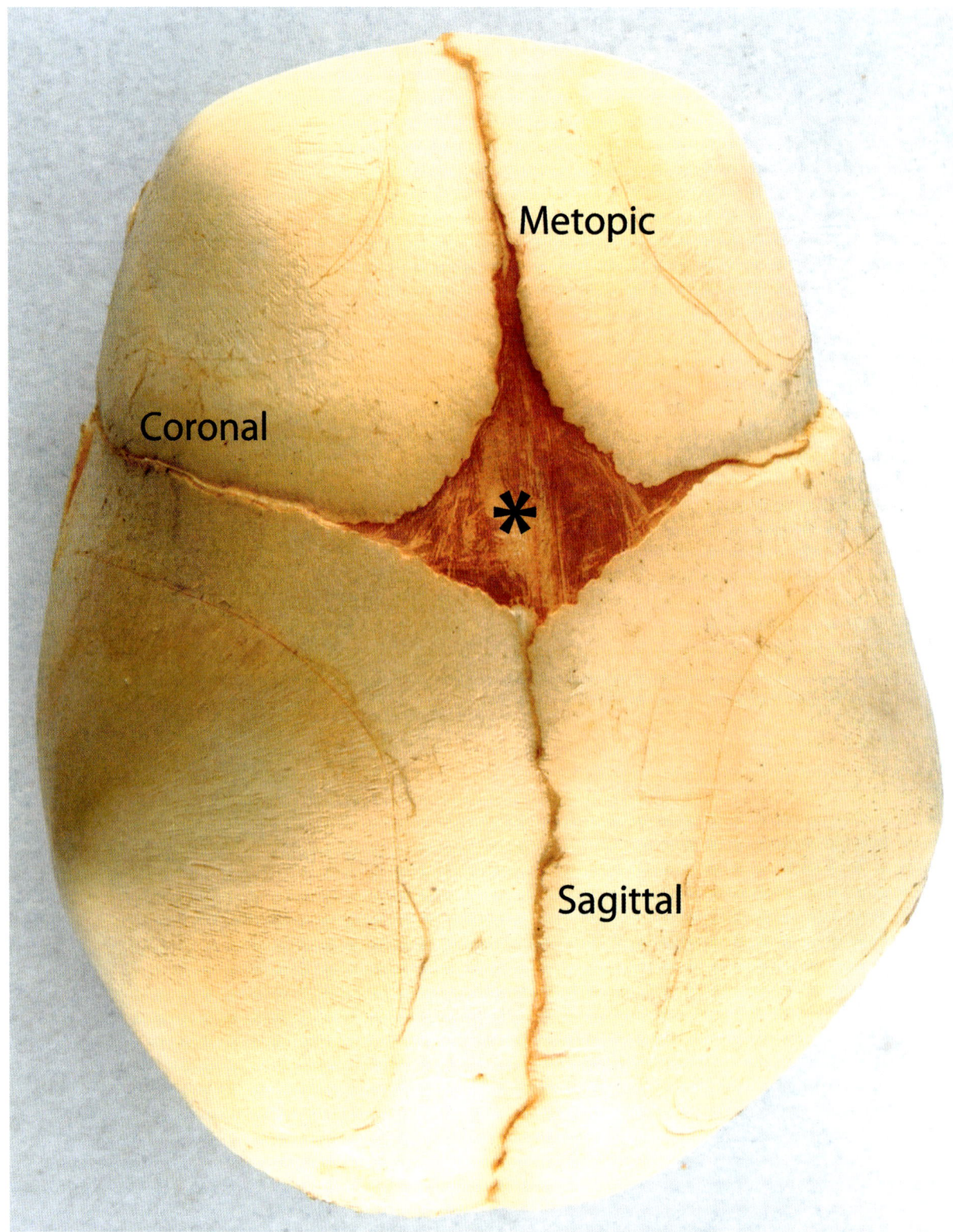

Figure 243. Morphology of the sutures and anterior fontanelle (*) in a newborn skull (CSC Oklahoma).

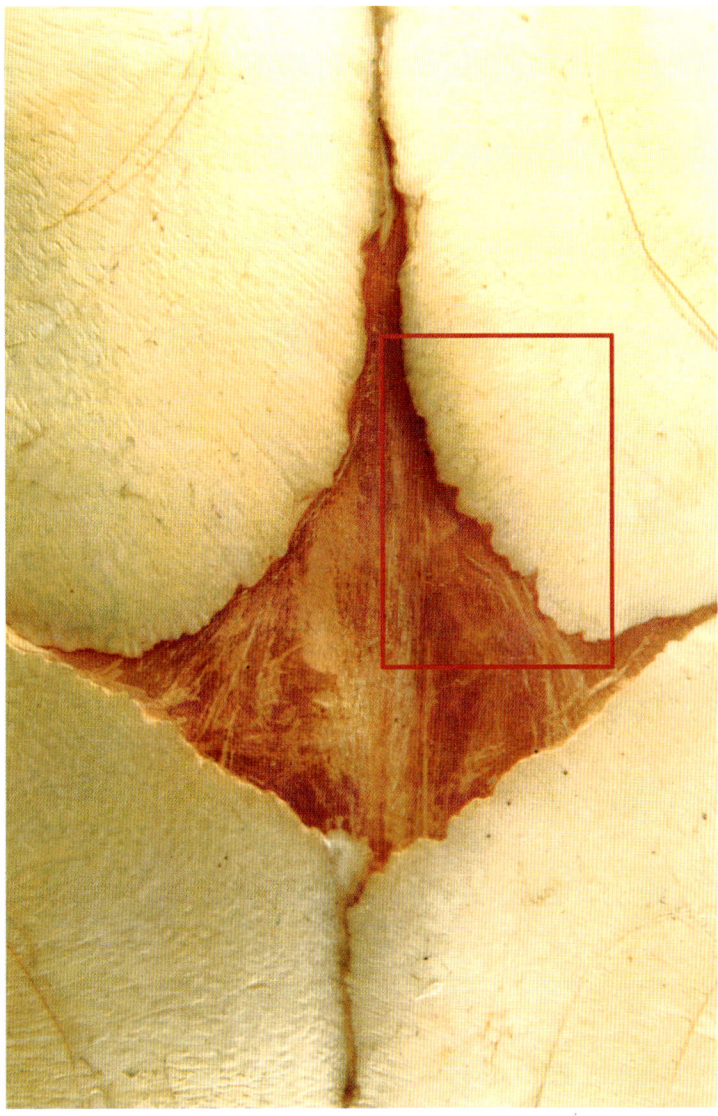

Figure 244. Close-up of the anterior fontanelle showing the dura mater (fibrous membrane) covering the fontanelle (CSC Oklahoma), the intersection of the coronal and sagittal sutures, and the wavy appearance of the interfrontal and coronal sutures in a newborn.

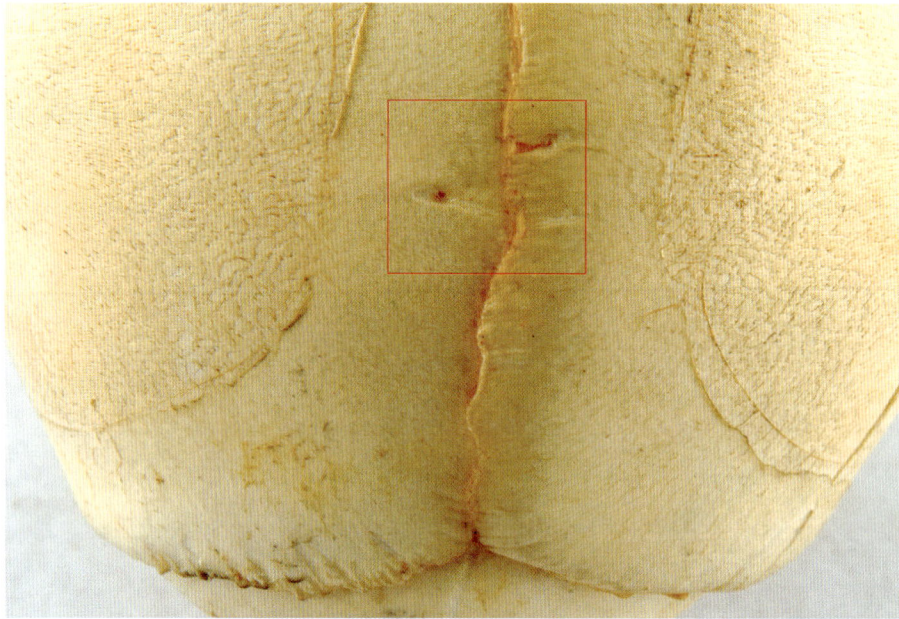

Figure 245. Obelion (square) where one or more parietal foramina may form. Note the adhering transparent fascia for attachment of the temporalis muscle and presence of a left parietal foramen in this cranium of a child. A right foramen may have formed in the right notch, known as the subsagittal suture of Pozzi (Breathnach 1965). Cf. Boyd (1930); Currarino (1976); Mann et al. (2009). See Yoshioka et al. (2006) for photos of vessels entering the parietal foramen.

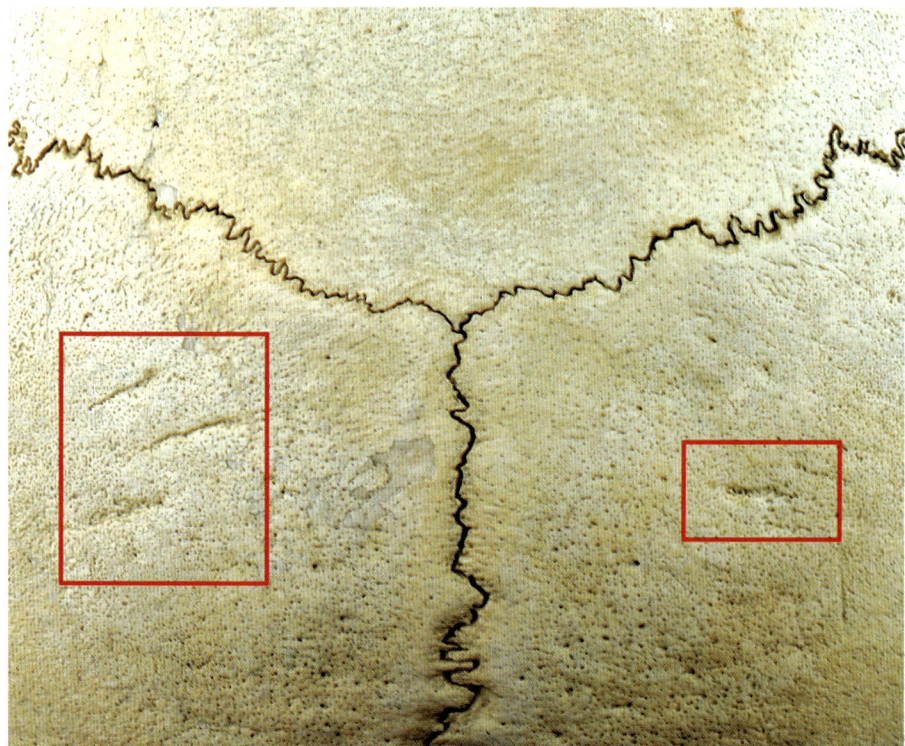

Figure 246. Parietal grooves in a subadult Thai skull (KKU). These grooves, of unknown etiology, can be misinterpreted as trauma to the skull or postmortem damage. Typical anatomical features in subadults and adults.

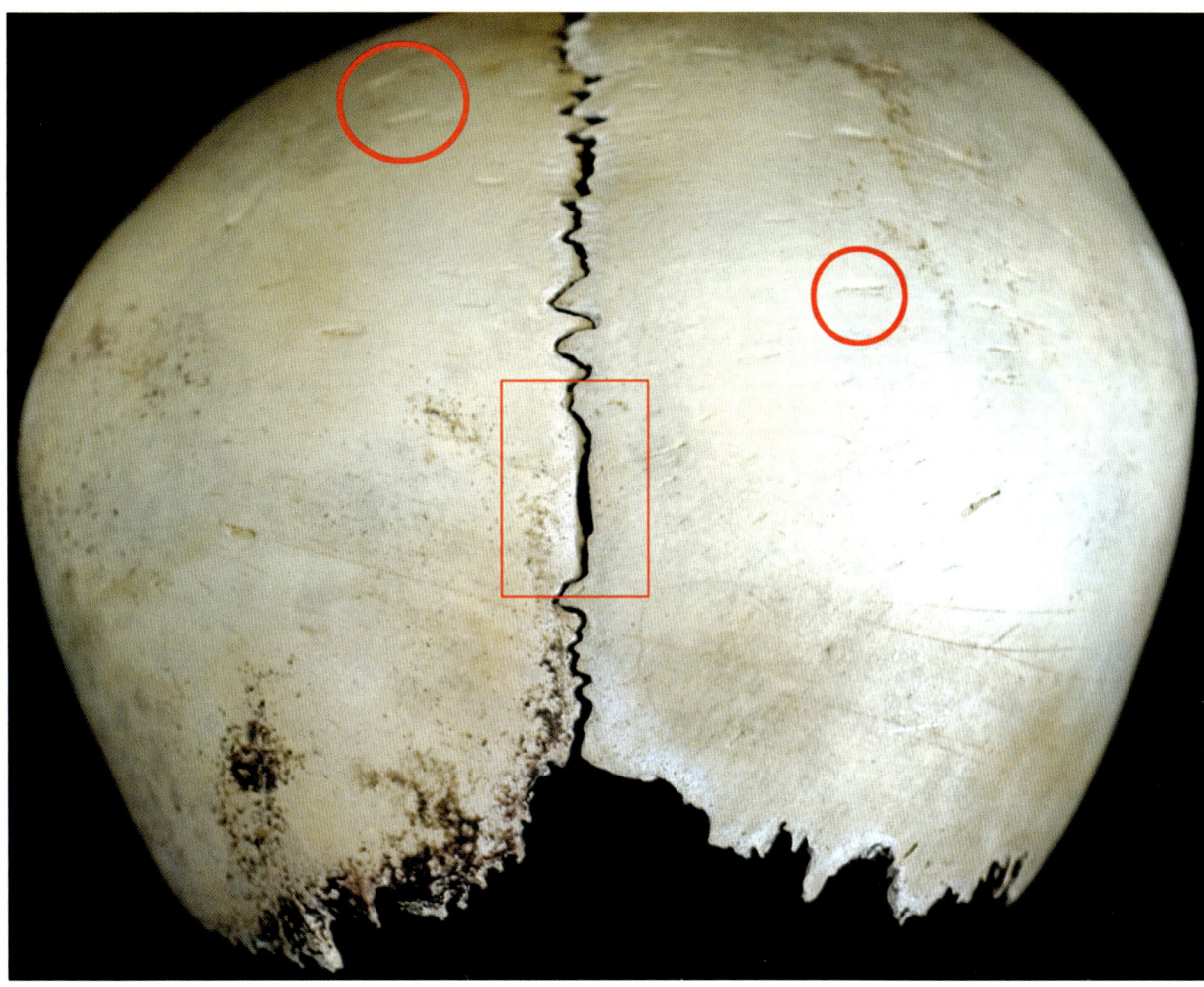

Figure 247. Simple Obelion (rectangle) without parietal foramina and numerous developmental lines/grooves (circles) in the outer table of the parietal bones in a child (SI 228838). These grooves, representing typical anatomical features, form during early childhood and may persist in adults. See Mann et al. (2009).

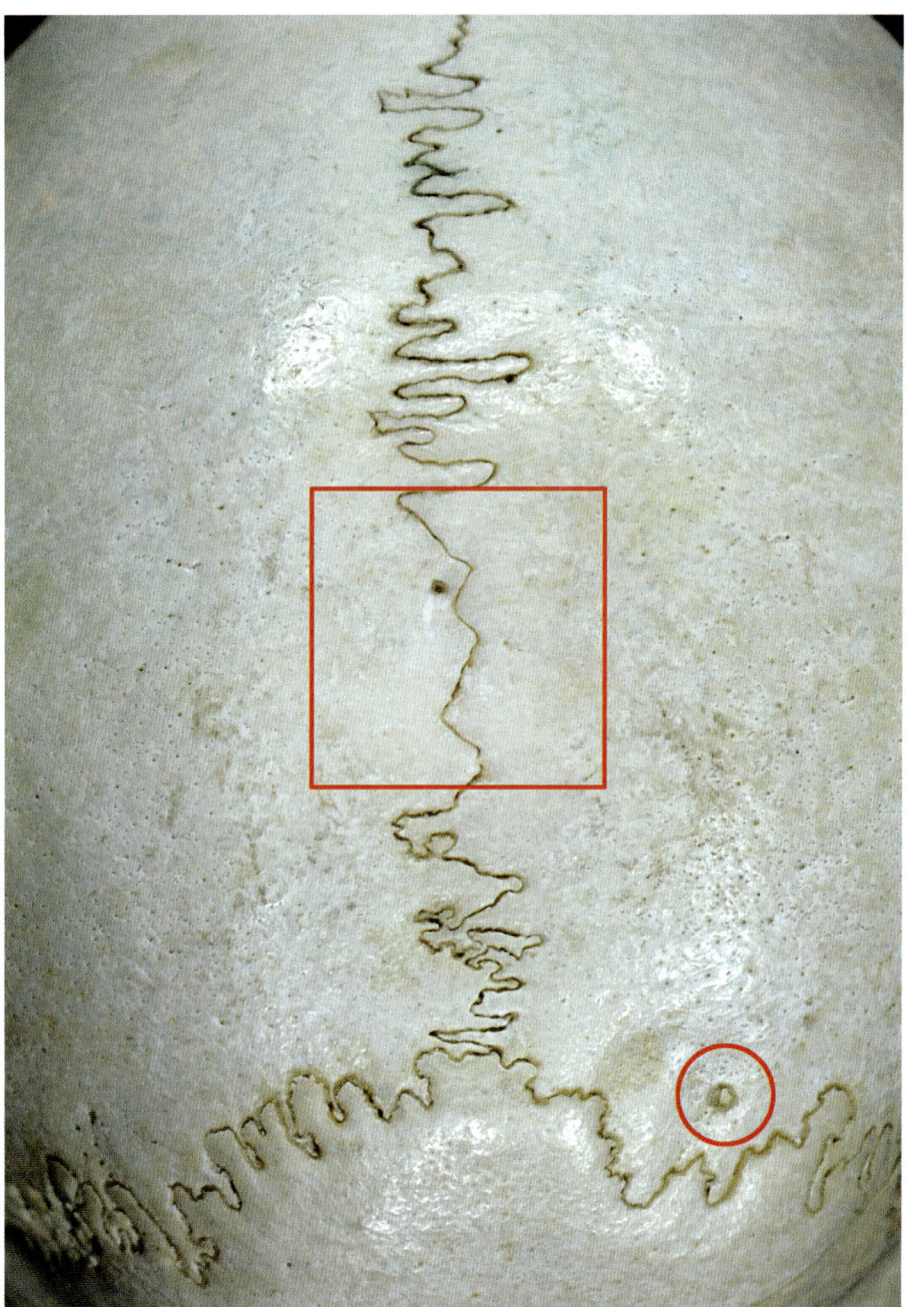

Figure 248. A relatively simple sagittal suture showing Obelion (square) and a single left parietal foramen as well as an unconnected small intercalary bone (bone island/ossicle; circle) superior to the lambdoidal suture (CSC). Obelion, which is the area along the sagittal suture that may contain none, one or several parietal foramina, is named for the Greek symbol Obelos (÷; the dots symbolize the parietal foramina to either side of the sagittal suture) (Dixon 1937). Obelion, with or without a parietal foramen, is almost always the simplest portion of the sagittal suture and first to obliterate along the sagittal suture. Suture morphology normal anatomy and bone island an uncommon finding. Cf. Boyd (1930) concerning the foramen; Mann et al. (2009) for complexity at Obelion.

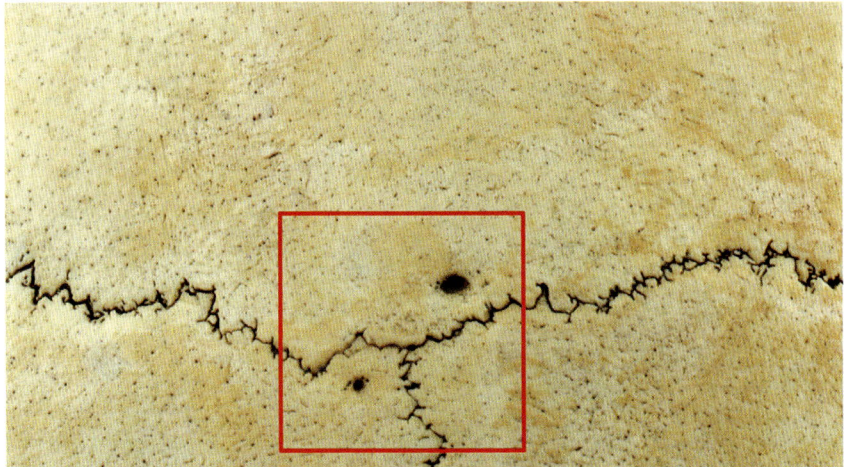

Figure 249. Two foramina near Bregma in a subadult. A large foramen is situated in the frontal bone and smaller one in the left parietal bone (KKU). Foramina in the region of Bregma are uncommon.

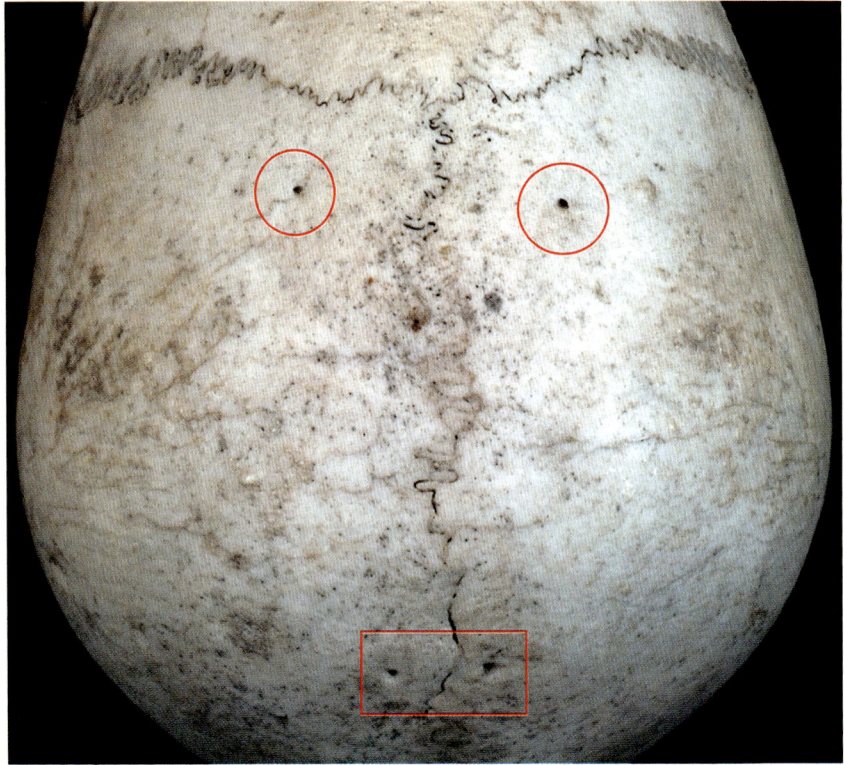

Figure 250. Typical anatomical position of the parietal foramina (rectangle) and "anterior" parietal foramina (circles) in a Black male cranium (SI P244059). Posterior foramina are common findings, while bilateral anterior foramina are common to uncommon. Cf. Boyd (1930) for parietal foramen; Hanihara and Ishida (2001b); Hauser and DeStefano (1989); Mann et al. (2009).

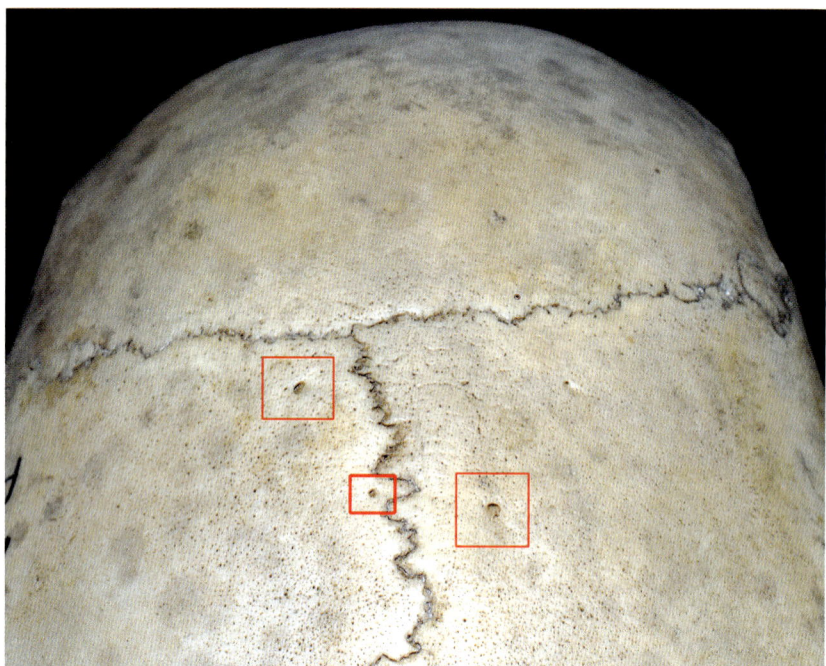

Figure 251. Three anterior parietal foramina (squares) in an adult cranium from Samoa (RV1492).

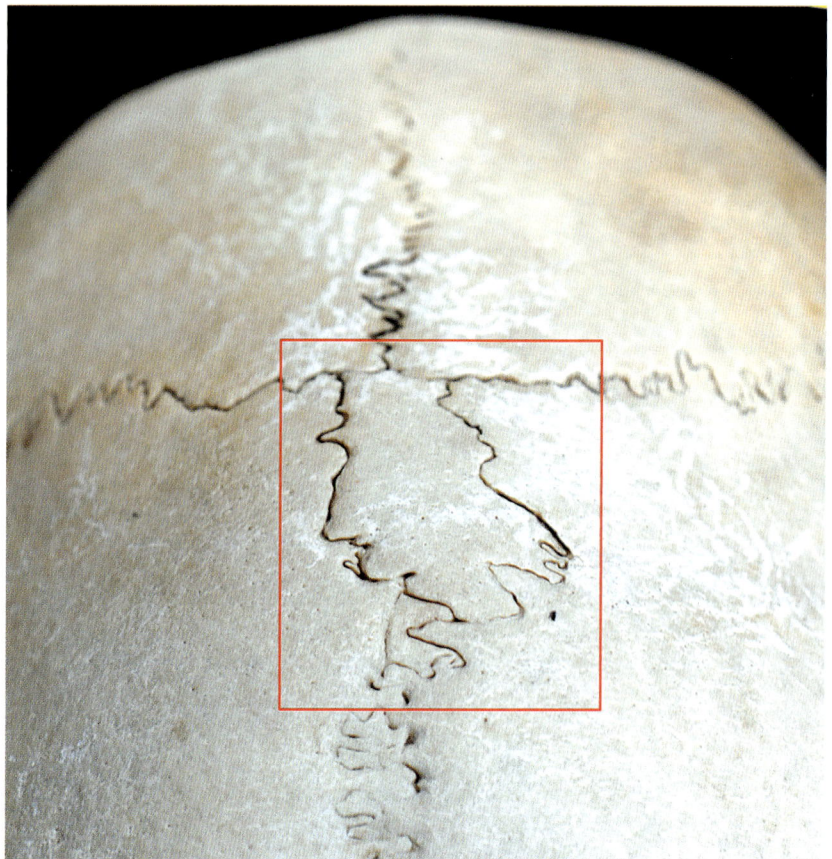

Figure 252. Large Bregmatic bone confined to the parietal bones (UHWO).

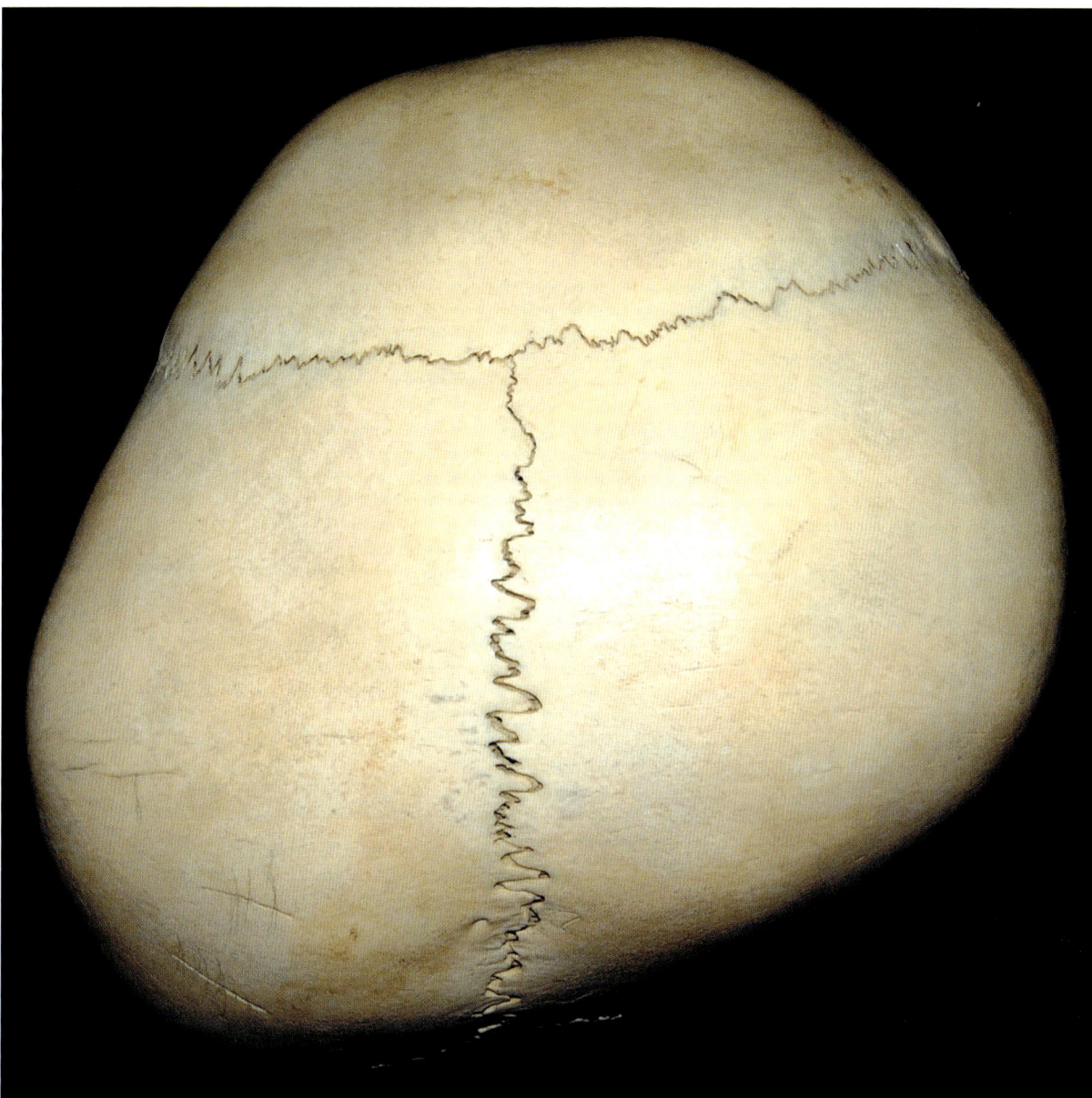

Figure 253. Artificial cultural (asymmetrical) cranial deformation or positional plagiocephaly in a child with all sutures patent (open) and no evidence of craniosynostosis (ancient Peruvian, SI). Note that the right parietal and occipital region is flattened and the right temporal region bulges more than the left due to cultural modification or positional activities (e.g., a baby's sleep position), not premature sutural closure. Flattening of one or both parietal regions and the frontal bone are common findings in some populations. Cf. O'Loughlin (2004); Van Arsdale and Clark (2012) for a discussion of cranial deformation and accessory ossicles. Sutures are the primary sites of cranial growth and act as shock absorbers that change their complexity in response to tension, compression and shearing forces/stresses.

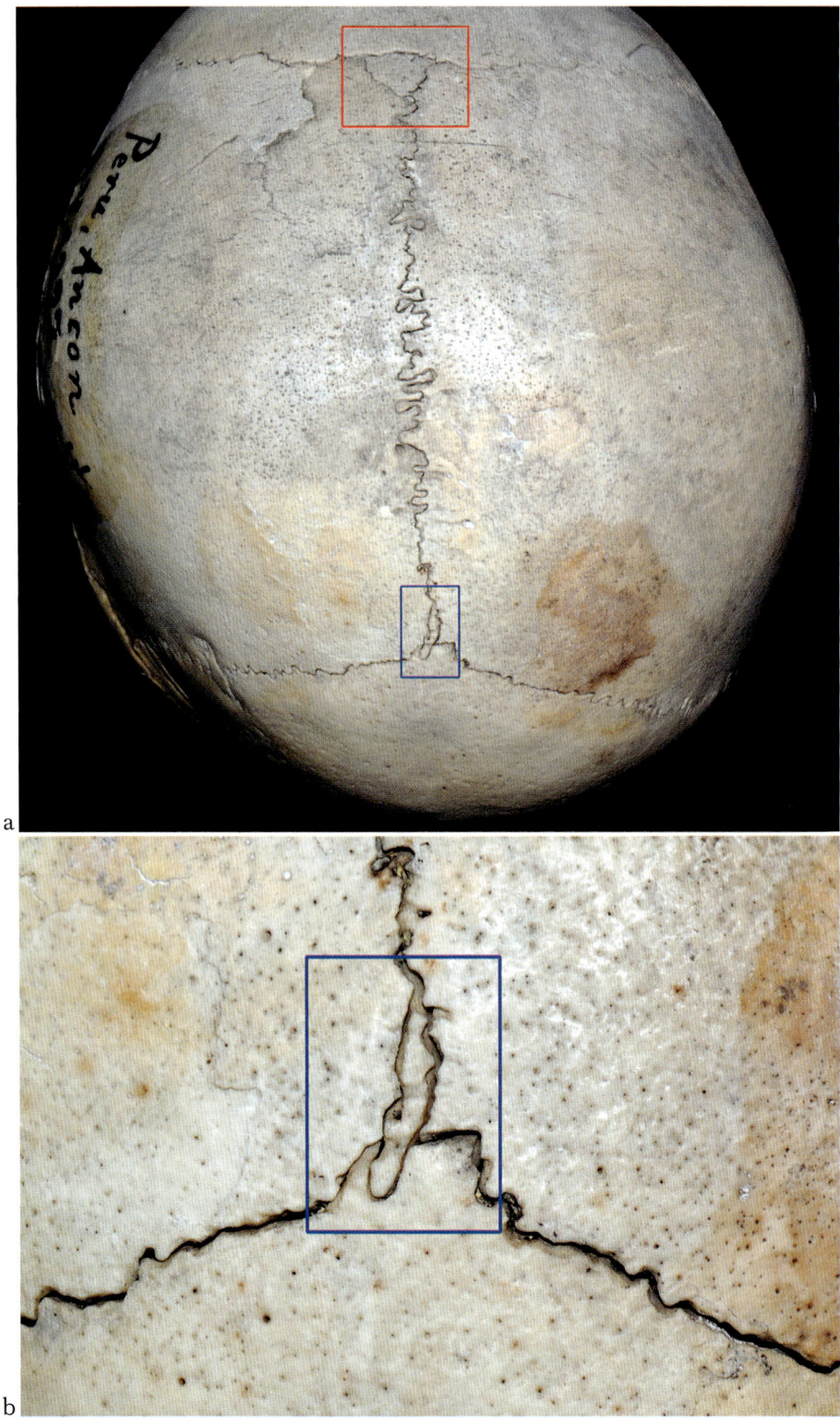

Figure 254a-b. Small ossicles at Bregma and Lambda in a 12–15-year-old Peruvian skull (RV1327). (a) Small bregmatic ossicle (red square) and elongated ossicle at Lambda (blue rectangle). (b) Higher magnification of the diminutive ossicle at Lambda (rectangle). These ossicles are usually larger and more oval or triangular shaped.

Superior View of the Skull

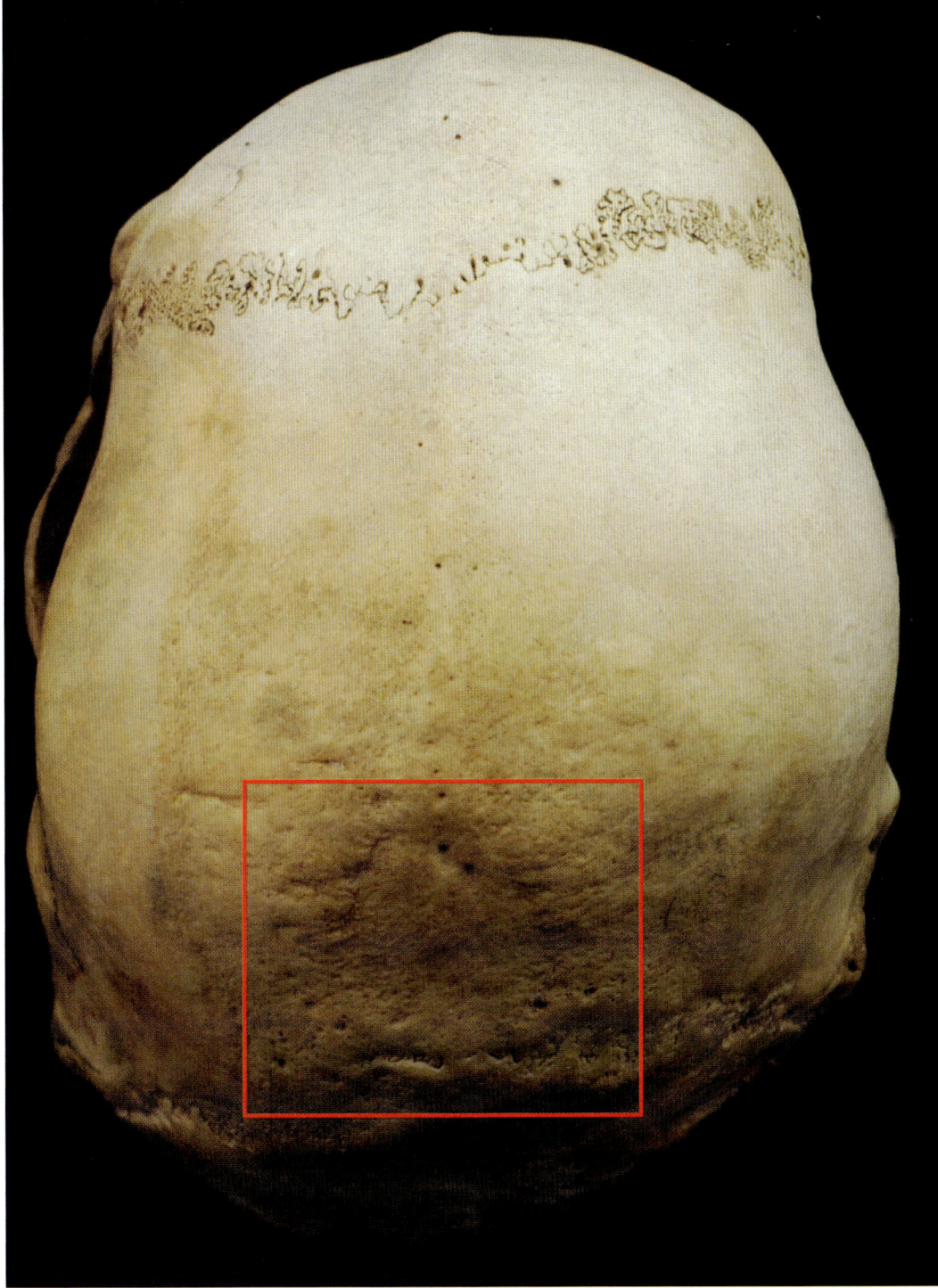

Figure 255. Scaphocephaly and keeling associated with premature craniosynostosis of the sagittal suture. Note trace of a large lambdoidal ossicle, ossicle at the Lambda (red square) (SI). Cf. Gopinathan (1992); Kohn et al. (1994); Weber et al. (2008).

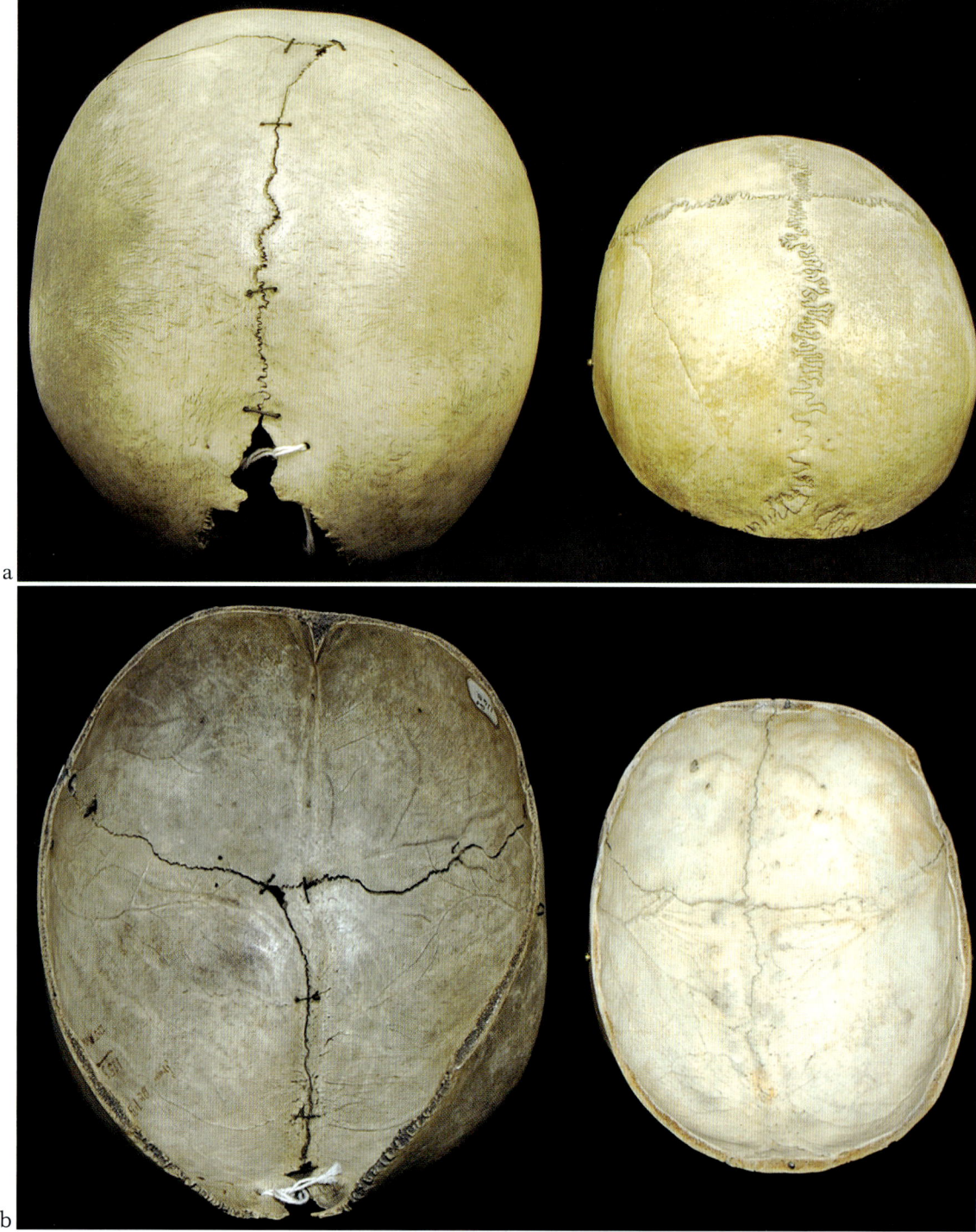

Figure 256a-b. Photograph of a macrocephalic/macrocrania calotte compared to a normal adult calotte (Mütter Museum). (a) Ectocranial and (b) endocranial views of a macrocephalic calotte (left in photo) compared to a normally-sized adult calotte. Note the sutures are less complex in the macrocephalic skull compared with the normal skull. Differences in sutural complexity are primarily due to differing rates of bone growth reflecting the distribution of forces and stresses that, in this macrocephalic individual with rapid growth, resulted in simple sutures. Macrocephaly is a rare finding in most skeletal collections.

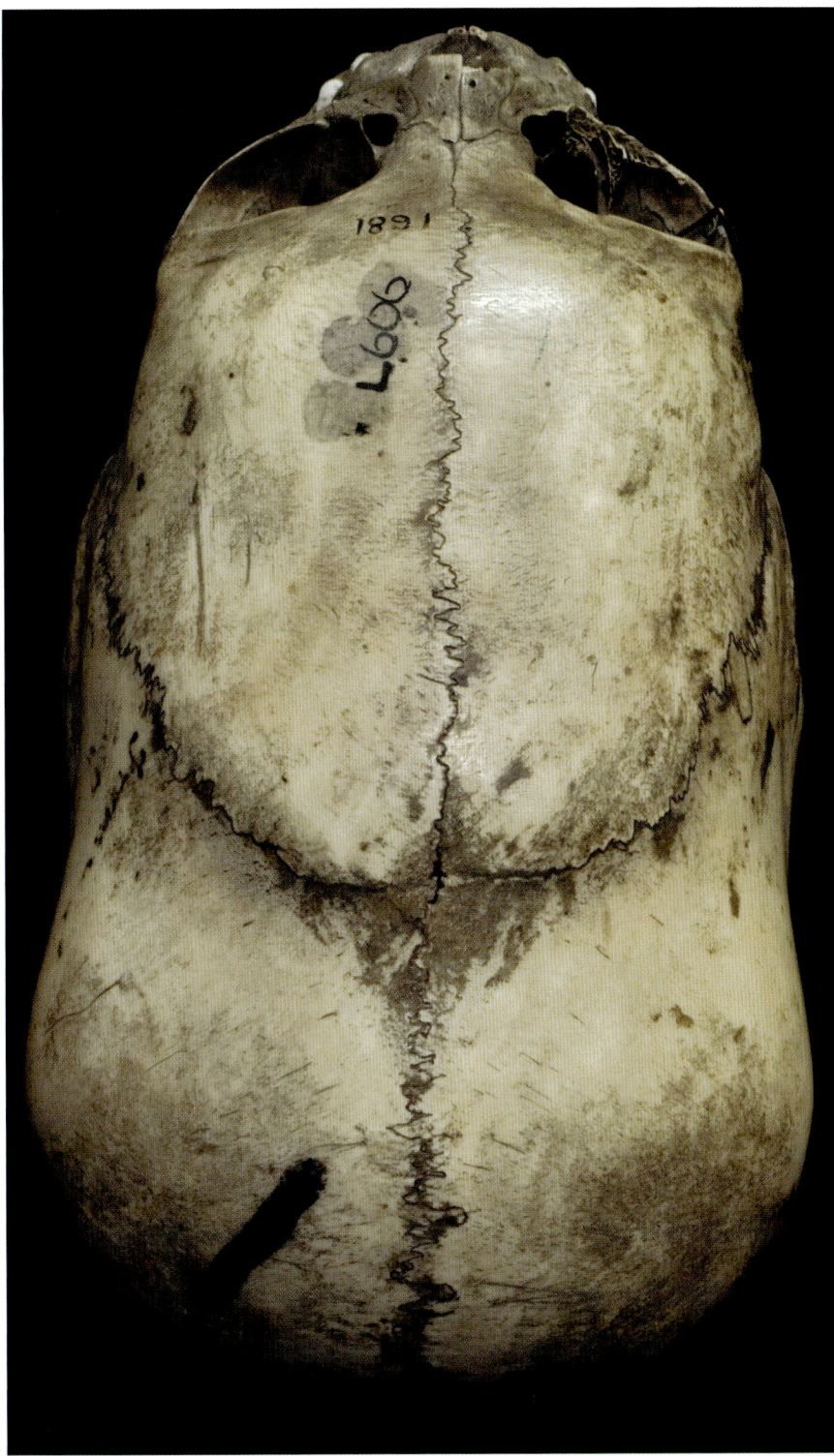

Figure 257. Artificial cranial deformation (wrapping) and metopism in a 3–5-year-old ancient Peruvian (UPenn L-606 1681). Note that the skull is "pinched" posterior to the coronal suture, where it was bound. Uncommon finding depending on group examined. Cf. O'Loughlin (2004) for more on cranial deformation and accessory ossicles.

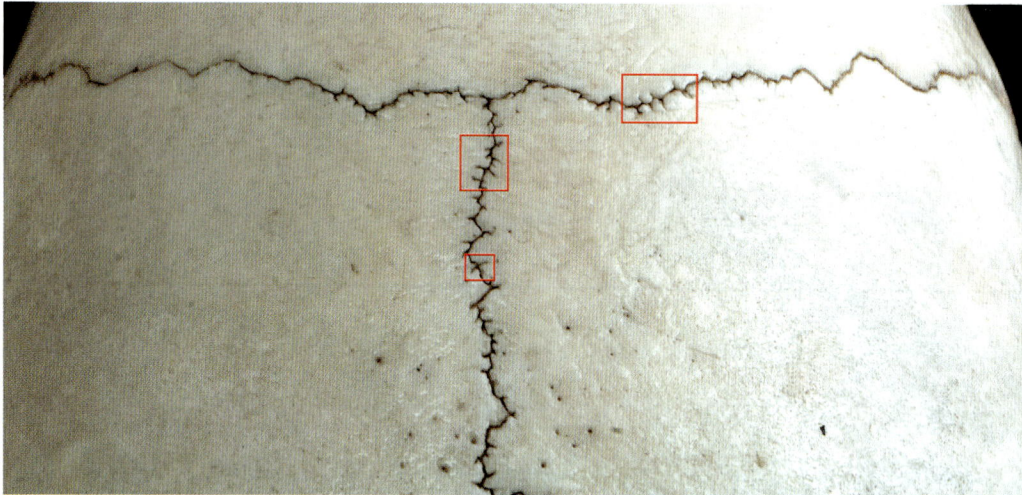

Figure 258. Sutural extensions (square), resembling baseball stitches, along the coronal suture in a Thai adolescent skull (KKU). These short, linear grooves or "stitches" are often present and clearly visible and sharply defined in subadults, but largely disappear, leaving small, shallow grooves in the adult cranium. The correlation of these extensions along the coronal and sagittal sutures and their usefulness as an indicator of age (subadult) warrants further research. Typical anatomy, but descriptions of these "stitches" in the literature remain unreported.

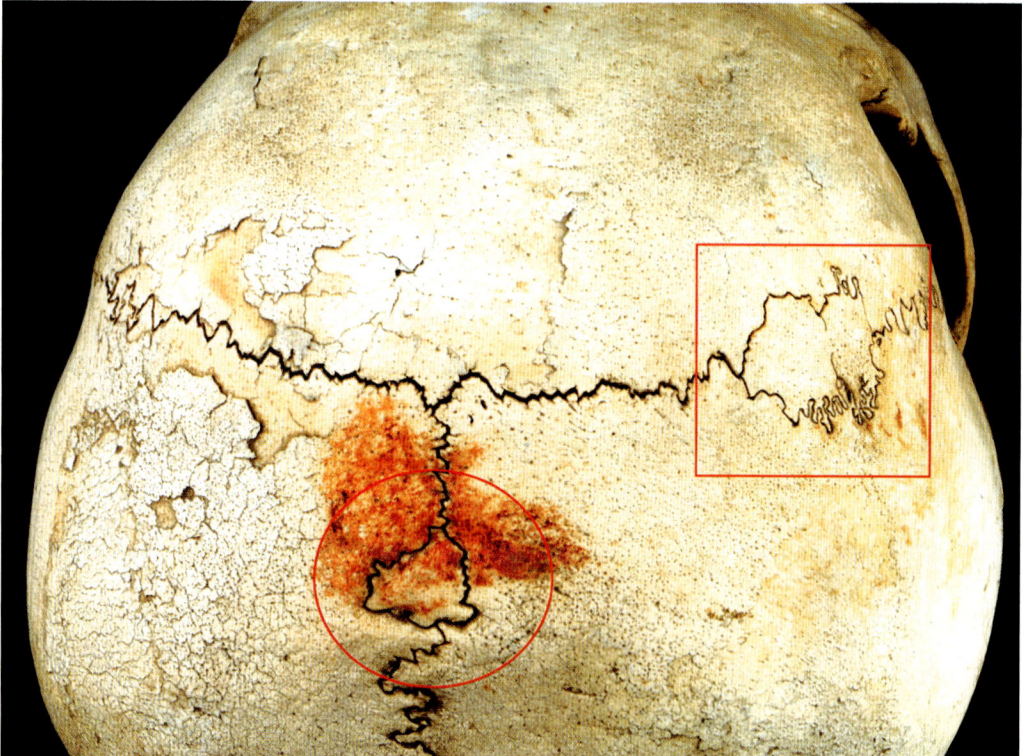

Figure 259. Sagittal ossicle (circle) and two coronal ossicles (square) in an adult Thai skull (KKU), both are uncommon findings. Flaking of outer table is postmortem taphonomic change. Cf. Hauser and DeStefano (1989).

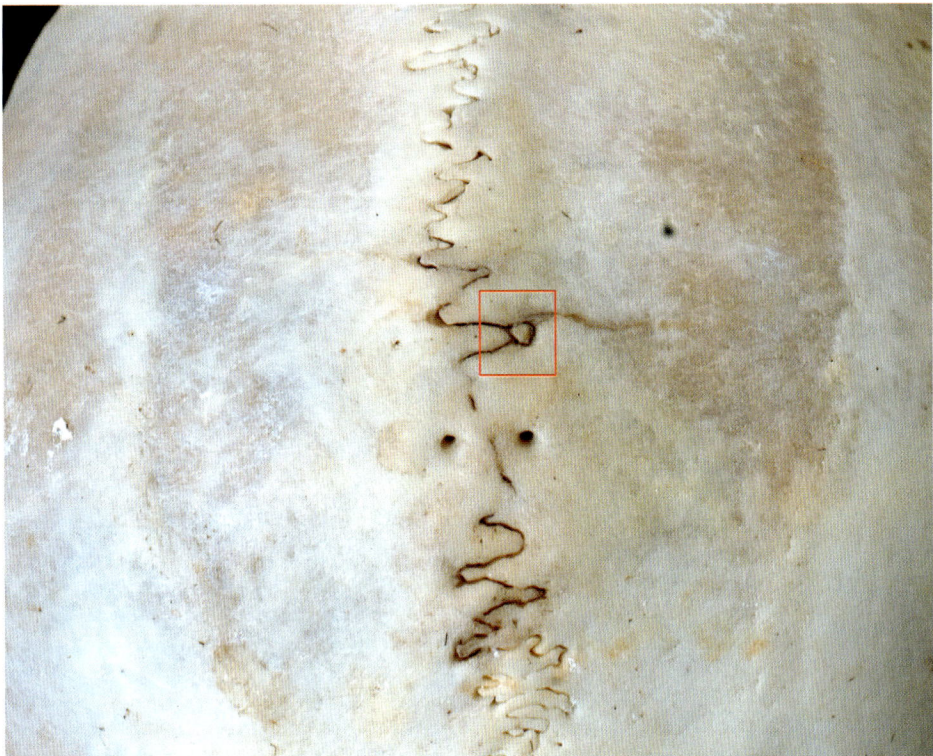

Figure 260. Tiny sagittal ossicle (square) superior to Obelion in a 70-year-old Thai male skull (CMU 5407120). Uncommon finding, but typical anatomy.

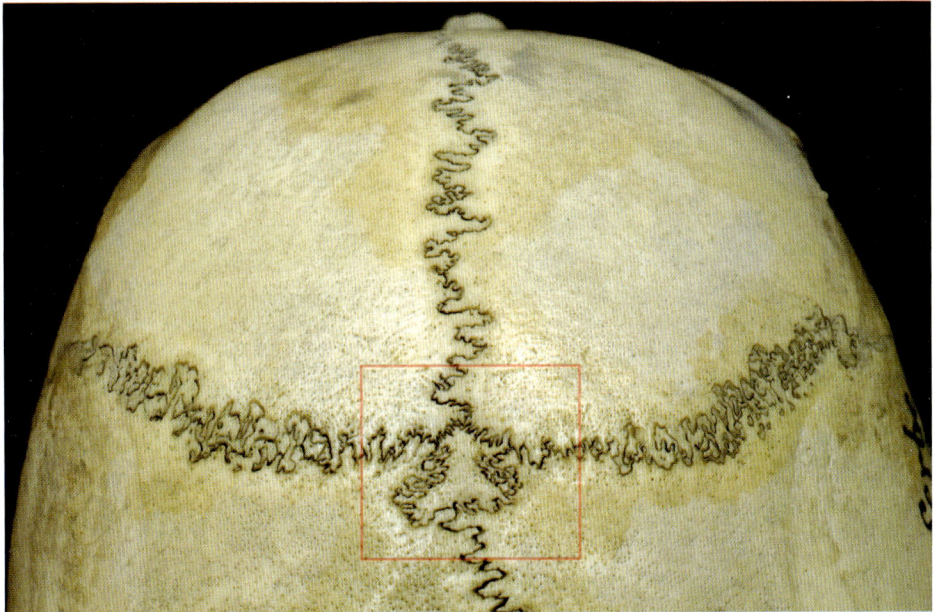

Figure 261. Bregmatic ossicle/fonticular bone (square), metopism and an unusually complex coronal suture in 25-year-old male (Mütter Museum 1006-090). See Barclay-Smith (1909) for ossicle at Bregma; Barberini et al. (2008); Hauser and DeStefano (1989) for all traits. Bregmatic ossicle is an uncommon, but typical variant.

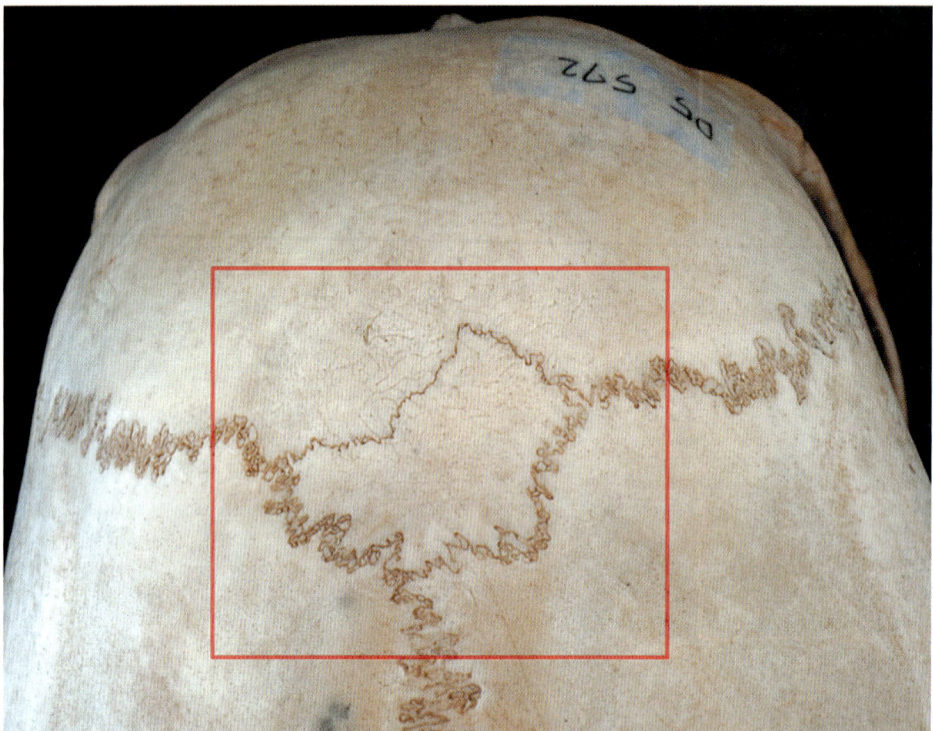

Figure 262. Unusually asymmetrical anterior fontanelle/fonticular bone (rectangle) anterior to the coronal suture and Bregma in an adult female (KKU 46-189). Cf. Barclay-Smith (1909); Barberini et al. (2008); Hauser and DeStefano (1989).

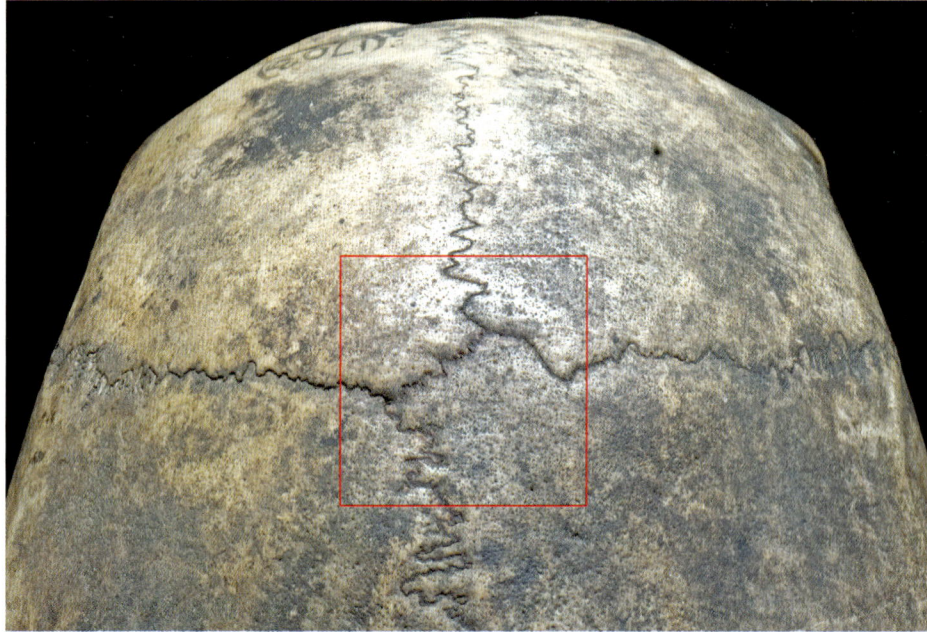

Figure 263. Misalignment of the metopic and sagittal sutures (square) (UPenn). Common finding.

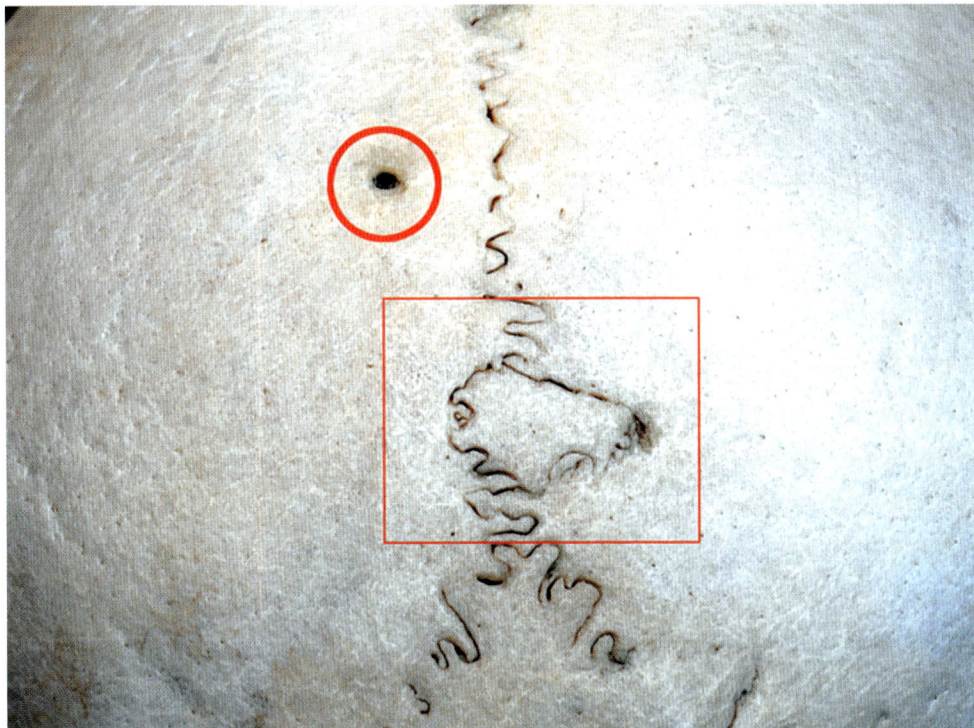

Figure 264. Sagittal suture ossicle (rectangle) and left parietal foramen (circle) in an Asian adult skull (UHWO). Parietal foramina are common findings and ossicles are uncommon to common findings depending on the group being examined. This ossicle is anterior to Lambda and, as such, would not be classified as an ossicle at Lambda, but as a sagittal suture ossicle. Parietal foramina transmit a vein and sometimes an arterial anastomosis between the middle meningeal and superficial arteries of the scalp. Parietal foramina were found in 20 of 40 parietal bones in 20 cadavers (Yoshioka et al. 2006). Cf. Hauser and DeStefano (1989).

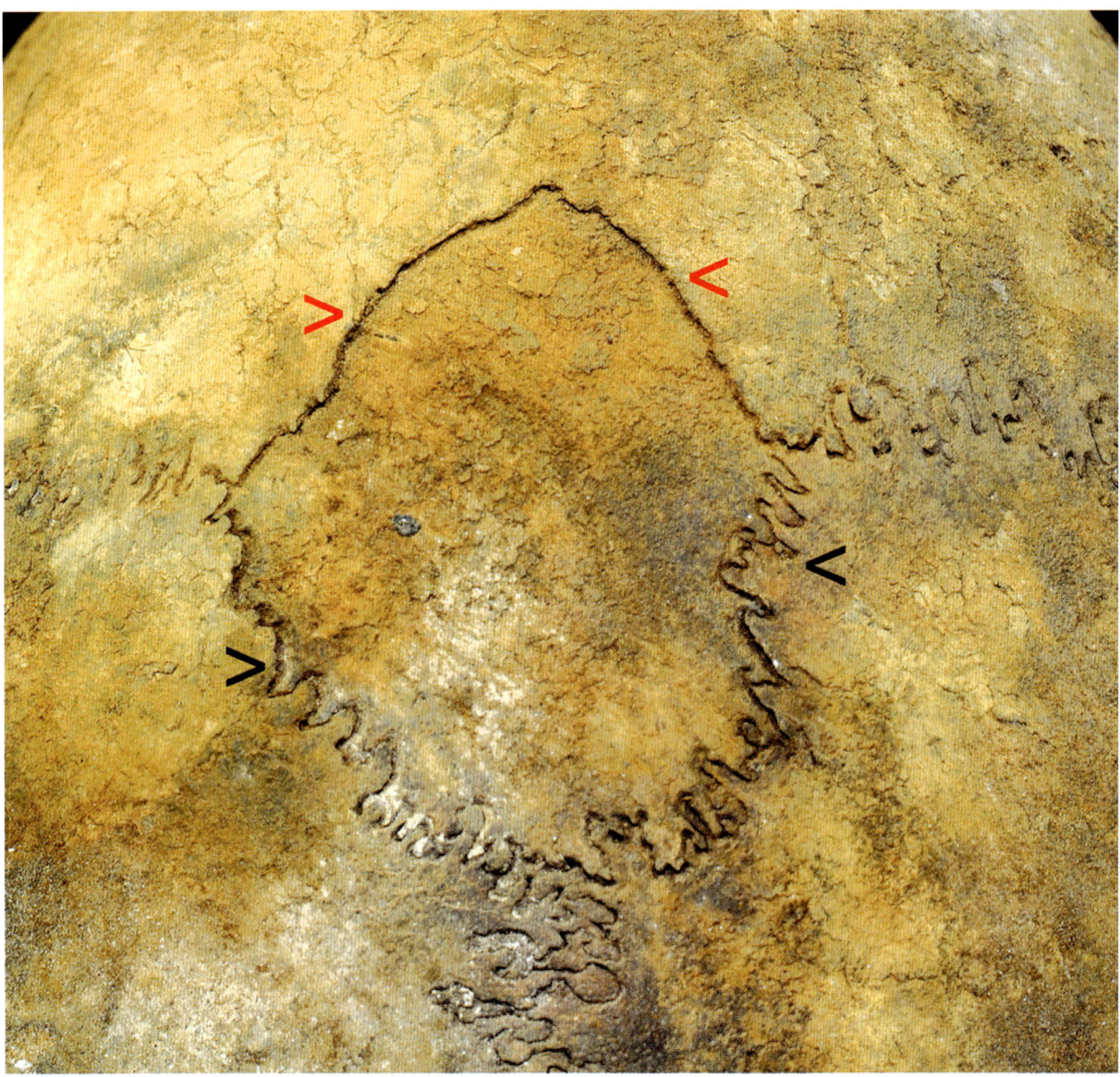

Figure 265. Large anterior fontanelle bone involving the frontal bone, in a young adult male from the XV to XVII centuries (Ospitale Maggiore, Milan; photo courtesy LABANOF, University of Milan). Note that the "V" portion of the suture joining the parietal bones (black <>) is more complicated and has more interdigitations than the frontal portion (red <>), suggesting that this ossicle, like others, typically assumes the complexity of the opposing and connecting suture. Uncommon to rare finding in most dry bone skeletons. Cf. Barberini et al. (2008); Girdany and Blank (1965).

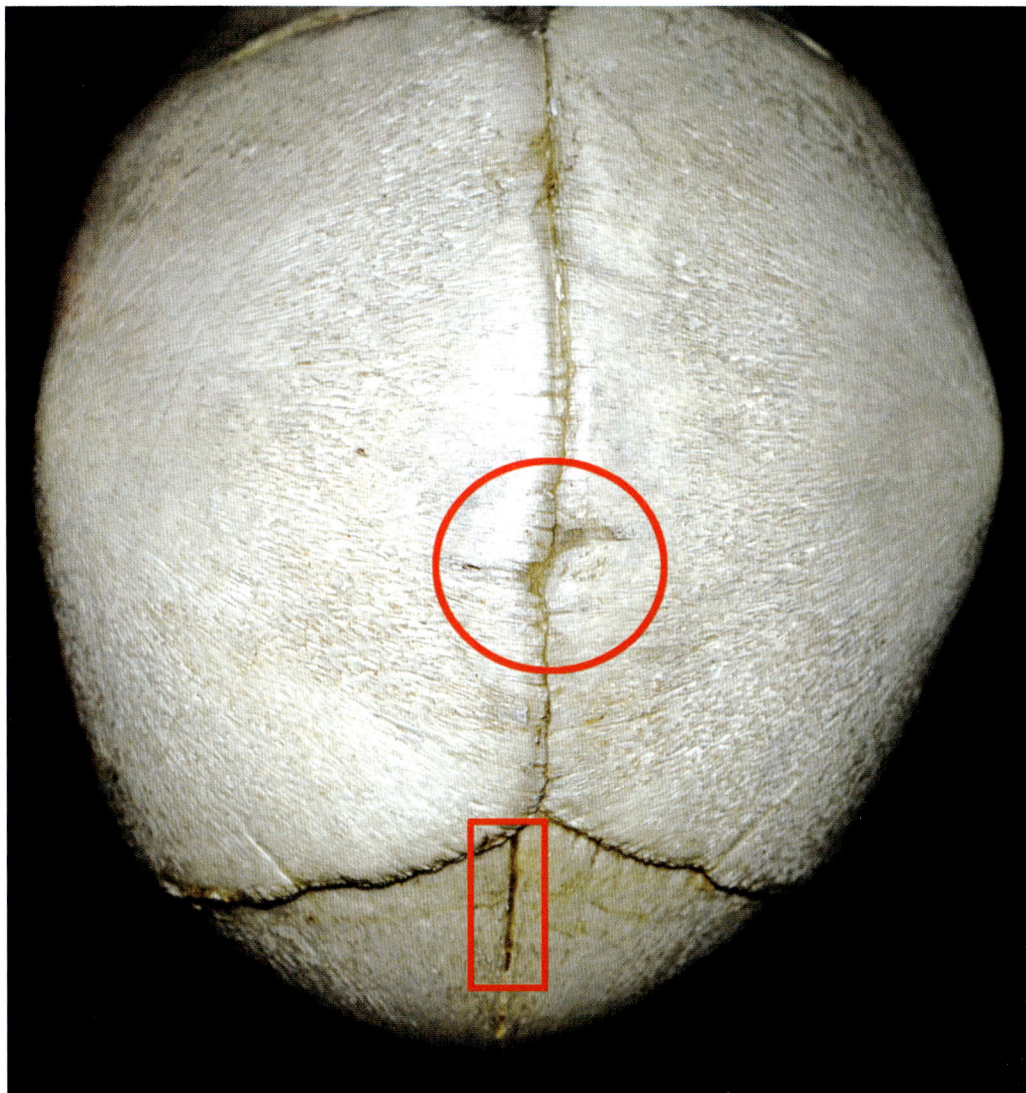

Figure 266. Defects in the region of Obelion (circle) that might have developed into parietal foramina and superior median fissure (rectangle) of the occipital bone in a newborn or infant skull (SI fetal anatomical). Note that the suture margins are relatively smooth (simple) and do not exhibit the complex interdigitations that will develop in an older child. Obelion is a craniometric point or landmark along the sagittal suture between the parietal foramina, when present.

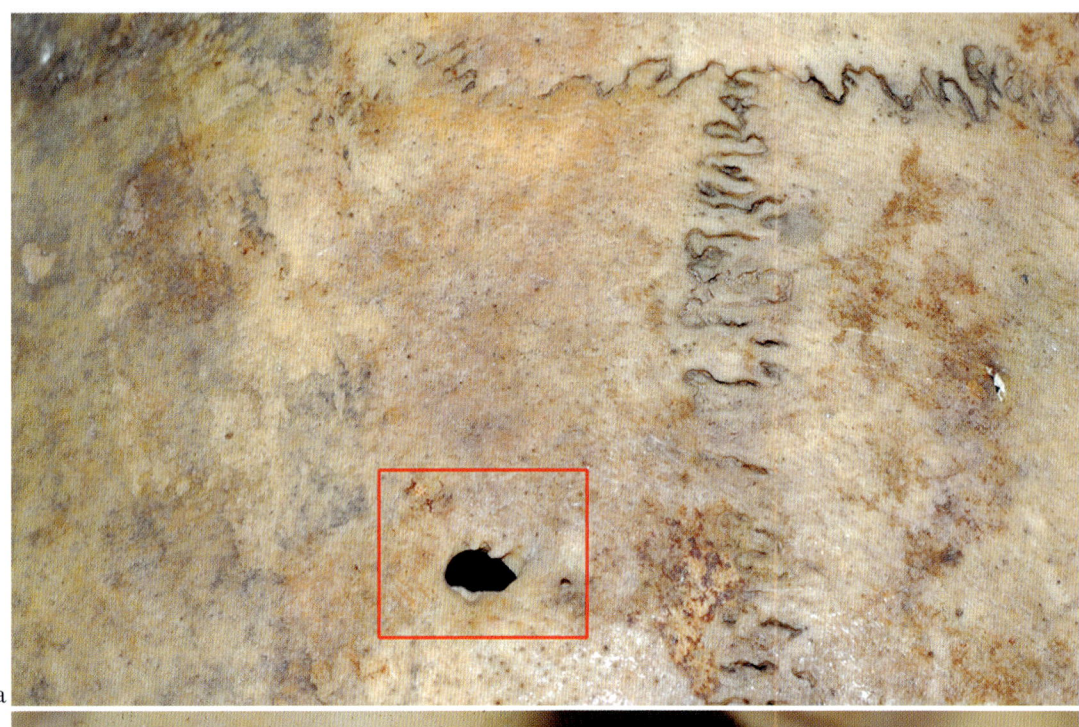
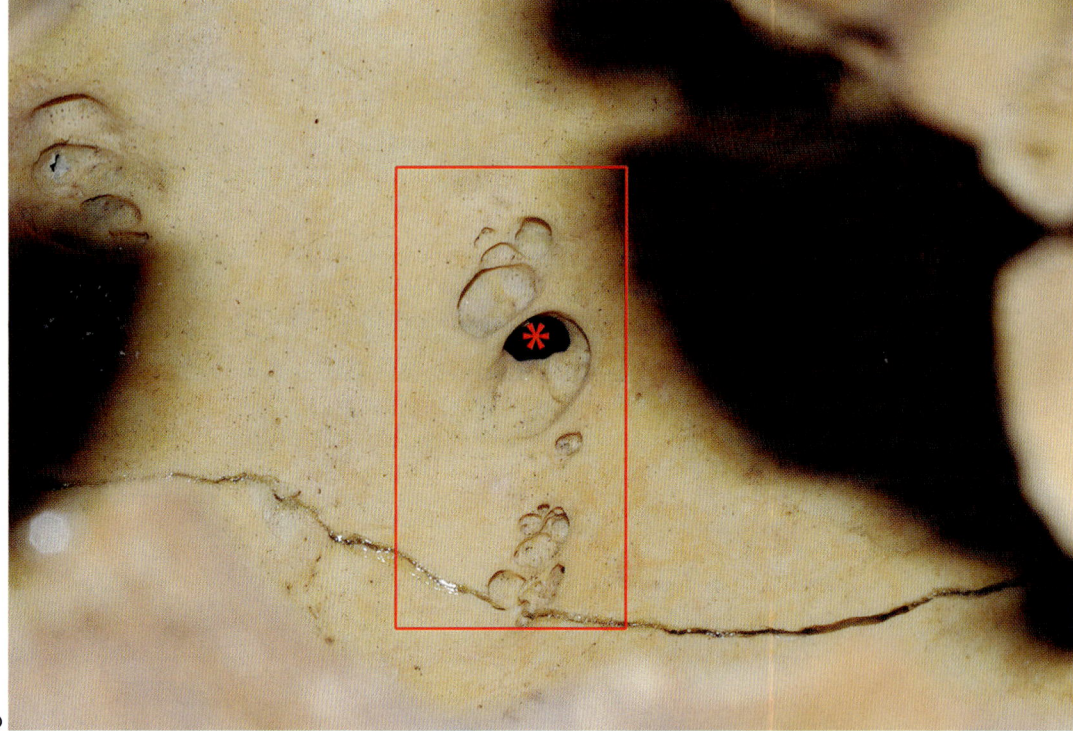

Figure 267a-b. Perforation of the outer plate/lamina of the left parietal bone due to erosion by arachnoid granulations in an elderly individual (RV500). (a) Ectocranial view showing perforation and remodeling (square) in the left parietal bone due to erosion by one or more arachnoid granulations. (b) Endocranial view showing multiple pits (rectangle) and erosion that resulted in perforation (*) of the cranium by arachnoid granulations, also known as Pacchionian bodies. Perforation of the outer table by these granulations is unusual, typically occurs in elderly individuals, and is not a typical variant, but an erosional process. Note the margin/edge of the perforation is blunt (remodeled) and darkly discolored indicating it occurred antemortem and not as a result of postmortem handling.

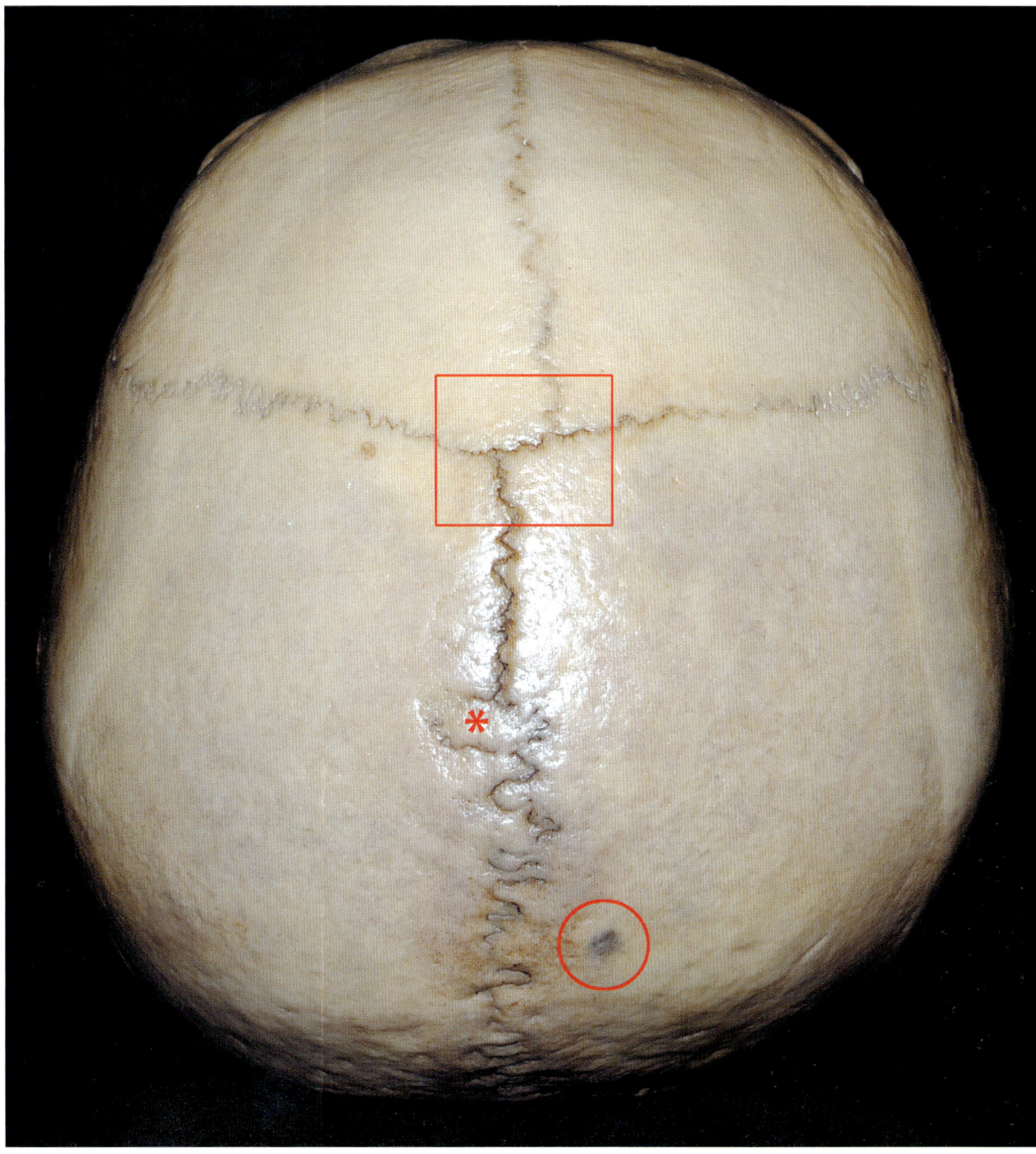

Figure 268. Slight misalignment of the metopic and sagittal suture (square), a sagittal ossicle (*) and paper-thin area (circle) where one or more arachnoid granulations have nearly perforated the outer table of the skull in an elderly Asian skull (JABSOM M02). Misalignment such as this is common, sagittal ossicle is uncommon, but not rare, and thinning or perforation of the outer table is common in elderly individuals (Cederlund et al. 1982; Phillips 2008).

Chapter 5

OCCIPITAL VIEW OF THE SKULL

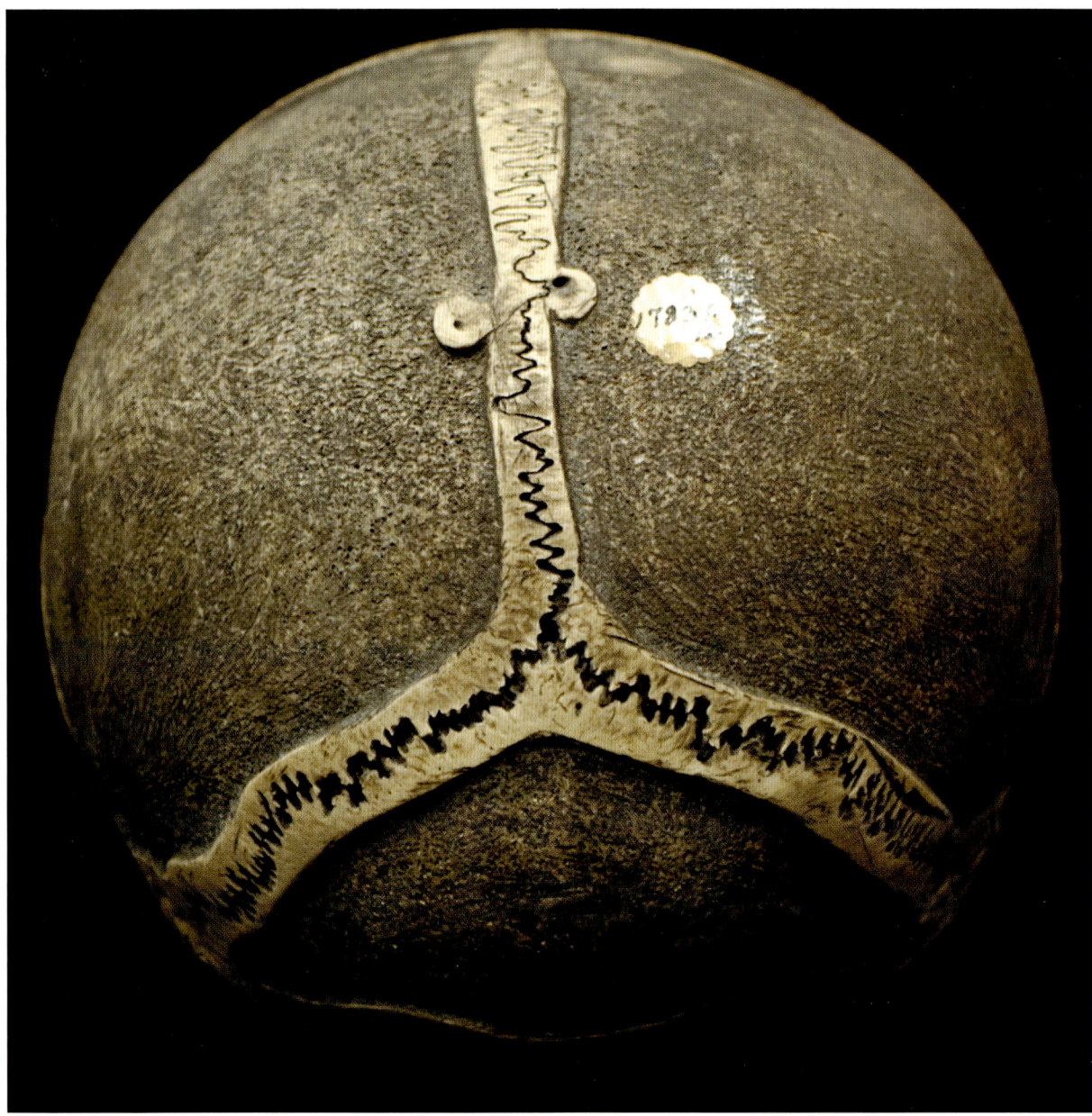

Figure 269. Ectocranial surface removed from around the sutures and parietal foramina exposing the sieve-like diploic area in a 4- to 5-year-old child (Mütter Museum 17831-12). Parietal foramen is a common and typical finding that transmits a vein (of Santorini) and sometimes an artery (Yoshioka et al. 2006).

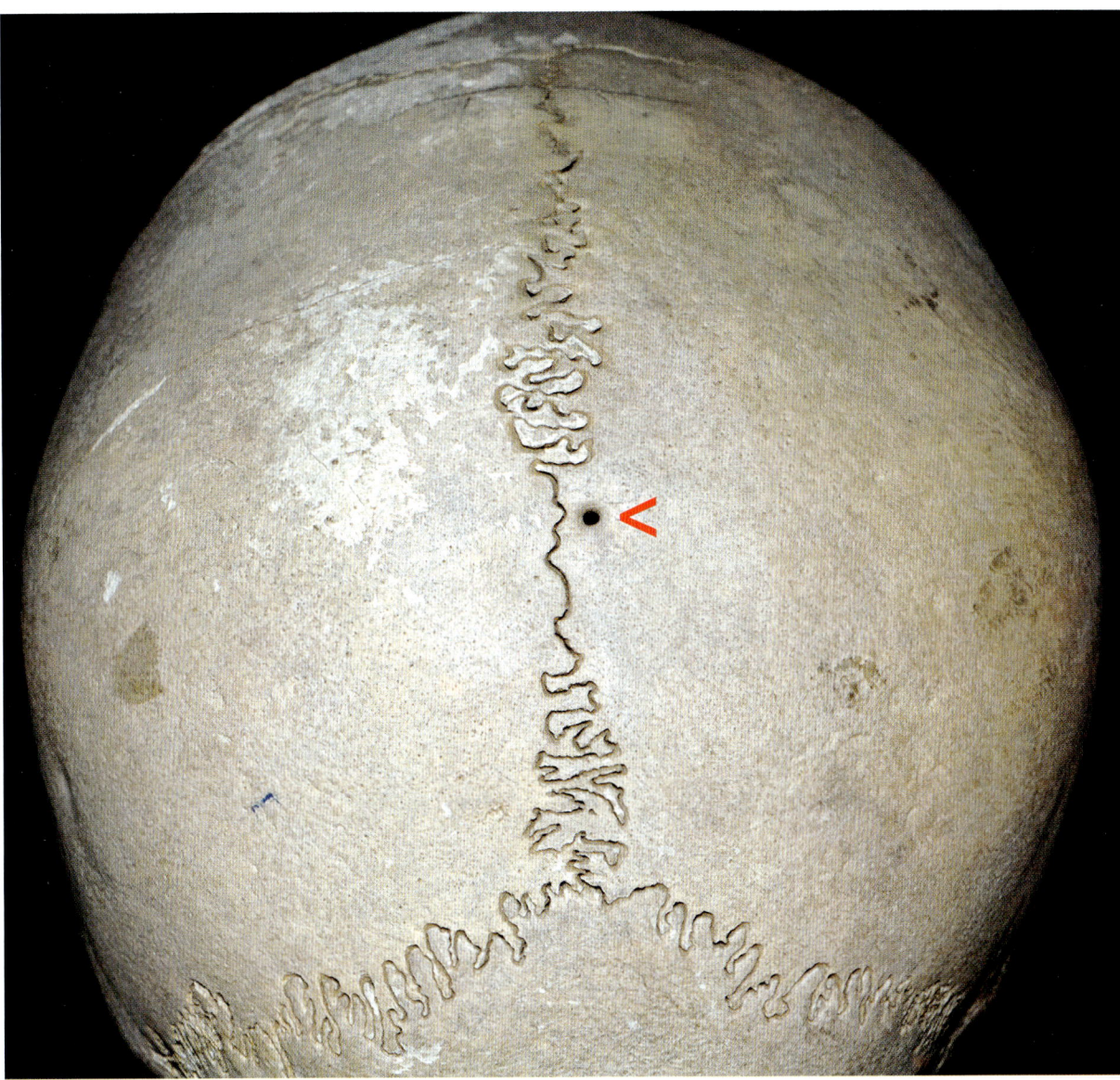

Figure 270. Single/unilateral right parietal foramen (<) and relatively simple sagittal suture showing that the straightest portion of this suture is nearly always in the region of Obelion (adult female; RV1124). Note that, as expected, the sagittal suture is more complex anterior and posterior to Obelion and its complexity takes the shape of the nearest suture. When referring to the coronal, sagittal and lambdoidal sutures, for example, the coronal suture typically is the least complex of the three. With this in mind, note that the sagittal suture posterior to Obelion becomes more tortuous (complex) as it approaches Lambda, more resembling the lambdoidal than the coronal suture. This general pattern of complexity likely reflects bone biomechanics of the sutures as they approach one another.

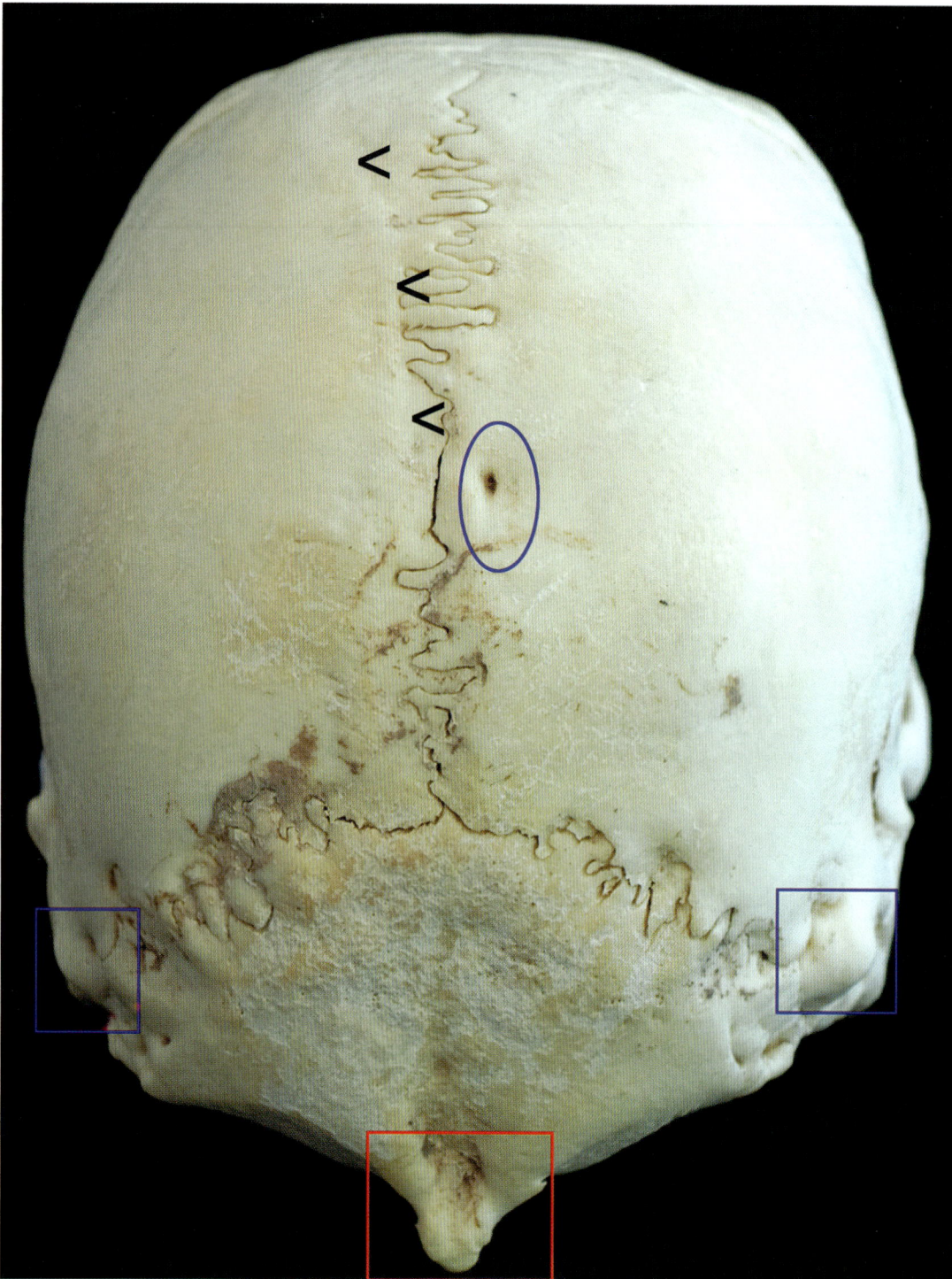

Figure 271. Unusual suite of traits including a metopic fissure, simple coronal suture (not shown), parietal foramen with a shallow groove leading into it (blue oval), highly developed retromastoid tubercles/processes (blue squares), a large occipital superstructure and Inion spike (red rectangle), and superior temporal lines (<) (temporalis muscle) best visualized in the left parietal and that nearly reach the sagittal suture. Although only the cranium is present, this is a robust, adult male with Asian features (CSC AS022). Cf. Hauser and DeStefano (1989); Heathcote et al. (2012); Yoshioka et al. (2006).

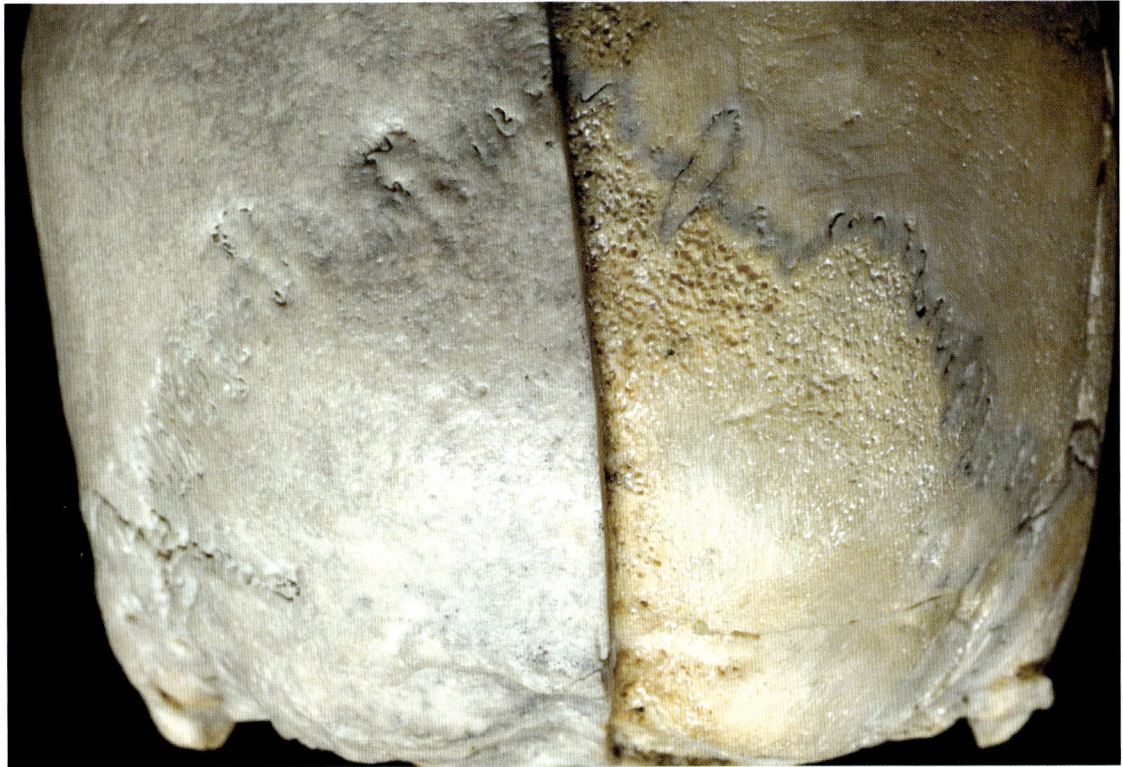

Figure 272. Outer table of the right half of the cranium removed to expose the diploë, lambdoidal suture and ossicles (UPenn 254). See Jivraj et al. (2009) for an MRI study on diploic anatomy.

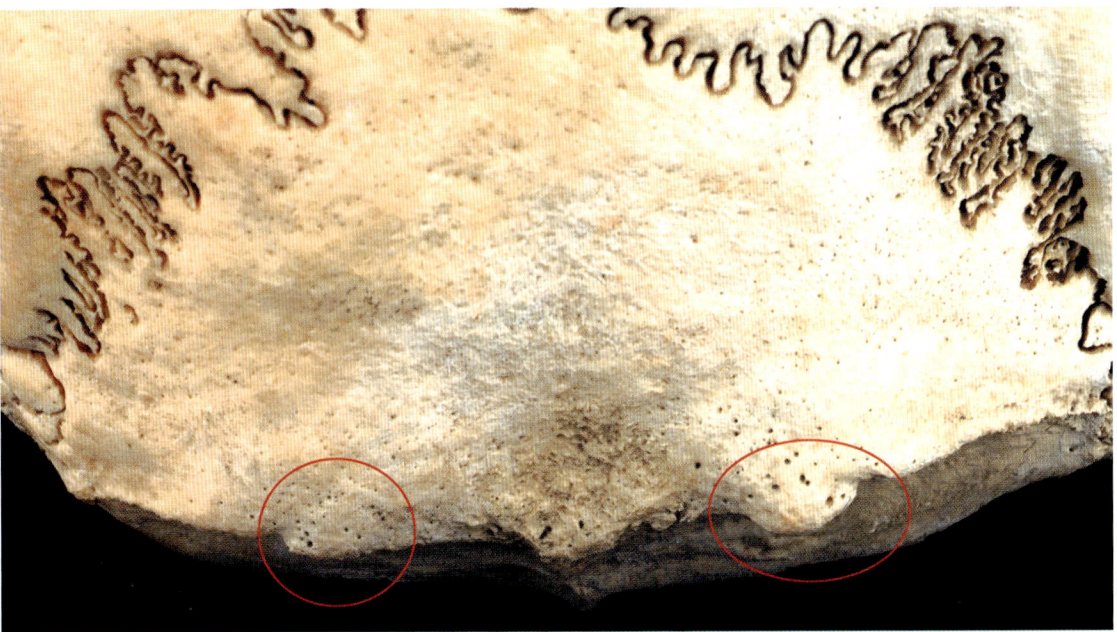

Figure 273. Rounded nodules (rectangles) for the attachment of muscles along the nuchal crest (superior nuchal line) in an adult Thai (KKU). Similar but much larger nodules have been reported in some Pacific Islander groups as possible occupational markers and repeated muscle use (Cf. Heathcote et al. 1992, 2012). Uncommon to common finding.

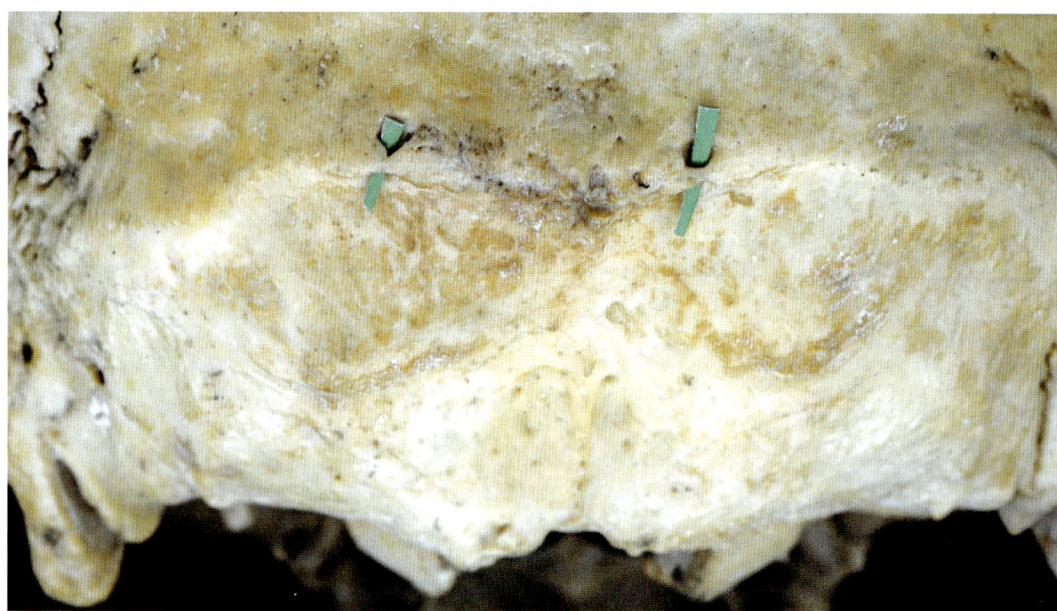

Figure 274. Bilateral "nuchal foramina" (green arrowheads) along the nuchal crest in an adult Thai male skull (KKU). Unknown frequency, but an uncommon to rare finding.

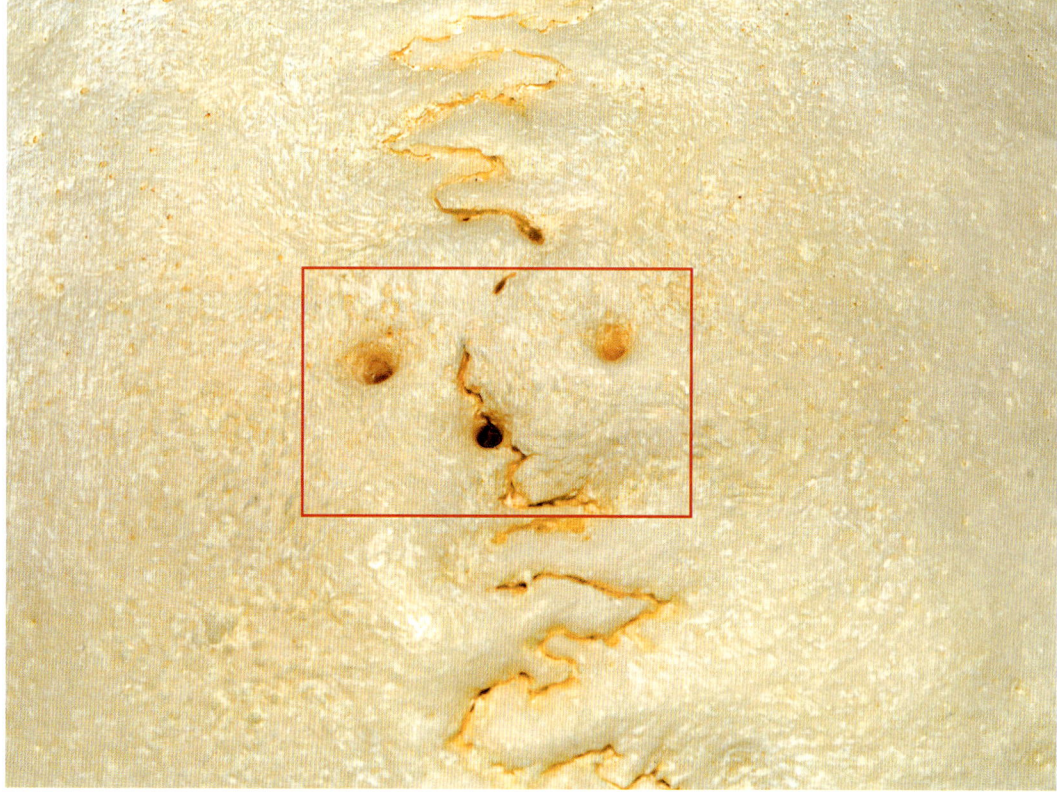

Figure 275. Obelion with three parietal foramina (rectangle), including one on the sagittal suture (CSC). Three or more parietal foramina are uncommon findings. The biomechanical relationship and impact stress exerted by one or more parietal foramina on the complexity of the sagittal suture is not fully understood (Mann et al. 2009). The parietal foramina in this individual are within the normal size variation of 5 mm or less in diameter (Tubbs et al. 2003).

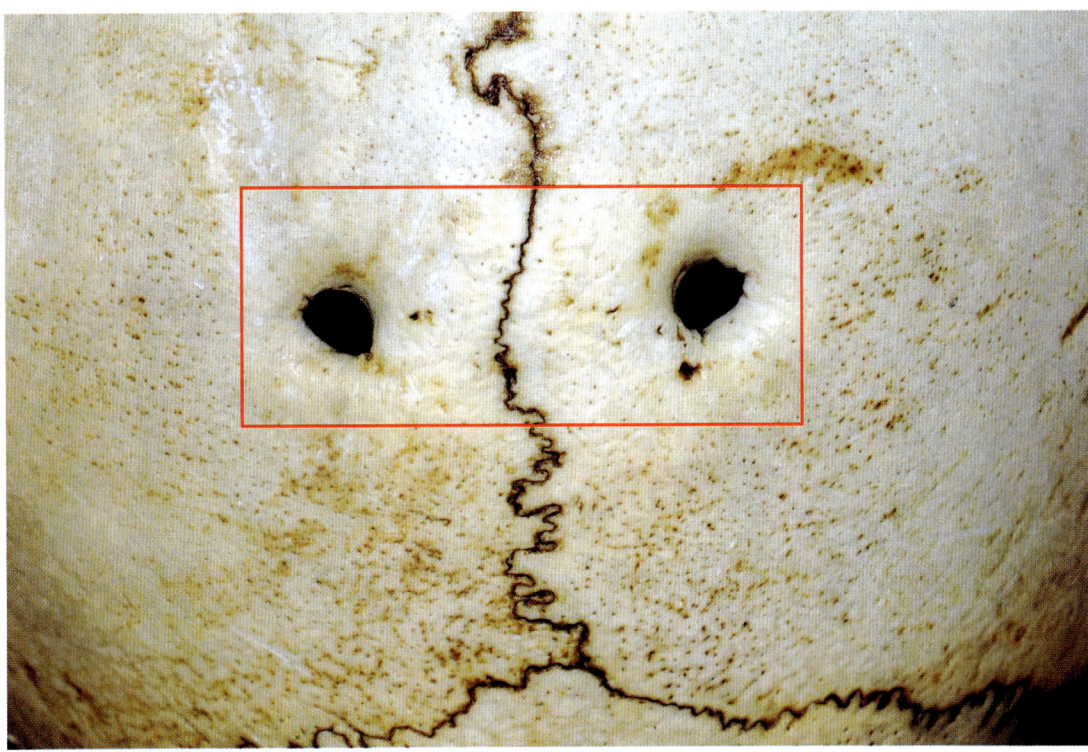

Figure 276. Enlarged parietal foramina (rectangle) in an African female (University of Pretoria).

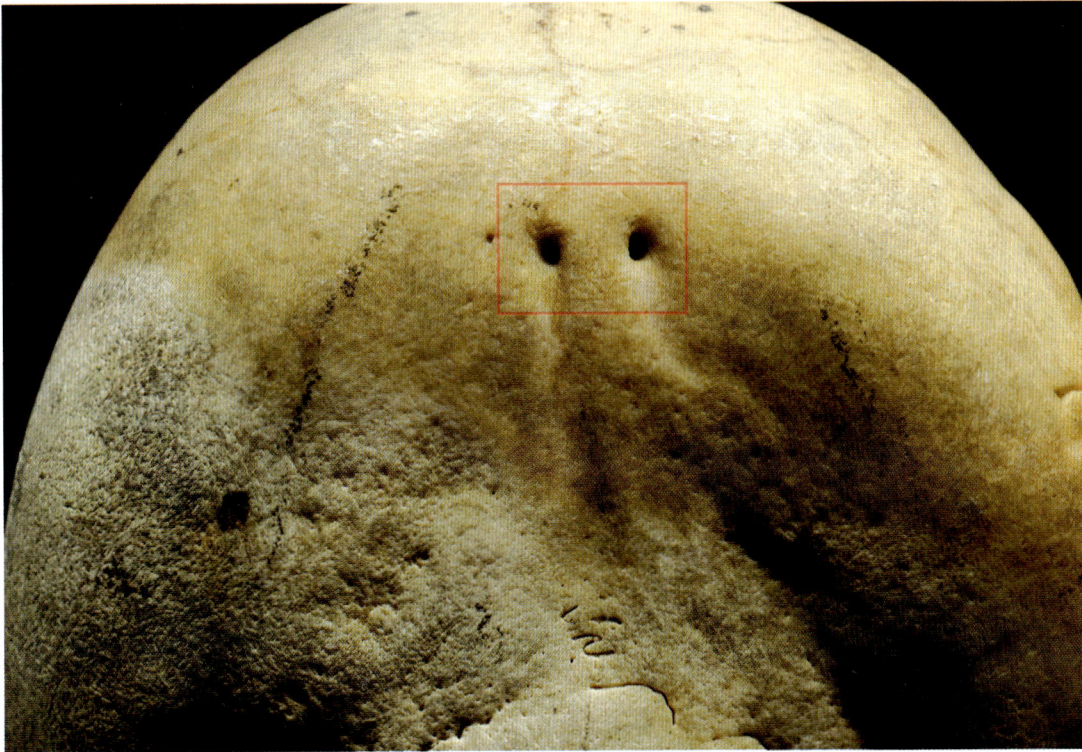

Figure 277. Enlarged but typical parietal foramina (rectangle) in an adult Peruvian skull with artificial cranial deformation and flattening (UPenn 29-144-13 L606) – note the faintly visible vessel grooves leading into the foramina.

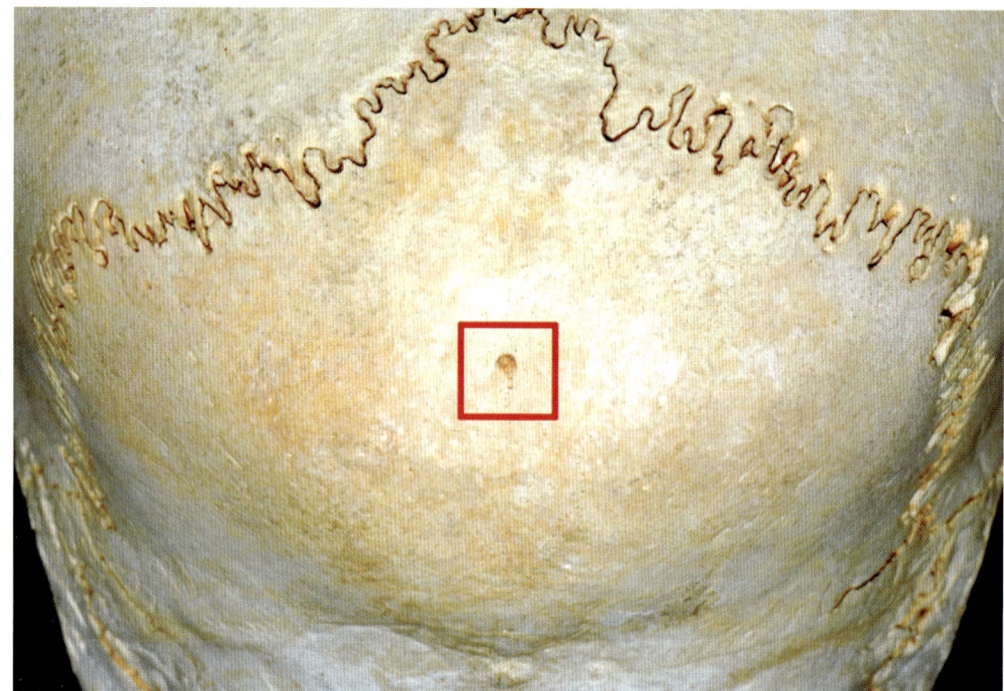

Figure 278. Emissary occipital foramen (square) in an ancient Peruvian child (SI). A foramen in this region of the occipital bone is an uncommon finding in most populations. Boyd (1930) reports presence of this foramen near Inion in 1.6% of skulls. Cf. Hauser and DeStefano (1989) and Vázquez et al. (2001).

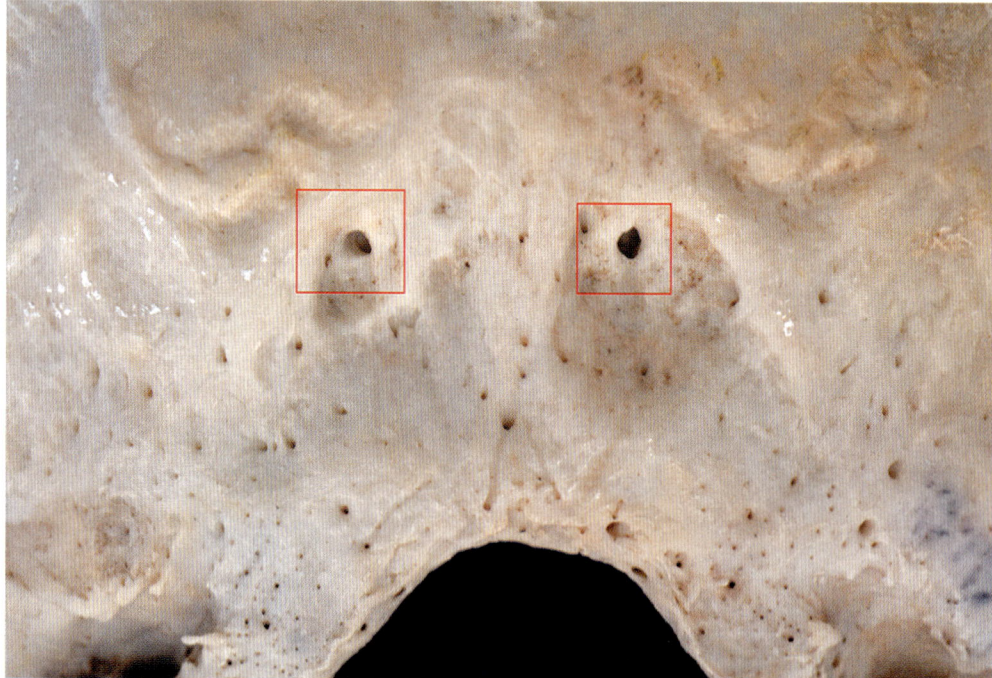

Figure 279. Double emissary occipital foramina (squares) in an adult Asian skull, probable male (CSC AC024). These foramina do not perforate the endocranium and do not communicate with one another.

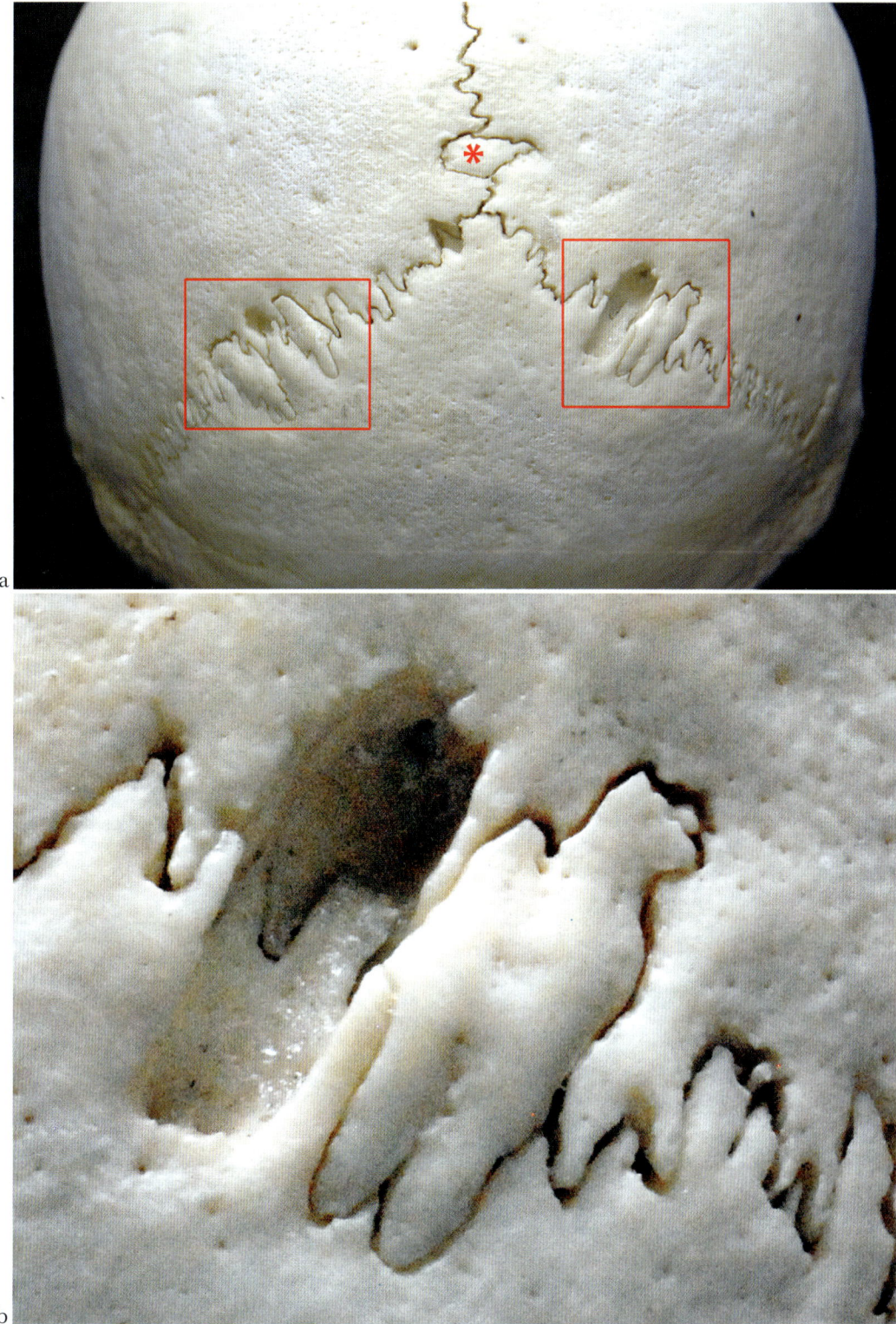

Figure 280a-b. Sagittal ossicle and lambdoidal ossicles in an adult (FSA DS043; Christopher Sciotto). (a) Small sagittal ossicle (*) near Lambda and elongated lambdoidal ossicles (rectangle and square). (b) Higher magnification showing that the lambdoidal suture is visible along the floor of the cavity formed by the missing ossicle, indicating that it formed as an island superficial to the suture.

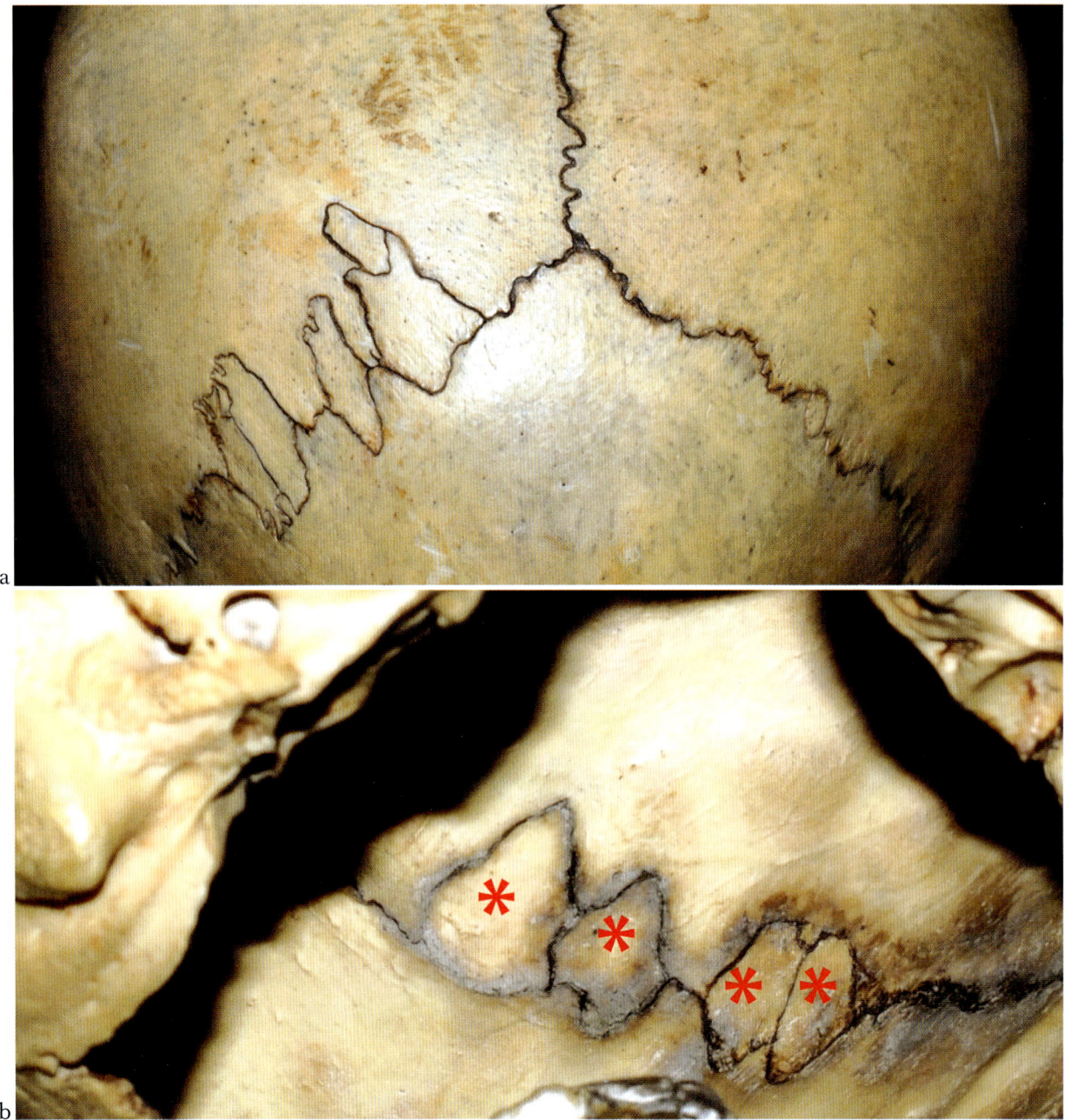

Figure 281a-b. Asymmetry of lambdoidal ossicles in an African child (University of Pretoria). (a) Ectocraniaum showing asymmetry of the lambdoidal suture with absence of ossicles along its right half. (b) Endocranial view showing that while five ossicles are visible ectocranially, only four (*) are visible endocranially.

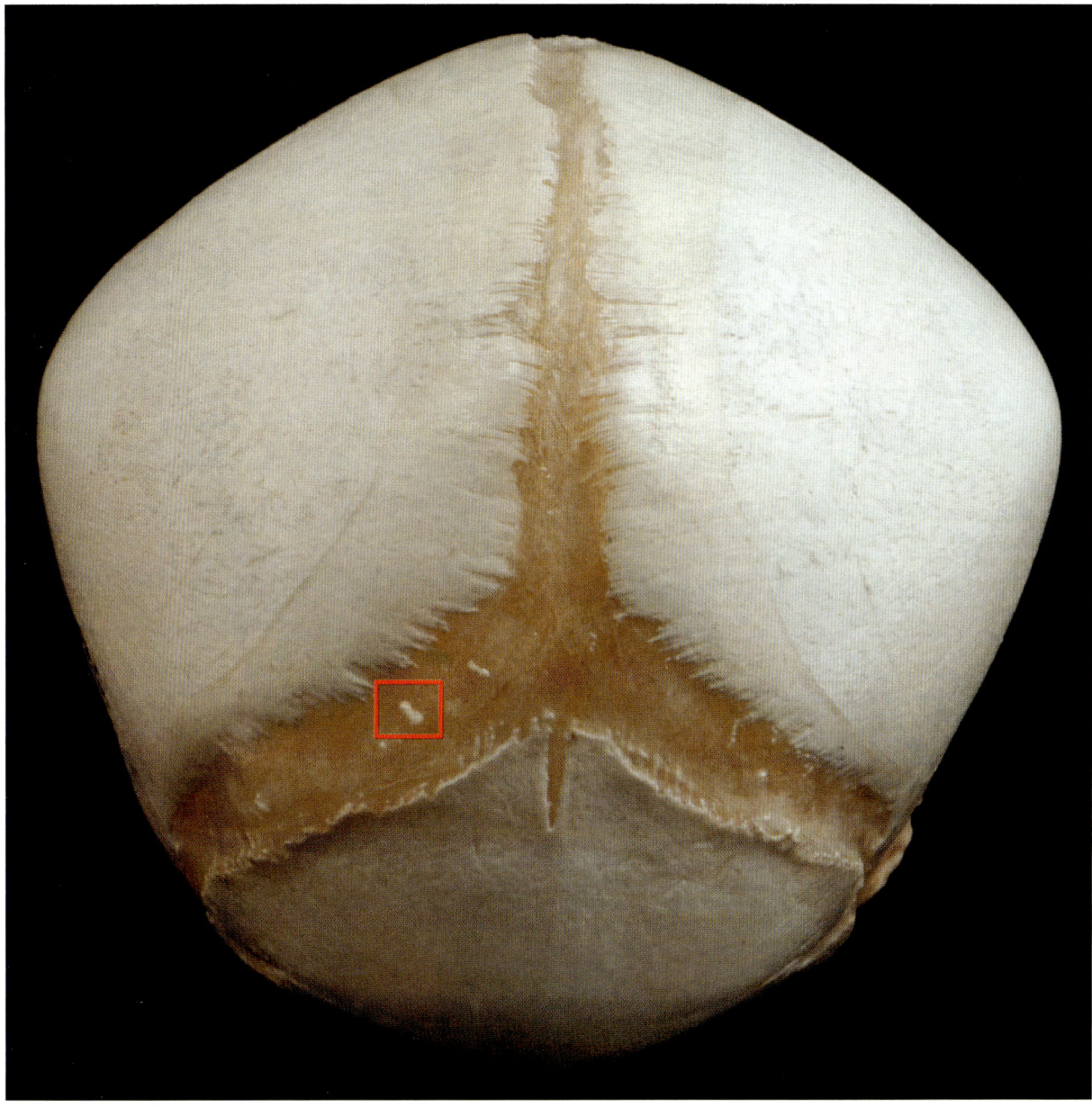

Figure 282. Small bone islands or accessory ossicles forming in the membrane along the lambdoidal suture of a neonatal skull (CSC AC 040). Typical anatomy and variant.

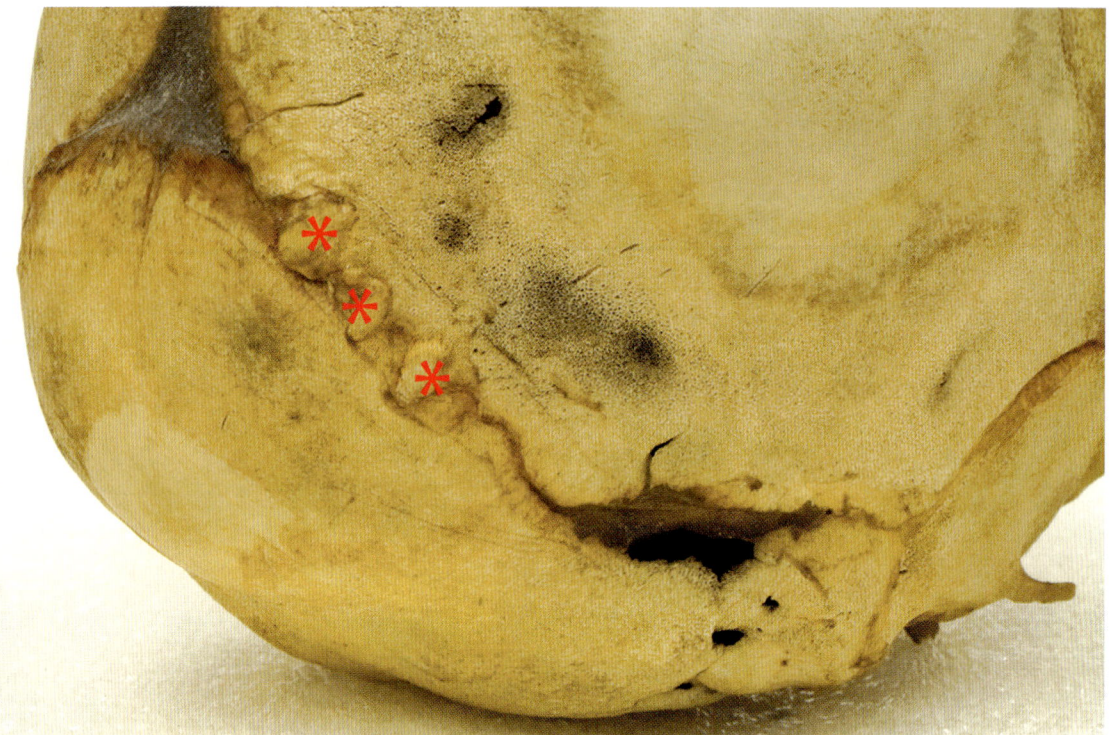

Figure 283. Lambdoidal ossicles (*) developing in a child (Mütter Museum).

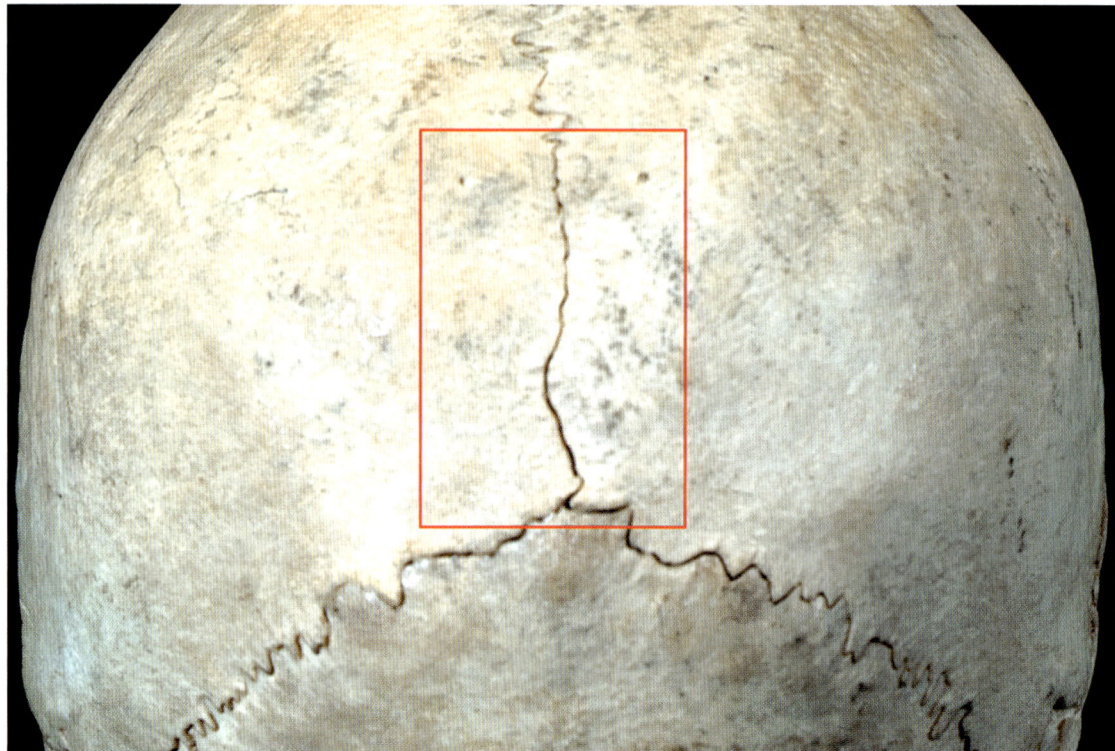

Figure 284. Unusually simple sagittal suture (rectangle) at and distal to Obelion in an adult Black male (SI 244071). While Obelion is typically the simplest portion of the sagittal suture, it is usually more complex than what is present in this individual. Typical anatomy and variant.

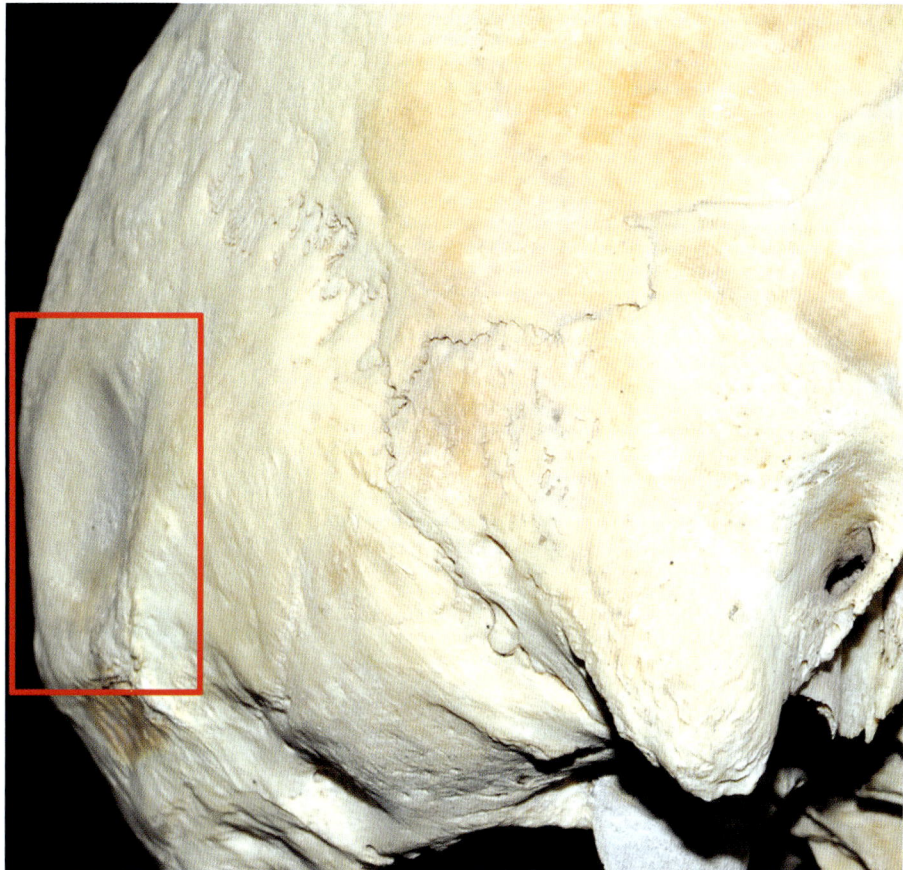

Figure 285. Large suprainion depression (rectangle) in an ancient adult Peruvian (SI). Uncommon finding often associated with artificial cranial deformation or alteration. Stewart (1976).

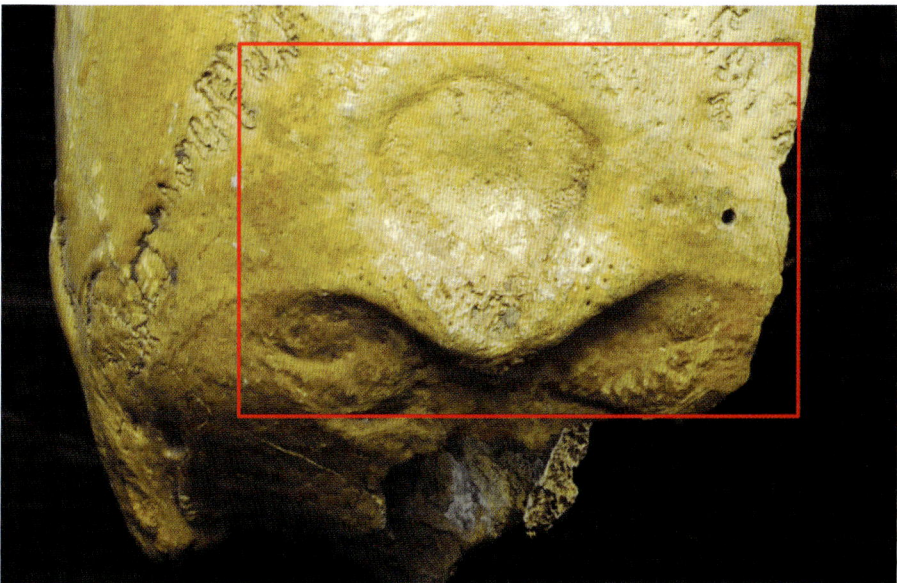

Figure 286. Large (40 mm S-I × 30 mm M-L) suprainion depression and large nuchal superstructure (massive superior nuchal line) (rectangle) in an adult Native American (Mütter Museum 1006.201). Uncommon finding, depending on the group. Stewart (1976).

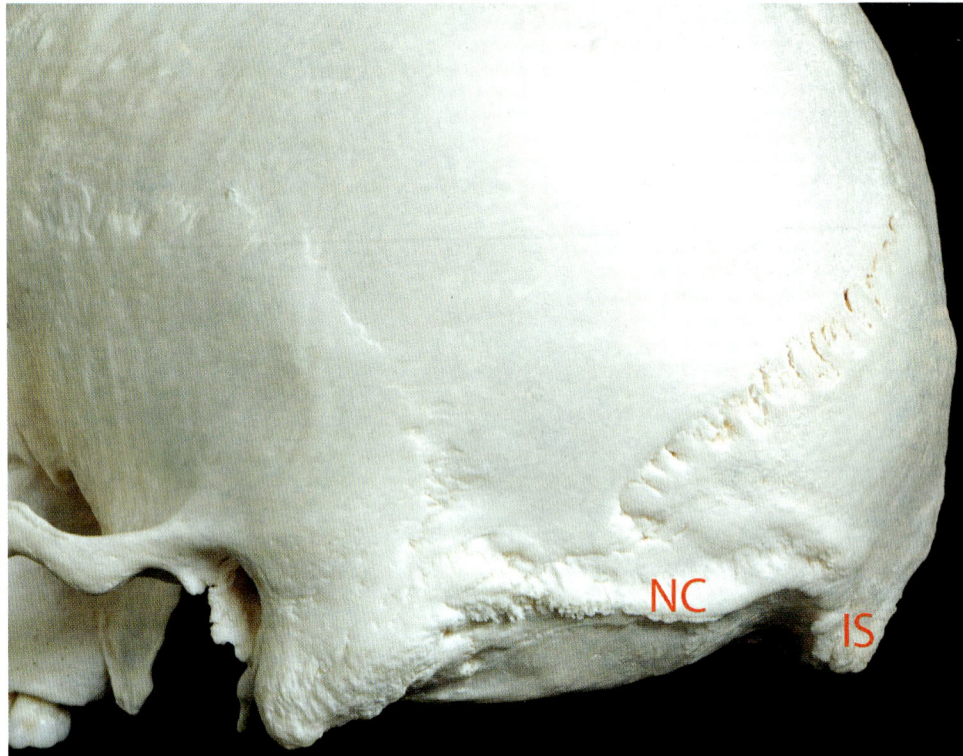

Figure 287. Unusually large and well-developed nuchal crest (NC) and Inion spike (IS) in a robust adult Asian male (CSC DS035). This crest is sometimes called the torus occipitalis transversus if highly developed and robust (Brash 1953). Cf. Heathcote et al. (2012); Mercer and Bogduk (2003) for muscle attachments in this region.

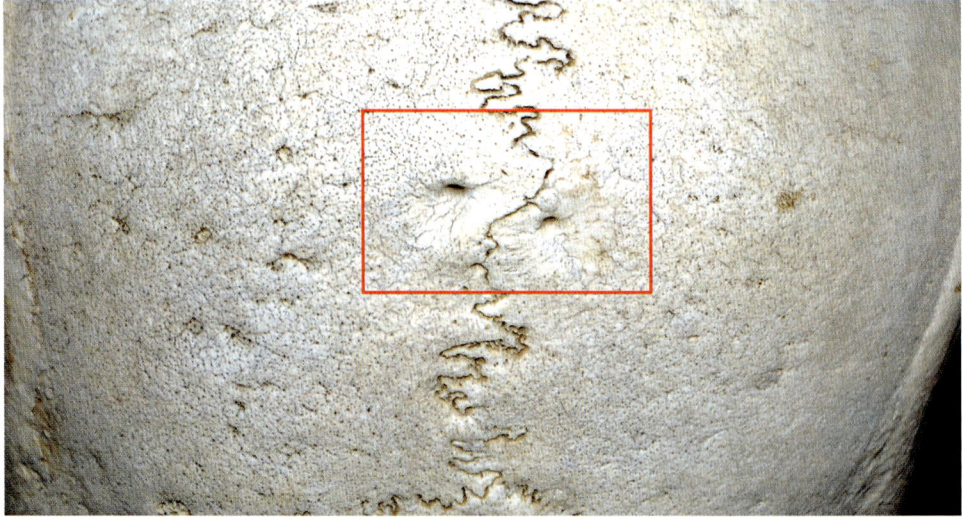

Figure 288. Adult Thai with bilateral parietal foramina and a simple sagittal suture at Obelion (rectangle) (KKU). Normal anatomy. Recent research suggests that the presence and number of parietal foramina affect the complexity of the sagittal suture at the Obelion (Mann et al. 2009).

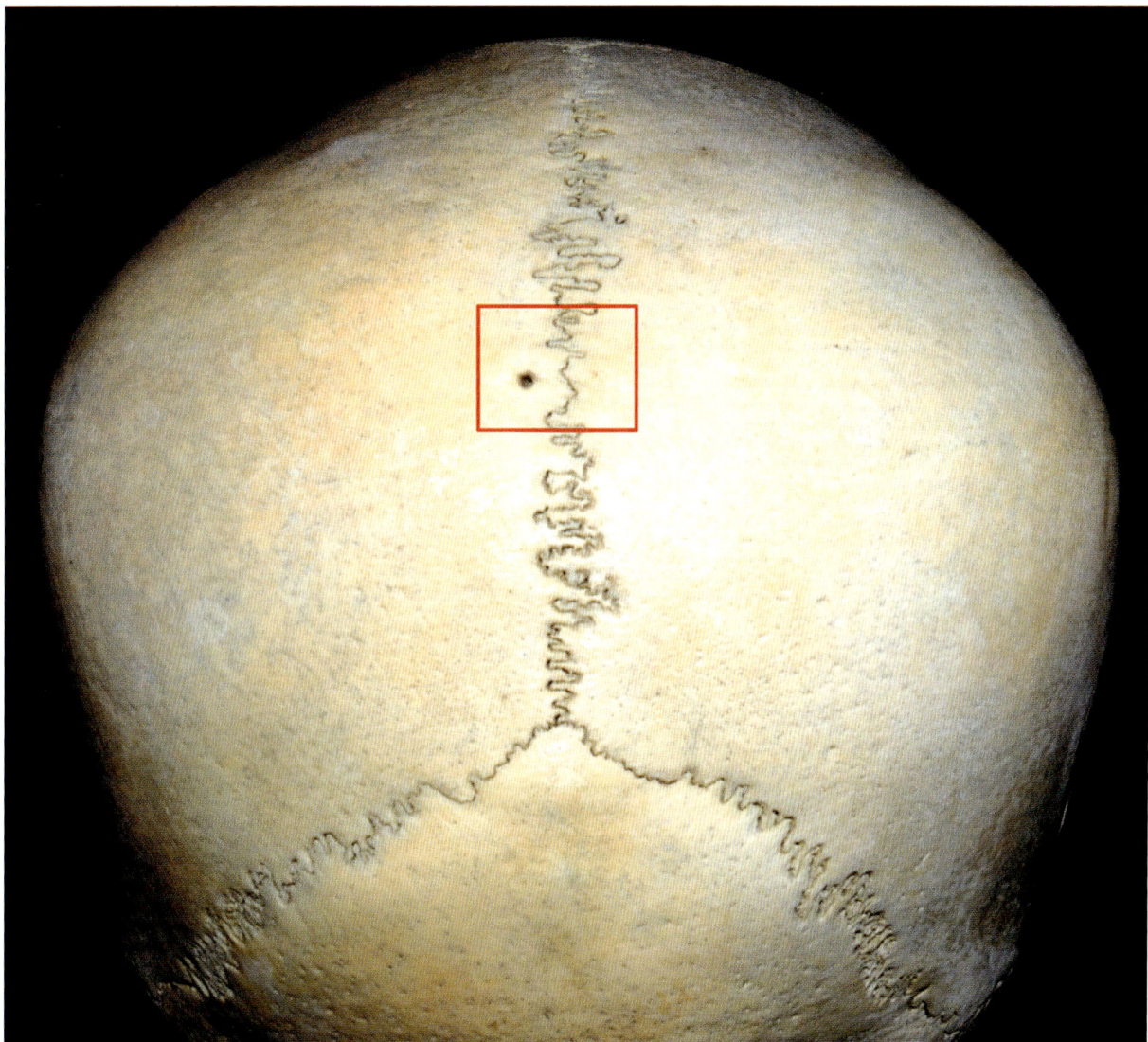

Figure 289. Relatively complex but typical sagittal suture with a single left parietal foramen that transmits an emissary vein (of Santorini) and/or artery at Obelion (rectangle) and a relatively simple lambdoidal suture. The lambdoidal suture typically is the most complex cranial vault suture.

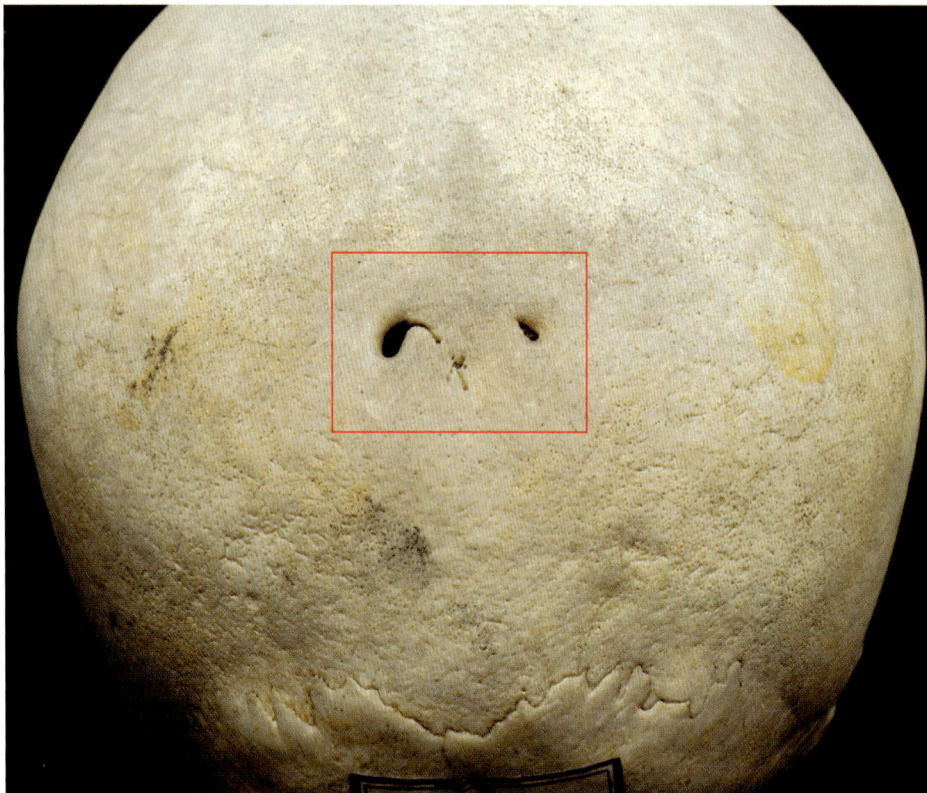

Figure 290. Asymmetrical, but normal sized parietal foramina (rectangle) and premature cranial synostosis of the sagittal suture in a 37-year-old adult Black male (Mütter Museum 1167.10). Common to uncommon findings.

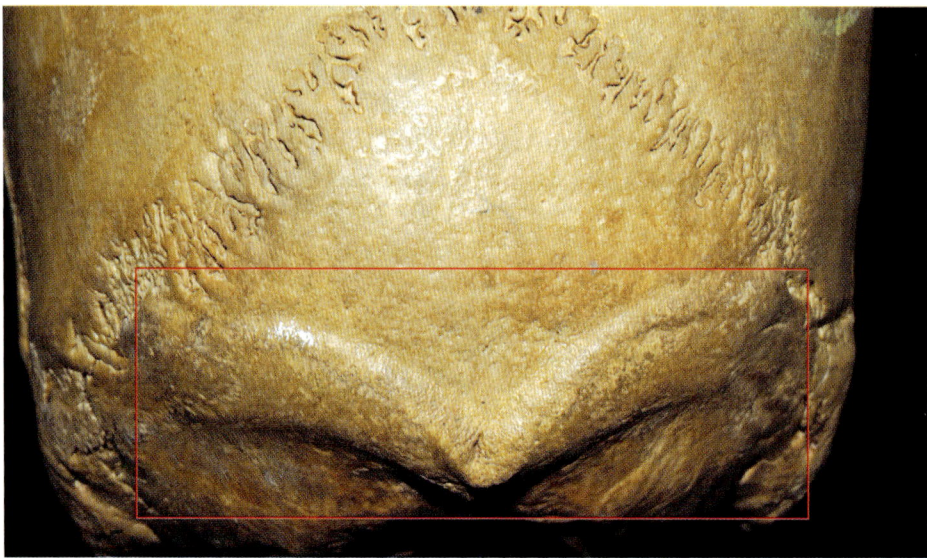

Figure 291. Highly developed occipital superstructure (rectangle; nuchal crest, superior nuchal line and small Inion spike or external occipital protuberance) in an adult Thai male (KKU). Large superstructures such as this are sometimes called torus occipitalis transversus (Brash 1953). Uncommon finding in most groups. Cf. Mercer and Bogduk (2003).

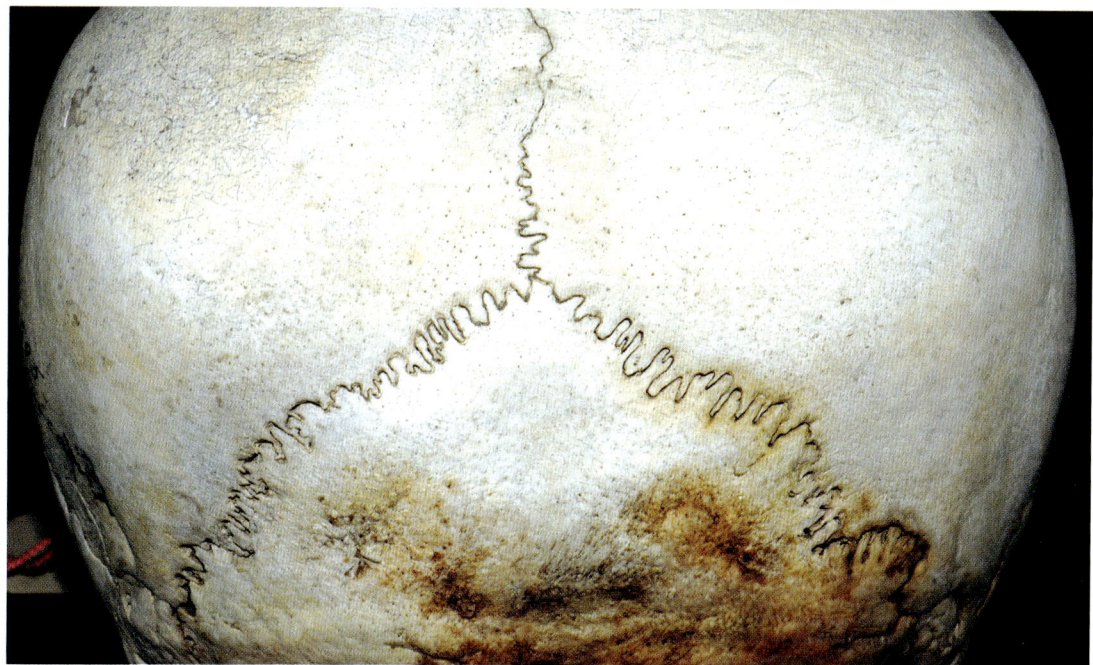

Figure 292. Unusually simple sagittal and lambdoidal sutures in an ancient Peruvian cranium (SI). As expected, the left half of the lambdoidal suture is simpler than the right half due to artificial cranial modification/deformation (flattening) to the left occipital region. Cf. Anton et al. (1992); Delashaw et al. (1991); Gottlieb (1978); O'Loughlin (2004) for deformation and ossicles.

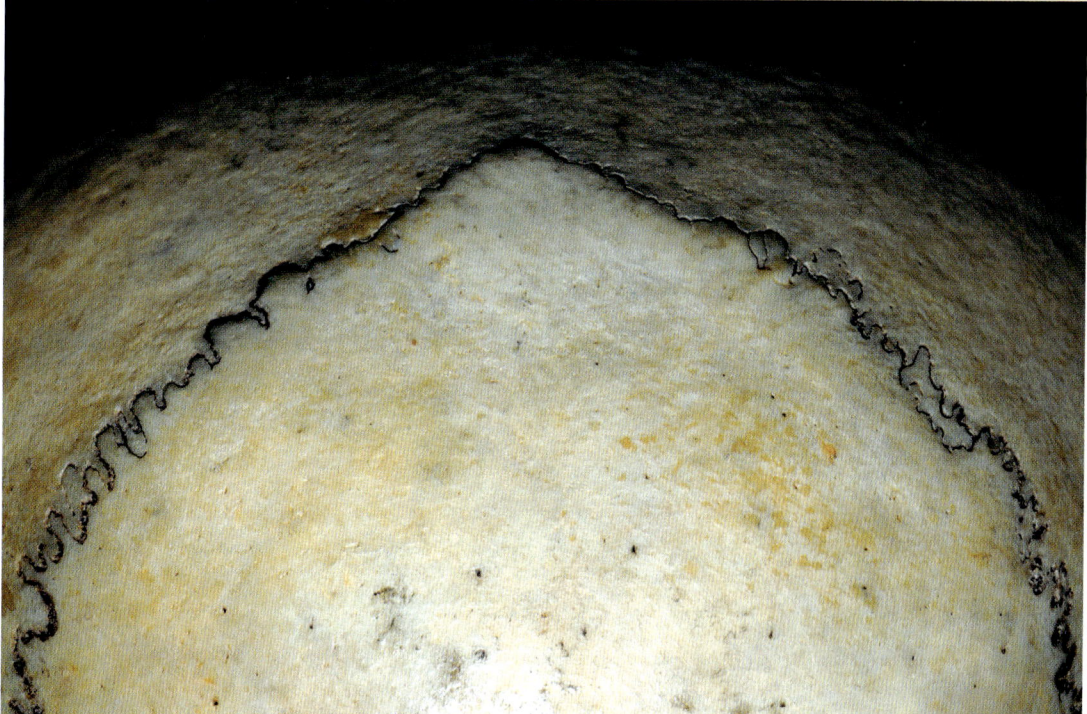

Figure 293. Unusually simple but normal lambdoidal suture in an adult Thai skull (KKU). The sagittal suture has completely obliterated in this individual. A simple lambdoidal suture is an uncommon finding.

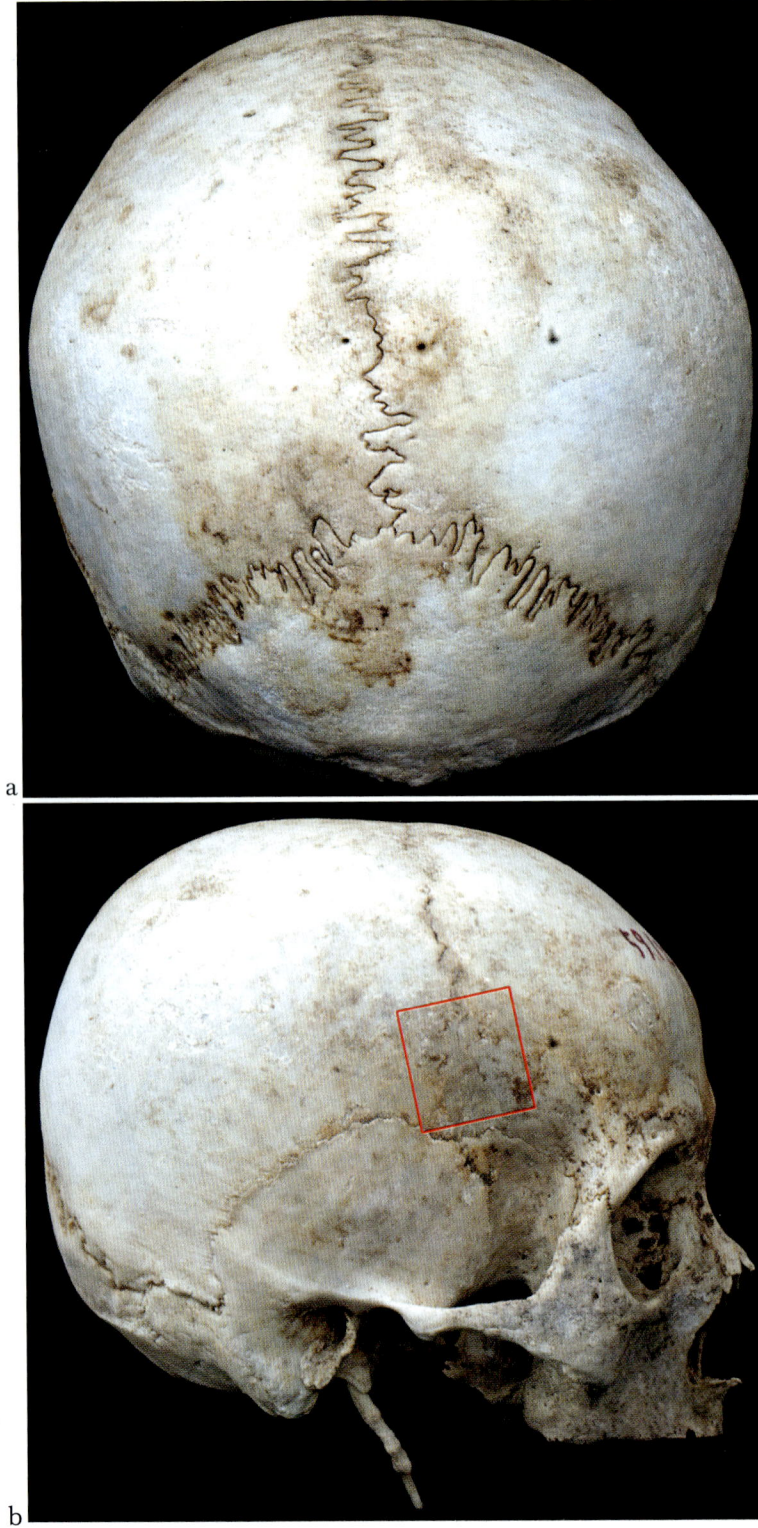

Figure 294a-b. Open sagittal and lambdoidal sutures and partial closure of the coronal suture bilaterally in an 82-year-old Thai female (CMU). (a) Occipital view of the open sagittal and lambdoidal sutures even at this elderly age. (b) Right lateral view showing obliteration of a portion of the coronal suture (square). Although vault sutures are one of the features commonly used to estimate age at death, there is great variation in their pattern and timing of closure. Note remarkable styloid process.

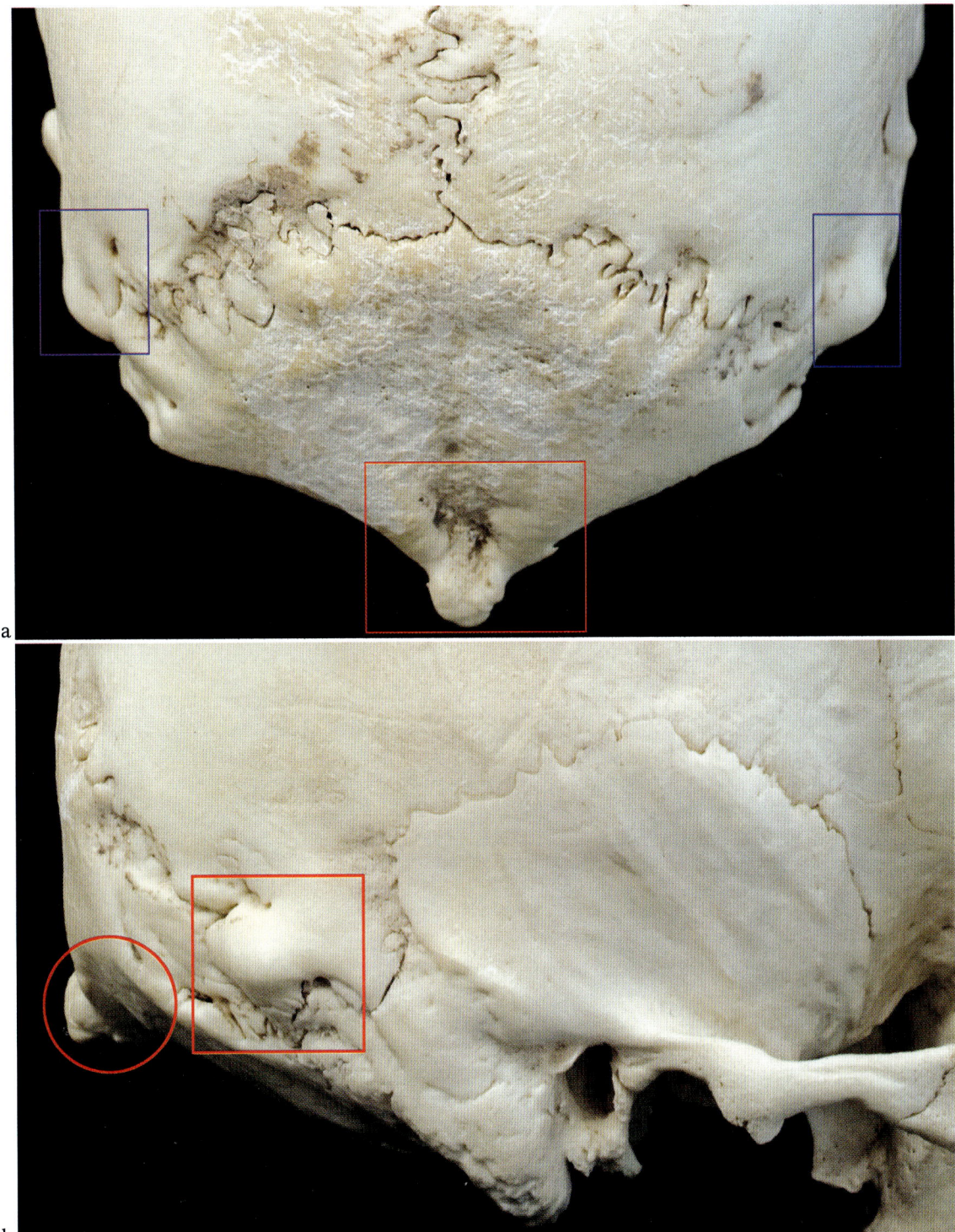

Figure 295a-b. Highly-developed occipital superstructure with a prominent nuchal spike and bilateral retromastoid tubercles/processes in an adult Asian male (CSC AS022). (a) Large, rounded retromastoid processes (blue rectangles) and a large nuchal spike (red square). (b) Right lateral view showing the nuchal spike (circle) and retromastoid tubercle (square). Cf. Hauser and DeStefano (1989); Heathcote et al. (2012).

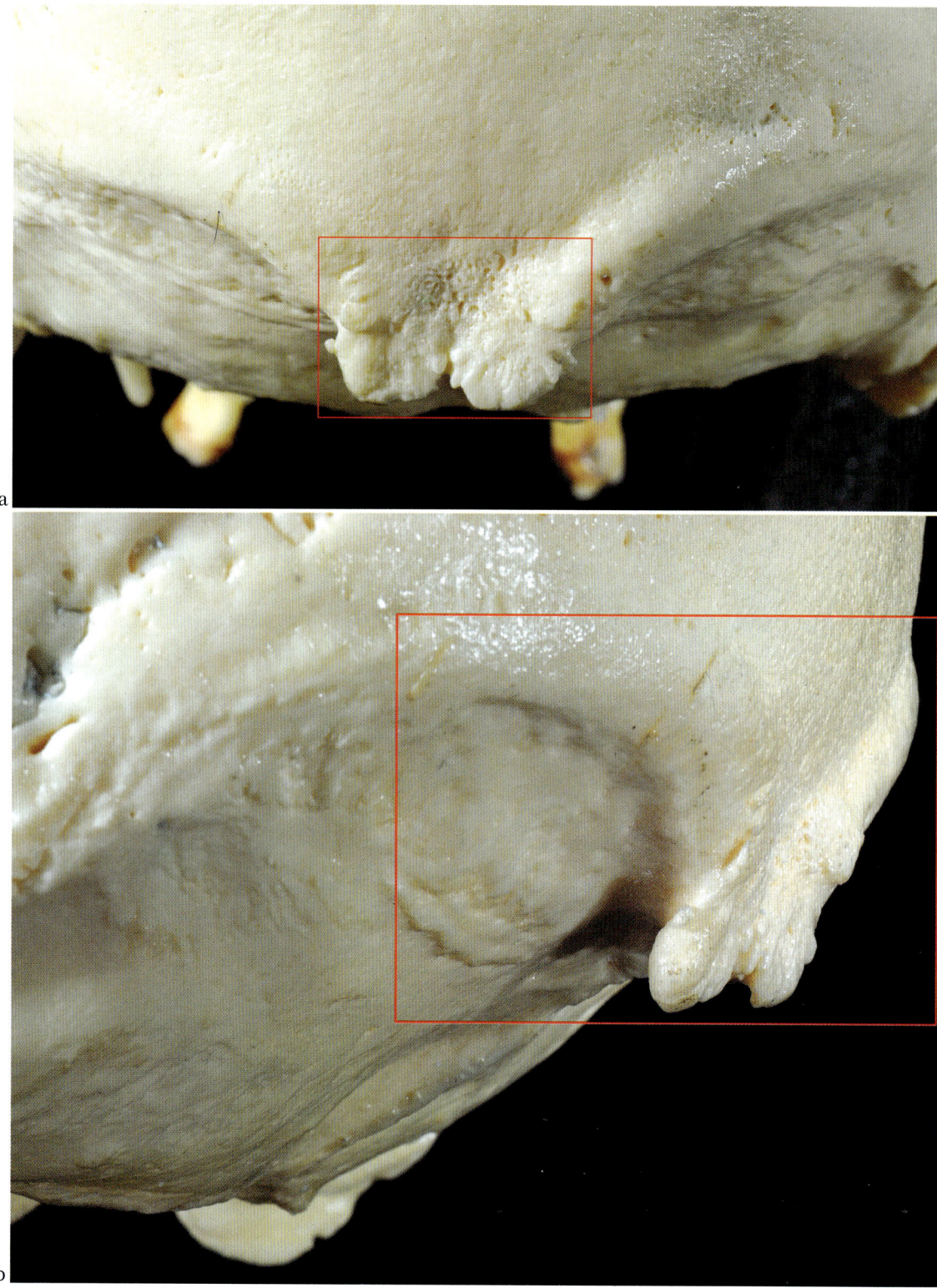

Figure 296a-b. Developed occipital superstructure and a large, bifurcated Inion spike/hook in an adult Asian male skull (CSC AC 001). (a) Occipital and (b) left oblique views of an unusually large Inion spike and a prominent nuchal crest/superstructure (rectangle). Uncommon finding.

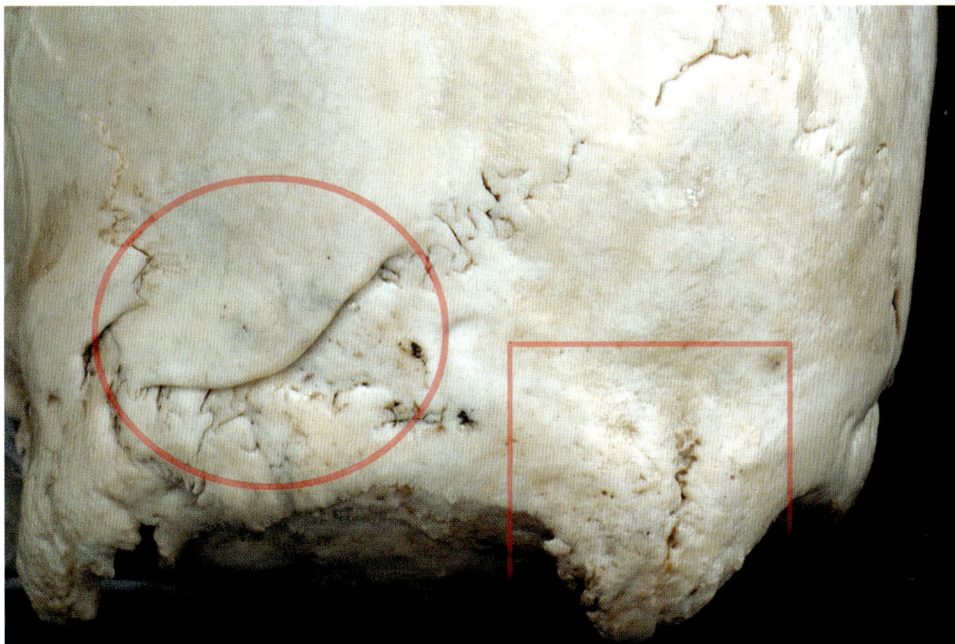

Figure 297. Unusually large nuchal superstructure and crest with a very rare vertically oriented suture (square) in a robust adult Thai male skull (KKU 1017-37). Note the "folded" nature of the bone along the left side (red circle) resembling flowing lava. This feature is occasionally present in robust skulls, but of unknown etiology (possibly hypermuscularity).

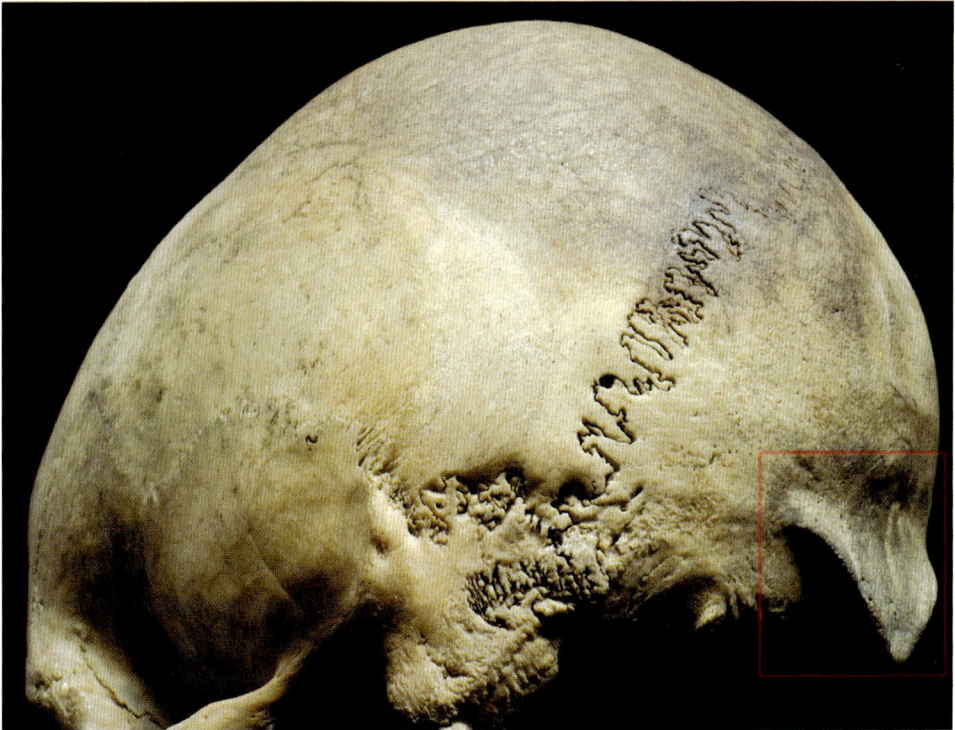

Figure 298. Unusually large and overhanging nuchal crest (rectangle) in an ancient Egyptian male (UPenn 814 L606).

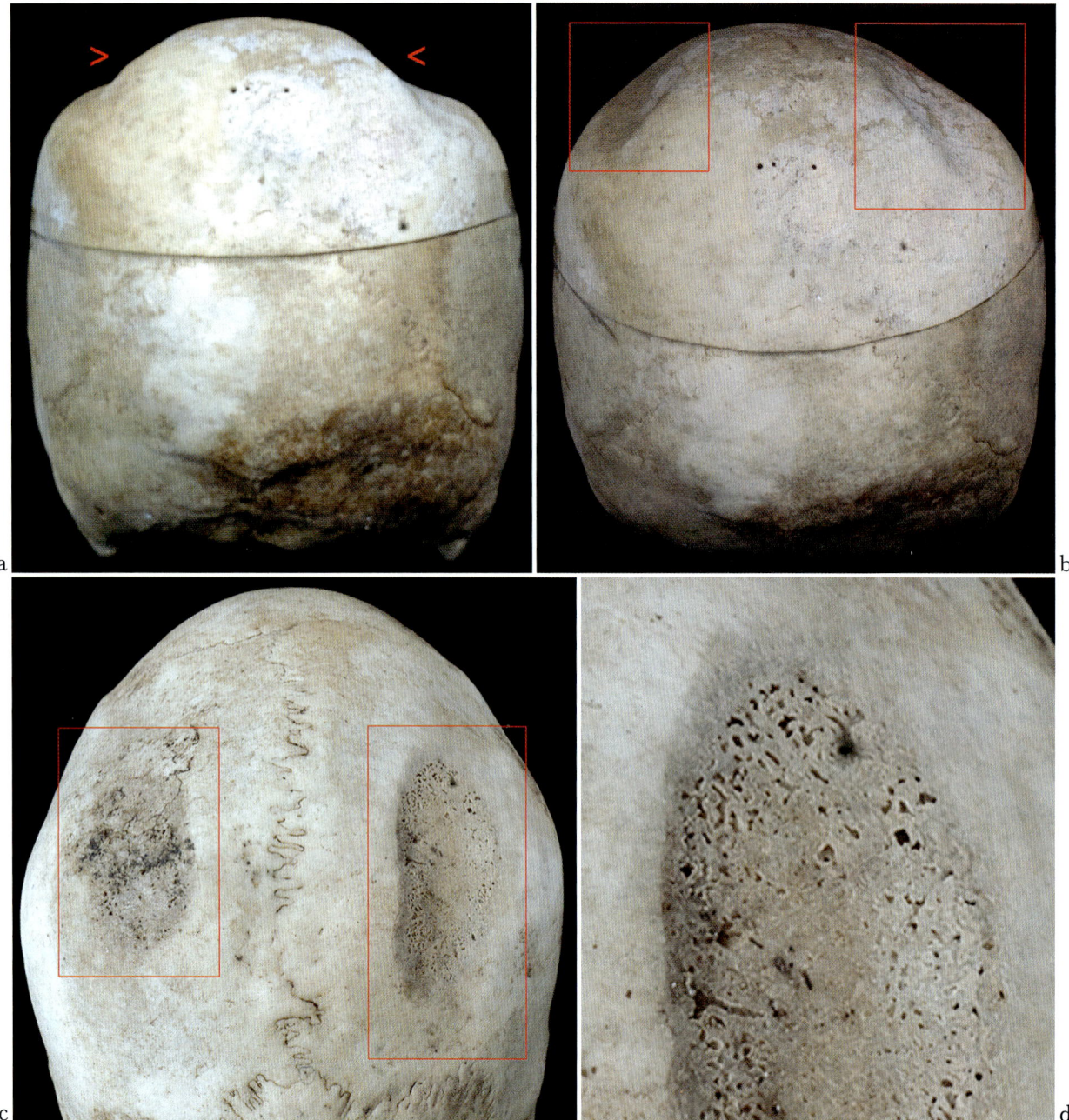

Figure 299a-d. Symmetrical osteoporosis (SO) (biparietal thinning, spongy hyperostosis biparietal osteodystrophy) in two adults (a-b) CMU 14 53; (c-d) CMU 7 53). (a-b) SO in an 87-year-old Asian female with resorption that does not involve the sutures and temporal lines. (c-d) Example of active SO in a 66-year-old Thai male skull. Note resorption of the outer table followed by exposure of the sieve-like diploë. Once the diploë resorbs, the floor becomes smooth. The inner table of the cranium is rarely affected by this process. SO reflects a pathological or age-related process (disease, anemia) and it is not a non-metric trait or typical variant. Cf. Mann and Hunt (2005, 2012) for references and Moseley (1965) for a description of the process; Cederlund et al. (1982); Phillips (2008).

Occipital View of the Skull 237

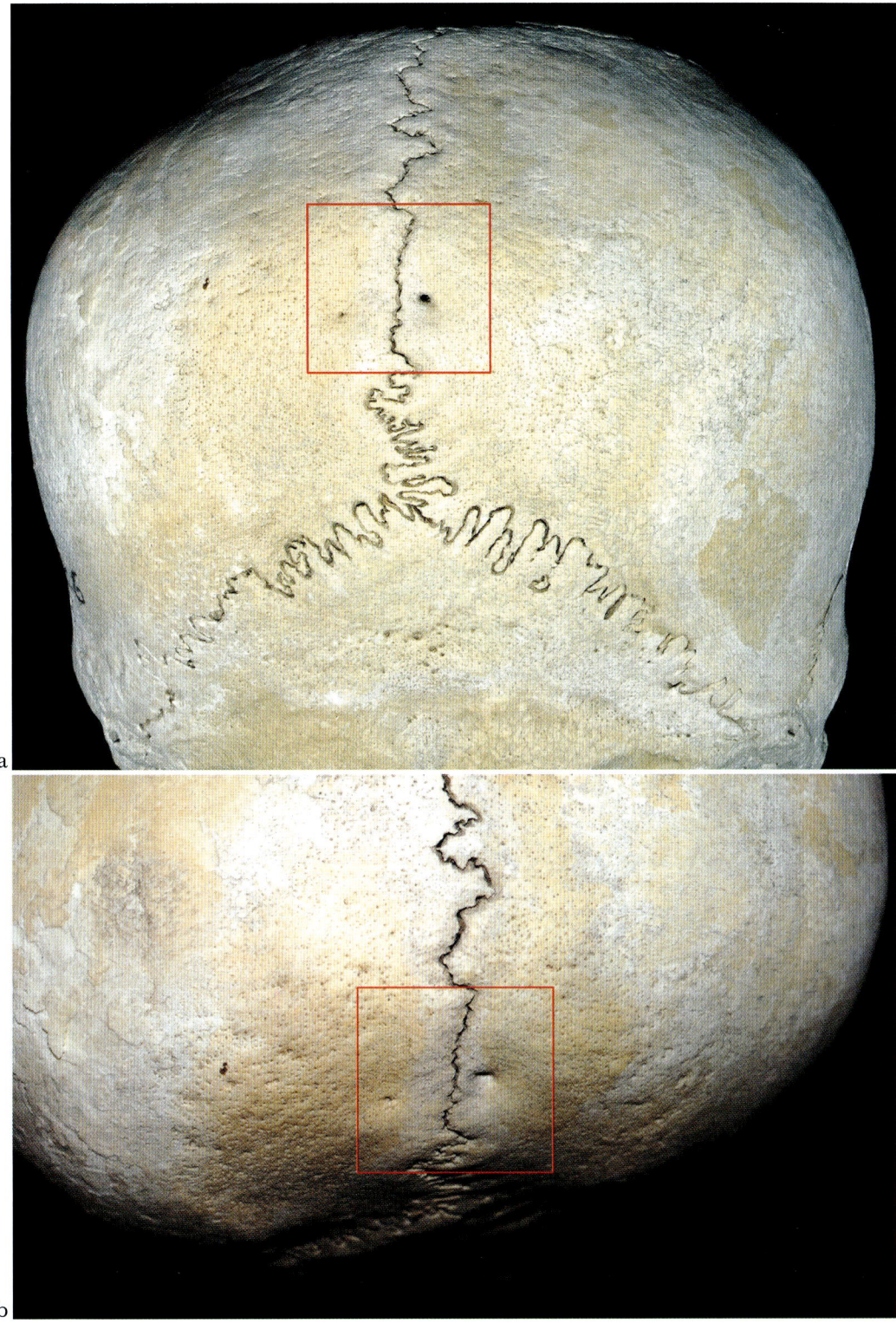

Figure 300a-b. Simple sagittal and lambdoidal sutures in an adult with asymmetrical parietal foramina. (a) Overview of the skull showing the morphology of the sagittal and lambdoidal sutures and parietal foramina (square). (b) Higher magnification of Obelion and the two parietal foramina (square). Typical anatomy and common findings. Cf. Hauser and DeStefano (1989); Mann et al. (2009).

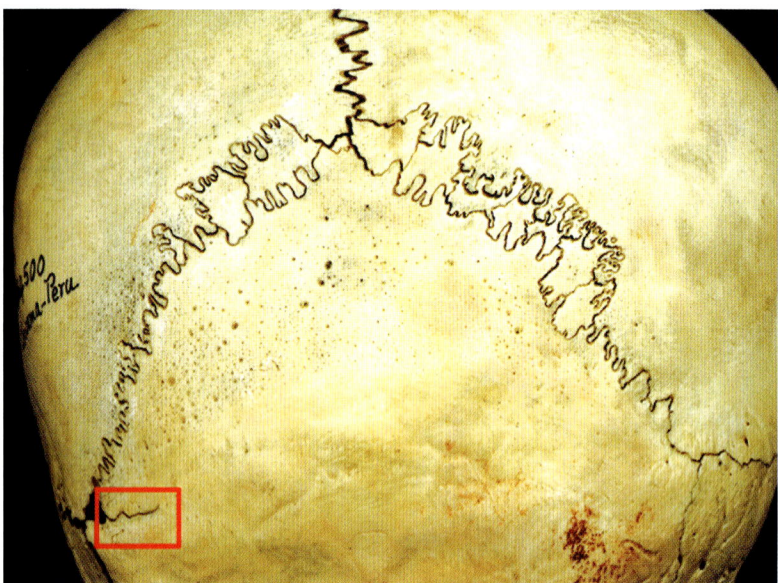

Figure 301. Trace left Mendosal/biasterionic suture (rectangle) and numerous lambdoidal ossicles in an ancient Peruvian child (SI). Although variable, the Mendosal suture usually closes by birth and obliterates between two and four years of age, but was found in 16% of 50 adult skulls (Tubbs et al. 2007) and 18 of 129 (14%) adult skulls (Tubbs et al. 2007). Cf. Fazekas and Kosa (1978); Kosa (1995); Schaefer et al. (2009); Scheuer and Black (2000); Shapiro and Robinson (1976).

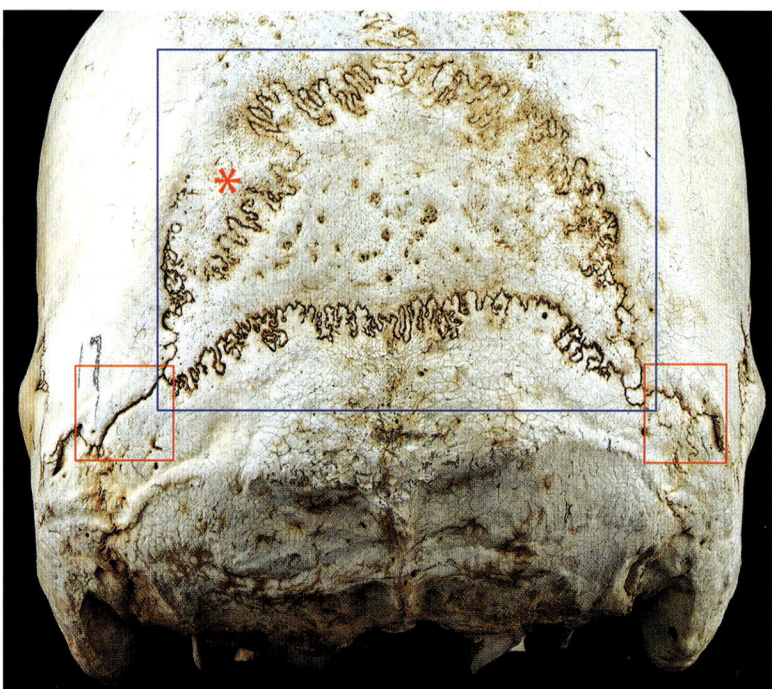

Figure 302. Trace Mendosal/biasteronic sutures (red square and rectangle) and an Inca bone (blue rectangle) with a lambdoidal ossicle (*) in an adult Thai male skull (SI). Note the Inca bone joins the Mendosal sutures (from Asterion to Asterion). The Mendosal suture may be at, above or below Asterion. Uncommon to common findings. Cf. Bhanu and Sankar (2011); Gayretli et al. (2011); Hanihara and Ishida (2001c); Hepburn (1908); Matsumura et al. (1993); Saheb et al. (2011); Srivastava (1977); Tubbs et al. (2007).

Occipital View of the Skull

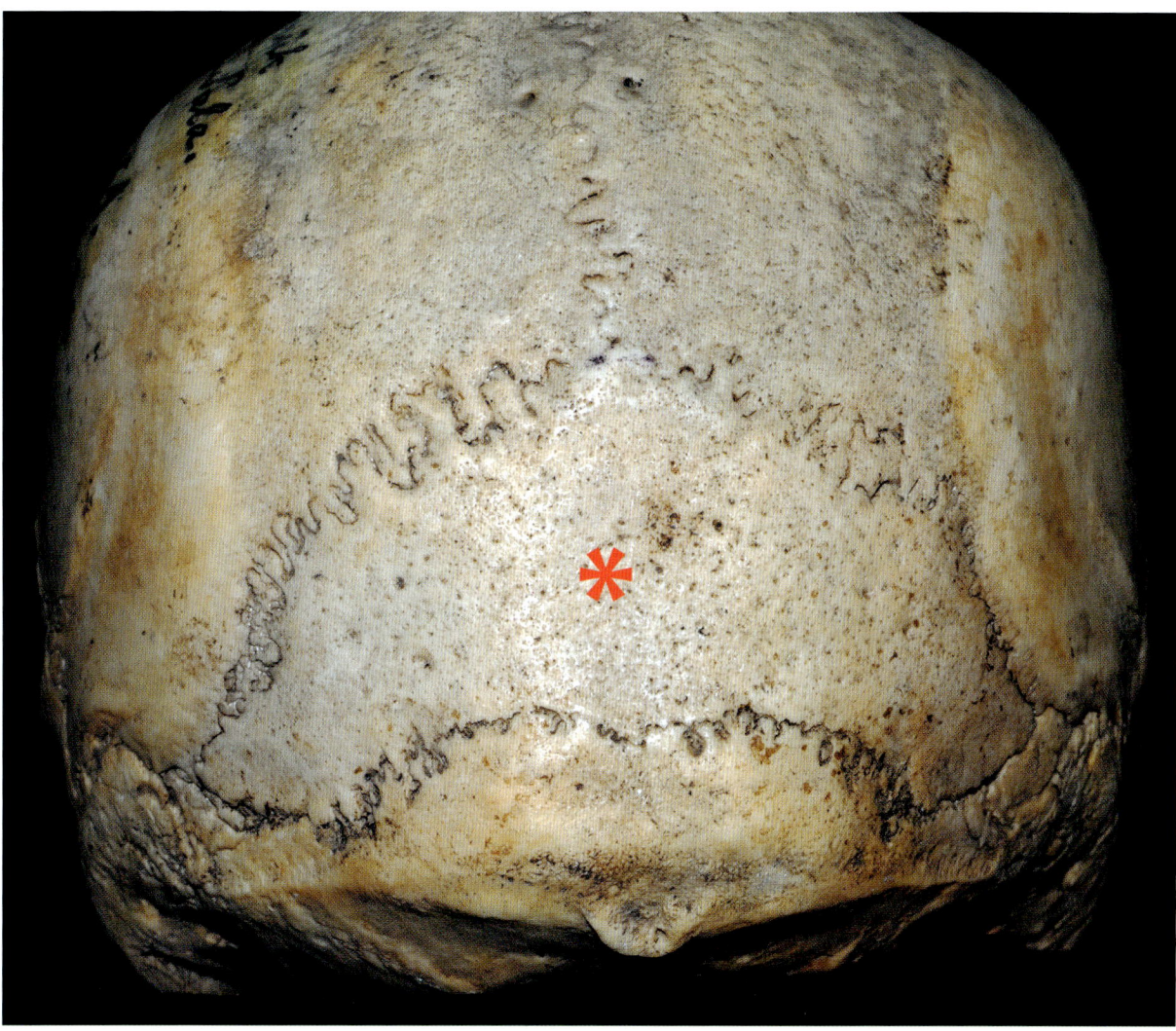

Figure 303. Inca bone (*) extending from Asterion to Asterion and dividing the occipital bone into upper and lower halves in an adult male skull (RV1061). Cf. Hanihara and Ishida (2001c). Hauser and Destefano (1989)

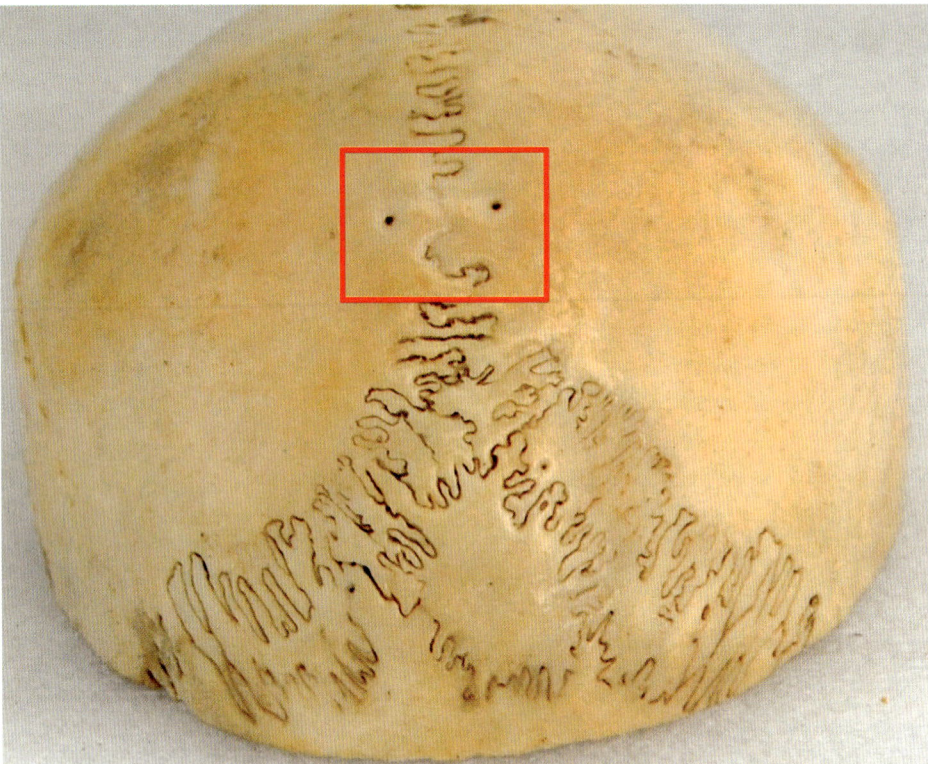

Figure 304. Bilateral parietal foramina (common finding), simple suture at Obelion (red rectangle) and unusually large and complex lambdoidal ossicles, all located posterior to Lambda. Cf. Hauser and DeStefano (1989).

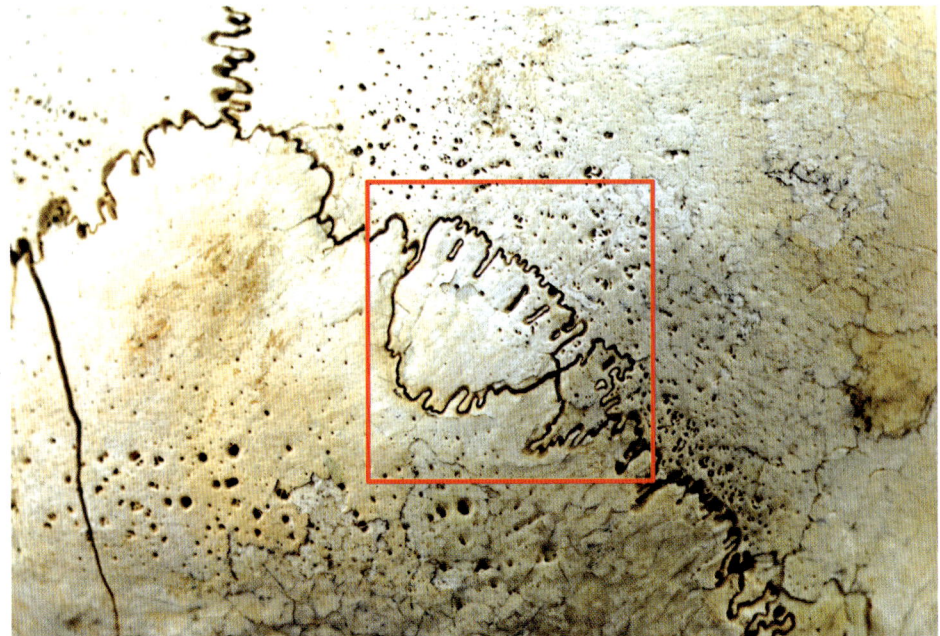

Figure 305. Lambdoidal suture with two unusual ossicles (square) and porotic hyperostosis (pitting) in an ancient Peruvian child (SI). The nearly vertical fracture occurred postmortem. Lambdoidal ossicles and porotic hyperostosis are common findings.

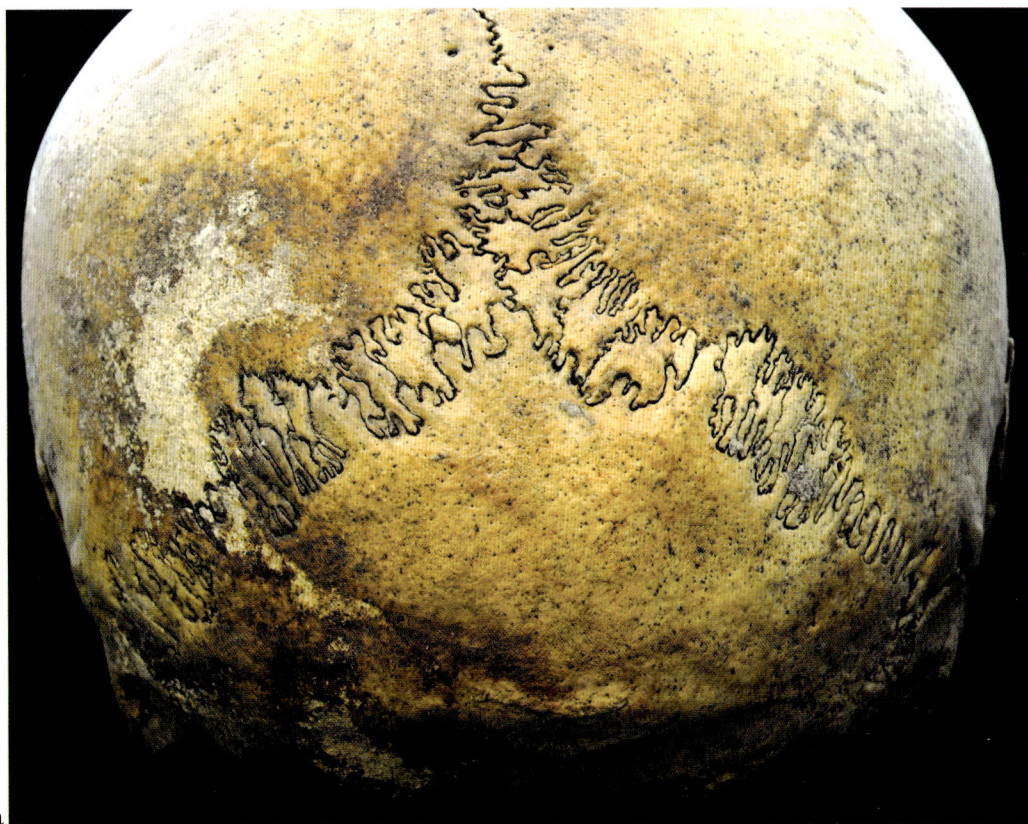

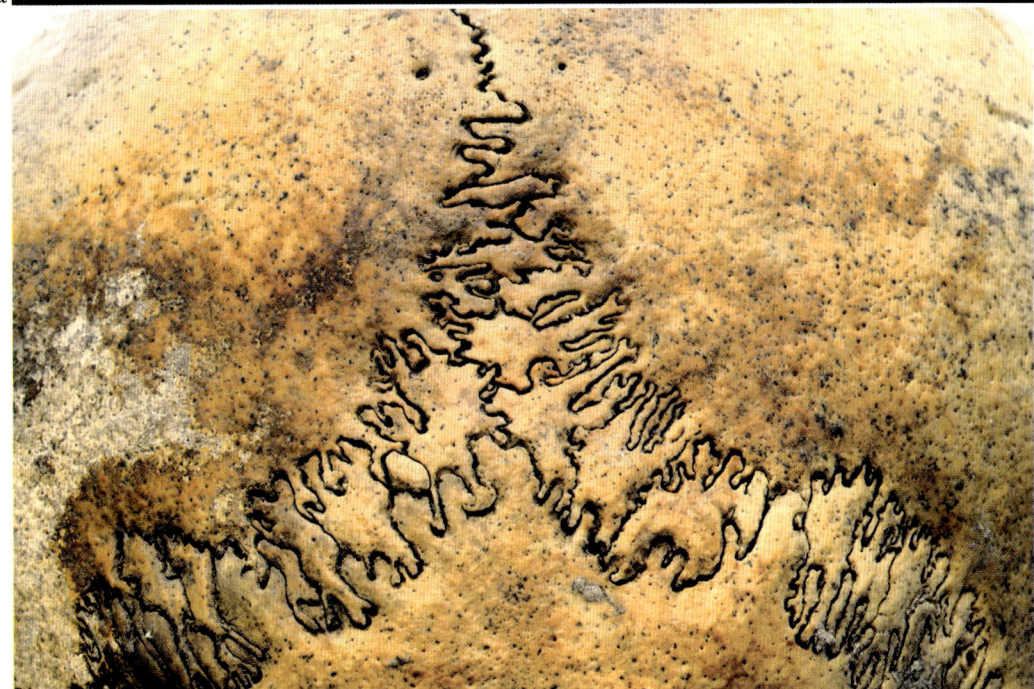

Figure 306a-b. Unusually high number of lambdoidal ossicles in an adult male. (a) Lambdoidal suture comprised almost entirely of ossicles extending into the sagittal suture to within about 1 cm of the parietal foramina in an adult male (RV1202). (b) Higher magnification showing the complexity of the ossicles. While subject to many variables, numerous lambdoidal ossicles as seen in this specimen are more commonly found in Asian crania. Ossicles extending into the sagittal suture are uncommon to rare.

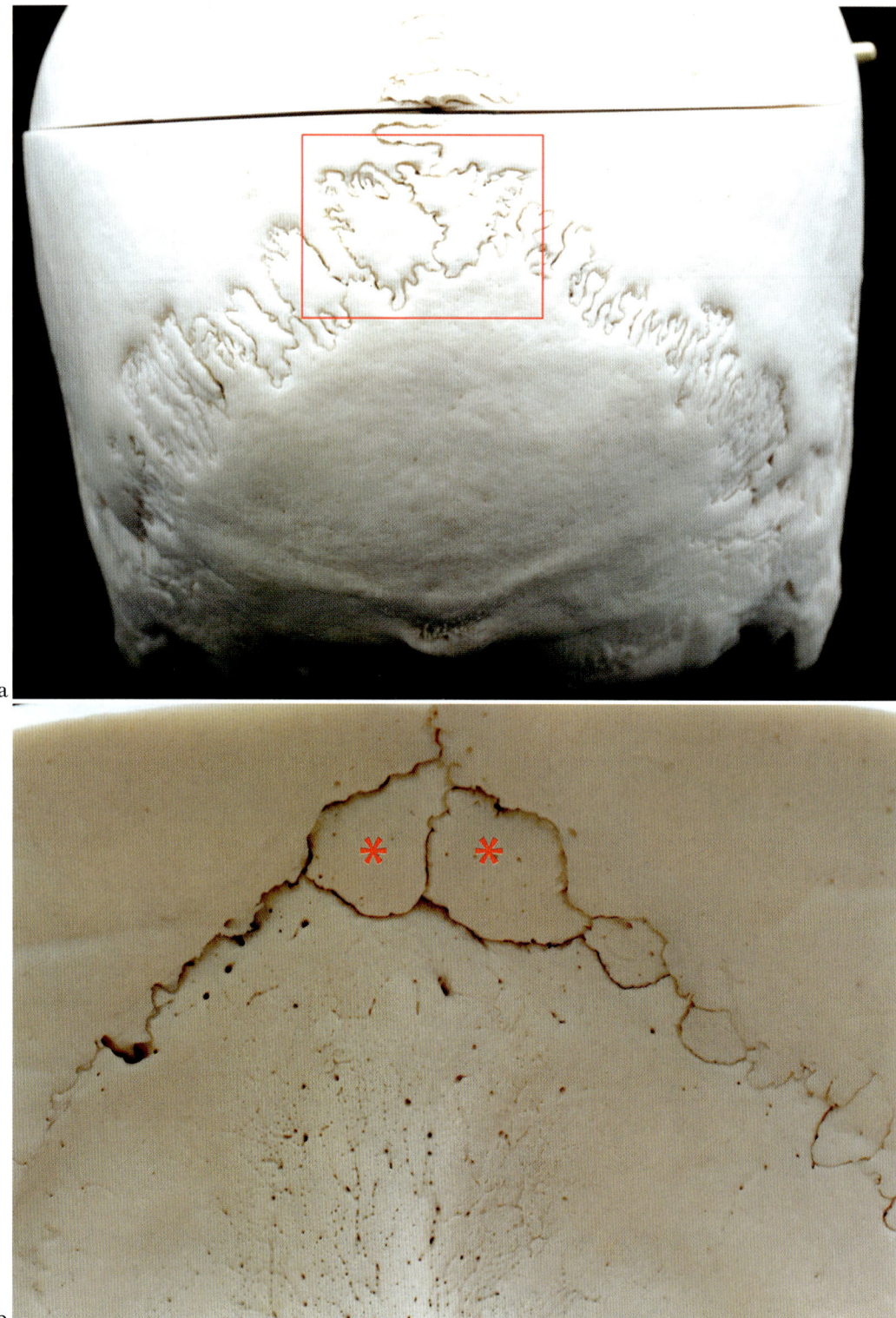

Figure 307a-b. Ectocranial view of lambdoidal ossicles and the two central ossicles. (a) Ectocranial view of the occipital region showing the differences in size, shape and complexity of lambdoidal ossicles in an adult male (FSA AC051). (b) Endocranial view of the morphology of the two largest ossicles (*). The ectocranial and endocranial morphology of ossicles differs, reflecting varying biomechanical stresses.

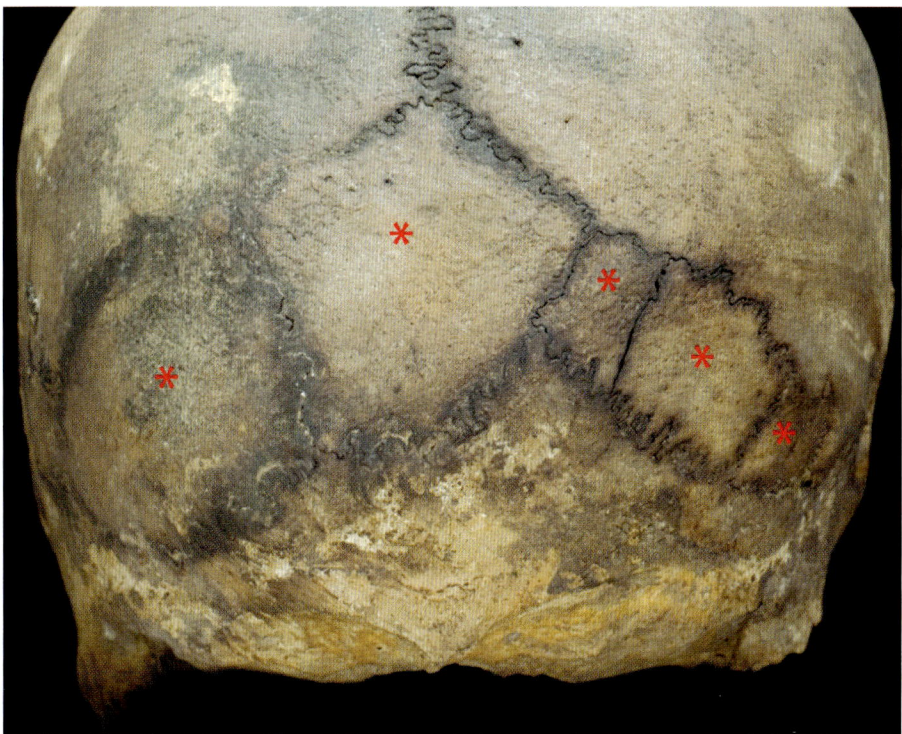

Figure 308. Large lambdoidal ossicles, sometimes referred to as interparietal bones (asterisks) (UPenn 808 L606).

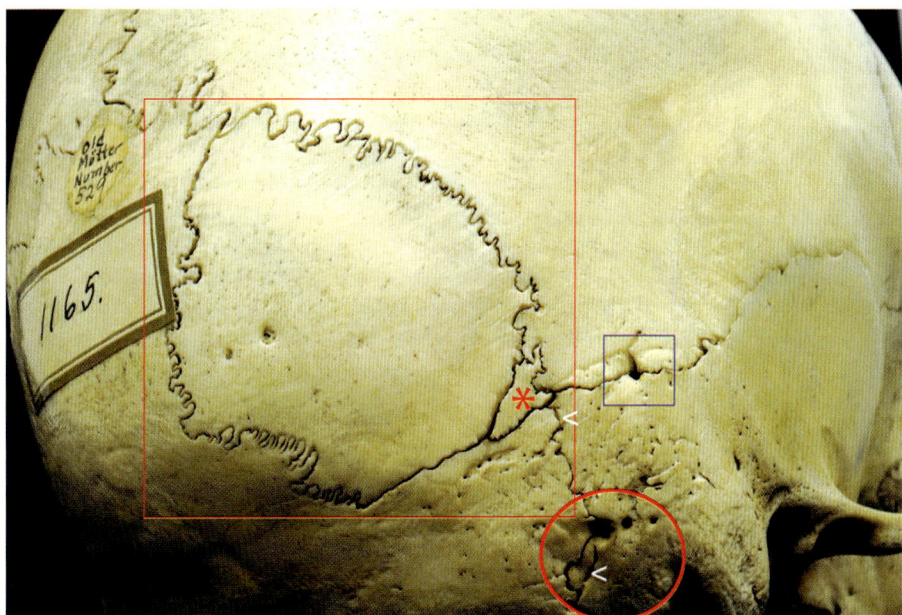

Figure 309. Asymmetric/bipartite Inca bone, sometimes called lateral pre-interparietal bone (red square) or bipartite occipital bone, and a small asterionic ossicle (*); supramastoid foramen in the squamosal suture (blue square); small ossicle (ossicle of Riolano; Vázquez et al. 2001) in the occipitomastoid suture (<); and mastoid foramina (circle; one sutural and two temporal) (Mütter Museum 1165.00). Cf. Bhanu and Sankar (2011); Berge and Bergman (2001); Boyd (1930); Hanihara and Ishida (2001a); Hauser and DeStefano (1989).

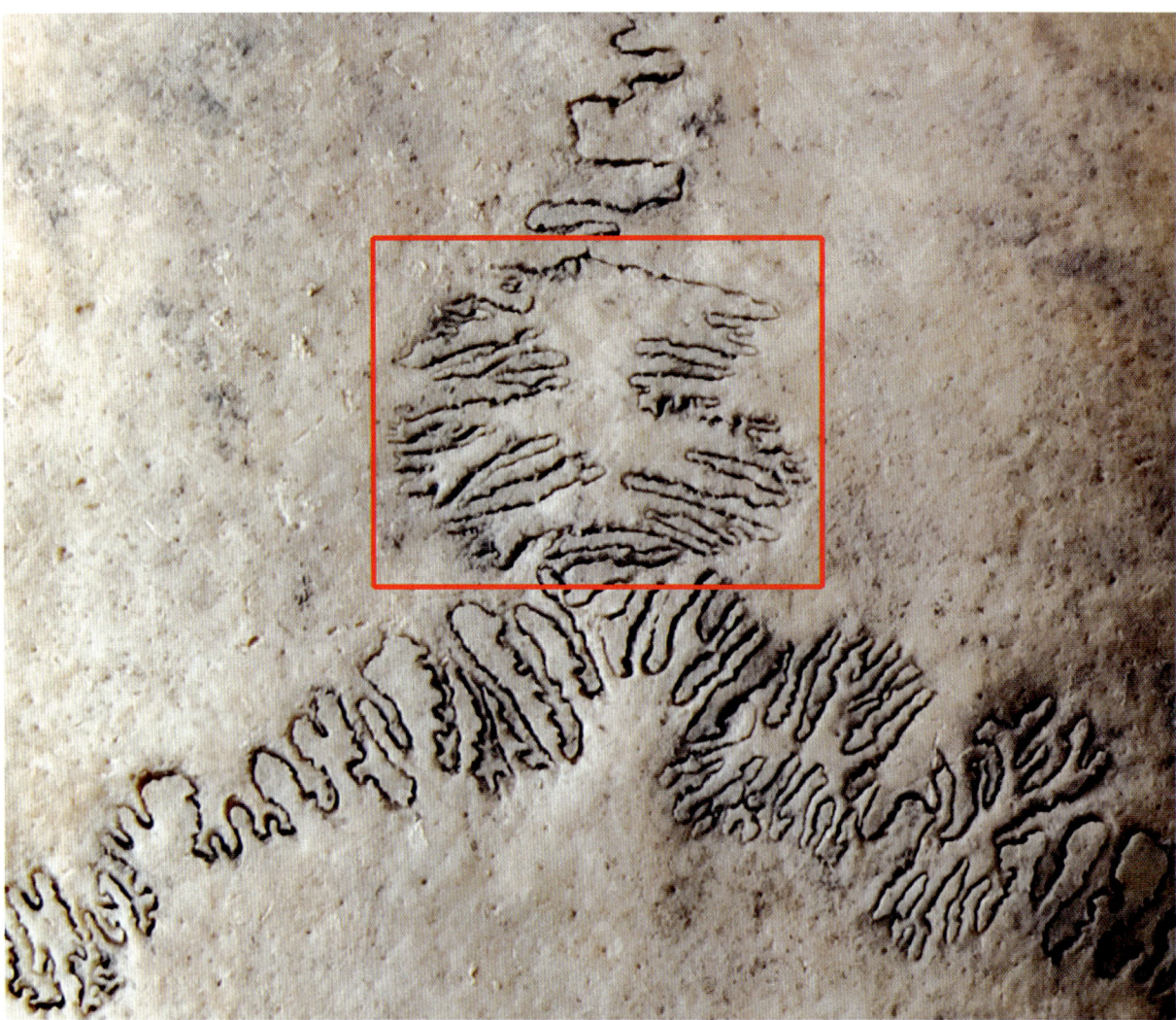

Figure 310. Supra-bregmatic ossicle/bone or sagittal ossicle (rectangle) connected, but anterior to the lambdoidal suture in a young adult (NHMH 2009.32.108). Note that the sutural complexity of this ossicle resembles the lambdoidal more than the sagittal suture. While few researchers draw the distinction, ossicles at Lambda may be superior ("supra" and part of the parietal bones) or inferior ("infra" and part of the occipital bone) to the apex of the lambdoidal suture. Sutures anterior to Lambda are less common than those that form along and part of the lambdoidal suture.

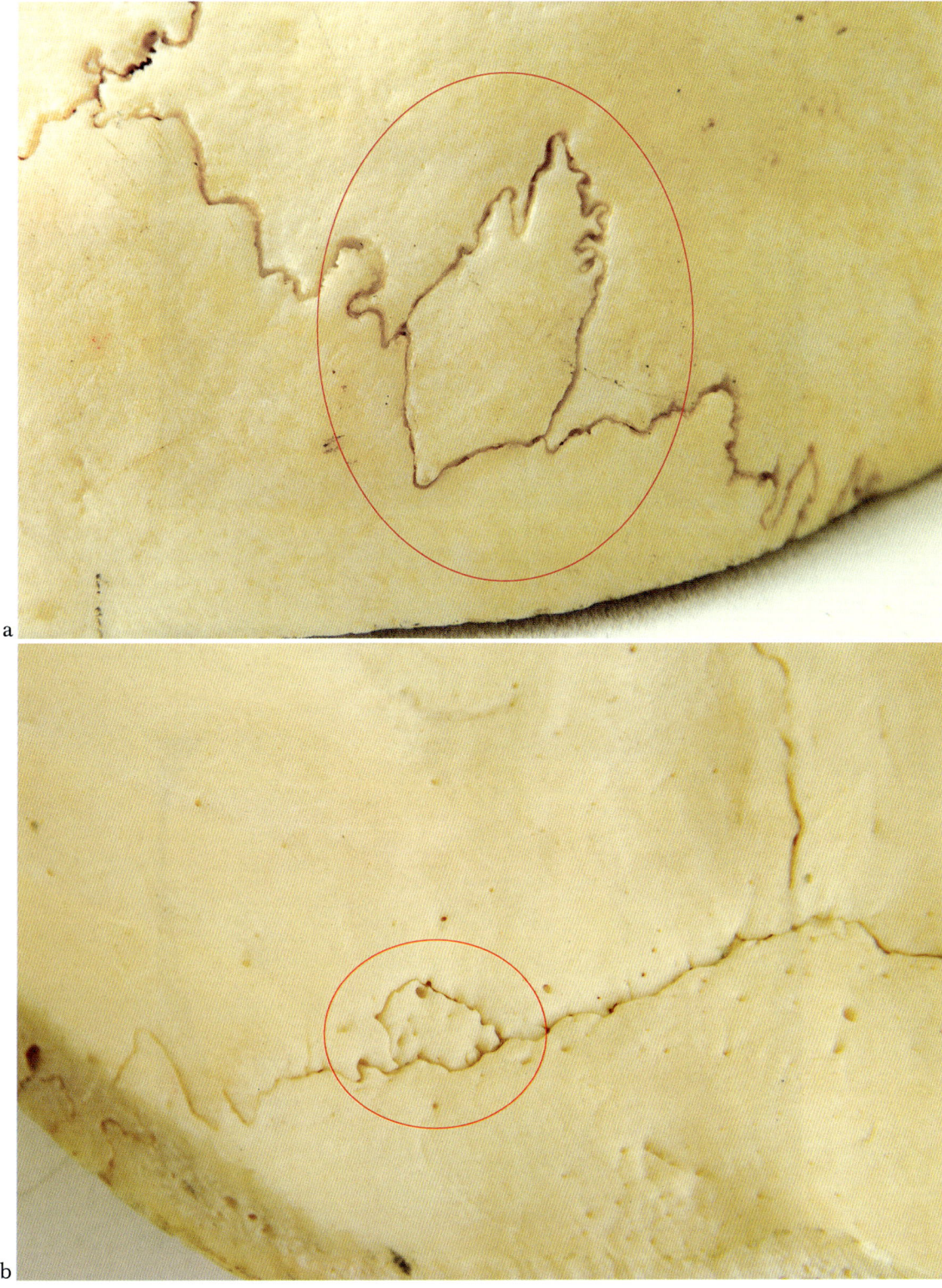

Figure 311a-b. Ectocranial and endocranial morphology of a lambdoidal ossicle. (a) Ectocranial and (b) endocranial views of a small lambdoidal ossicle (oval) demonstrating differences in size, shape and sutural complexity in the outer and inner vault. Most ossicles are smaller and more simple endocranially than ectocranially. Typical anatomy and common finding.

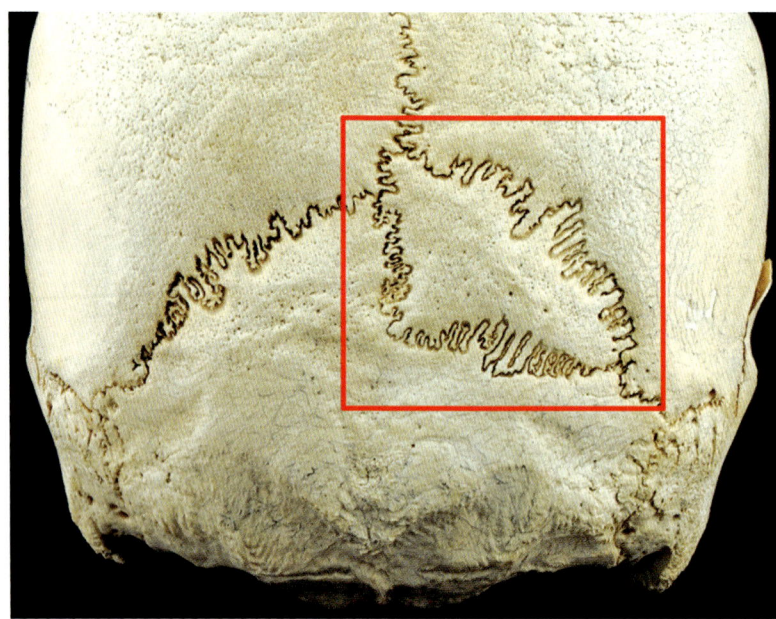

Figure 312. A large asymmetric right lambdoidal ossicle (square) might also be identified as a single pre-interparietal bone, bipartite occipital bone, or partial Inca bone because of its connection to the right Mendosal/asterionic suture (KKU). A true Inca bone is the result of a persistent Mendosal/biasteronic suture and spans bilateral Asterion points, via both Mendosal sutures. Uncommon finding. Cf. Hanihara and Ishida (2001c); Hauser and DeStefano (1989); Shapiro and Robinson (1976); Matsumura et al. (1993) on pre-interparietal bone; Srivastava (1977); Tubbs et al. (2007) on the Mendosal suture; Weinberg et al. (2005).

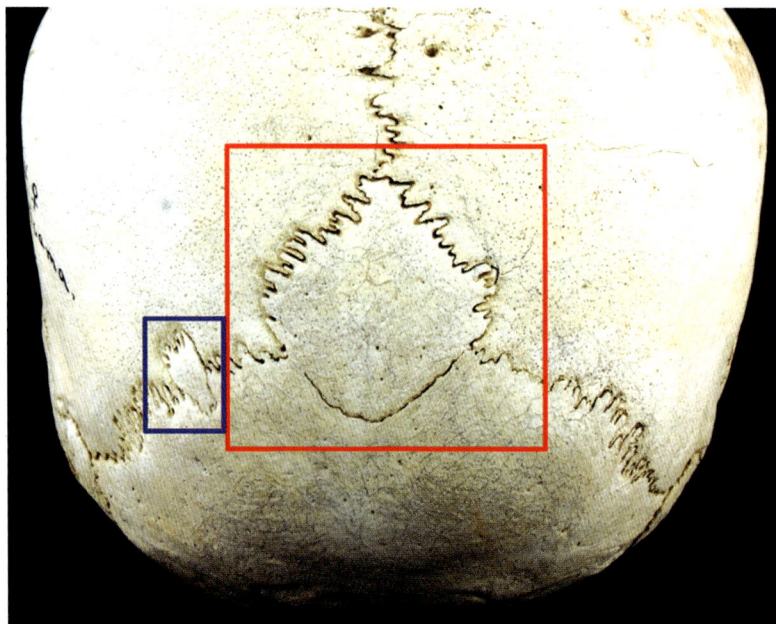

Figure 313. Diamond-shaped ossicle at Lambda/apical bone/pre-interparietal bone (red square) and a small lambdoidal ossicle (blue rectangle). Note the lambdoidal part of the large ossicle is much more simple than the parietal portions. (SI ancient Peruvian). The large ossicle is an uncommon finding. Cf. Gopinathan (1992); Hanihara and Ishida (2001a).

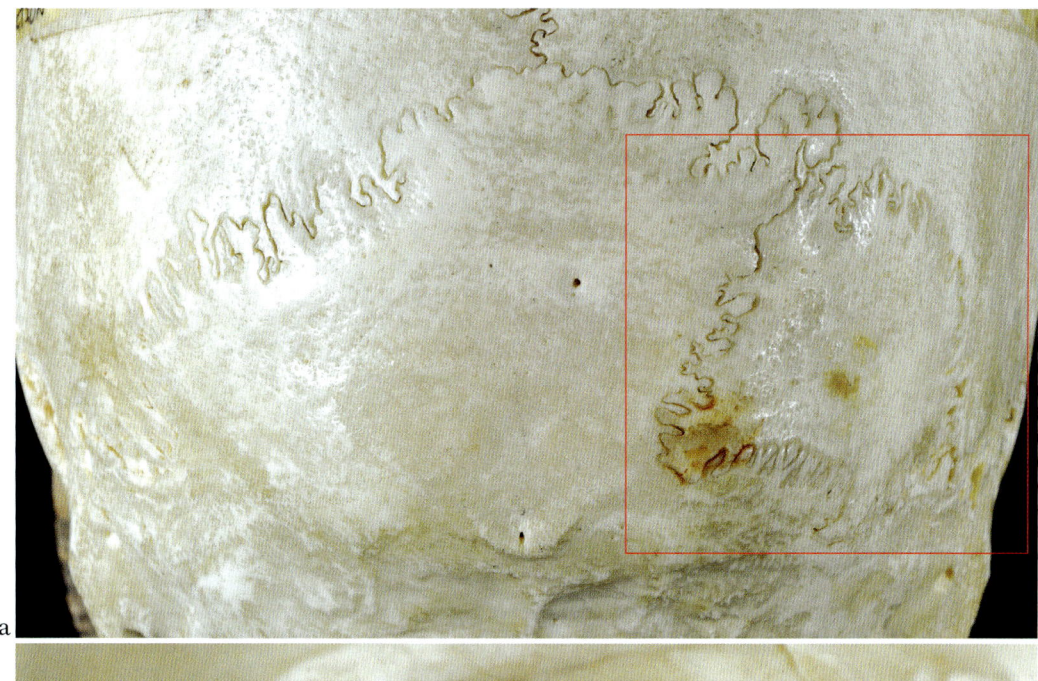

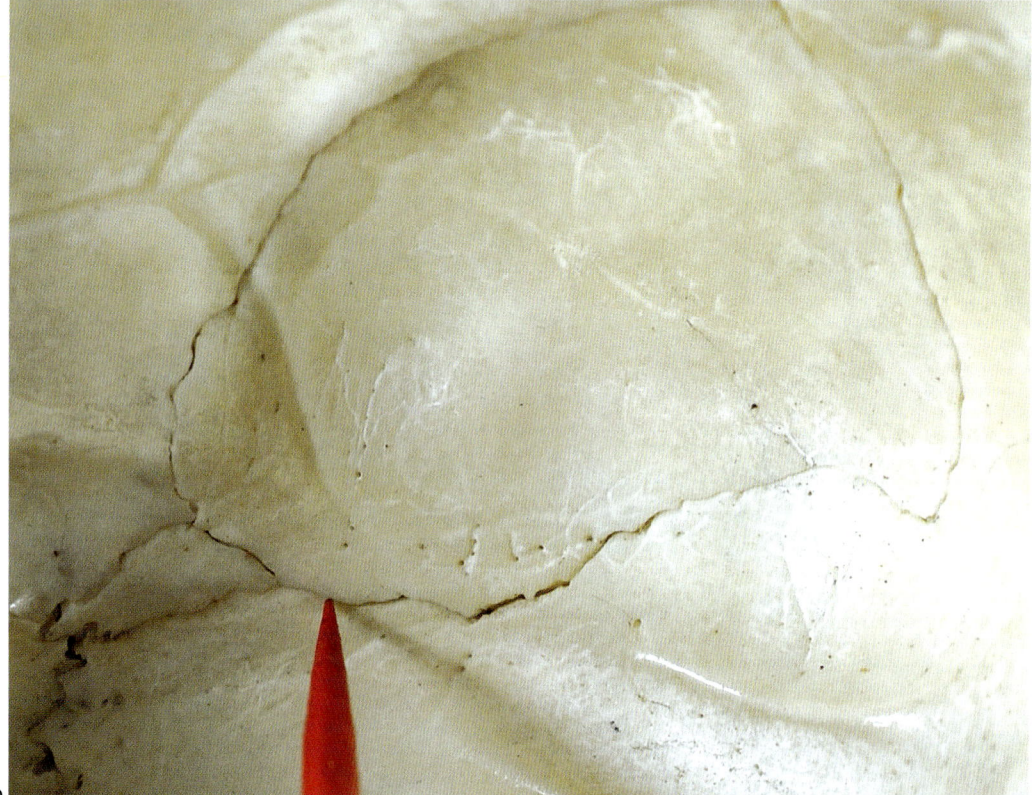

Figure 314a-b. Ectocranial and endocranial views of an asymmetric ossicle along the right lambdoidal suture in an adolescent Asian female skull (CSC AC 007). (a) Photograph demonstrating that the morphology of the suture comprising the ossicle (square) is much more complex ectocranially than (b) endocranially (red probe), a condition typical of most sutures and ossicles. Uncommon finding in most groups. Cf. Bhanu and Sankar (2011), Hanihara and Ishida (2001a). This ossicle may possibly be referred to as a lambdoidal ossicle since it is found along the lambdoidal suture.

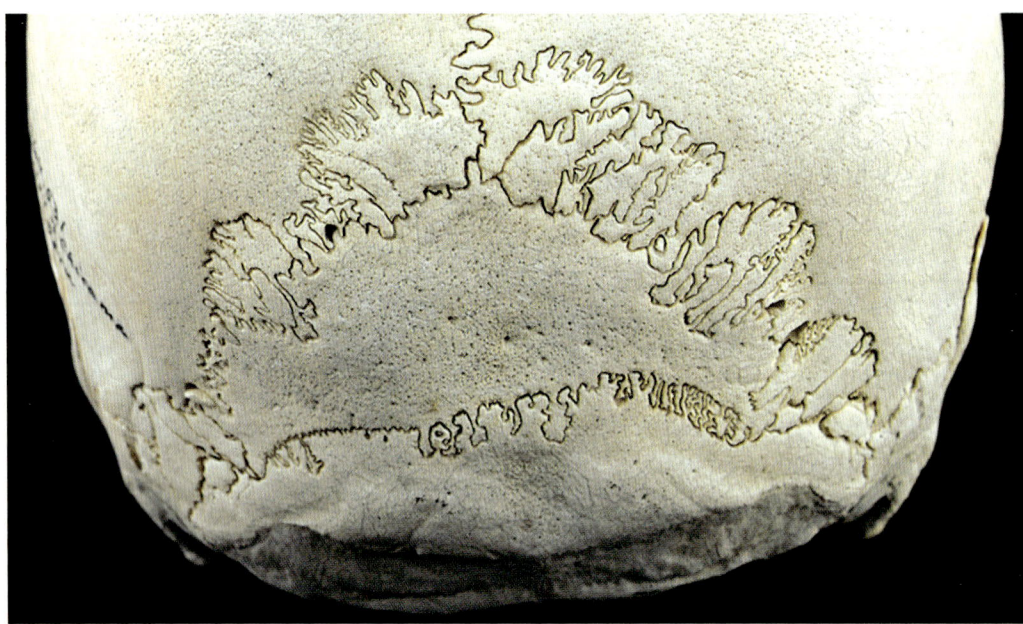

Figure 315. Asymmetrical Inca bone with numerous lambdoidal ossicles (ancient Peruvian, SI). Uncommon finding in most groups. Cf. Bhanu and Sankar (2011); Dorsey (1897); Hanihara and Ishida (2001c); Srivastava (1977).

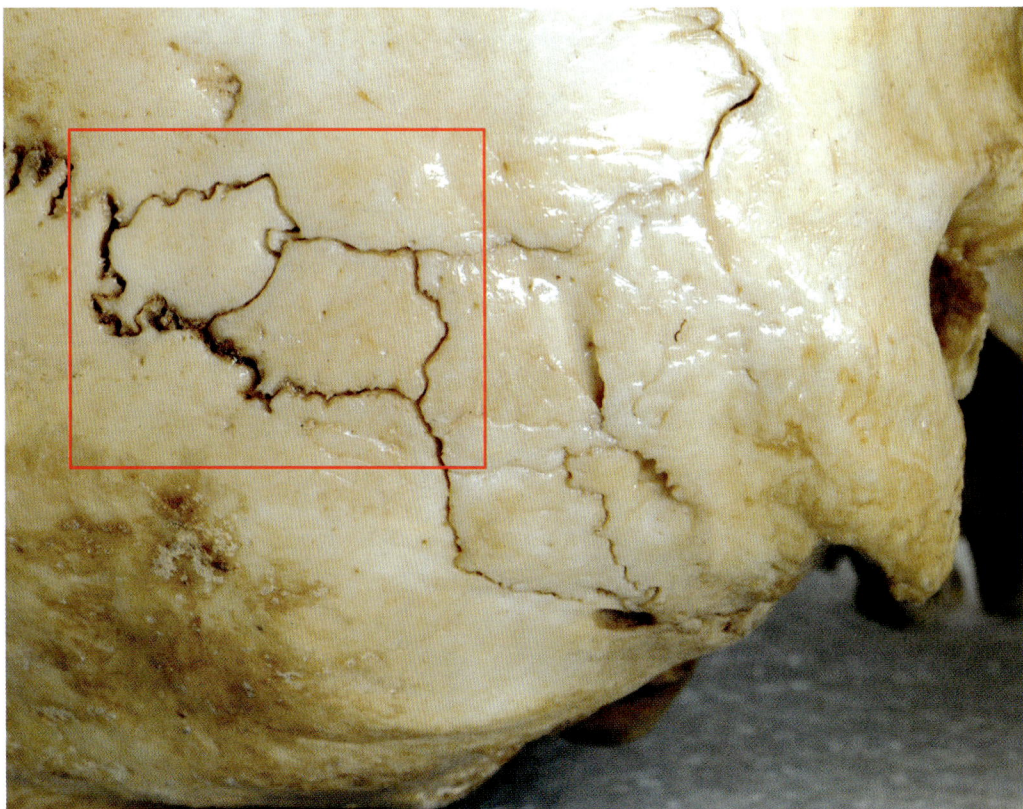

Figure 316. Two asterionic ossicles/bones (rectangle) in an adult Thai (KKU). Common finding. Cf. Hanihara and Ishida (2001a); Hauser and DeStefano (1989).

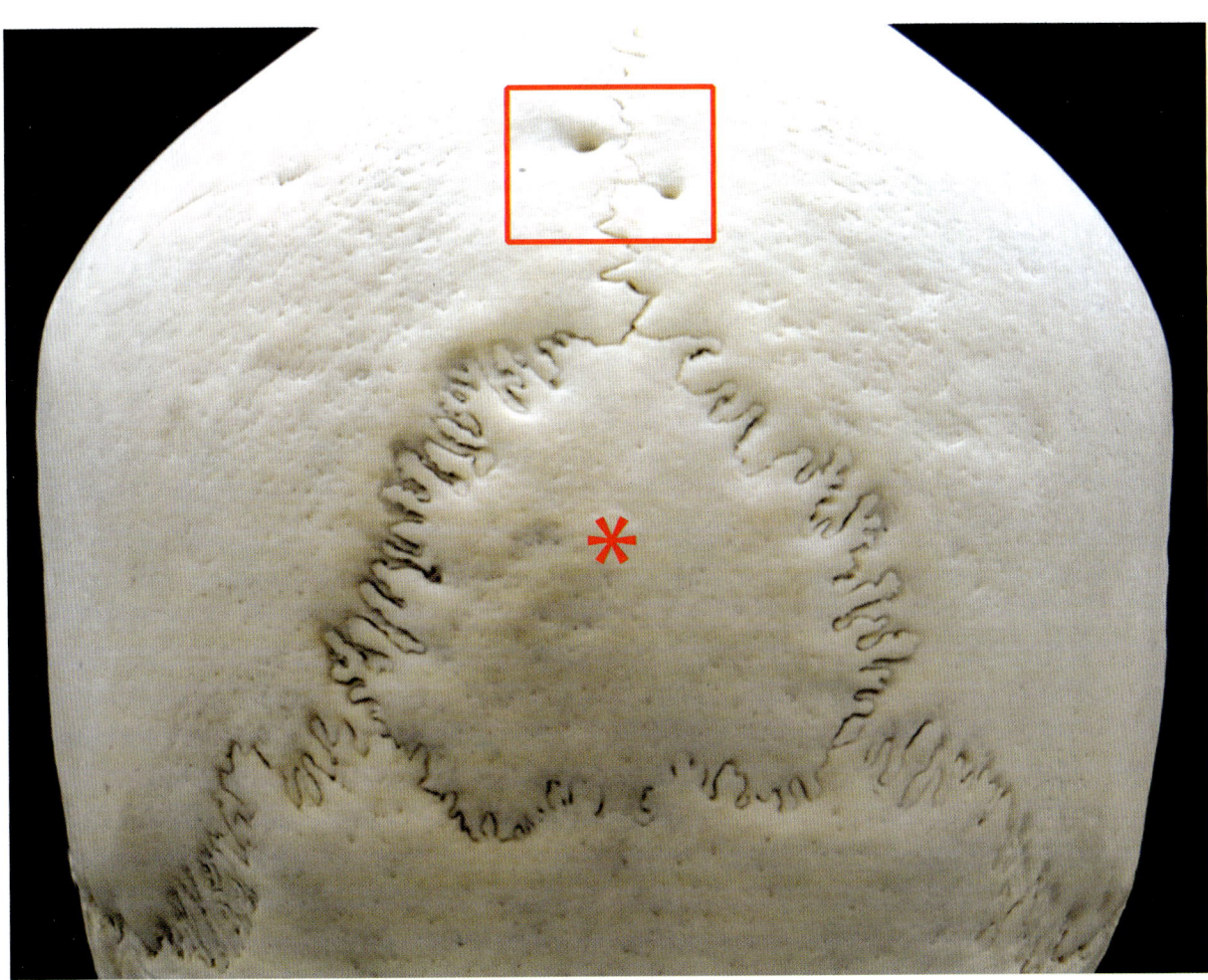

Figure 317. Large central pre-interparietal bone (*) or Inca bone and bilateral parietal foramina (rectangle) in an adult Asian skull (FSA AC032; photo by Christopher Sciotto). Cf. Pal (1987).

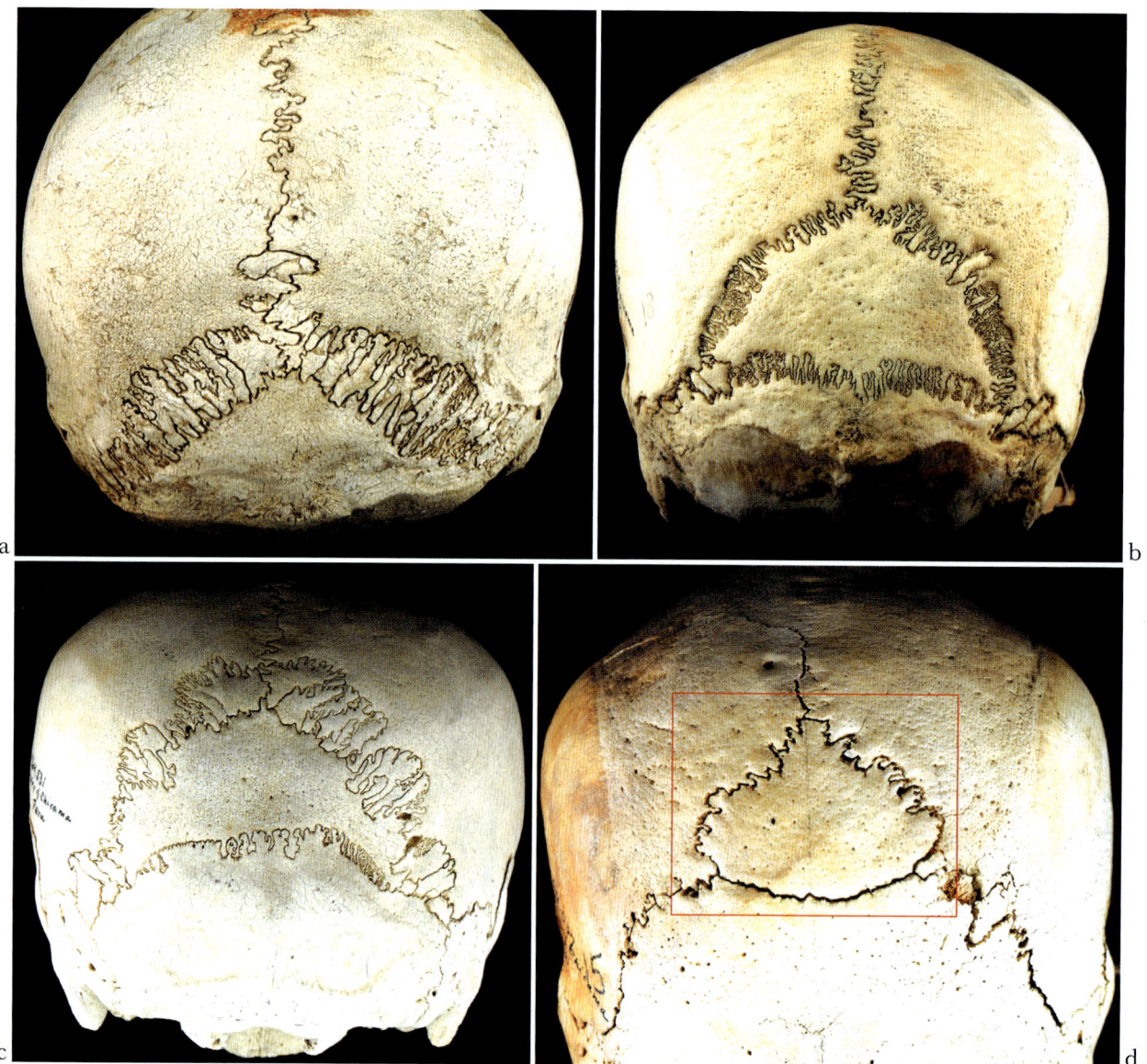

Figure 318a-d. Variation in size and complexity of the lambdoidal suture in four individuals. (a) Unusually complex lambdoidal sutures. (b) Inca bone. (c) Inca bone with numerous lambdoidal ossicles. (d) Central pre-interparietal bone (KKU). Note that the large ossicle in the top right image involves large portions of the parietal bones. There are many different variants, forms and classifications of ossicles, Inca bones, bipartite bones and pre-interparietal bones (see Bhanu and Sankar 2011, Matsumura et al. 1993, Pal 1987, Saxena et al. 1986 for more on pre-interparietal bones). Cf. Gopinathan (1992); Hanihara and Ishida (2001a,c); Hauser and DeStefano (1989); Srivastava (1977); Dorsey (1897); O'Loughlin (2004); Van Arsdale and Clark (2012); Wilczak and Ousley (2009) for discussion of the effect of cranial deformation and the formation of accessory ossicles.

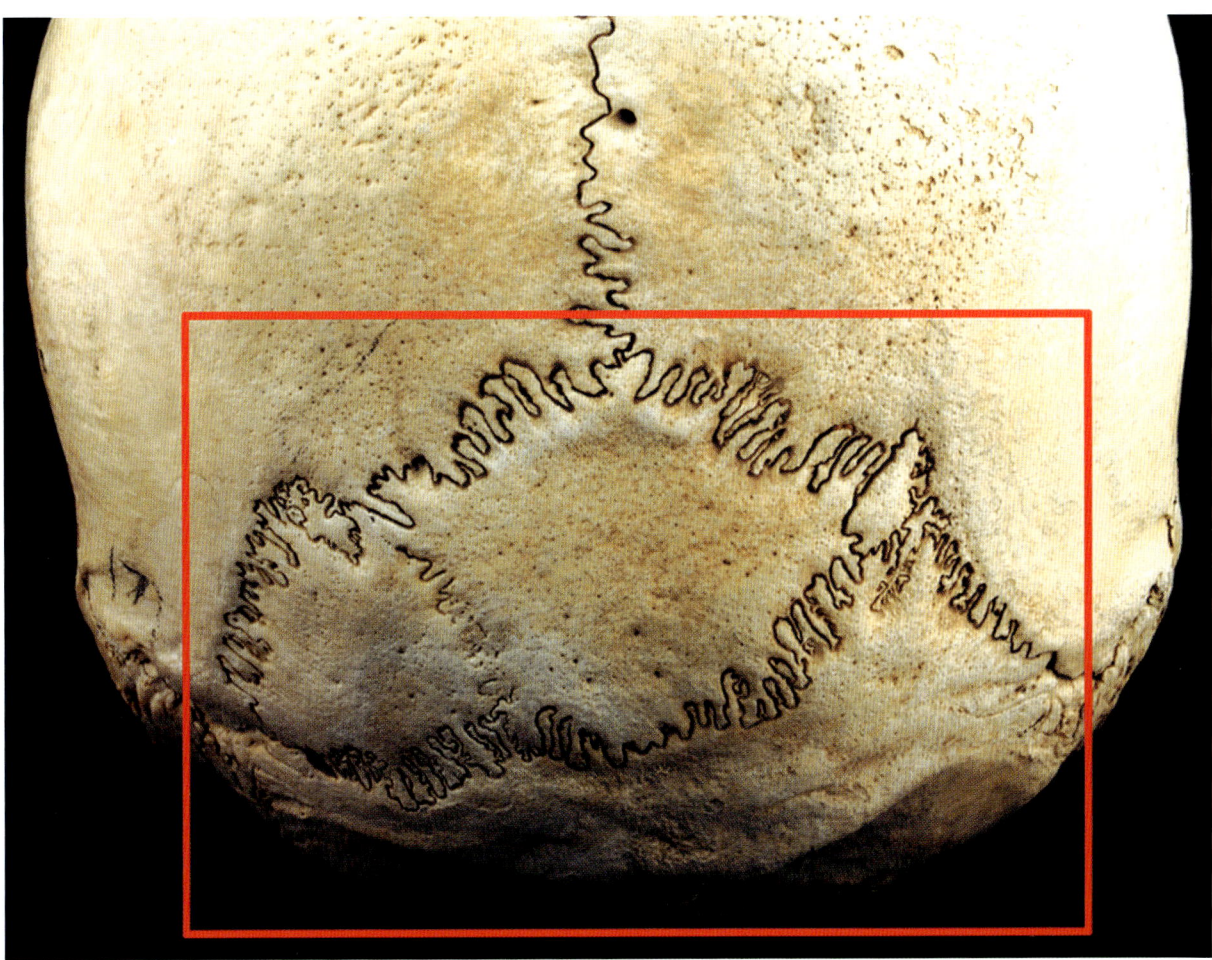

Figure 319. Type II Inca bone (rectangle) consisting of two ossicles of differing sizes (KKU), but what could also be termed pre-interparietal bones. The few smaller ossicles are insignificant, but could be scored as present. Note relative simplicity of the sagittal suture at Obelion. Cf. Bhanu and Sankar (2011); Hanihara and Ishida (2001c).

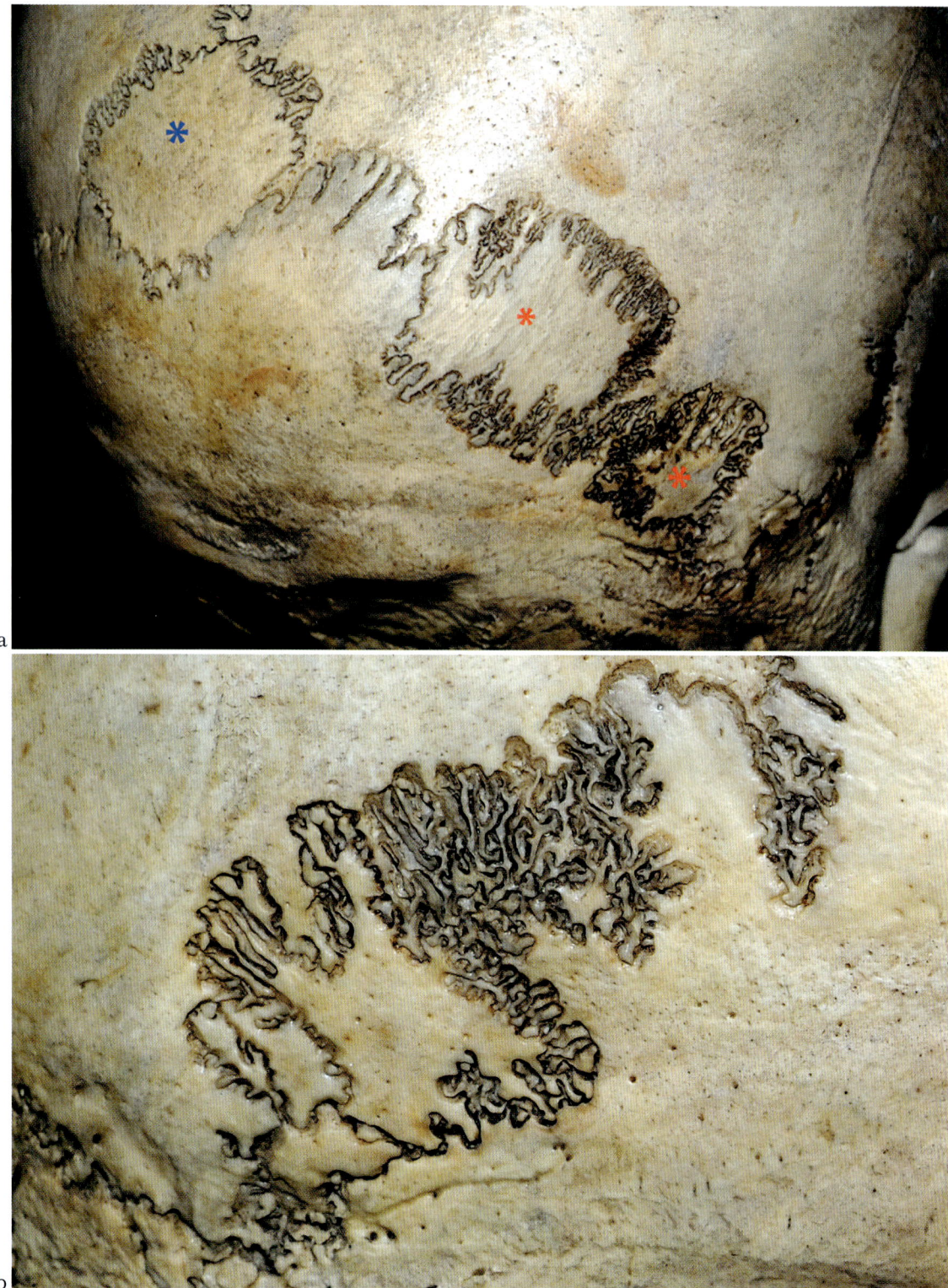

Figure 320a-b. Unusually complex lambdoidal suture and ossicles. (a) Right half of the lambdoidal suture and multiple ossicles (*) with unusually complex suture margins. (b) Higher magnification of the complexity of a portion of the left lambdoidal suture near Asterion. This complexity reveals compressive, tensile and shearing stresses in the posterior portion of the cranium.

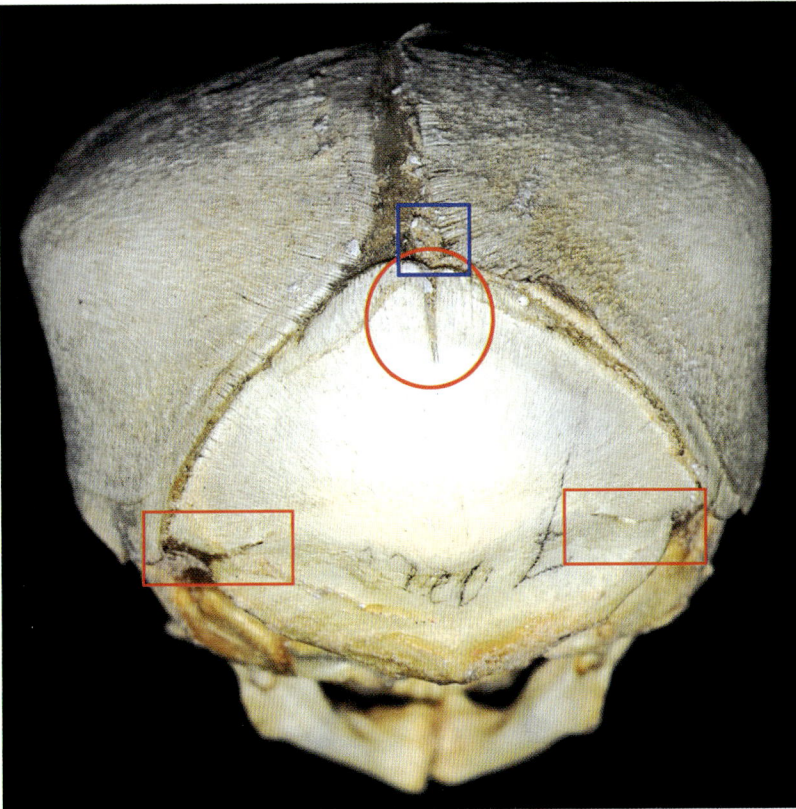

Figure 321. Trace Mendosal/biasterionic sutures (rectangles), superior fissure (circle) and a small lambdoidal ossicle (square) in a fetal skull (KKU). Typical anatomy. Cf. Fazekas and Kosa (1978); Gayretli et al. (2011); Hrdlička (1903); Kosa (1995); Hauser and DeStefano (1989); Shapiro and Robinson (1976); Tubbs et al. (2007); Weinberg et al. (2005).

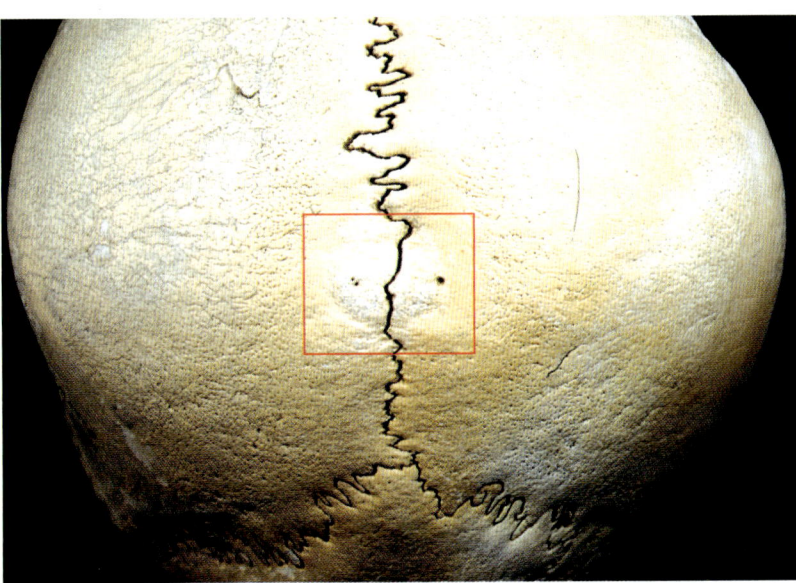

Figure 322. Obelion (red square) and bilateral parietal foramina in an ancient Peruvian cranium. Note that the sagittal suture is simple in the area of Obelion that also includes a faintly, circular depression (uncommon). The biomechanics at Obelion may result in it being flat, raised or depressed (ancient Peruvian, SI). Cf. Mann et al. (2009).

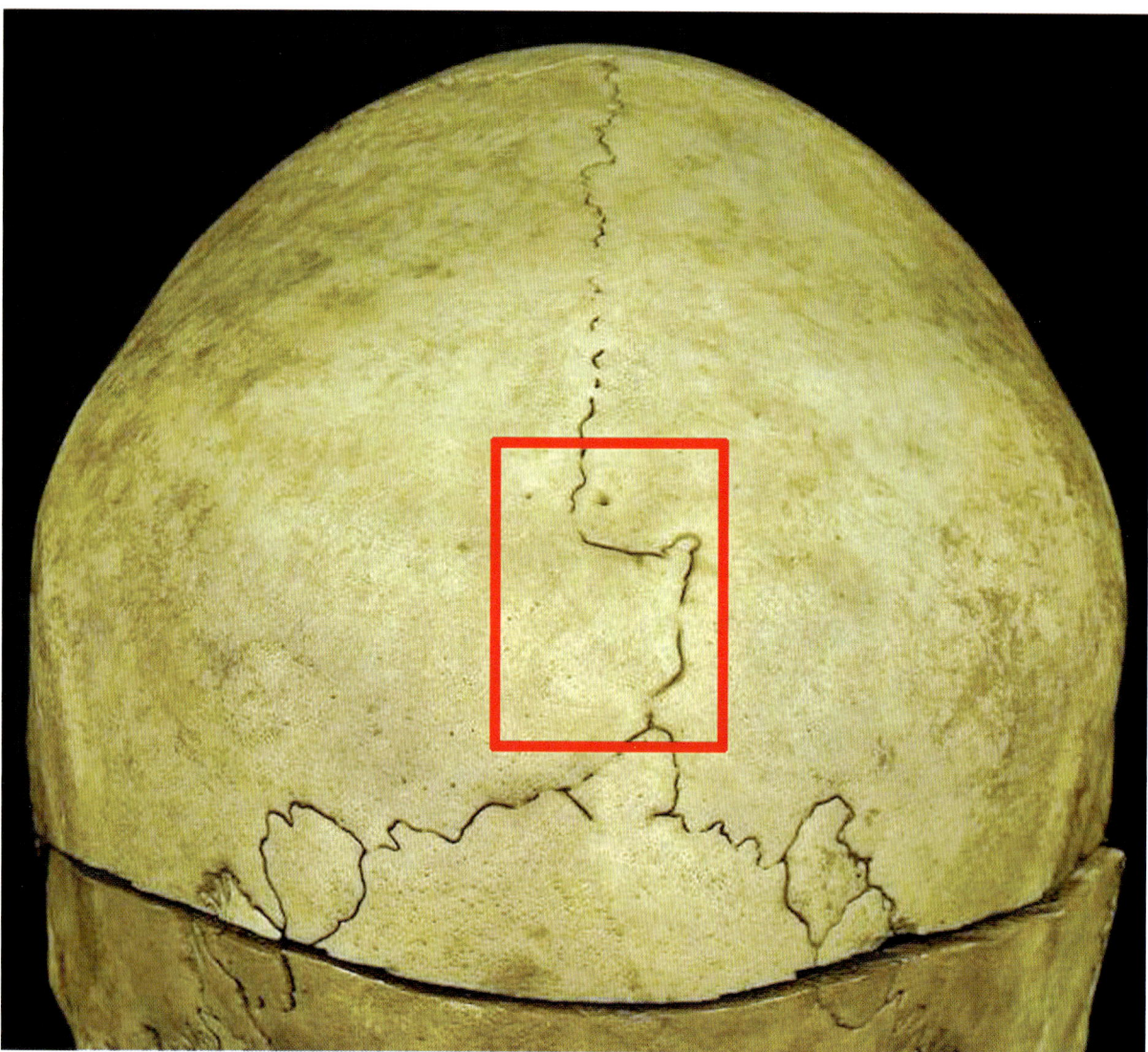

Figure 323. Rare deviation (rectangle) and simple posterior portion of the sagittal suture in an adult Peruvian skull (UTK; Hefner). This sagittal suture is unusually simple along its entirety.

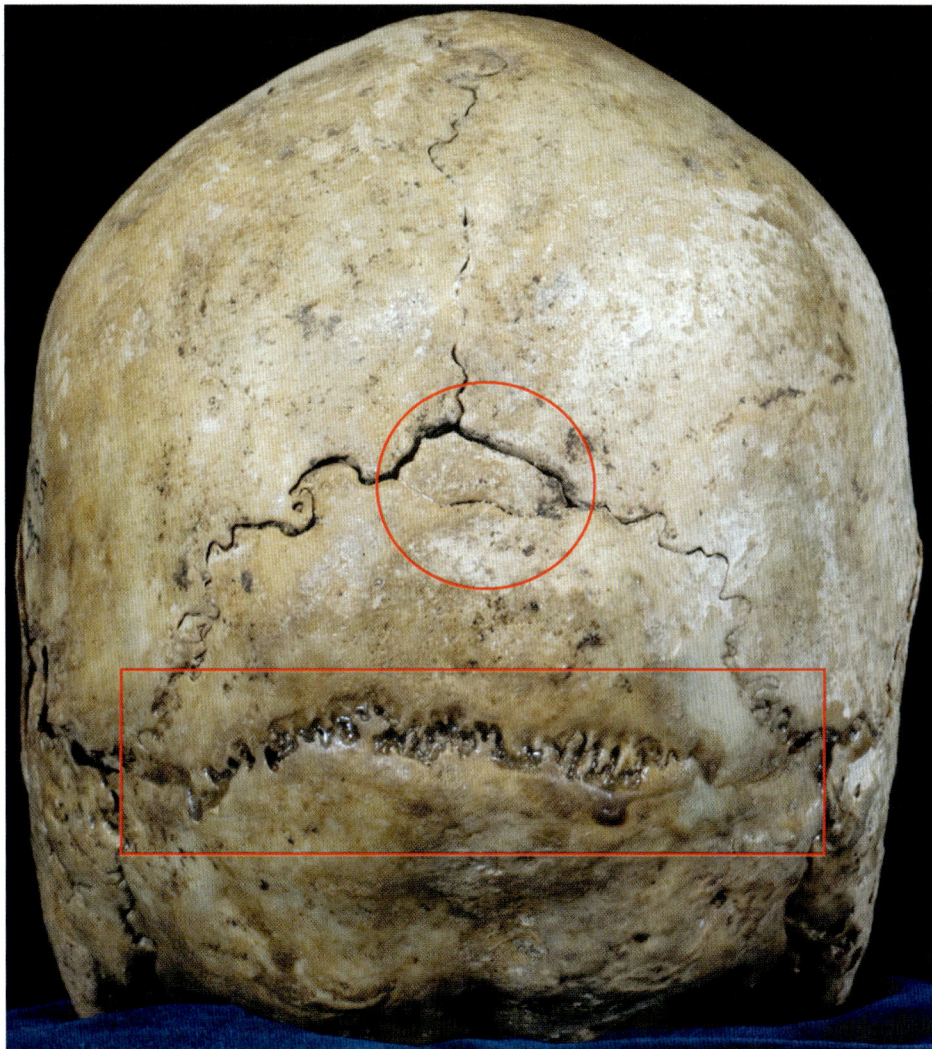

Figure 324. Inca bone/single median interparietal bone/central interparietal bone in an adult Black male cranium (SI 244085). Note that the transverse suture (rectangle) separating the superior and inferior portions of the occipital bone is more complex than the lambdoidal suture; also note the partially closed/synostosed Lambdoidal ossicle (circle). Cf. Bhanu and Sankar (2011); Hauser and DeStefano (1989); Pal (1987); Saxena et al. (1986) for more on Inca and pre-interparietal bones.

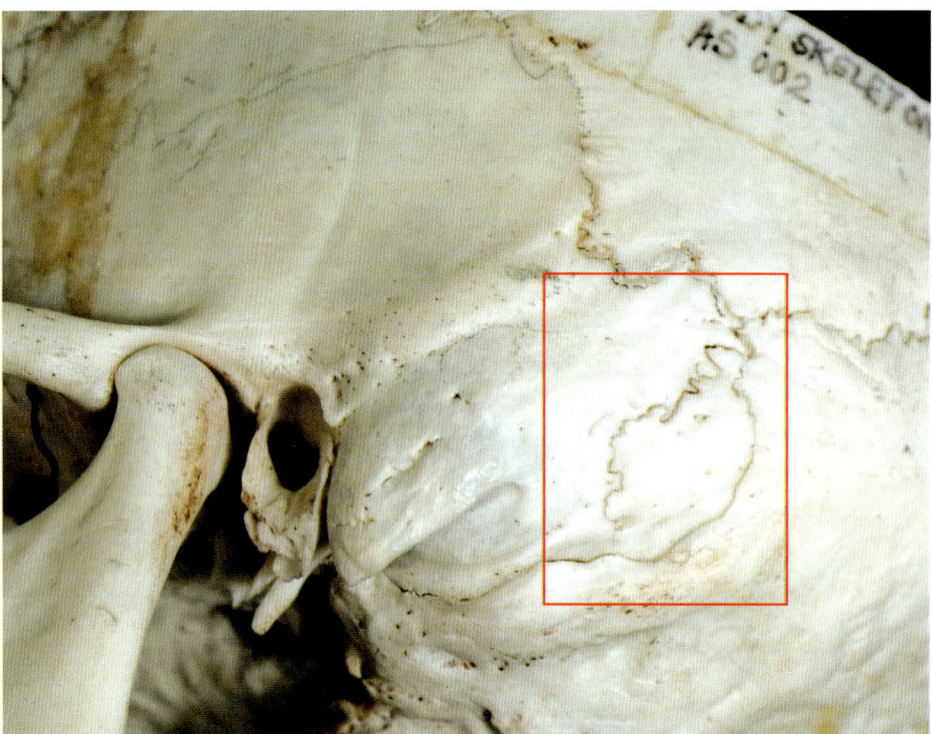

Figure 325. Occipito-mastoid ossicle (rectangle), sometimes referred to as ossicle of Riolano (Vázquez et al. 2001), in an adult Asian female skull (CSC AS 002). Cf. Hauser and DeStefano (1989).

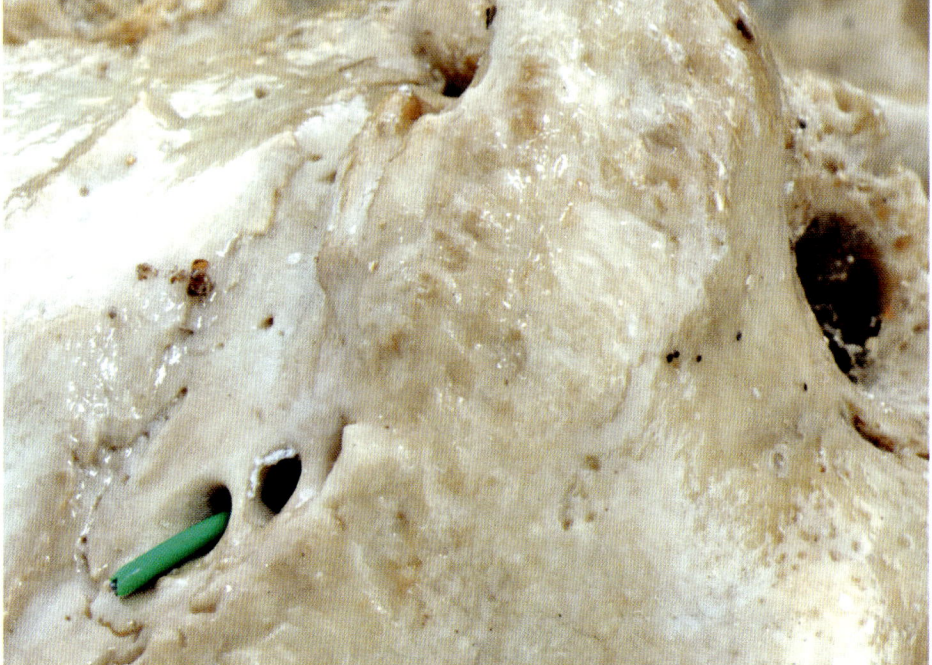

Figure 326. Vertically divided or "double," left mastoid foramen (KKU 4096-43). Note that the green probe is visible through both external foramina communicating with only one internal canal. Cf. Boyd (1930); Hauser and DeStefano (1989); Vázquez et al. (2001).

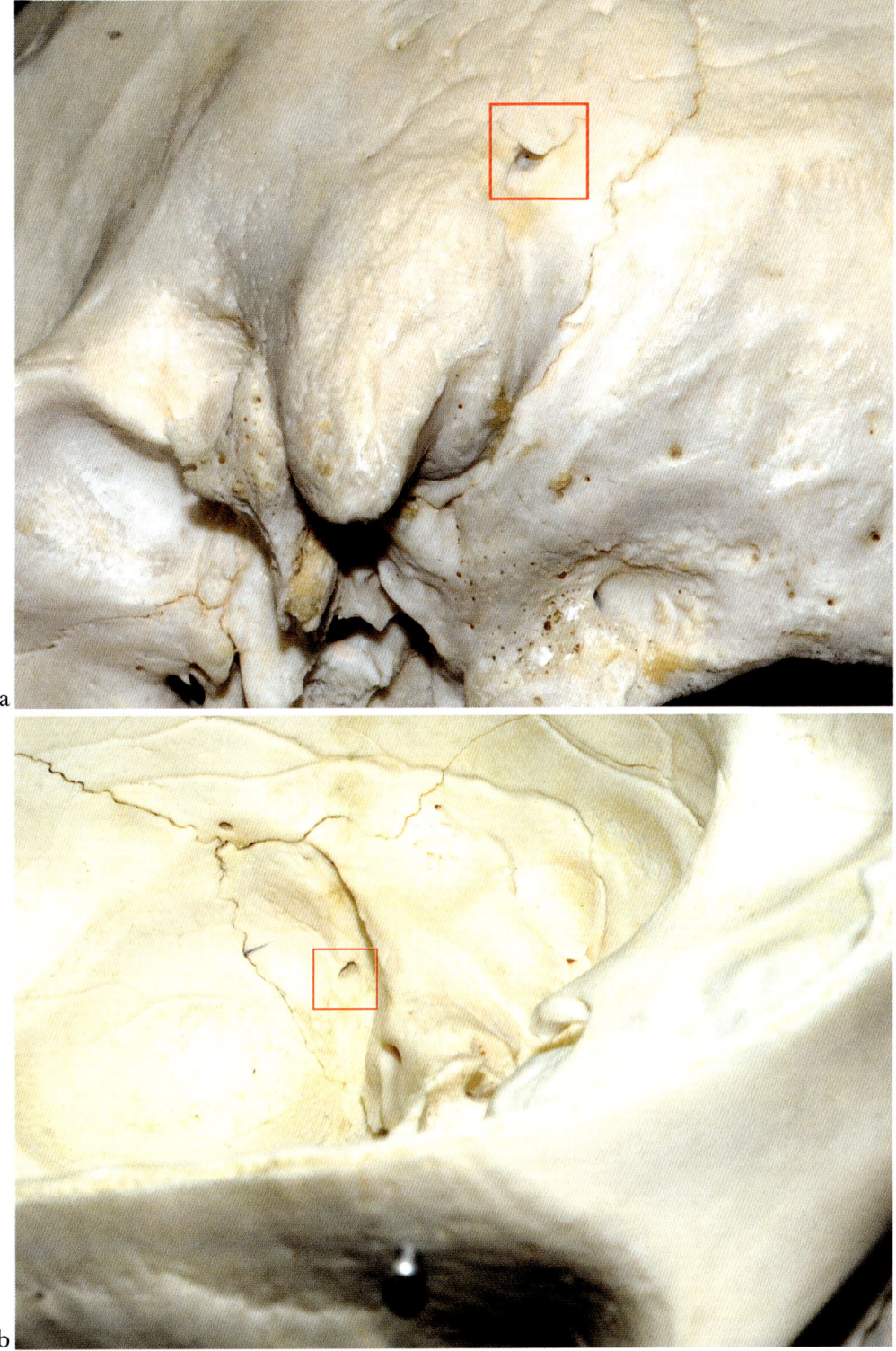

Figure 327a-b. Ectocranial and endocranial views of a mastoid foramen. (a) Ectocranial and (b) endocranial views showing the location of a left mastoid foramen (square) as it communicates with the sigmoid sinus in an adult, probable Asian female (FSA AS044). Most mastoid foramina lie along or near the occipitomastoid suture.

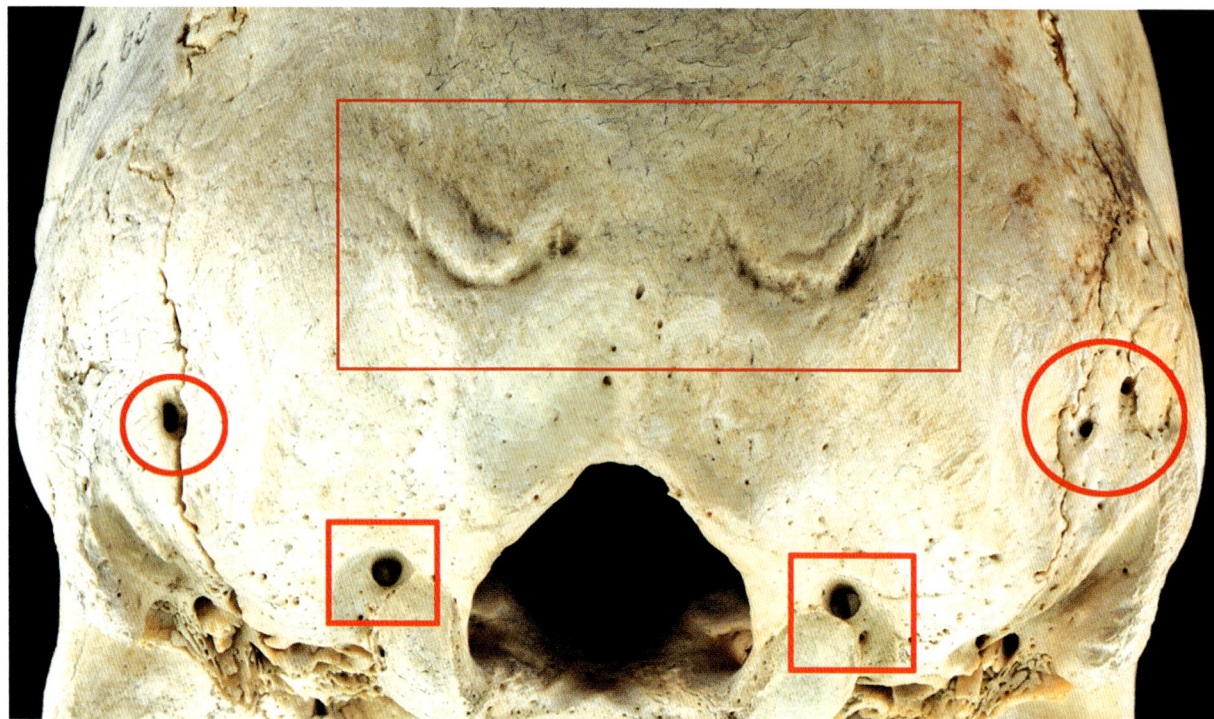

Figure 328. Nuchal "waves" (large rectangle) for attachment of muscles along the inferior nuchal crest (nuchae) in a subadult. These "waves" are uncommon findings, since the nuchal crest is usually much straighter. Note the left mastoid foramen along the suture (small circle), double right mastoid foramina exsutural (large circle) and posterior condylar canals (small squares) (ancient Peruvian, SI). Cf. Berge and Bergman (2001); Boyd (1930); Ginsberg (1994); Hauser and DeStefano (1989); Vázquez et al. (2001) for posterior condylar canals and mastoid foramen.

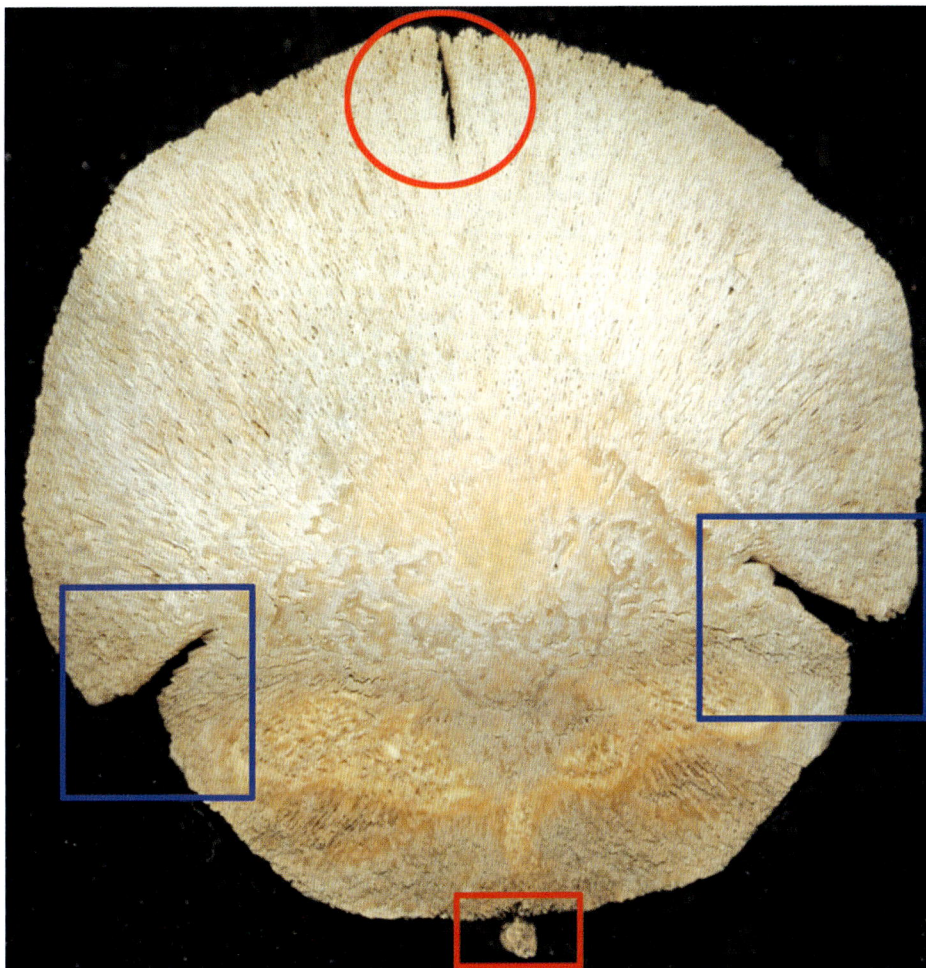

Figure 329. Process of Kerckring (Kerckring's center, bone or process, manubrium squamae occipitalis, opisthial process; red rectangle), Mendosal sutures (blue square and rectangle) and vertical fissure (red circle) in a fetal occipital bone (SI – fetal anatomical). The Kerckring's center, which commonly appears as a small tongue of bone resembling the tail of a skate or ray, may occasionally appear as one or two small separate islands of bone. This ossicle is a separate center of ossification along the midline that fuses with the supraoccipital portion within a few days or weeks of birth (Madeline and Elster, 1995). This tongue of bone is not usually visible or present in adults. Mendosal sutures usually obliterate by age 4–6 years postnatal, but are found in some adults. Cf. Fazekas and Kosa (1978); Freyschmidt et al. (2002); Gray (1901); Kosa (1995); Madeline and Elster (1995); Scheuer and Black (2000); Schaefer et al. (2009); Shapiro and Robinson (1976); Sperber (2001); Tubbs et al. (2007); Weinberg et al. (2005). Typical anatomy.

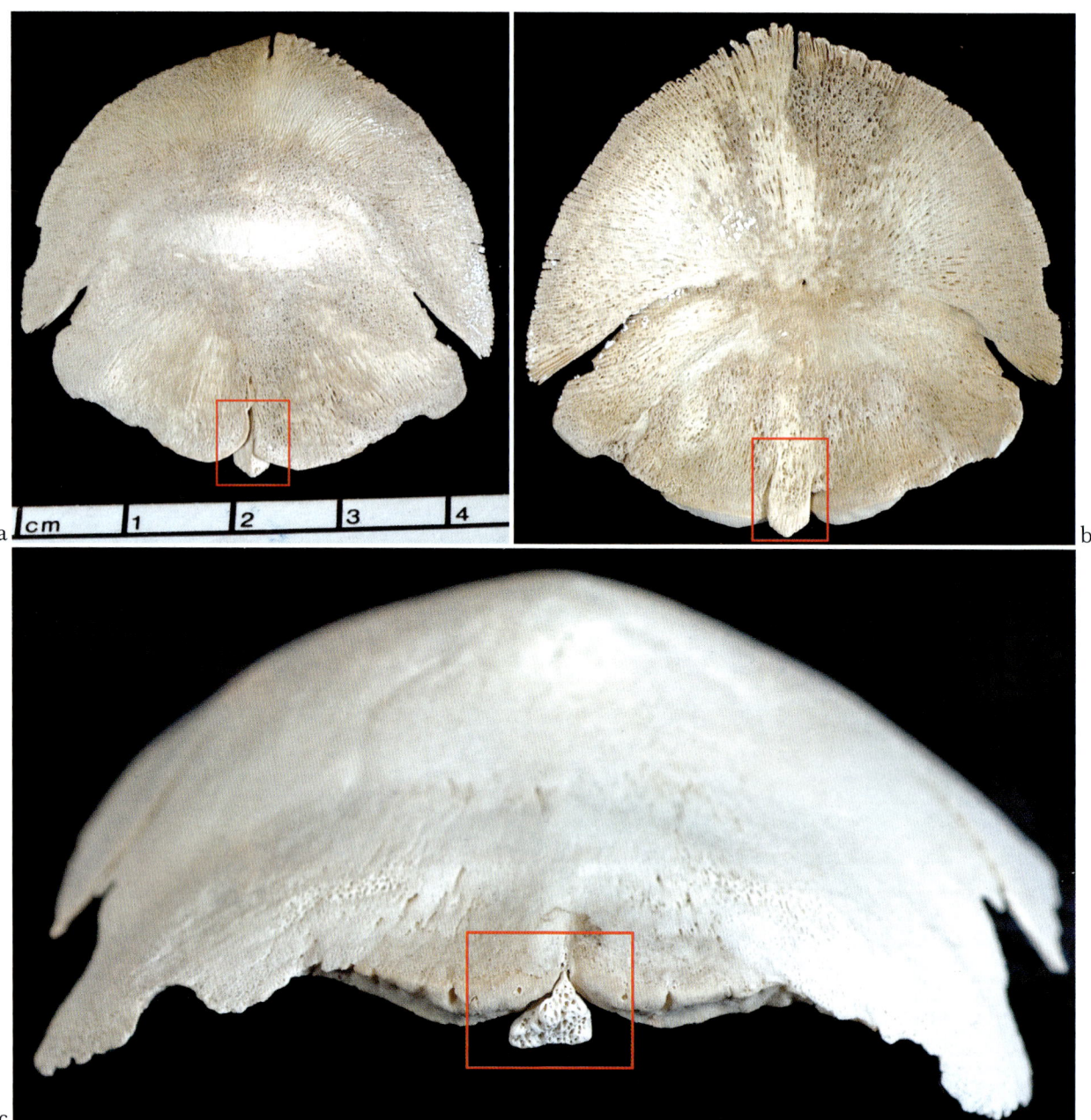

Figure 330a-c. Kerckring's process/bone in a fetal squama (SI 228826). (a) Ectocranial view of Kerckring's process (rectangle), a tongue-like segment of bone along the inferior midline of the occipital bone (i.e., posterior margin of the foramen magnum) that appears about five months' intrauterine and, if separate, fuses to the squama before birth (Gray 1901) or soon thereafter (Madeline and Elster, 1995). (b) Endocranial view of the Kerckring's process (rectangle). (c) Inferior view of the process (rectangle) showing how it fits into a small V-shaped notch in the occipital squamous. Typical anatomy. Cf. Freyschmidt et al. (2002); Fazekas and Kosa (1978); Kosa (1995); Shapiro and Robinson (1976); Weinberg et al. (2005). Shapiro and Robinson (1976) studied 125 skulls of 8- to 40-week-old fetuses and found Kerckring's in only two skulls.

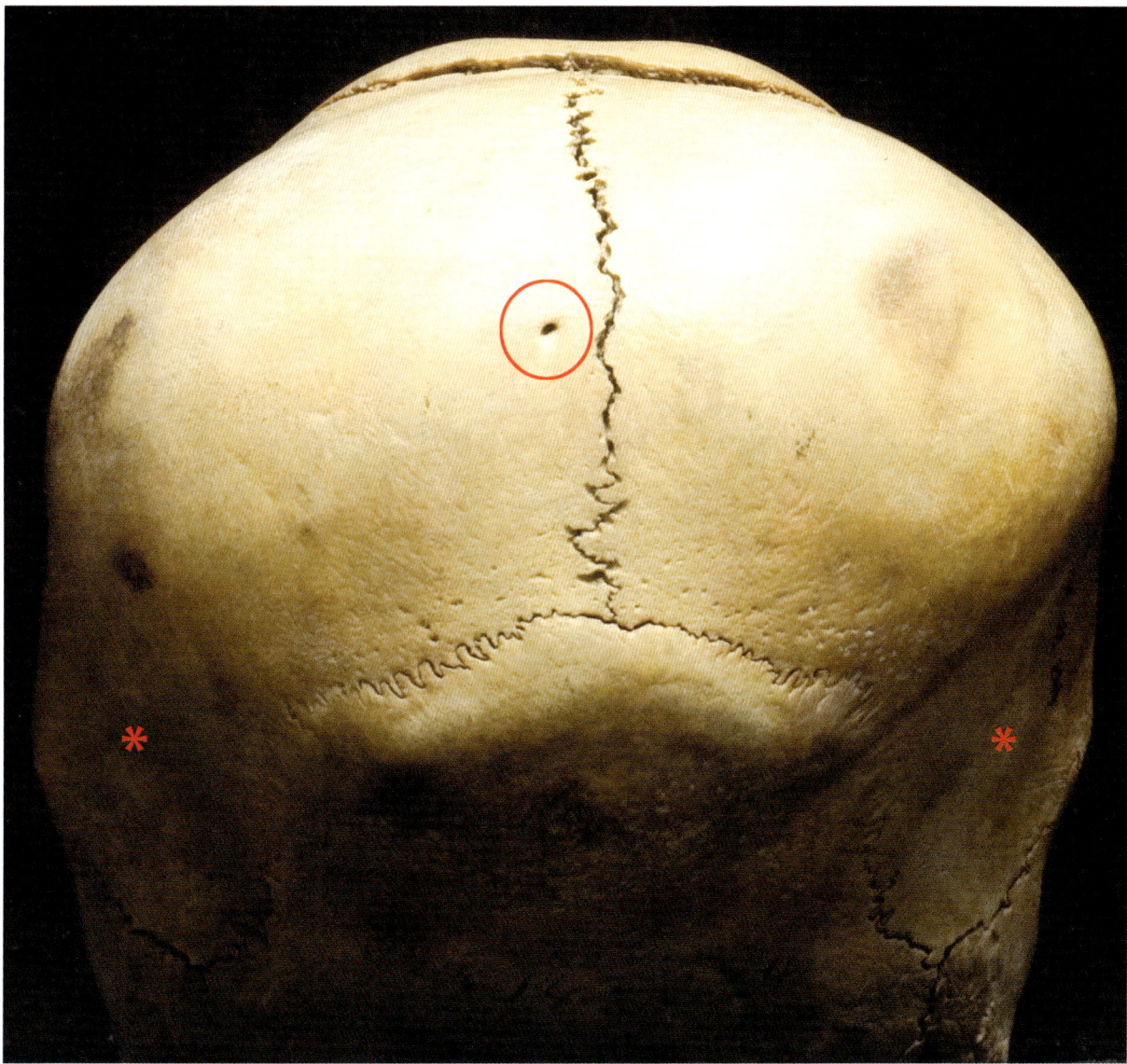

Figure 331. Artificial cranial deformation resulting in constriction and flattening of the lateral portions of the skull (*) in an ancient Peruvian, about 12–15 years old at death (UPenn 24-142-224). Also note the simple nature of the sagittal suture and presence of a left parietal foramen (circle).

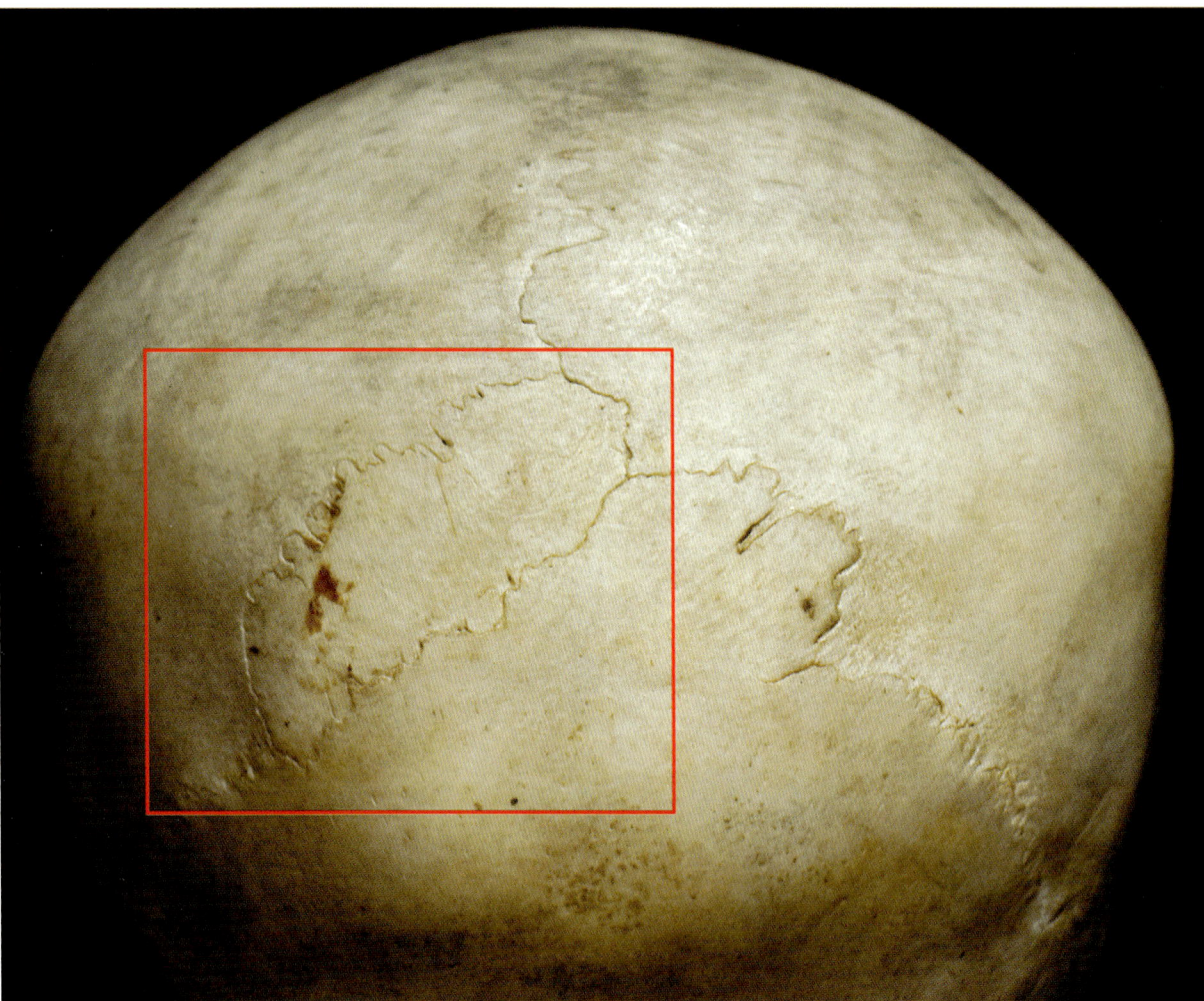

Figure 332. Large, elongated left interparietal/lambdoidal ossicle (rectangle) in a child of about 4 years of age (UPenn L606 88). Note that this accessory ossicle primarily occupies the left parietal bone, not the occipital bone. While this bone formed at Lambda, it appears to be an accessory ossicle along the lambdoidal suture and it is not a divided or bipartite parietal bone formed by an accessory suture.

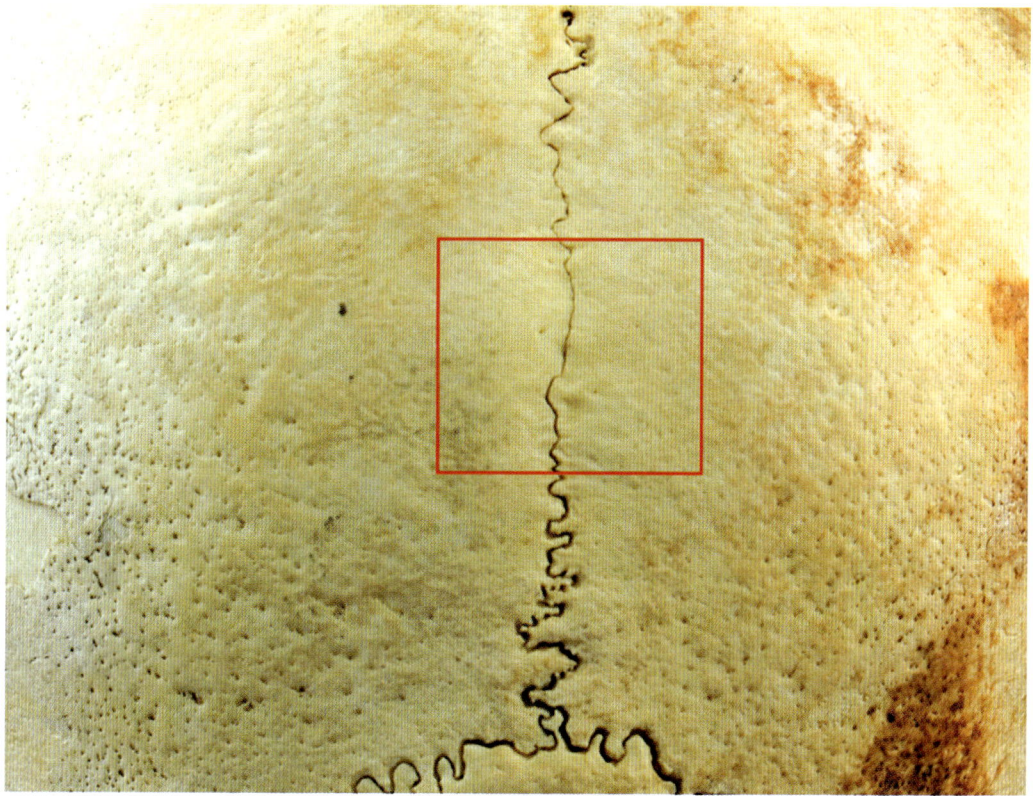

Figure 333. Example of the simple nature of the sagittal suture (square) at Obelion, without the presence of a parietal foramen.

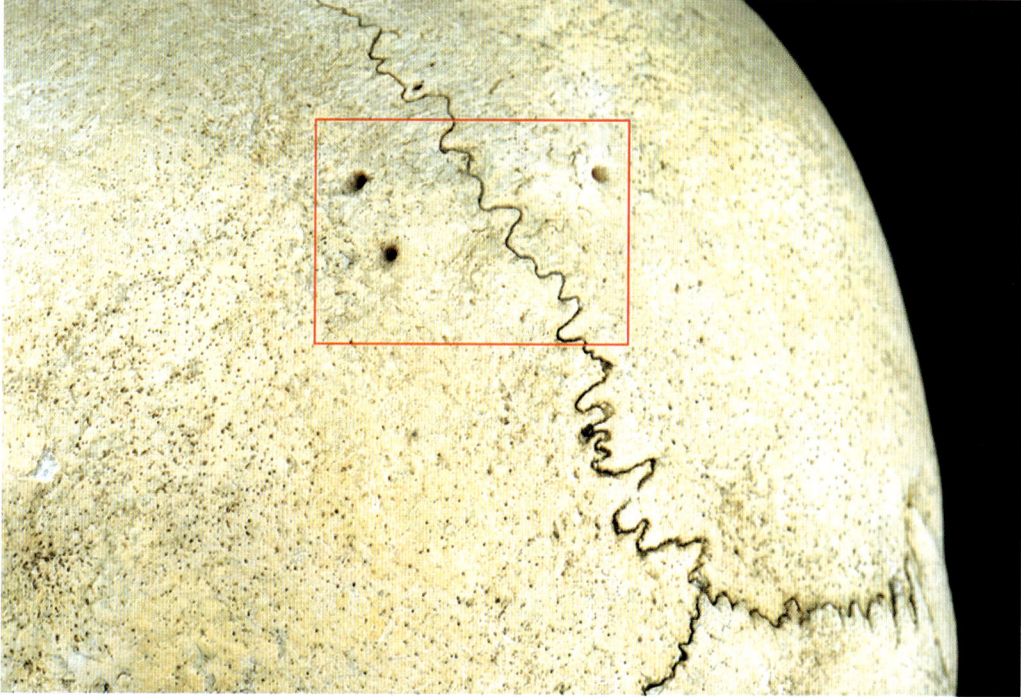

Figure 334. Two left and one right parietal foramina (rectangle) in an adult.

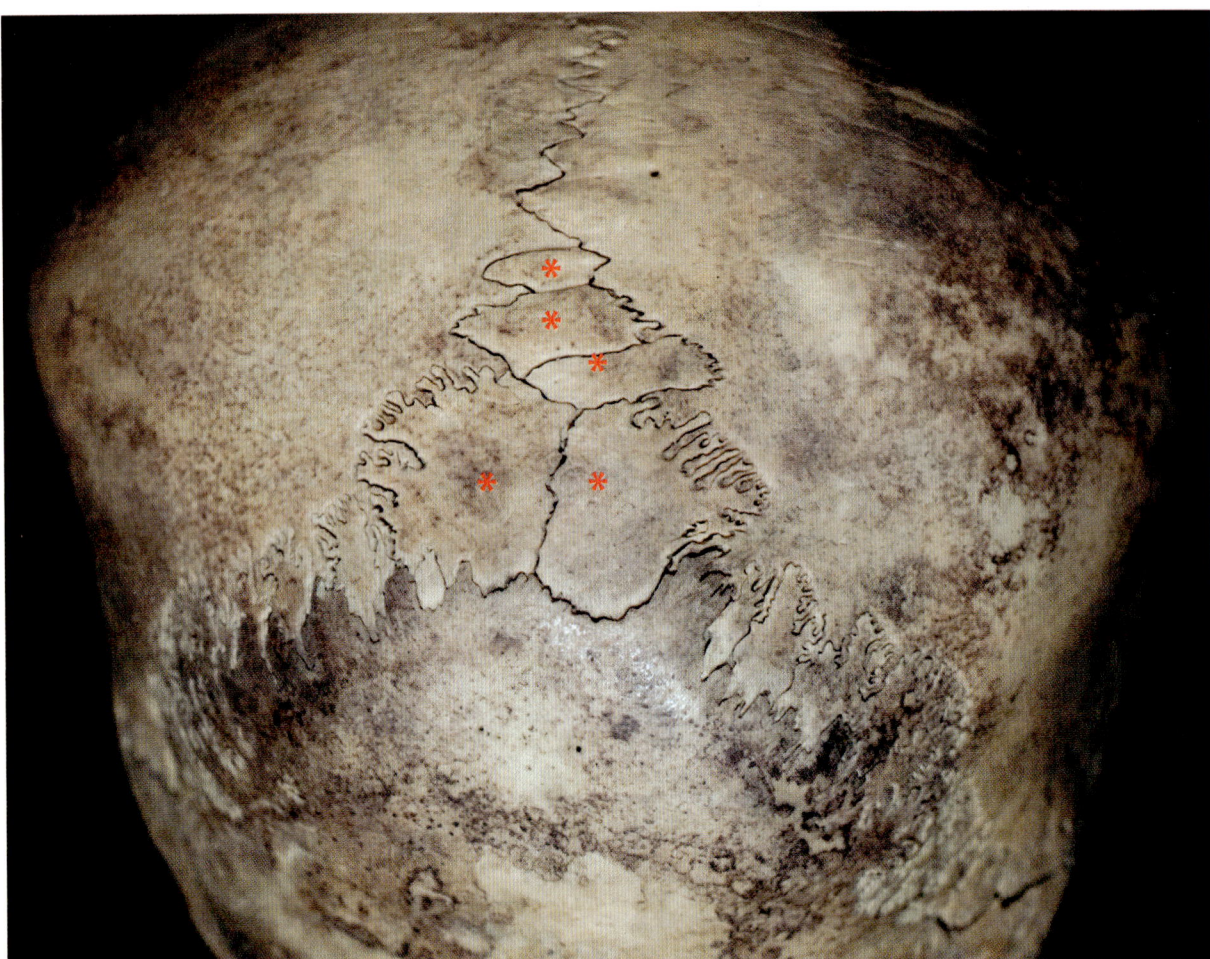

Figure 335. Multiple, large ossicles (*) at Bregma in a 4–6-year old-child. Note that these ossicles occupy portions of the parietal bones, not the occipital bone, along the sagittal suture (UPenn L606 29-142).

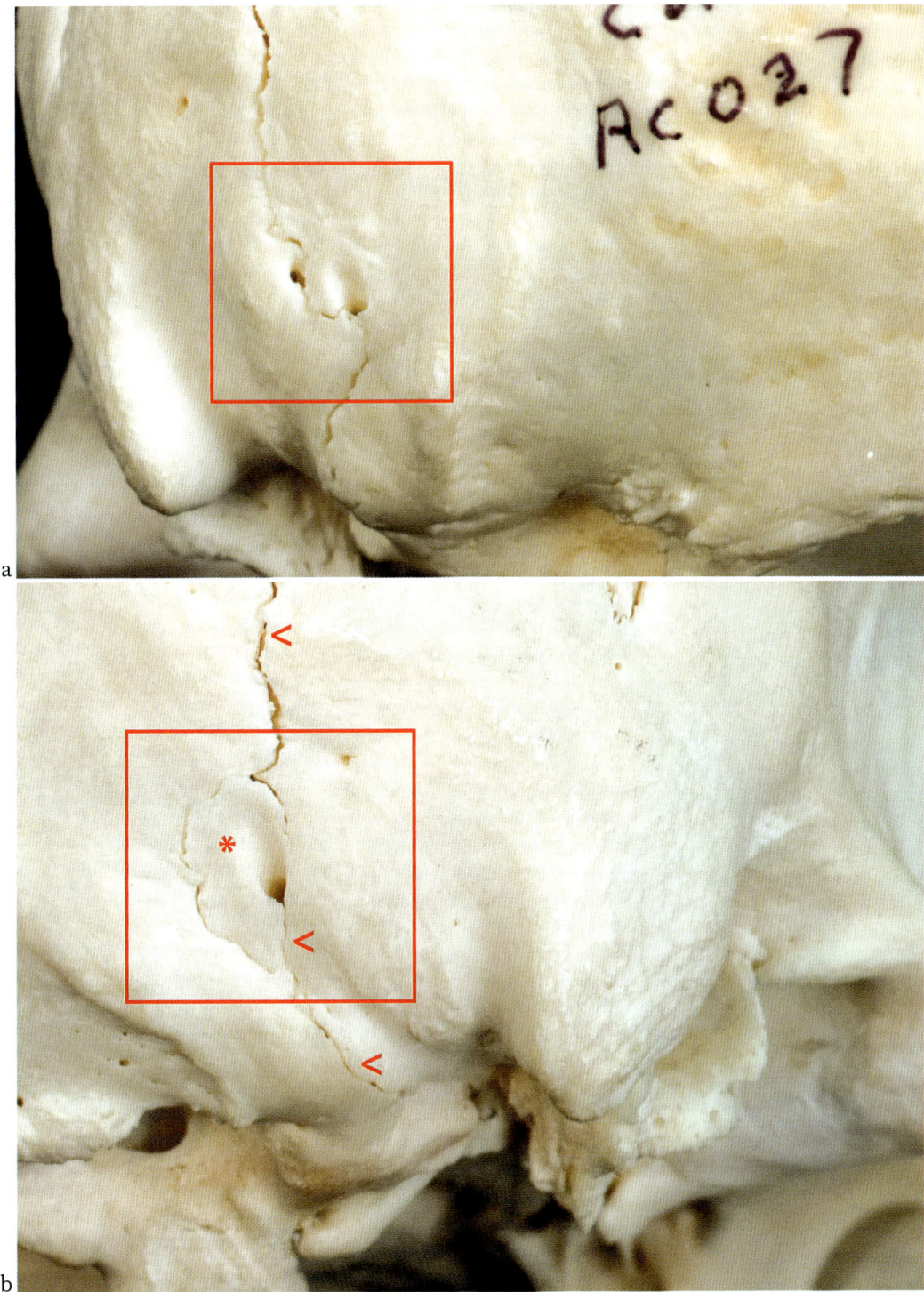

Figure 336a-b. Left and right mastoid foramina located on or adjacent to the occipitomastoid suture (AC027). (a) Two foramina (square) leading directly into the suture. (b) An asterionic bone (*) with a foramen leading directly into the suture (<) and a smaller foramen that is lateral (exsutural) to the suture. Most researchers refer to foramina on, along, or in the suture as sutural, as opposed to foramina that are exsutural, not directly in the suture. See Hauser and DeStefano (1989). All are common findings.

Chapter 6

ENDOCRANIAL VIEW OF THE SKULL

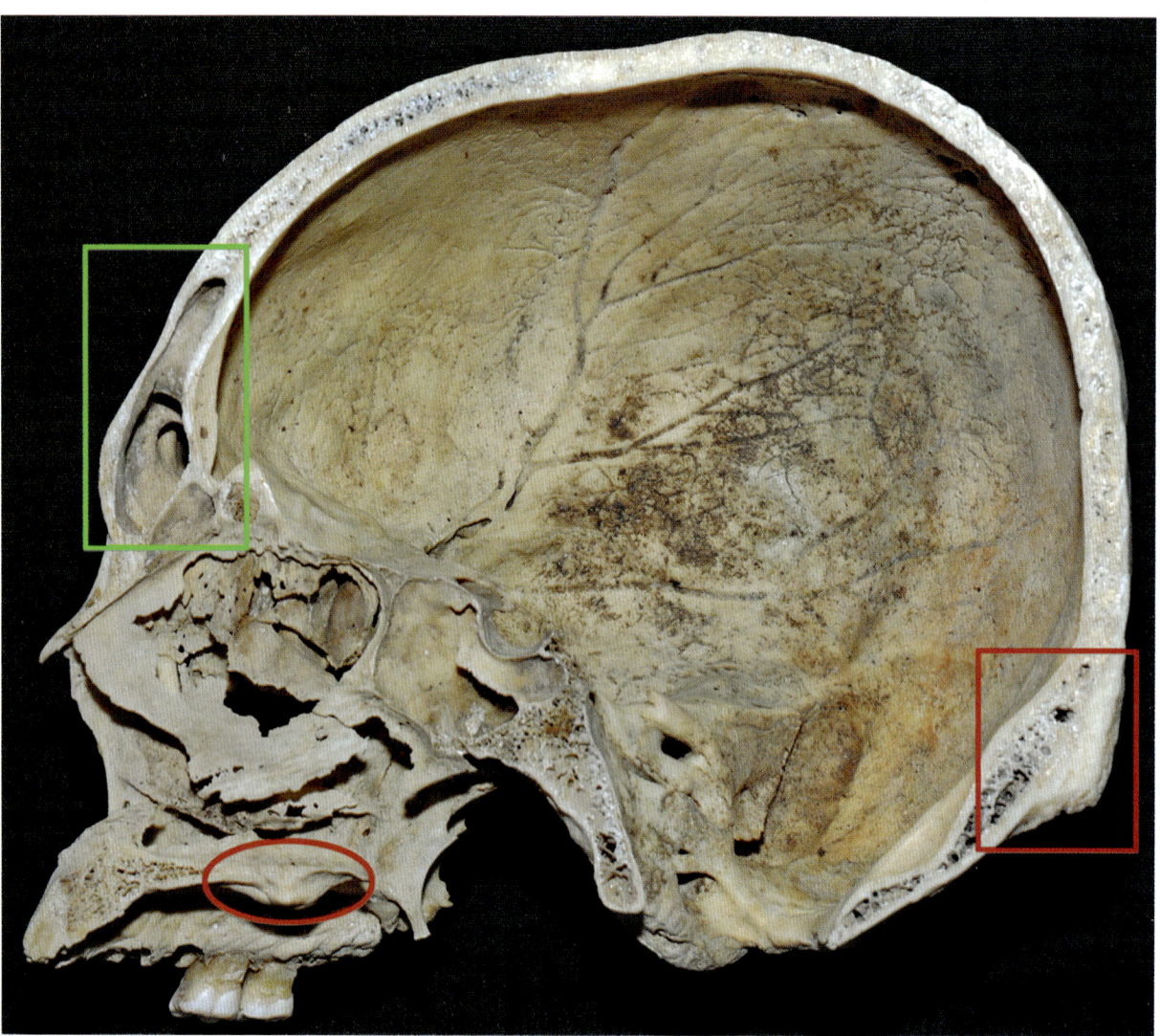

Figure 337. Frontal and ethmoidal sinuses (green), maxillary torus (red circle) and small Inion spike (red rectangle) in an adult Thai male skull (KKU). The frontal sinuses vary in size and shape, sometimes being absent even in adults. The maxillary tori (palatal exostosis) are solid and dense hyperostotic growths along the midline of the palate that lack diploë. The large external occipital protuberance, or Inion spikes, form as dense bone in response to muscle stresses, activity and development. This Asian adult exhibits a prominent postbregmatic depression, a feature often attributed to someone of Negroid ancestry. Also note the extensive meningeal groove pattern extending posterosuperiorly.

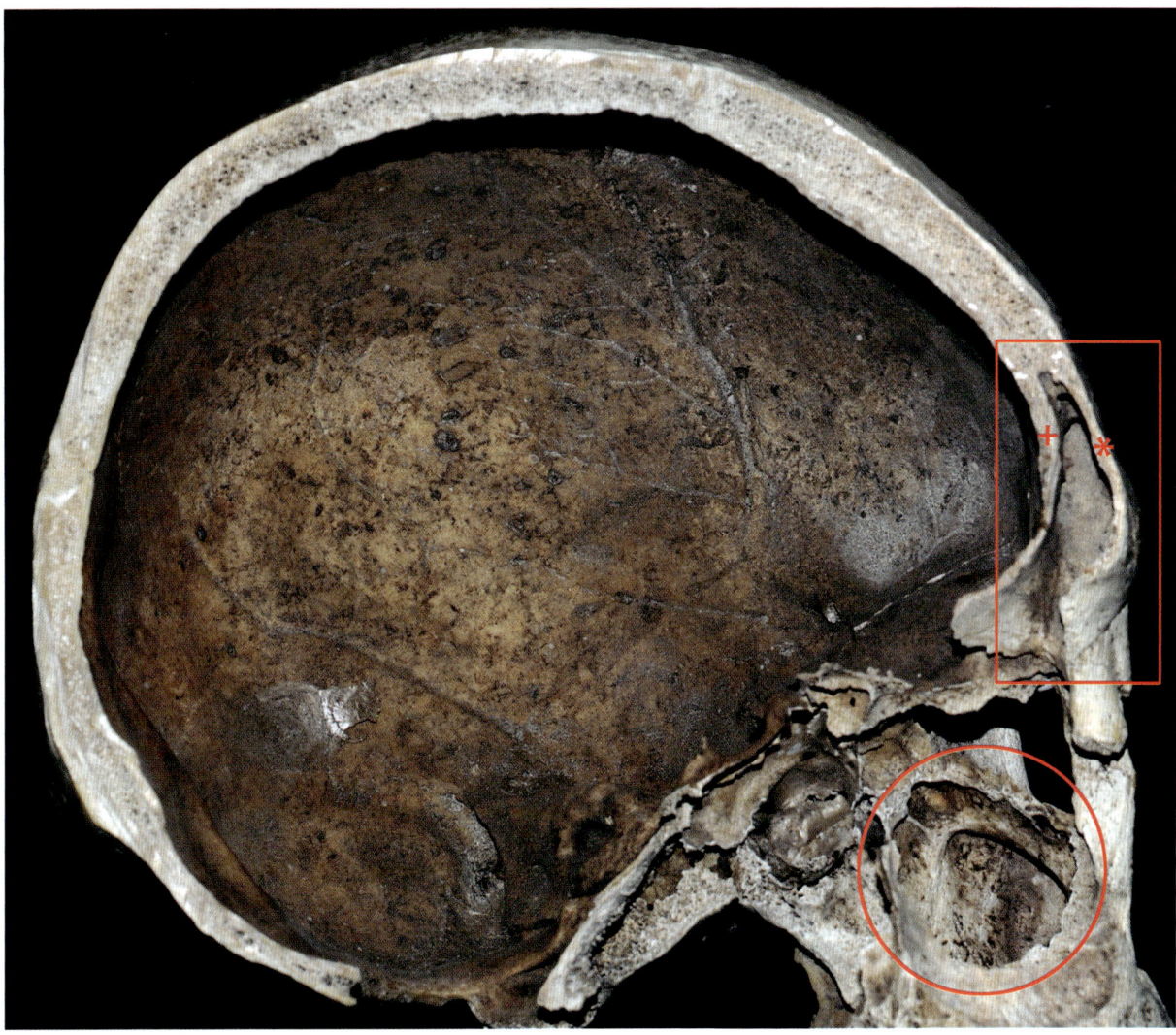

Figure 338. Sagittally sectioned adult skull showing large frontal sinuses (rectangle), maxillary antrum (circle), outer table of the frontal bone (*) and inner table of the frontal bone encompassing the frontal sinuses in an adult, probable male (teaching specimen).

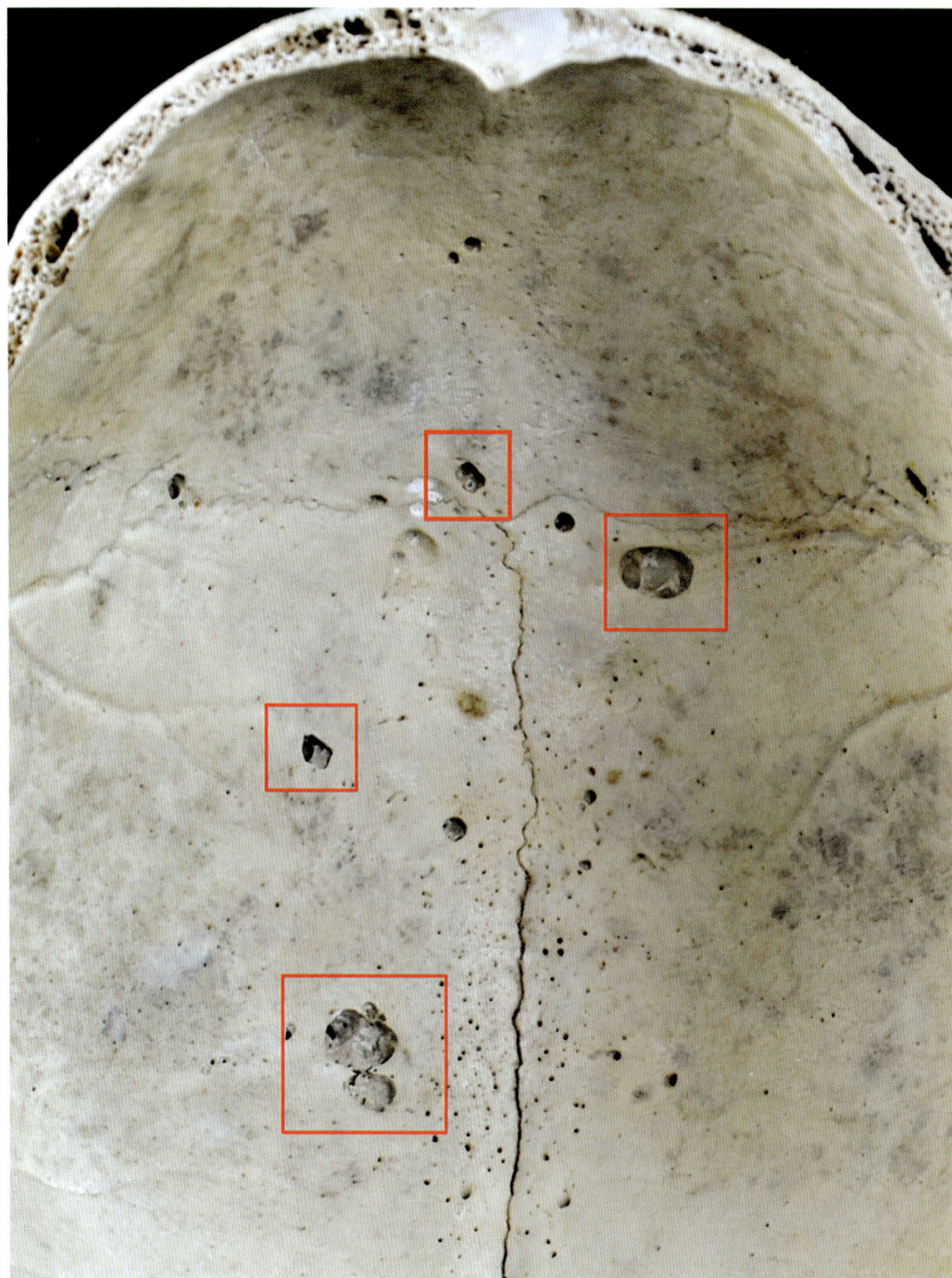

Figure 339. Pacchionion pits/impressions (square) in the parietal and frontal bones of an adult Thai skull (KKU). These pits contain clusters of arachnoid granulations that filter and regulate the flow of cerebrospinal fluid into the venous system. Pacchionian pits increase in size and depth in middle-age and older and may perforate the outer table. They are absent at birth and may be absent in young adults. While their relationship to disease is not fully understood they typically are present in the parietal as well as the occipital bones. Common finding that are sometimes scored as pathological, not a non-metric trait. Cf. Grossman and Potts (1974); Le Gros Clark 1920; Lu et al. (2012); Roche and Warner (1996).

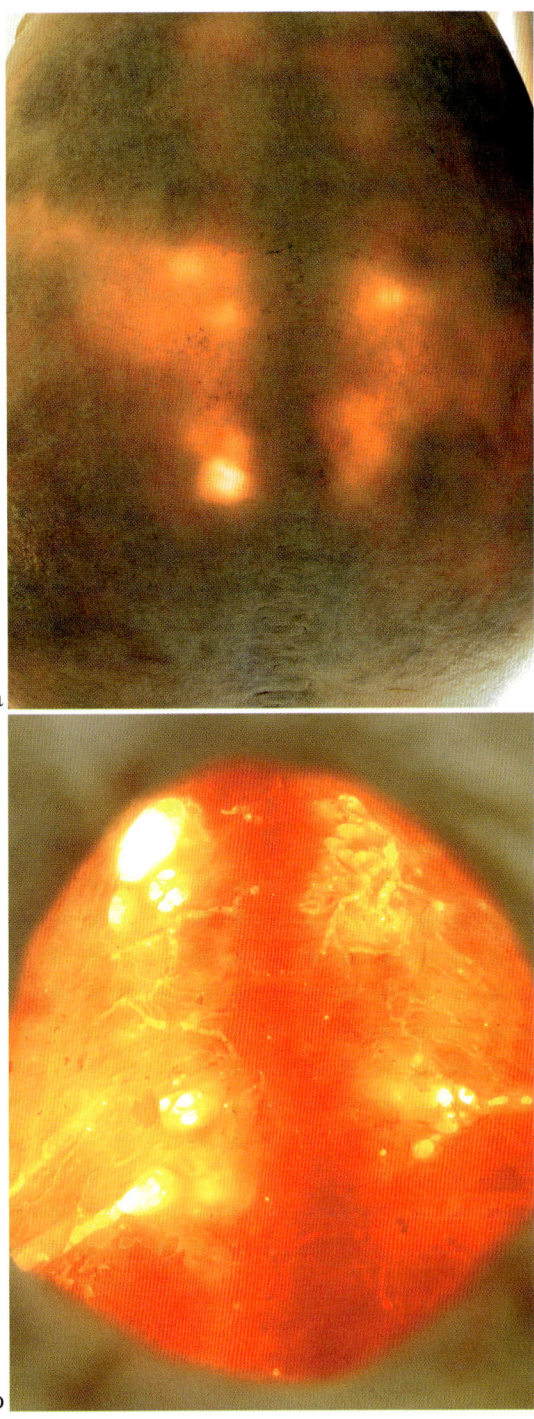

Figure 340a-b. Backlighting to show thin areas associated with arachnoid granulations. (a) Ectocranial and (b) endocranial views through the foramen magnum of arachnoid granulations (Pacchionian pits) and thinned meningeal grooves along either side of the sagittal suture in an elderly Thai (KKU). Arachnoid granulations may erode and herniate the inner table and diploë in the frontal, parietal, and temporal bones. Herniations through the occipital and temporal bones may mimic lytic lesions. Radiographic studies typically record these pits at lower frequencies than dry bone studies. For more information on arachnoid granulations see Bayrak et al. (2009). Cf. Leach et al. (1996); Liang et al. (2002); Roche and Warner (1996).

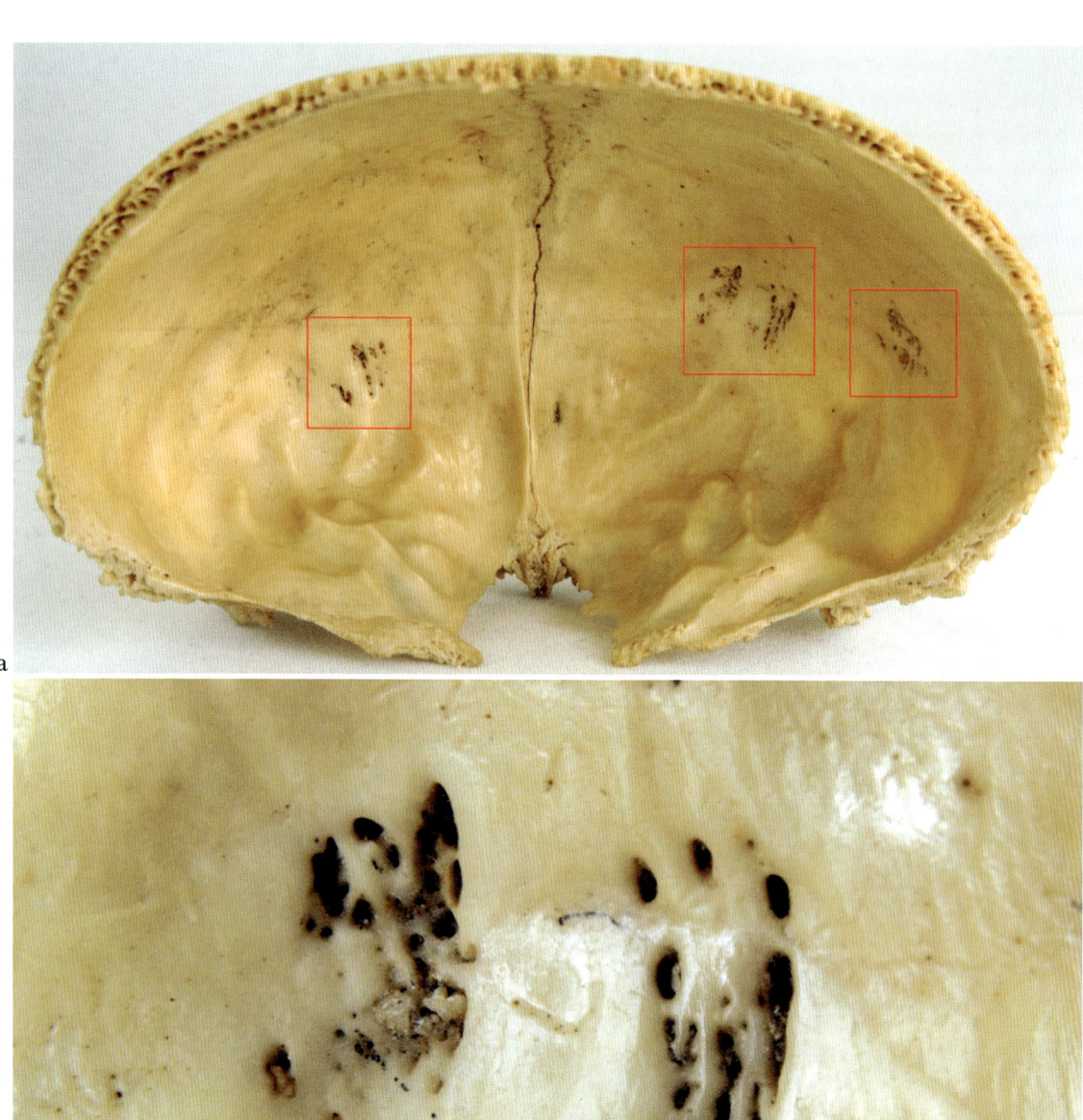

Figure 341a-b. "Frozen waves" of the orbital plates and Pacchionian pits. (a) Endocranium of a child showing an open interfrontal/metopic suture, "frozen waves" (personal communication, William Bass 1983) of the orbital plates and Pacchionian pits (circles). (b) Endocranial magnification of Pacchionian pits that house arachnoid granulations showing perforation of the inner lamina of the vault (KKU) and represents typical anatomy.

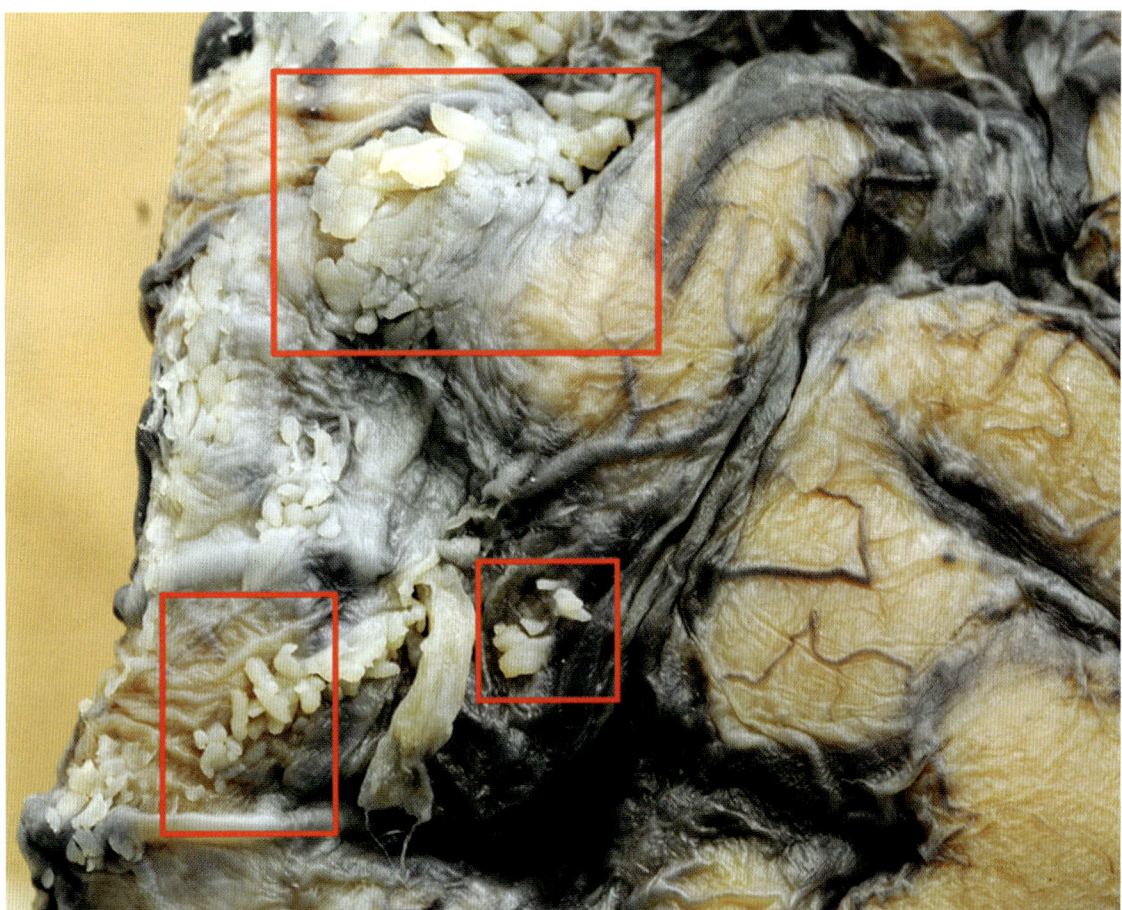

Figure 342. Arachnoid granulations (red squares and rectangles) are absent at birth, first become visible by about 18 months, are rarely found in children younger than 9 years, and continue to increase in size and number thereafter. These granules ossify in middle-age and older individuals, can form bony pits and impressions along the inner table of the cranium, and are often associated with deepened venous grooves primarily along the sagittal suture in the parietals, as well as the frontal bones (sometimes the occipital bone). There is disagreement whether these pits increase in number and depth in response to disease, or if they can be used to ascertain age at death. Cf. Barber et al. (1995); Le Gros Clark (1920); Freyschmidt et al. (2002); Grossman and Potts (1920); Köhler and Zimmer (1968); Leach et al. (1996); Taveras and Wood (1964); Roche and Warner (1996).

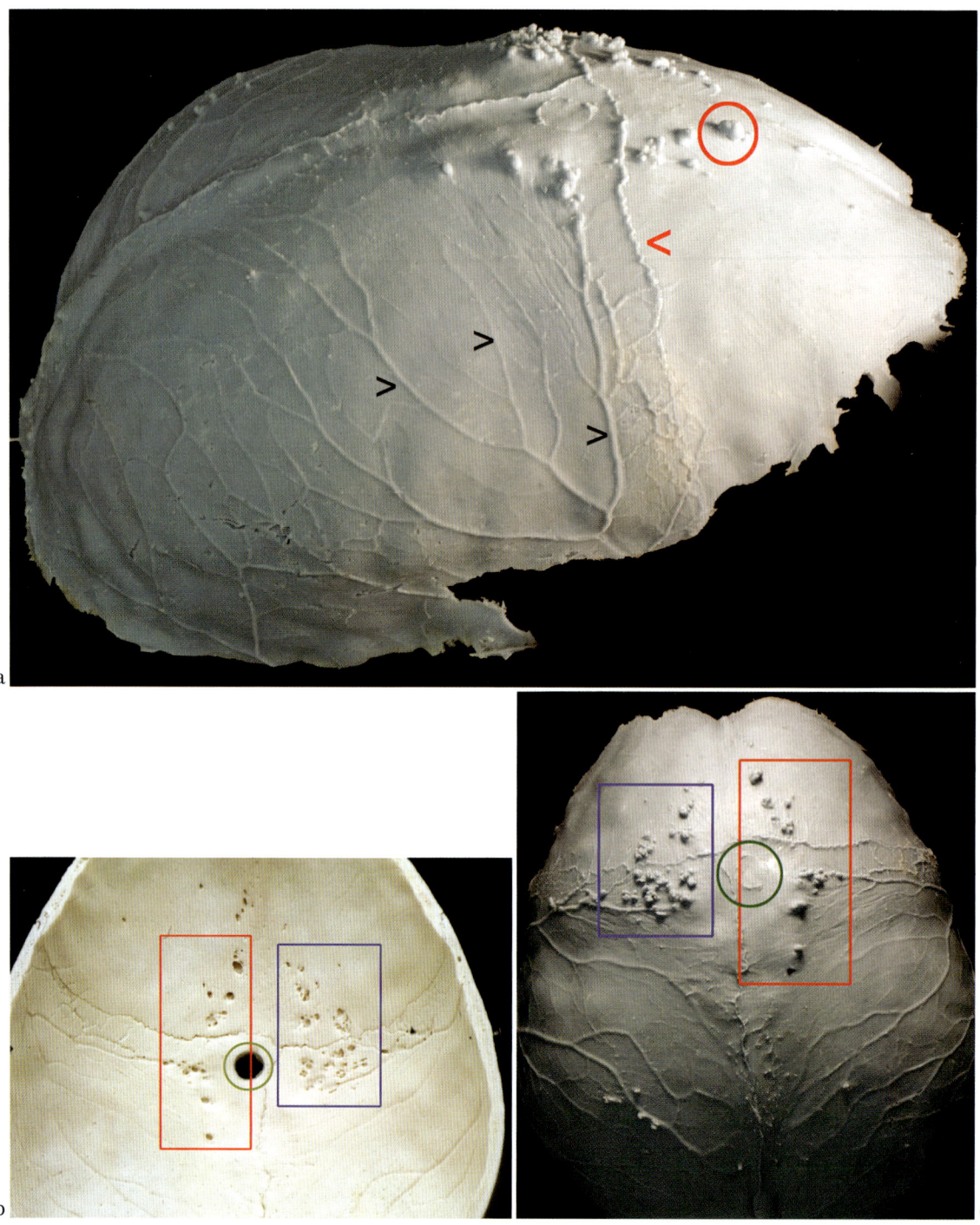

Figure 343a-c. Endocast of Pacchionian pits. (a) Cranial endocast of clusters of Pacchionian bodies (circle), coronal suture (<) and the meningeal arteries (>) of an adult skull (FSA AC039) using a flexible silicone-based impression material (polyvinylsiloxane). (b) Distribution of Pacchionian pits in the right endocranium (red rectangle) and left endocranium (red rectangle). The green circle is the hole where the skull was articulated with the cervical spine as a teaching/hanging skeleton. (c) Using this impression material allows visualization of the size and shape of Pacchionian bodies (blue and red rectangles) deep within the diploë. Pacchionian pits are usually scored as pathological, and not as a non-metric trait. (Endocranial cast made by Cortland Sciotto.)

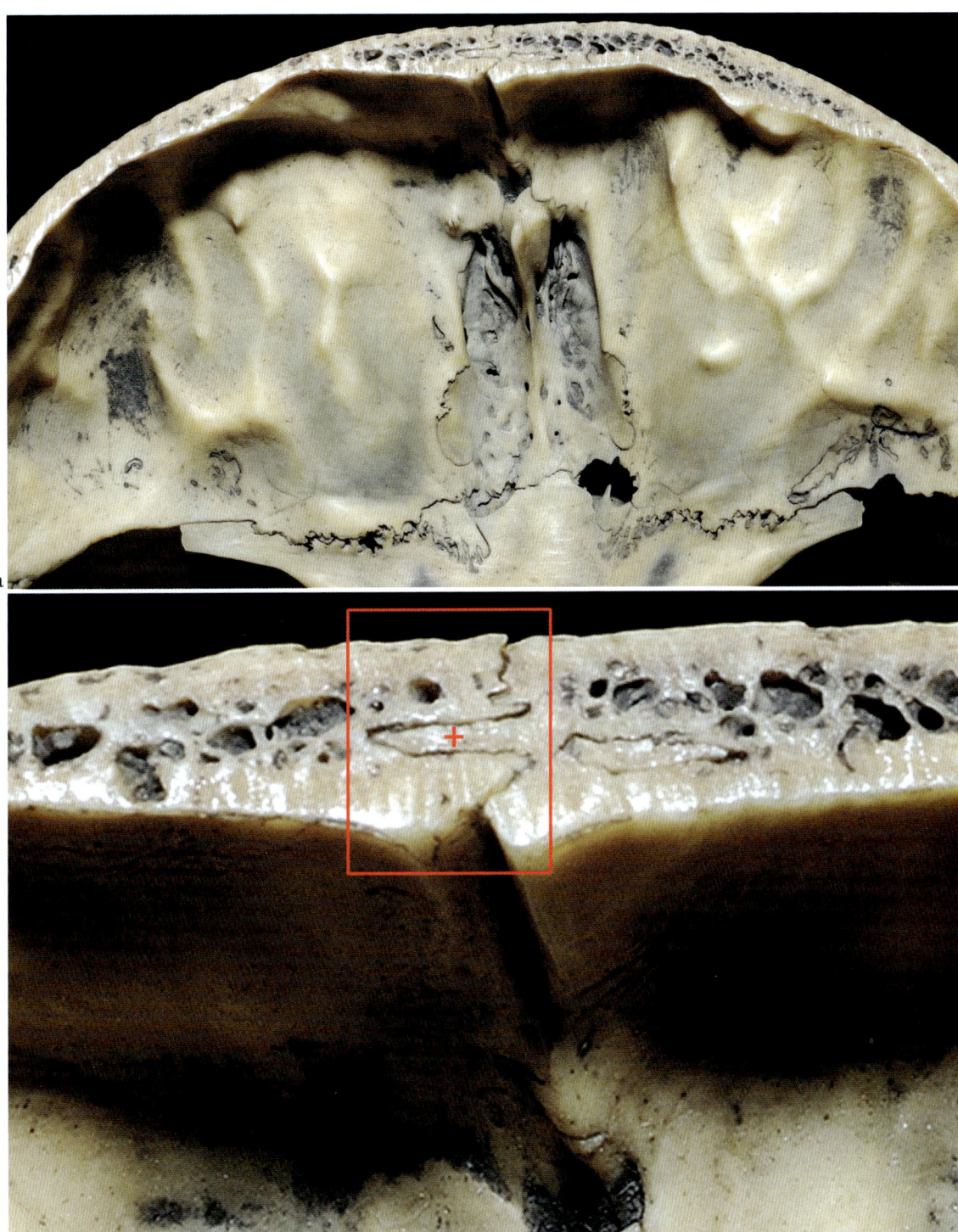

Figure 344a-b. Cerebral ridges ("frozen waves") and open metopic suture in an adult (Mütter Museum 1979.1006.73A). (a) Endocranium displaying the cerebral ridges and depressions of the superior orbital plates that fit the convolutions (i.e., gyri and sulci) of the brain. (b) Diploë between the inner and outer tables and the open metopic suture (rectangle) depicting the cross-sectional anatomy of the suture with a long finger-like extension of bone (+). Complexity of a suture increases its surface area and ability to dissipate stresses. Typical anatomy.

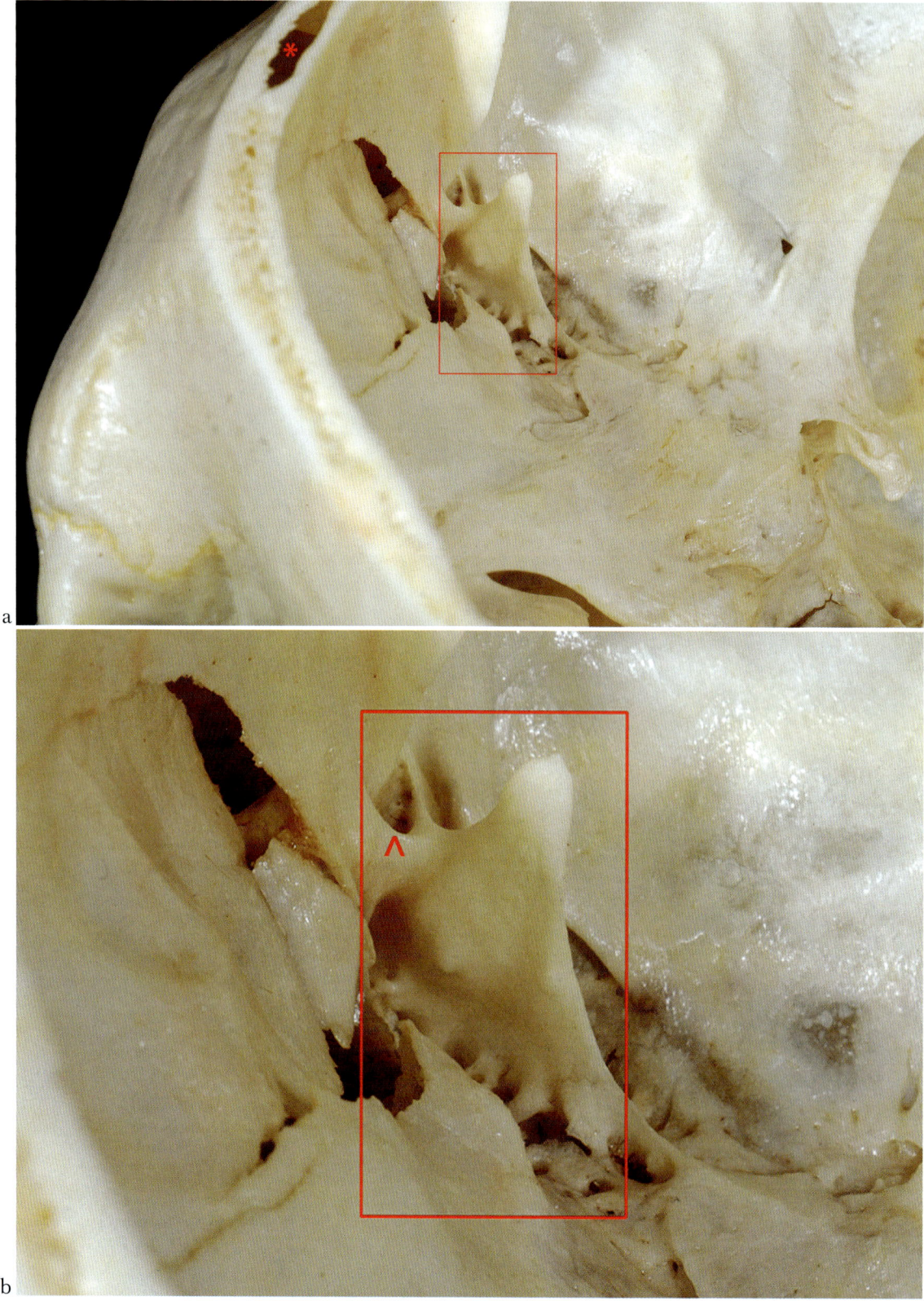

Figure 345a-b. Large crista galli in an adult. (a) Left oblique view of an unusually large crista galli (rectangle) and opening into the frontal sinuses (*) (JABSOM 609). (b) Close-up of the crista galli and foramen cecum (∧).

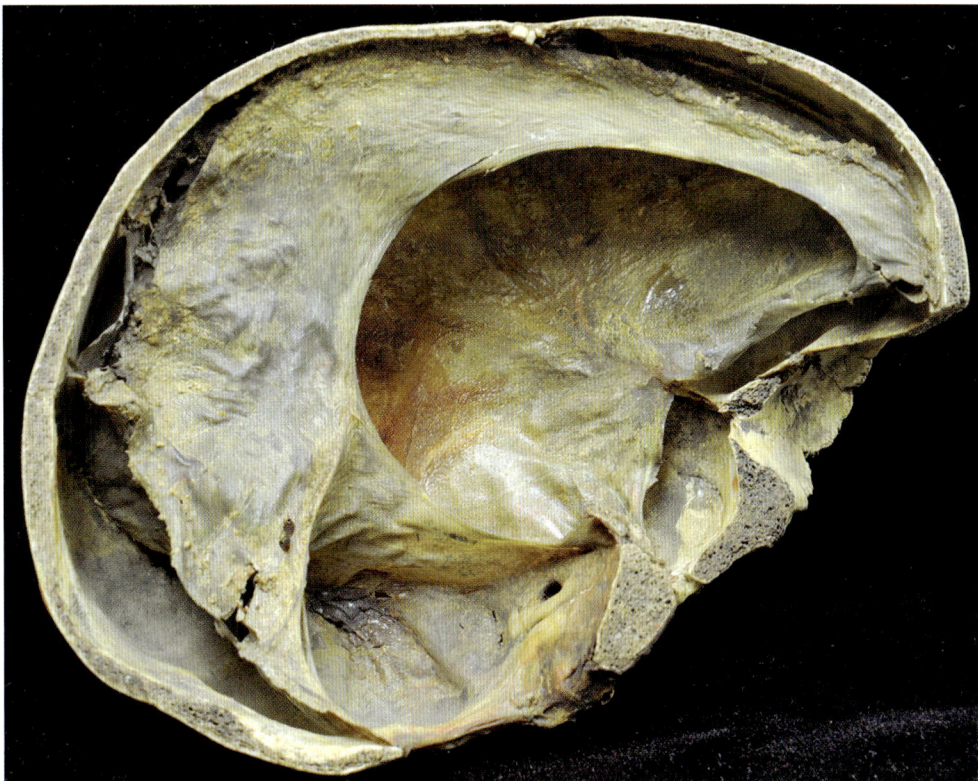

Figure 346. Sagittal section of a subadult skull showing attachment of the dura mater throughout the skull and falx cerebri that separated the right and left hemispheres along the midline (Mütter Museum 1008.26). Normal anatomy.

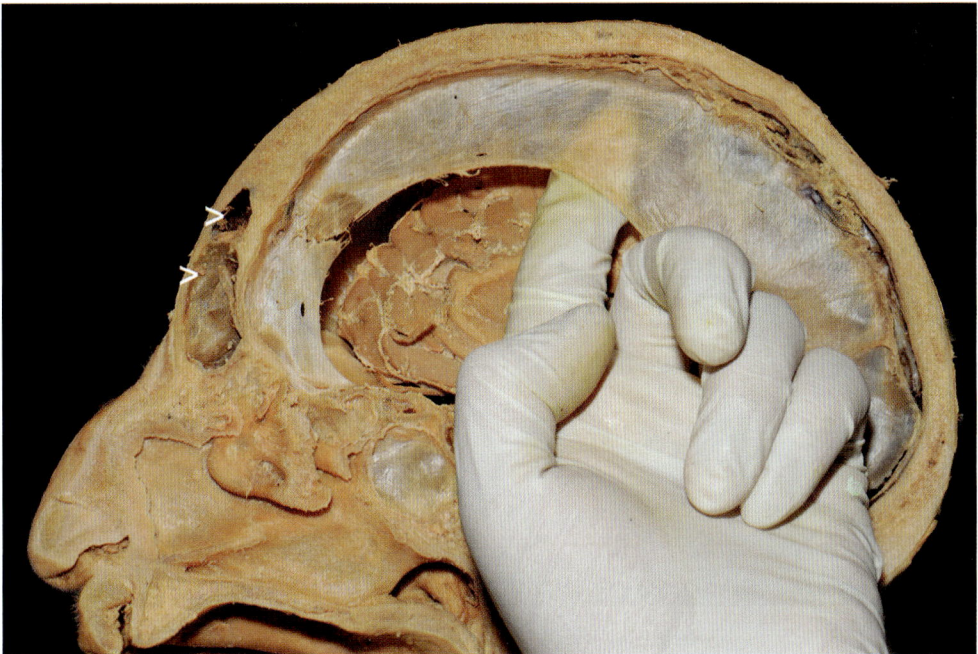

Figure 347. The translucent falx cerebri and frontal sinuses (>) with adhering soft tissue in an elderly male (JABSOM).

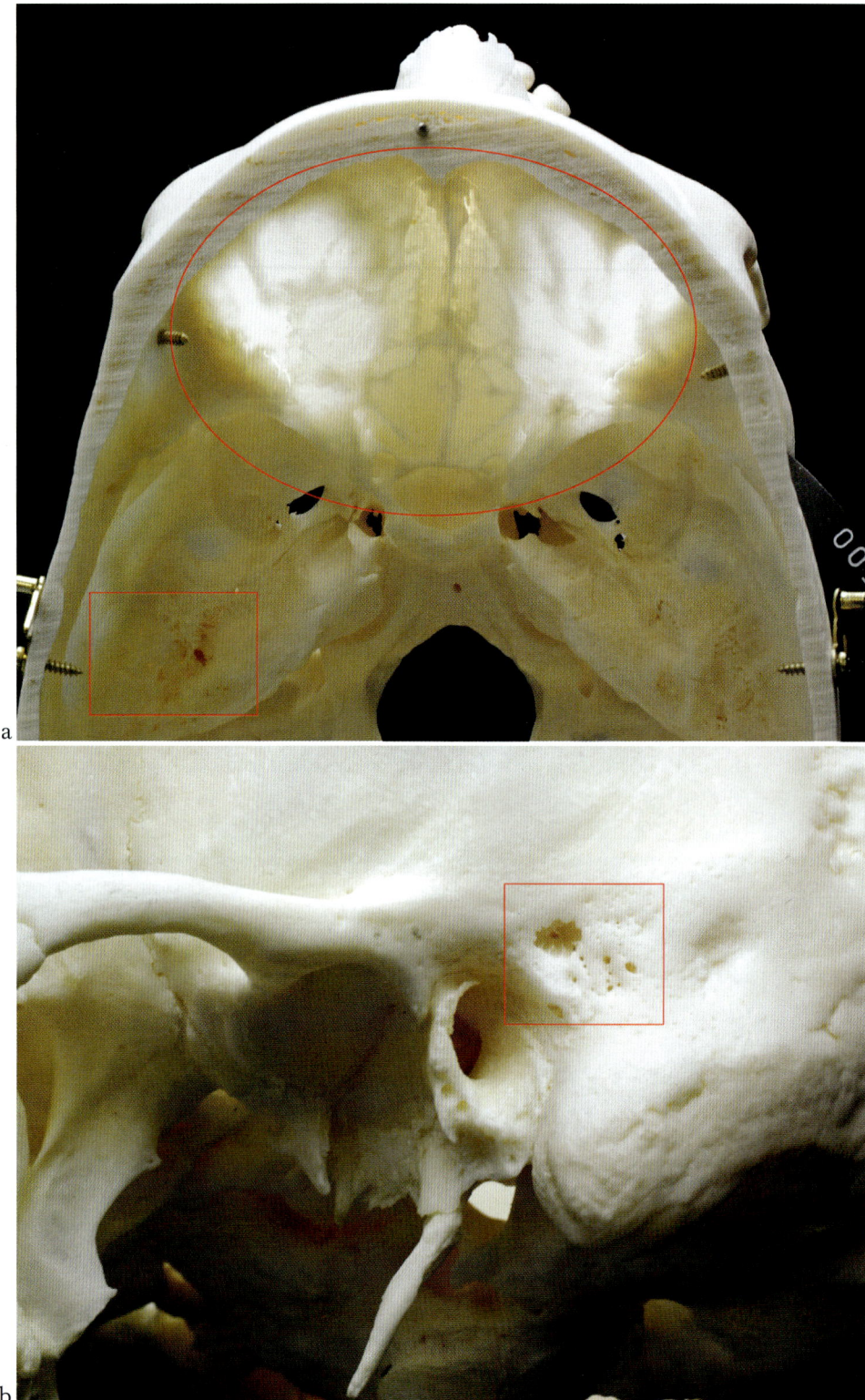

Figure 348a-b. Thin orbital plates and tegum dehiscence. (a) Endocranium showing unusually osteoporotic and thin orbital plates (oval) and a tegmun dehiscence (rectangle) that communicates with (b) several perforated lesions in the left temporal bone (square).

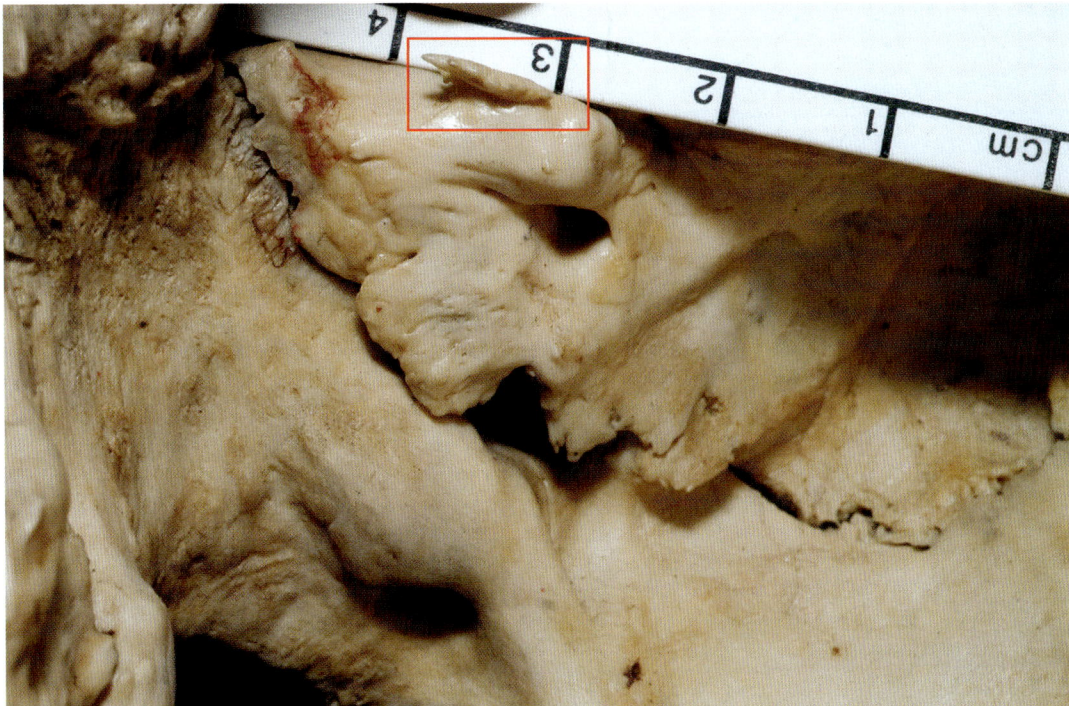

Figure 349. Small spiked projection of calcification (exostosis) along the ridge of the right petrous bone superior to the internal auditory meatus (SI Terry 522, young adult Black male). Most of these projections measure 5-8 mm in length, but may be longer, straight, curved or hooked. Common finding in the elderly and appears to have largely gone unreported in the literature.

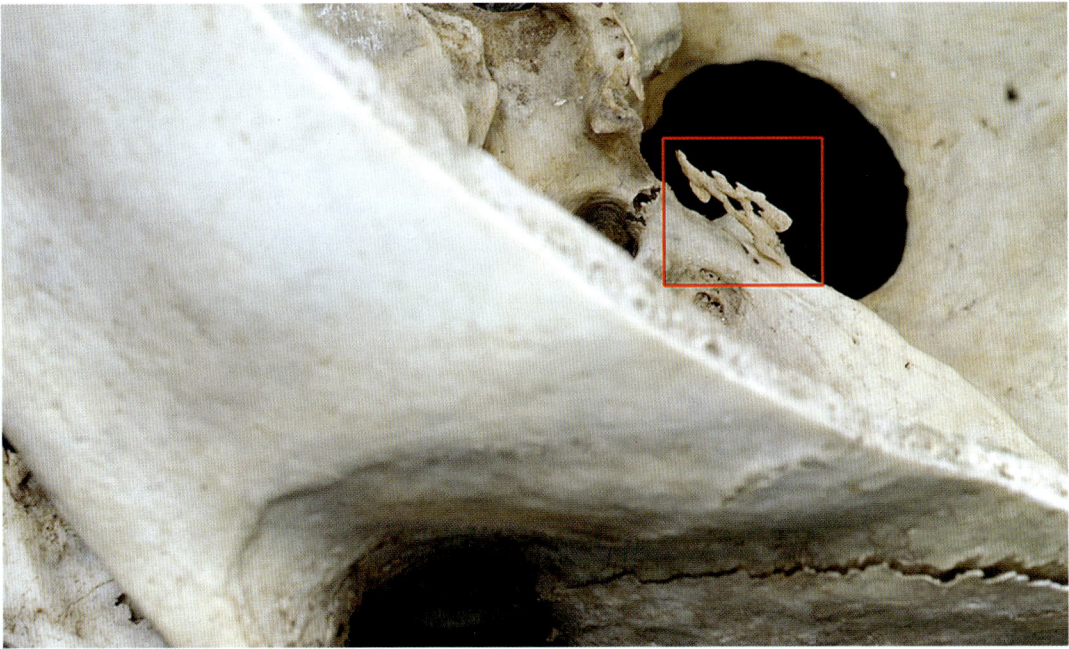

Figure 350. Calcification (square) beneath the tentorium cerebelli along the superior petrosal sinus of the temporal bone in an elderly male (CMU 113 52). Unusual "lightning bolt" shape, but projections at this location are common in the elderly.

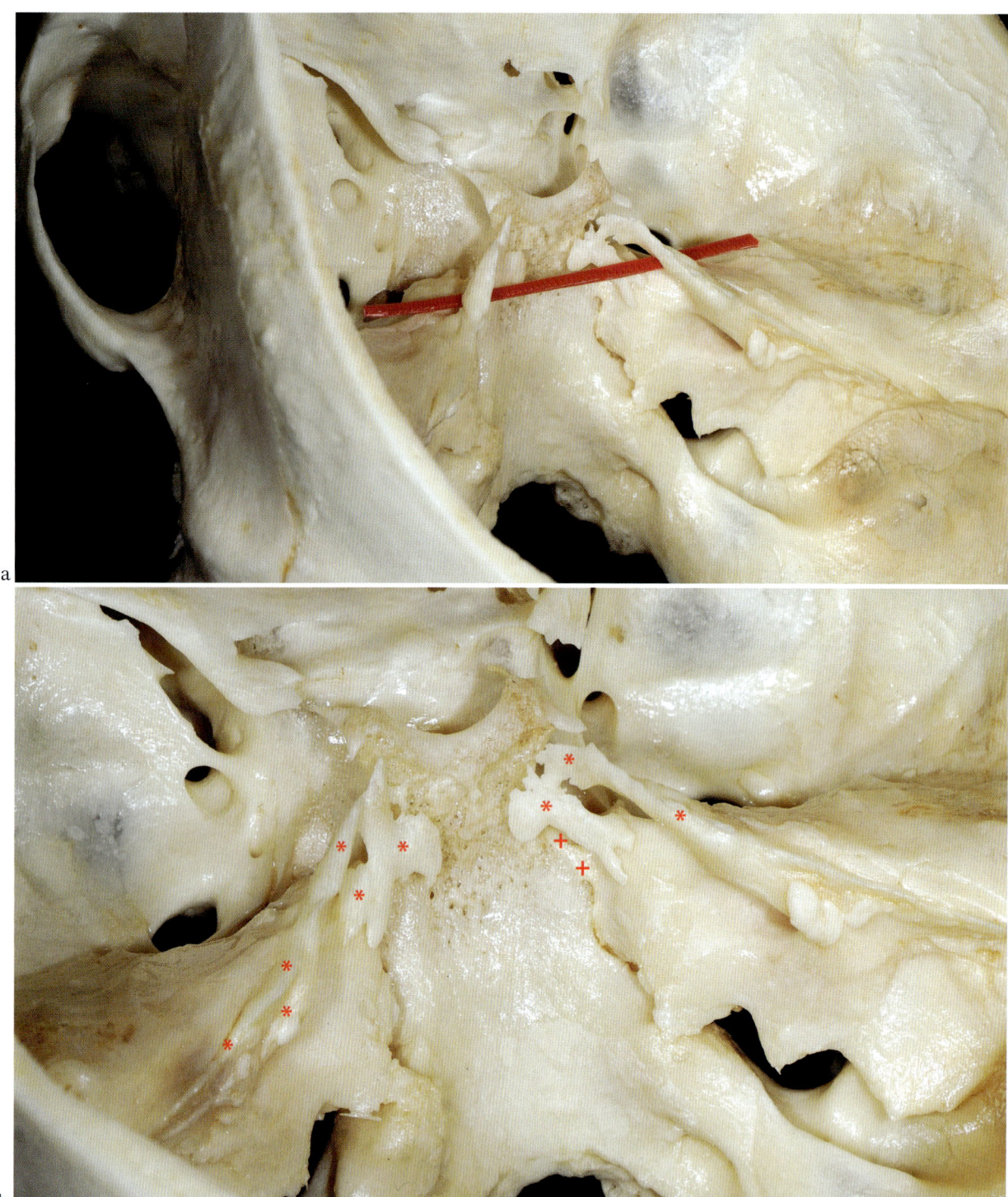

Figure 351a-b. Subdural calcifications in a 60-year-old African American male (JABSOM 1079). (a) Bilateral calcificiation (red probe) beneath the dura mater, along either side of the superior petrosal sinus (*). (b) Numerous bar-like calcifications, possibly of the petrosphenoid ligament (of Gruber), along the temporal bone. The literature reveals different descriptions for attachment of Gruber's ligament, either along the petrous ridge or its apex. See Aggarwal et al. (2012) and Tubbs et al. (2013a) for more on ossification of the petrosphenoid ligament, a rare feature. Ossification or calcification along the superior petrosal sinus, however, is common among elderly individuals.

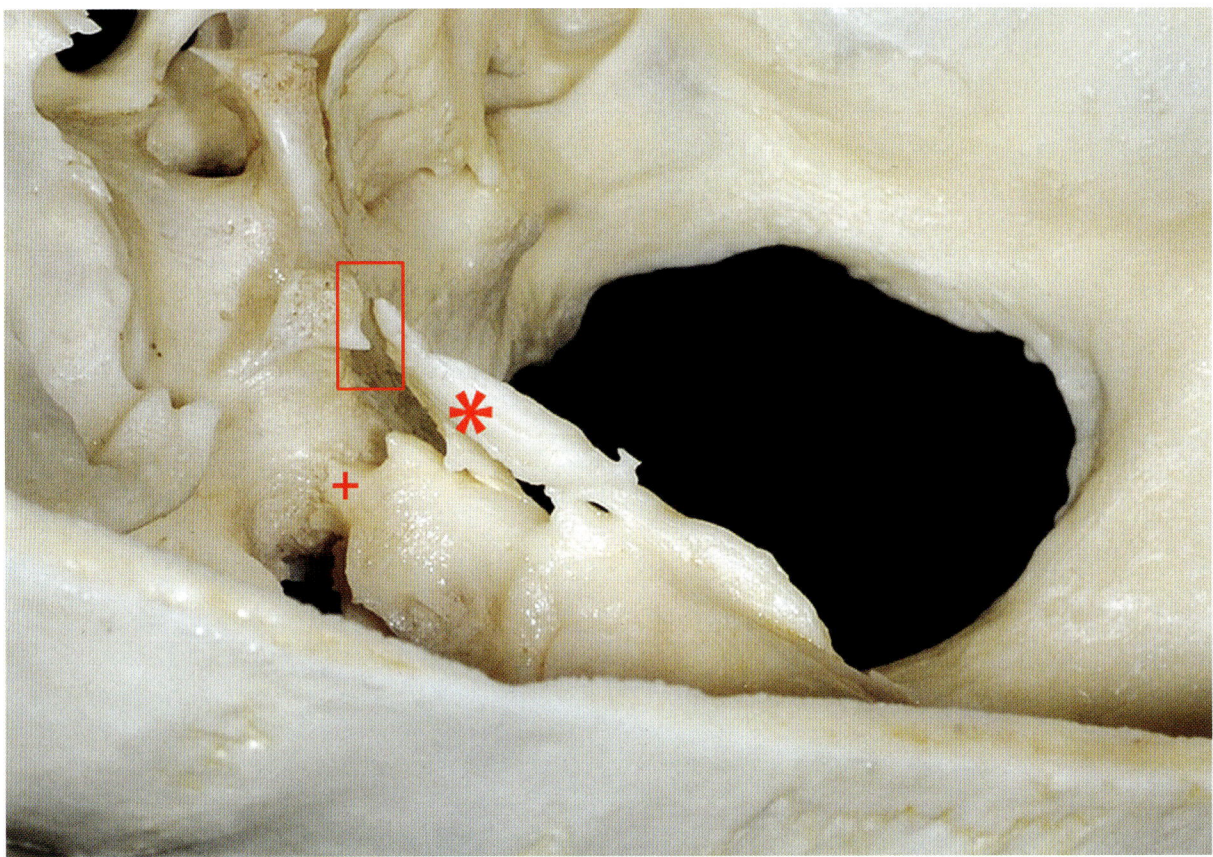

Figure 352. Magnification of calcifications (*) along the left superior petrosal sinus showing incomplete bridging with the clivus (rectangle) of the sphenoid and calcification (+) of the petrosphenoid ligament (of Gruber) spanning from the petrous apex and clivus in a 60-year-old African American male (JABSOM 1079). Calcification along the petrous ridge, beneath the osteogenic layer of the dura mater, is common in elderly individuals, while calcification of the petrosphenoid ligament (of Gruber) is rare.

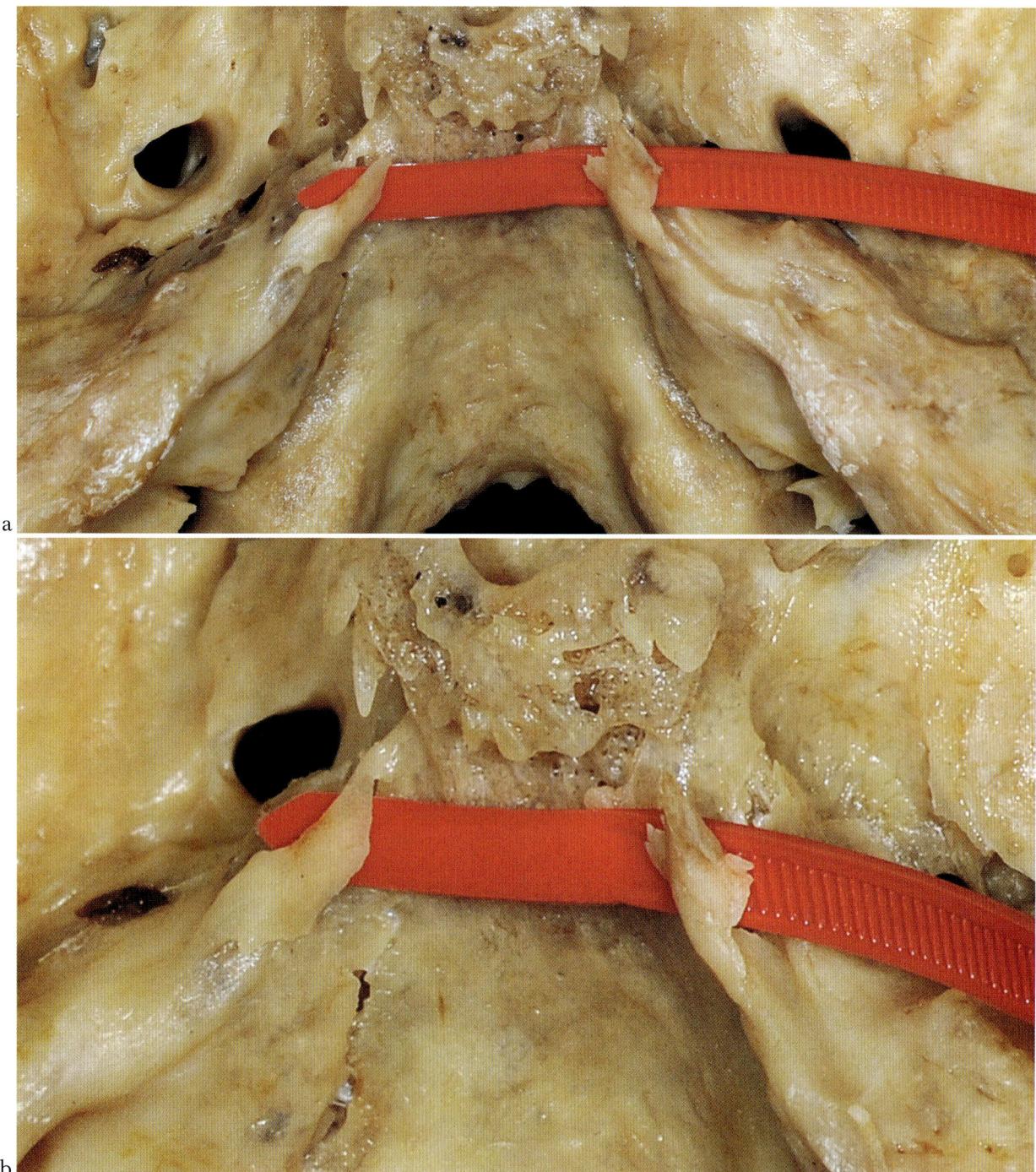

Figure 353a-b. Calcification along the petrous ridge and superior petrosal sinus of the temporal bone. (a) Bilateral calcifications (red) along the petrous ridge and superior petrosal sinus in a 54-year-old Asian male (JABSOM 1198). (b) Slightly enlarged view of the calcifications showing that they extend beyond the petrous processes (red probe). Aggarwal et al. (2012) report a similar example of calcification along the petrous ridge and identify it as ossified petrosphenoid ligament (of Gruber). See Tubbs et al. (2013a), however, for details on ossification of the petrosphenoid ligament (a rare trait) spanning the apex of the petrous bone, but not along its ridge. The present degree of development is an uncommon to rare finding.

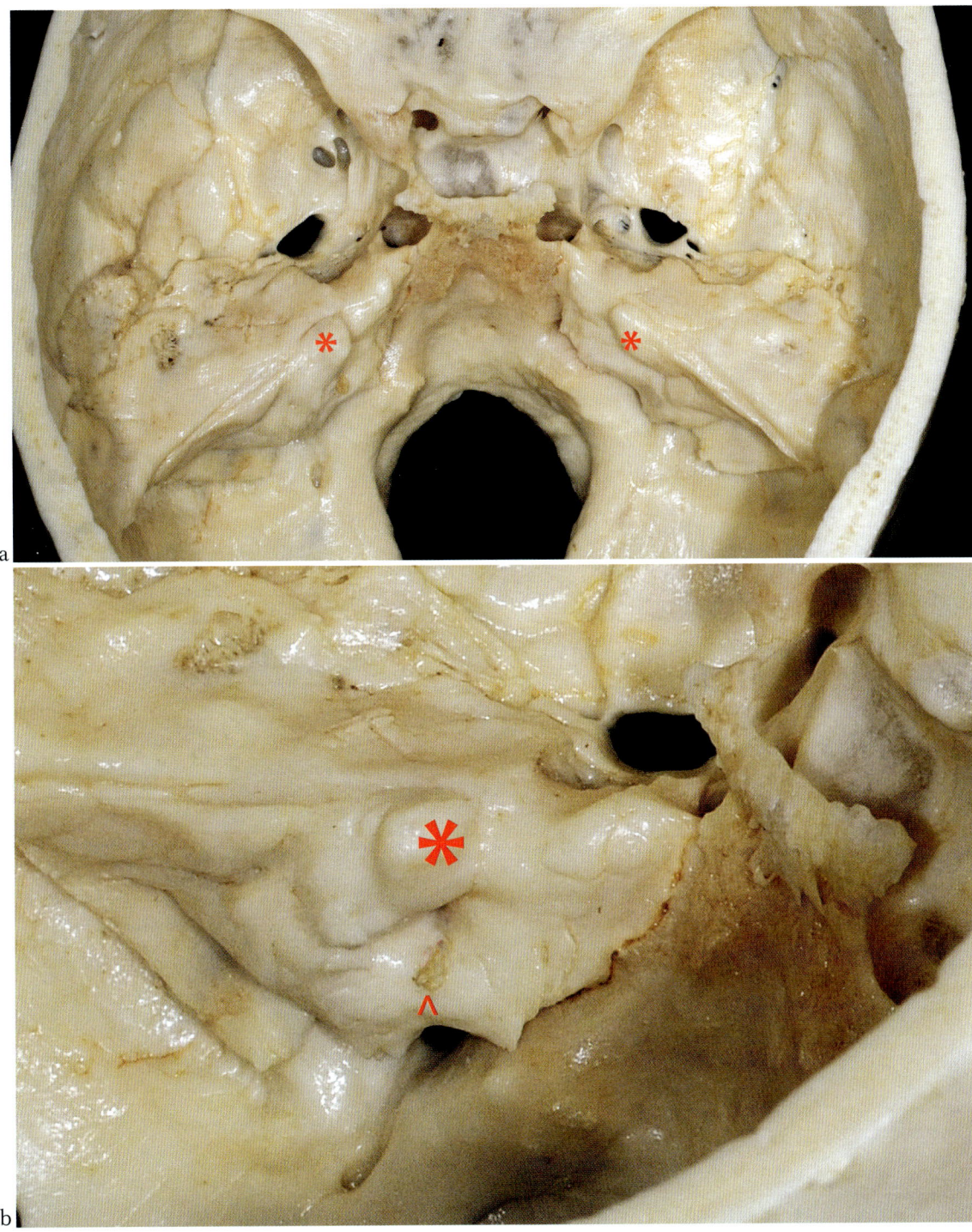

Figure 354a-b. Bony growth eminences along the superior petrosal sinus. (a) Bilateral bony growths (*) in a 76-year-old Caucasoid male with hyperostosis frontalis interna (HFI) (JABSOM 1068). Bony growths and spiked projections in this location are common in elderly individuals, especially those with HFI. These growths are likely associated with increased age and/or a pathological condition and not typical variants. (b) Bony eminence (*) and cranial nerve VII (∧) present in the left internal auditory meatus.

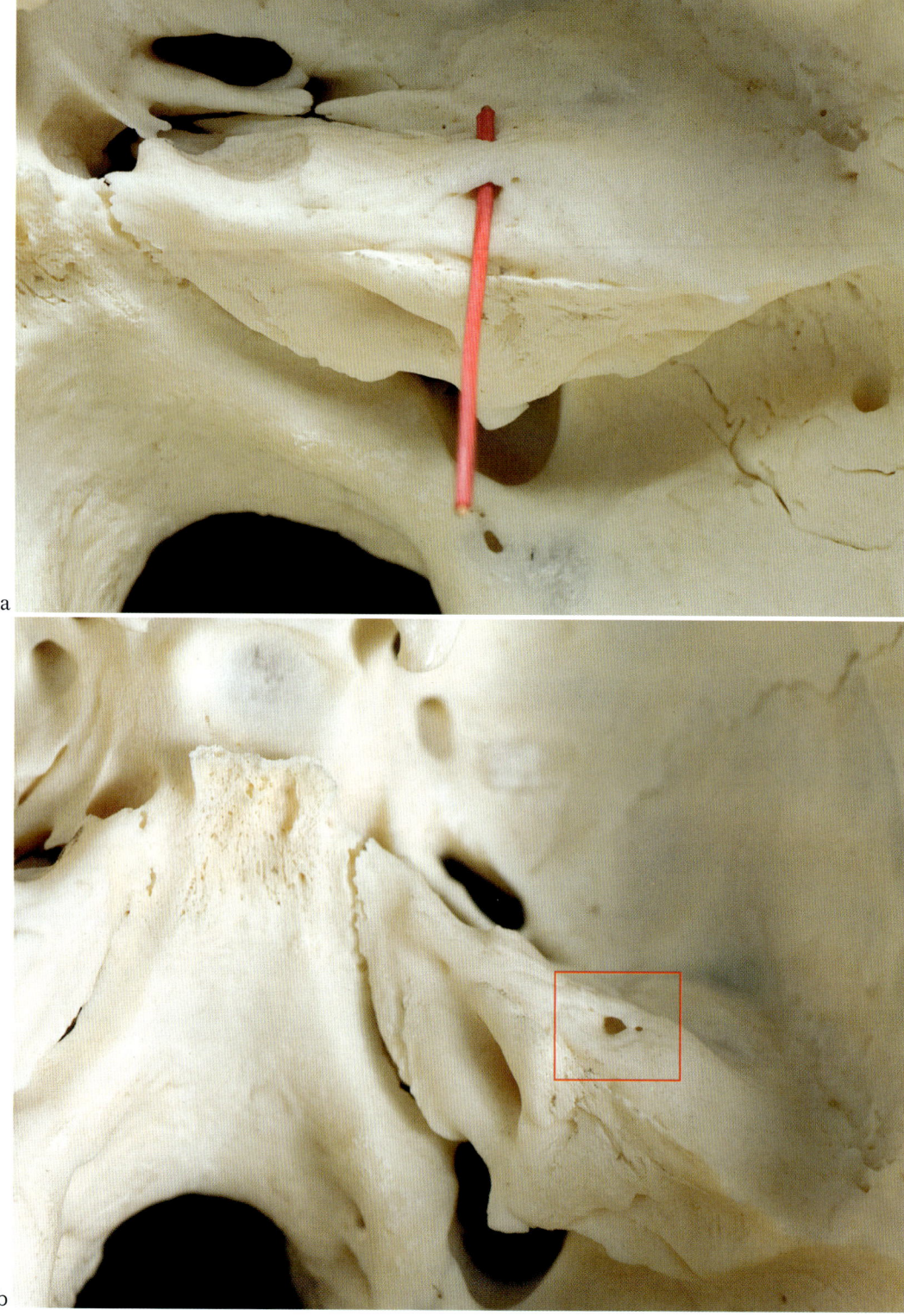

Figure 355a-b. Foramen along the right petrous ridge. (a) Unilateral foramen (red probe) and (b) a tiny lateral accessory foramen to its right, possibly the hiatus canalis facialis in the pyramidal process of the right temporal bone in an Asian adult skull. (CSC AC027). When compared to the anatomy of the left petrous bone, this large foramen does not appear to be the result of soft tissue bridging. Uncommon finding of unknown frequency.

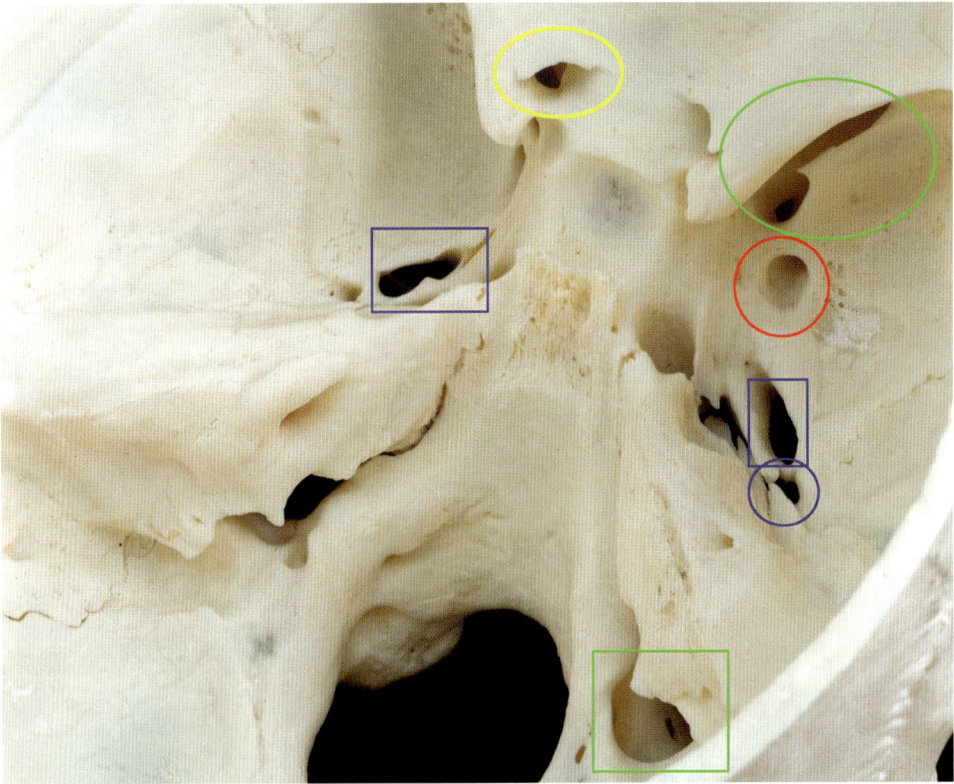

Figure 356. Normal anatomy and typical foramina: optic foramen (yellow), superior orbital fissure (green oval), foramen rotundum (red), foramen ovale (blue rectangles), foramen spinosum (blue circle) and jugular foramen (green square) (CSC AC027). Cf. Boyd (1930); Berge and Bergman (2001); Kale et al. (2009a); Kodama et al. (1997); Krayenbühl et al. (2008); Lanzieri et al. (1988); Rossi et al. (2010); Shapiro and Robinson (1967); Wood-Jones (1931).

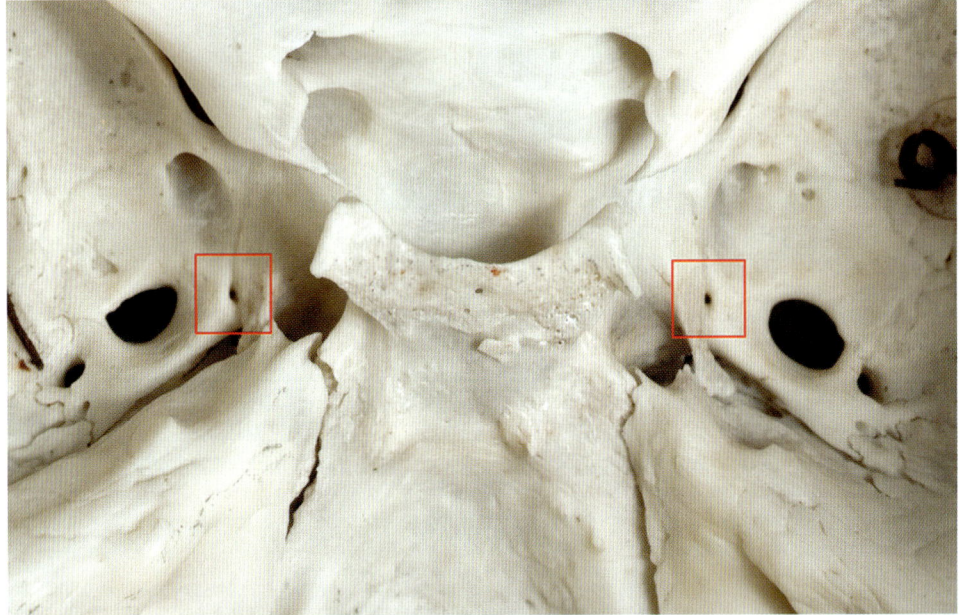

Figure 357. Bilateral foramen of Vesalius (squares) in a young adult Asian female skull (CSC AS002). Wood-Jones (1931) reported this foramen is found only in humans and no other primates.

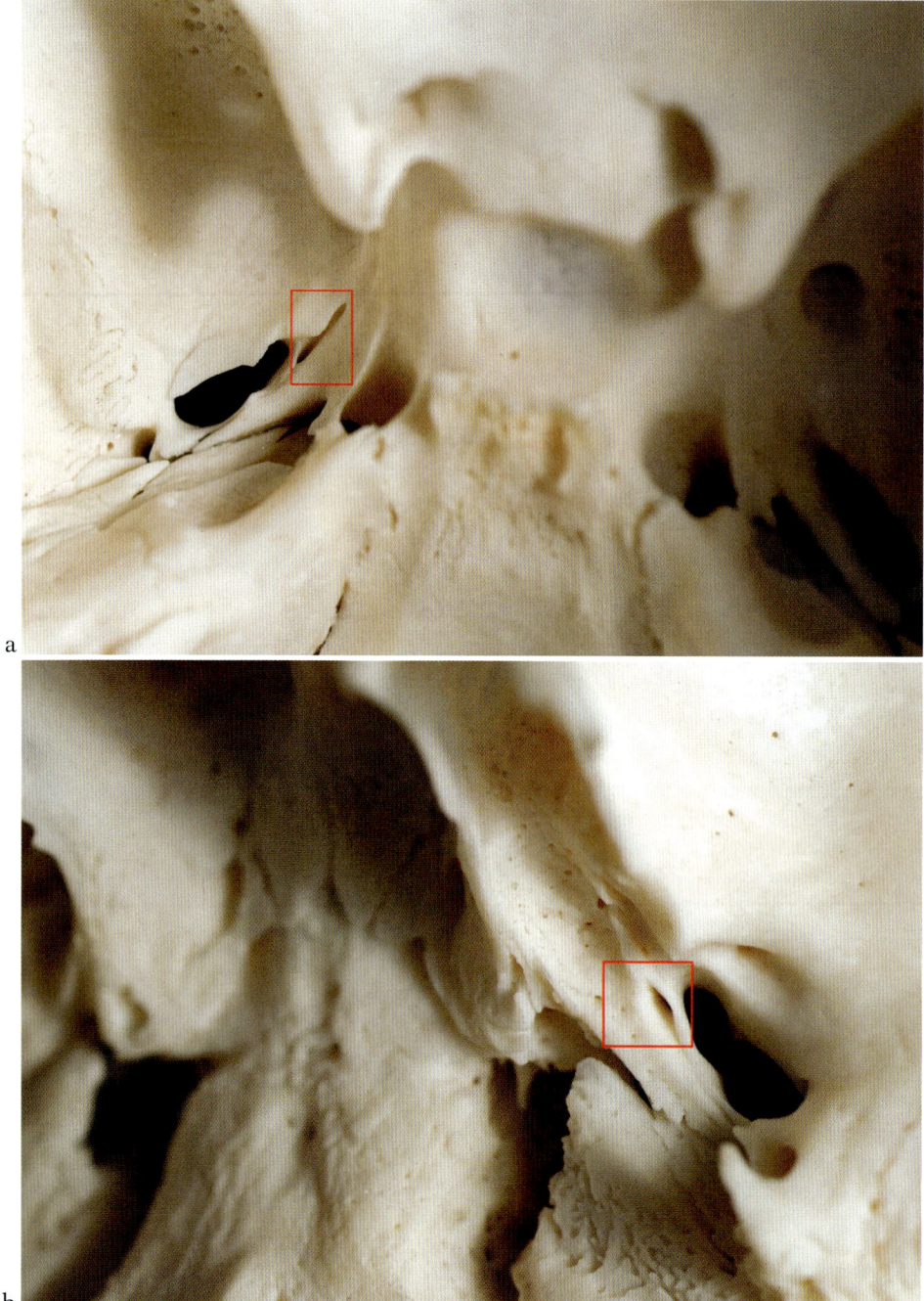

Figure 358a-b. Foramen of Vesalius in an adult Asian female skull (CSC AC027). (a) Endocranial and (b) ectocranial views of a slit-like single left foramen of Vesalius. This feature was bilateral in this individual. Foramen of Vesalius (FV) was found in 135 of 400 (33.75%) adult skulls; absent on both sides in 265/400; unilateral in 18% and bilateral in 15.5% of the skulls examined by Shinohara et al. (2010). Chaisuksunt et al. (2012), in comparison, found FV in 16.1% of 377 Thai skulls, of which 23.6% (89 of 377 skulls) were unilateral and 14.0% (53 of 377 skulls) were bilateral. This foramen is sometimes called the sphenoidal emissary foramen (Brash 1953) and may be doubled (or divided) on the same side (Kale et al. 2009a). Cf. Shinohara et al. (2010).

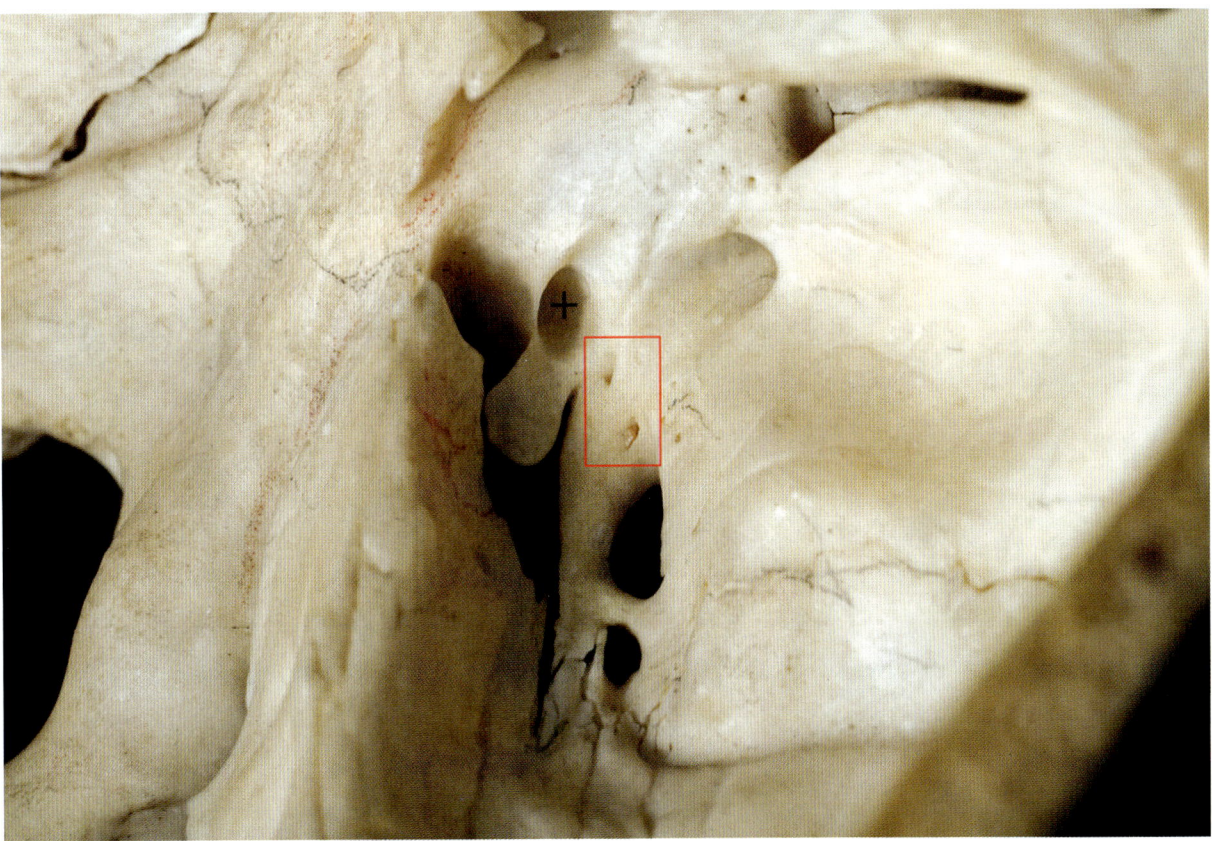

Figure 359. Possible double right foramen of Vesalius (rectangle) in an adult female (CSC AS007). The tongue-shaped portion of bone (circle) to the left of the two foramina is the lingula sphenoidalis. Note the fossa (+) in the right sphenoid that is not present on the left side. This fossa contains a pinpoint-sized foramen and warrants further research. Cf. Baert et al. (2010); Wood-Jones (1931); Kale et al. (2009a); Steele and Bramblett (1988); Shinohara et al. (2010) for more on the foramen of Vesalius.

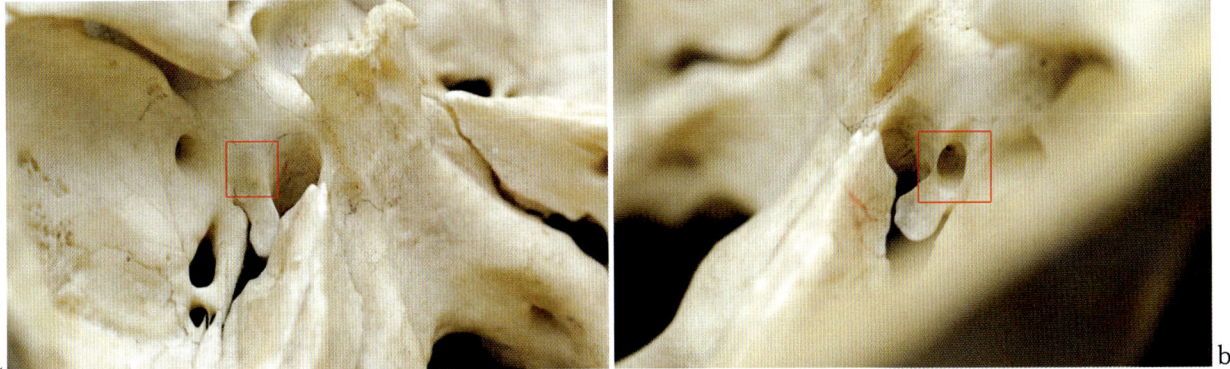

Figure 360a-b. Foramen of unknown etiology and origin in the sphenoid bone. (a) Absence of a fossa and foramen on the left side (square) above the lingual sphenoidalis (CSC AS007). (b) Fossa containing a small foramen of unknown origin. This fossa and foramen warrant further research regarding their origin and frequency in different ethnic and geographical groups.

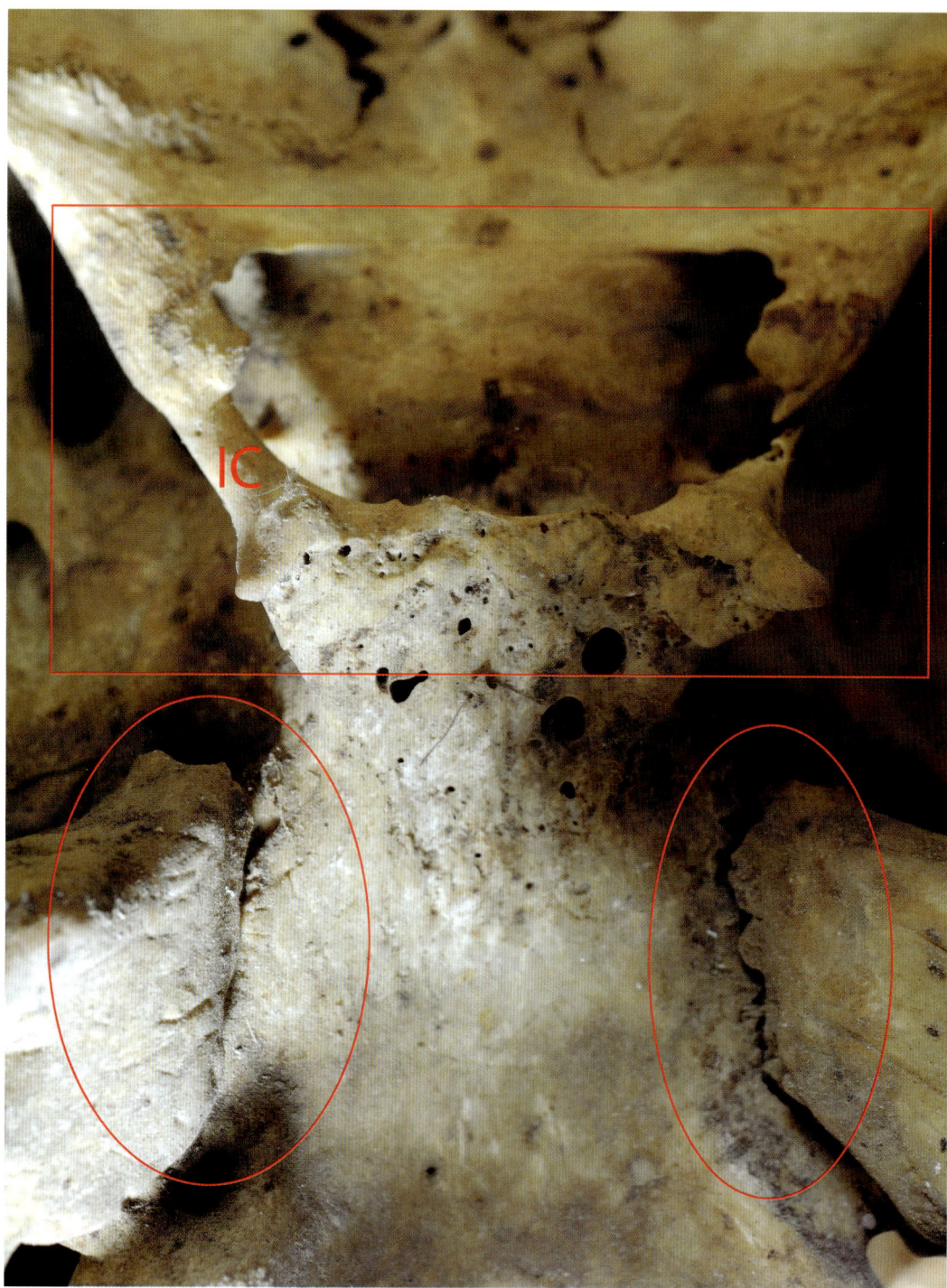

Figure 361. Bridging of the anterior and posterior clinoid processes. Clinoid bridging of the anterior and posterior clinoid processes by calcification of the interclinoid ligaments (ICL) and incomplete fusion of the petrous bones (sphenoid tubercles) with the basilar process at the level of the basilar synchondrosis (ovals) in a Thai (KKU). Note complete bridging of the left ICL forming the caroticoclinoid foramen and incomplete or partial bridging of the right interclinoid ligament. Higher magnification of incomplete fusion of the petrous bones with the basilar process (rectangles). Ossification or calcification of the ICL may be bilateral or unilateral, occurs in about 8% of skulls (Keyes 1935) and may be symptomatic. Radiographic study revealed 3 of 325 healthy patients (1%) with petroclinoid ligament calcifications (Tetradis and Kantor 1999). Some researchers record calcified ICL as an ancillary anomalous finding (Cederberg et al. 2003).

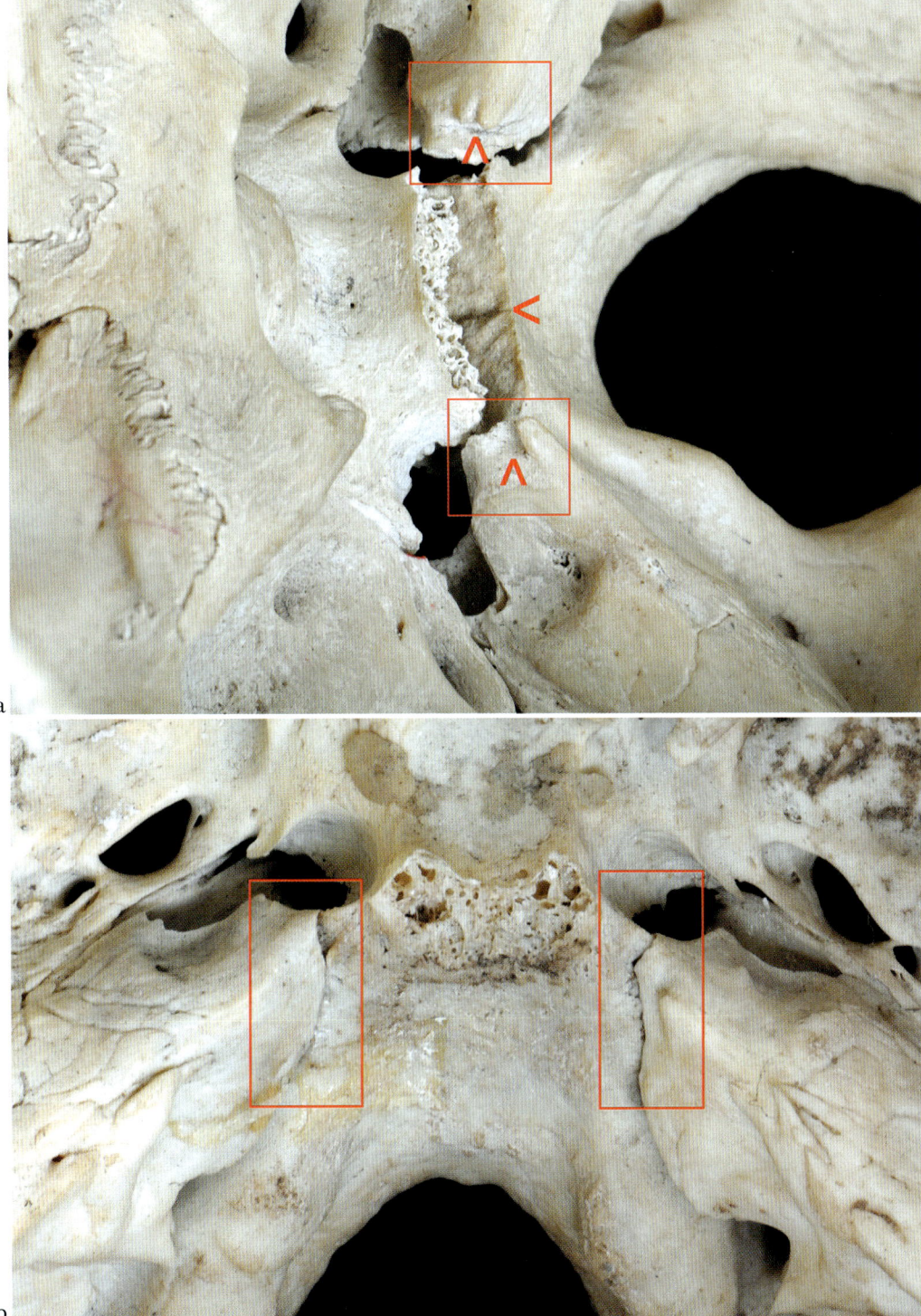

Figure 362a-b. Petrous portions of the temporal bone in two individuals. (a) Oblique view of the petrous bones in a child showing where they attach (square and rectangle) to the basilar bone. Note the open basilar synchondrosis (<). Note the "V"-shaped notch (∧) at the medial end of the petrous process where a small bar of loose bone called the sphenoid tubercle forms a bridge across this junction (rectangles) in subadults and fuses in adults. (b) Petrous and basilar bones in a Thai adult (KKU).

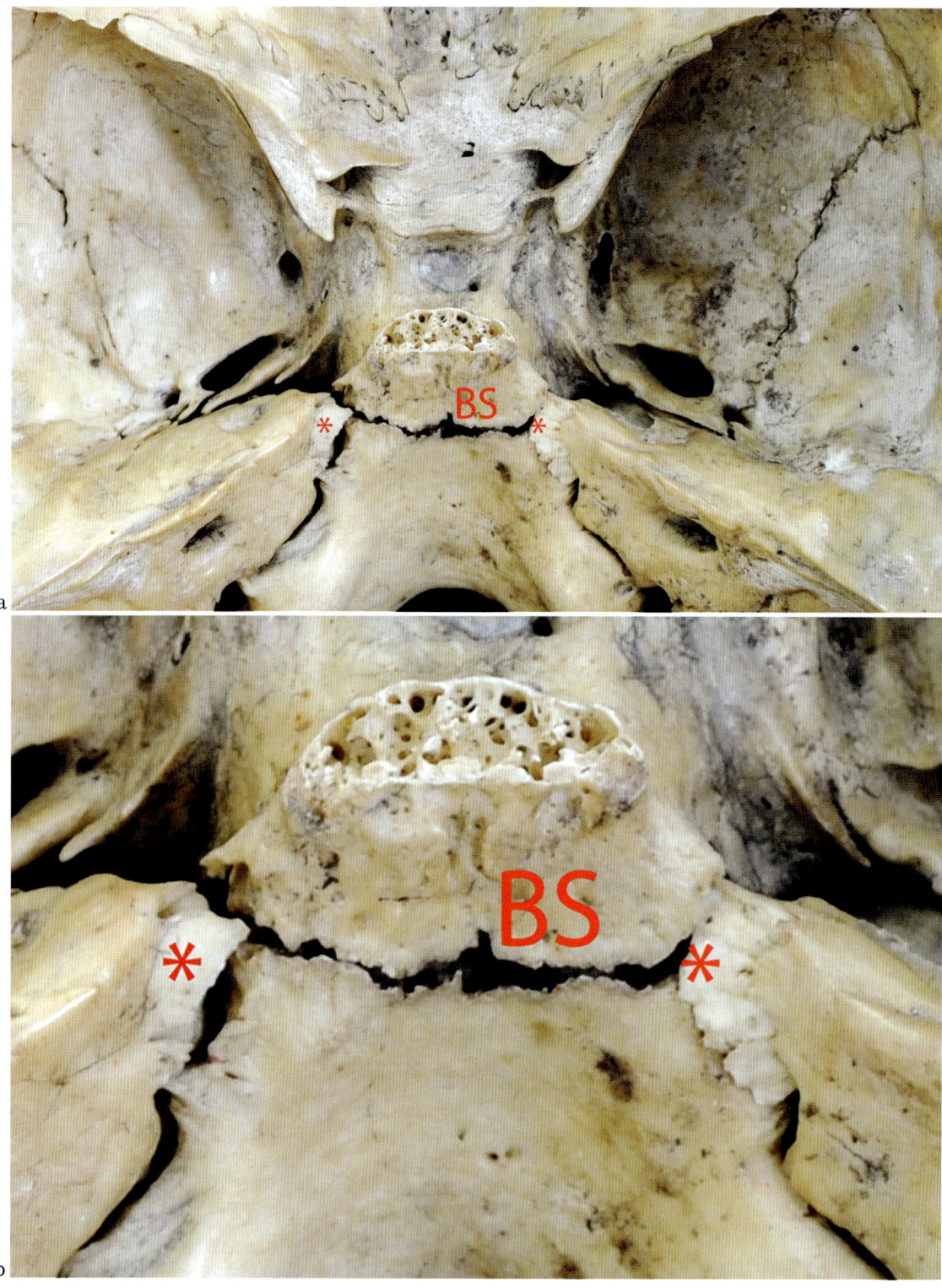

Figure 363a-b. Basilar synchondrosis and bony islands of the petrous bone. (a) Basilar synchondrosis (BS) and bony islands (*) of the pyramidal portions of the petrous bone. Note the white "scalloped" bone (*) present in the right and left pyramidal portions joining the petrous bone with the basilar in a subadult Thai skull (KKU). This isthmus of bone, actually a synchondrosis, warrants study as an indicator of age. Typical anatomy.

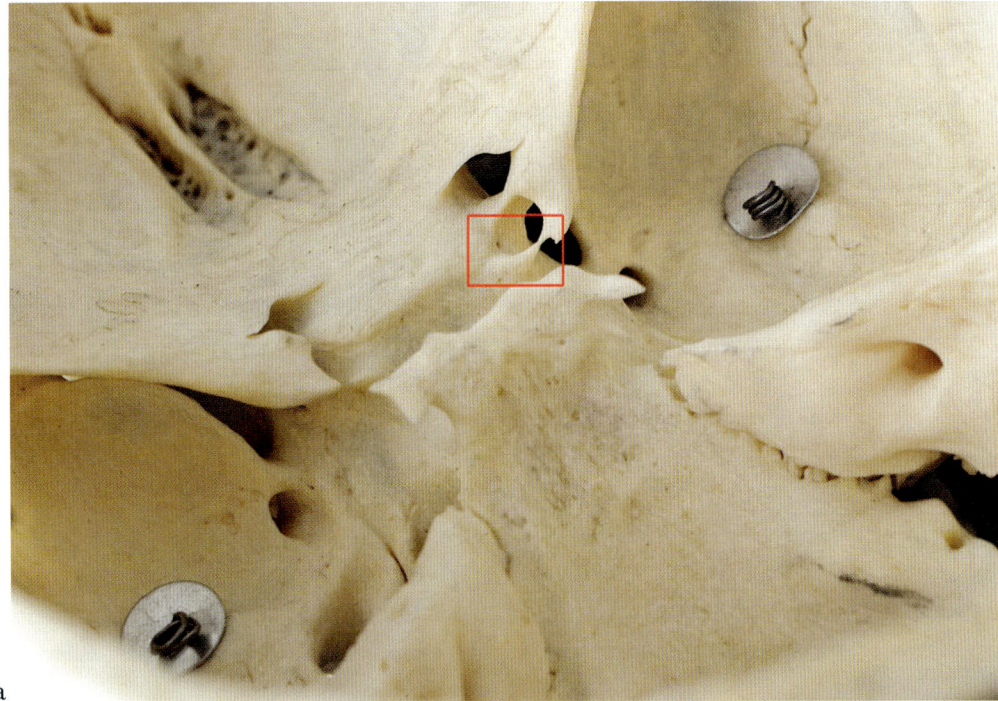
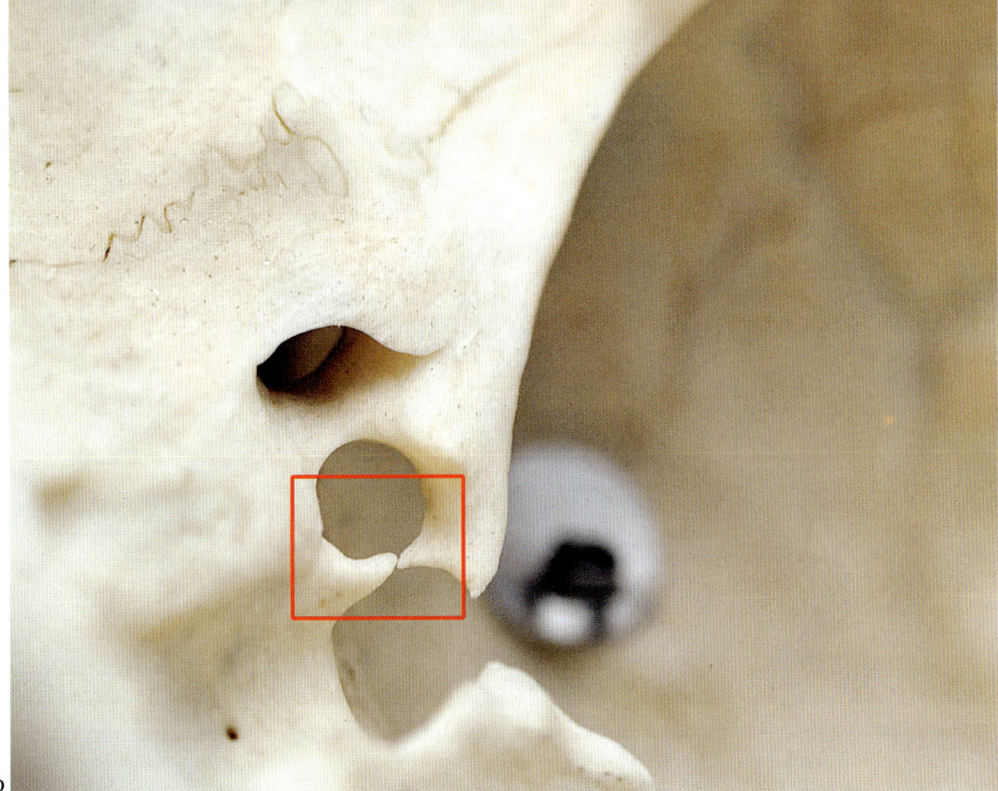

Figure 364a-b. Caroticoclinoid foramen. (a) Right caroticoclinoid foramen (rectangle) in a young adult Asian male skull (FSA AS008). (b) Note that bridging of the anterior and middle clinoid processes resulted in a nearly complete and closed right foramen. Examination of 80 Brazilian human skulls revealed 8.5% skulls with at least one foramen (Freire et al. 2011). Cf. Ertuck et al. (2004); Freire et al. (2010).

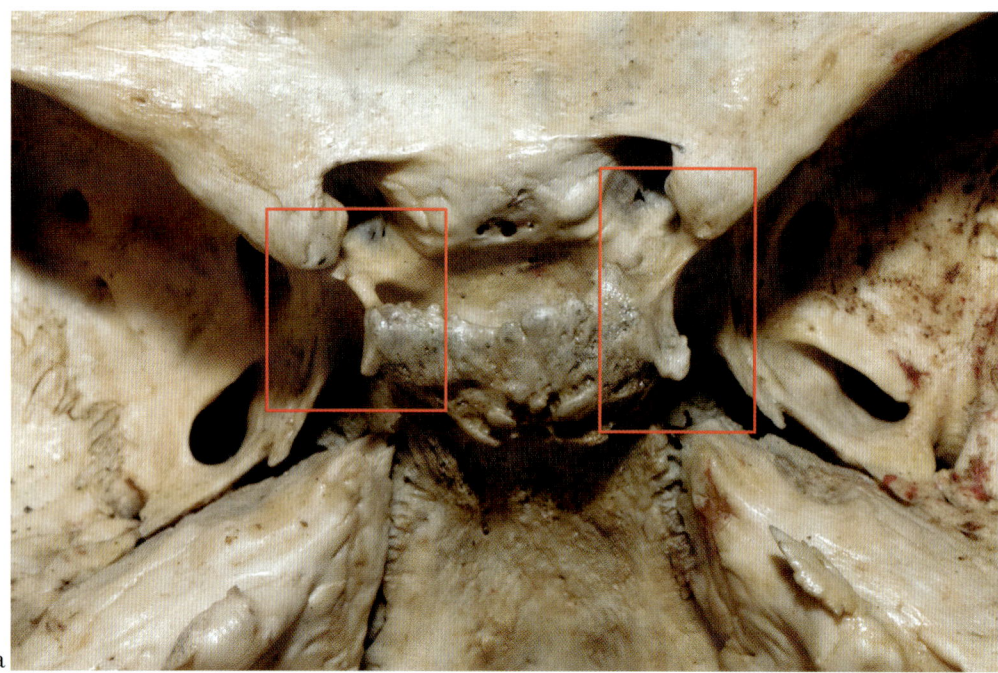

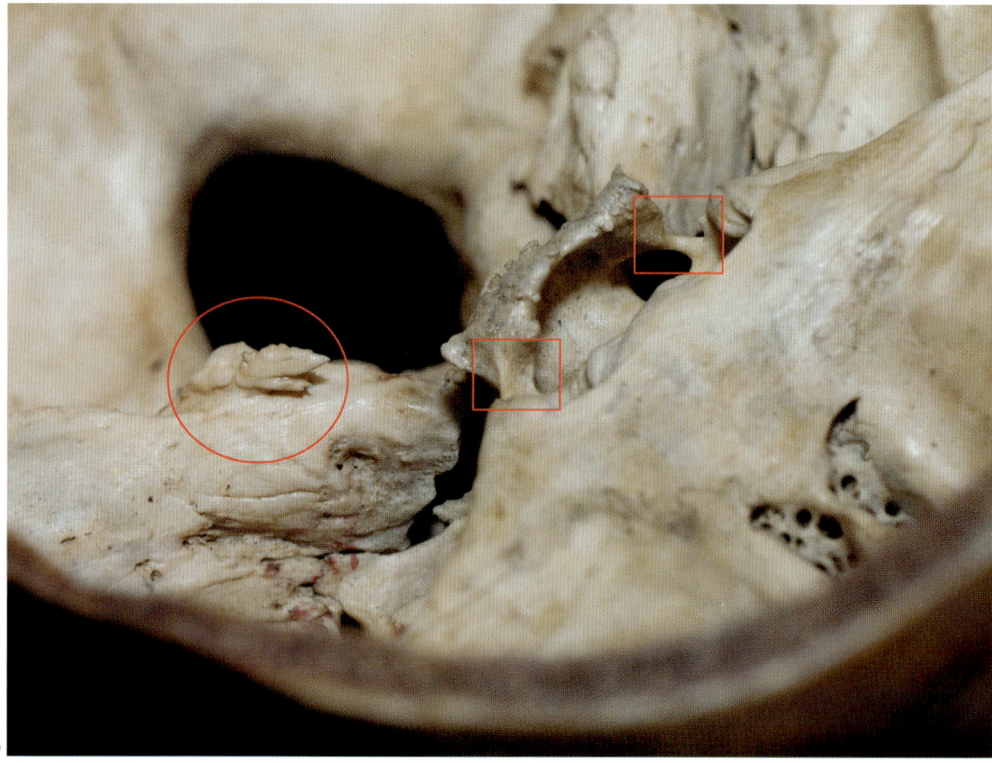

Figure 365a-b. Bridging of the clinoid, calcification of the interclinoid ligaments and petrosal exostosis. (a) Bridged clinoid with calcified interclinoid ligaments (square and rectangle), resulting in a small gap between the left anterior clinoid process and posterior processes and complete fusion resulting in a caroticoclinoid foramen between the right clinoid processes (SI Terry522) in a young adult Black male. (b) Note the exostosis (circle) along the ridge of the right temporal bone. This osseous projection is of unknown origin, but likely provides attachment for the tentorium cerebelli. Common findings. For clinoid bridging see Antonopoulou et al. (2008). Cf. Erdogmus et al. (2009); Erturk et al. (2004); Galdames et al. (2010); Rosa et al. (2010); Rossi et al. (2011); Saunders and Popovich (1978); Skrzat et al. 2006a; Freyschmidt at al. (2002) for exostosis.

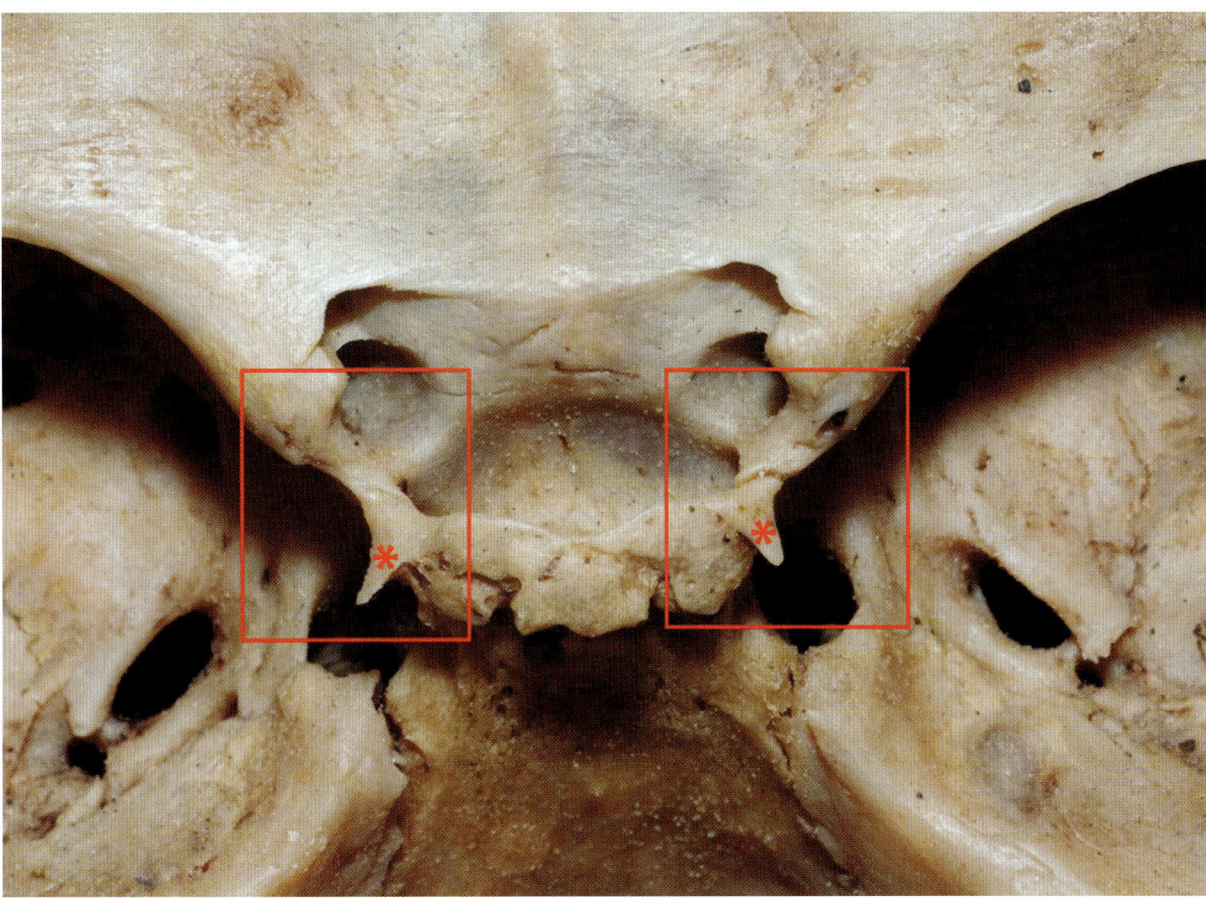

Figure 366. Osseous clinoid/sellar bridging (squares) and typical anatomy of the posterior clinoid process resulting in small bony spikes (*) in an elderly Black female (SI 171R). Ossification of the petrosphenoid ligament, also known as the ligament of Grüber, is an unusual finding that forms the Dorello's canal (Tekdemir et al. 1996) for passage of the abducens nerve that can become compressed in this canal. See Aggarwal et al. (2012). Leonardi et al. (2009) found an increased prevalence between palatally displaced canine teeth (PDC) and interclinoid bridging or sella turcica bridge ossification or calcification, ponticulus posticus and posterior arch deficiencies.

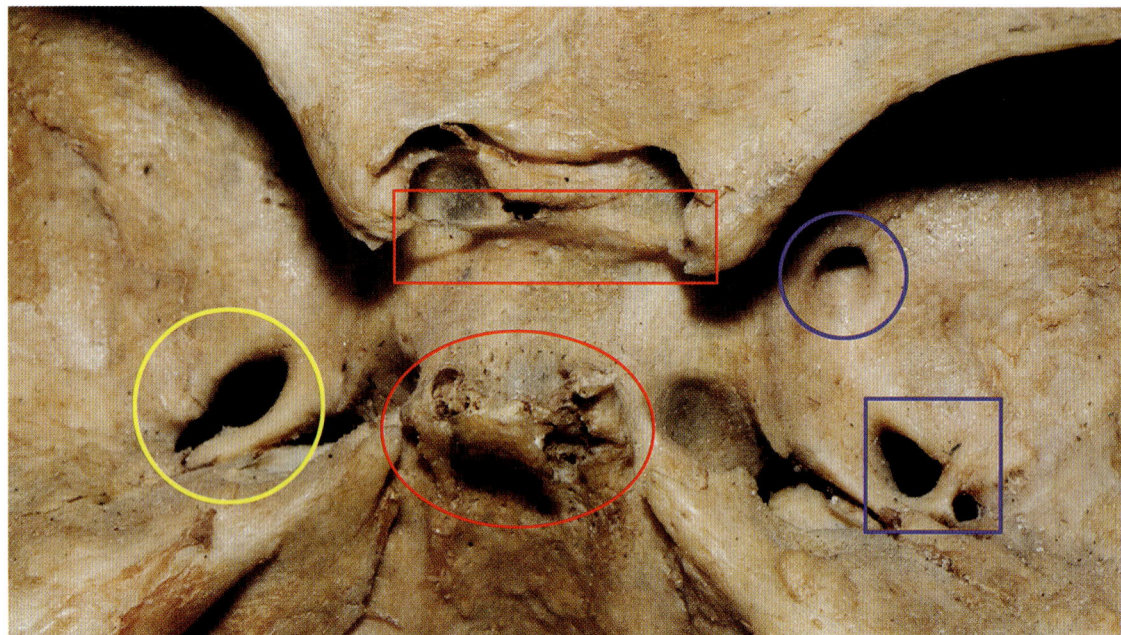

Figure 367. Ossification (rectangle) resulting in a thin band and "wall" joining the left and right anterior clinoid processes (ACP) with the middle clinoid processes (65-year-old Black female; SI 662R). This is not the typical form of clinoid bridging between the ACP and posterior clinoid processes (PCP) where bridging occurs "front to back" joining the apex of the ACP to the PCP. As is often the case, the PCP and portion of the clivus in this individual are misshapen (red oval), appearing as if diseased or lytic even though this is not the case. Note normal foramen rotundum (blue circle), right foramen ovale and foramen spinosum (large and small foramina in blue square, respectively) and non-divided left foramen ovale and foramen spinosum (yellow circle). Cf. Berge and Bergman (2001); Kale et al. (2009b); Krayenbühl et al. (2008); Saunders and Popovich (1978).

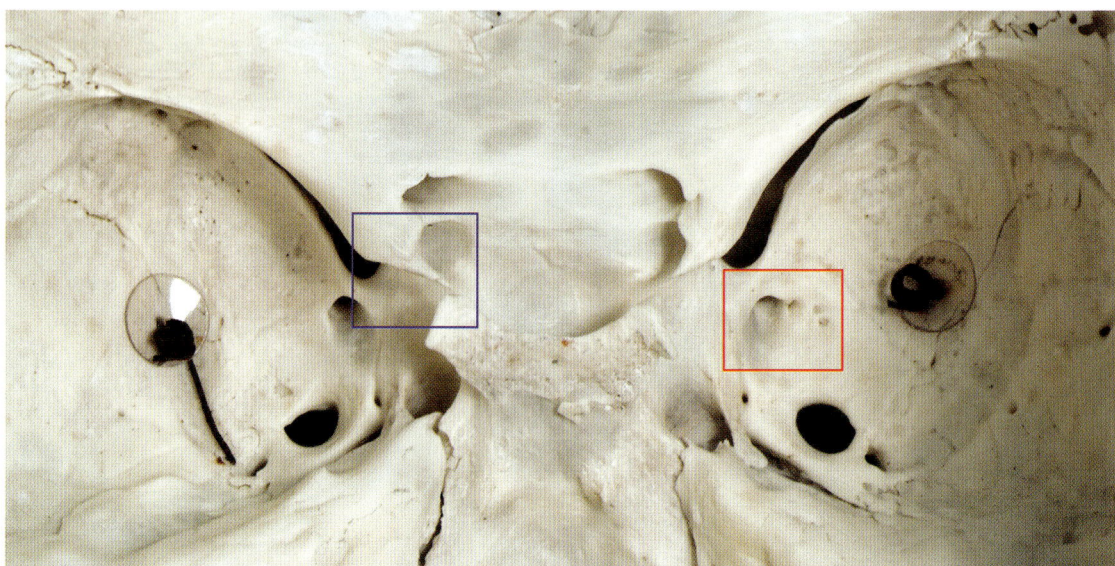

Figure 368. Partial bridging of the left anterior clinoid process (blue square) and a foramen rotundum and three small accessory foramina (red square) in an adult Asian female skull (CSC AS 002). Cf. Saunders and Popovich (1978) for more on clinoid bridging.

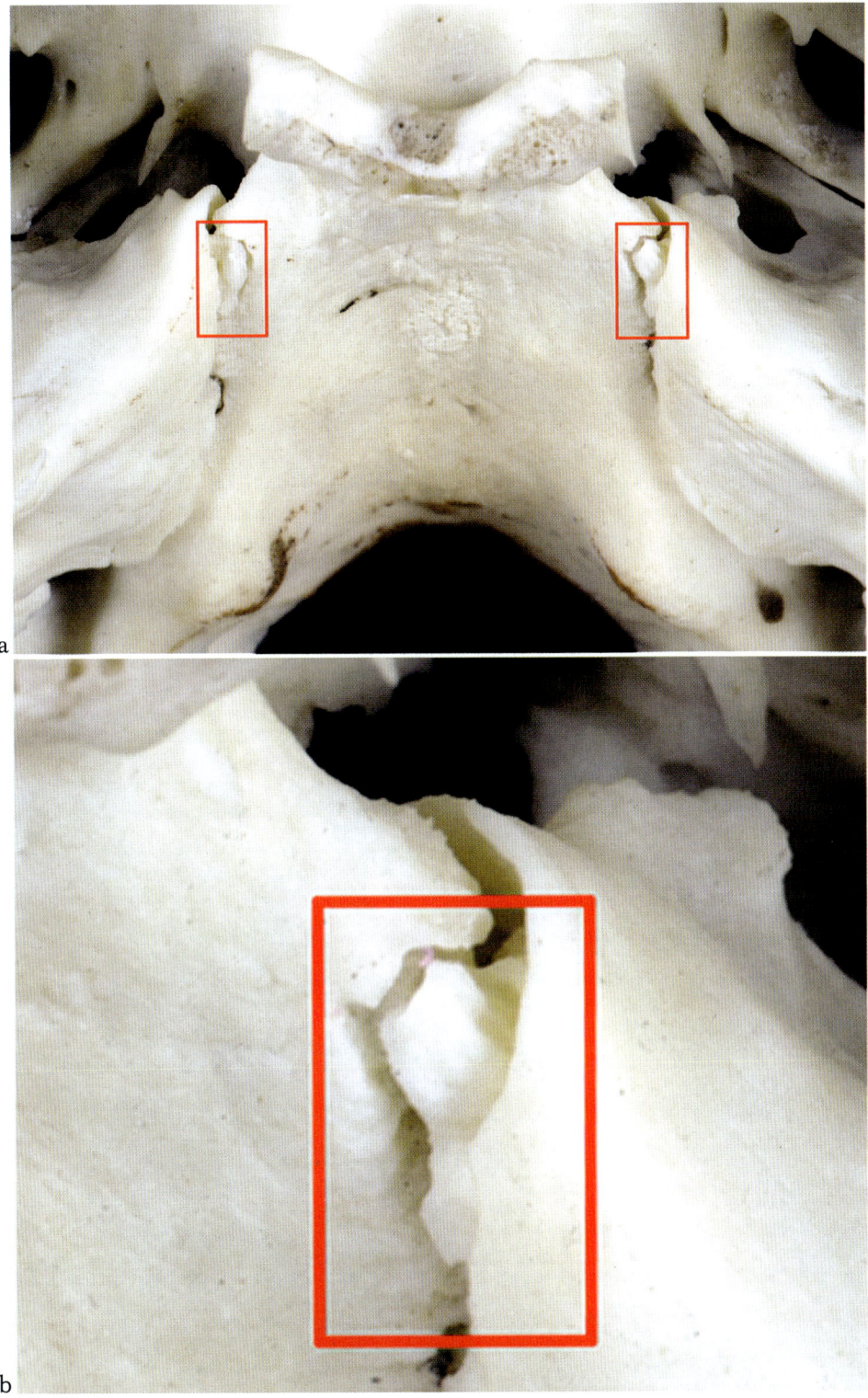

Figure 369a-b. Bony islands and synchondroses joining the sphenoid and temporal bones in an adult of unknown sex and ancestry (CSC AS003). (a) Endocranium displaying the right and left synchondroses and (b) close-up of the synchondrosis between the right petrous bone and basilar bone.

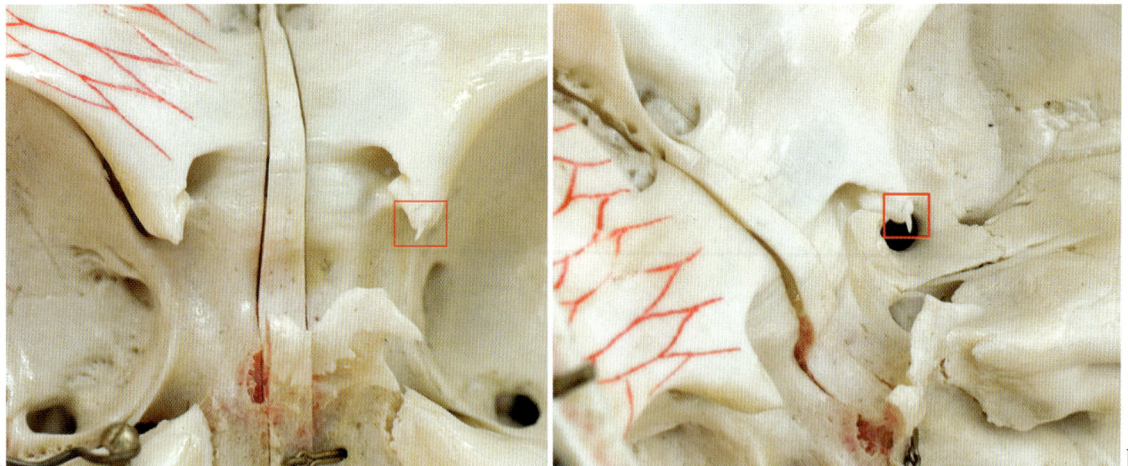

Figure 370a-b. Early-stage calcification of the interclinoid ligament in a young adult (CSC AC 039). (a) A small, pointed projection (square) illustrating early development of the right clinoid bridge. (b) Oblique view of the small finger-like projection representing clinoid bridging. This teaching specimen was sagittally sectioned and marked with red ink. Uncommon finding. Saunders and Popovich (1978) reported that clinoid bridging often appears on an average age of 7 years and does not simply reflect soft tissue ossification.

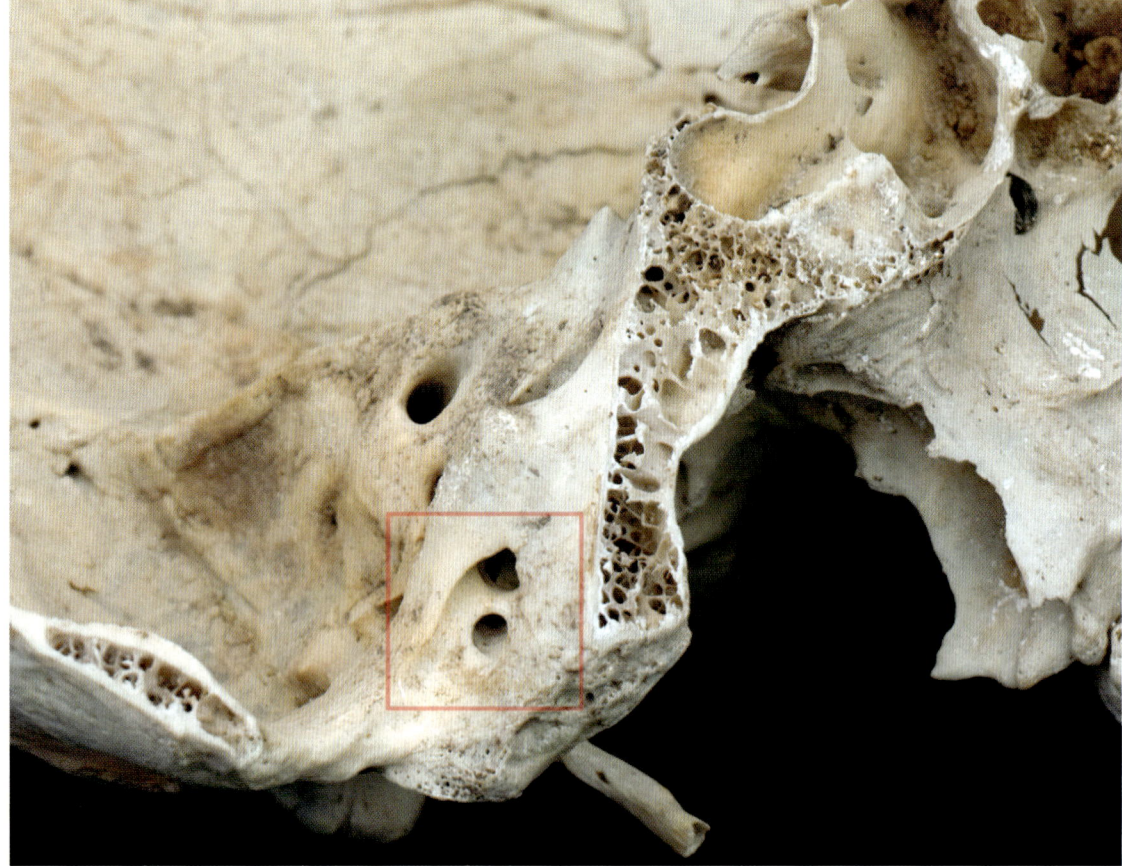

Figure 371. Internal/endocranial view of a divided/double left hypoglossal canal (square) in an adult Thai (KKU 2591-41). The bony bridge reportedly separates the meningeal artery from the hypoglossal nerve (Berge and Bergman 2001). Cf. Hanihara and Ishida (2001b); Hauser and DeStefano (1989). Common finding.

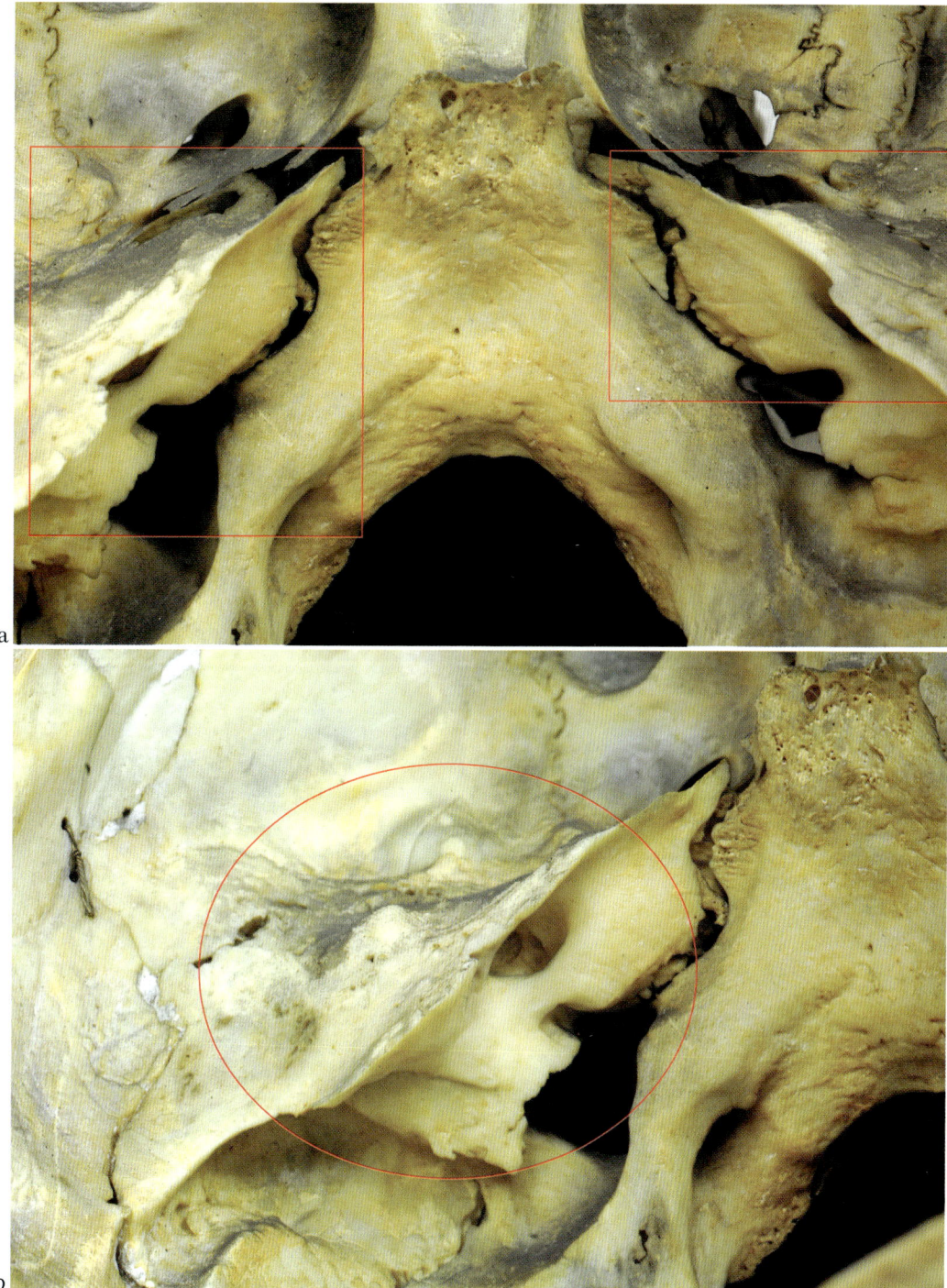

Figure 372a-b. Sharp superior margin of the petrous portion giving it an overhanging appearance with respect to the superior petrosal sinus in an adult White male (Mütter Museum 1008.48). (a) Endocranial view showing a wave-like, sharp ridge (rectangles) running the length of the petrous ridges. (b Higher magnification of the ridge (oval) along the left petrous bone. Note its position in relation to the internal auditory meatus. This overhanging ridge is an unusual condition and a new feature to the authors. While the frequency of this condition is unknown, it appears to be an uncommon to rare finding that warrants further research.

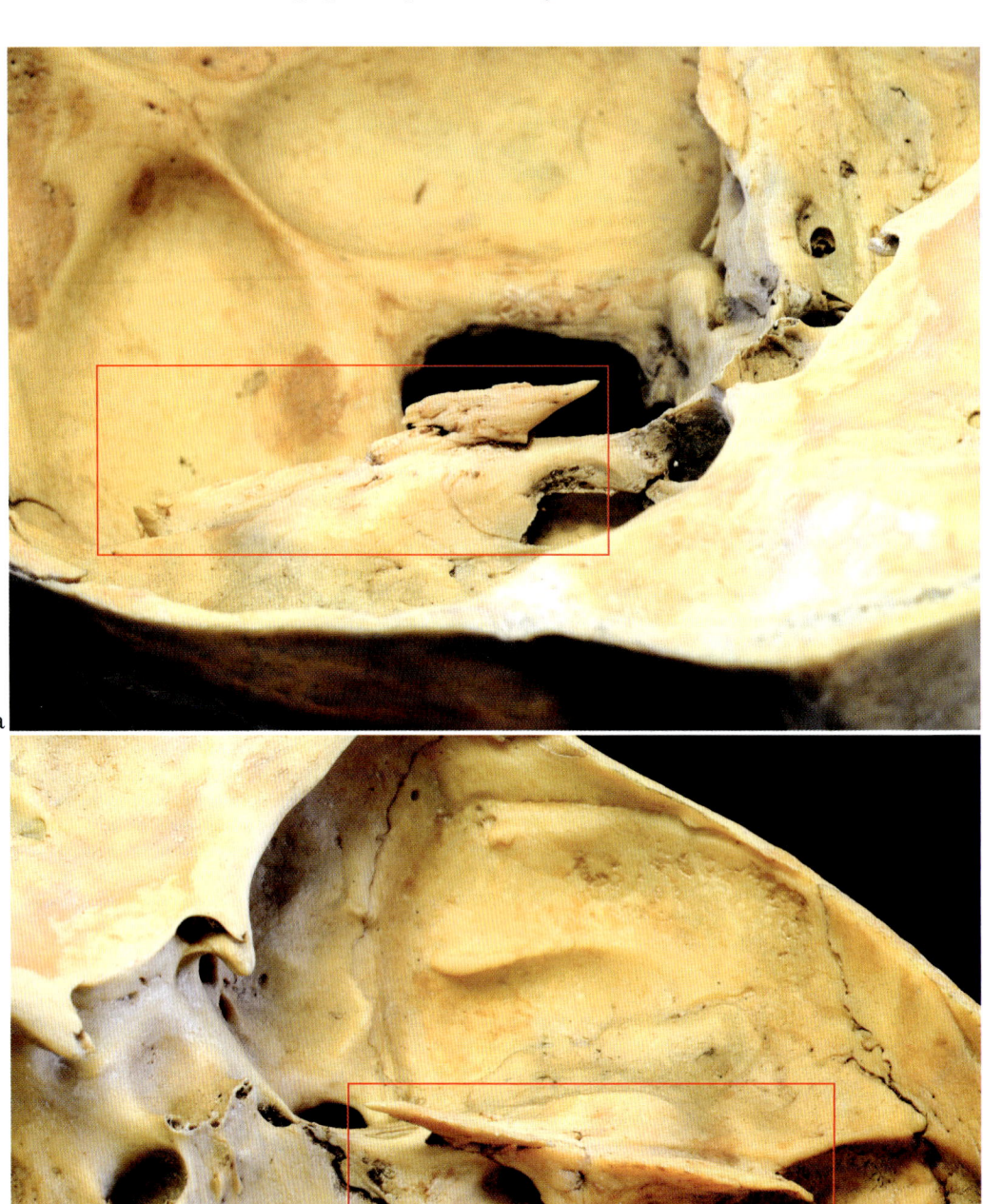

Figure 373a-b. Bilateral calcifications along the petrous bones. (a) Small osteophyte (rectangle) along the right petrosal ridge in an adult African (University of Pretoria). (b) Asymmetrically-shaped linear calcification (rectangle) forming an unusually long and ridge-like osteophyte along the right petrous process.

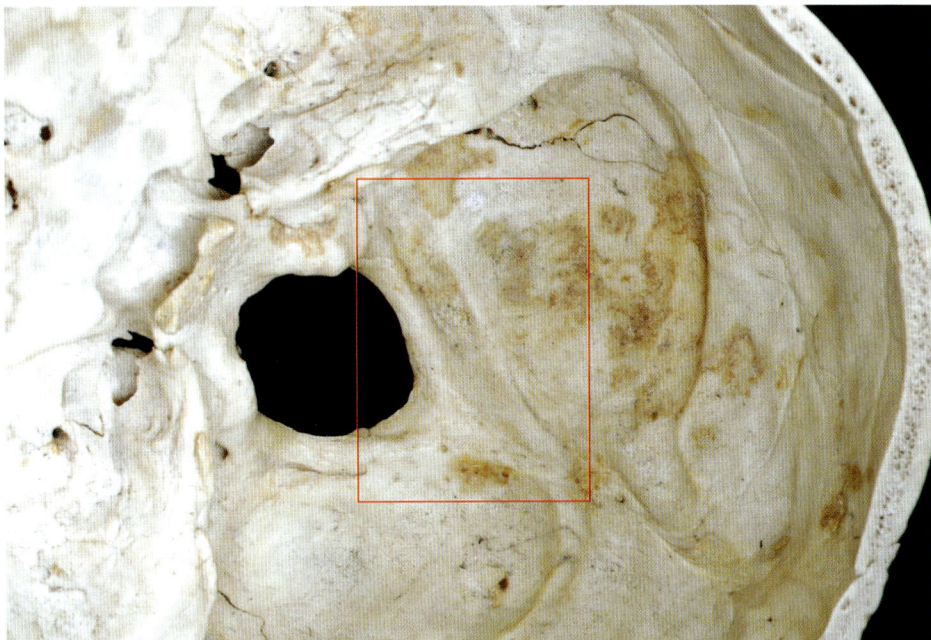

Figure 374. Variant of the occipital fossa and marginal sinus (red rectangle) in the form of a groove extending along the right side of the foramen magnum in an adult Thai skull (KKU). These fossae are not present in all individuals (see http://neuroangio.org/VenousAnatomyBrain.aspx) with a reported frequency of 0.9% (1 of 112 skulls; Vázquez et al. 2001). Cf. Kale et al. (2008); Toldt (1928) for variants of the vermian fossa.

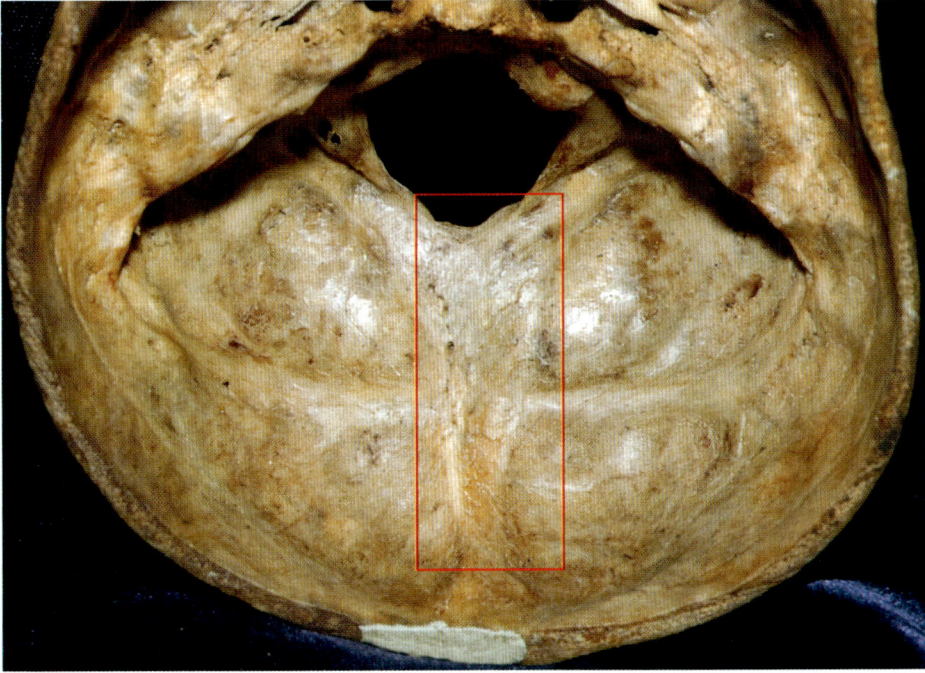

Figure 375. Variant for the sulcus (rectangle) sometimes known as the Fosita Torcular (Vázquez et al. 2001) for the occipital sinus in a 70-year-old White male (SI Terry 1176). Although this is typical anatomy, there are many variants of these bony sulci.

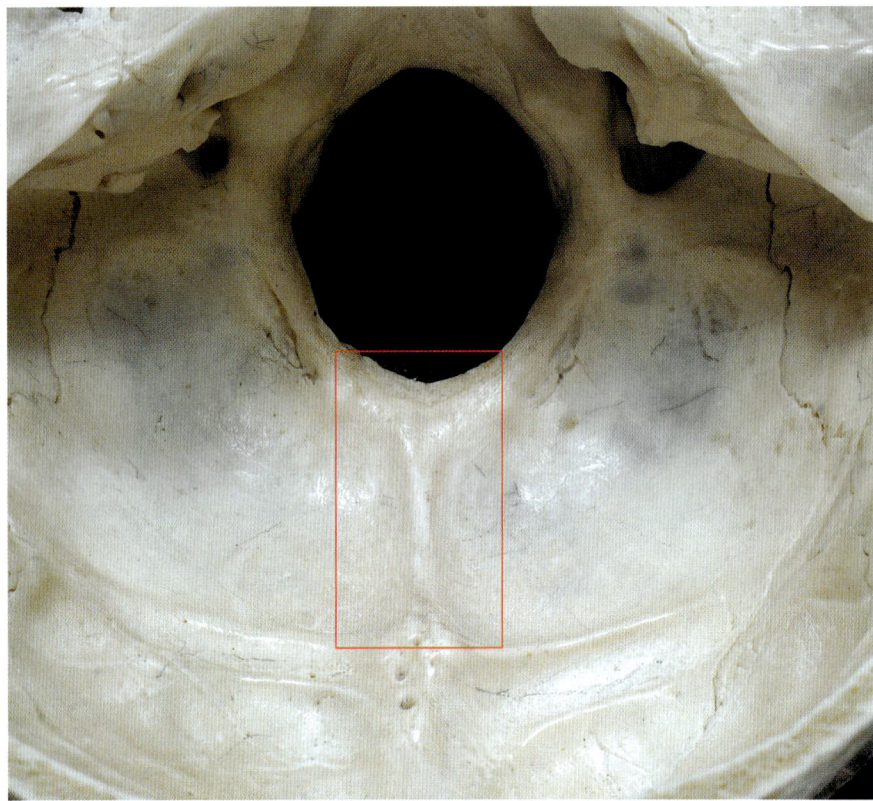

Figure 376. Common form of the internal occipital crest and absence of a sulcus in the occipital fossa (rectangle) in an adolescent Asian female (CSC AC 007). Compare with Figure 374-375.

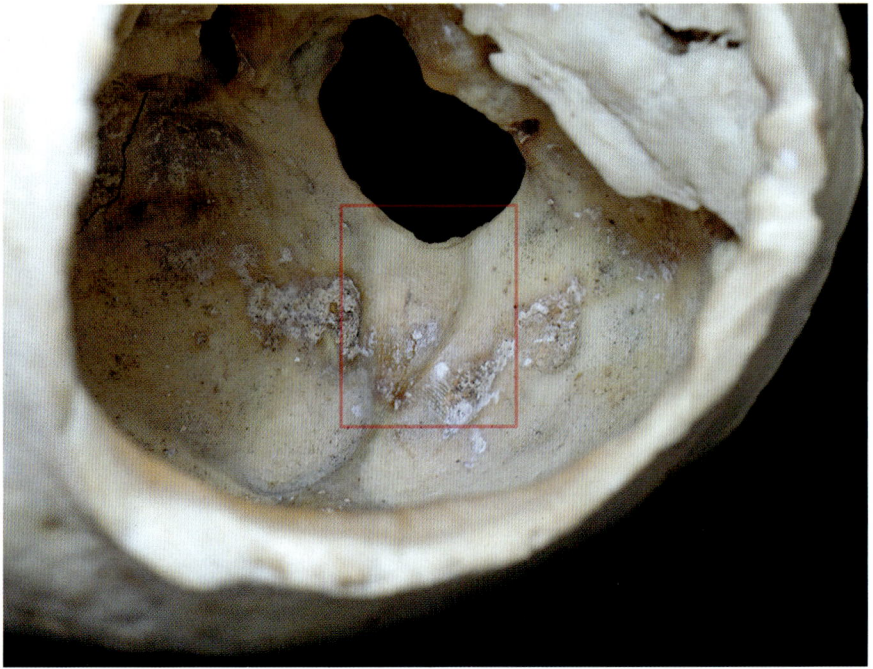

Figure 377. Vermian fossa (rectangle; inside the "V") in an adult Thai male (KKU 1109-44). Note the fossa opens along the posterior margin of the foramen magnum. Cf. Kale et al. (2008).

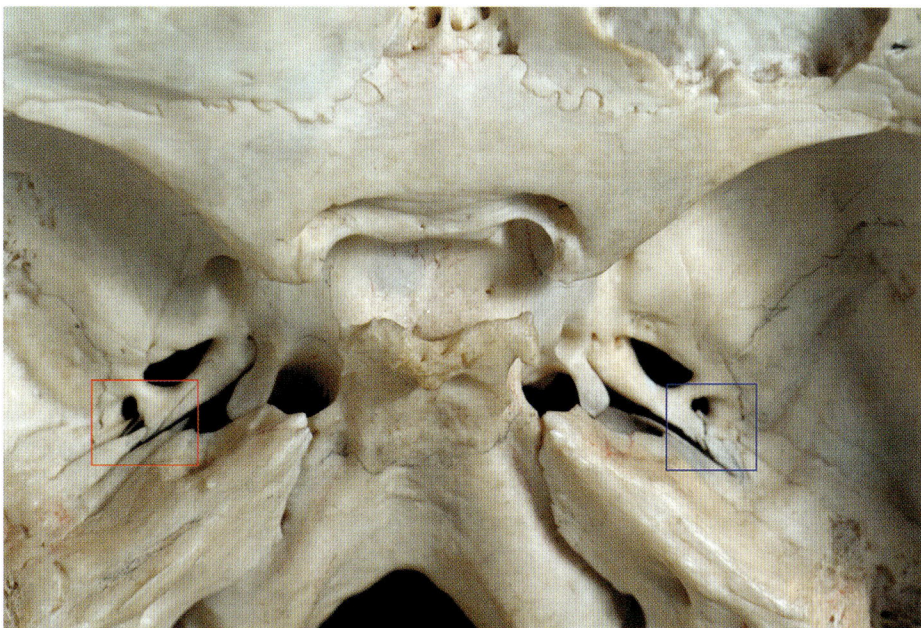

Figure 378. Two types of bridging of the left (red) and right (blue) foramen spinosum in a 17- to 20-year-old Asian female (CSC AS 007). Note that the medial wall of the left foramen spinosum is open (incomplete) while that of the right is nearly continuous (complete), but exhibits a thin gap between its anterior and posterior segments where they join. This trait is often scored as complete and incomplete. Cf. Shapiro and Robinson (1967) for foramina in the middle fossa.

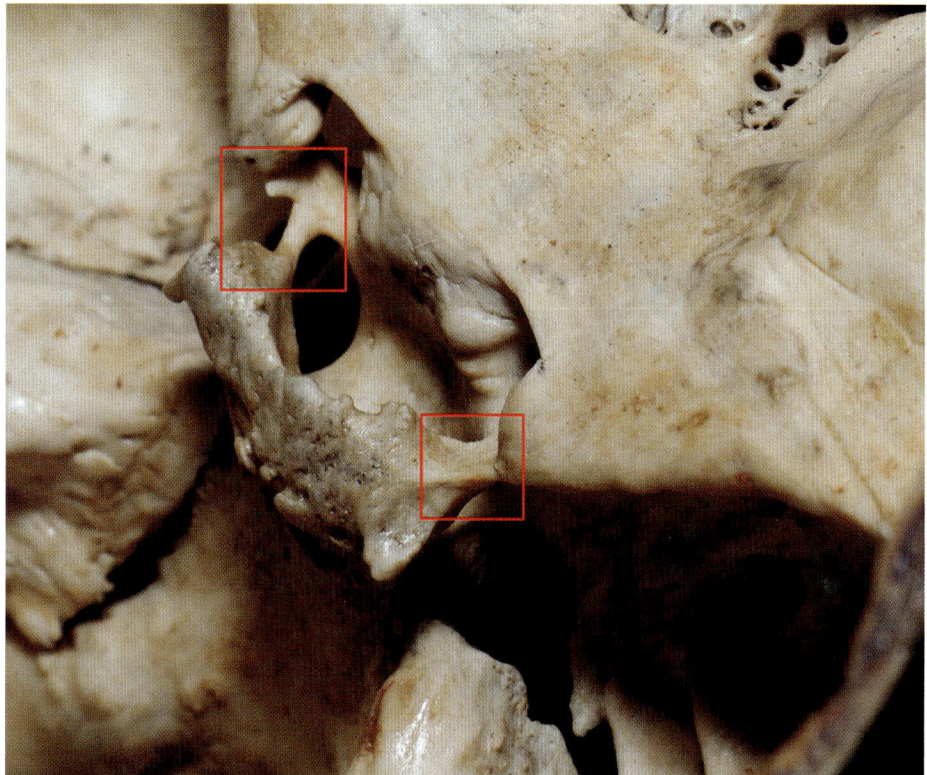

Figure 379. Bilateral petroclinoid bridging (squares) in a young adult Black male (SI Terry 522).

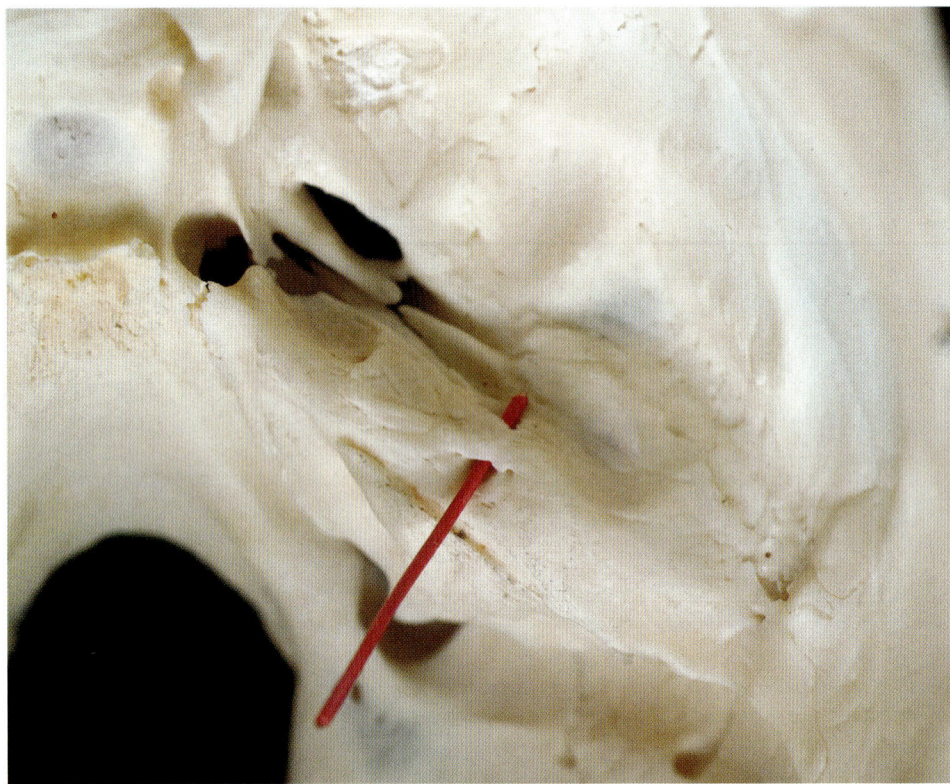

Figure 380. Calcification along the right petrous ridge resulting in a foramen (red probe) in an adult See Figure 355) (CSC AC027).

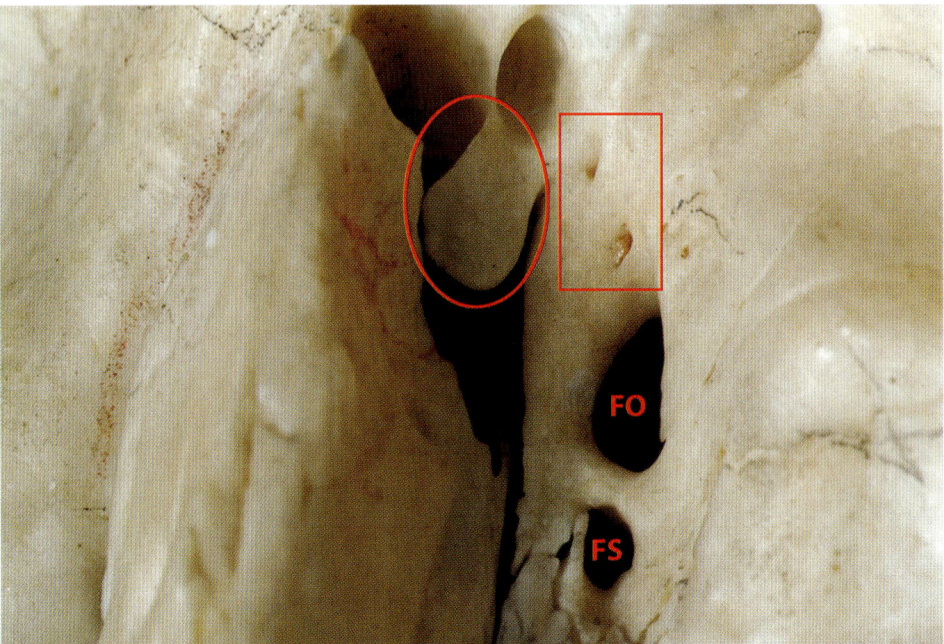

Figure 381. Double foramen of Vesalius (rectangle) and lingual sphenoidialis (oval) in an adult Asian female (CSC AS007). FO is the foramen ovale and FS is the foramen spinosum, both relatively constant foramina. Double foramen of Vesalius is an uncommon to common typical variant.

Chapter 7

BASILAR (INFERIOR) VIEW OF THE SKULL

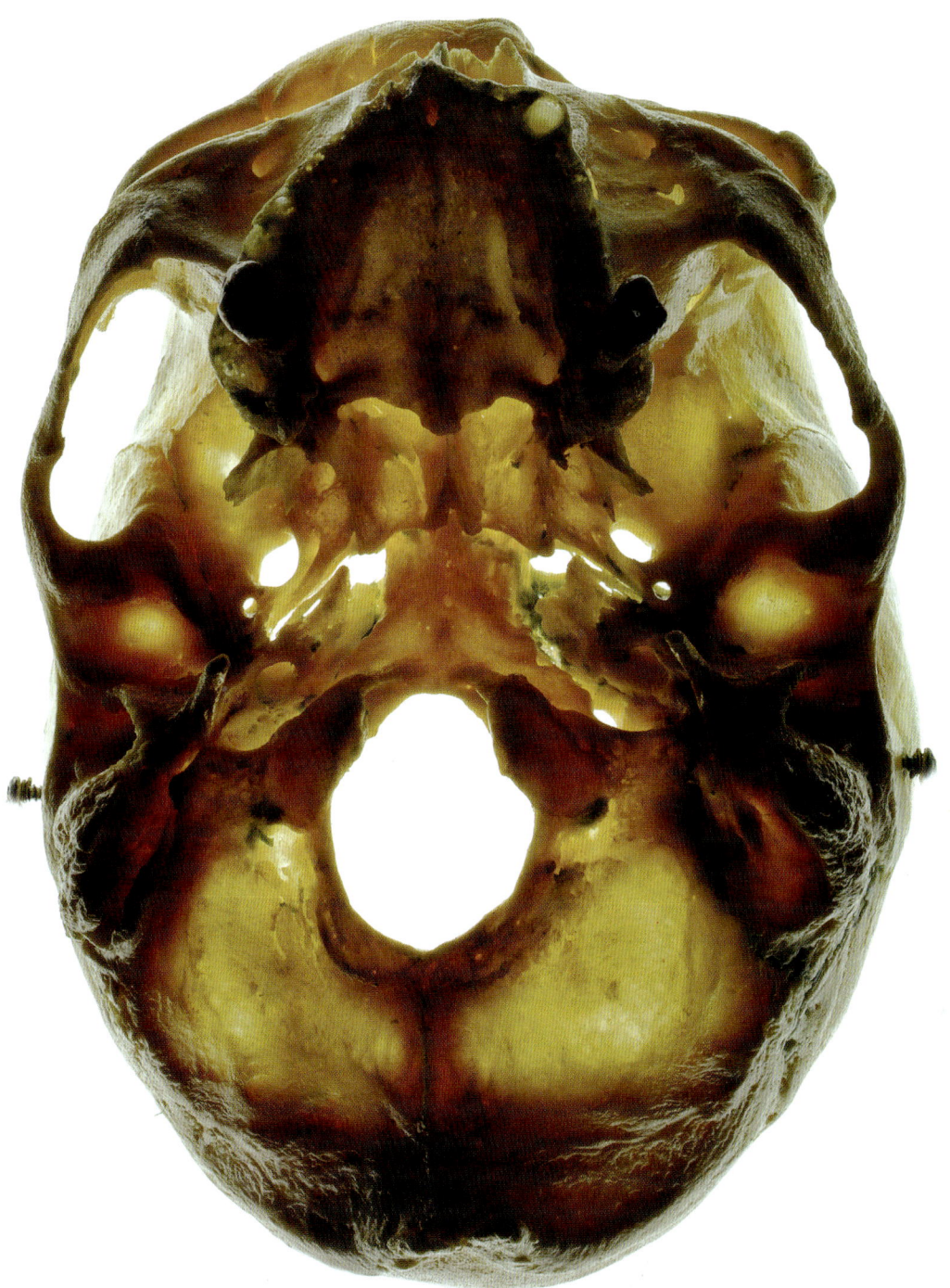

Figure 382. Backlighting showing varying thickness of the cranial base (CSC). The paper-thin translucent areas do not have diploë.

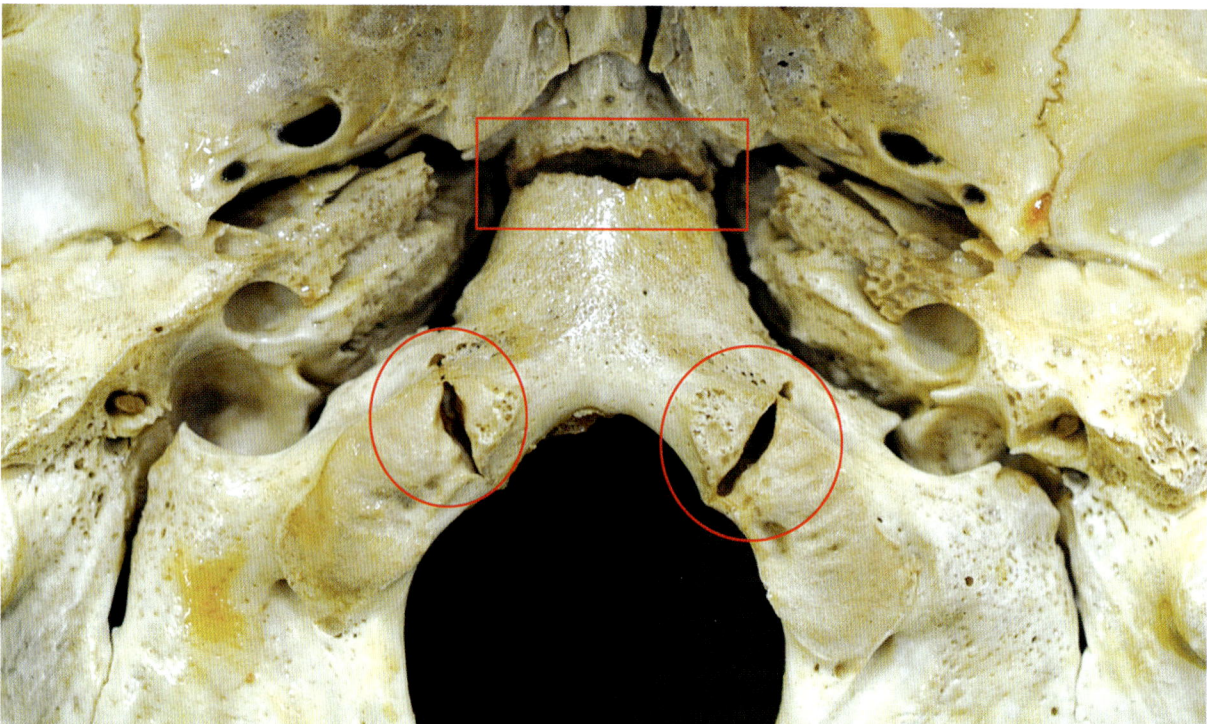

Figure 383. Open basilar synchondrosis (rectangle) and fusing condylar portions (circles) with the basilar bone in a subadult Thai skull (KKU). The basilar synchondrosis, also known as sphenobasilar and spheno-occipital syncondrosis, sometimes leaves a remnant line where it closed, while the lines of fusion of the condylar portions (basioccipital) do not. The reported age of closure of this syncondrosis varies greatly by researcher. Typical anatomy.

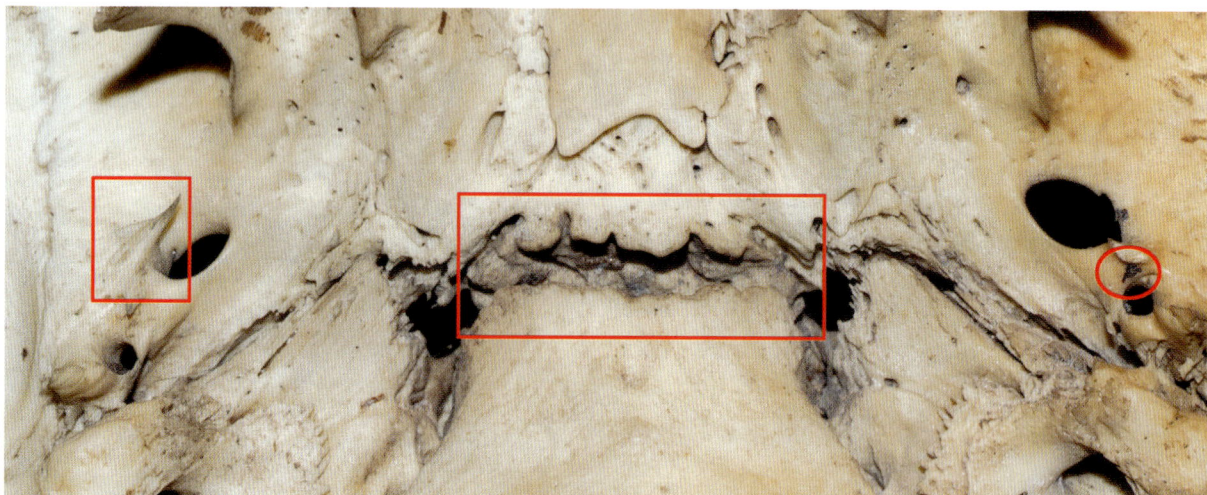

Figure 384. Open basilar synchondrosis (rectangle), trace right pterygoalar ligament (square) and possible foramen of Arnold (oval) situated between the foramen ovale and foramen spinosum in a 12–16-year-old probable female (TM 107, Ditsong Museum). Skrzat et al. (2012) reported a rare accessory osseous spine, probably asymptomatic, within the opening of the left foramen ovale. The pterygoalar bridge is formed by small spike-like bony projections that calcify along the lateral pterygoid plate and greater wing of the sphenoid and extend towards one another, meeting in the approximate middle of the pterygoalar ligament. In this individual, only the alar portion of the ligament has developed and calcified (square), pointing towards the pterygoid plate.

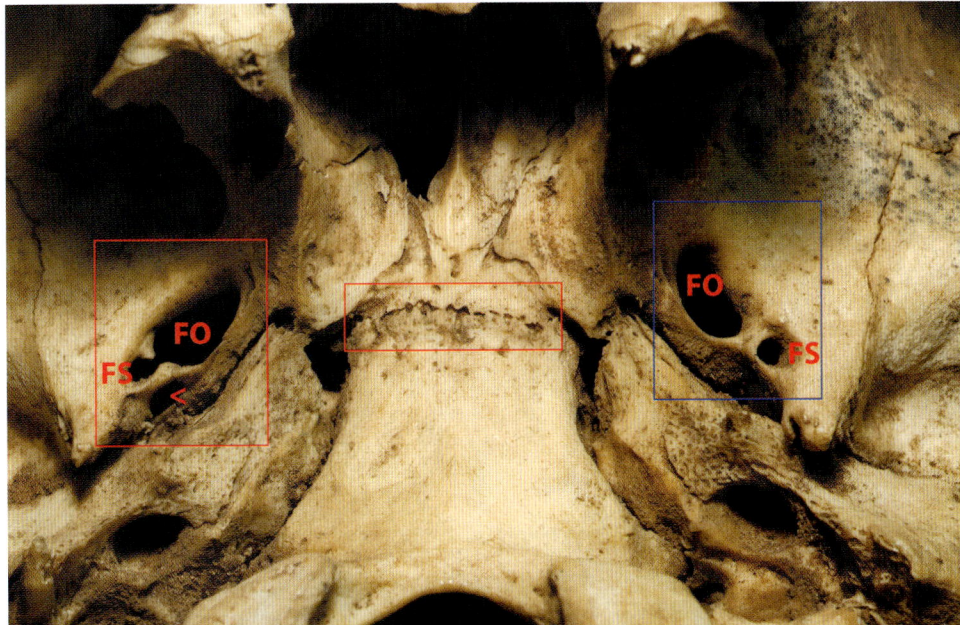

Figure 385. Non-divided, communicating right foramen ovale (FO) and foramen spinosum (FS) (<, red square). A divided left FO and FS (blue square) and a trace of the basilar synchondrosis (rectangle) in a young adult African female (TM 35, Ditsong Museum). A trace of the basilar synchondrosis may be visible in elderly individuals even if fully fused or united.

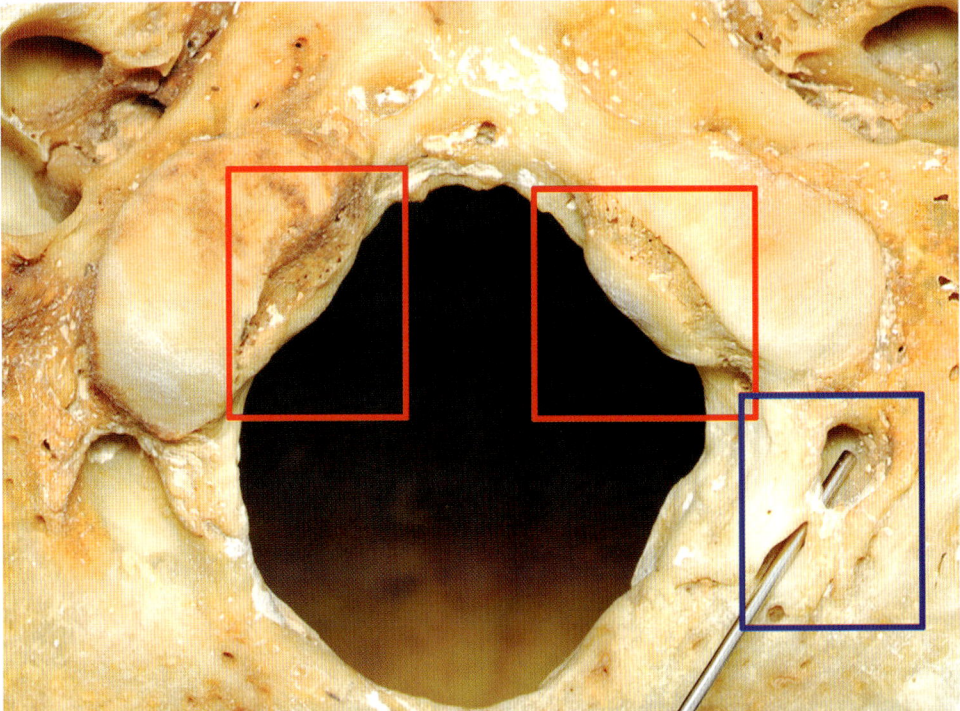

Figure 386. Bridged left postcondyloid foramen (posterior condyloid; blue rectangle) and condylar dysplasia encroaching on the occipital condyles (red squares) in an adult Thai skull that could result in stenosis (KKU). Note the cloverleaf shape of the foramen magnum. Uncommon to common findings. Cf. Boyd (1930) for the foramen; Freyschmidt et al. (2002) for condylar dysplasia; Taitz (2000).

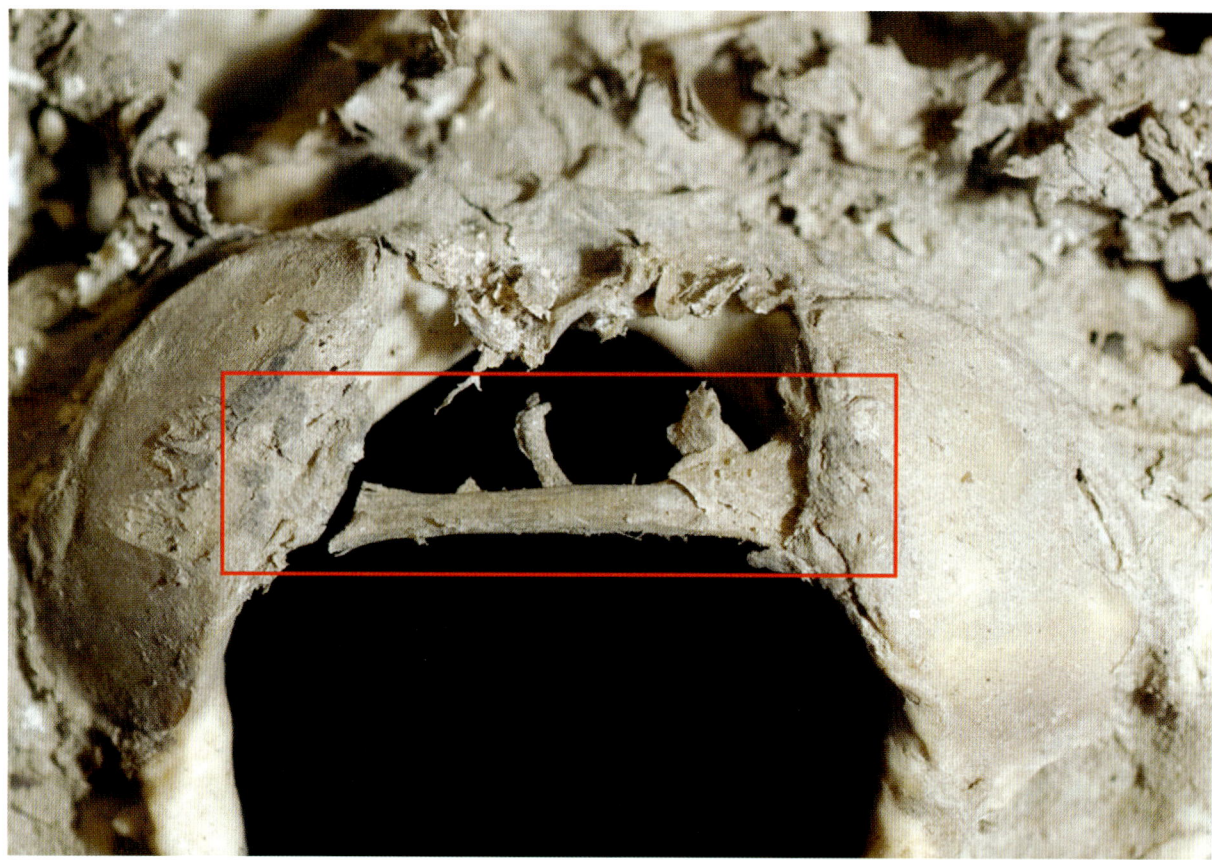

Figure 387. Dessicated, but not calcified, alar ligament of the cranial base in a 12–16-year-old probable female (DSC 7405, UPenn). This ligament spans across two tubercles medial to the occipital condyles.

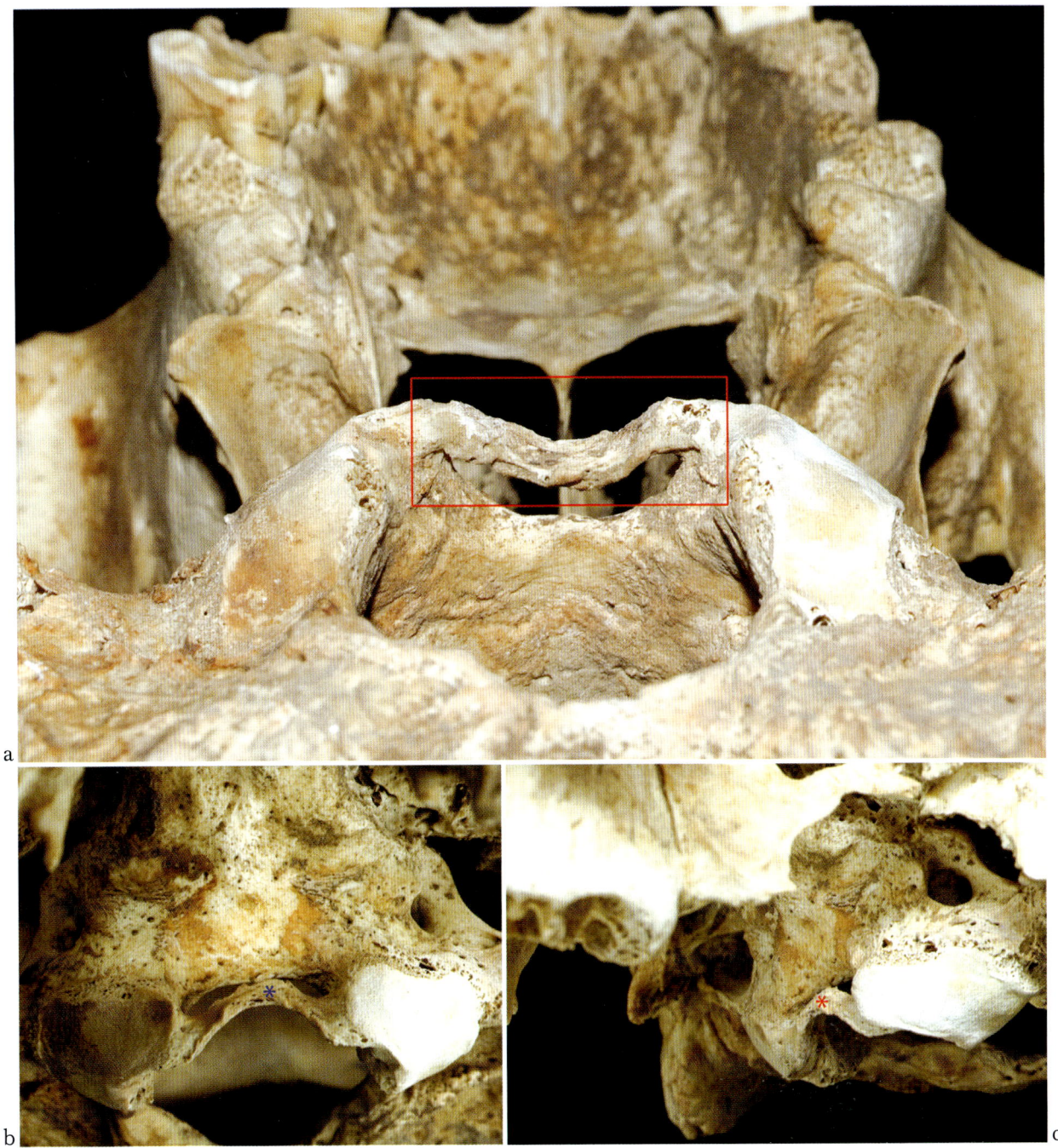

Figure 388a-c. Calcified alar ligament. (a) Posterior view of a calcified alar ligament (red rectangle) attached to the medial tubercles of the occipital condyles (UPenn). (b) Inferior perspective of the alar ligament (*). (c) Left oblique view of the ligament (*). Calcification of this ligament is an uncommon to rare finding in most skeletal collections.

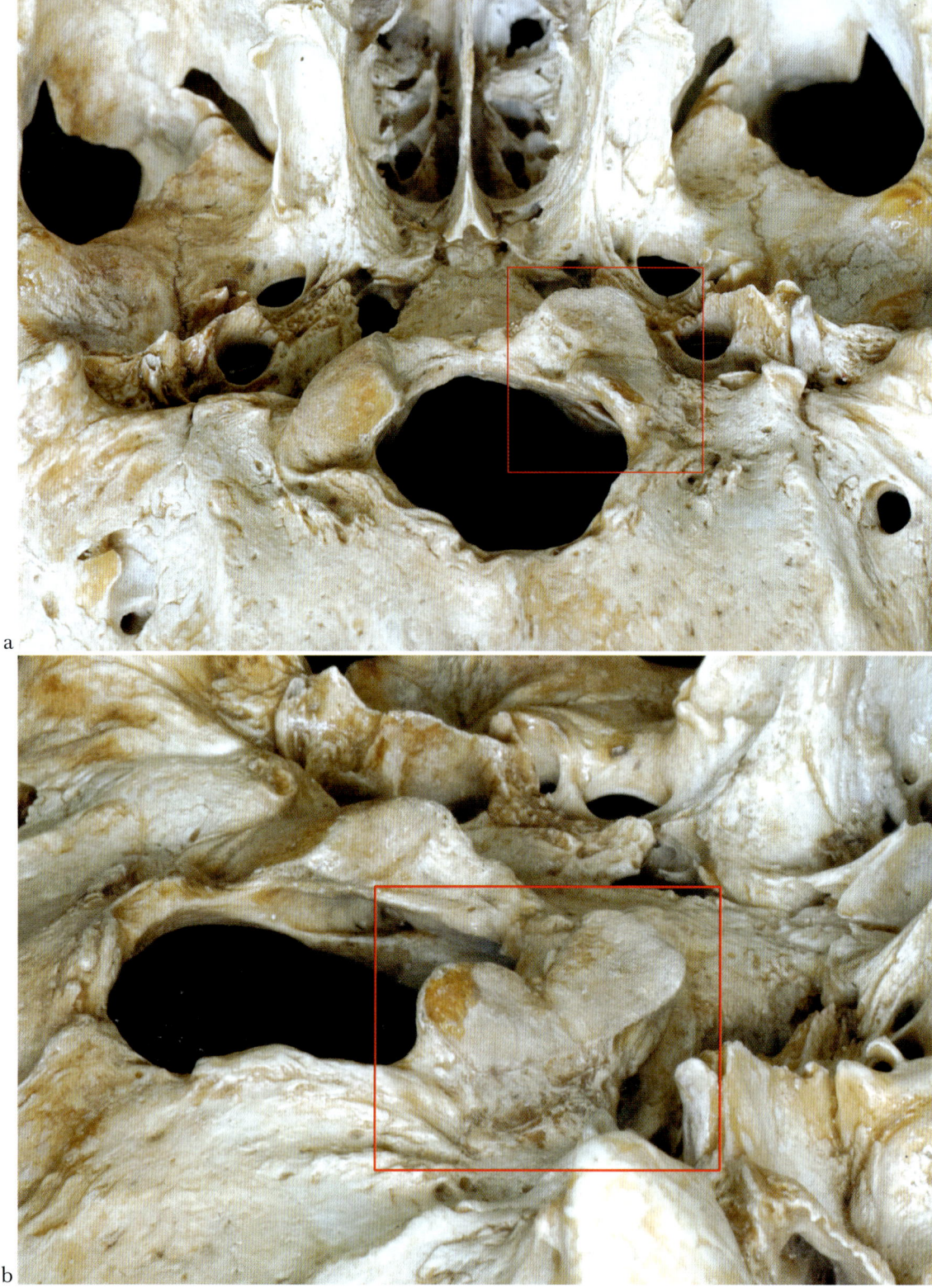

Figure 389a-b. Concave and partially divided left occipital condyle. (a) Concave left occipital condyle (square) resulting in a downward slope of the facets in an adult Thai skull (KKU 12 31). (b) Partial separation of the occipital condyle into two facets (square).

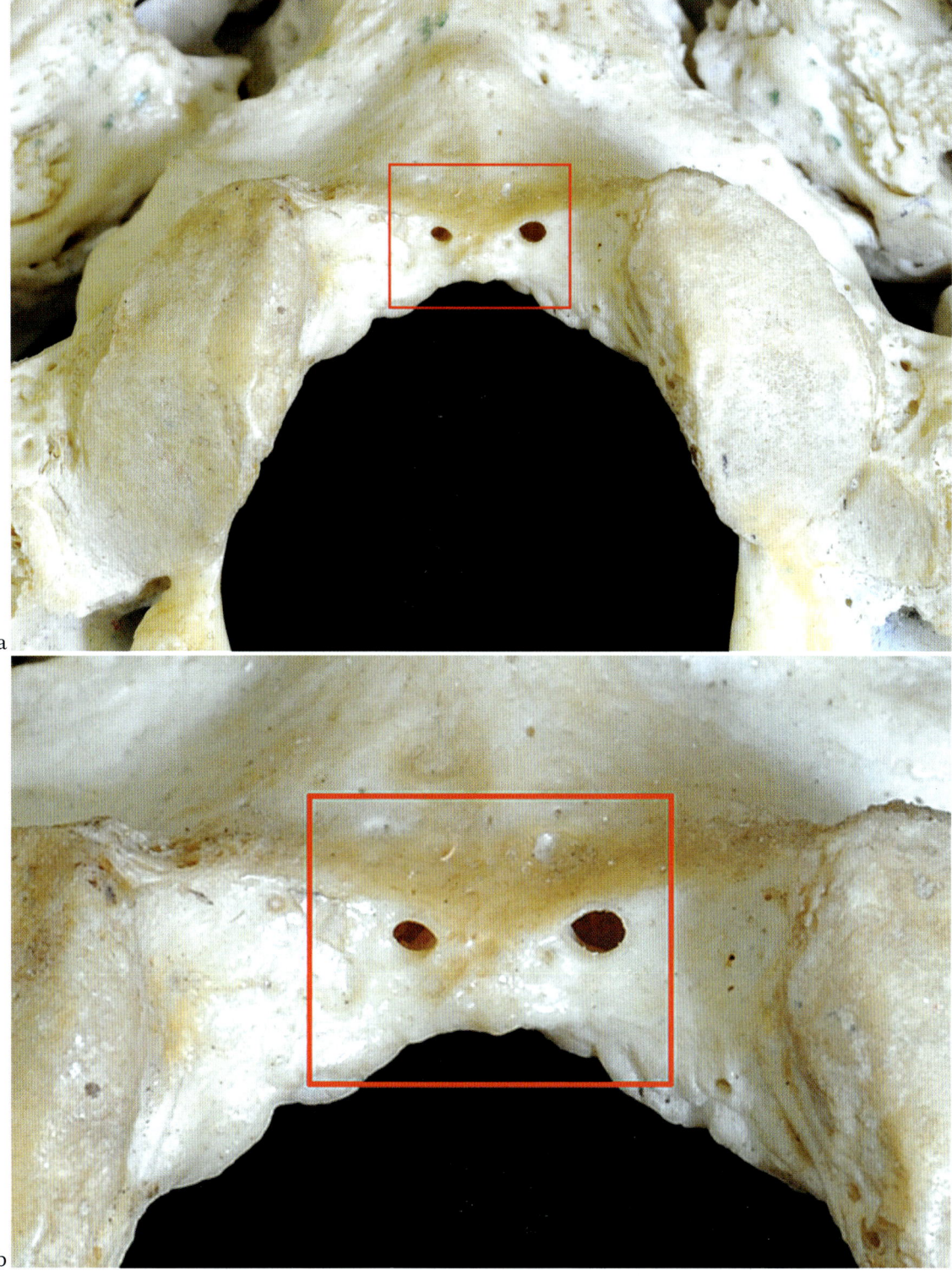

Figure 390a-b. Bilateral median basioccipital canals. (a) Bilateral and asymmetrical median canals (rectangle) in adult Thai skull (KKU). (b) Higher magnification showing the size differences and oval-shape of the two foramina (rectangle). These canals often communicate with one another. Double foramina such as this are uncommon to common findings. Cf. Hauser and DeStefano (1989); Naderi et al. (2005); Vázquez et al. (2001).

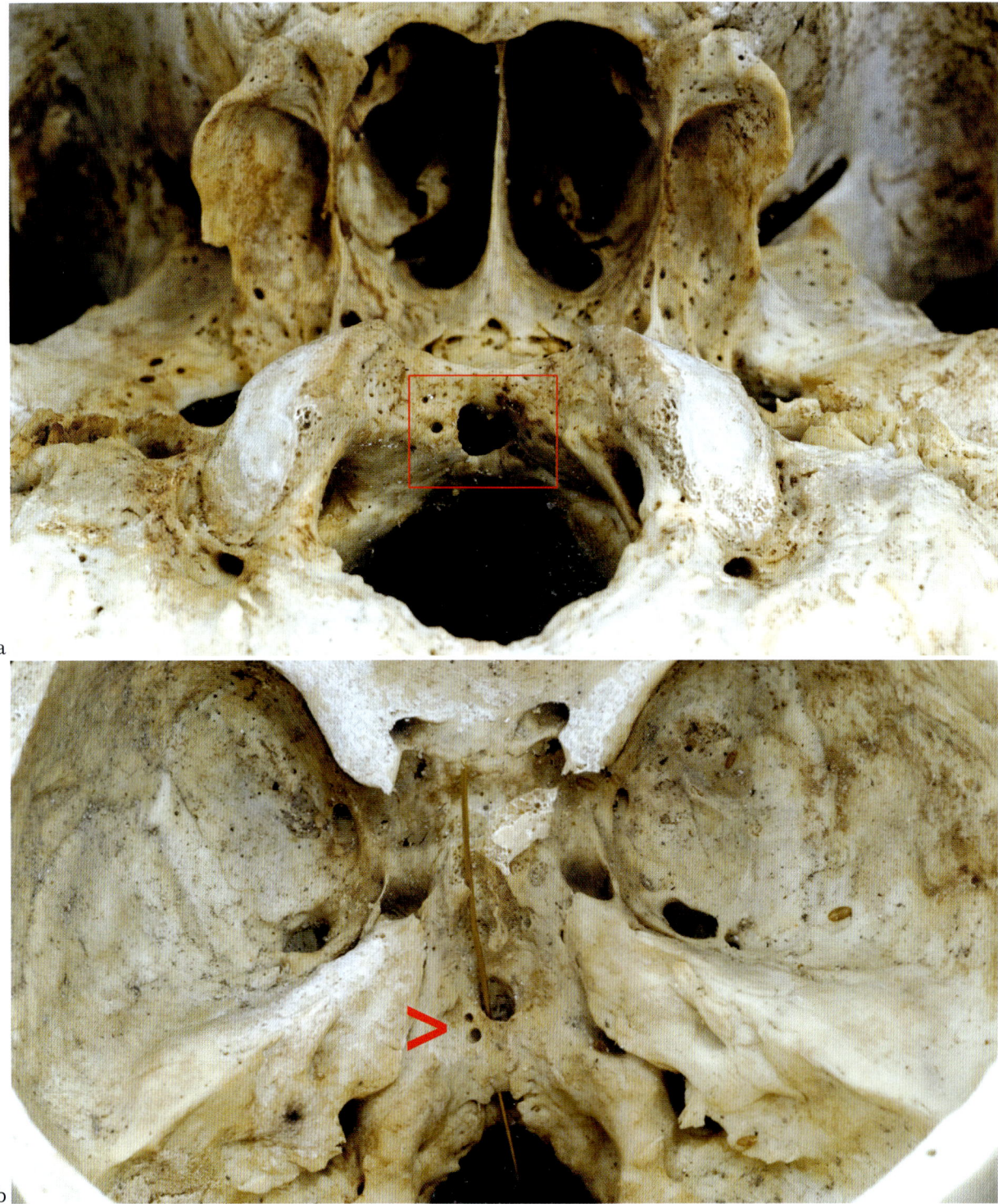

Figure 391a-b. Unusually large median canal. (a) Ectocranial views of an unusually large median canal (rectangle) in a 66-year-old Thai male (CMU 9 50). (b) Note that the two small foramina (>) communicate with the large central foramen (probe).

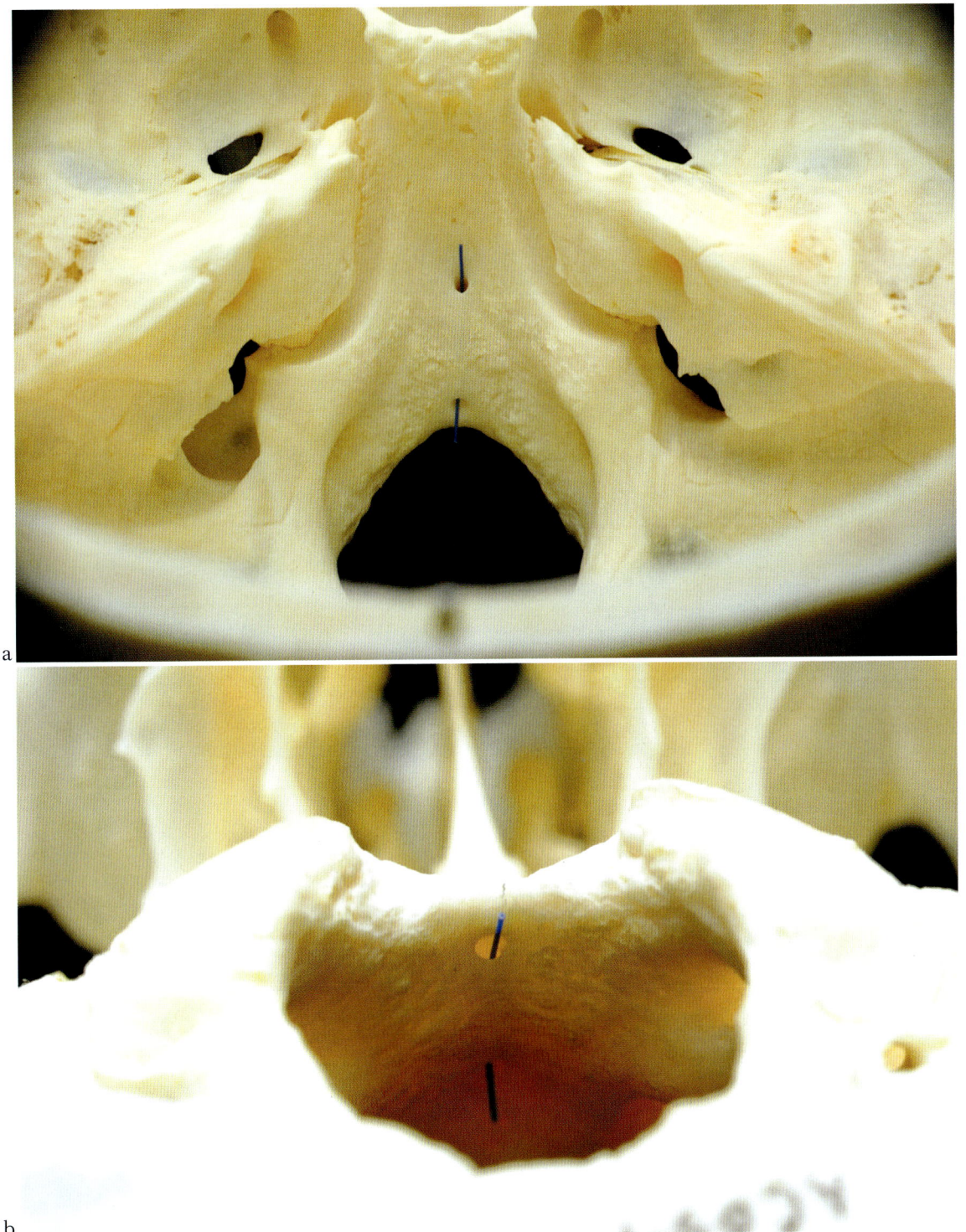

Figure 392a-b. Median canal in an elderly individual (FSA AC054). (a) Endocranial and (b) basilar views of the canal (probe).

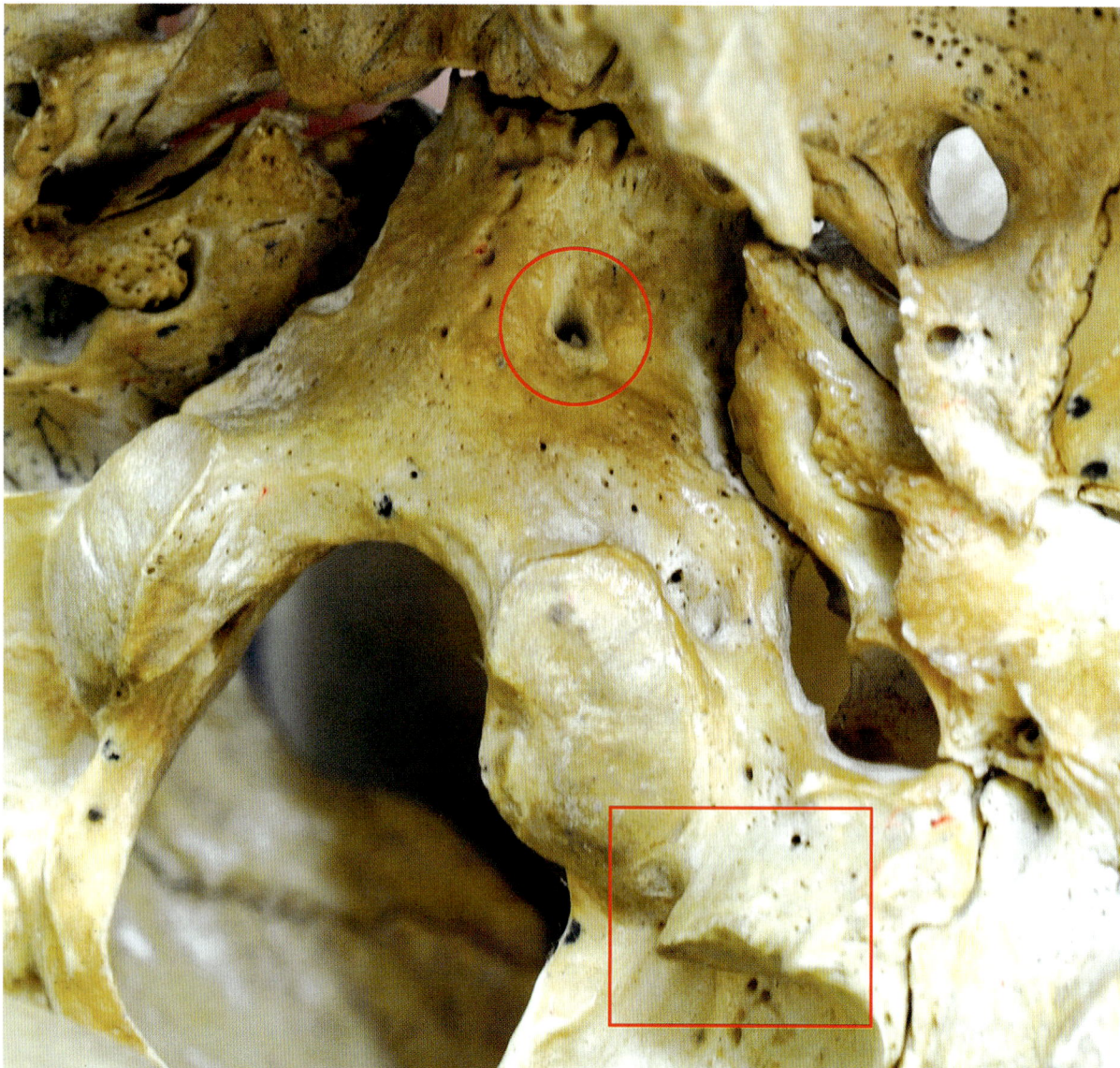

Figure 393. Median canal (circle) in parasagittal plane, possibly a craniopharyngeal foramen (Wood 2012) and paracondylar process (square) in a subadult Thai (KKU). Paracondylar process, sometimes referred to as paramastoid process in older literature, is a rare congenital anomaly of the craniovertebral junction and cervicooccipital region (de Graauw et al. 2008). The paracondylar process ranges in frequency from 0.125% to 4% (Prescher et al. 1996). Cf. Corner (1896); Hauser and DeStefano (1989); McCall et al. (2010); Prescher (1997); Vázquez (2001); Stathis et al. (2011) for the paracondylar process.

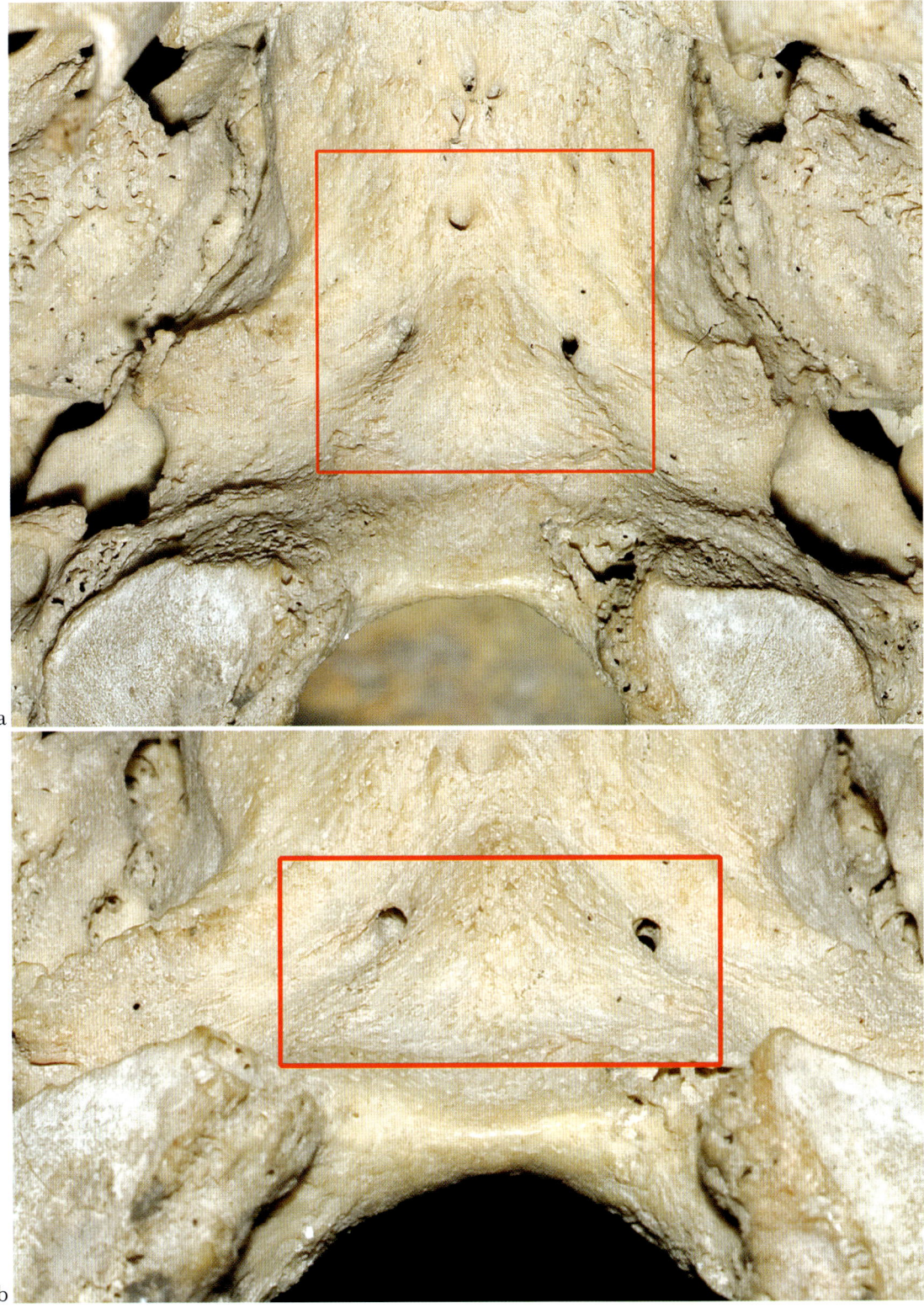

Figure 394a-b. Triple median foramina. (a) Triple median foramina (square) in an adult (UPenn). (b) Higher magnification of two of the foramina along either side of the pharyngeal tubercle of the basilar bone. These foramina do not appear to communicate with one another. Cf. Hauser and DeStefano (1989).

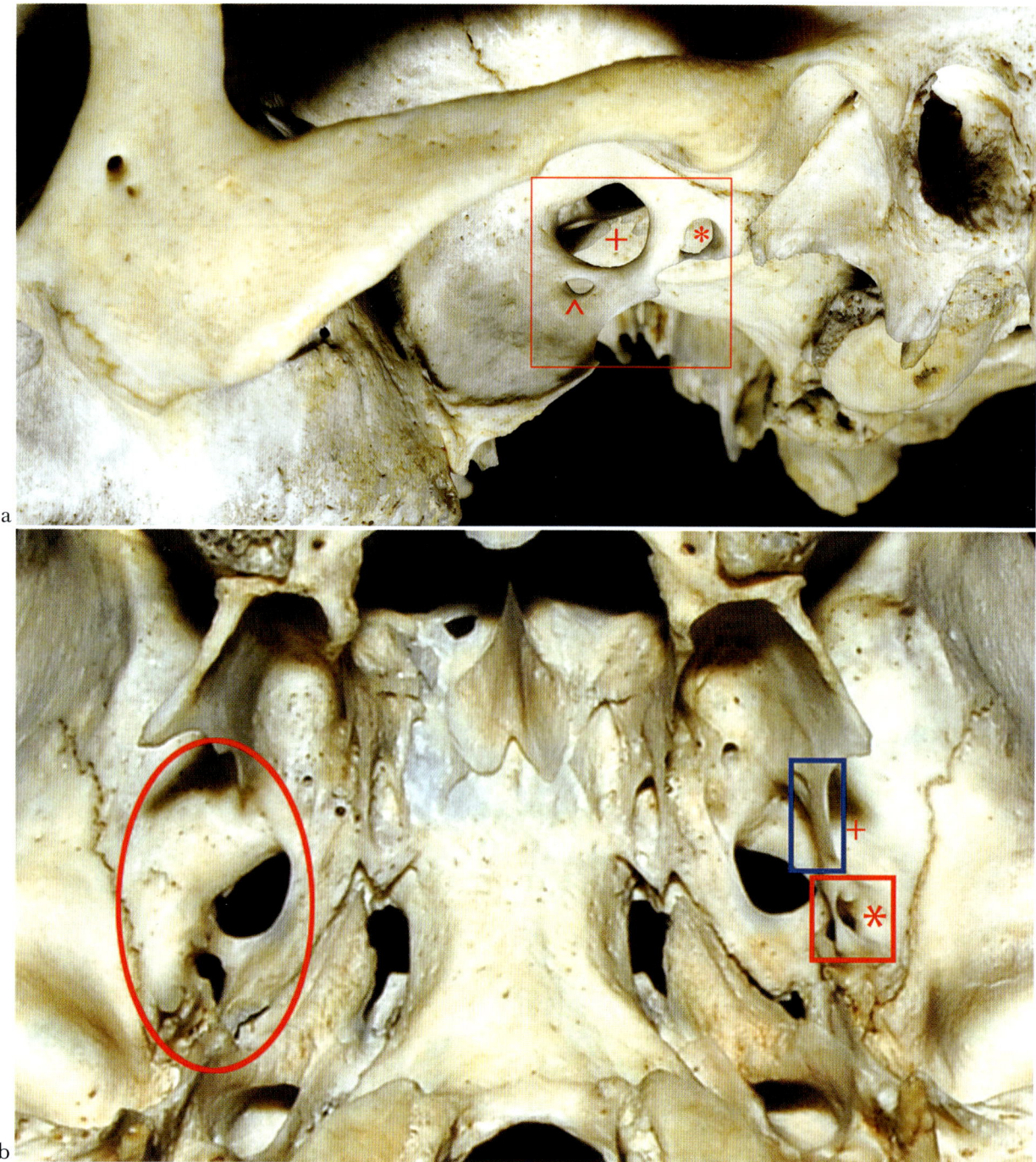

Figure 395a-b. Pterygospinous bridge and foramen and pterygoalar bridge and foramen. (a) Pterygospinous bridge and foramen (*), also known as Foramen of Civinini and pterygoalar bridge and foramen resulting in a large Porus crotaphitico-buccinatorium foramen, the Foramen of Hyrtl (+). The small anterior foramen (∧) was formed by the pterygoalar bar and elongation through calcification of two spines of bone along the posterior margin of the lateral pterygoid plate. (b) Ptery-gospinous bridge (red square and *) and pterygoalar bridge/bar (blue rectangle and +). Note absence of bridging on the right side (oval). Cf. Chouke (1946); Chouke and Hodes (1951); Daimi et al. (2011); Hauser and DeStefano (1989) for more on basal sphenoid bridges; Peuker et al. (2001); Saran et al. (2013); Skrzat et al. (2005); Tubbs et al. (2009).

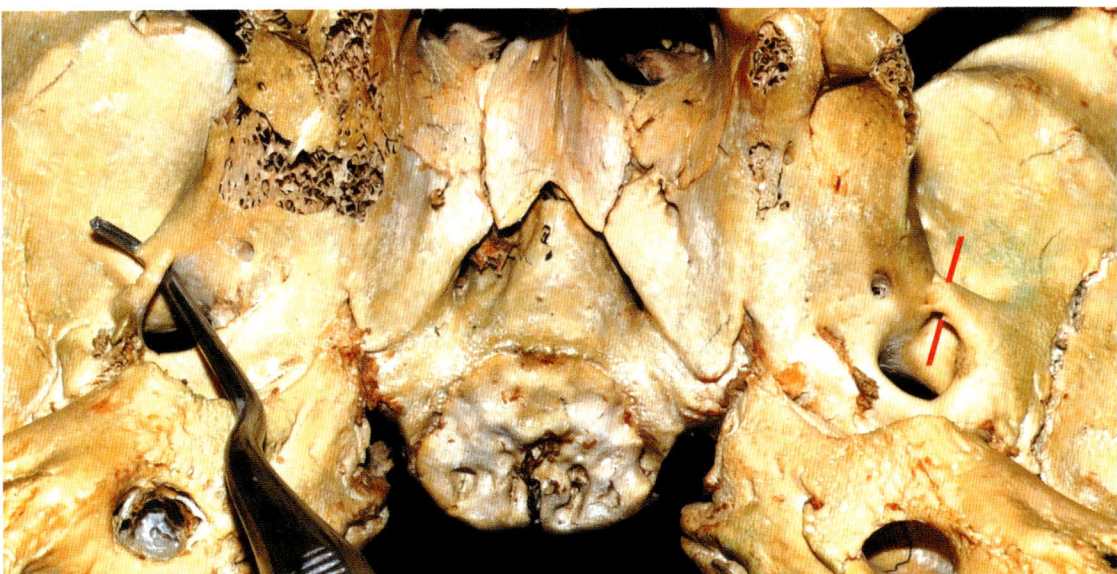

Figure 396. Pterygoalar bridges (metal probe and red line) in a 1- to 2-year-old African child (University of Pretoria). This specimen is noteworthy since it shows that the pterygoalar ligaments, that always form lateral to the foramen ovale, may calcify/ossify in children, not only adults.

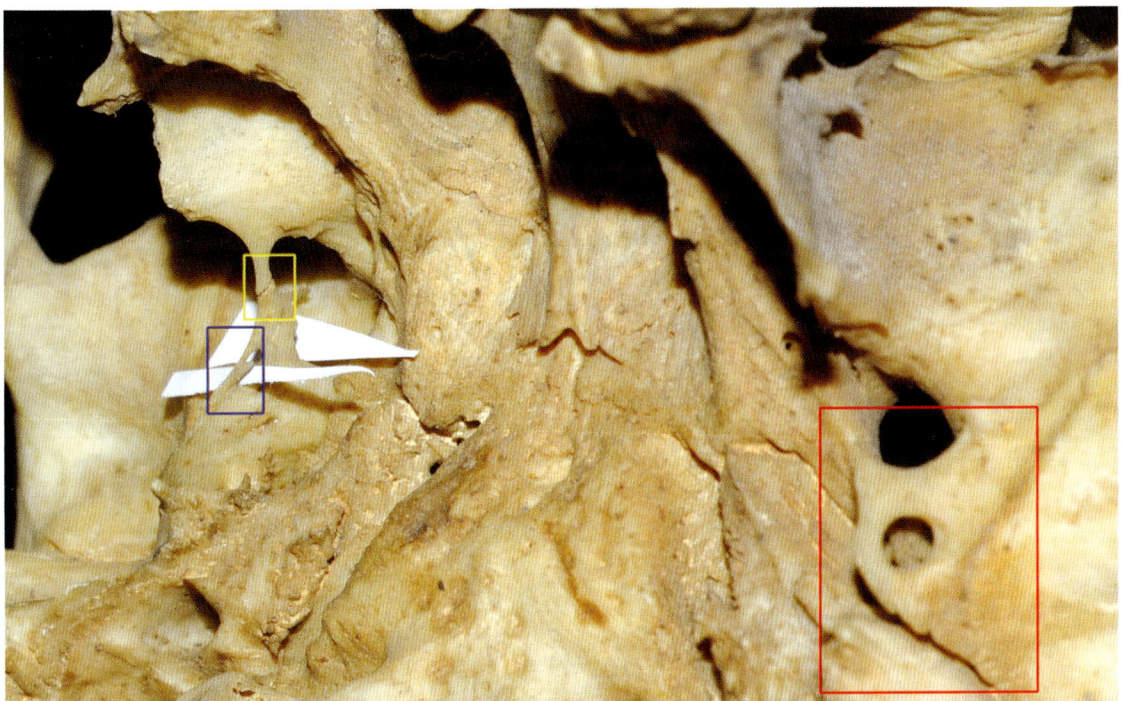

Figure 397. Two right foramina (White arrowheads) in a 13–16-year-old subadult (RV125) and a left pterygospinous foramen (red rectangle). The two right foramina were formed as a result of calcification and bridging of the pterygospinous (blue rectangle; foramen of Civinini) and pterygoalar (yellow rectangle; foramen of Hyrtl) ligaments. The left pterygospinous foramen (red rectangle) formed on top of the foramen spinosum. Calcification of these ligaments, due to their wide variety of expressions, is sometimes difficult to identify. Cf. Saran et al. (2013).

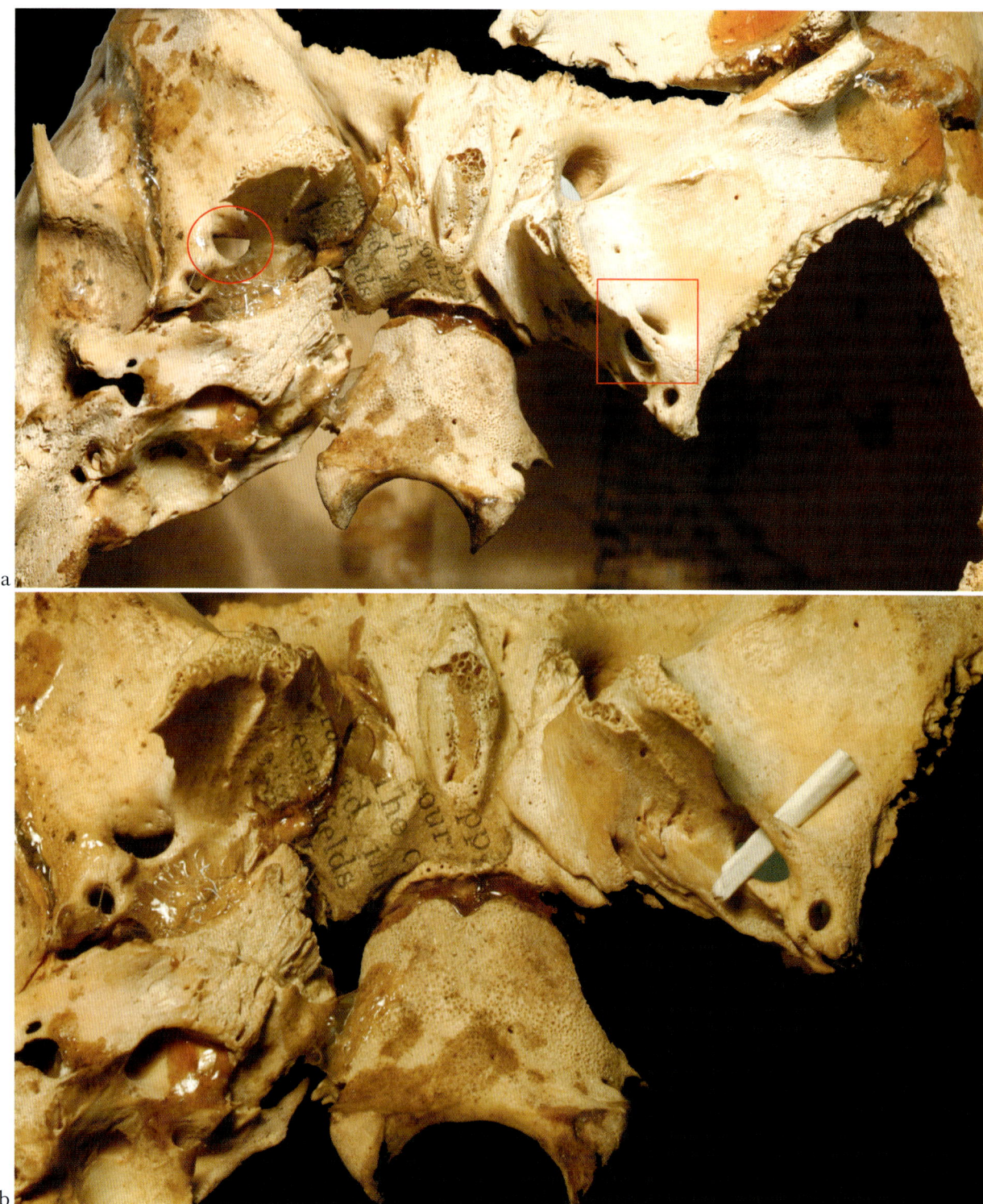

Figure 398a-b. Pterygoalar bridge and trace pterygoalar bridge in a 1- to 2-year-old African child (TM 42, Ditsong Museum, San Bushman). (a) Left pterygoalar bridge (square) with absence of right pterygoalar bridging (circle). Pterygoalar bridging typically occurs lateral to the foramen ovale, whereas pterygospinous bridging results in a bridge across the foramen ovale. (b) Probe passed through the foramen formed by calcification of the pterygoalar ligament. Calcification of the alar ligament is usually believed to begin in adulthood, although examples of this condition have been found in very young children.

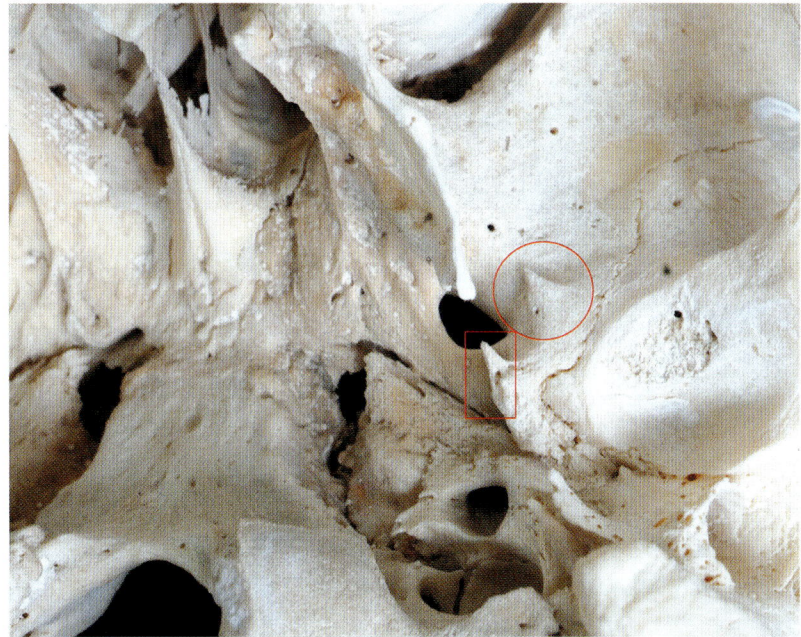

Figure 399. Pterygoalar spine (circle) and partial pterygospinous bridging (rectangle). Note the alar ligament is lateral to the foramen ovale, while the sphenoid spinous ligament is medial to foramen ovale. These are the hallmark positions (lateral or medial) in relation to ovale that distinguish the two traits from one another. Cf. Hauser and DeStefano (1989); Rossi et al. (2011); Rosa et al. (2010); Skrzat et al. (2005, 2006b).

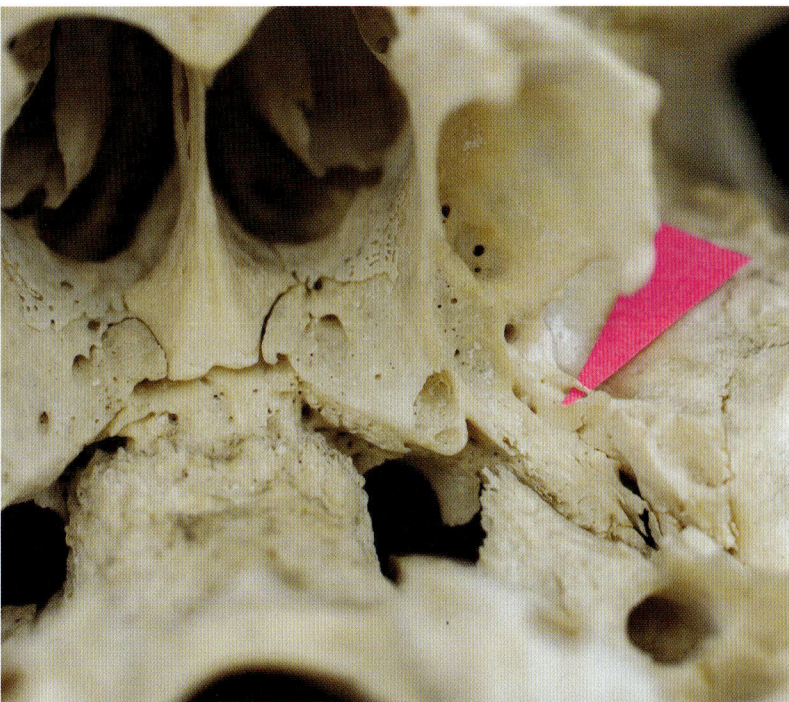

Figure 400. Small left pterygospinous bridge (pink arrowhead) in an adult male (FSA DS043). The bridge or bar of bone in this specimen is thin, fragile and could easily be broken postmortem or during excavation or handling. Note that the trait is sometimes written as two words as "pterygo spinous," in the literature.

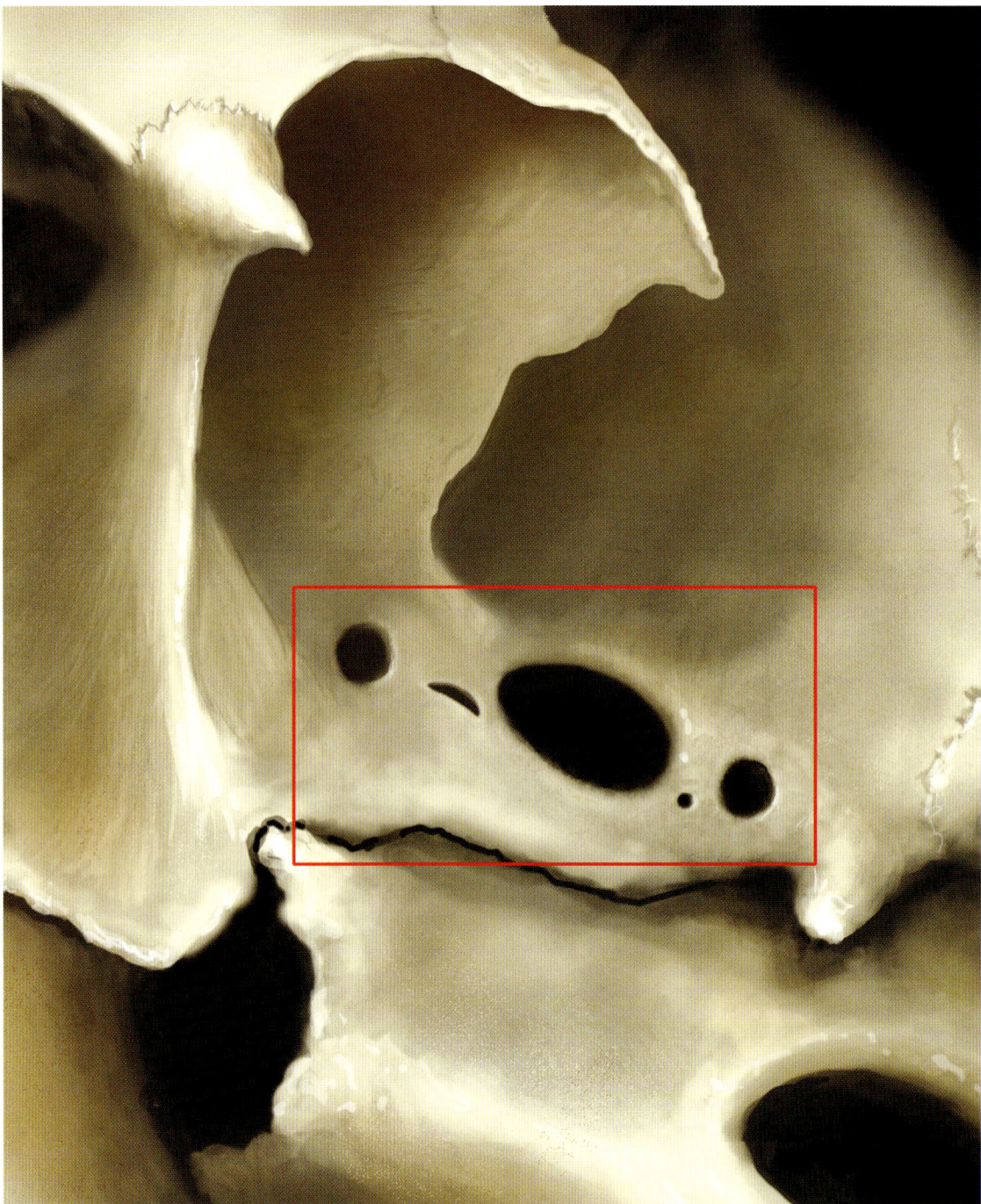

Figure 401. Typical appearance and position of foramina in the cranial base (Illustration by Beth Lozanoff). From left to right (rectangle): cavernous foramen, foramen of Vesalius (slit-like), foramen ovale, foramen of Arnold (also known as canaliculus innominatus) and foramen spinosum. Foramen ovale and foramen spinosum are present in most skulls, but may vary in size and shape and are sometimes double or divided. Cavernous foramen, foramen of Vesalius and foramen of Arnold are often but not always present and vary greatly in size, shape and position in relation to foramen ovale. Numerous additional foramina may be present in this region to transmit vessels or as the result of osteoporosis or disease.

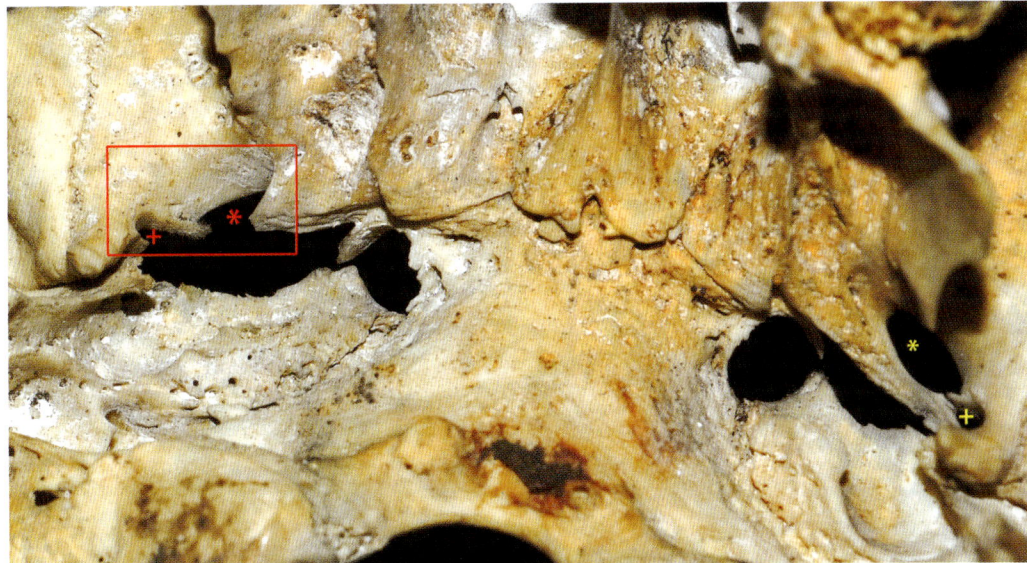

Figure 402. Open medial walls (rectangle) in the right foramen ovale (*) and foramen spinosum (+) compared to closed foramen ovale (yellow asterisk) and foramen ovale (yellow plus sign) on the left side in an adult male (RV795).

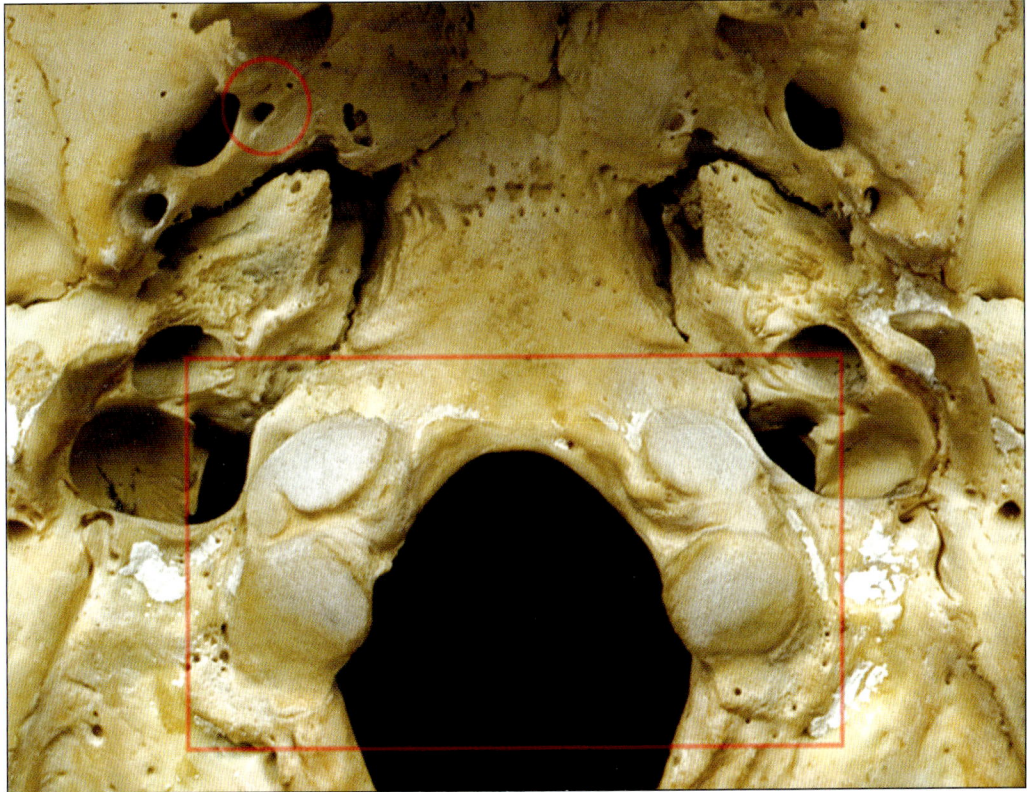

Figure 403. Divided occipital condyles (rectangle) and large foramen of Vesalius (circle) in a 24-year-old male skull (Mütter Museum 1006-090). Naderi et al. (2005) examined 404 occipital condyles in 202 Turkish skulls and found oval condyles to be most common, followed by kidney-shaped, S-like, figure-8 like, triangular, ring-like, two-portioned and deformed. The rarest type was the two-portioned condyle (0.8%), as seen in this figure. Cf. Lanzieri et al. (1988) for foramen of Vesalius.

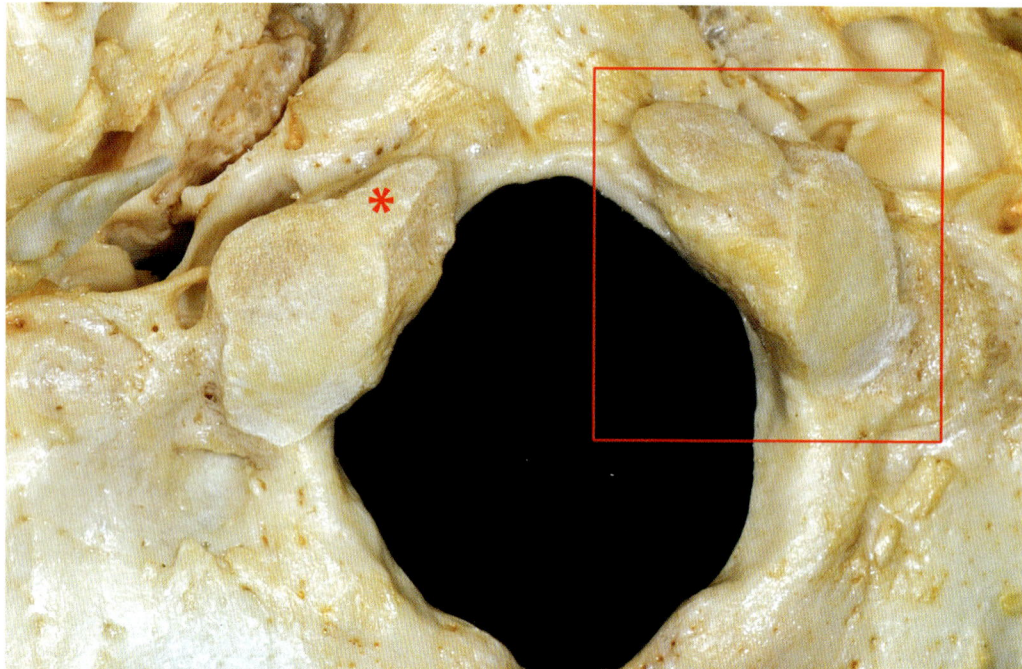

Figure 404. Divided left (square) and asymmetrically shaped right (*) occipital condyle in a 68-year-old Caucasian male skull (JABSOM 881).

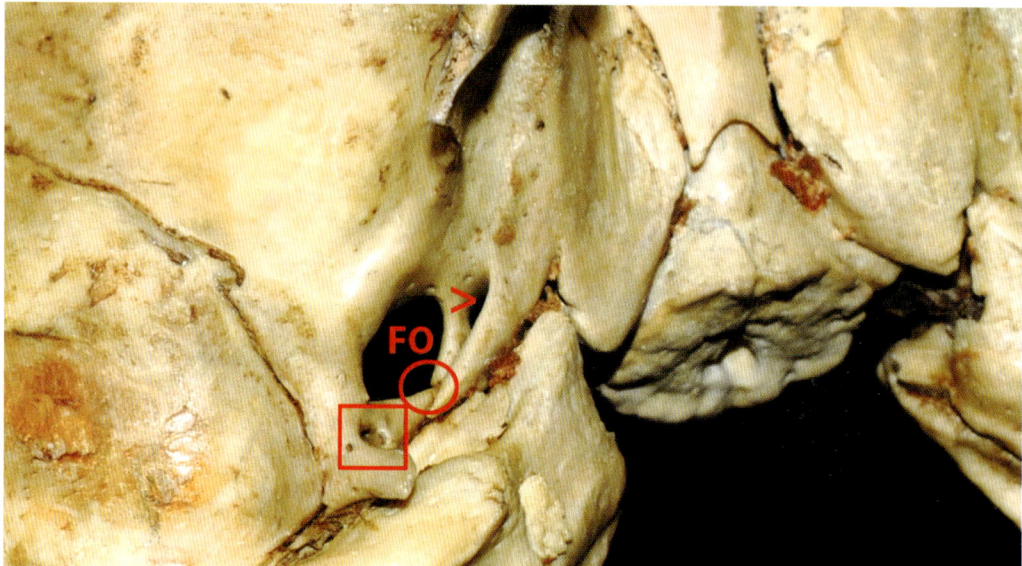

Figure 405. Foramen ovale (FO) and divided medial wall (circle), foramen spinosum (square), and large slit-like foramen of Vesalius (>) in an African child (University of Pretoria). Foramen of Vesalius is often larger ectocranially than endocranially.

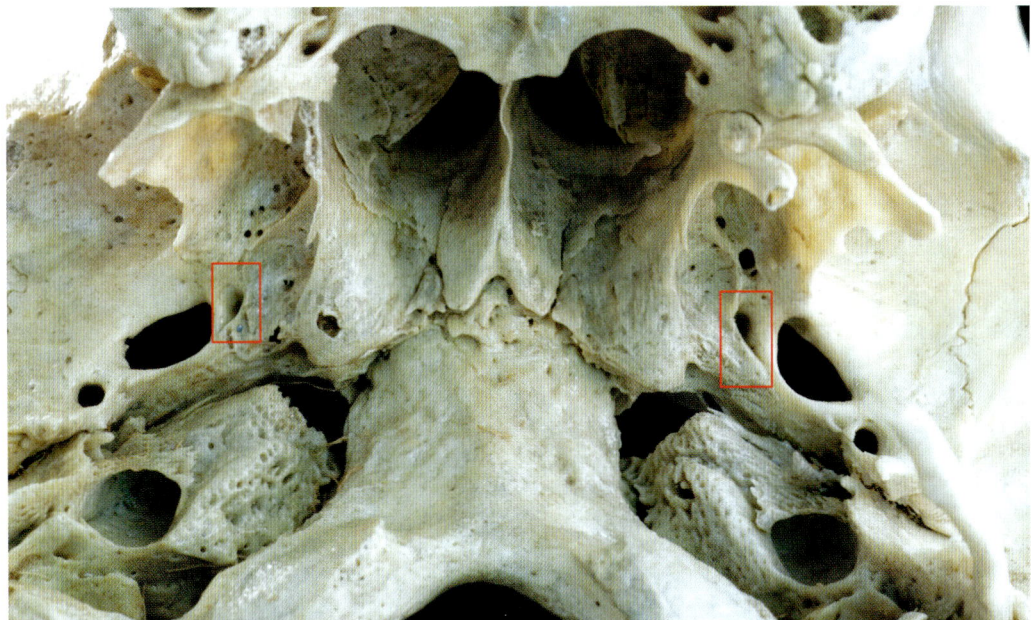

Figure 406. Bilateral foramen of Vesalius (rectangles) in an adult Asian female (CSC AC027). When present, these small, often slit-like foramina are located medial and anterior to the foramen ovale. Cf. Hauser and DeStefano (1989).

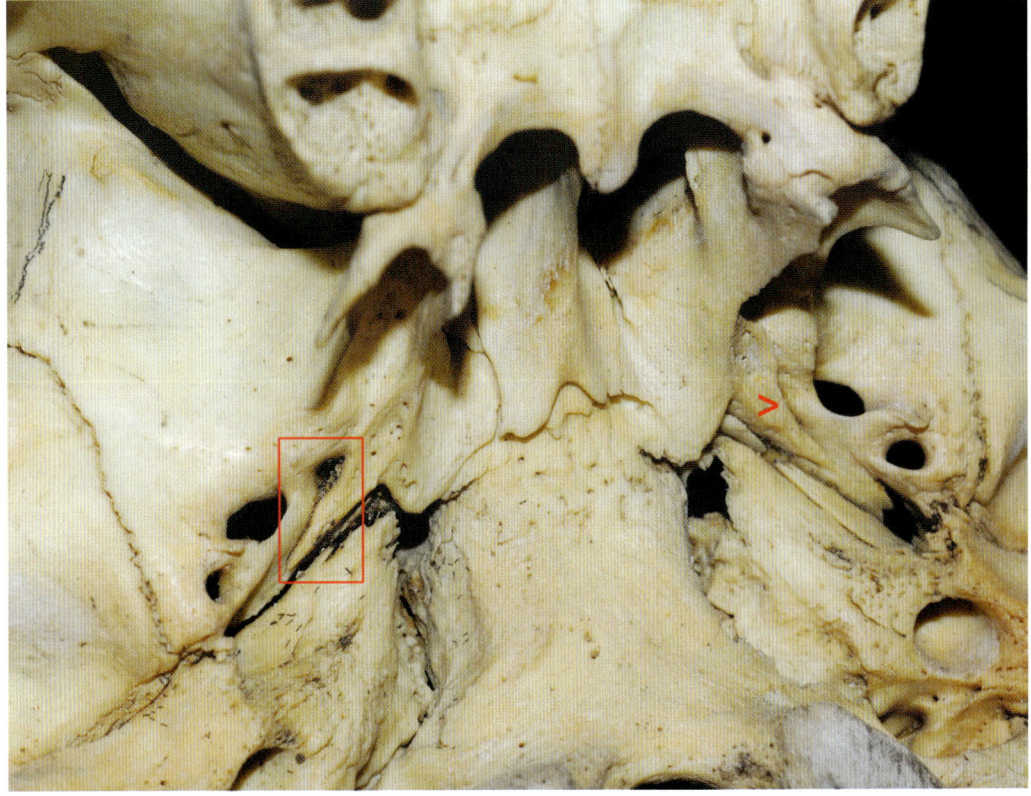

Figure 407. Unusually long and slit-like foramen of Vesalius (rectangle, right and >, left) (RV61).

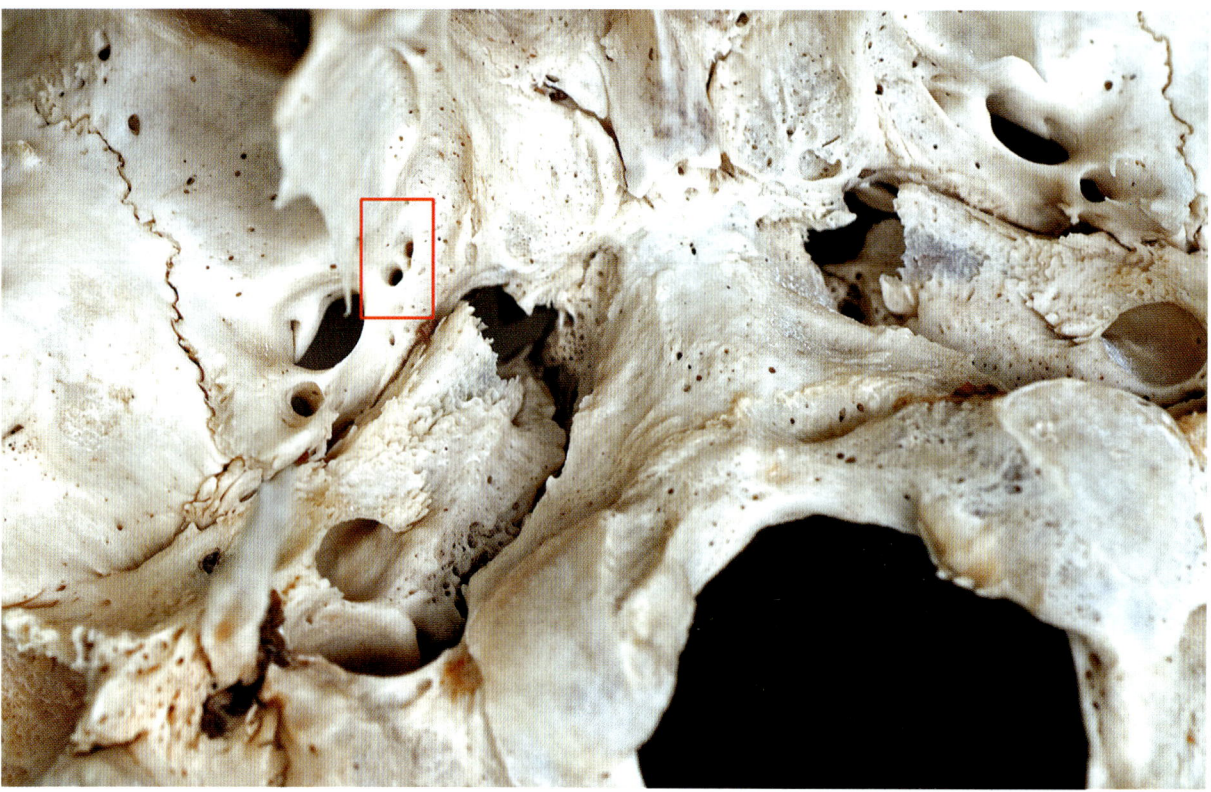

Figure 408. Double/divided right foramen of Vesalius (rectangle) in an adult Thai skull (KKU 44 1363). Cf. Kale et al. (2009a) for frequency of double foramen of Vesalius in Turkish skulls.

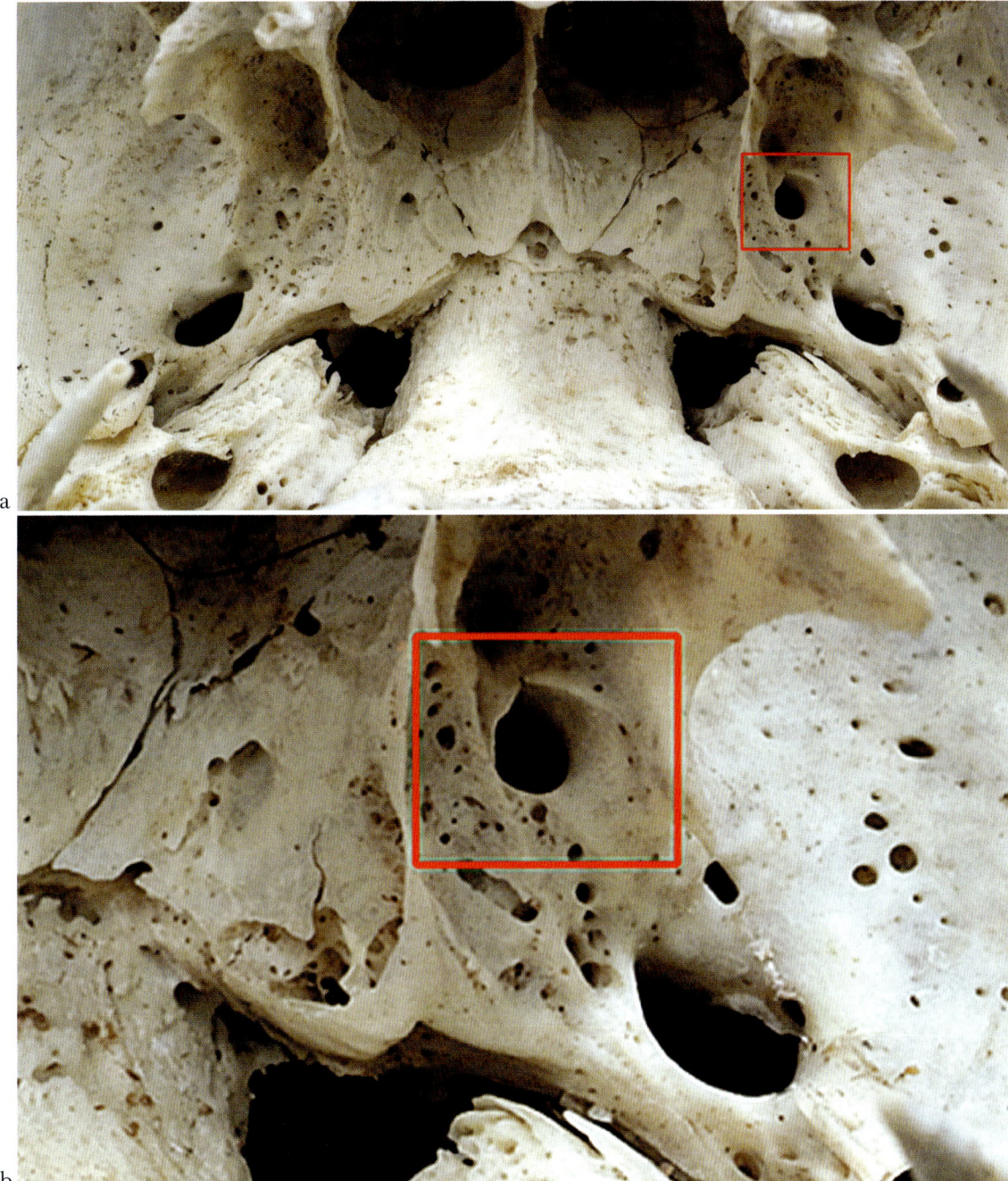

Figure 409a-b. Large cavernous foramen. (a) Unusually large cavernous foramen (square) in the left sphenoid bone (absent in the right side) of a 78-year-old Thai male (CMU 128/46) with diffuse pitting that is consistent with osteoporosis. (b) View of the cavernous foramen (square). Osteoporotic pitting differs from vessel foramina in that the latter often has sloping margins and exhibits grooves (for vessels) into one or more foramina. While subject to debate, the cavernous foramen may transmit a diploic or an emissary vein and is often overlooked or mistaken for another foramen. Its anteromedial position and distance from the foramen ovale, large size and circular shape distinguish it from the more posteromedially positioned foramen of Vesalius (Cf. Reymond et al., 2005 for more on the cavernous foramen). This foramen is a common finding in most groups. See Lanzieri et al. (1988), and Shinohara et al. (2010) for more on the foramen of Vesalius.

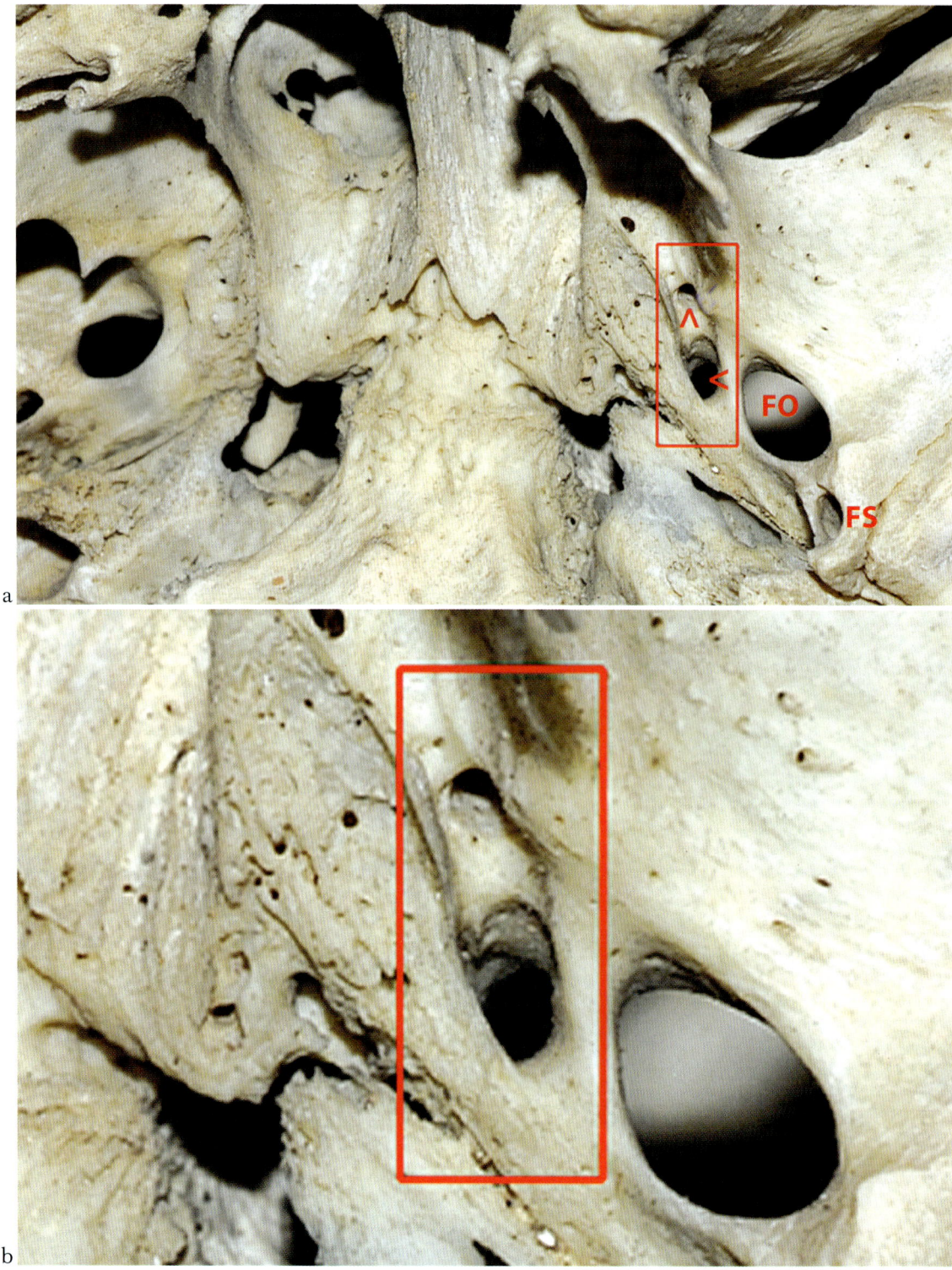

Figure 410a-b. Large and funnel-like left foramen of Vesalius and cavernous foramen in an adult (RV69). (a) Unusually large and funnel-like left foramen of Vesalius (< and rectangle) and cavernous foramen (∧). (b) Higher magnification of the foramen of Vesalius and cavernous foramen (rectangle). The bar of bone separating the foramen of Vesalius and foramen ovale (FO) probably does not represent a divided FO, since this would have been a division of an exceptionally large foramen.

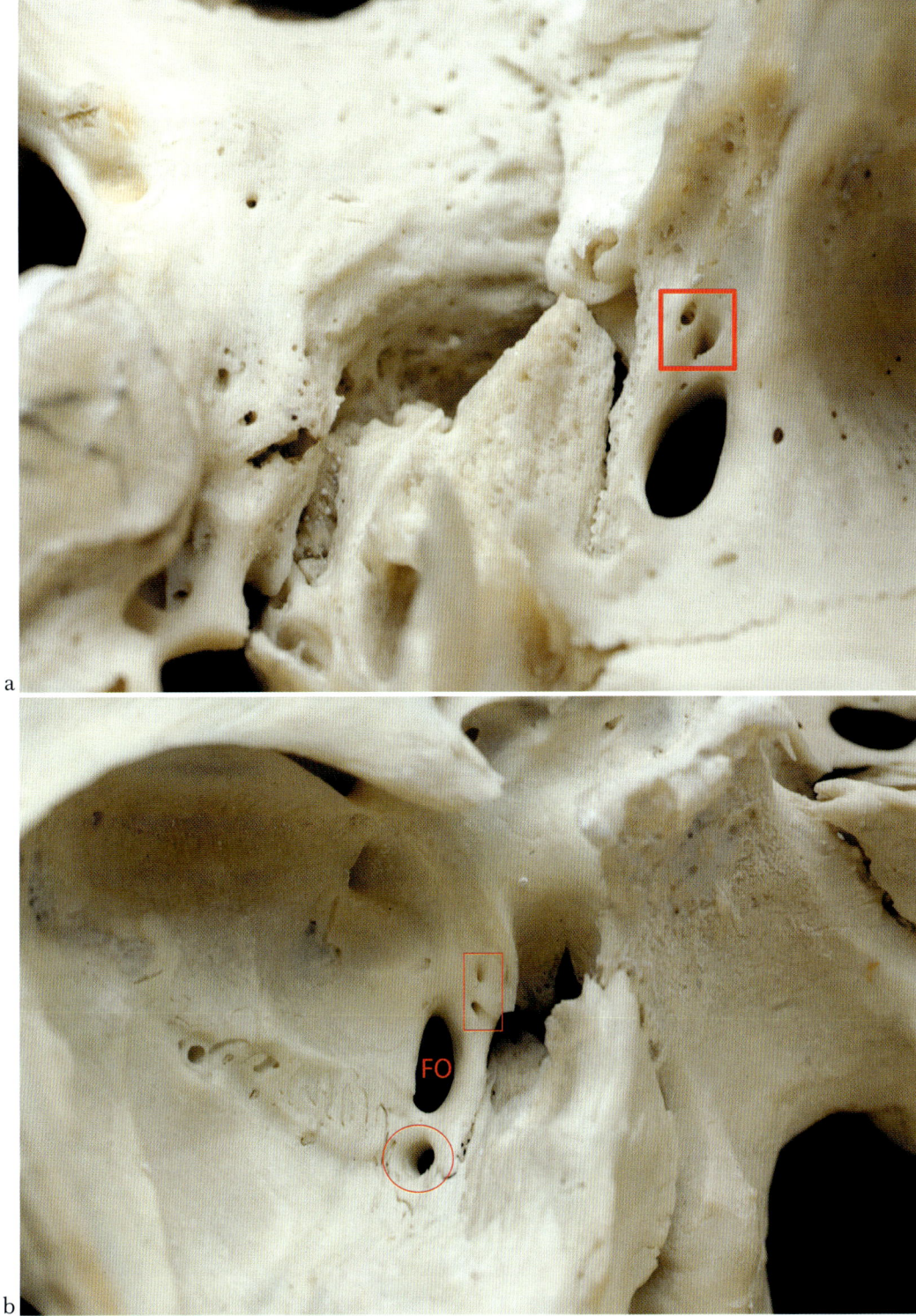

Figure 411a-b. Double left foramen of Vesalius. (a) Ectocranial and (b) endocranial views of double left foramina of Vesalius (square and rectangle, respectively) in an adult male skull (FSA DS043). Bottom photo shows the position of the foramen ovale (FO) and foramen spinosum (circle) endocranially. Chaisuksunt et al. (2012) found the foramen of Vesalius in 25.9% (ectocranially) and 10.9% (endocranially) of 377 skulls. Cf. Lanzieri et al. (1988).

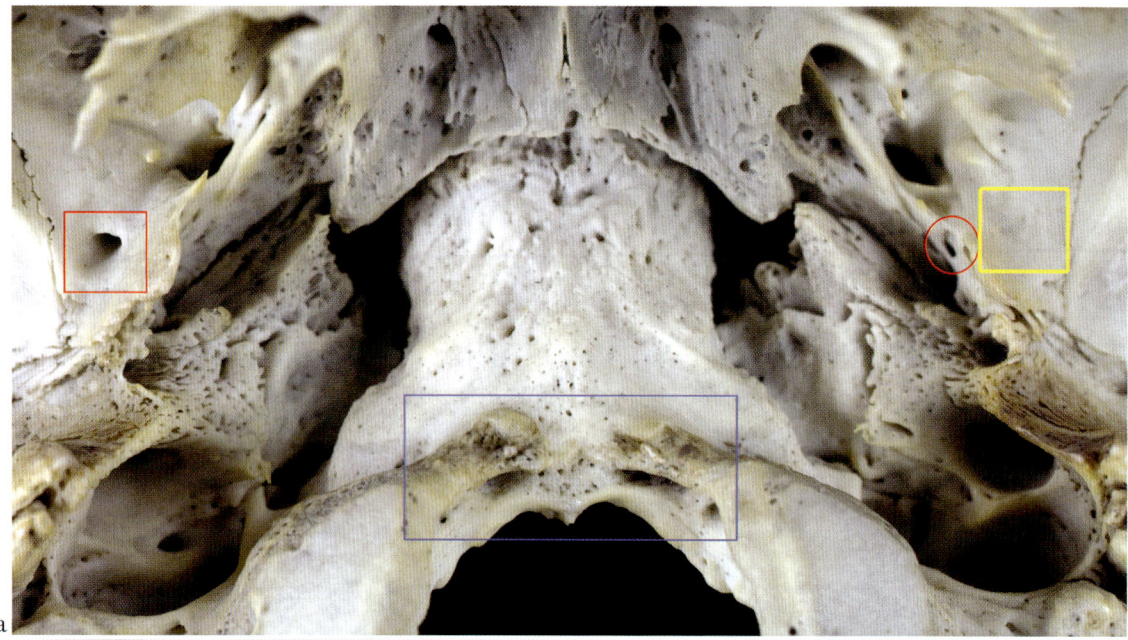

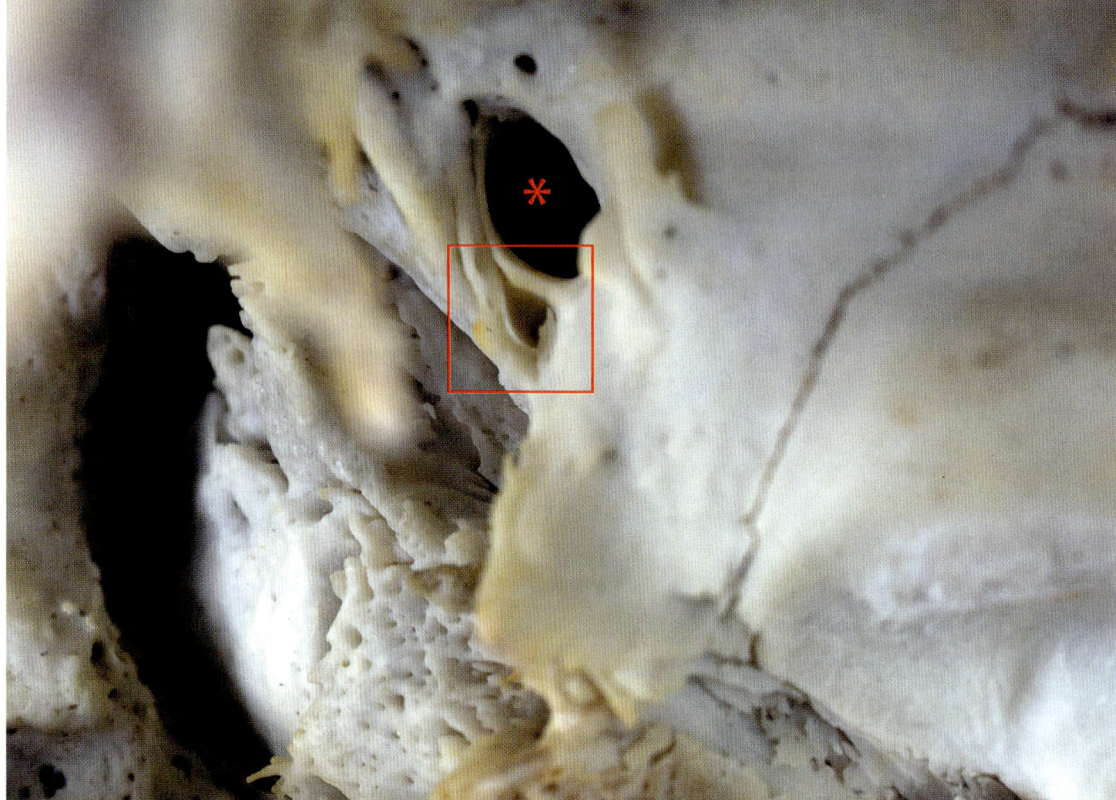

Figure 412a-b. Precondylar tubercles and canaliculus innominatus. (a) Precondylar tubercles or pedestals (rectangle) that are continuous with the occipital condyles, anteriorly oriented right foramen spinosum (FS) (square) and left canaliculus innominatus (circle) – note absence of the left FS in its usual position posterior and/or lateral to the FO (yellow square) (CIL 2002-097). (b) Left foramen ovale (*) with confluent FS (square) along the medial border of the FO. The position of the FS this far medial to the FO is unusual. See Lindblom (1936) and Nikolova et al. (2012) for examples of absent FS. Cf. Berge and Bergman (2001); Hauser and DeStefano (1989).

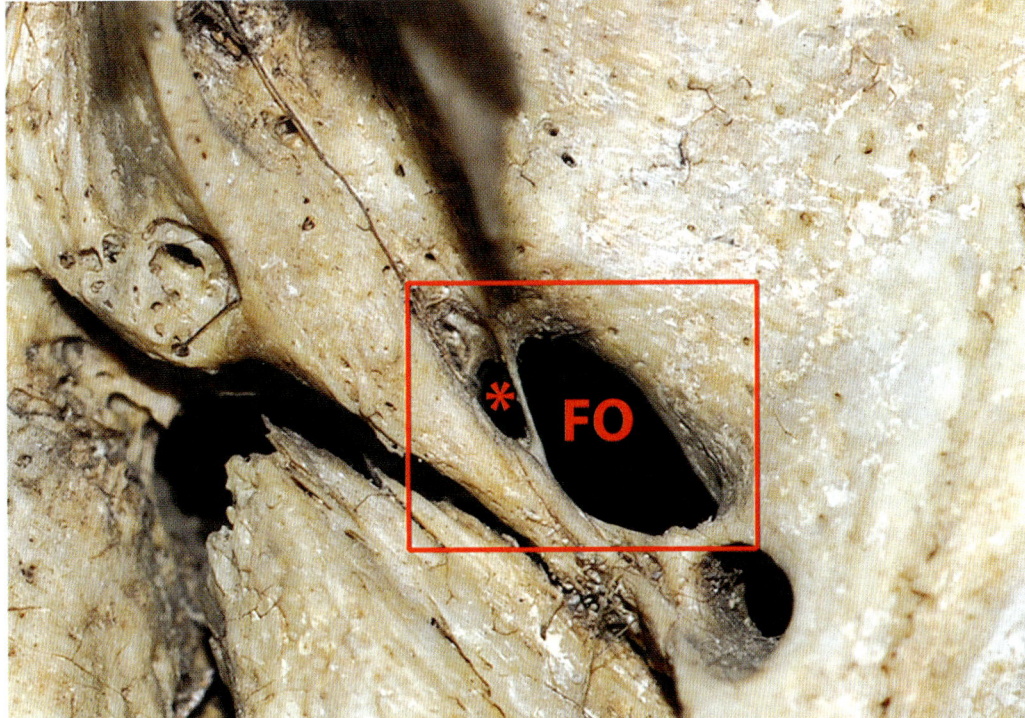

Figure 413. A thin bar of bone separates what could either be a left foramen of Vesalius (*) and foramen ovale (FO, rectangle) or a divided foramen ovale and absence of a foramen of Vesalius (RV78).

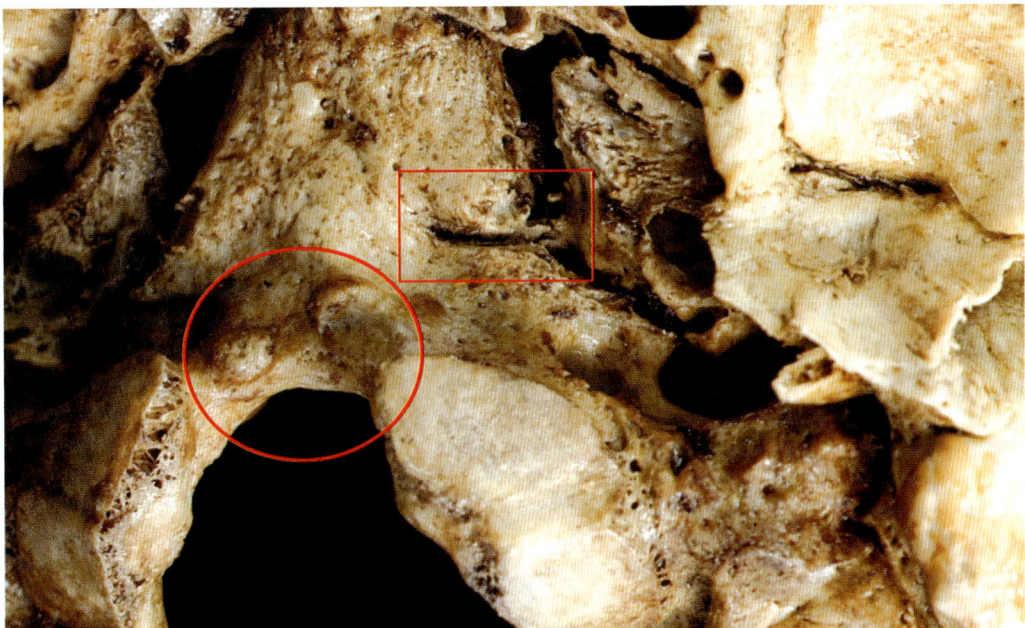

Figure 414. Unilateral basilar transverse cleft (Sauser's fissure; canalis hypoglossi bipartitus) (rectangle) in an adult Asian skull (CSC DS009) reflecting cranial shifting. Note small right precondylar tubercle and elongated basilar process (circle) anteromedial to the left occipital condyle. Precondylar tubercle is a common finding and basilar clefting is rare. Cf. Anderson (2000); Broman (1957); Freyschmidt et al. (2002); Gupta et al. (1981); Marshall (1955); Oetteking (1923); Prescher (1997); Scheuer and Black (2004); Vasudeva and Choudhry (1996).

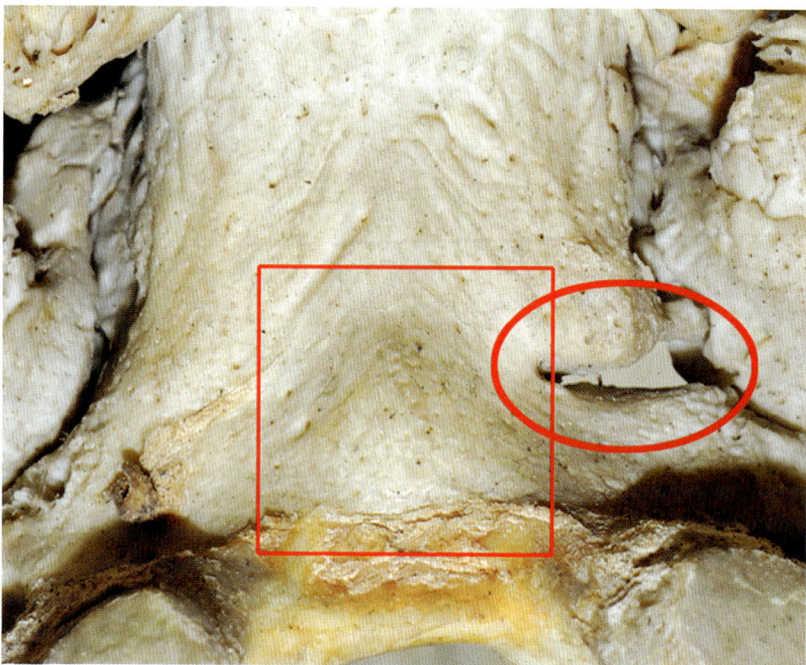

Figure 415. Unilateral basilar cleft (oval) and a pharyngeal tubercle (square) in an adult cranium (RV488 from Romania).

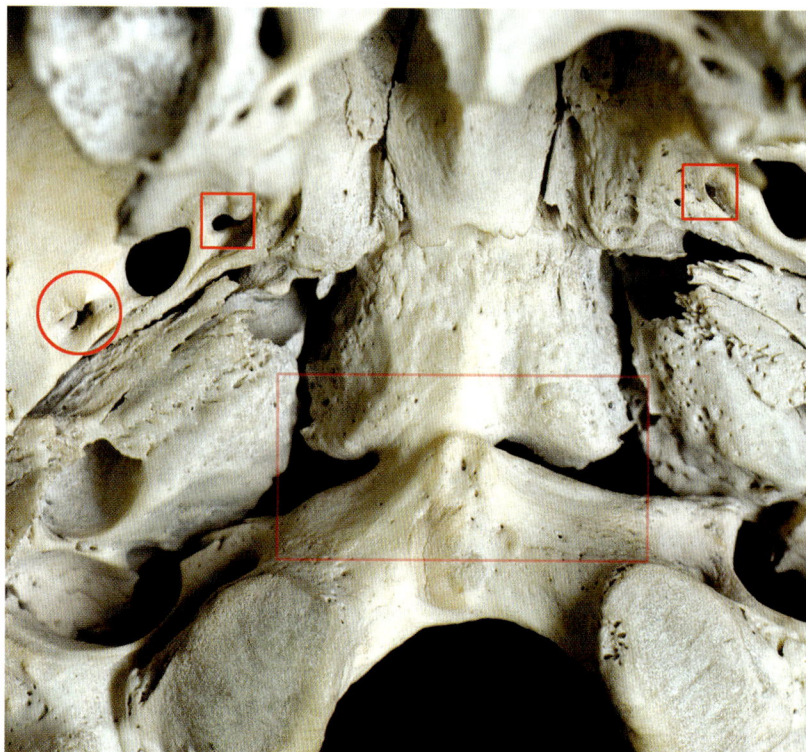

Figure 416. Bilateral basilar cleft/fissures (rectangle) representing incomplete segmentation of the basi-occipital in an adult Asian skull (UPenn, Wistar 254). This rare condition has a reported frequency of about one per thousand individuals (Wackenheim 1985). Note the basilar synchondrosis has fully closed and the right foramen spinosum (circle) is small and irregularly shaped. Cf. Barnes (1994); Madeline and Elster (1995); Prescher et al. (1996); Prescher (1997).

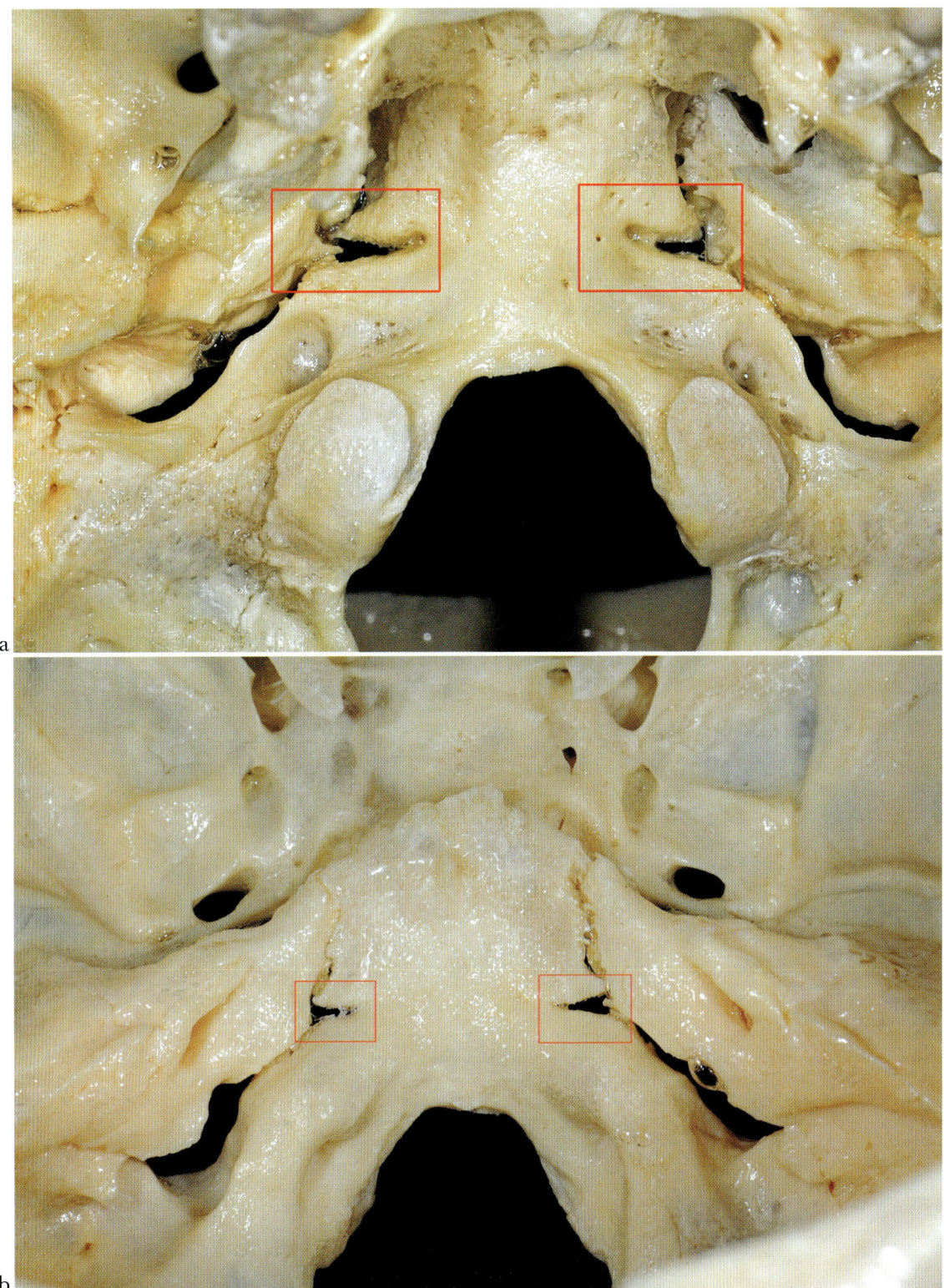

Figure 417a-b. Bilateral basilar fissures. (a) Ectocranial and (b) endocranial views of bilateral basilar fissures (rectangles) in an adult (JABSOM SK15). Note that the V-shaped fissures are roughly symmetrical endocranially and ectocranially.

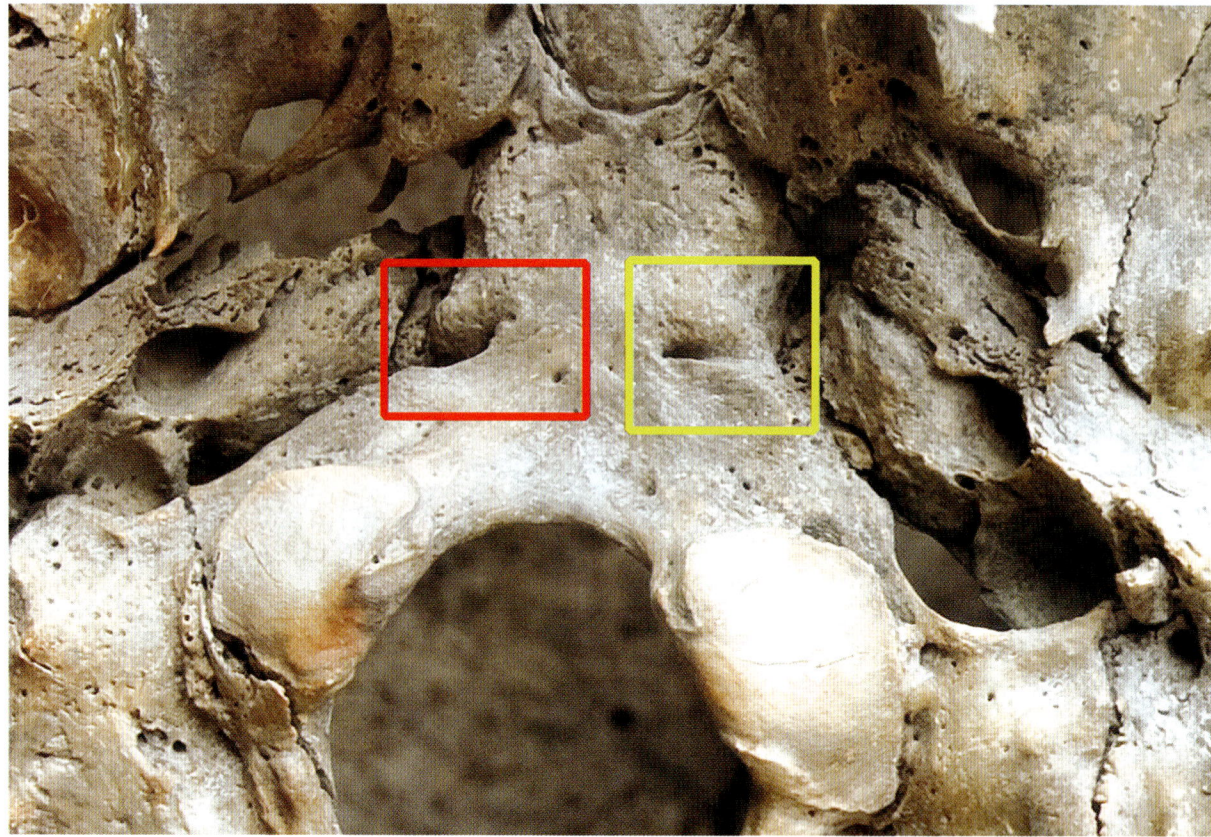

Figure 418. Bilateral basilar fissures (basioticum variant) in a young adult Hungarian skull (NHMH 65.6.13 21). The right fissure perforated the basilar bone, while the left fissure was only a few millimeters deep. These congenital traits represent cranial shifting of the somites of the occipitocervical border. Cf. Barnes (1994, 2008); Madeline and Elster (1995).

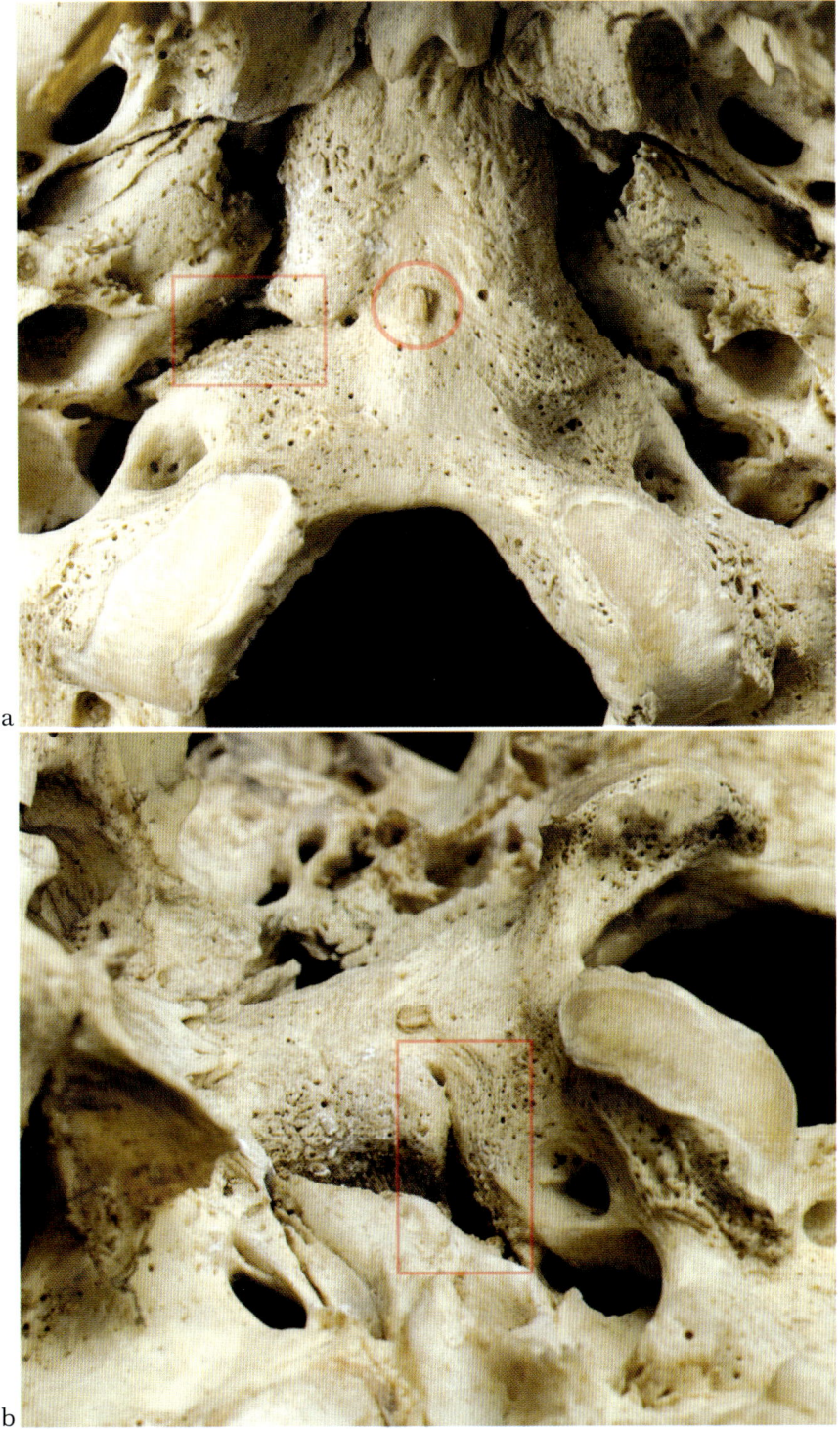

Figure 419a-b. Basilar transverse fissure and pharyngeal tubercle. (a) Right unilateral basilar fissure (rectangle) and a small pharyngeal tubercle (circle) in an adult male (UPenn 1331 L606). (b) Higher magnification of the basilar transverse fissure (rectangle). See Barnes (1994); Madeline and Elster (1995); Prescher et al. (1996); Prescher (1997); Wackenheim (1985) for more on the basilar transverse fissure. Uncommon to rare trait.

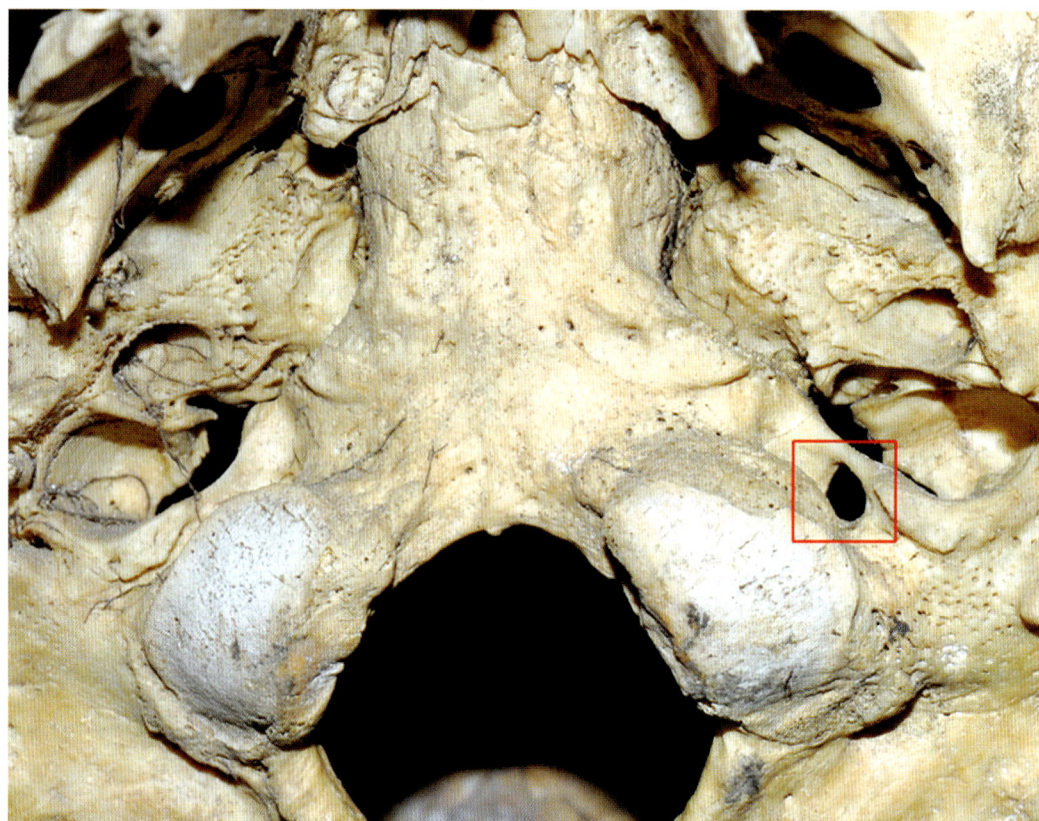

Figure 420. Unilateral (left) paracondylar foramen (square) resulting in a superior-inferiorly oriented foramen posterior to the jugular foramen and lateral to the hypoglossal canal (HC) in an adult (RV1234). Note absence of a right paracondylar foramen. Manjunath (1998) noted this foramen unilaterally in four of 118 skulls.

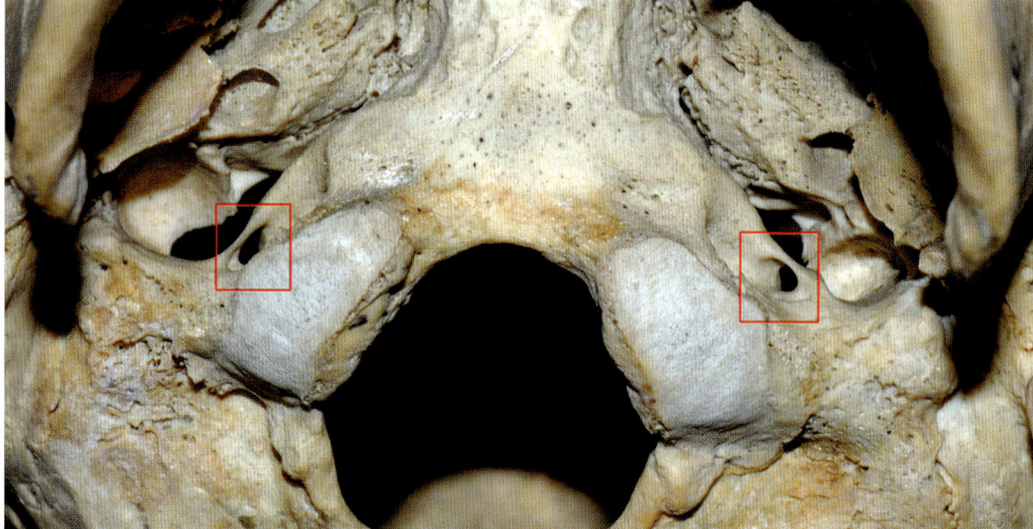

Figure 421. Bilateral paracondylar foramina (rectangles) (RV801) located posterior to the jugular foramen and lateral to the hypoglossal canals, possibly for transmission of the hypoglossal nerve. Bilateral foramina such as this are uncommon to rare. Cf. Manjunath (1998).

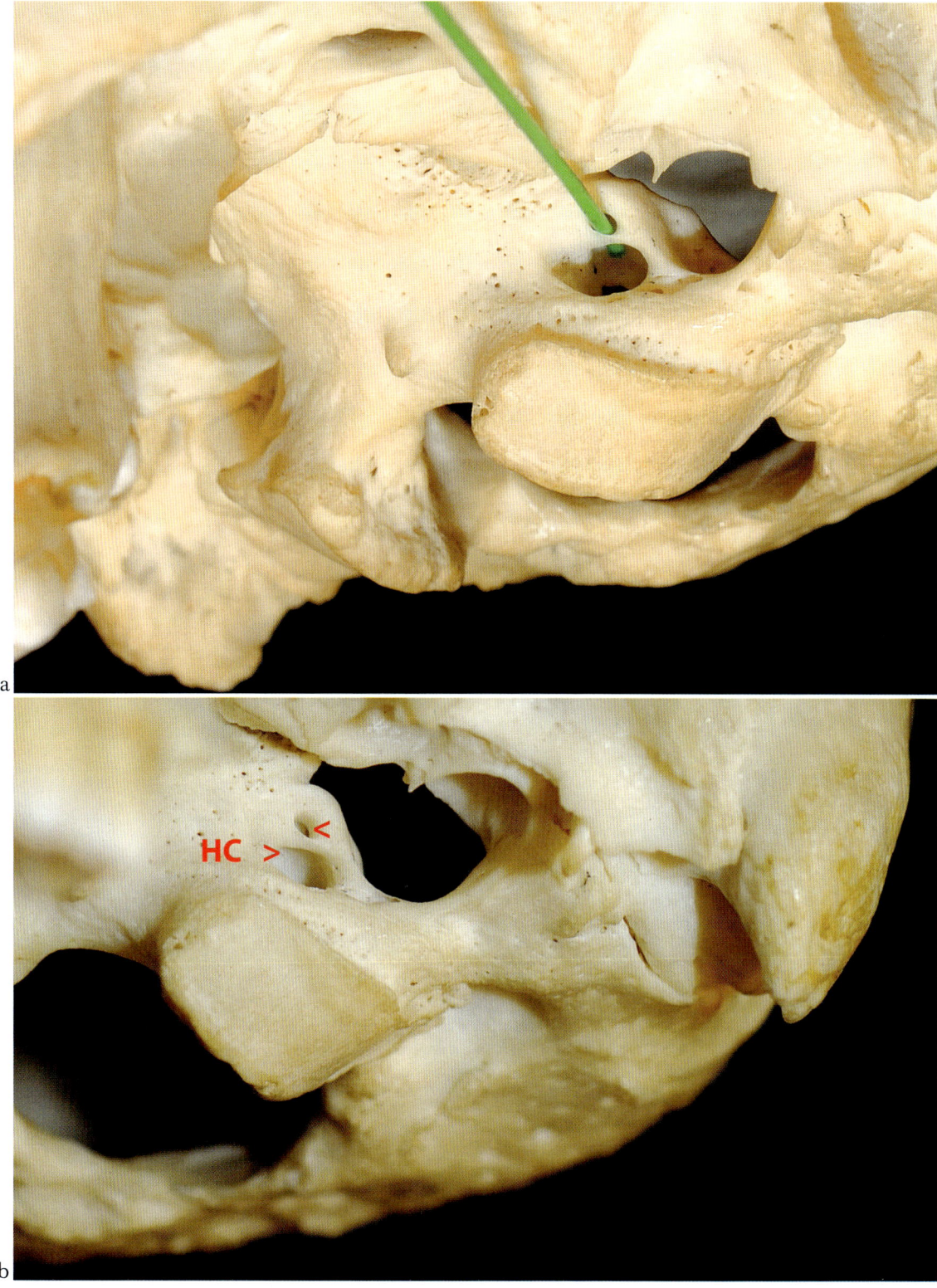

Figure 422a-b. Left paracondylar foramen. (a) Inferior view of a left paracondylar foramen (green probe and <) in an adult male (JABSOM). (b) Note that the paracondylar foramen communicates with the hypoglossal canal (HC>). The right hypoglossal canal does not exhibit a paracondylar foramen.

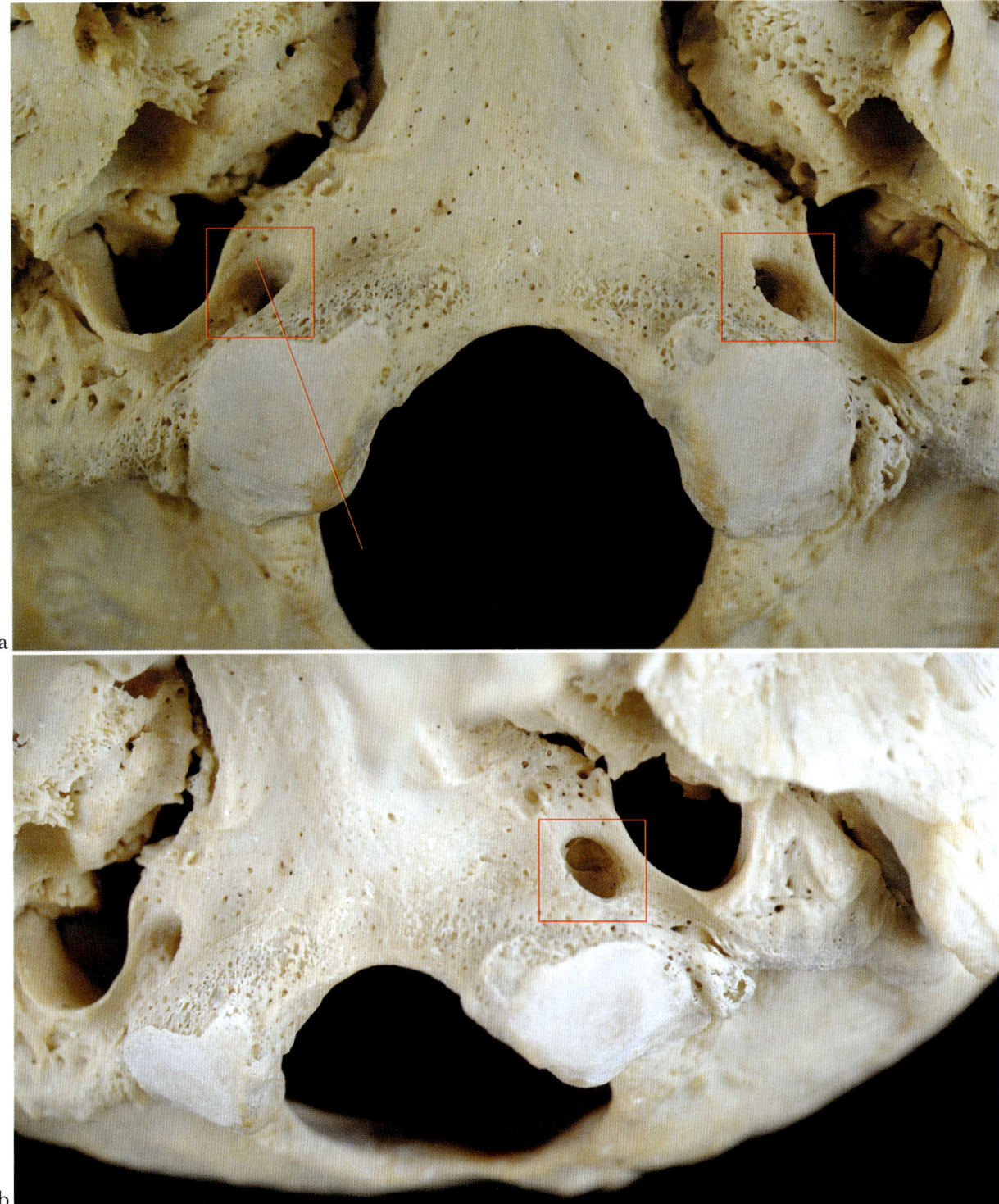

Figure 423a-b. Lateral openings of the hypoglossal canals. (a) Depiction of the direction and orientation of the hypoglossal canals (squares) in an adult male without a paracondylar foramen. The red line shows the direction of the right hypoglossal canal internally and externally. (b) Morphology and orientation of the external opening of a hypoglossal canal (square) that did not perforate the floor of the fossa (FSA AC-030).

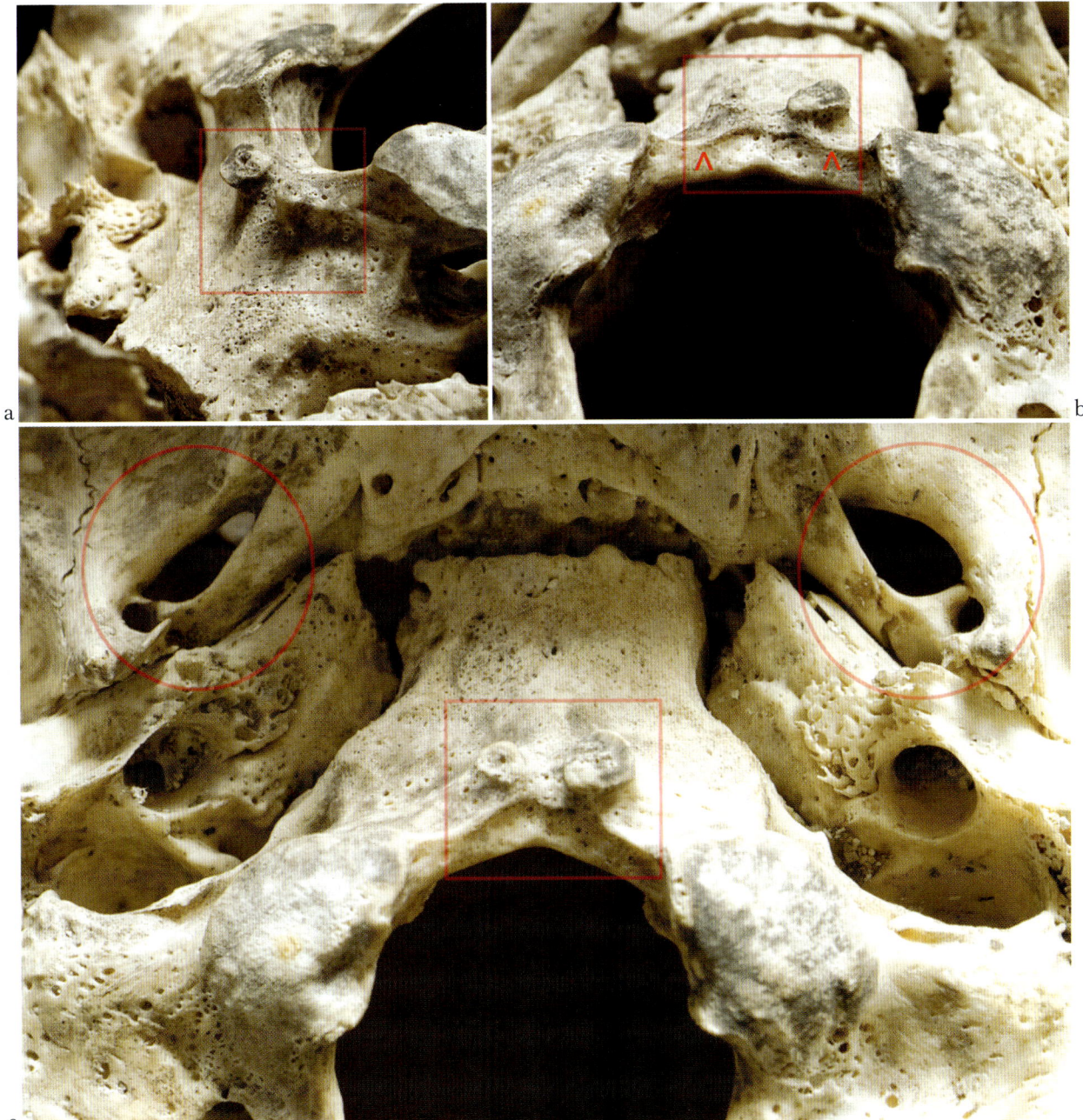

Figure 424a-c. Pedestaled precondylar tubercles. (a) Pedestaled precondylar tubercles (rectangle) with flat articular surfaces and bilateral bridged foramen ovale and foramen spinosum (circles) in a 12- to 16-year-old African subadult (UPenn 969 L606). (b) Bone bridges (rectangle and ∧) connecting the anterior occipital condyles with the two tubercles. (c) Inferior view illustrating differences in the size and shape of the two tubercles. Precondylar tubercles, representing caudal or downward shift in the developmental field, often articulate with the anterior arch (tubercle) of the atlas, resulting in a beak-like curved extension directed toward the base of the skull. The anterior arch and precondylar tubercle may have contacted when the head is tightly flexed. Travan et al. (2008) reported on two saddle-shaped basilar processes in a medieval skeleton that articulated with the anterior arch of the atlas. There are at least nine variants of precondylar tubercles ranging from spines to faceted pedestals, as in this example. Cf. Barnes (1994, 2008); Broman (1957); Hanihara and Ishida (2001b); Hauser and DeStefano (1989); Marshall (1955); Oetteking (1923).

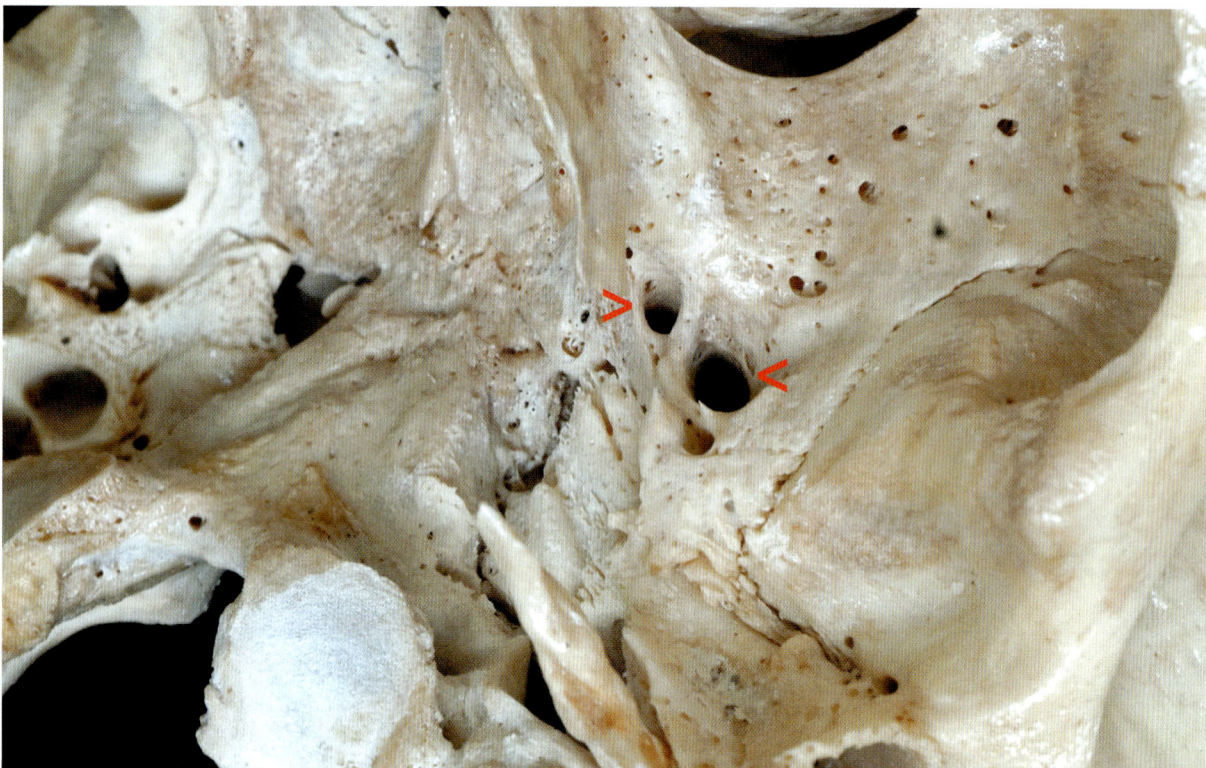

Figure 425. Ectocranial view showing an atypically round left foramen of Vesalius (>) anterior to the foramen ovale (<). The right foramen of Vesalius is slit-like (KKU). Cf. Lanzieri et al. (1988) and Shapiro and Robinson (1967) for foramina in the middle cranial fossa.

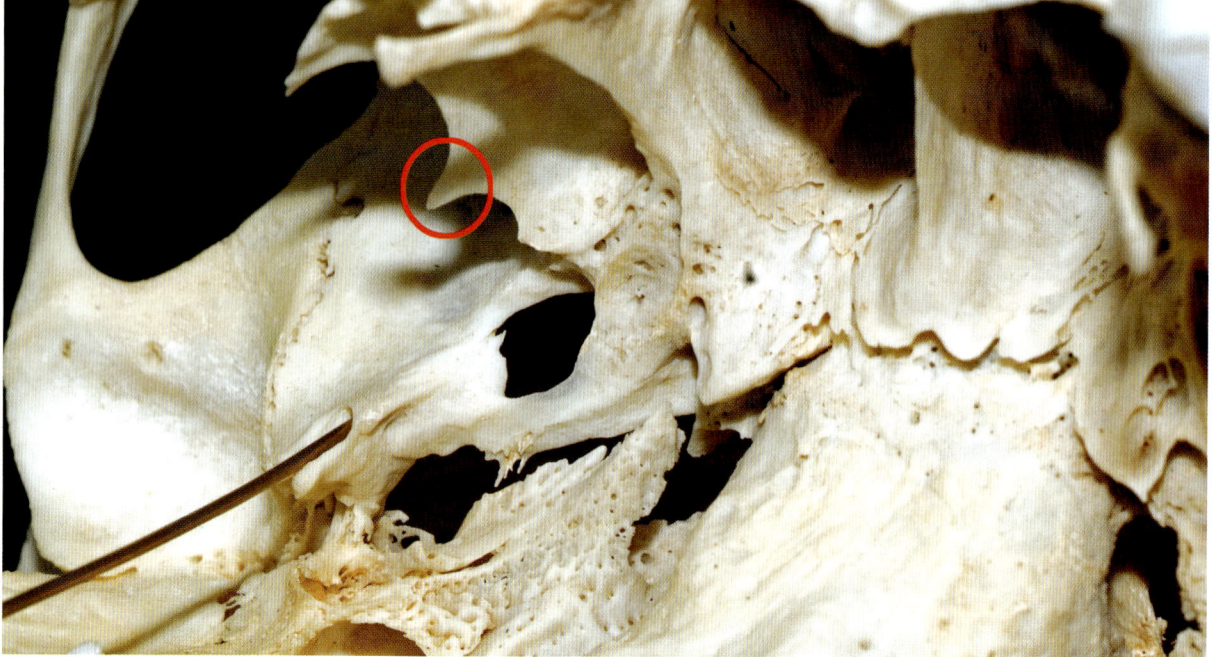

Figure 426. Tunnel-like right (probe) and left foramen spinosum in 66-year-old male (CMU 74 51). This foramen is usually oriented perpendicular to the cranial base. Note the right spine of Civinini (circle) (Saran et al. 2013).

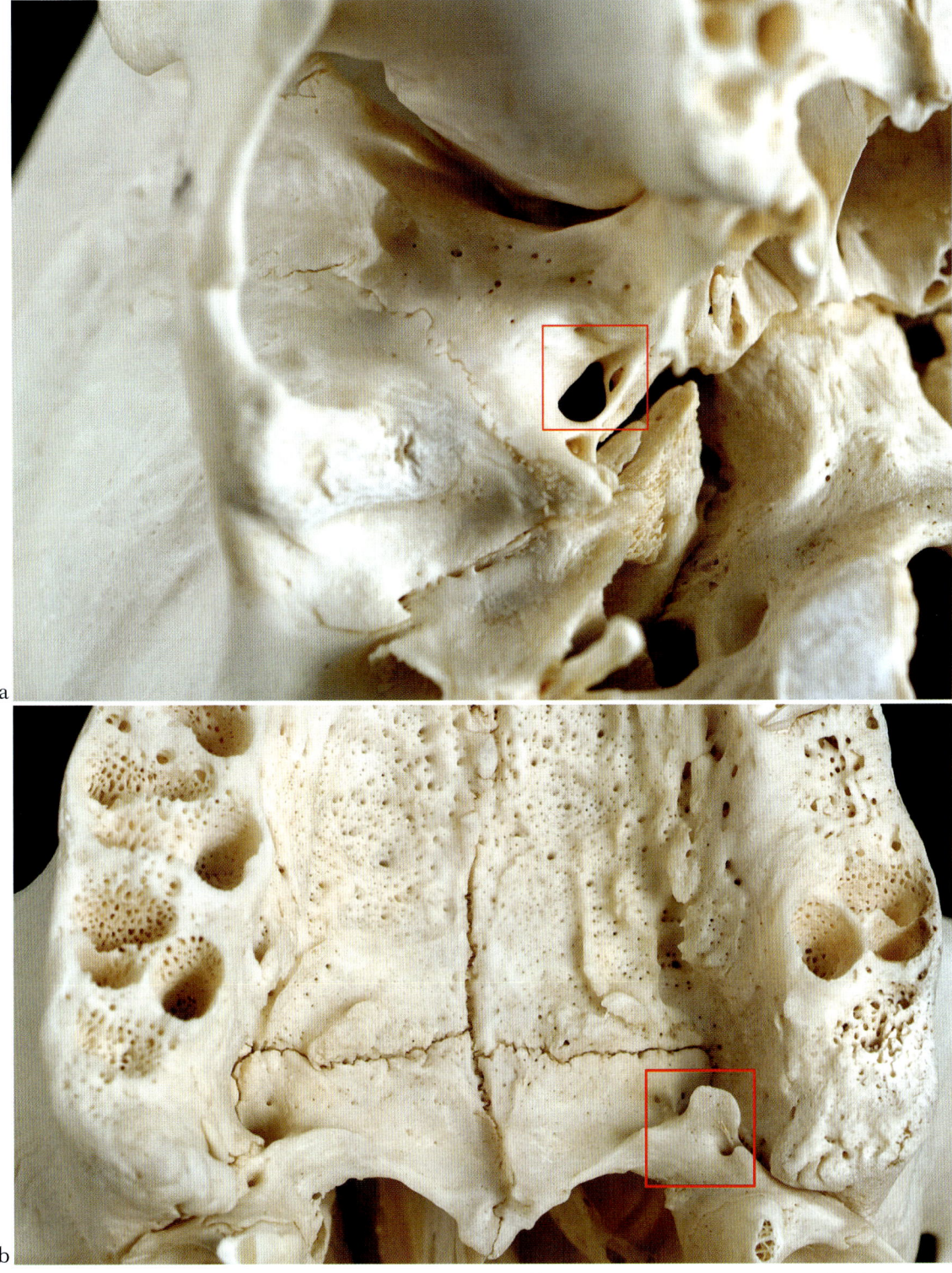

Figure 427a-b. Divided foramen ovale or foramen of Vesalius. (a) Divided right foramen ovale, or a slit-like foramen of Vesalius positioned very close to the foramen ovale. (b) Note the tongue-shaped projection of bone along the left palatine crest and posterior to the palatine foramen in a young adult Asian skull, probable male (CSC AC 026). Note porous nature of the molar dental alveoli indicating remodeling after loss of the teeth antemortem. Cf. Shinohara et al. (2010) for foramen of Vesalius.

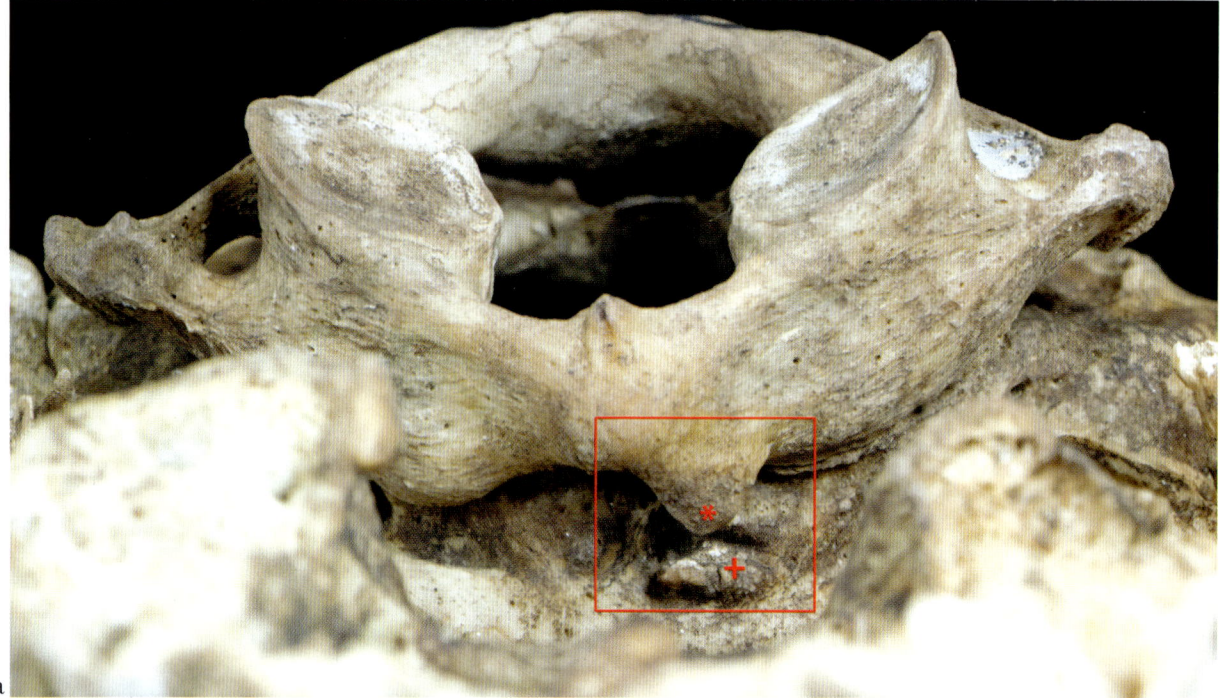

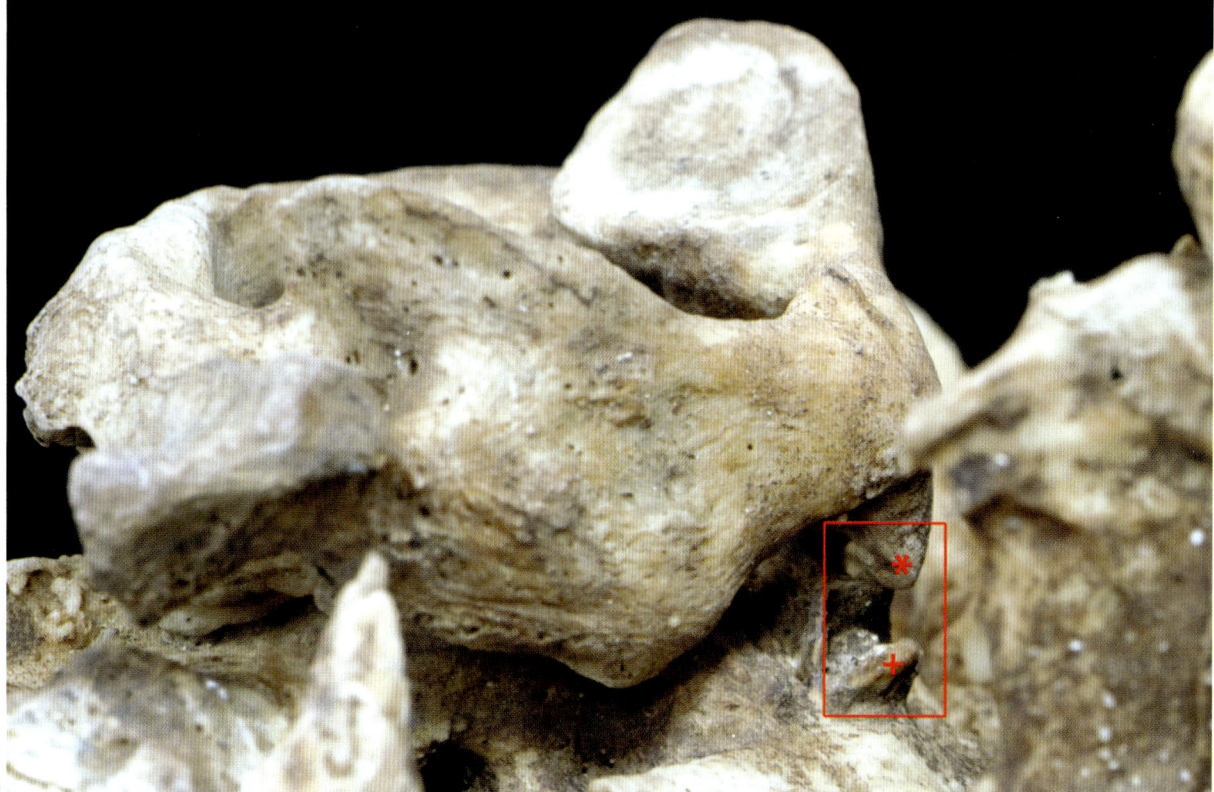

Figure 428a-b. Precondylar tubercle of the occipital base. (a) Photograph of a precondylar tubercle (rectangle and +) in close proximity with a bony projection (*) along the anterior arch of the atlas (rectangle) (CMU). (b) The two tubercles (rectangle, * and +) may have achieved contact during some movements of flexion.

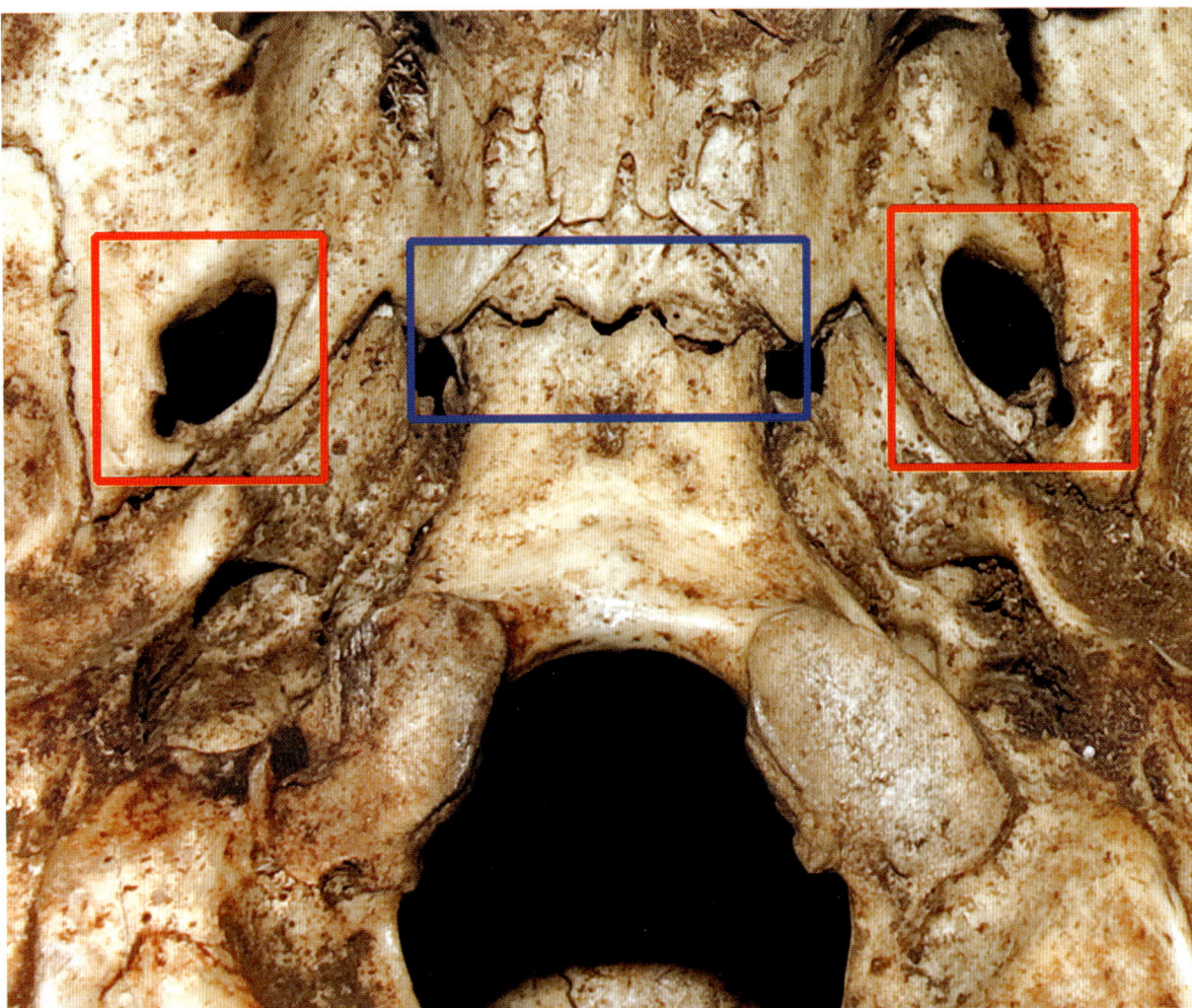

Figure 429. Bilateral undivided foramen ovale and foramen spinosum (red squares) and open basilar synchondrosis (blue rectangle) in a subadult from Hungary (NHMH Maszaj Koponya). Cf. Burdan et al. (2011); Hauser and DeStefano (1989); Krayenbühl et al. (2008); Osunwoke et al. (2010); Wood-Jones (1931) for more on these foramina. Abd Latiff et al. (2009) found one accessory left foramen ovale in 15 adult Malaysian skulls. The tiny accessory foramen was medial to the normal foramen ovale. Cf. Gluncic et al. (2002) for accessory foramen opticum, accessory foramen ovale and accessory foramen spinosum in a 71-year-old man; see Krmpotic-Namanic et al. (2001) for an accessory oval foramen.

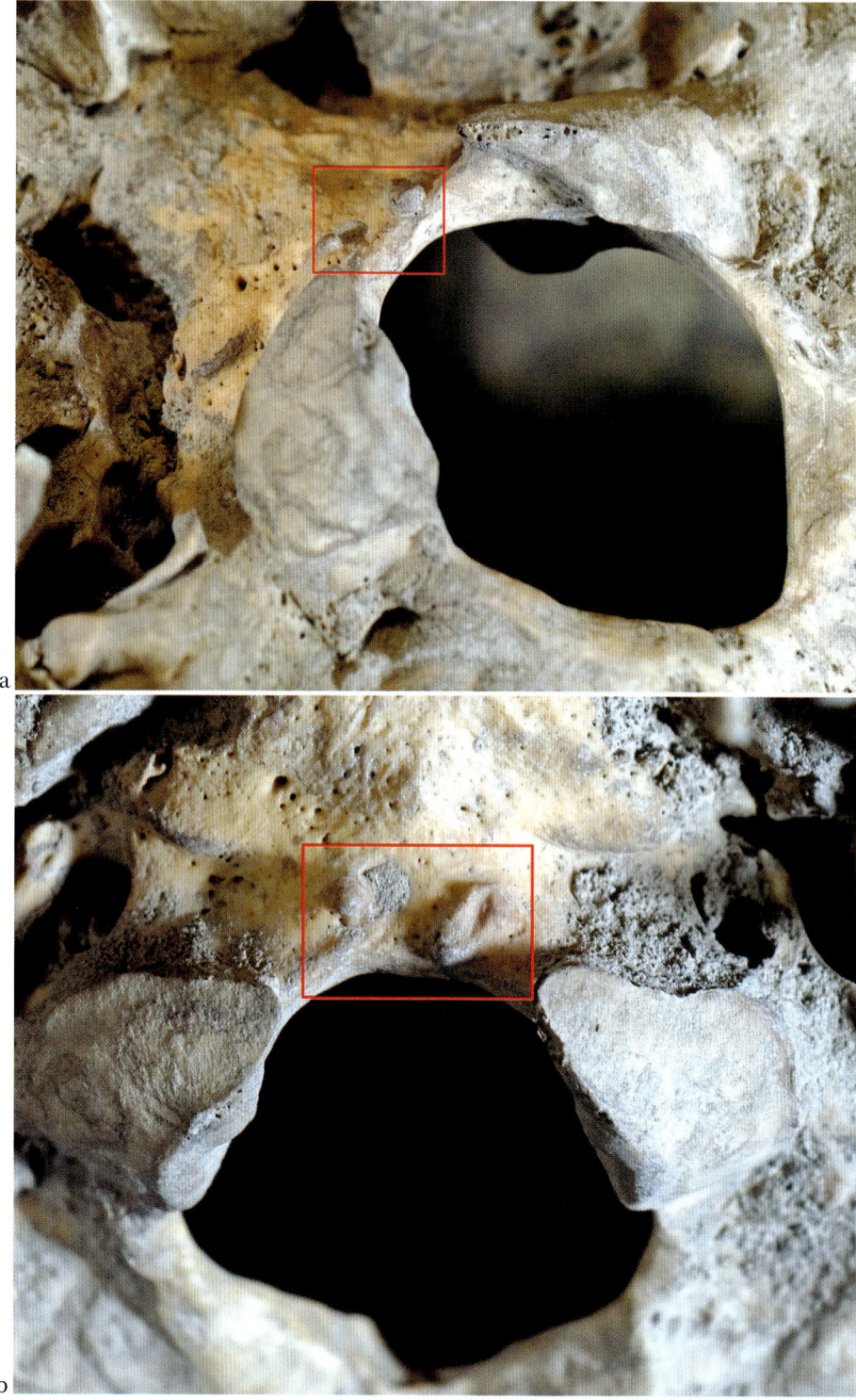

Figure 430a-b. Bilateral and asymmetrical precondylar tubercles. (a) Bilateral and asymmetrical precondylar tubercles (rectangle) in an adult, probable female (SI 243944). (b) Higher magnification showing that the two tubercles are not connected to the occipital condyles nor to one another and that the left tubercle is larger than the right. Uncommon finding. Cf. Agrawal et al. (2010); Barnes (1994); Broman (1957); Gupta et al. (1981); Hanihara and Ishida (2001b); Hauser and DeStefano (1989); Kale et al. (2009b); Marshall (1955); Oetteking (1923); Vasudeva and Choudhry (1996).

Basilar (Inferior) View of the Skull 339

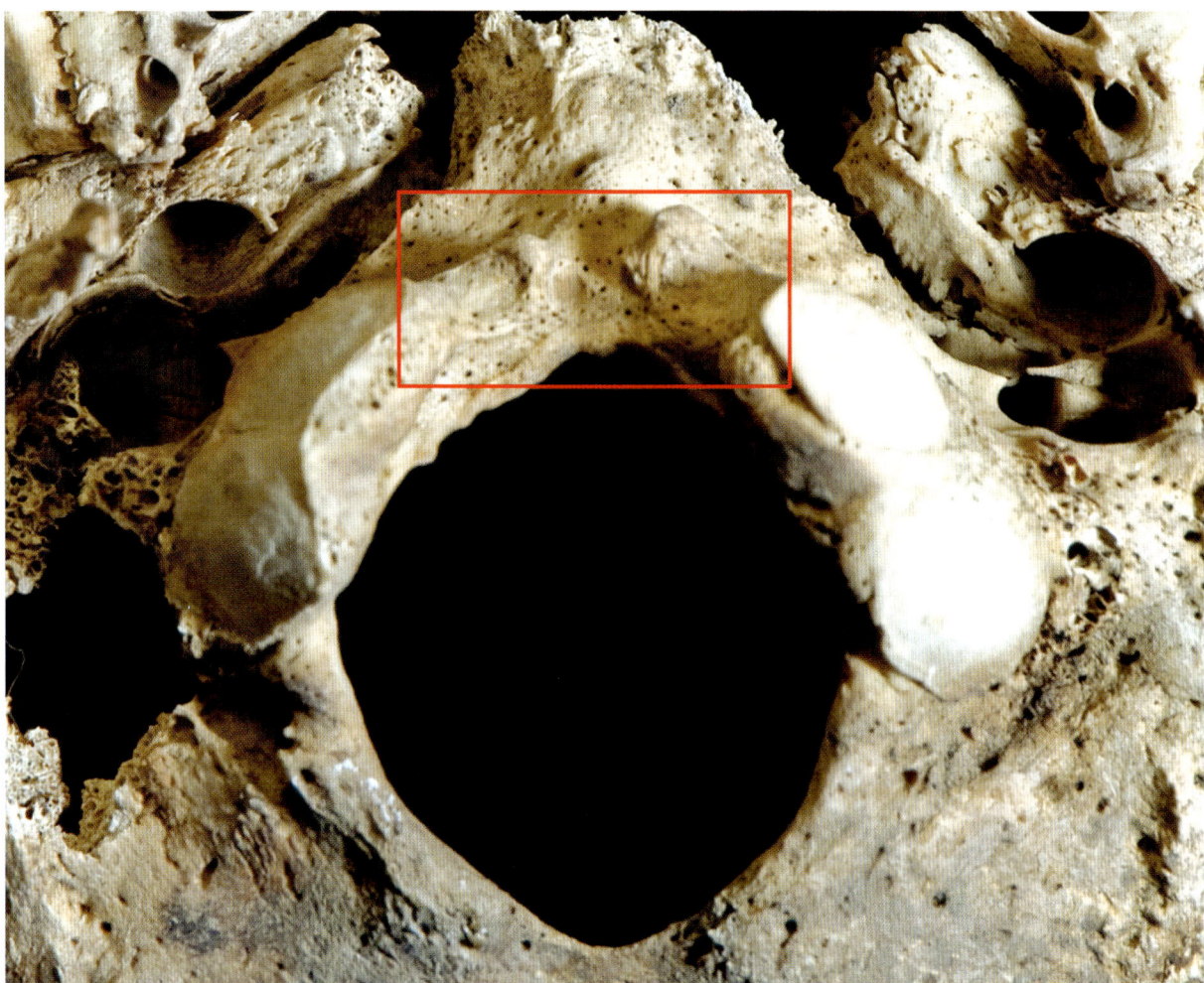

Figure 431. Bilateral basilar processes (rectangle), occasionally referred to as labia foraminis magni, anterior to the occipital condyles in an adult probable male (SI 243950). Also note that the left occipital condyles are divided, resulting in two separate facets. Cf. Barnes (1994); Kale et al. (2009b); Oetteking (1923); Prescher et al. (1996).

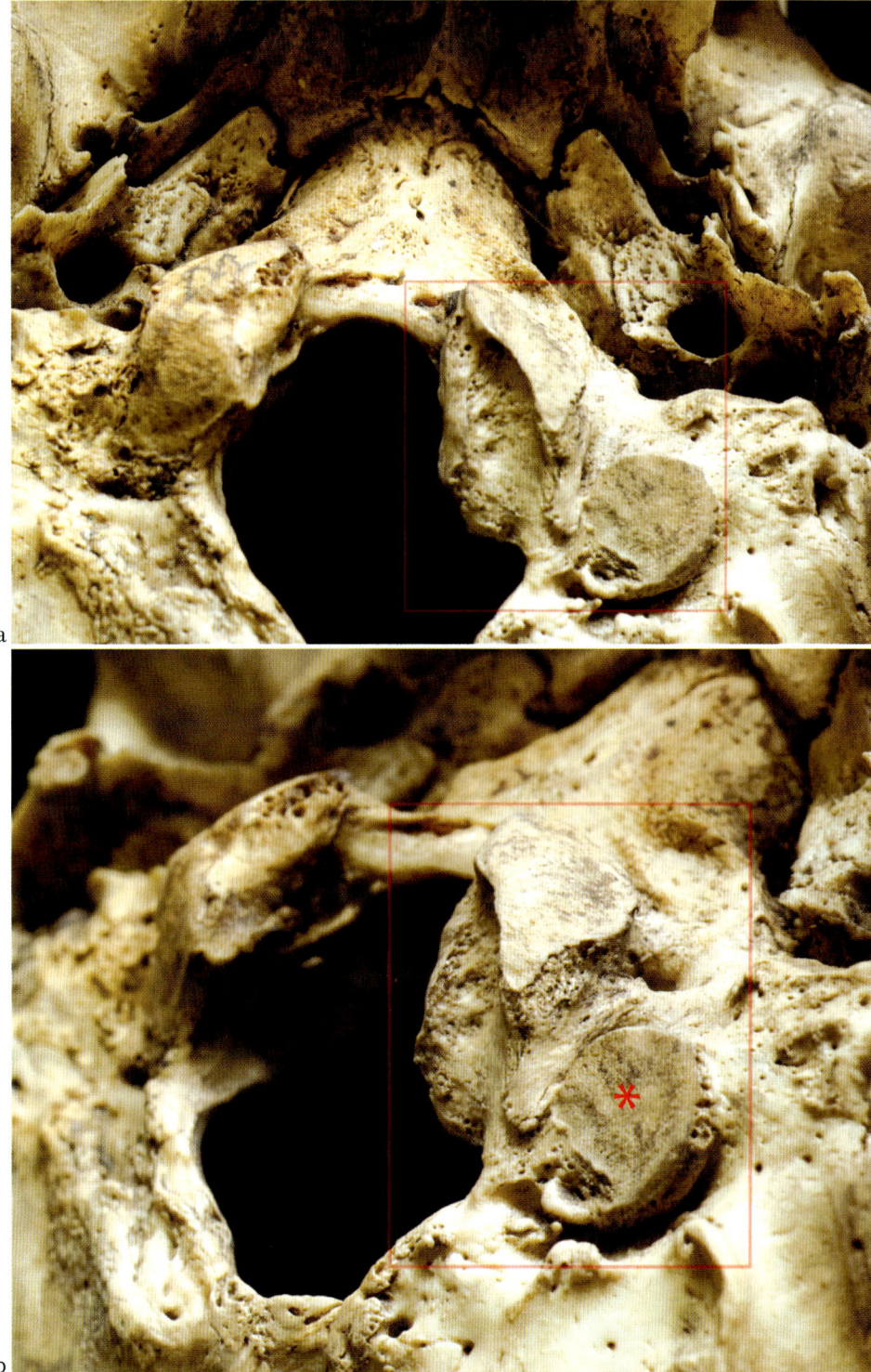

Figure 432a-b. Postcondylar or paracondylar process. (a) Unusual morphology of the left occipital condyle (square) possibly representing a postcondylar, or paracondylar process, and an asymmetrical foramen magnum in a subadult African male (UPenn 1224 L606). (b) Oblique view of the condyle and postcondylar process (*). This example could also be a divided left occipital condyle (no vertebrae are present for examination). Rare trait. Cf. Prescher (1997); Naderi et al. (2005).

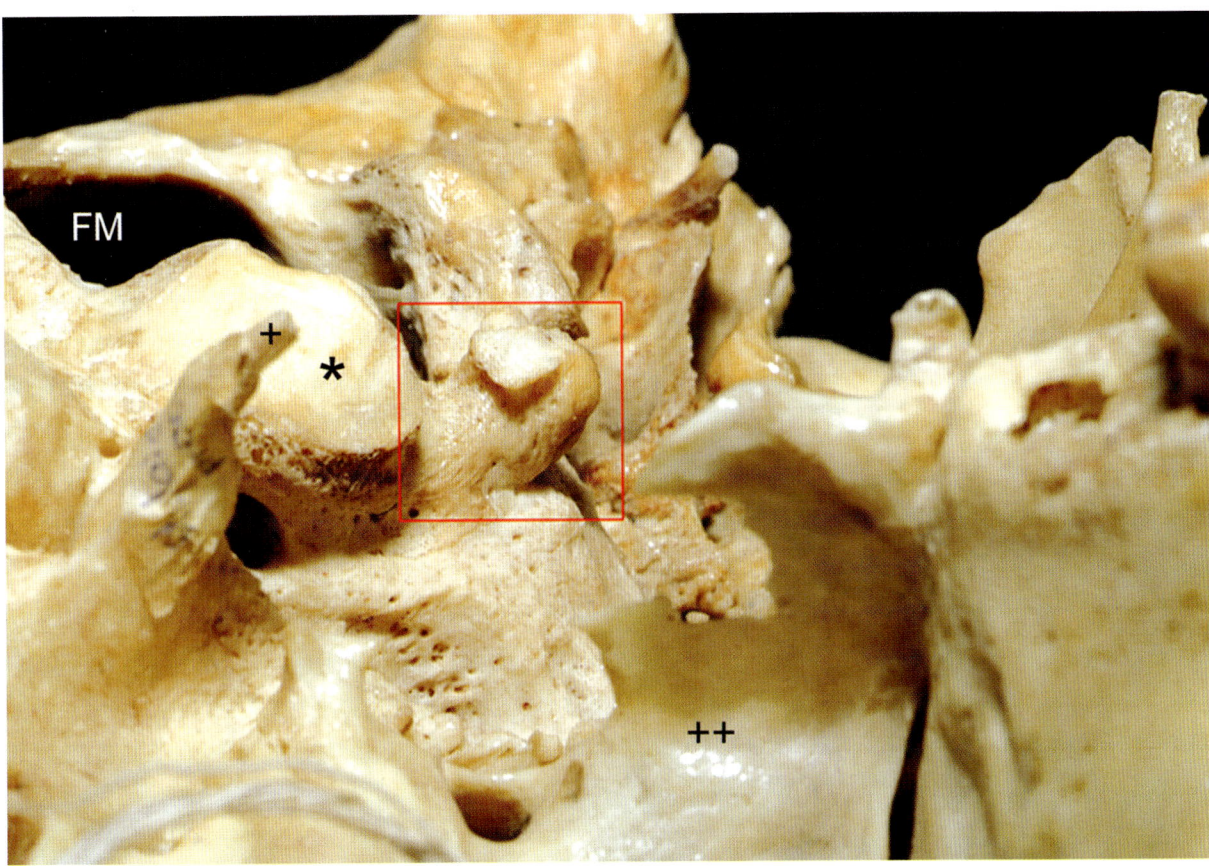

Figure 433. An unusually large, faceted precondylar tubercle (square), tertiary condyle, or third occipital condyle in an adult Thai male skull (KKU) viewed from the inferolateral perspective with the skull inverted to emphasize the large groove between articular surfaces. For anatomical positioning note foramen magnum (FM), left temporal styloid process (+), left occipital condyle and left lateral pterygoid plate (++). Uncommon finding. Cf. Oetteking (1923); Vasudeva and Choudhry (1996).

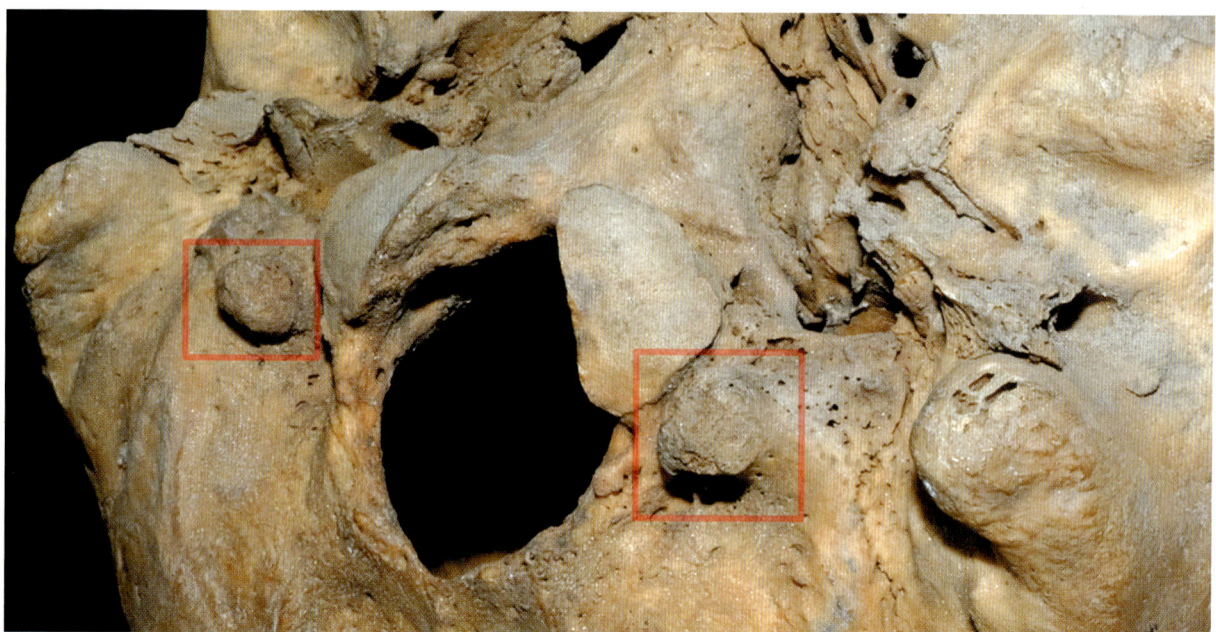

Figure 434. Bilateral paracondylar tubercles (squares) (UPenn). Cf. Corner (1896); Hauser and DeStefano (1989).

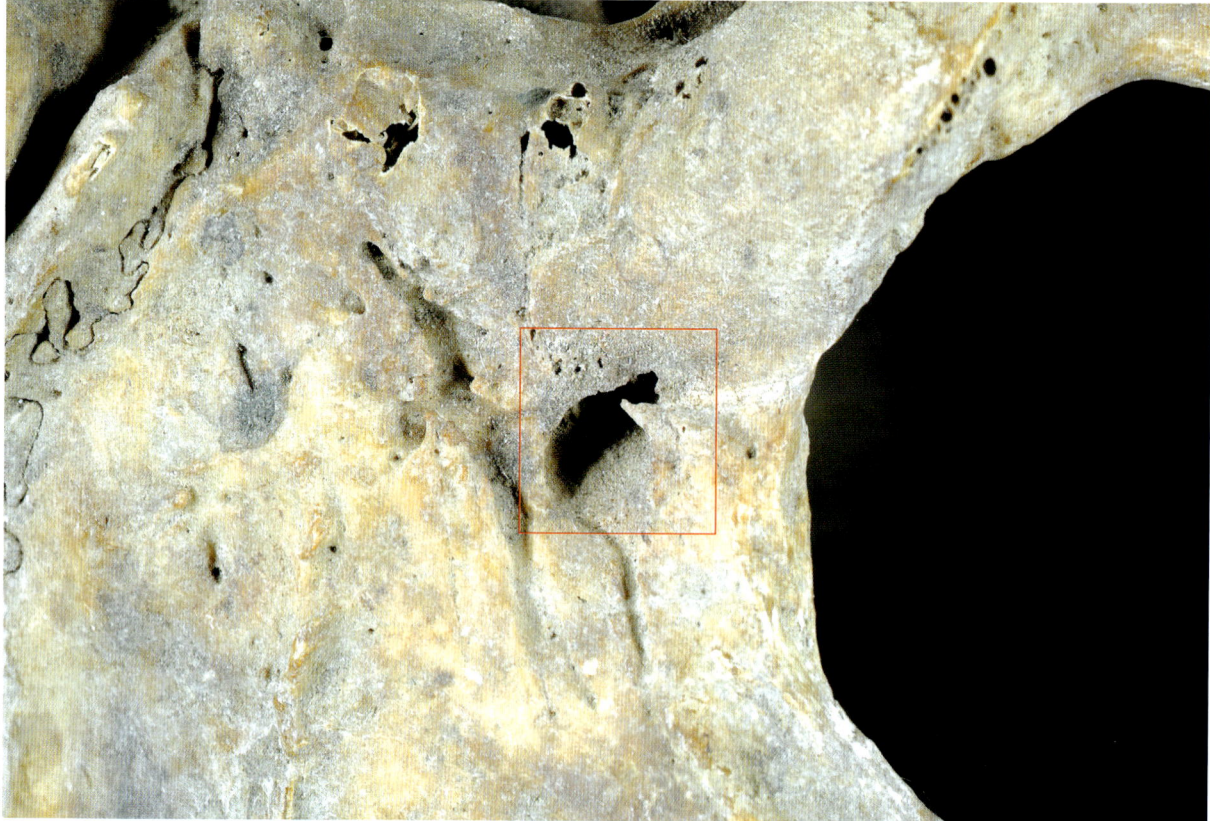

Figure 435. Partial bridging (square) of the right postcondylar fossa/canal in the form of a small spike of bone in an adult Asian skull (CIL). Uncommon finding. Cf. Berge and Bergman (2001).

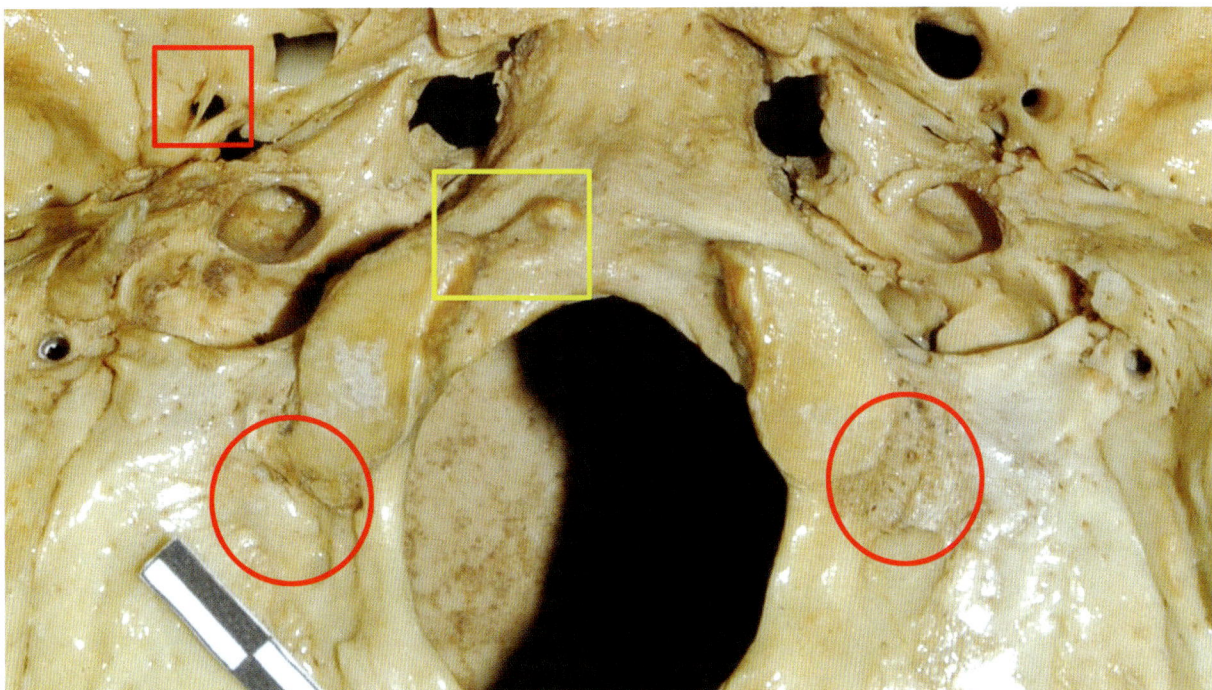

Figure 436. Bar of bone (red square) extending across the right foramen spinosum from the sphenoid spine to the region of the alar ligament. Also present is a right precondylar tubercle (yellow square) and bilateral absence of the postcondylar canals (red circles) in an adult Thai skull(KKU 1304 36). Cf. Oetteking (1923) for drawings of tubercles and ossifications on the cranial base; Ginsberg (1994); Wood-Jones (1931).

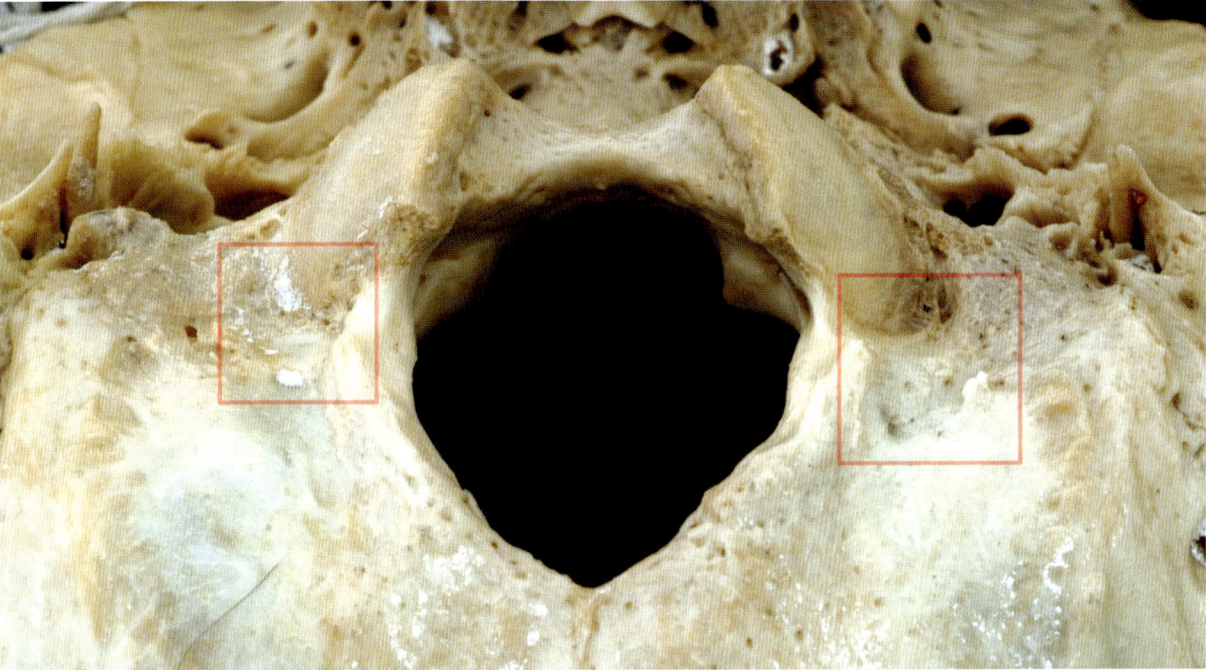

Figure 437. Absence of postcondylar canals (squares) in an adult skull (KKU 46-306). Boyd (1930) reported this canal as present unilaterally in 30.3% of crania and absent bilaterally in 23.1% of crania. Berge and Bergman (2001), in comparison, found the posterior condylar canal present in 54% of crania, present unilaterally in 36% of crania and absent bilaterally in 10% of crania. Cf. Ginsberg (1994).

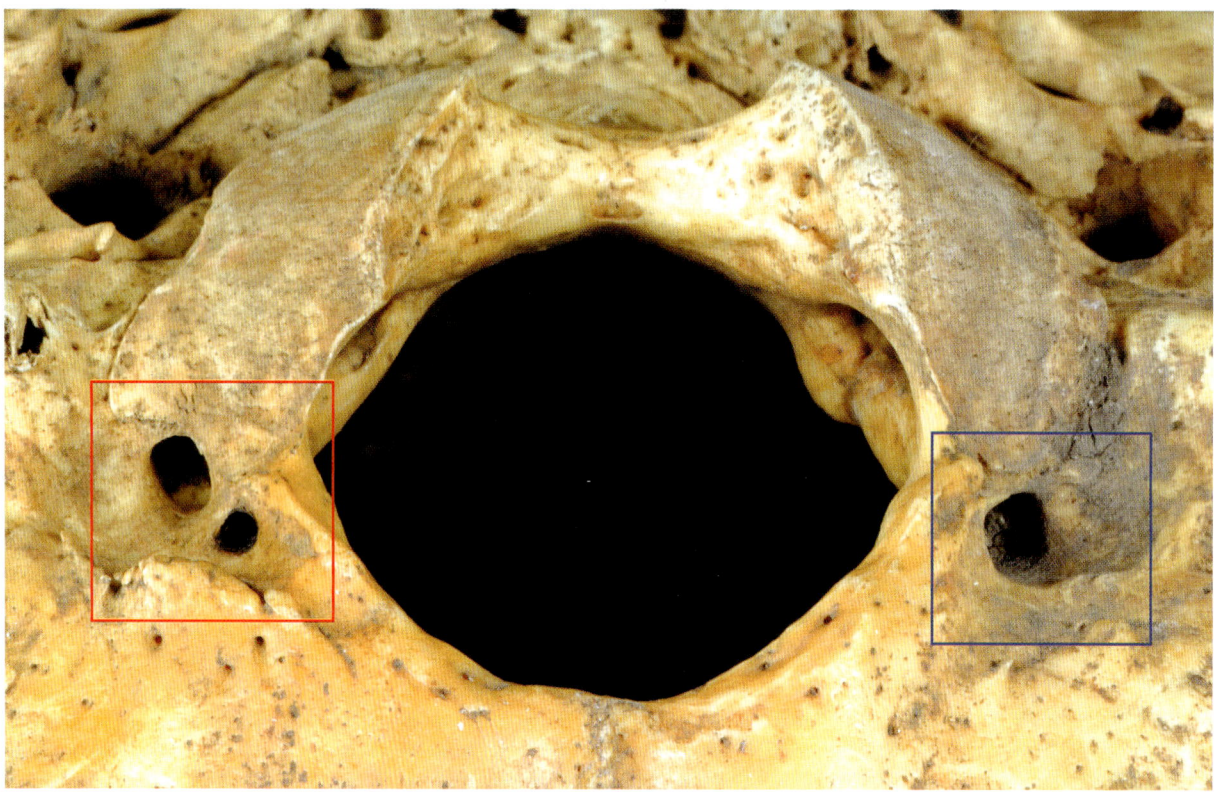

Figure 438. Double right/divided (red square) and single left (blue square) postcondylar foramina in an adult Asian male skull (CSC AC 005). Common to uncommon findings. Berge and Bergman (2001); Boyd (1930); Ginsberg (1994); Hanihara and Ishida (2001b). The postcondylar canal was present in 81% (94 of 116) patients (Ginsberg 1994).

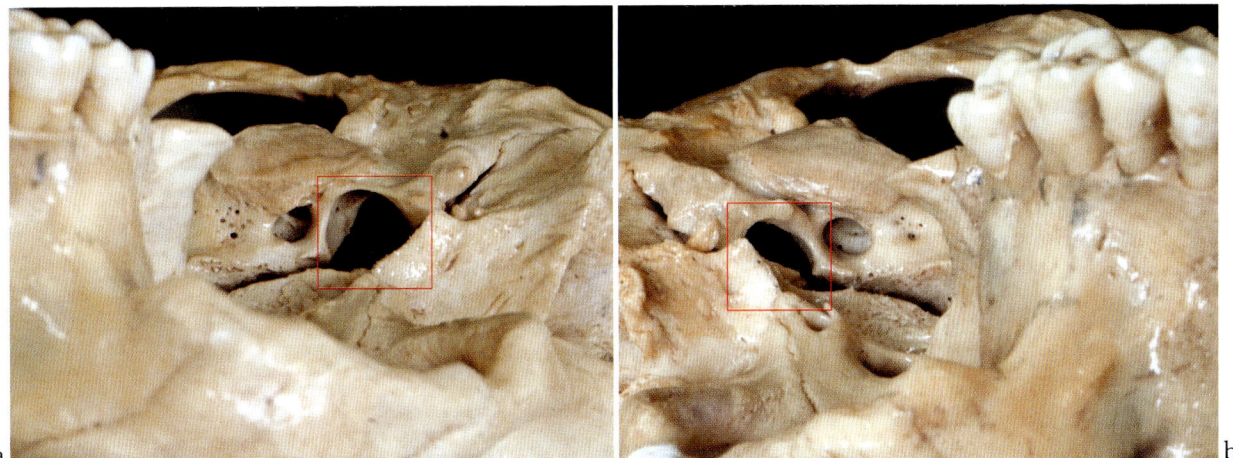

Figure 439a-b. Asymmetry of the jugular foramen. (a) Asymmetrical jugular foramen resulting in a much larger left fossa than (b) the right fossa in an adult male with congenital os odontoideum, an upward or cranial shift of the occipitocervical border (KKU 0202). Jugular foramen dominance has been shown to be correlated to hand preference (Adams et al. 1997), although other researchers have found no statistically significant correlation in symmetry of the jugular foramen with long bones of the arms (e.g., Glassman and Bass 1986). See Barnes (1994 and 2008) for more on the os odontoideum.

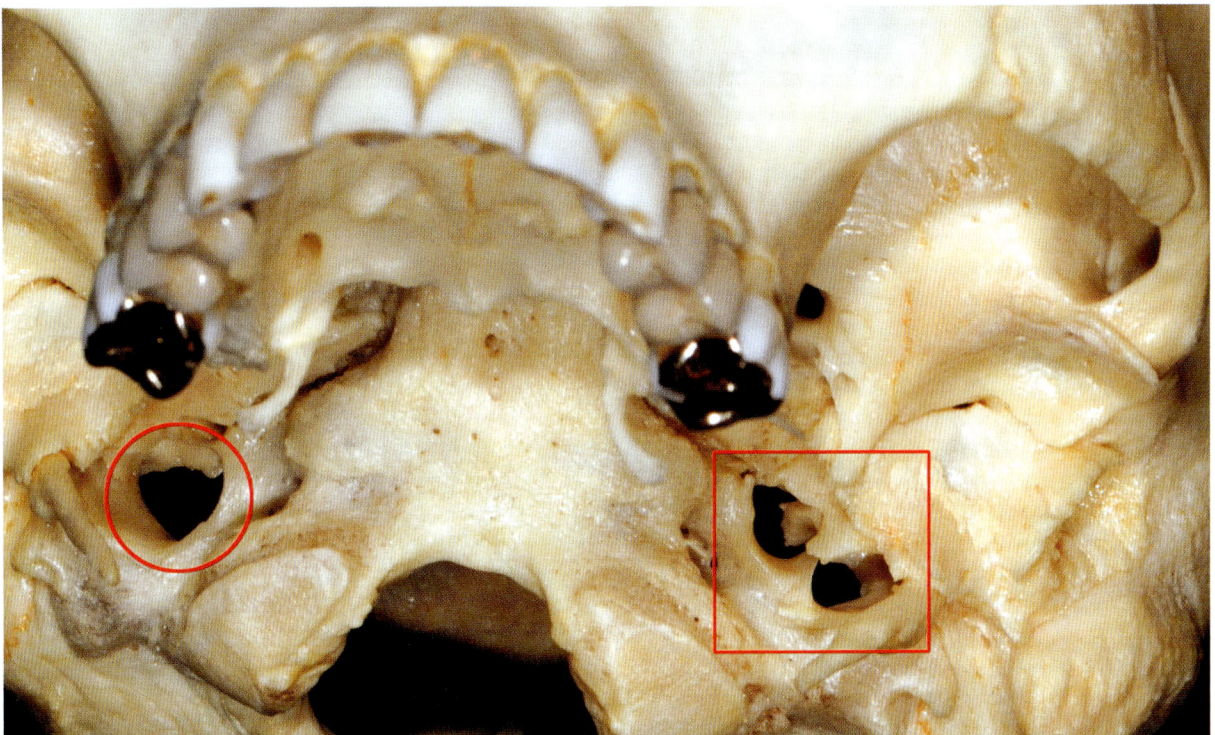

Figure 440. Divided left (square) and single right (circle) jugular fossa in a 54-year-old White female (JABSOM 1056). Both are common variants.

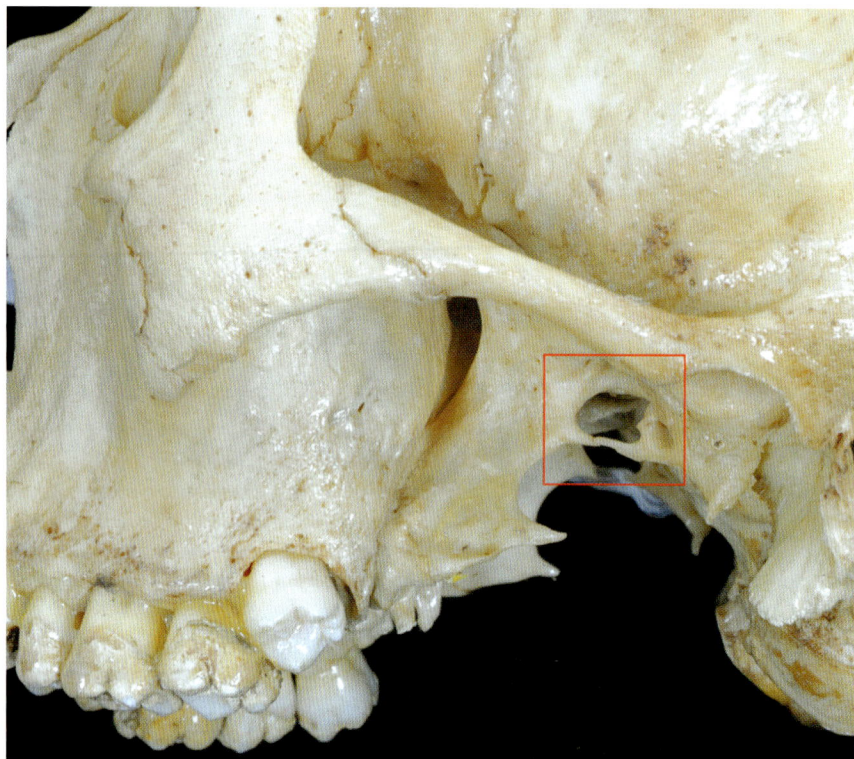

Figure 441. Pterygoalar bridge/bar and foramen (rectangle) in a young adult Thai skull (KKU). Pterygoalar foramen is present in about 1% of individuals (Shaw 1993). Cf. Antonopoulou et al. (2008); Chouke (1946); Chouke and Hodes (1951); Galdames et al. (2010); Hauser and DeStefano (1989); Peuker et al. (2001); Rosa et al. (2010); Rossi et al. (2011); Tubbs et al. (2009).

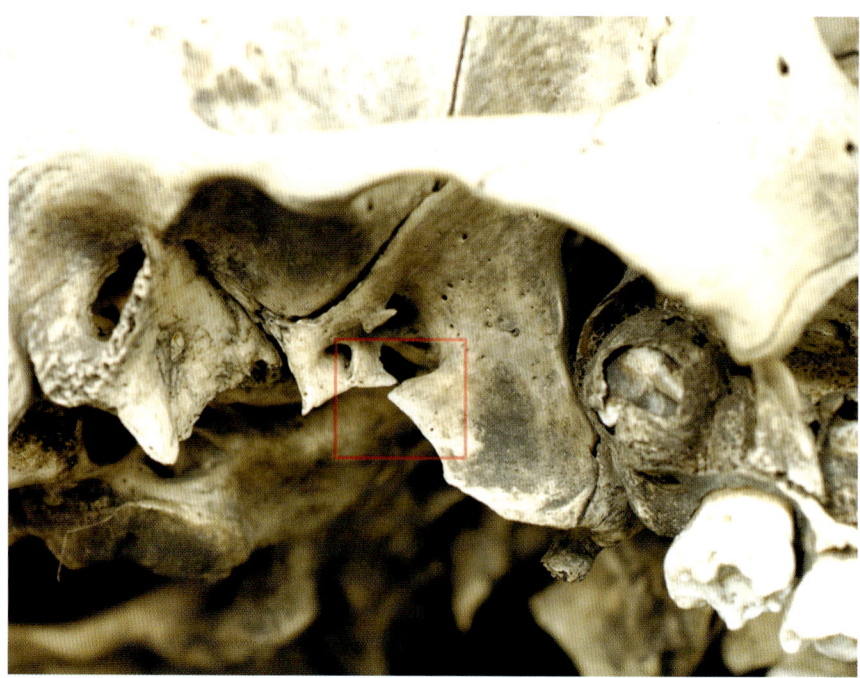

Figure 442. Partial pterygoalar (square) bridging in a 4- to 5-year-old child (Mütter Museum 17831-12). Cf. Skrzat et al. (2005).

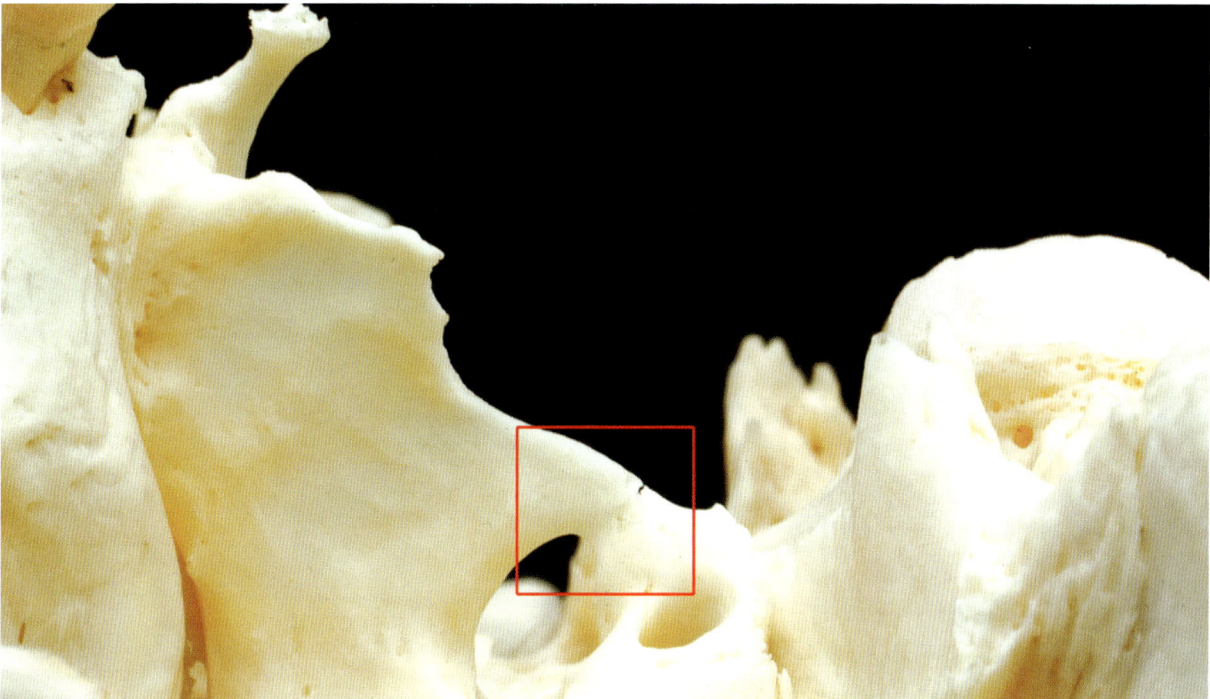

Figure 443. Right pterygosphenoid bridge and foramen (of Civinini) showing a faint line of fusion (square) of the two ligaments in an adult Asian (CSC AC042).

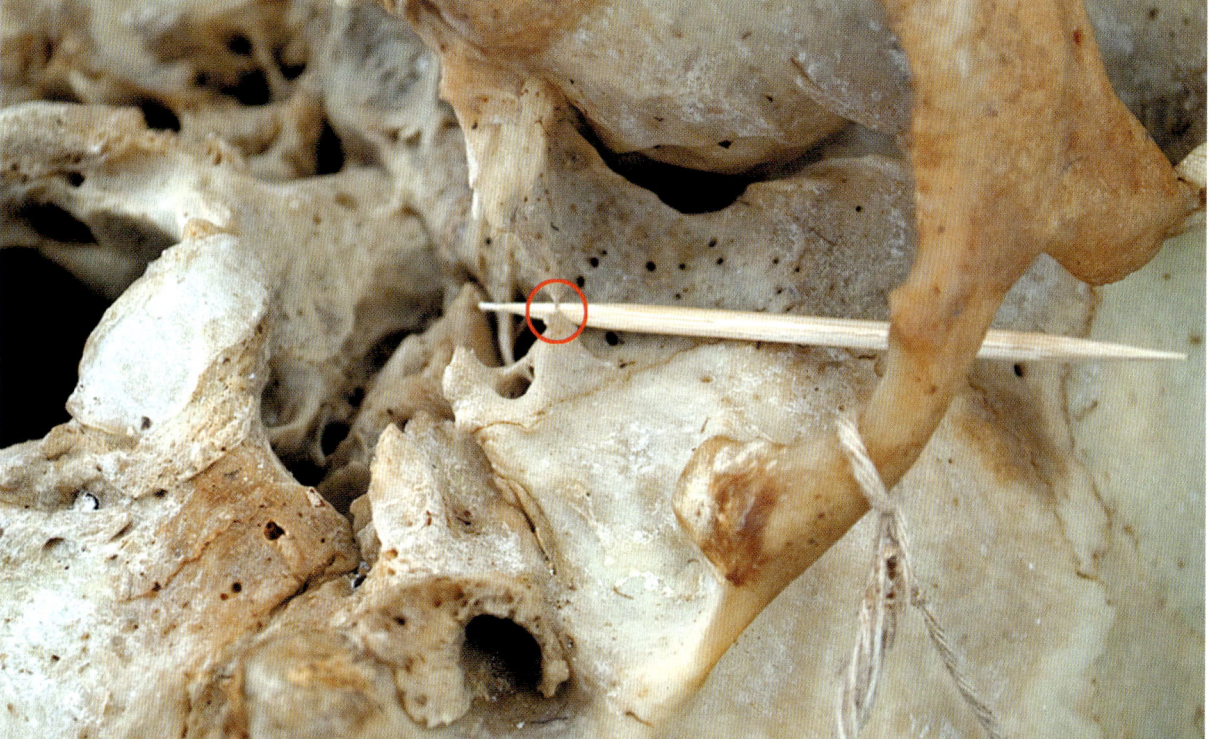

Figure 444. Small left pterygoalar bridge forming a foramen (toothpick and circle) in an adult Thai male skull (KKU 0675). This osseous bridge, when complete, is known as the foramen of Hyrtl and forms lateral to the foramen ovale. Cf. Hauser and DeStefano (1989); Peuker et al. (2001); Rosa et al. (2010); Rossi et al. (2011).

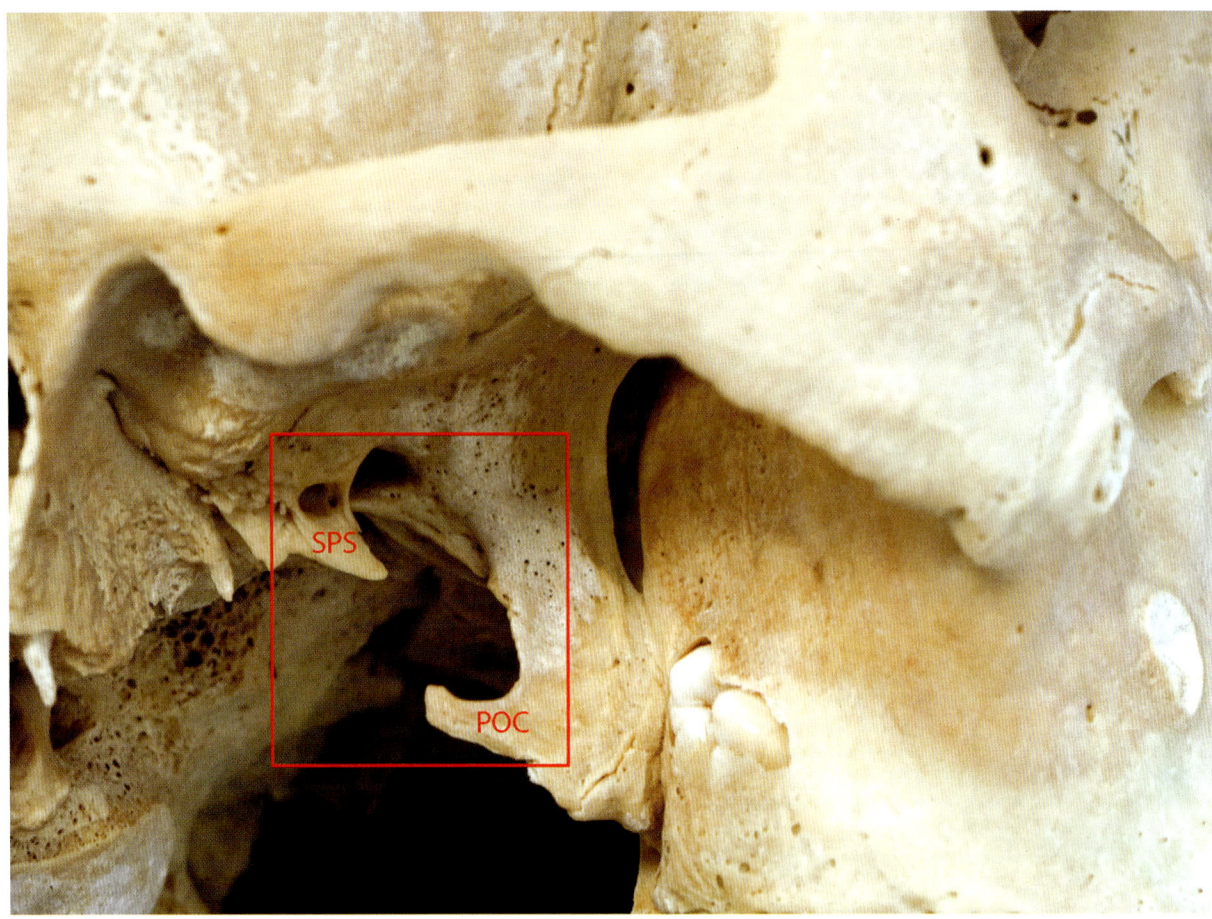

Figure 445. Partial pterygospinous bridging in an adult Asian female skull (CSC AC036). Lateral view showing calcification and formation of calcified spines extending from the spine of the sphenoid (SPS) and the process of Civinini (POC). If these two spines join, the resulting foramen is known as the foramen of Civinini (POC). Chouke (1946) noted pterygospinous bridging in 7.9% of 6,000 crania. Cf. Antonopoulou et al. (2008); Chouke and Hodes (1951); Hauser and DeStefano (1989); Peuker et al. (2001); Rosa et al. (2010); Rossi et al. (2011); Tebo (1968).

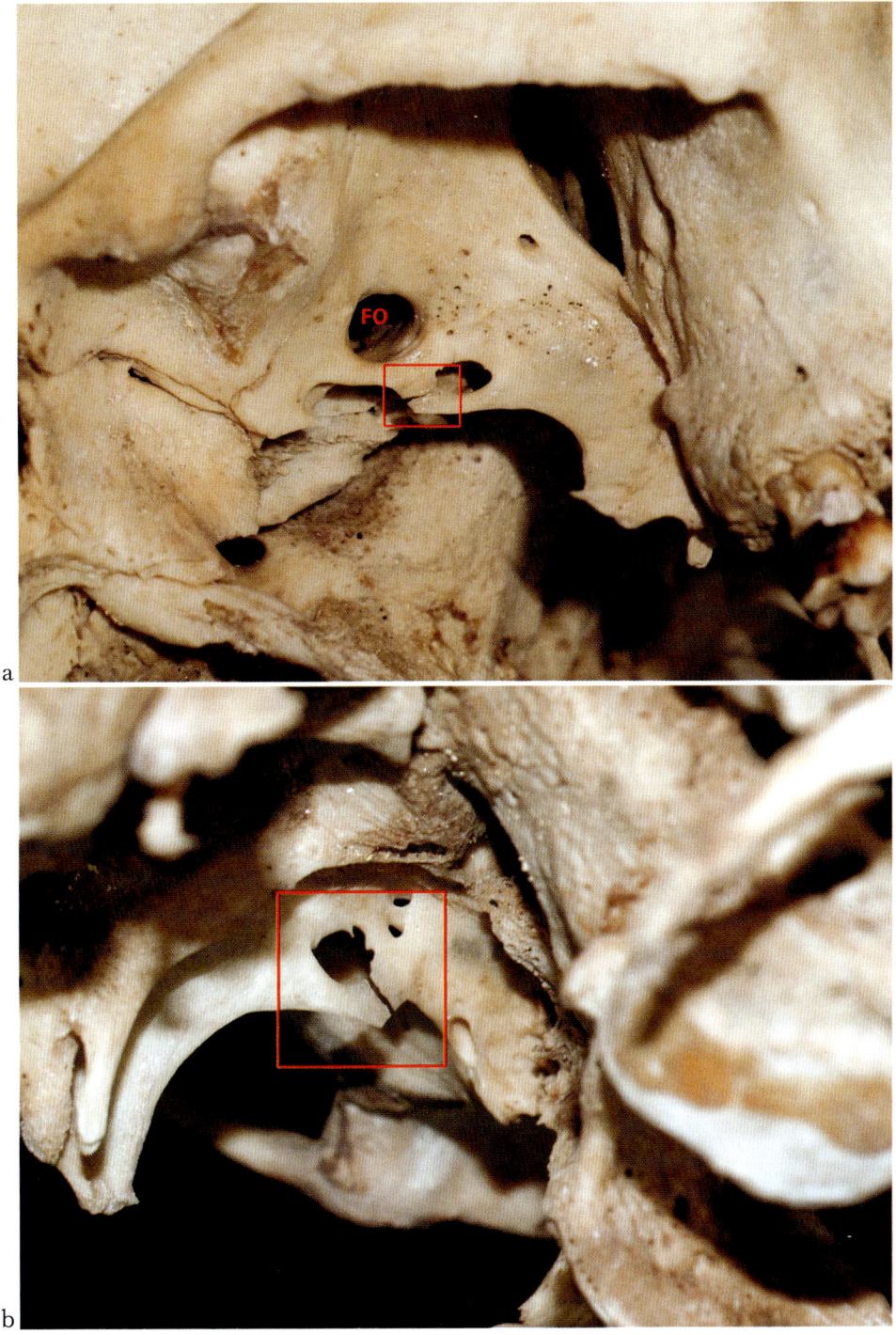

Figure 446a-b. Calcification of the right pterygospinous ligament. (a) External and (b) internal views of right pterygospinous ligament (square) in an adult Asian (KKU) (FO = foramen ovale). Note the opposing edges where the ligaments nearly meet are almost identical in size and shape as they ossify towards one another (also note the two small accessory foramina). Skrzat et al. (2006b) reported on a similar specimen with a laterally facing and laterally visible FO (a), which they called the oval canal (canalis ovalis), a rare finding. This is a complicated region of the skull that warrants additional research.

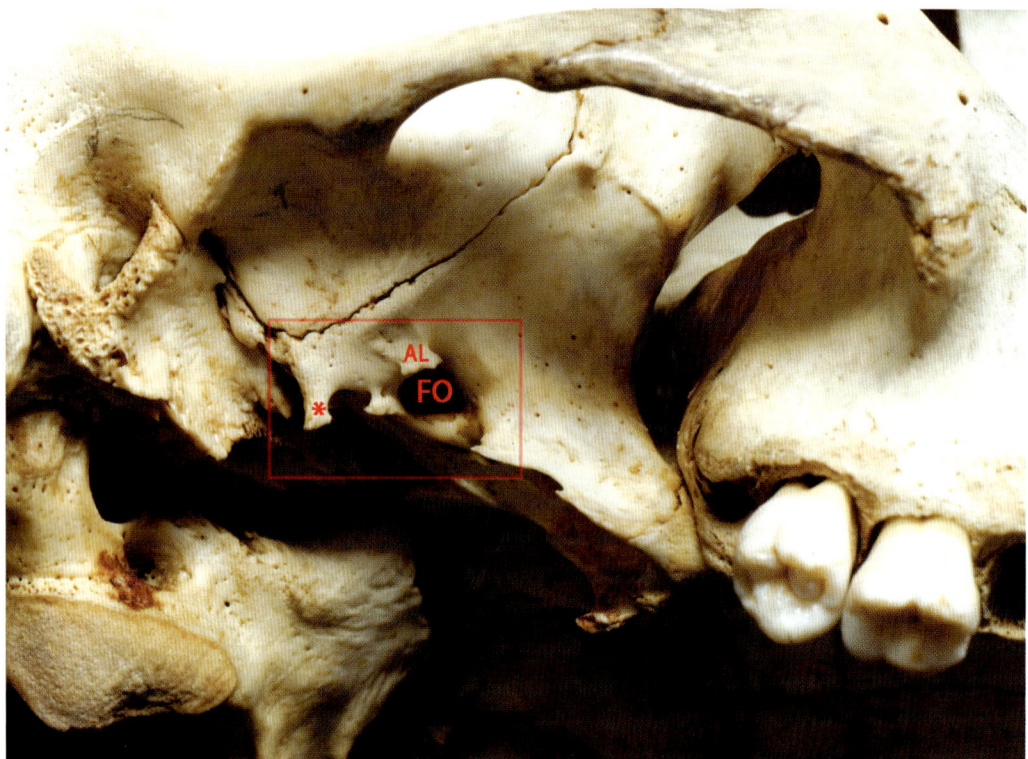

Figure 447. Foramen ovale (FO), trace ossification and partial bridging of the pterygolar ligament (AL) and partial bridging of the sphenoid ligament (*) across the foramen spinosum (UPenn).

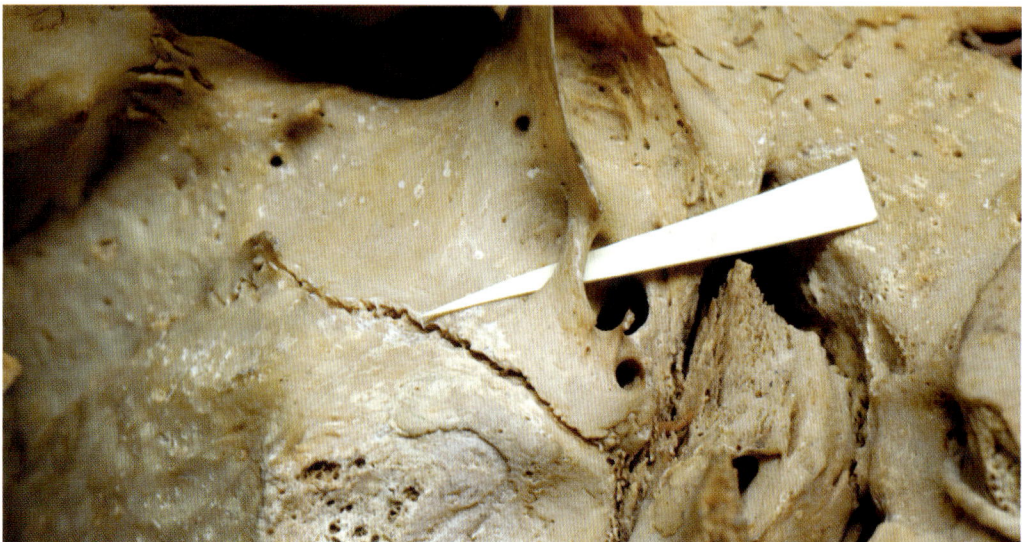

Figure 448. Right pterygoalar bridging/bar and foramen of Hyrtl (arrowhead) in an adult (UPenn 15498). Note the ossified ligament connecting to the lateral pterygoid plate is lateral to the foramen ovale, indicating it is the pterygoalar, not the pterygospinous ligament. Cf. Chouke (1946); Chouke and Hodes (1951); Daimi et al. (2011); Hauser and DeStefano (1989).

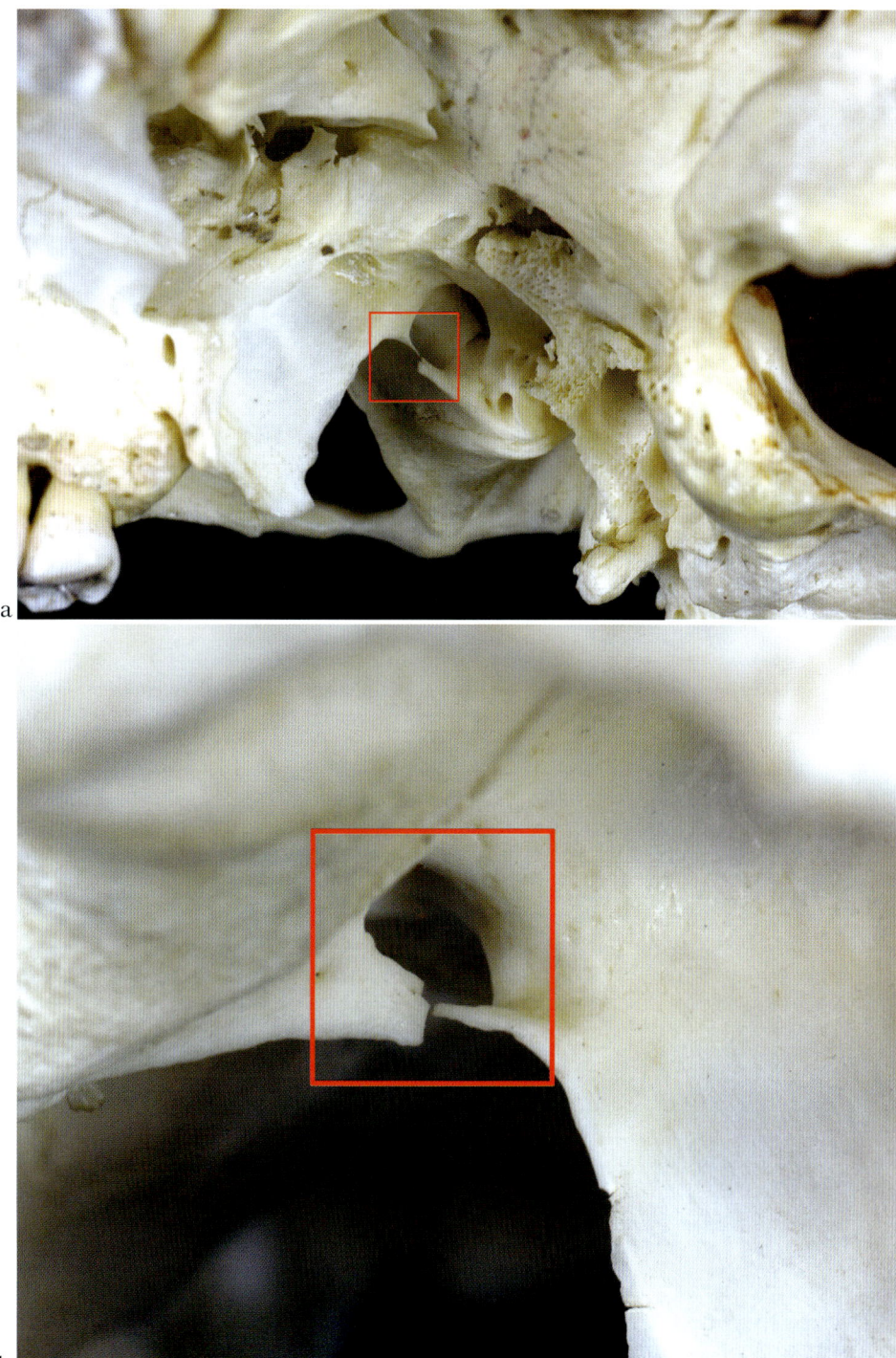

Figure 449a-b. Partial right pterygoalar bridging in an adult (Photo Daniel Herrera; CSC AS003). (a) Internal view demonstrating incomplete bridging (square) on the right side and complete osseous bridging with formation of a pterygoalar foramen on the left side. Note the small spiked projection emanating from the lateral pterygoid plate. There is a slight gap between the pterygoid and alar ligament projections. (b) Higher magnification from the lateral and external perspective of the ossified or calcified right pterygoalar ligament (square).

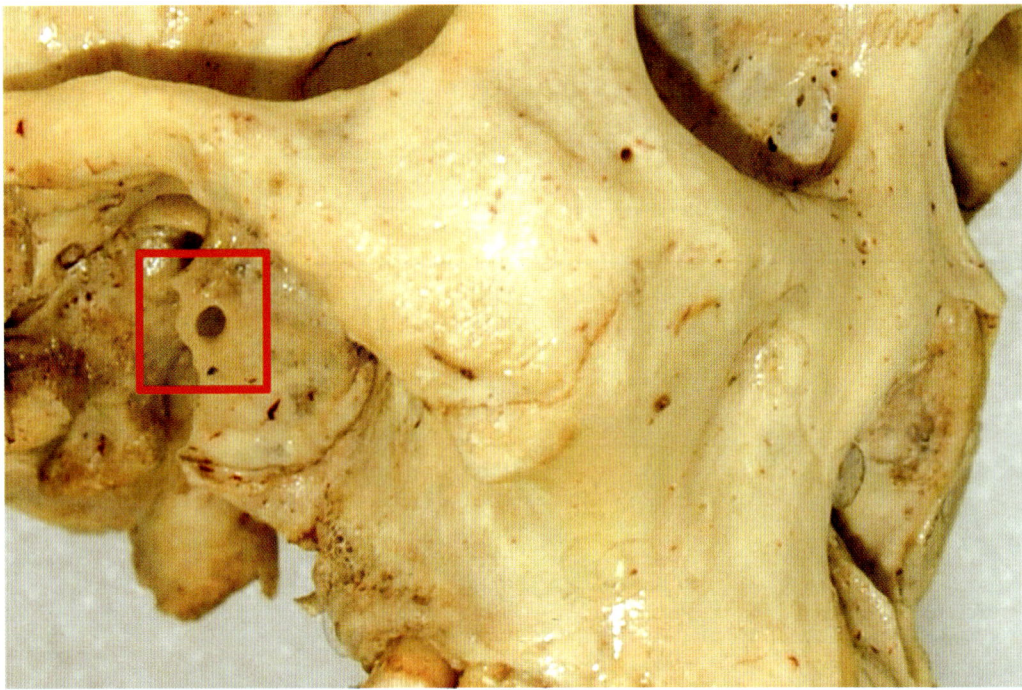

Figure 450. Right pterygospinous bridge and small foramen, often referred to as the Foramen of Civinini (square) in an adult Thai skull (KKU). Ossification of this ligament is a common finding. Rossi et al. (2011) found complete or partial ossification of the pterygoalar ligament in 5 (2.73%) of 183 Brazilian adult crania 30 to 60 years of age. Note that calcification of the pterygospinous ligament occurs posterior to the foramen ovale (FO) and crosses over the FO, while ossification of the pterygoalar ligament is lateral to the FO. Cf. Antonopoulou et al. (2008); Chouke (1946); Galdames et al. (2010); Nayak et al. (2007); Peker et al. (2002); Rossi et al. (2011); Skrzat et al. (2005). Ossification and calcification are often used synonymously.

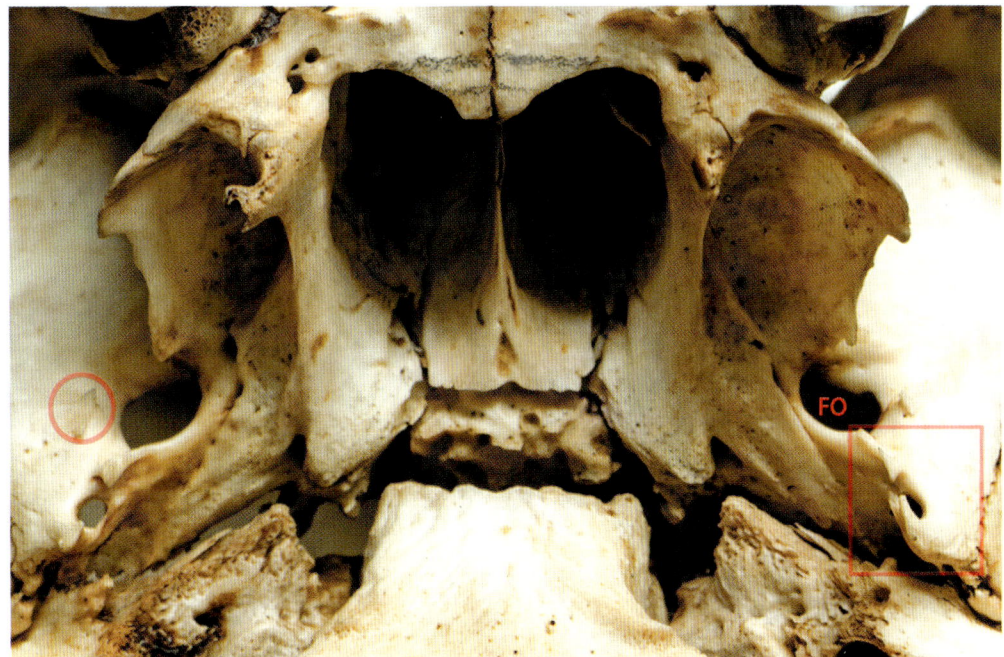

Figure 451. Partial bridging (spinous) over the left foramen spinosum (square) and trace ossification of the right pterygoalar ligament (circle) in a subadult (UPenn). FO is the foramen ovale. Cf. Chouke (1946); Chouke and Hodes (1951); Daimi et al. (2011); Hauser and DeStefano (1989).

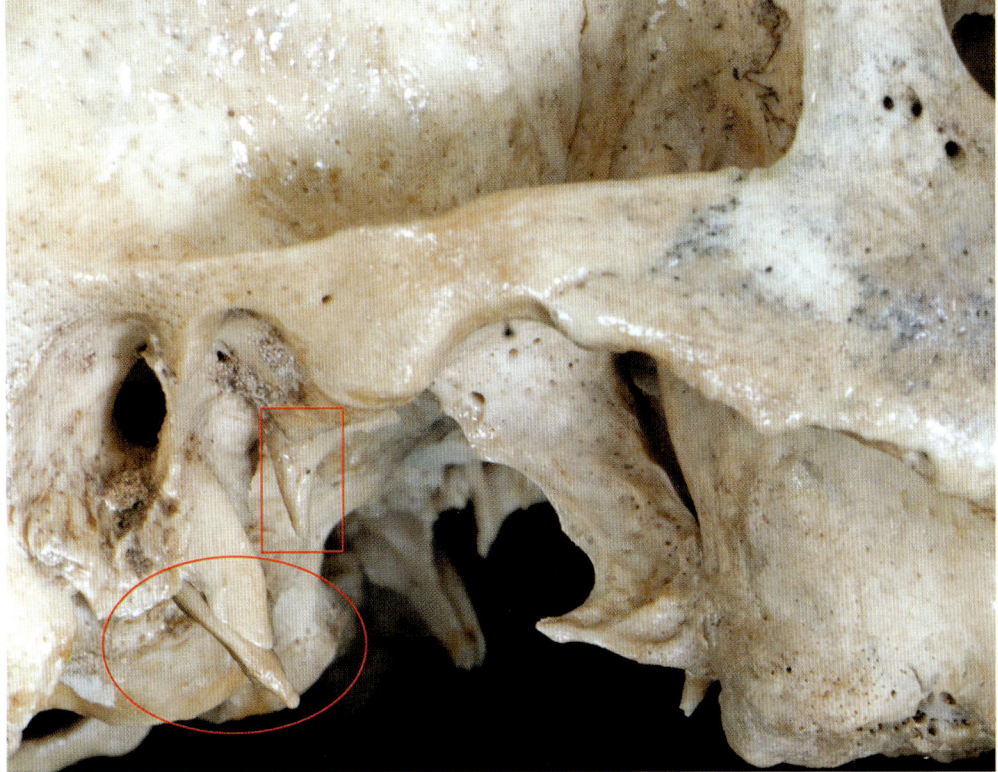

Figure 452. Unusually long and inferiorly directed right angular spine of the sphenoid (rectangle) compared to typical temporal styloid process (oval) in an adult Thai skull (KKU 688 38 B2 203).

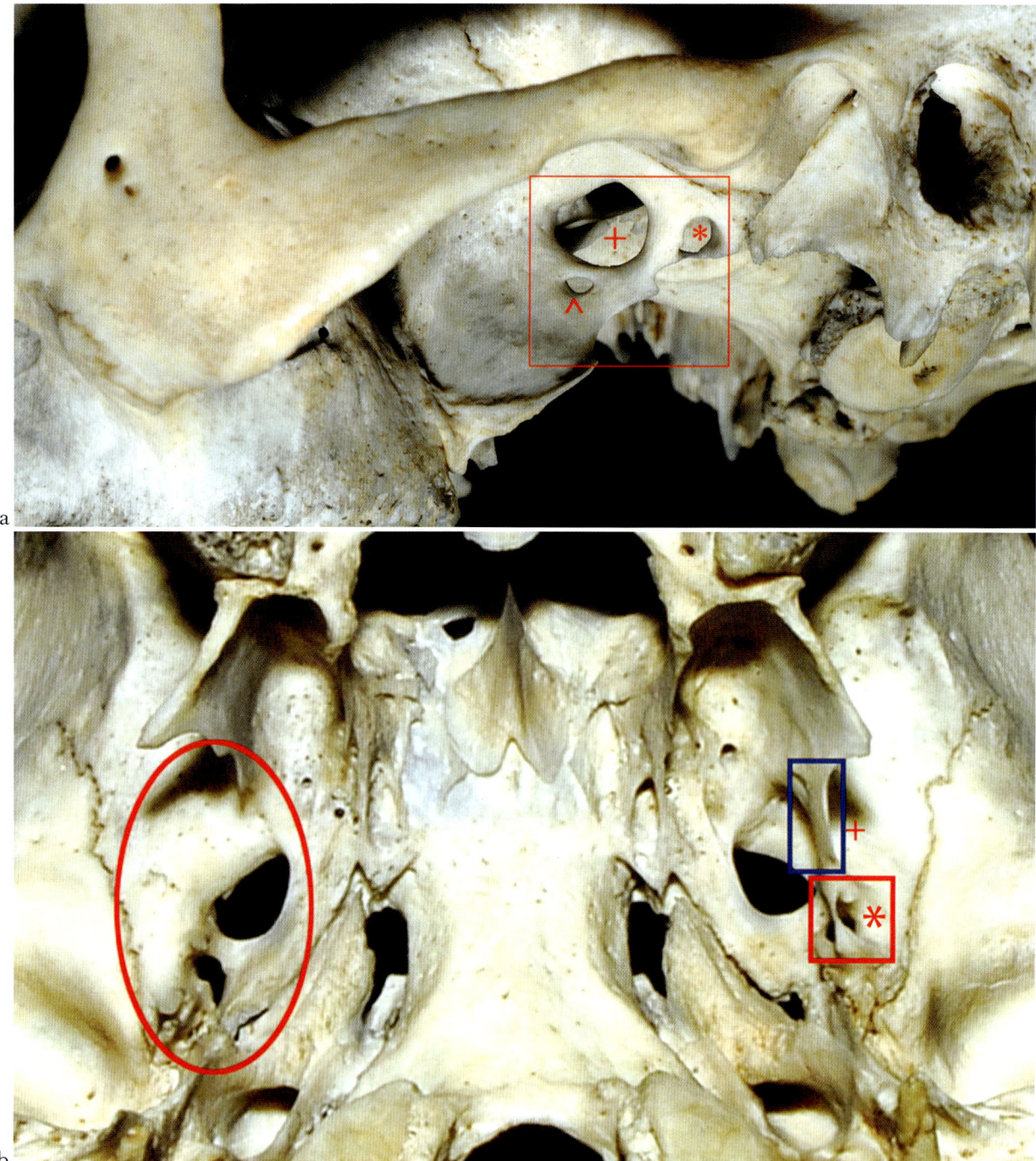

Figure 453a-b. Pterygospinous and pterygoalar bridges. (a) Left pterygospinous bridge (red square) and foramen (*), also known as Foramen of Civinini, and pterygoalar bridge and foramen (+) resulting in a large porus crotaphiticobuccinatorium foramen, also known as foramen of Hyrtl. The small accessory anterior foramen (∧) was formed by the pterygoalar bar and enlongation through ossification of two spines of bone along the posterior margin of the lateral pterygoid plate. (b) Ptery-gospinous bridge (red square and *) extends across the foramen spinosum; pterygoalar bridge indicted by blue rectangle and +. Note absence of bridging on the right side (red oval). Cf. Chouke and Hodes (1951); Daimi et al. (2011); Hauser and DeStefano (1989); Peuker et al. (2001); Skrzat et al. (2005); Tebo (1968); Tubbs et al. (2009). See Singh and Anand (2009) for position of the foramen spinosum as well as spinous bridging across the foramen spinosum.

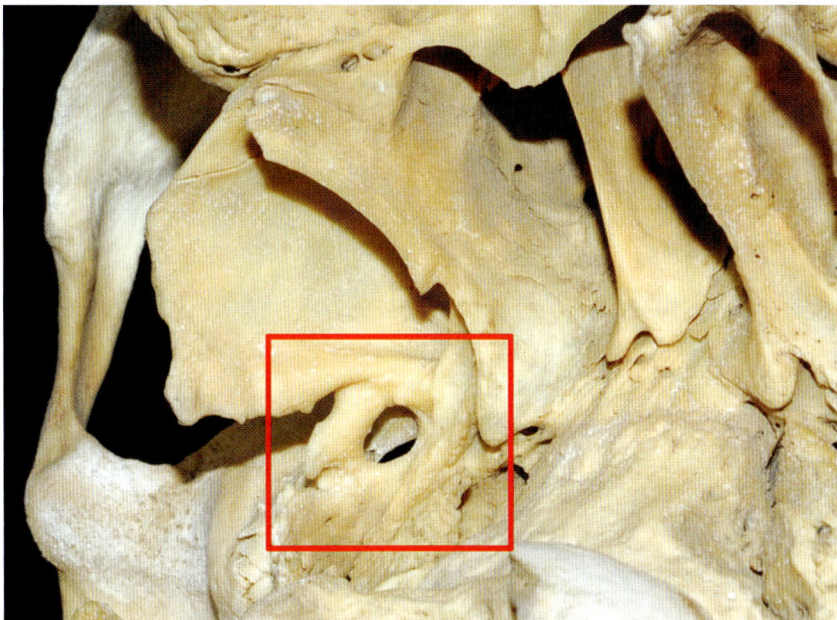

Figure 454. Pterygospinous bridge and foramen (of Civinini) in an ancient Peruvian (UPenn). Note the large size and "elephant-ear" shaped right lateral pterygoid plate. The foramen is formed by ossification and extension of the uppermost spine of the lateral pterygoid plate with the spinous ligament of the sphenoid. Cf. Daimi et al. (2011); Hauser and DeStefano (1989); Peuker (2001); Rosa et al. (2010); Rossi et al. (2011); Tebo (1968).

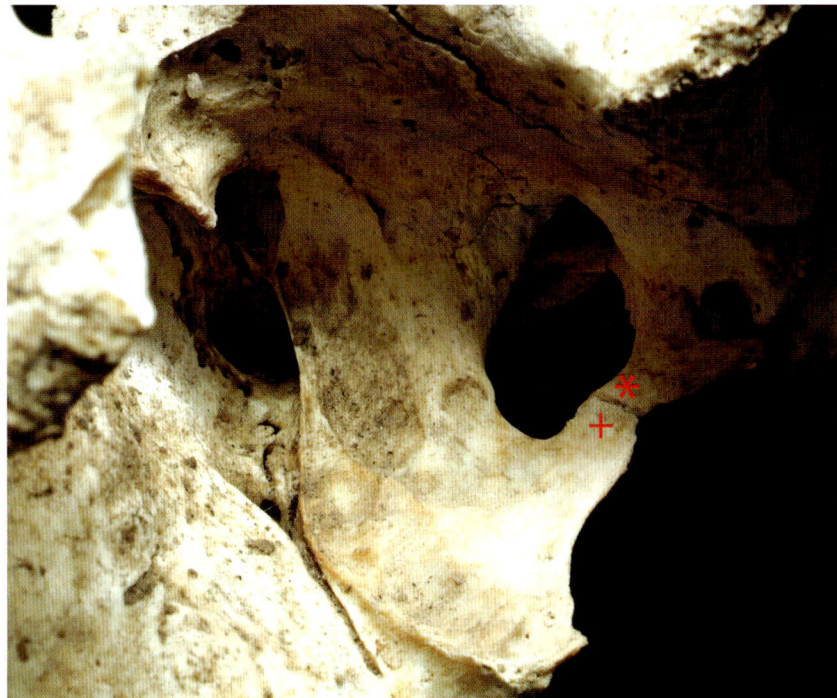

Figure 455. Junction of the ossified left pterygoid plate (+) and sphenoid spine (*) forming the pterygospinous bridge and foramen of Civinini (UPenn). The junction of these two spines, usually near the middle of the foramen, ranges from a pointed spike to a blunt bar of bone such as in this individual. Antonopoulou et al. (2008); Chouke (1941); Chouke and Hodes (1951); Galdames et al. (2010); Hauser and DeStefano (1989); Peuker et al. (2001); Rosa et al. (2010); Rossi et al. (2011); Tubbs et al. (2009).

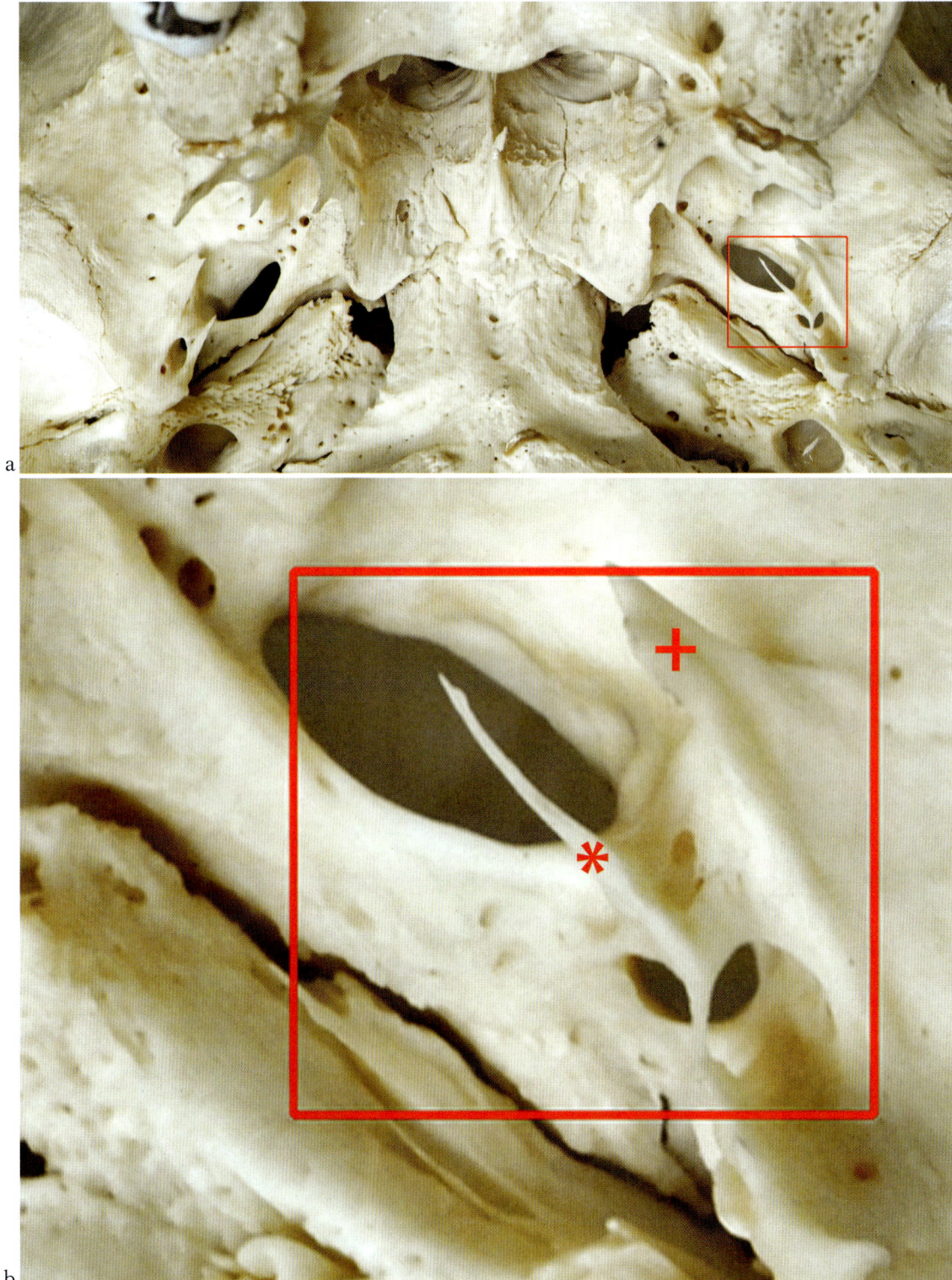

Figure 456a-b. Slender calcified spines in the left sphenoid bone. (a) Basilar view of a slender osseous projection (square) extending from the left foramen spinosum and partially spanning the foramen ovale. (b) High magnification of the left pterygospinous ligament (*) and the thicker pterygoalar ligament (+) in an adult Asian (KKU). Note that the calcified spinous projection (*) crosses, but is not lateral to the foramen ovale. This example illustrates an unusually thin and delicate spinous ligament.

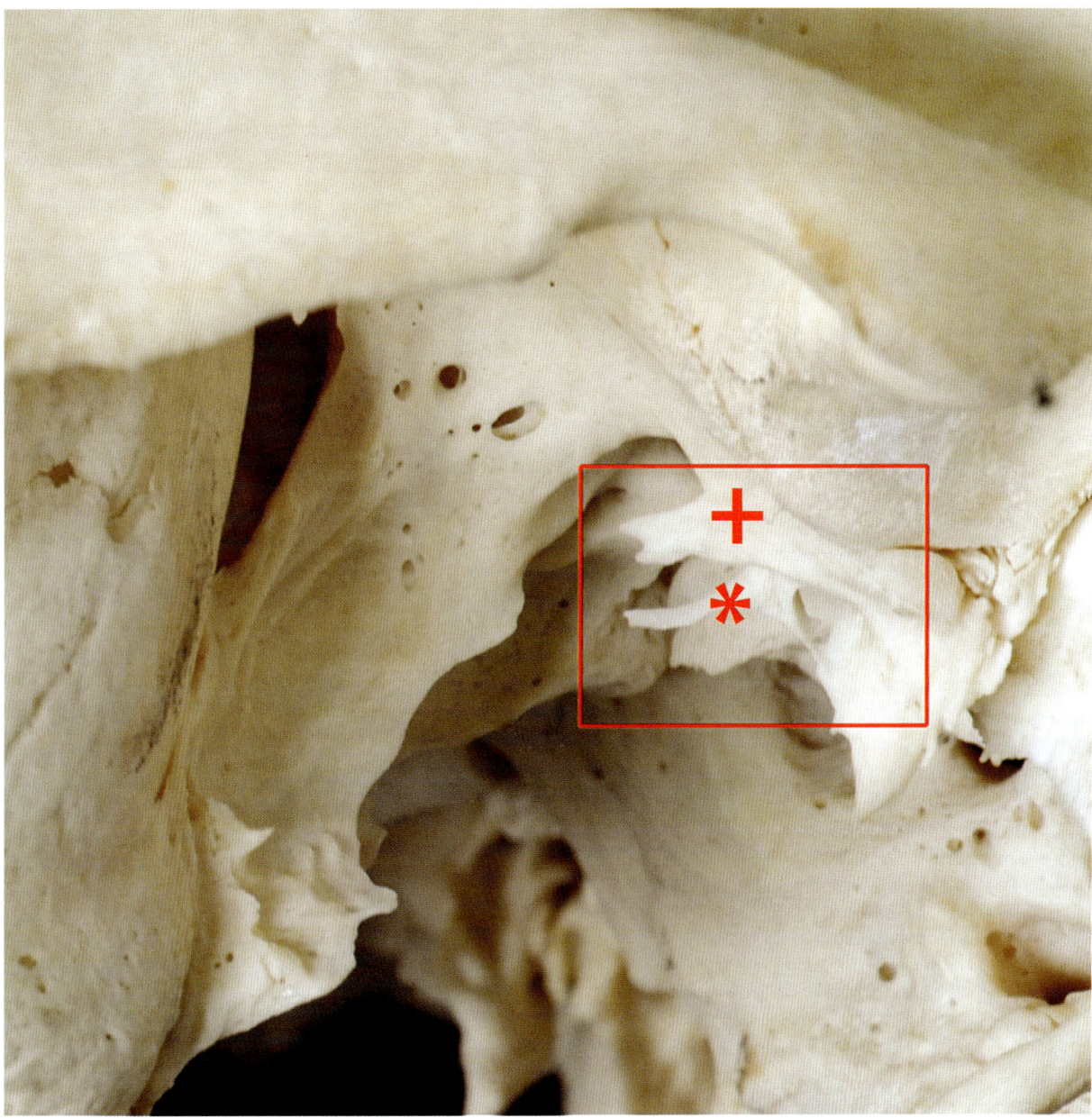

Figure 457. Left lateral view of calcification and partial bridging of the pterygoalar ligament (+) above the thinner pterygospinous ligament (*) in an adult Thai (KKU) (see Figure 456a-b for more views of this specimen). Antonopoulou et al. (2008); Chouke (1941); Chouke and Hodes (1951); Galdames et al. (2010); Hauser and DeStefano (1989); Peuker et al. (2001); Rosa et al. (2010); Rossi et al. (2011); Skrzat (2005); Tubbs et al. (2009). See Singh and Anand (2009) for more on bridging across the foramen spinosum.

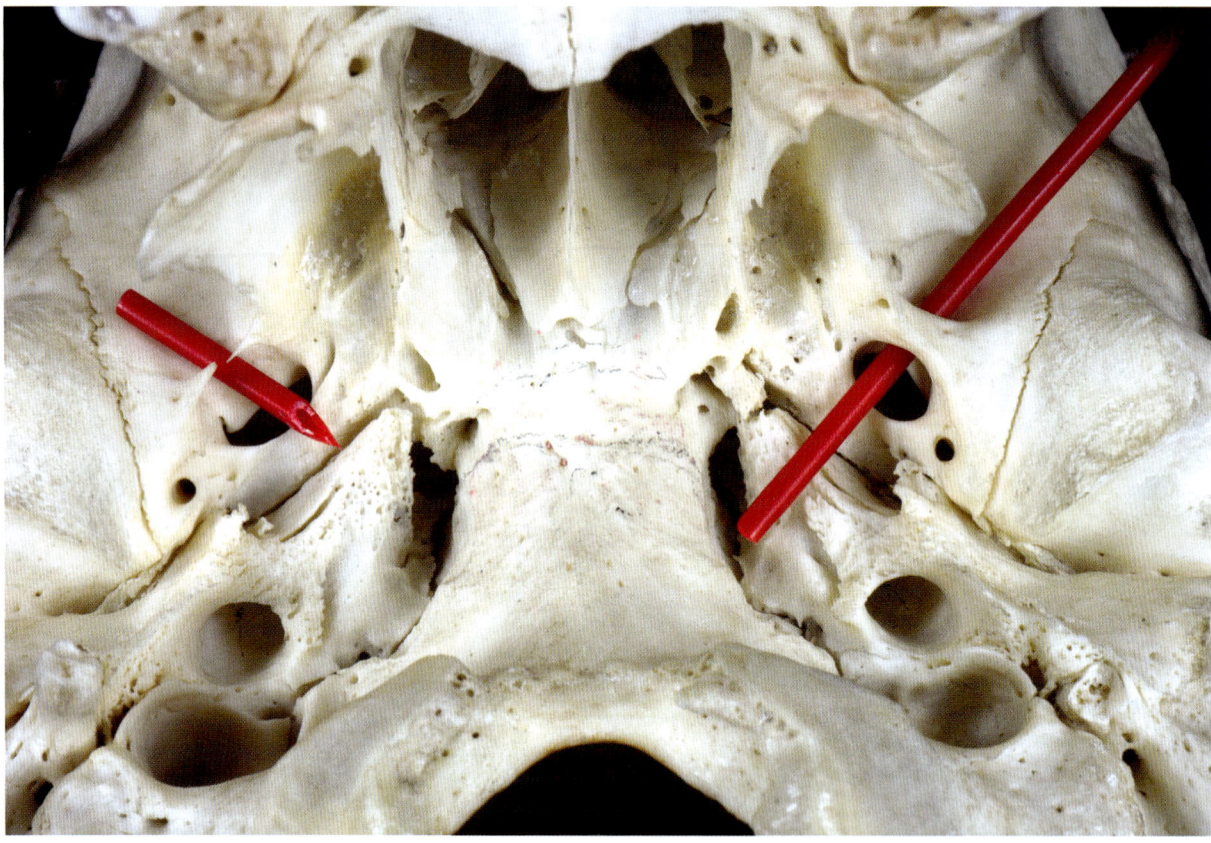

Figure 458. Classic example of partial bridging of the right pterygoalar ligament (short probe) and complete osseous bridging of the left pterygoalar ligament (long probe) resulting in formation of a foramen of Hyrtl in an adult (CSC AS003, Daniel Herrera). Similar bridging may be present in children between one and two years of age. Note that the pterygoalar spines and osseous bridges are positioned lateral to the foramen ovale. Bony bridges and spines that lie medial to the foramen ovale are pterygospinous (ligament and foramen; bar of Civinini) while those lateral to the foramen ovale are the pterygoalar ligament and, if fully bridged, the foramen of Hyrtl. This example shows bilateral asymmetry reflecting differing rates of side-to-side development of bridging. Cf. Antonopoulou et al. (2008); Chouke (1941); Chouke and Hodes (1951); Galdames et al. (2010); Hauser and DeStefano (1989); Peuker et al. (2001); Rosa et al. (2010); Rossi et al. (2011); Skrzat et al. (2005); Tubbs et al. (2009).

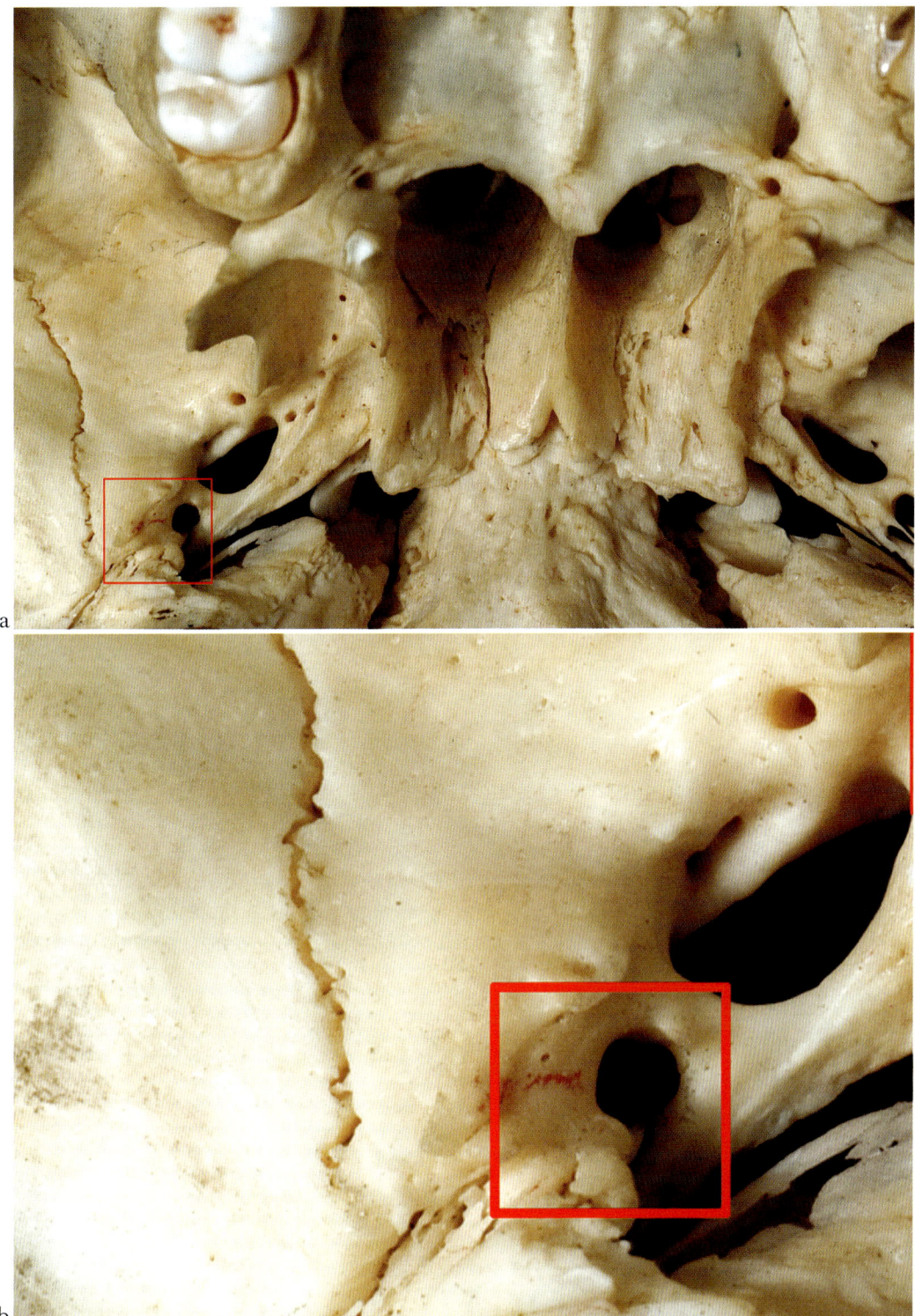

Figure 459a-b. Partial bridging of the foramen spinosum (CSC AC 027). (a) Low and (b) High magnification of basilar views of partial bridging of the right foramen spinosum (square) resulting in a slight gap between the nearly joined ends in an adult Asian female skull. Common finding. Cf. Hauser and DeStefano (1989); Singh and Anand (2009) for more on the position of the foramen spinosum.

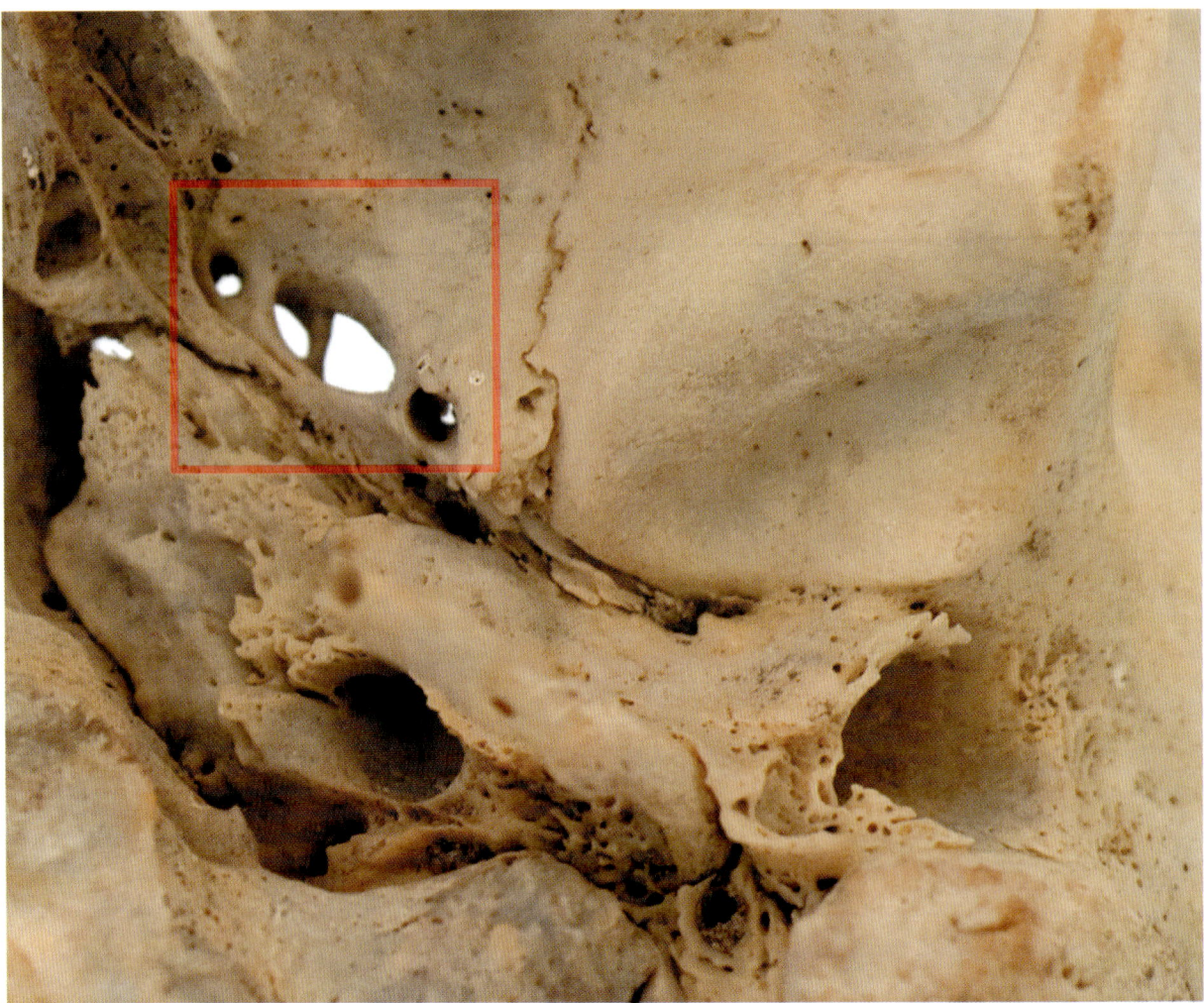

Figure 460. Ectocranial view of (square; from left to right) a foramen of Vesalius, divided foramen ovale and foramen spinosum in an adult Thai (KKU 2591-41). These foramina are typically arranged in a semi-circular/arc manner. Cf. Ginsberg et al. (1994); Hauser and DeStefano (1989); Lanzieri et al. (1988).

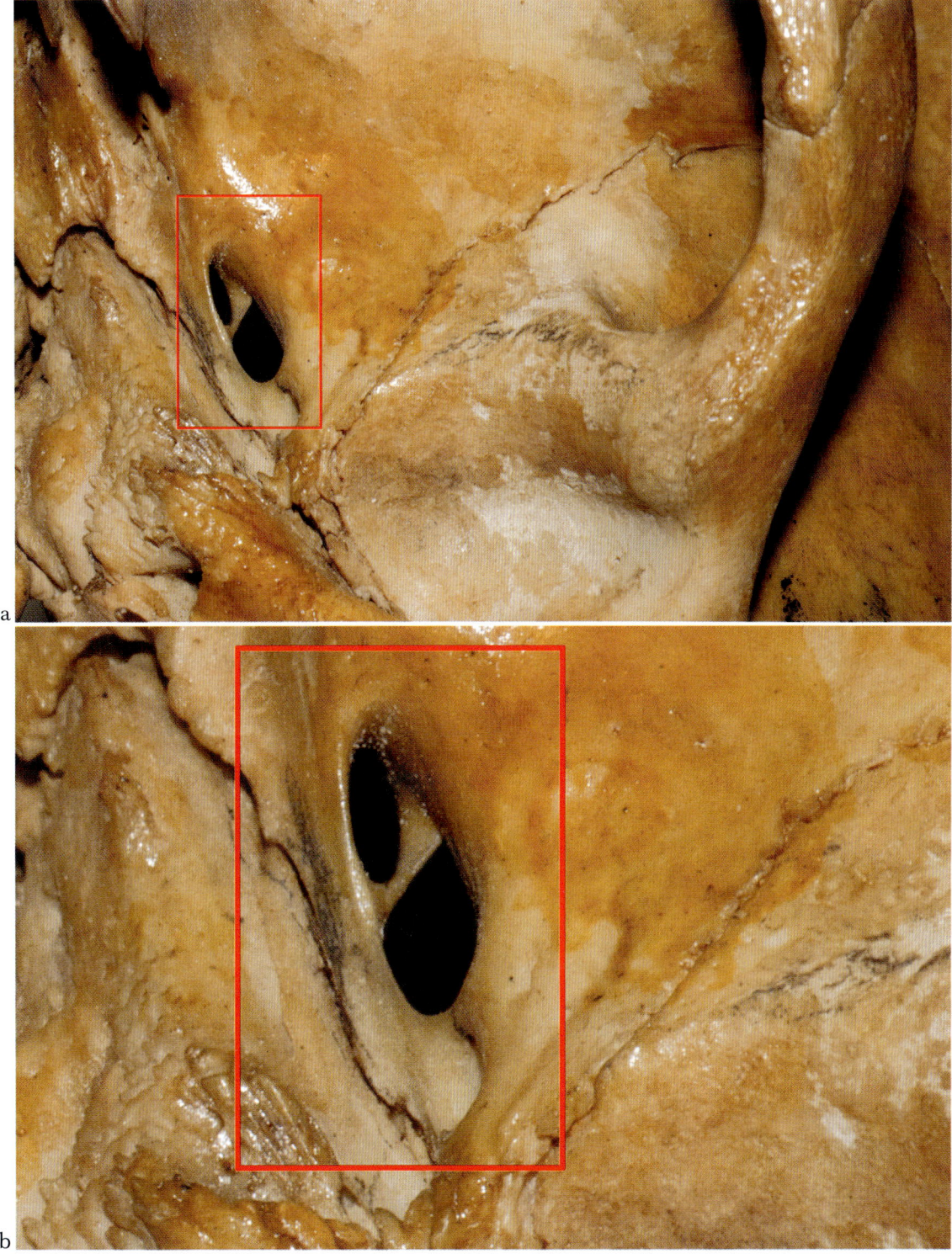

Figure 461a-b. Divided left foramen ovale. (a) Divided left foramen ovale (rectangle) in an adult African skull, probable female (TM 38, Ditsong Museum). (b) Higher magnification of the division. Absence of a foramen spinosum was also noted suggesting that the middle meningeal artery ran endocranially through this opening. See Hauser and DeStefano (1989) and Singh and Anand (2009) for more on the foramen spinosum. Common to uncommon finding.

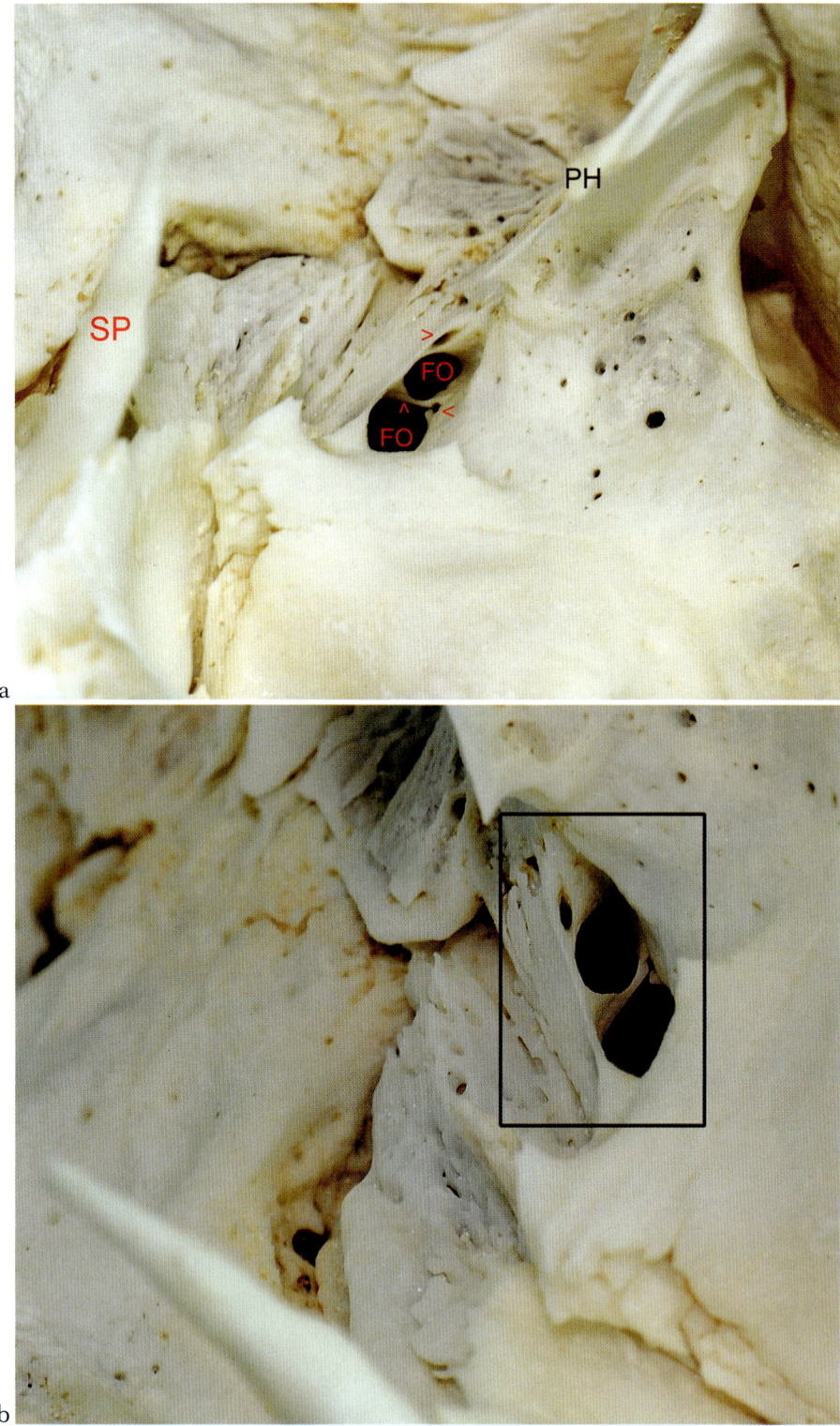

Figure 462a-b. Divided foramen ovale with internal foramina. (a) Divided left foramen ovale (FO) with a foramen of Vesalius (>) and small foramen (<) of unknown etiology within the sloping borders of foramen ovale (PH is the pterygoid hamulus and SP is the spinous process of the temporal bone) in a 36-year-old Thai female (CMU FO-805/57-023). (b) Higher magnification of these foramina.

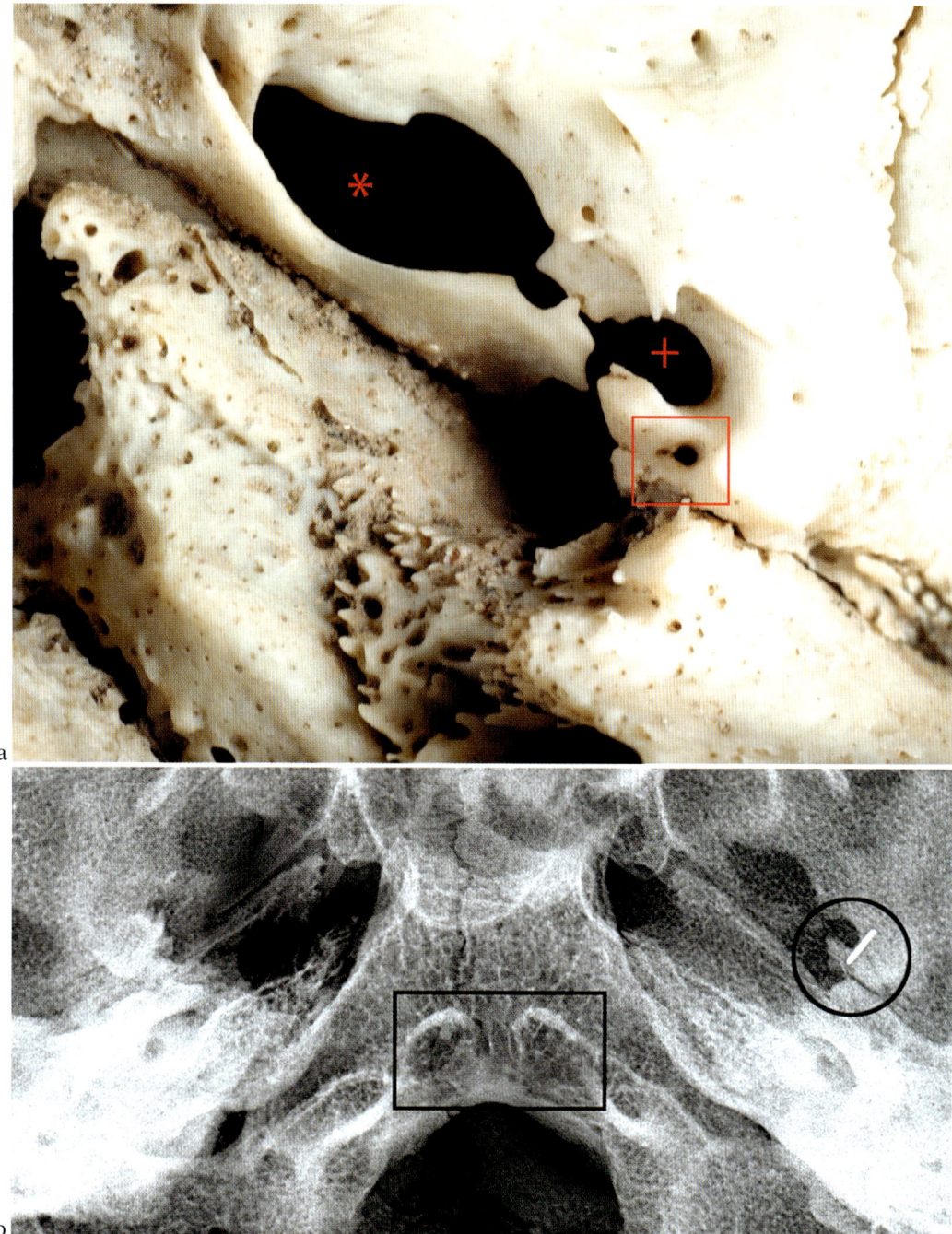

Figure 463a-b. Possible canaliculus innominatus. (a) Ectocranial view of a possible variant of canaliculus innominatus (CI) posterior and medial to the foramen spinosum (+) which has a medial wall defect (* is the left foramen ovale; CSC AC018). (b) X-ray showing bilateral precondylar tubercles (rectangle) and wire probe (circle) in the left CI, revealing its directionality. The clinical, anatomical and anthropological literature reveals considerable disagreement as to the location of the CI. Some researchers identify the CI as between the foramen ovale and spinosum, while others report that it is positioned medial, or posterior to foramen spinosum or "the interval between the great wing of the sphenoid and the petrous part of the temporal bone" (Bast and Anson 1949:23). Ginsberg et al. (1994) examined (CT) 123 adult patients and found 20 individuals with CI (1 bilateral), placing it between the foramen ovale and foramen spinosum. The CI is not mentioned in many anatomical texts.

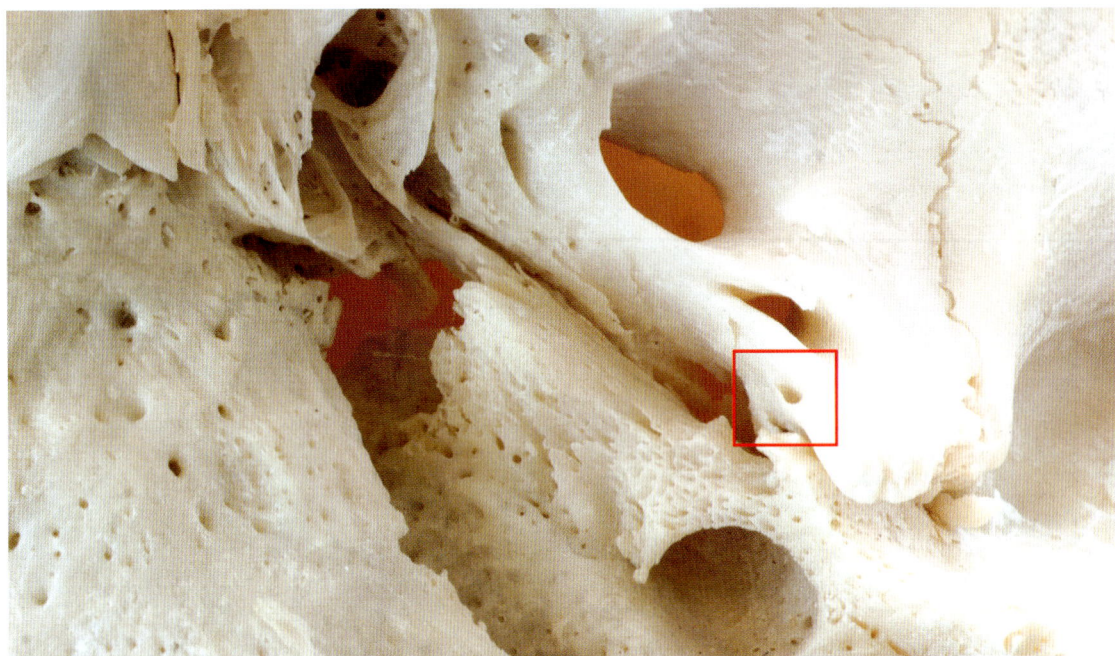

Figure 464. Possible variant of canaliculus innominatus (CI), also known as foramen of Arnold (square) or foramen petrosum, in an adult male skull (CSC033). This occasional foramen, which transmits the lesser petrosal nerve, has been described as (1) in the bar of bone between the foramen ovale and foramen spinosum (Ginsberg et al. 1994; Hasan and Pratap 2009); (2) medial, or posterior to the foramen spinosum (Kakizawa et al. 2007); and (3) between and posterior to the foramen ovale and foramen spinosum, when present (Berge and Bergman 2001). The many normal and occasional accessory foramina in the middle cranial fossa often make it difficult to distinguish the CI from other minor foramina. The location and frequency of this foramen warrants additional research. Cf. Reymond et al. (2005) for a description and photographs of foramina.

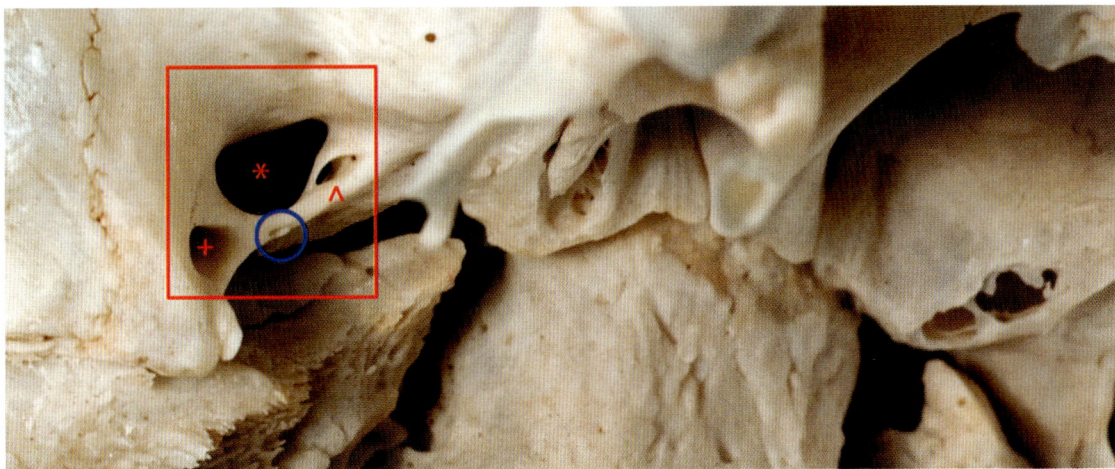

Figure 465. Right foramen of Vesalius (∧) medial to the foramen ovale (*), normal position of the foramen spinosum (+) and variant of canaliculus innominatus (blue circle) medial to the foramen ovale and foramen spinosum. Typical anatomy, although the foramen of Vesalius may vary in location, symmetry and number (CSC AC026). Cf. Shinohara et al. (2010). Vázquez et al. (2001) identified this foramen (Foramina Nervorum) at this location in 8 of 509 (1.5%) crania.

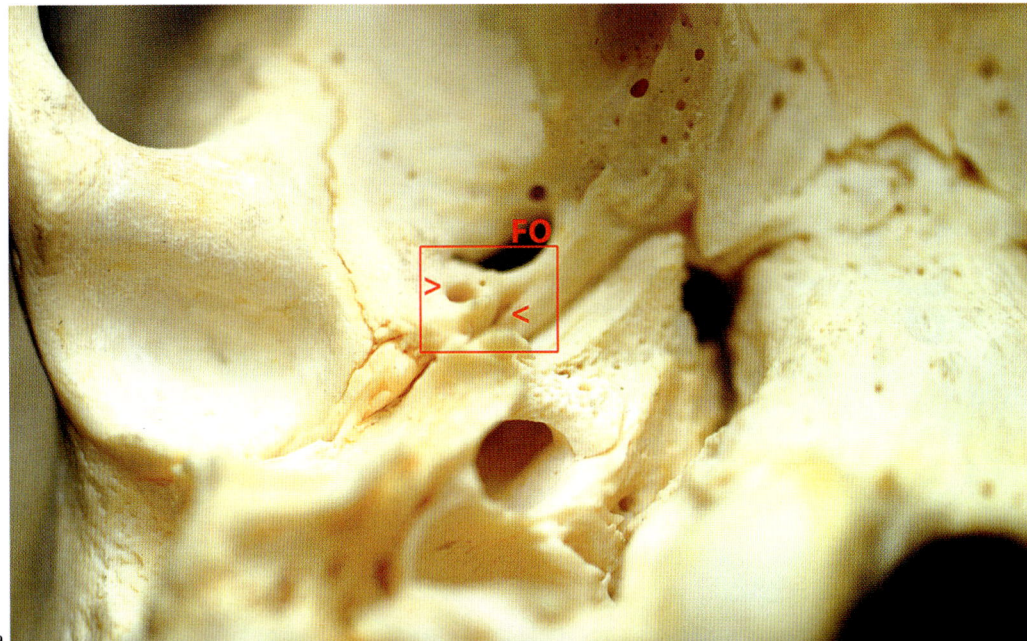

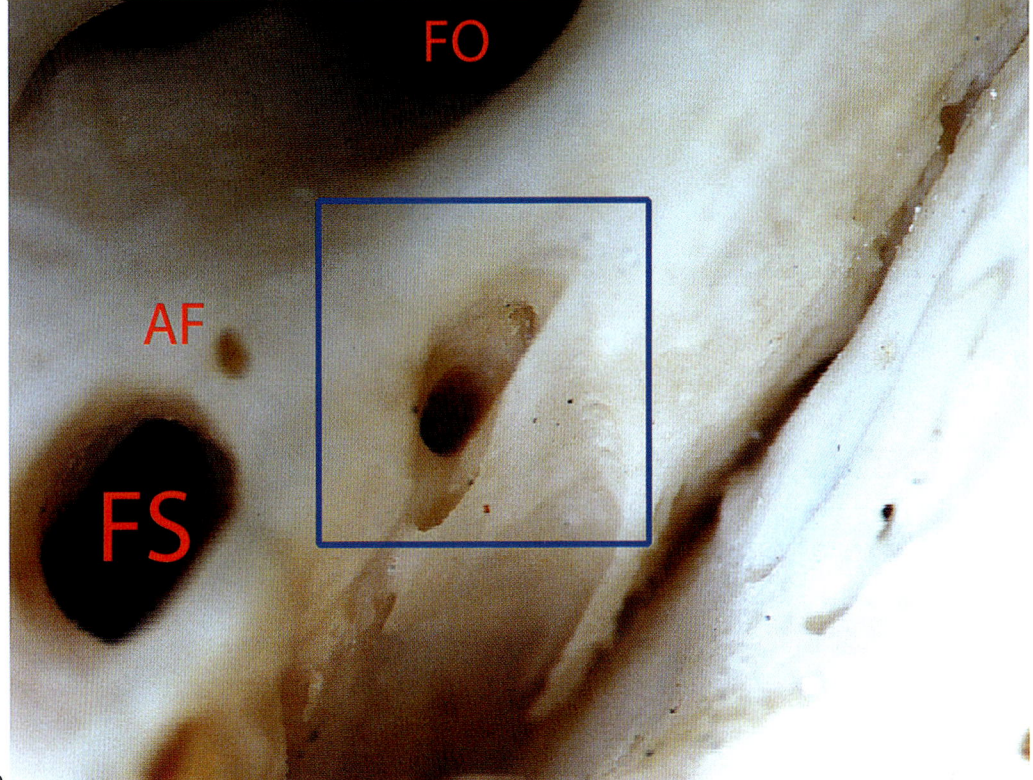

Figure 466a-b. Foramina in the area (red rectangle) of the foramen ovale (FO). (a) Right FO, foramen spinosum (>) and possible foramen of Arnold (<) in an adult Asian skull (FSA DS044; Christopher Sciotto). (b) Higher magnification of the possible foramen of Arnold (blue square) showing that its slit-like entrance becomes a round foramen deep within (variable, but typical anatomy) positioned lateral to the foramen spinosum (FS) and a small accessory foramen (AF).

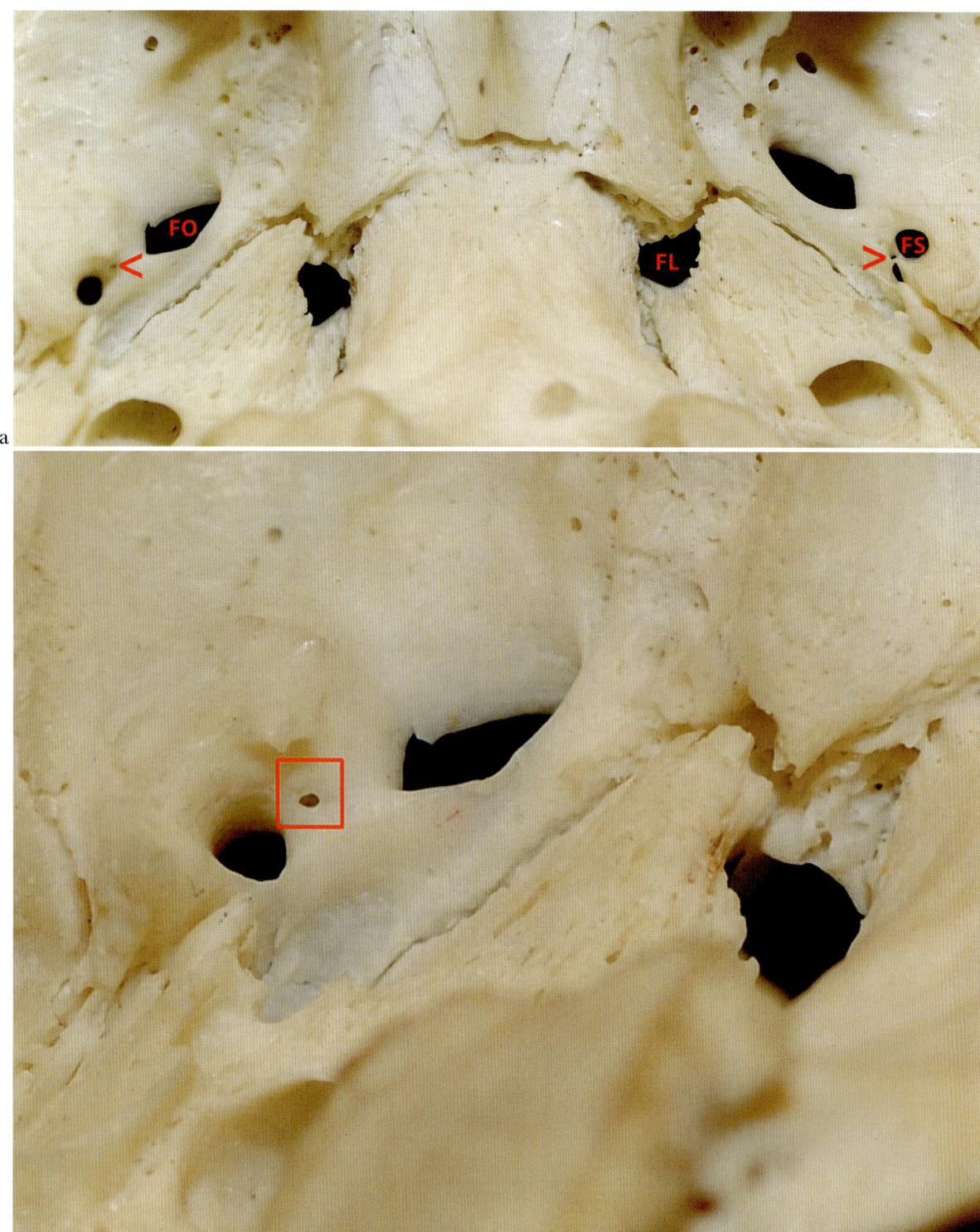

Figure 467a-b. Foramina of the middle cranial fossa. (a) Ectocranial and (b) endocranial views of left canaliculus innominatus (foramen of Arnold; square) in an elderly adult (JABSOM). The foramen of Arnold (< and >) are visible in relation to the foramen ovale (FO), foramen spinosum (FS) and foramen lacerum (FL). (Bottom) In this individual the left foramen of Arnold (square) enters the middle cranial fossa between the FO and FS.

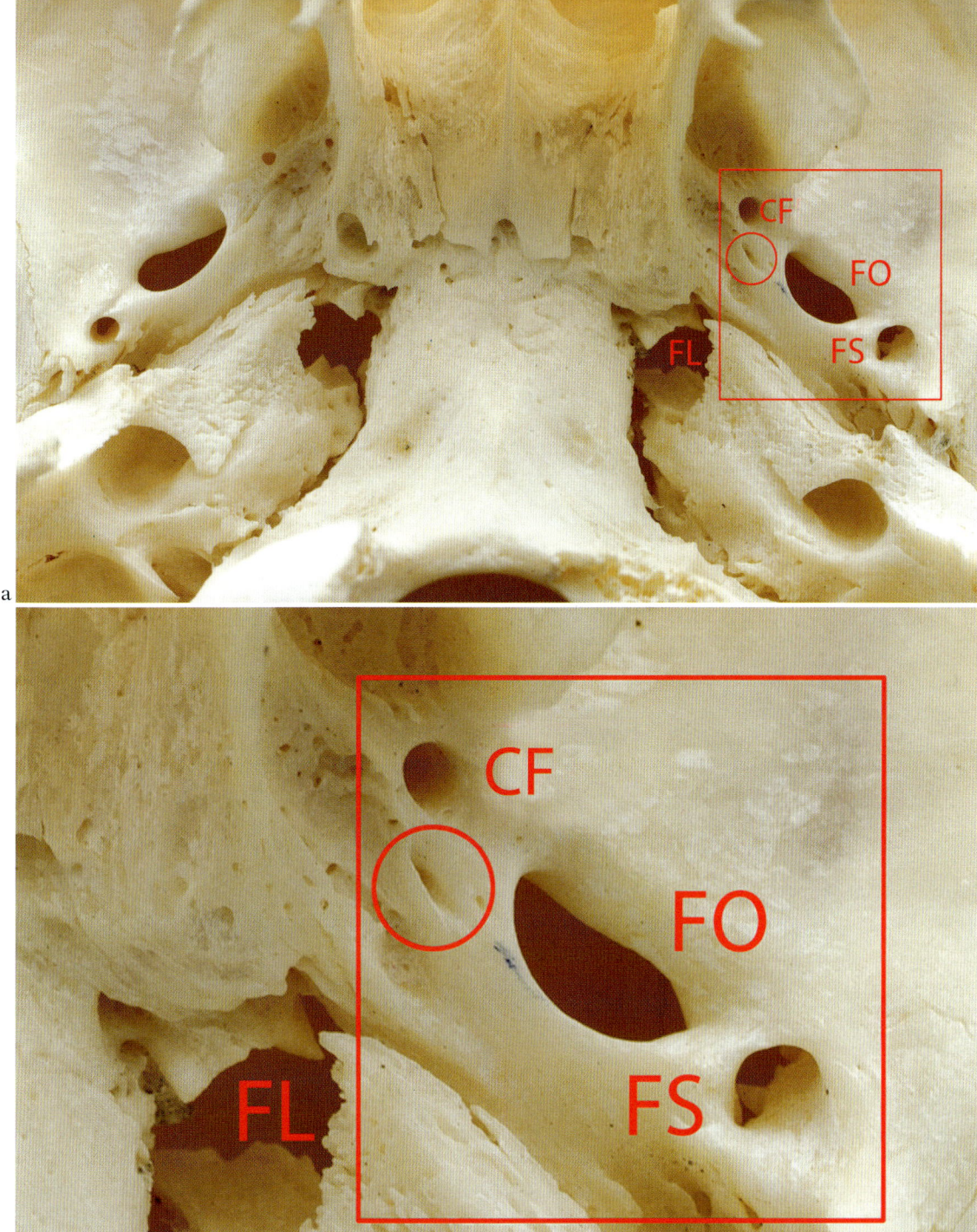

Figure 468a-b. Cavernous (CF) and other foramina of the cranial base. (a) Foramen of Vesalius (circle), foramen ovale (FO), foramen spinosum (FS) and foramen lacerum (FL) in an adult female skull (FSA AC050). (b) Higher magnification of the foramina. Cf. Reymond et al. (2005) for more on the cavernous foramen, which may be single or multiple. See Ginsberg et al. (1994) and Lanzieri et al. (1988) for foramen of Vesalius.

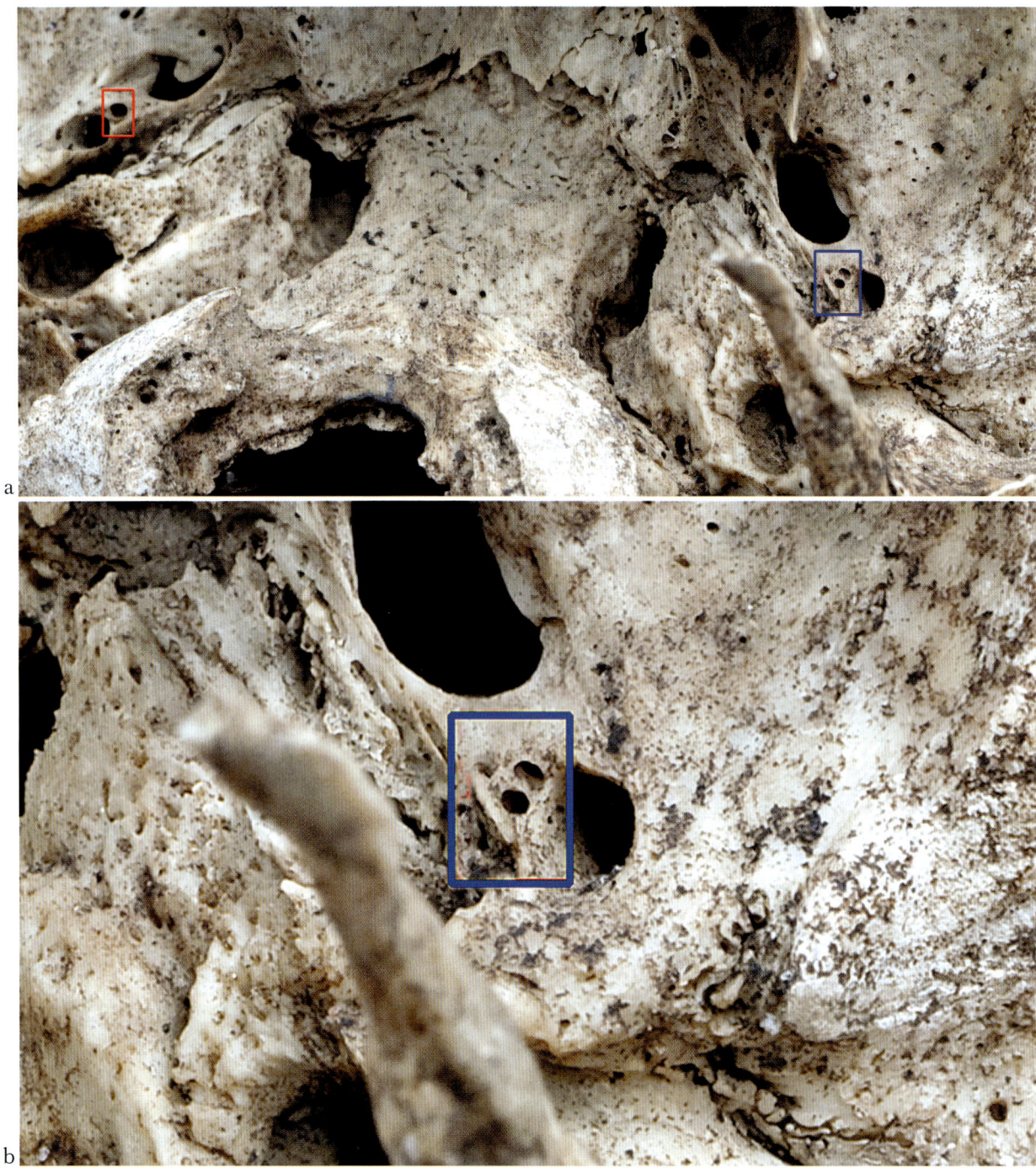

Figure 469a-b. Foramen of Arnold. (a) Single right (red rectangle) and double left (blue rectangle) foramen of Arnold in an elderly Thai female skull (CMU 32 51). (b) Higher magnification of the double left foramen of Arnold (blue).

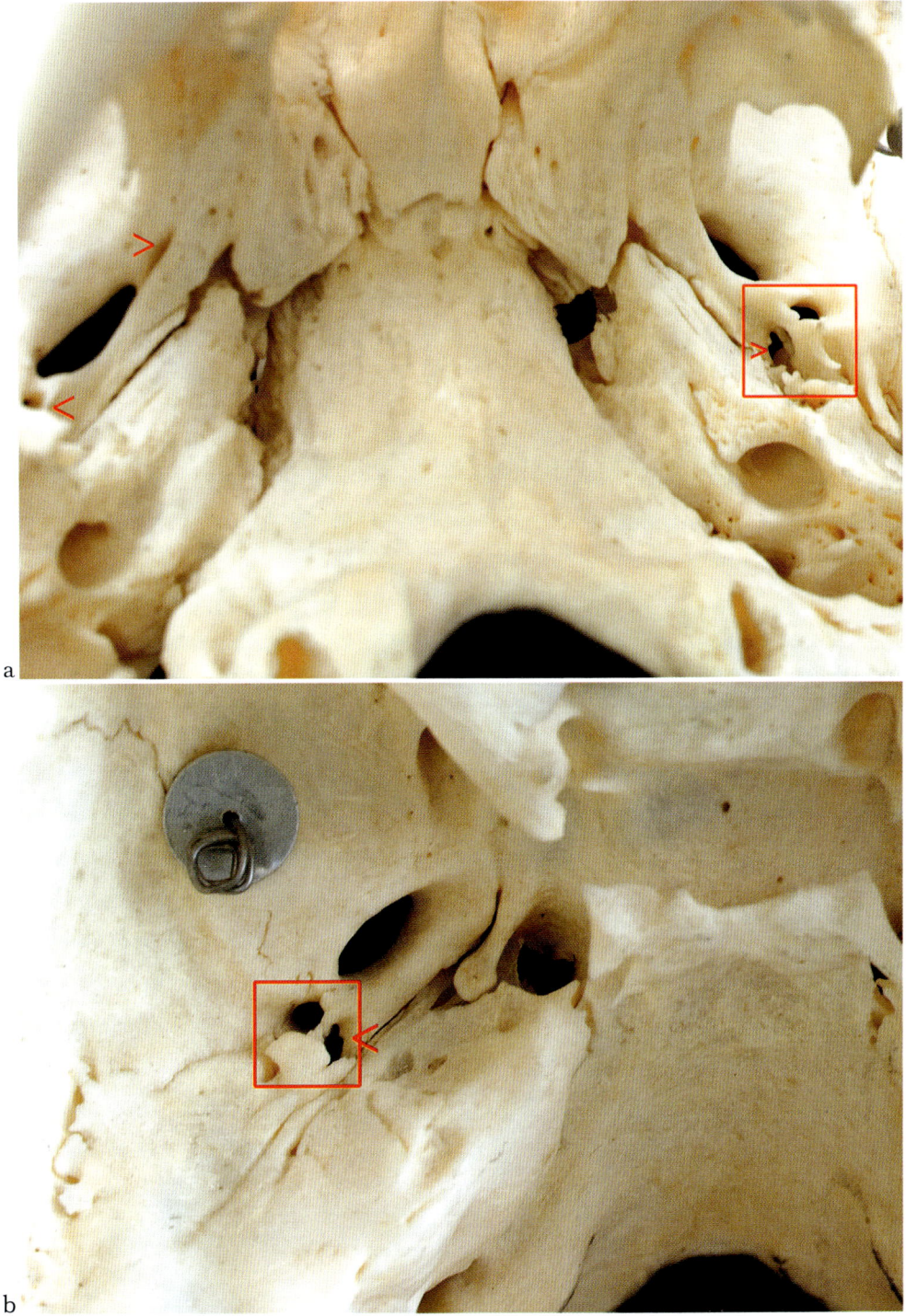

Figure 470a-b. Canaliculus innominatus and foramen of Vesalius. (a) Ectocranial and (b) endocranial views of canaliculus innominatus (CI) (square and <) and foramen of Vesalius (>) in a young adult Asian (FSA AS008). The large CI (<) in this example is medial to the round foramen spinosum (square). A search of the literature revealed considerable disagreement in the location of the CI in relation to the foramen ovale and foramen spinosum. Cf. Sampson et al. (1991) for an example of the CI in this location; Vázquez et al. (2001); Singh and Anand (2009) for more on foramen spinosum.

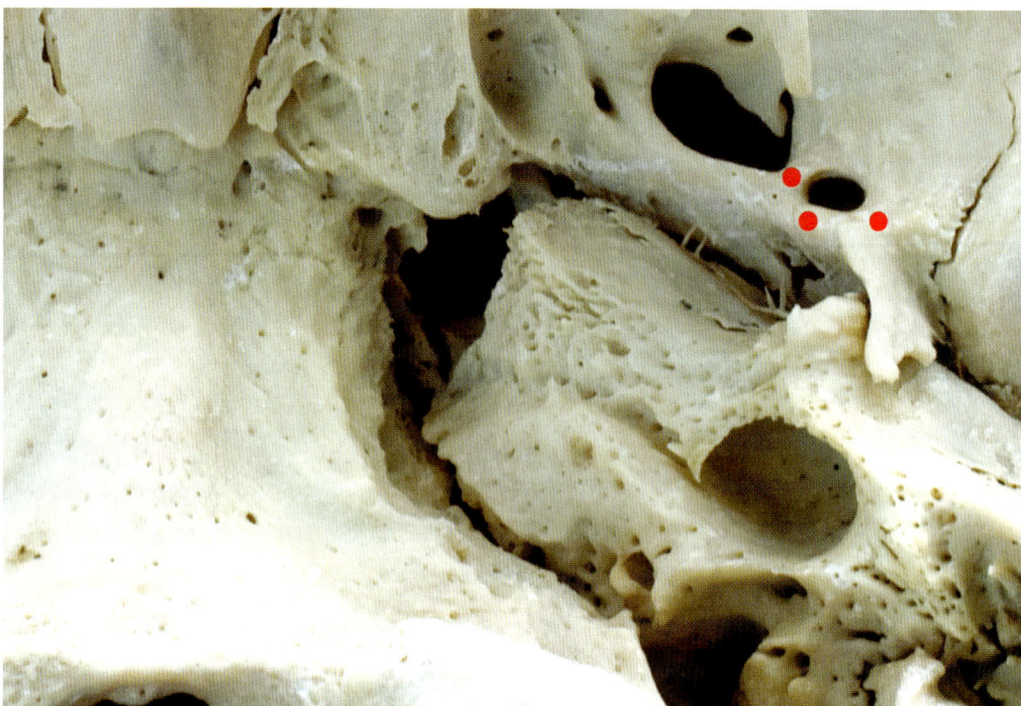

Figure 471. Position of the canaliculus innonimatus (red dots) in the left sphenoid bone, as reported by authors in the clinical, radiological and anatomical literature.

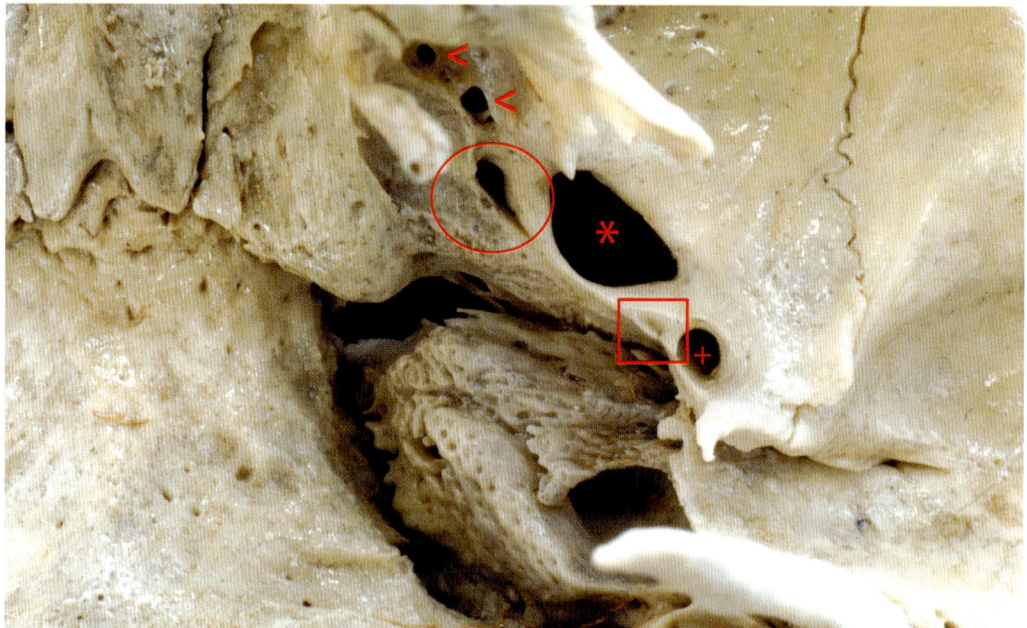

Figure 472. Foramen ovale (*), foramen spinosum (+), slit-like foramen of Vesalius (circle), faintly visible canaliculus innominatus (square) and two possible cavernous foramina (<) in an Asian adult (FSA CSC DS008). Reymond et al. (2005) noted 68 of 100 skulls (36 males and 32 females) with one or more cavernous foramina.

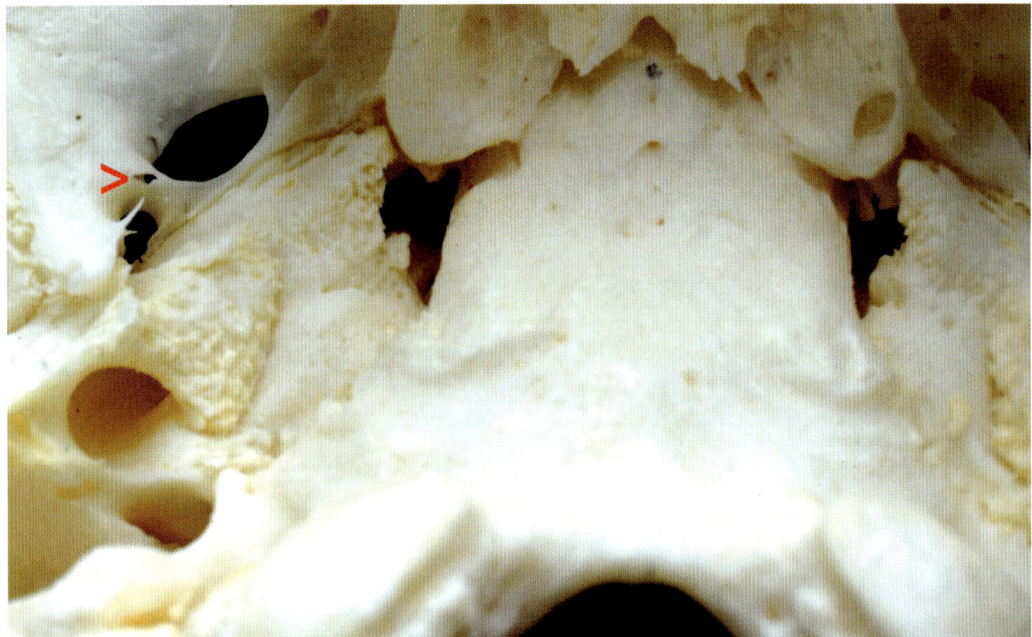

Figure 473. Probable right canaliculus innominatus (>), aka the foramen of Arnold, in an adult (FSA AC054). While researchers have identified this inconstant foramen in a variety of locations near the foramen ovale, this is the location generally accepted.

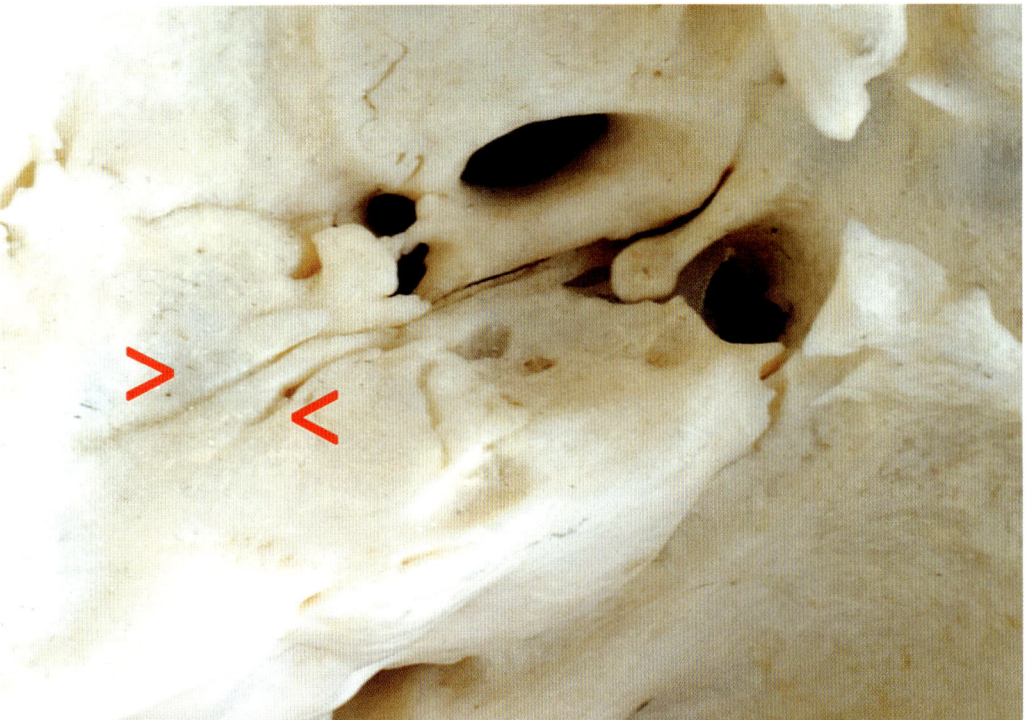

Figure 474. Grooves for the greater (<) and lesser (>) petrosal nerves in the left petrous bone (FSA AS008).

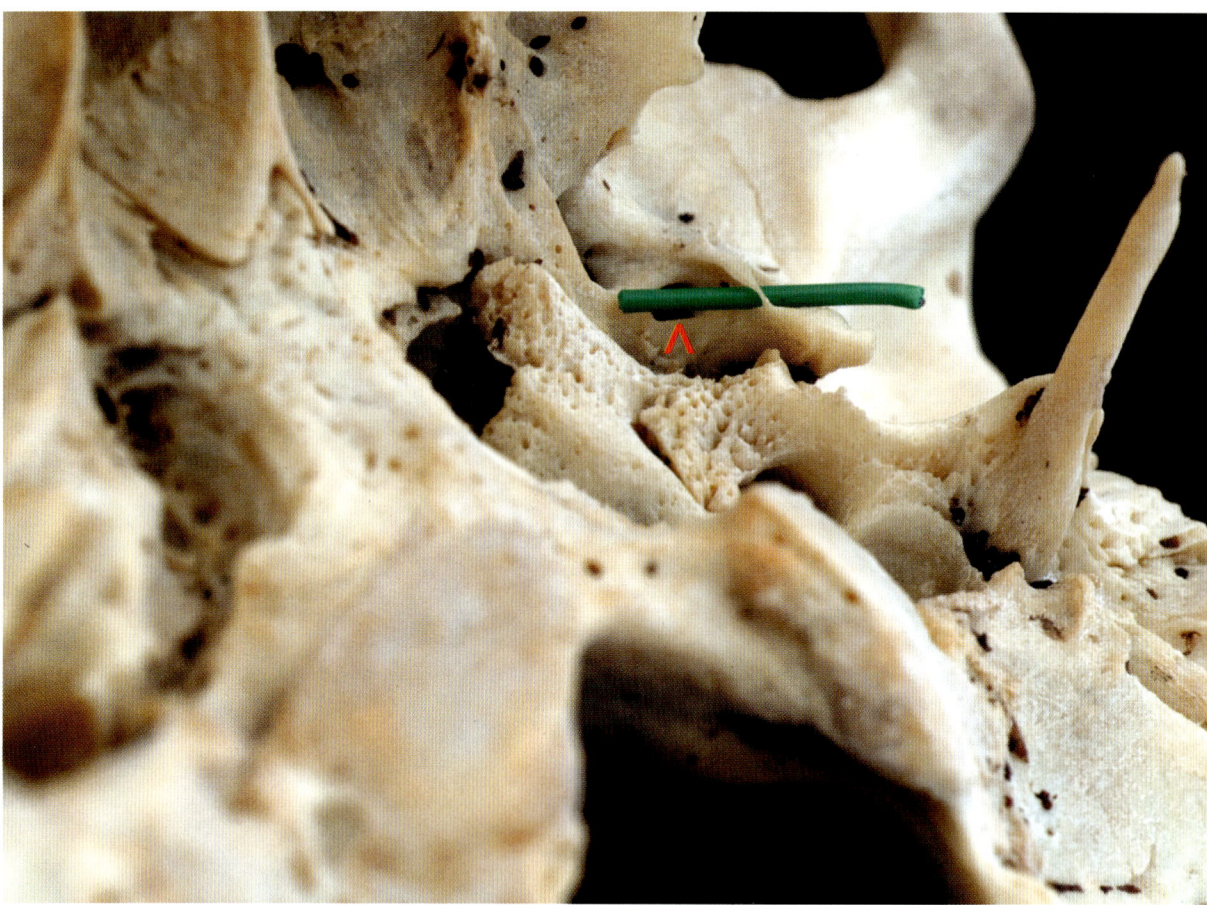

Figure 475. Bridged left foramen spinosum (green wire) forming a partial tunnel above the foramen in a Thai adult (48-1590). See Singh and Anand (2009).

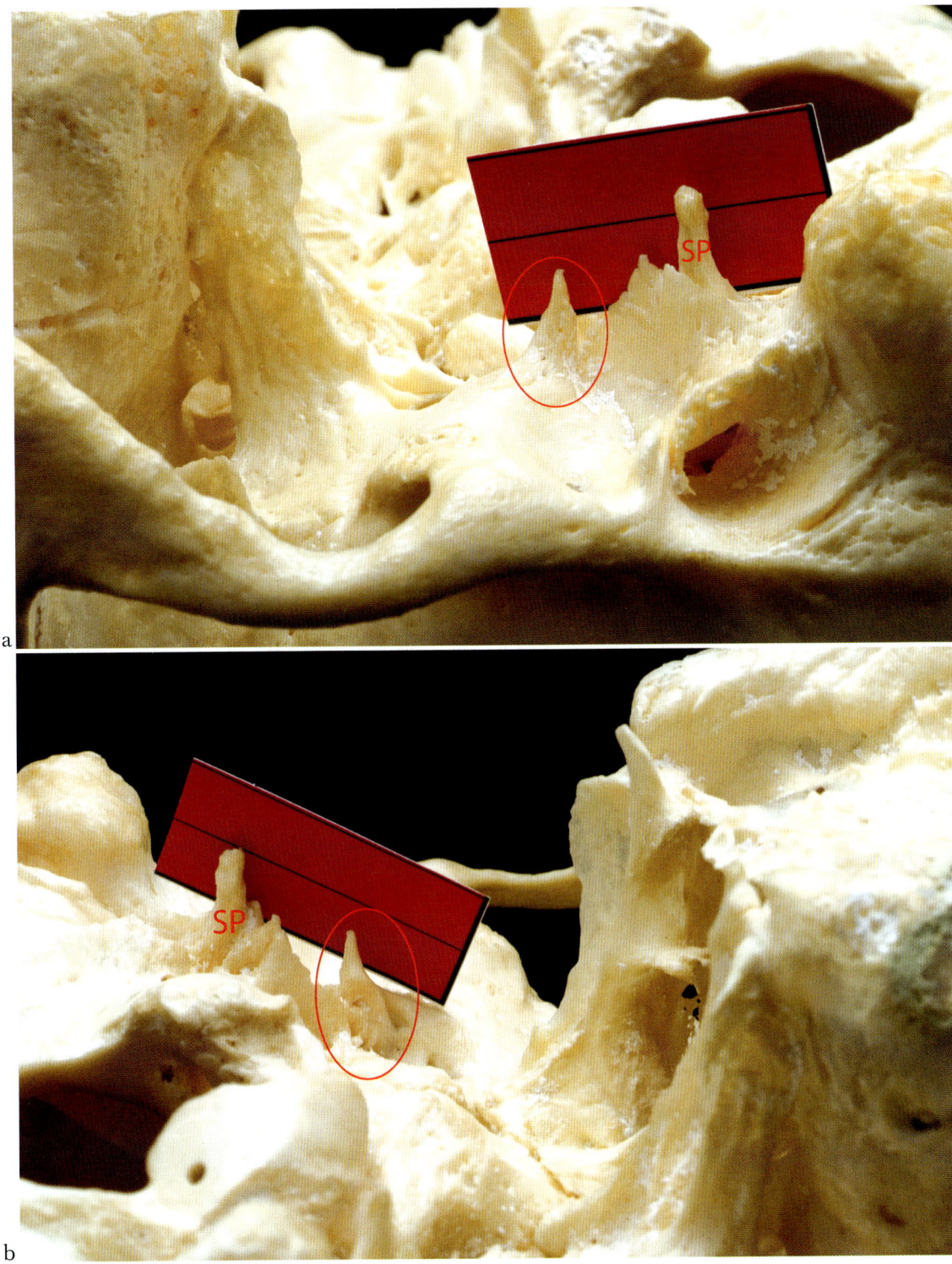

Figure 476a-b. Elongated and calcified sphenoid spine. (a) An elongated and calcified sphenoid spine (red oval), sometimes known as the angular spine of the sphenoid, in a robust adult male; SP denotes the styloid process (SP) of the temporal bone (CSC FSA DS006). (b) Higher magnification of the spine (oval) and SP. Typical anatomy.

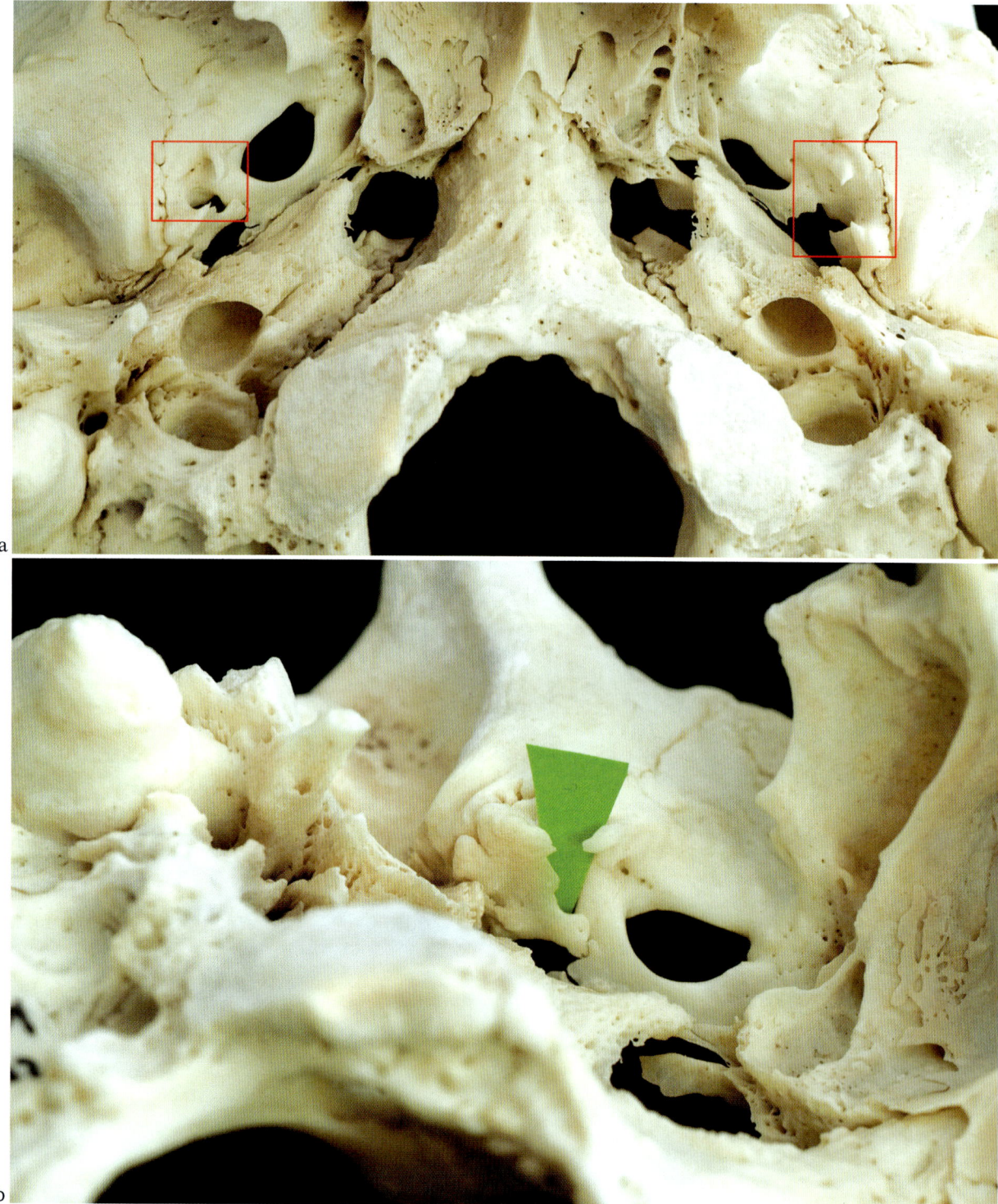

Figure 477a-b. Bilateral partial bridging of the foramen spinosum. (a) Basilar view of bilateral partial bridging of the foramen spinosum (squares) in an adult Asian male skull (CSC AS022). (b) Note the hook-like projections directed towards one another (green arrowhead) and incomplete formation of the canal. The medial wall of this foramen is typically open in fetuses, but usually closes. To designate as a trace of pterygoalar bridging, the bony spike must be directed toward the lateral pterygoid plate. See Hauser and DeStefano (1989) and Singh and Anand (2009).

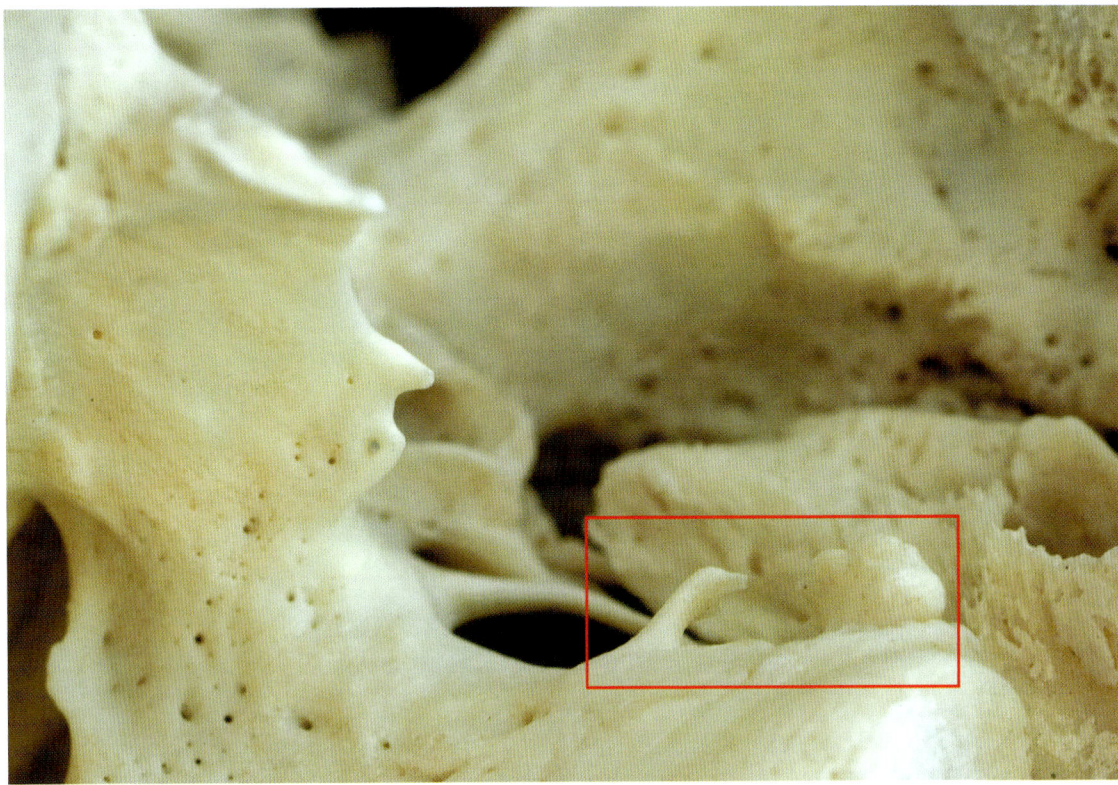

Figure 478. Bilateral partial bridging of the foramen spinosum in an adult Asian male. Note the two hook-like projections directed towards one another (rectangle) and not toward the lateral pterygoid plate (bottom photo, rectangle) (CSC AS022). Uncommon to common finding depending on the group being studied.

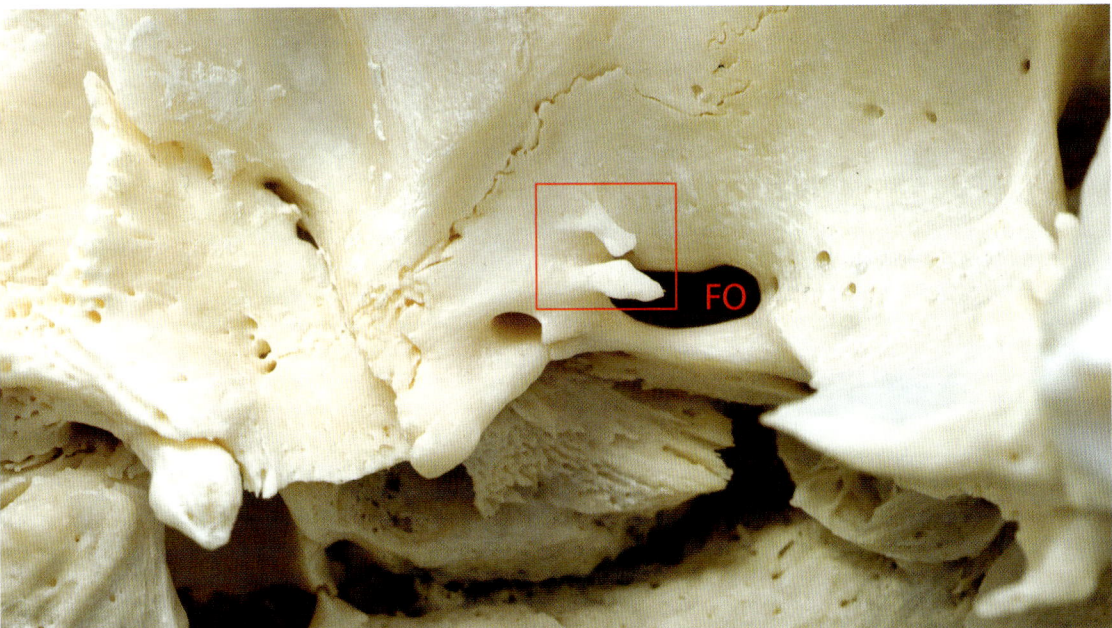

Figure 479. Two small exostoses, likely calcified pterygospinous and pterygoalar ligaments (square) extending partially across the right foramen ovale (FO) in a robust adult Asian male (CSC DS033).

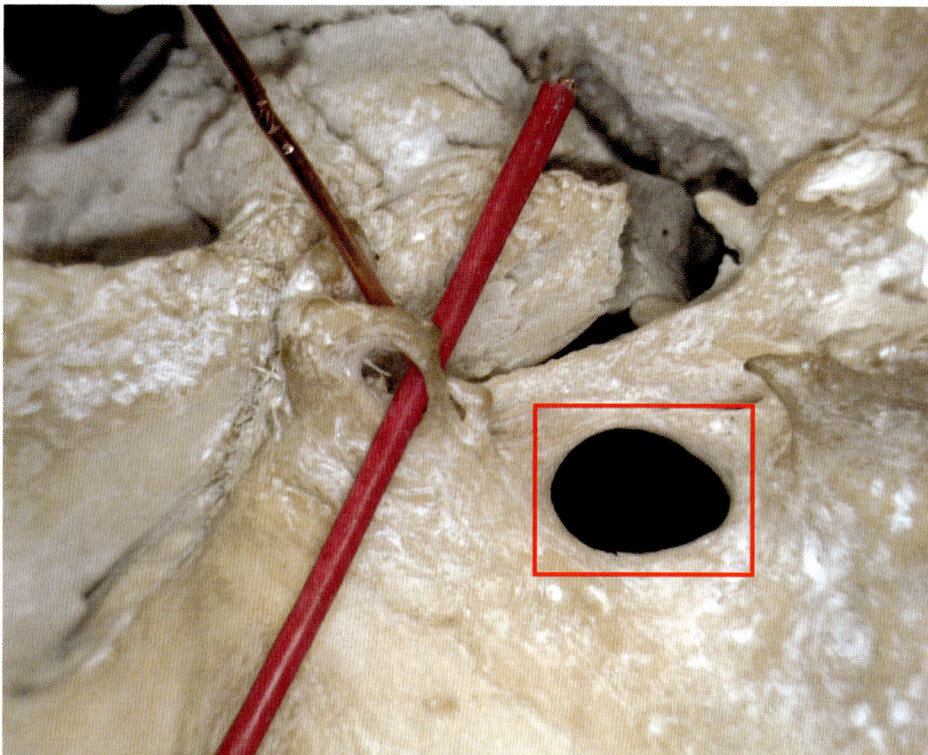

Figure 480. Lateral view of bridged left sphenoid spine (red wire passing through it) and orientation of the foramen spinosum (copper wire inserted) posterior to the foramen ovale (red rectangle) in an adult White male skull. The bridge across foramen spinosum is an uncommon to common finding and may be a variant of ossified pterygospinous bridging.

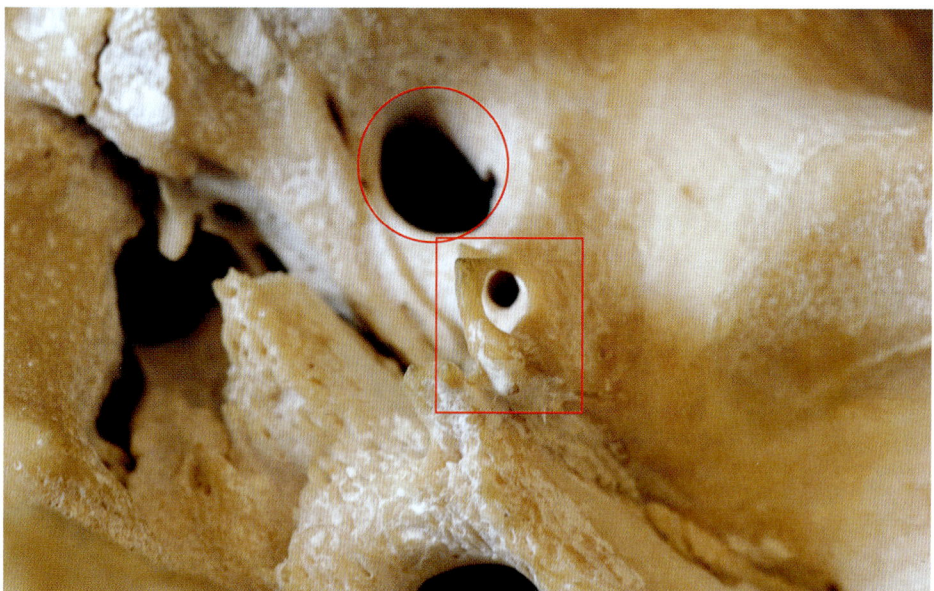

Figure 481. Inferior view showing the bridged left sphenoid spine (red square) spanning the foramen spinosum (red square). The bridge is posterior to the foramen ovale (red circle) and foramen spinosum warranting further research. The tunnel formed within the square is likely a variant of ossified pterygospinous bridging.

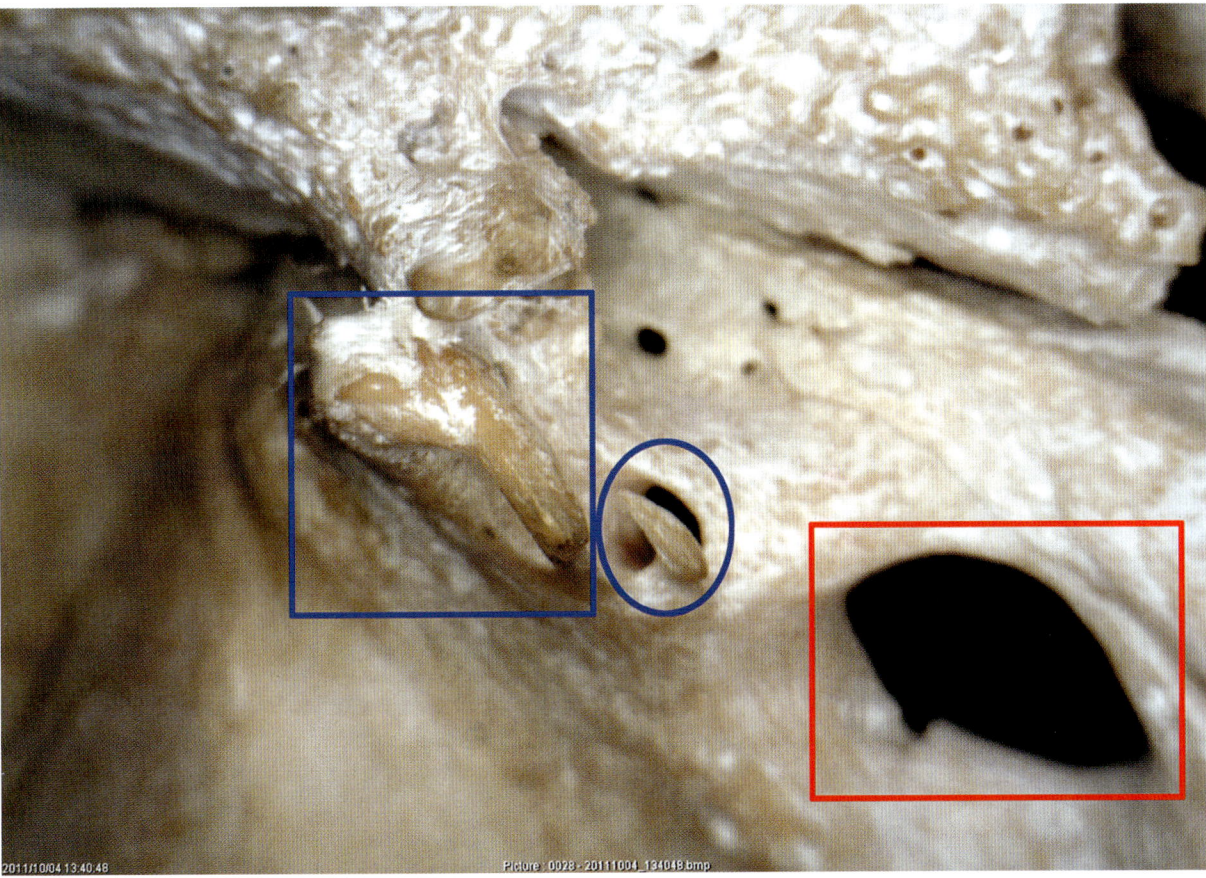

Figure 482. Foramen ovale (red rectangle), bridged left sphenoid spine (blue square; possibly a variant of pterygospinous bridge) and a small hook-like exostosis (oval) along the anterolateral margin of the foramen spinosum in an adult White male skull. The spine of the sphenoid serves for attachment of the sphenomandibular ligament and is located posterior to the foramen spinosum, hence the term "sphenoid spine." This spine is an uncommon to common finding that warrants additional research. See Singh and Anand (2009) for varying position as well as some variants of foramen spinosum.

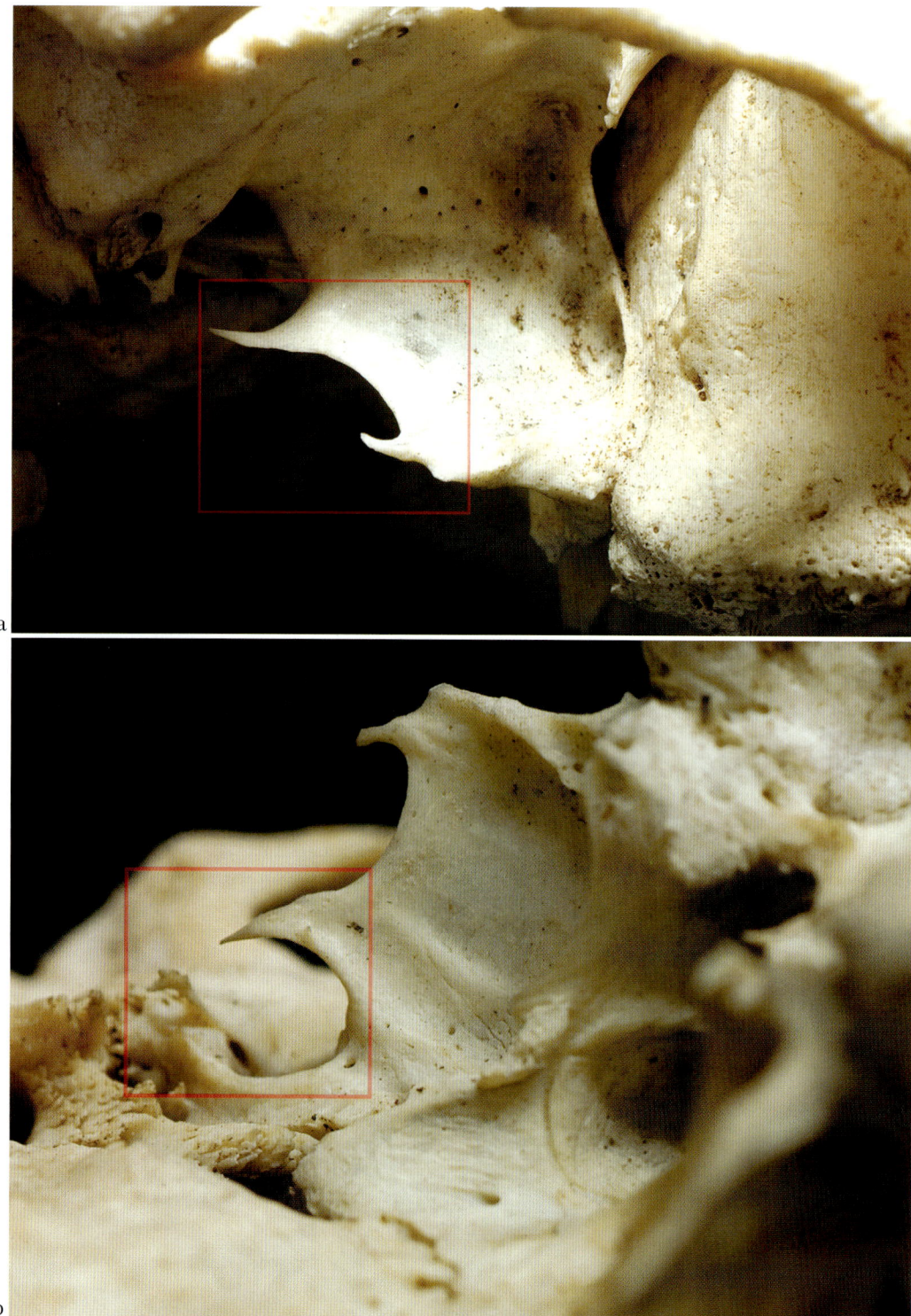

Figure 483a-b. Partial bridging by a calcified right pterygospinous ligament. (a) Lateral view of unusually long extensions (rectangles) resulting in partial bridging in an adult Polynesian (UPenn 15710). (b) Note that the delicate bony spines are directed toward one another. Although speculative, these spines may have bridged and formed a foramen if this individual had lived longer.

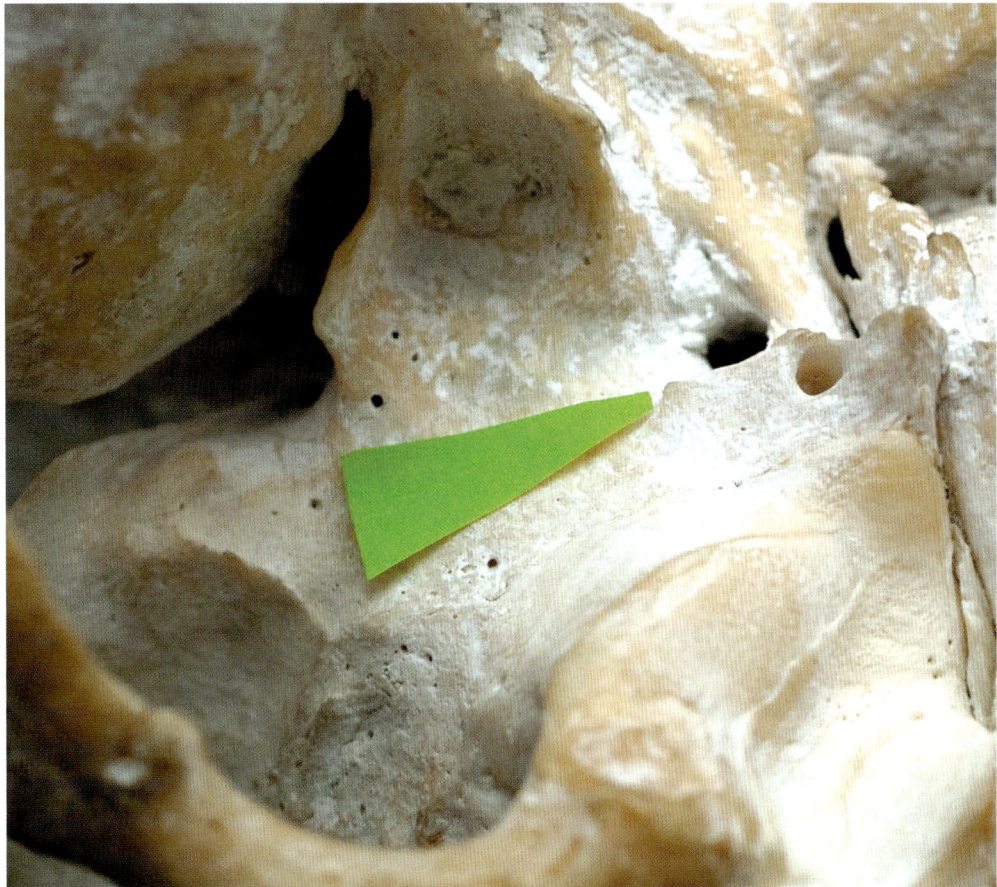

Figure 484. Trace right pterygoalar bridge (tip of green arrowhead) in an adult male. This is an example of trace development of the alar ligament that, in some individuals, ossifies and joins the lateral pterygoid plate resulting in a pterygoalar bridge (Mann personal collection). There appears to be some terminological confusion when it comes to identifying and classifying small calcifications located adjacent to the spine of the sphenoid and the foramen ovale. Regardless, pterygoalar bridging refers to projections that are lateral or posterolateral to foramen ovale. Pterygospinous bridging refers to projections that originate precisely at the spine of the sphenoid. Cf. Antonopoulou et al. (2008); Galdames et al. (2010); Hauser and DeStefano (1989).

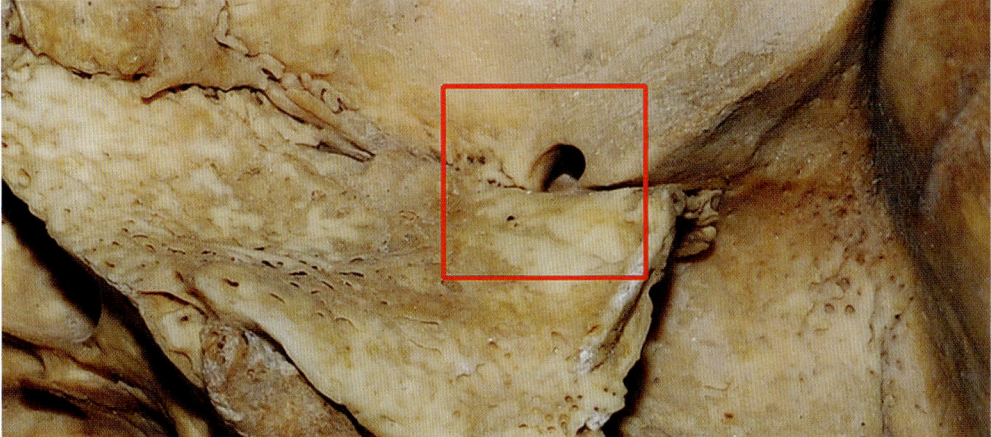

Figure 485. Foramen (square) in the left Glaserian fissure of the temporal bone (PAVN Forensic Institute) for transmission of the chorda tympani. Common finding of varying size.

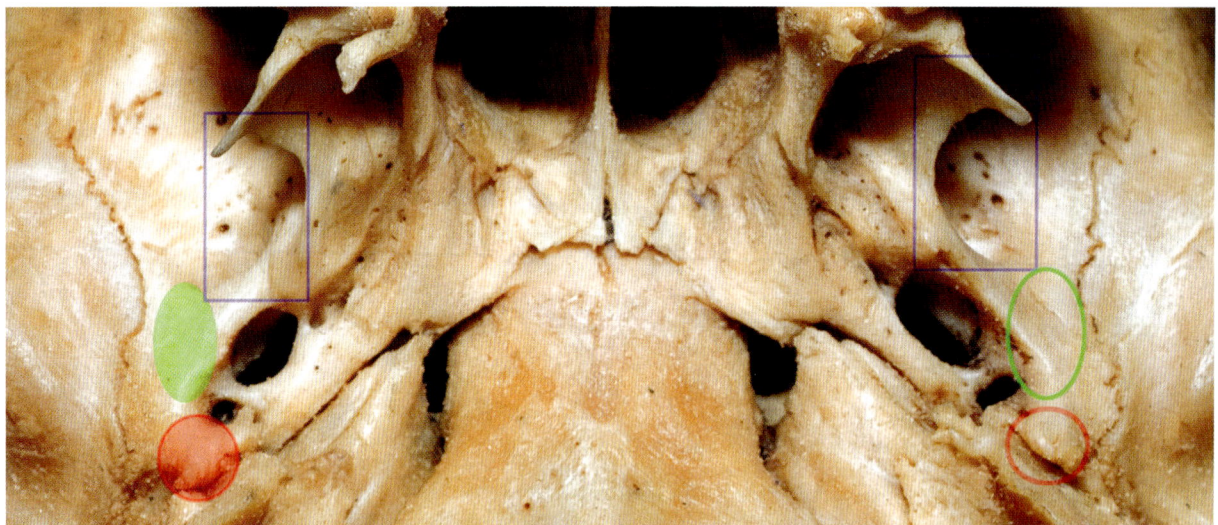

Figure 486. Attachment sites for the pterygospinous ligament or bridge (red), pterygoalar ligament or bridge (green) and the lateral pterygoid plate (blue) of the cranial base (SI Terry 171R).

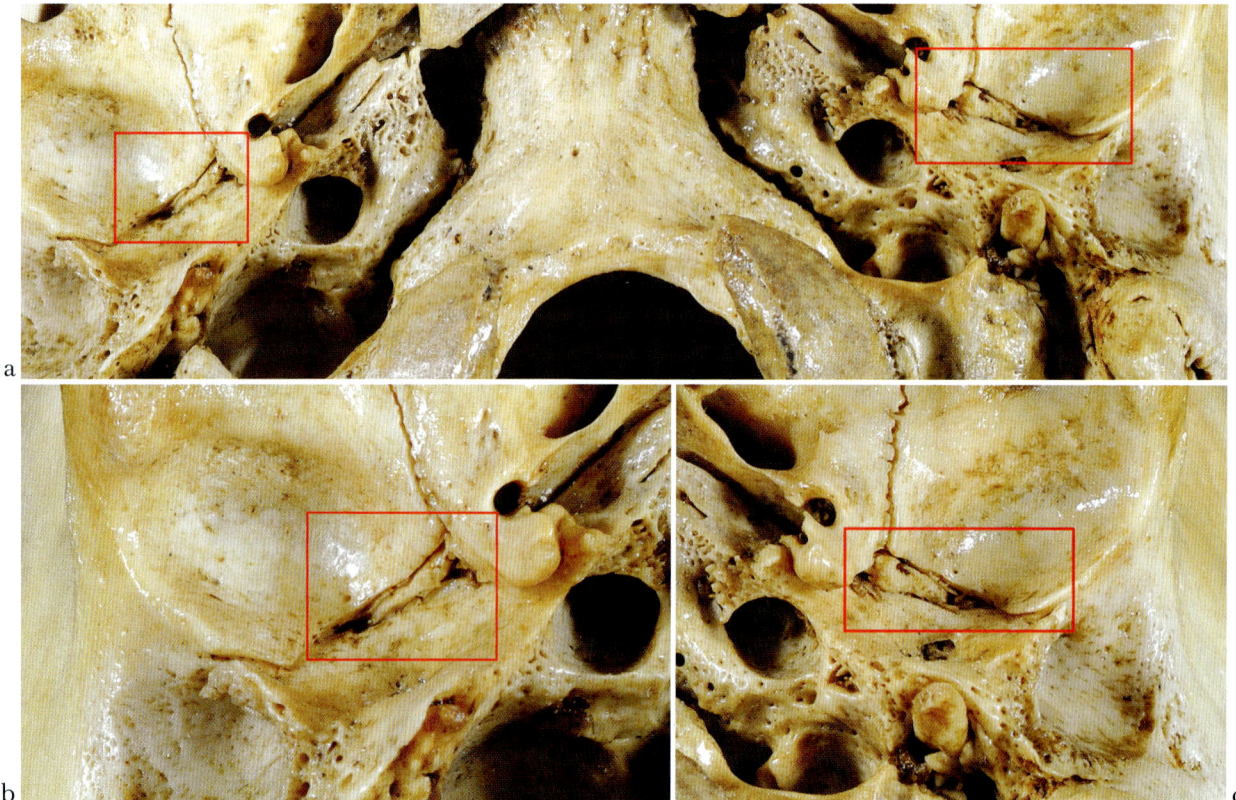

Figure 487a-c. Small slivers of bone (rectangles) along the Glaserian fissure (petrotympanic fissure) in a young adult Asian skull (CSC AC011). (a) Slender bone "islands" known as tegman tympani are visible in the left and right fissures. (b) Higher magnification of the right and (c) left Glaserian fissures. Each of these slender "islands" of bone forms the roof of the middle ear cavity and is part of the anterior portion of the petrous portion of the temporal bone. Typical anatomy.

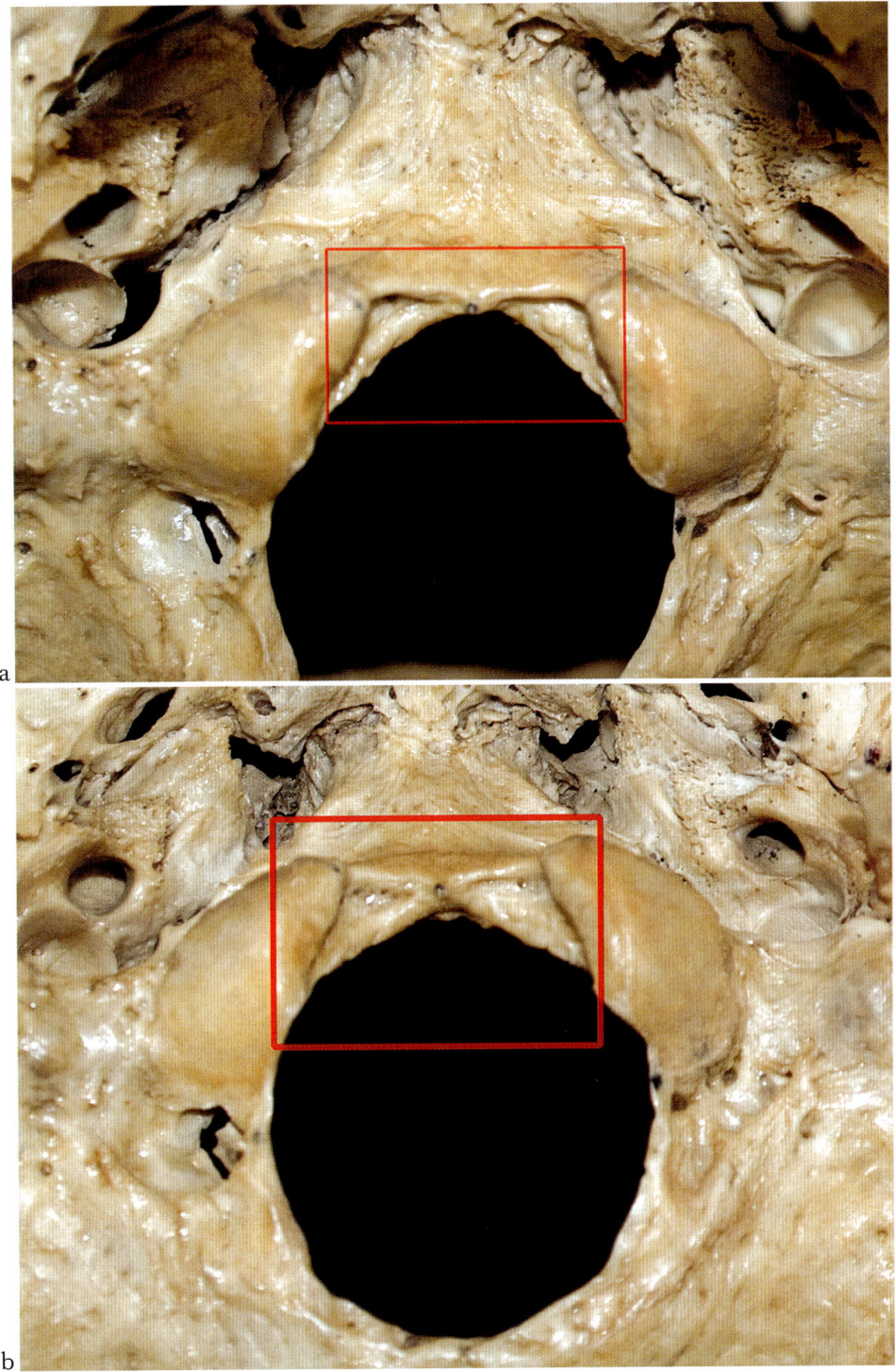

Figure 488a-b. Hypochordal arch. (a) The hypochordal arch (rectangle), part of the proatlas, in an adult Thai male (KKU 0014) – note the position of Basion at the apex of the midline, previously marked with a pencil for measurement. (b) Slightly different view showing the "bowtie" shape of the hypochordal arch. Cf. Pang and Thompson (2011); Prescher et al. (1996).

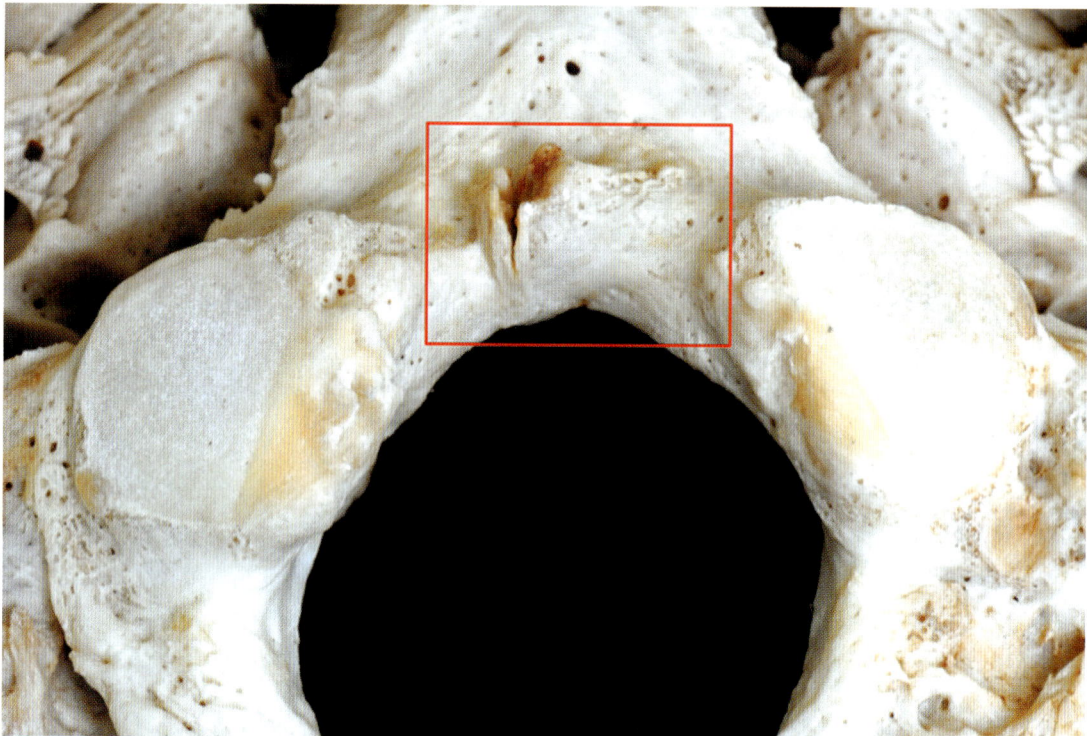

Figure 489. Precondylar tubercle (rectangle) along the midline. This morphology could be interpreted variously such as fused condyles, ossified apical ligament of the odontoid process, or possibly, as a tertiary or third condyle, in an adult Thai skull (KKU). Rare finding. Hauser and DeStefano (1989); Oetteking (1923); Prescher et al. (1996).

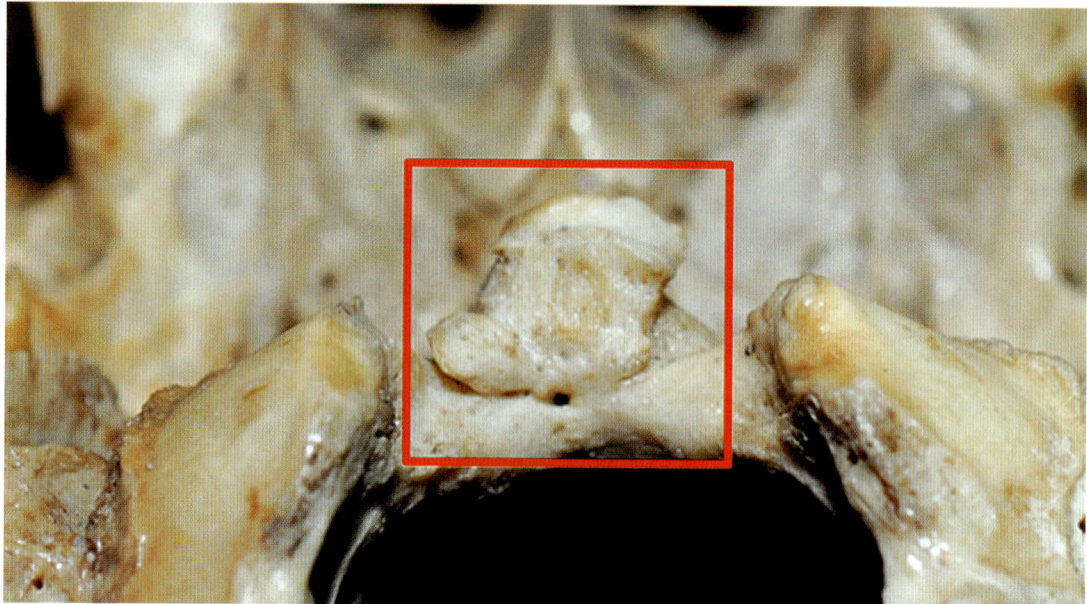

Figure 490. A tertiary (third) occipital condyle (square), also known as condyles tertius, a precondylar tubercle for articulation with the dens of the axis or calcified alar and cruciate ligament of the dens in an adult Thai skull (KKU). Rare finding. Cf. Broman (1957); Hanihara and Ishida (2001b); Oetteking (1923); Prescher et al. (1996); Prescher (1997); Smoker (1994); Von Ludinghausen et al. (2005); Taitz (2000).

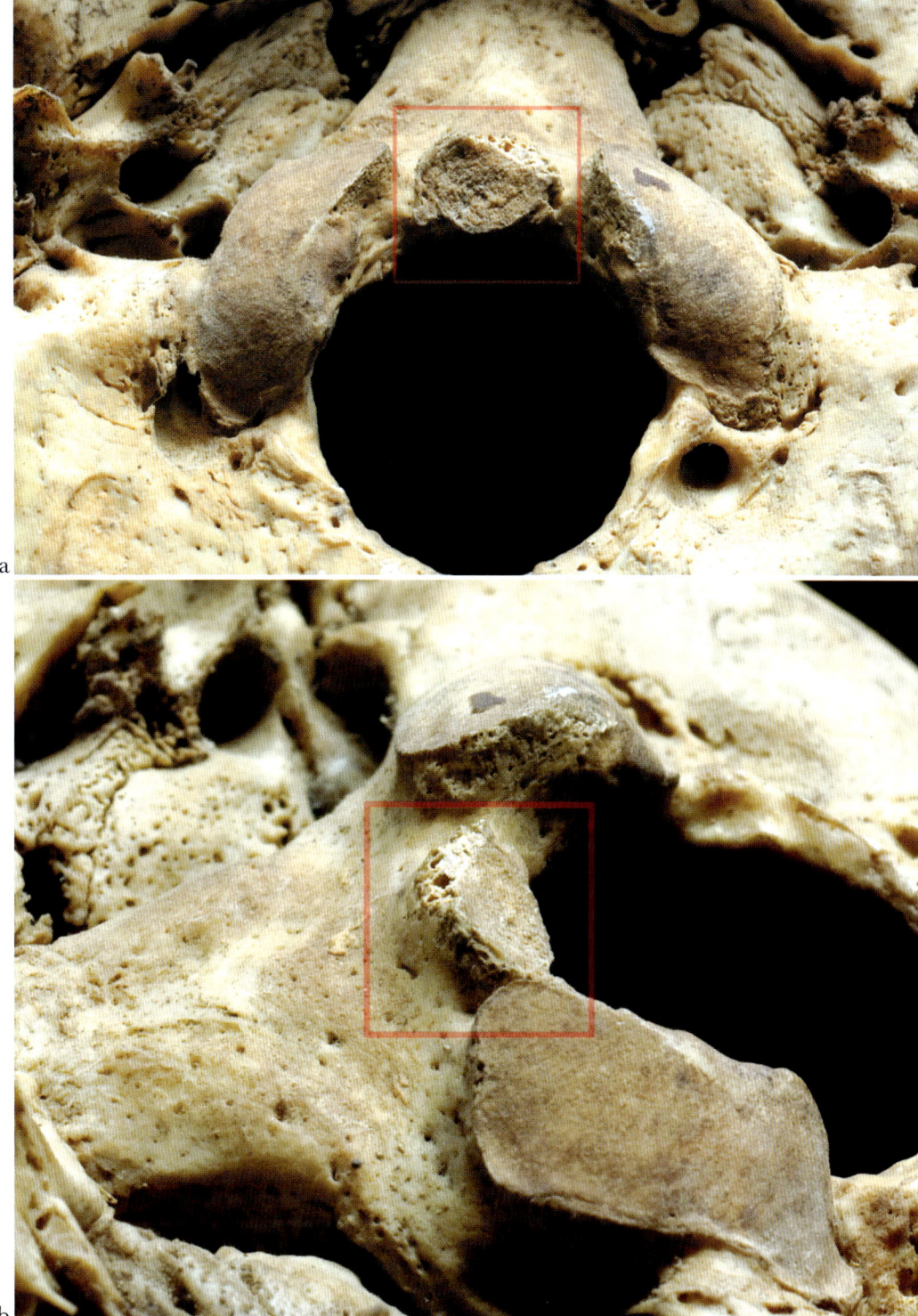

Figure 491a-b. Tertiary condyle. (a) Classic tertiary/third occipital condyle (square) in a 30- to 40-year-old Peruvian female skull (UPenn 631 L606). Cf. Hanihara and Ishida 2001(b). (b) Oblique view showing the morphology of the third condyle (square) in relation to the other two occipital condyles. Tertiary condyles are rare and form if the medial part of the hypochordal arch/bow (of the proatlas) persists (Pang and Thompson 2011; Prescher et al. 1996; Prescher 1997). Cf. Oetteking (1923); Smoker (1994).

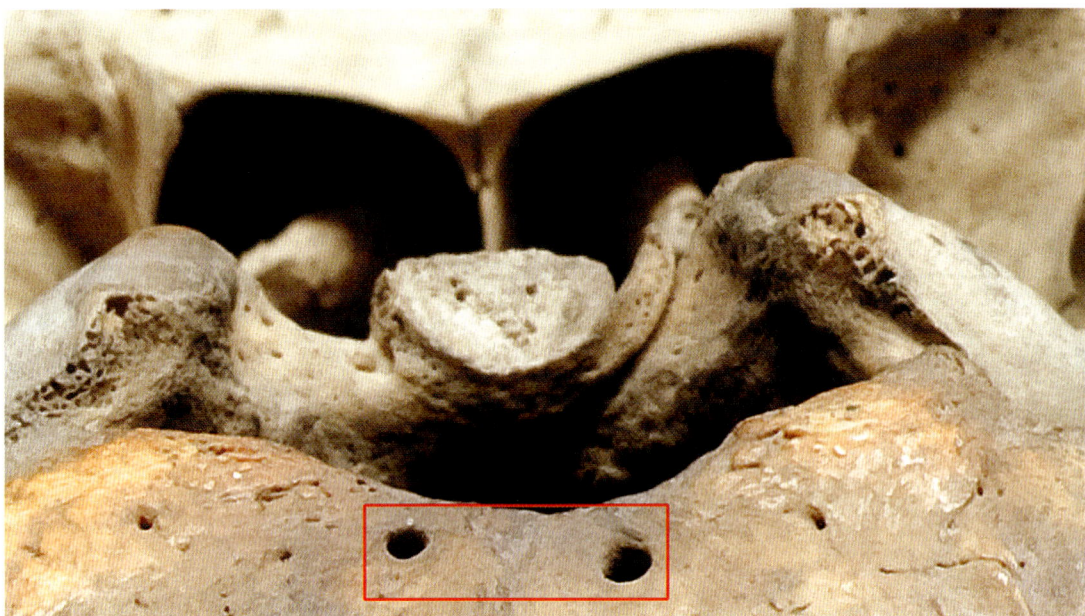

Figure 492. Tertiary condyle in a 30–40-year-old Peruvian female skull (UPenn 631 L606). Tertiary occipital condyles may be in the midline or offset to either side. Note the two unusually large foramina (rectangle) along the posterior margin of the foramen magnum.

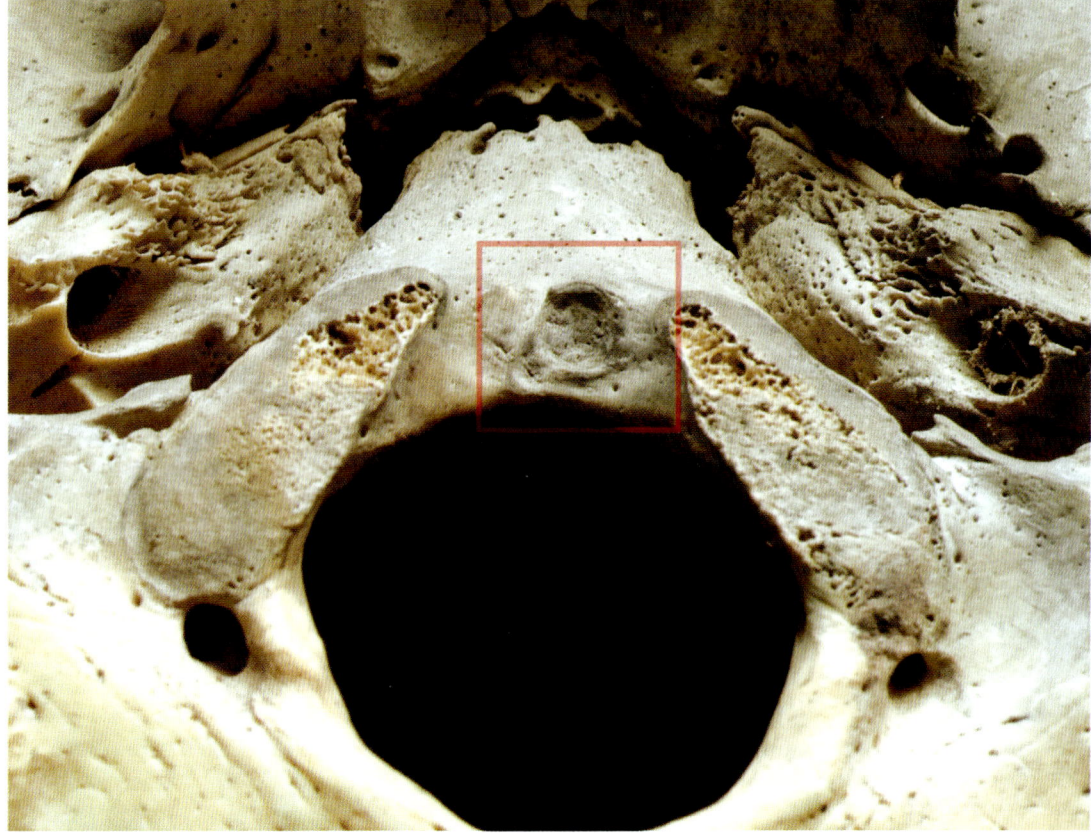

Figure 493. Rare tertiary condyle (square) in a 6–10-year-old Peruvian child (UPenn 569 L606). Cf. Oetteking (1923); Prescher et al. (1996); Prescher (1997); Smoker (1994).

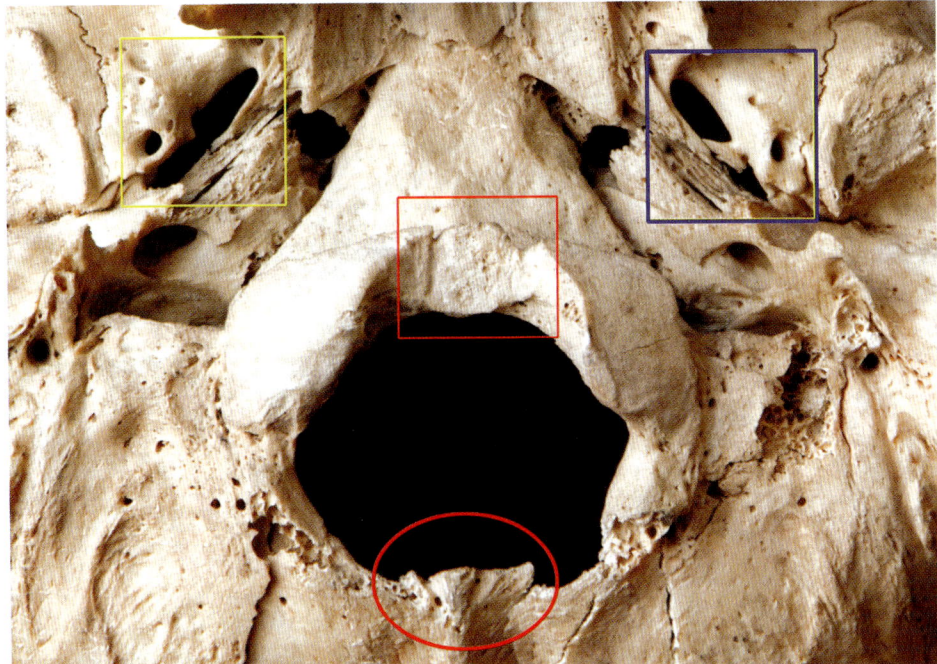

Figure 494. Tertiary condyle (red square) that is an extension of the occipital condyles, elongated and incomplete right foramen ovale (yellow square), double/divided left foramen ovale (blue square) and probable Kerckring's process (oval) in an adult Australian (NHMH 13 on frontal bone and 8911 on left temporal). Kerckring's process usually fuses with the occipital bone within the first month following birth (Madeline and Elster 1995).

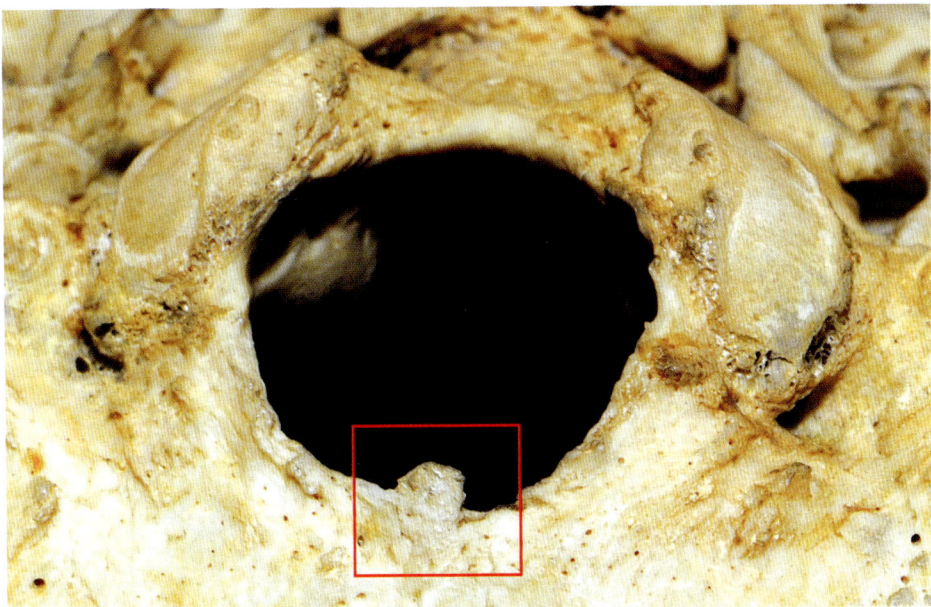

Figure 495. Kerckring's process/bone or center (square) in an adult skull (Mütter Museum 1008.68). Although Weinberg et al. (2005) found the Process of Kerckring in 33 of 63 (52%) Black and White perinatal individuals, the present authors have seen this feature in only a few adults. The purpose of this feature remains unknown (Weinberg et al. 2005). Cf. Fazekas and Kosa (1978); Freyschmidt et al. (2002); Kosa (1995); Madeline and Elster (1995). See Shapiro and Robinson (1976) for drawings, x-rays and description in fetuses.

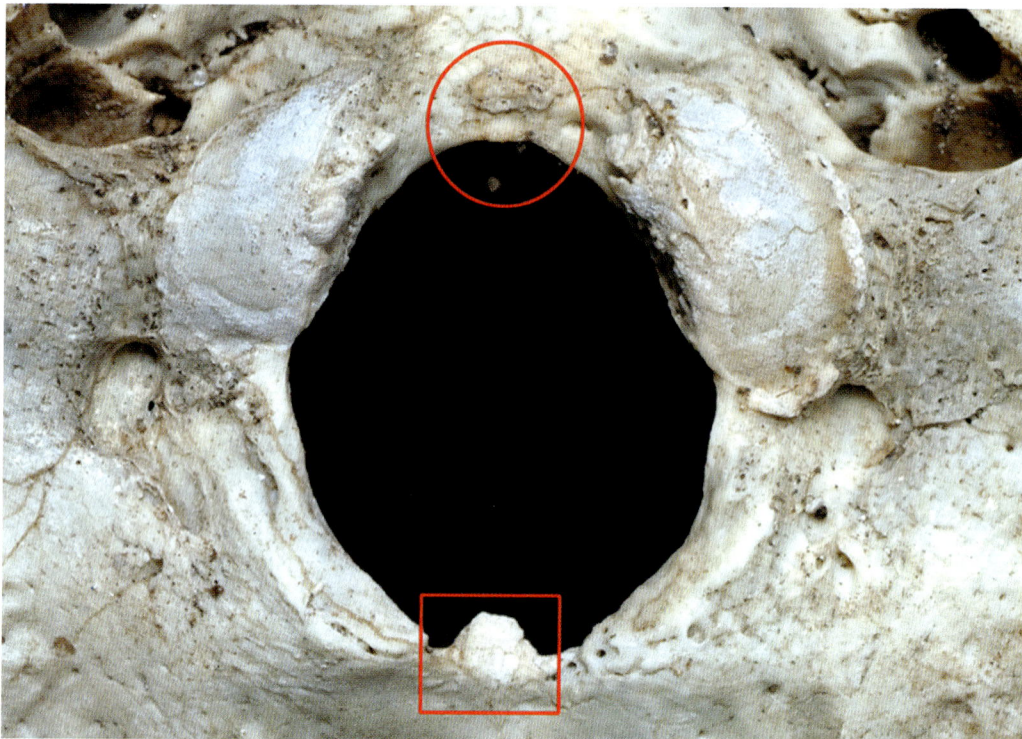

Figure 496. Kerckring's process (square) and precondylar tubercle (circle) in an 84-year-old Thai female skull (CMU 43 52). Cf. Hauser and DeStefano 1989.

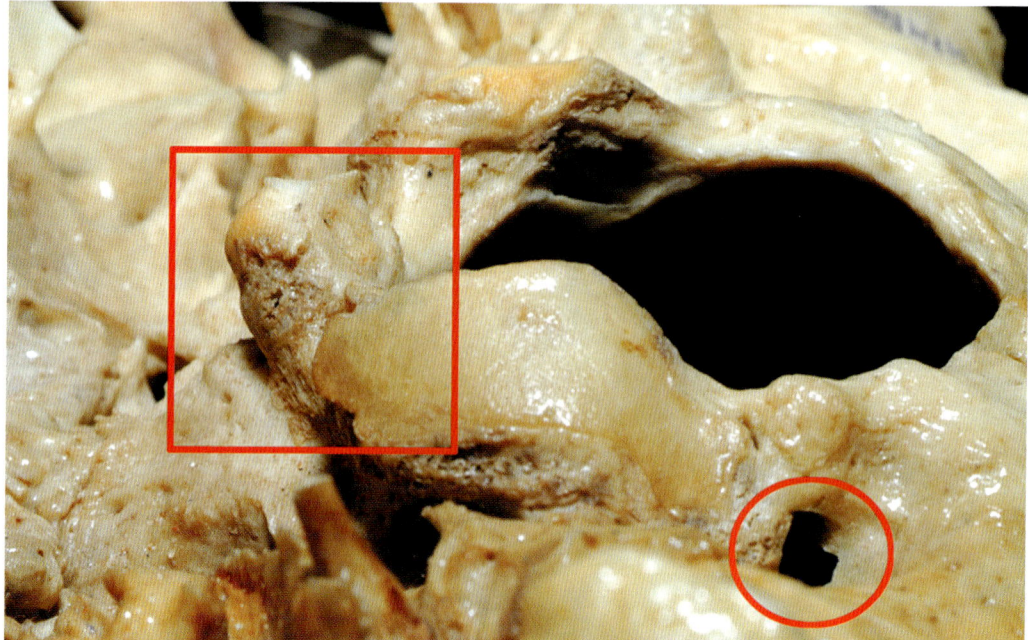

Figure 497. Peg-shaped tertiary occipital condyle (precondylar process) (square) in an adult Thai skull (KKU). Tertiary condyles are uncommon findings and those that are peg-shaped are rare. Cf. Oetteking (1923); Broman (1957). Agujero retrojugular de Serrano (circle) that communicates with the interior of the skull, with a reported frequency of 0.1% (1 of 540 Spanish skulls) (Vázquez et al. 2001).

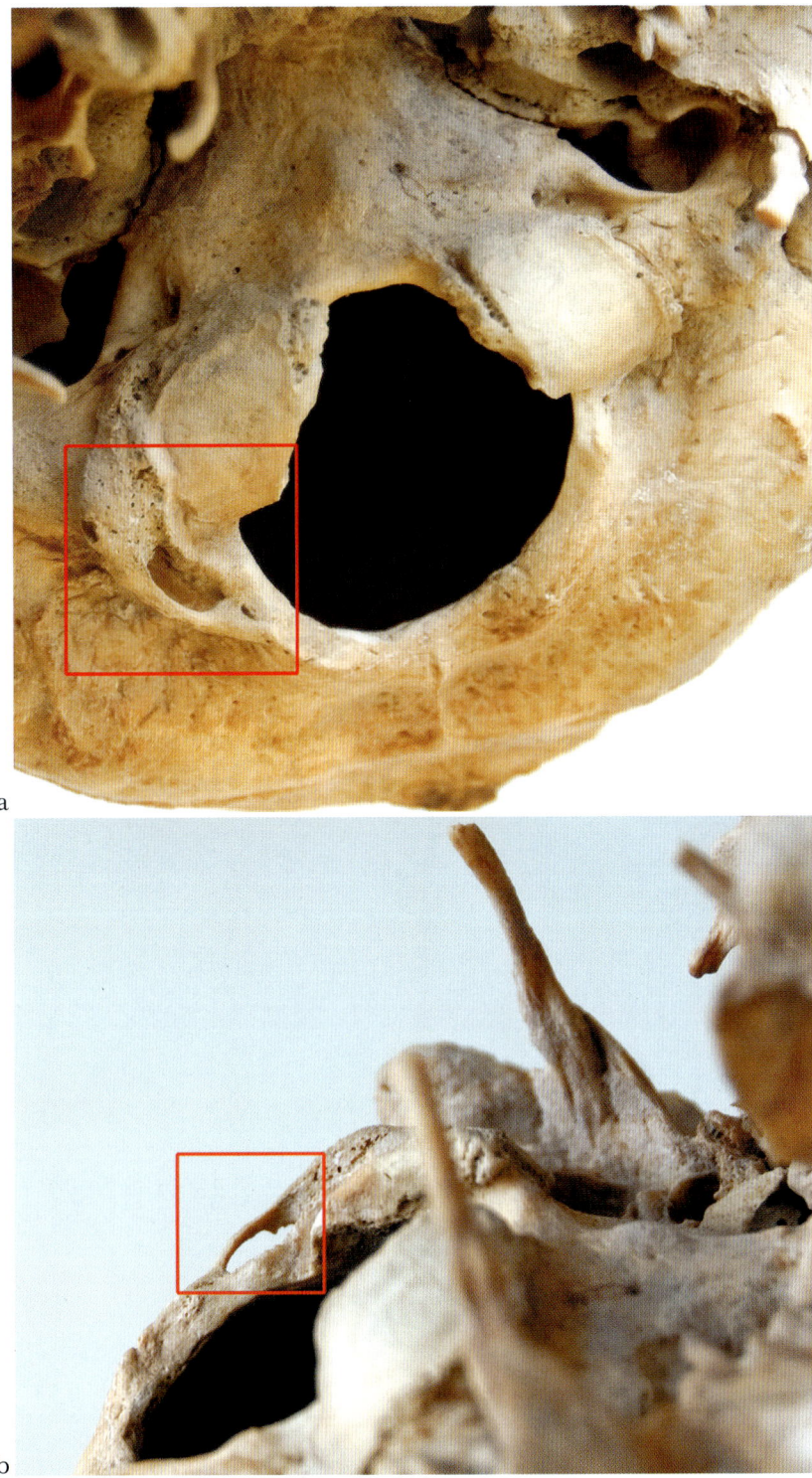

Figure 498a-b. Calcified bridge of bone. (a) Basilar view of a small, calcified bridge of bone (intermediate condylar canal bridging) spanning from the lateral portion of the right occipital condyle (square) in an adult probable male (NHMH Larlotalva 232, Kopanya). (b) Right lateral view of the calcified bridge (square). Vázquez et al. (2001) reported 33 of 544 skulls (6%) with this feature (canalis condylaris intermedius). Cf. Hauser and DeStefano (1989).

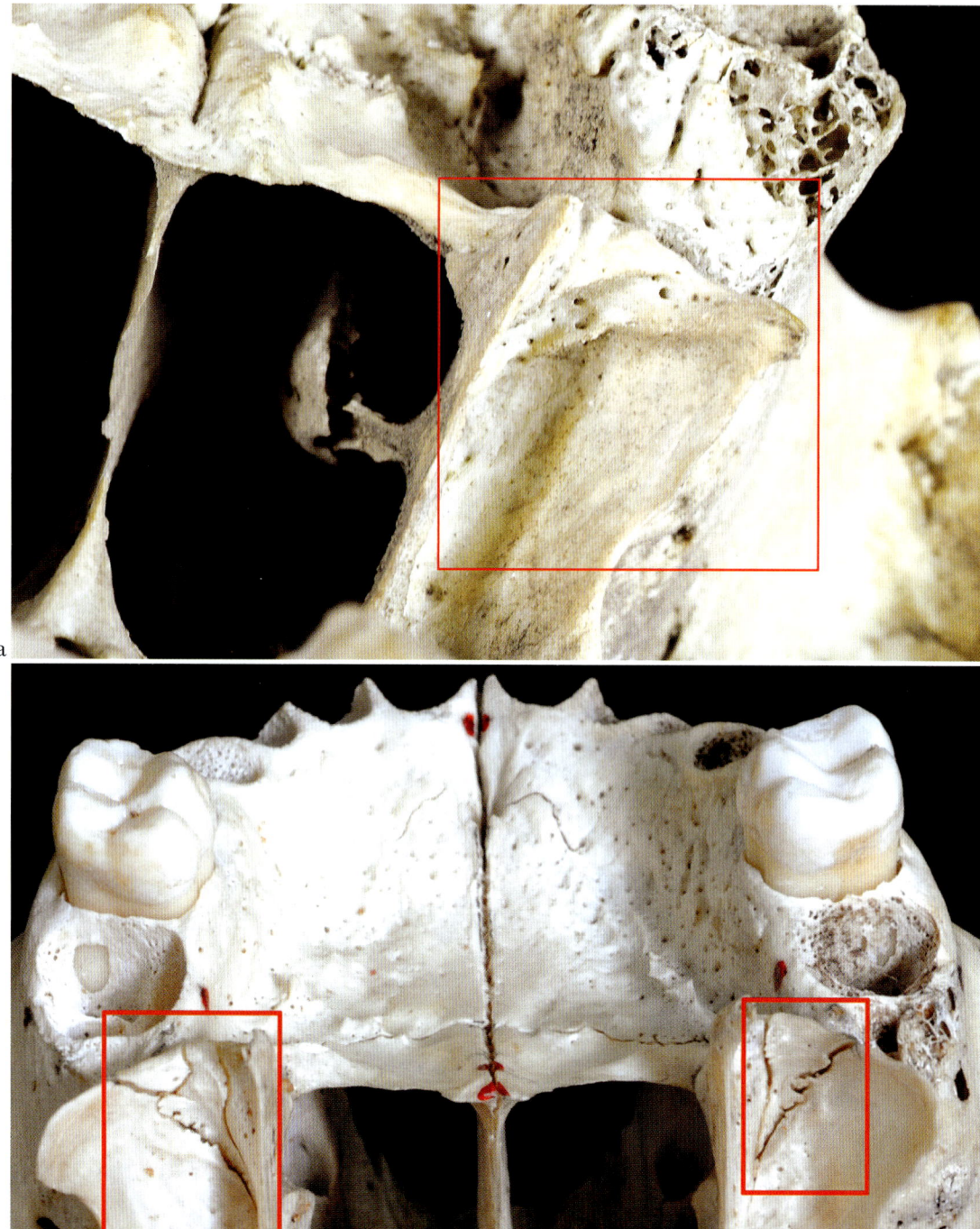

Figure 499a-b. The sphenomaxillary suture (*sutura sphenomaxillaris*), sometimes referred to as the pterygopalatine, pterygomaxillary or pterygopalatomaxillary suture. (a) Obliterated left sphenomaxillary suture (square) in an elderly Thai male. (b) Open sphenomaxillary sutures in a Thai child (rectangles) (KKU). In the child, what is actually a single bone filling the right notch appears to be two "ossicles" (palatine part of the maxilla). The V-shaped sphenomaxillary suture has an age-related growth component to its closure or obliteration much like the vault and maxillary/palatal sutures. The sphenomaxillary suture is present (Dauber 2007; Pick 1999; Remmelink 1988, 1993; Schiel 2007) in all individuals, is a growing suture (Vacher et al. 2010), is visible (not obliterated) in adolescence, and usually obliterates in middle-age and older adulthood. The sphenomaxillary suture and junction warrants further research regarding its utility as an indicator of age.

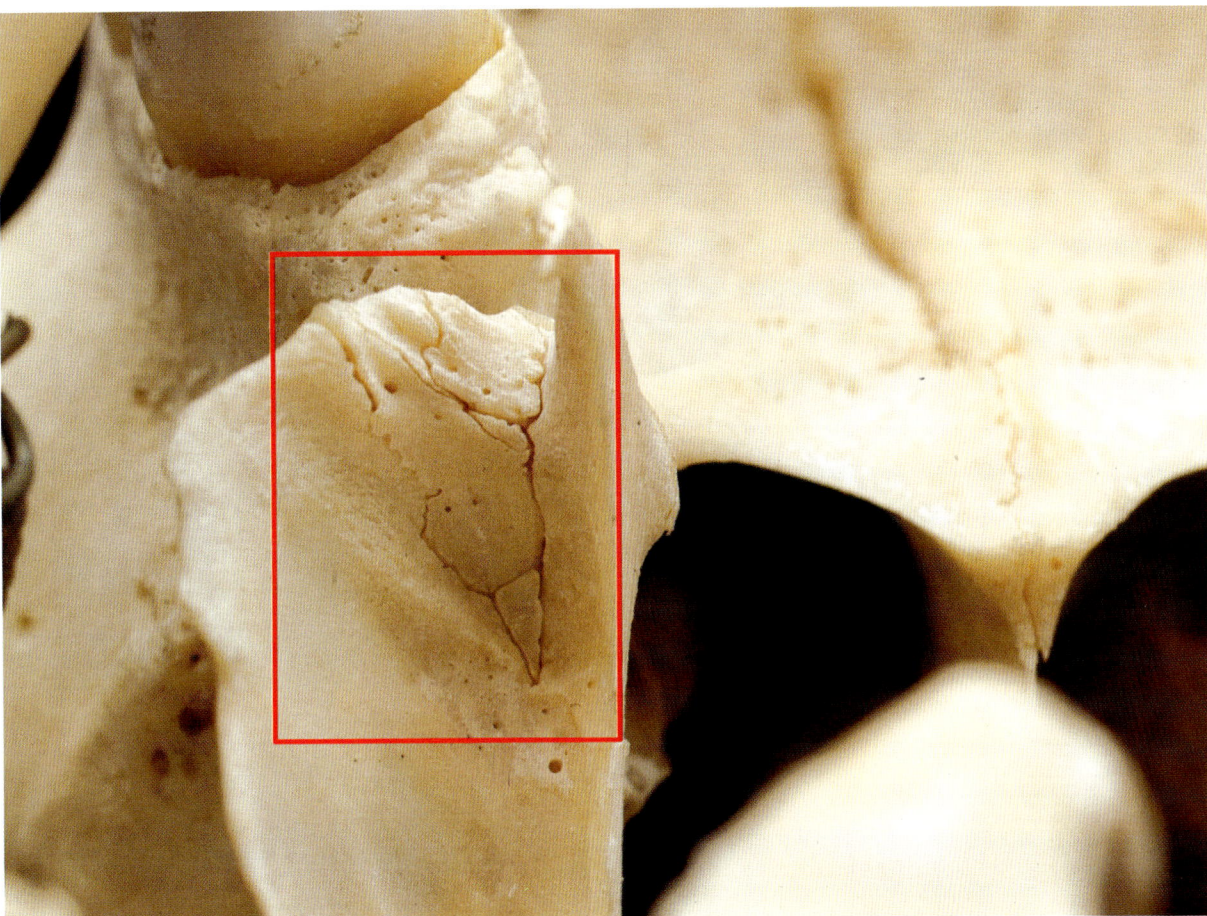

Figure 500. What appears to be a five-segmented right sphenomaxillary suture (rectangle), but is actually a single bone in an adult male (FSA DS043). The "ossicles" are usually just the ridges in the palatine part of the maxilla. This is the site where the sphenoid and maxillary bones are surgically separated (sphenomaxillary dysjunction) for some Le Fort osteotomies (Dauber 2007; Pick 1993; Remmelink 1988, 1993; Schiel 2007 for more on the V-shaped pterygoid notch, fossa and fissure as well as the sphenomaxillary suture (Vacher et al. 2010). Obliteration of the sphenomaxillary suture (aka pterygopalatomaxillary suture) appears to be correlated to age (Mann, Lozanoff and Byrd, unpublished observations). This relationship is revealed in that the entire V-shaped suture is visible in subadults, begins to obliterate in early adulthood, and typically obliterates partially or completely in middle-age and older individuals. These preliminary findings are supported by the research of Melsen and Ousterhout (1987) who reported that disarticulation of the pterygomaxillary region in Le Fort I procedures was possible only during the infantile period, with fractures occurring in older juveniles and adolescents. Melsen and Ousterhout further noted an increasing association of interdigitations between the palatine and adjacent bones with increasing age. Typical anatomy in subadults as well as young and middle-age adults.

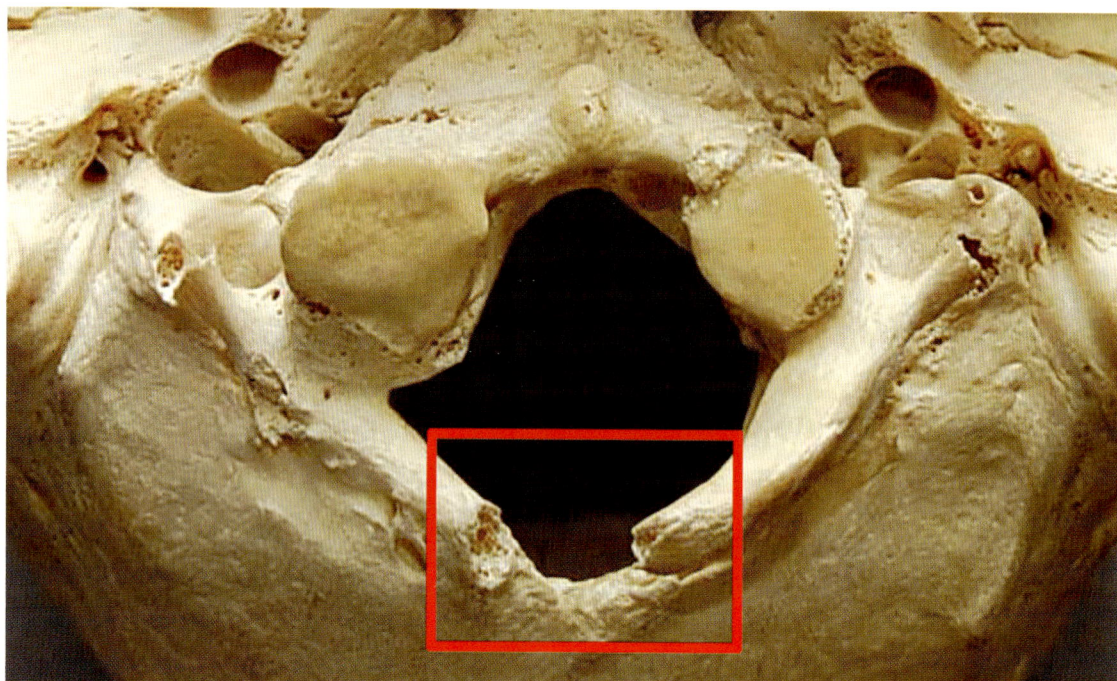

Figure 501. Atlanto-occipitalization, bifid posterior arch (rectangle) and asymmetrically sized and shaped inferior articular facets of the atlas (C1) in an adult Thai skull (KKU). Uncommon finding in most groups. Cf. Agrawal et al. (2010); Al-Motabagani and Surendra (2006); Gladstone and Wakeley (1925); Macalister (1893).

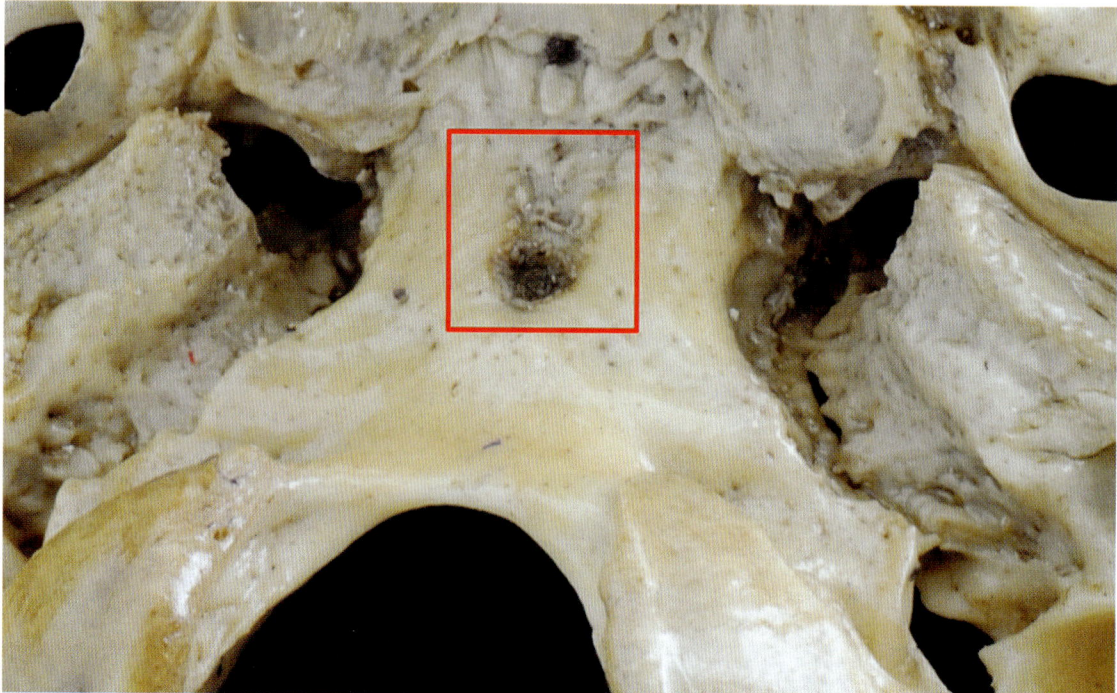

Figure 502. Large pharyngeal foveola or pit, also known as fossa navicularis (Cankal et al. 2004) in an adult Thai skull (KKU). Common to uncommon finding. Cf. Hauser and DeStefano (1989).

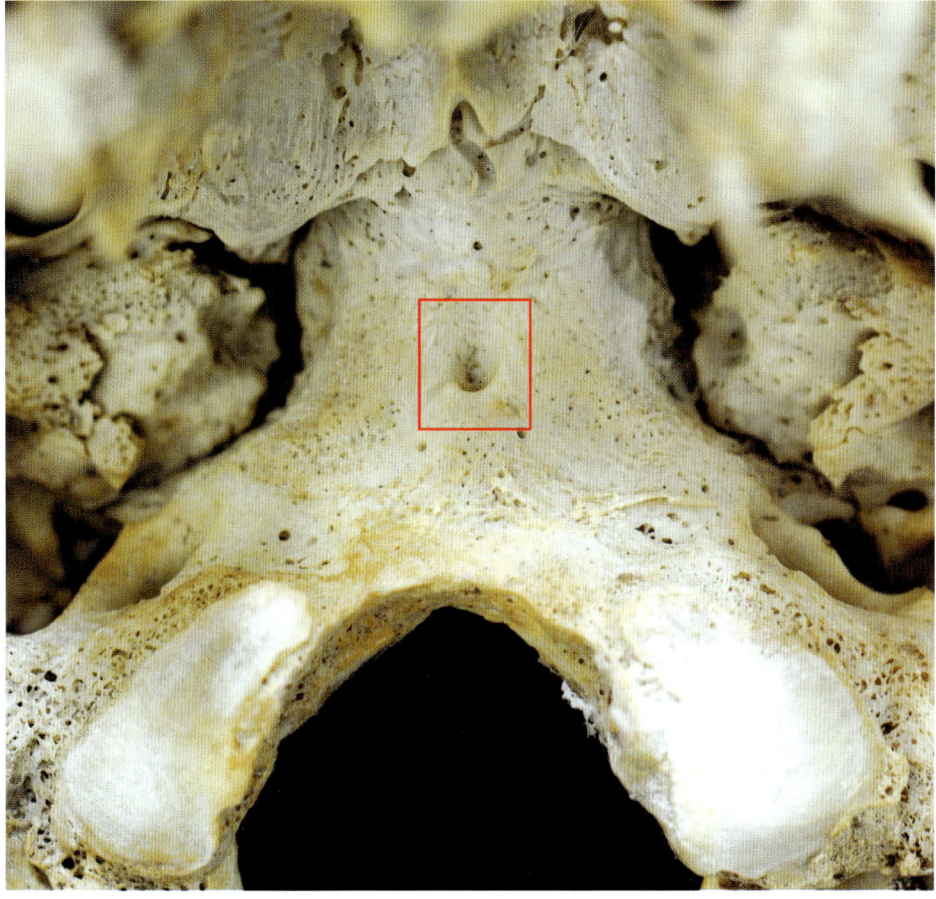

Figure 503. Small pharyngeal foveola/fossa navicularis (square) in adult Thai skull (KKU). Common to uncommon finding. Cf. Cankal et al. (2004); Hauser and DeStefano (1989); Vázquez et al. (2001).

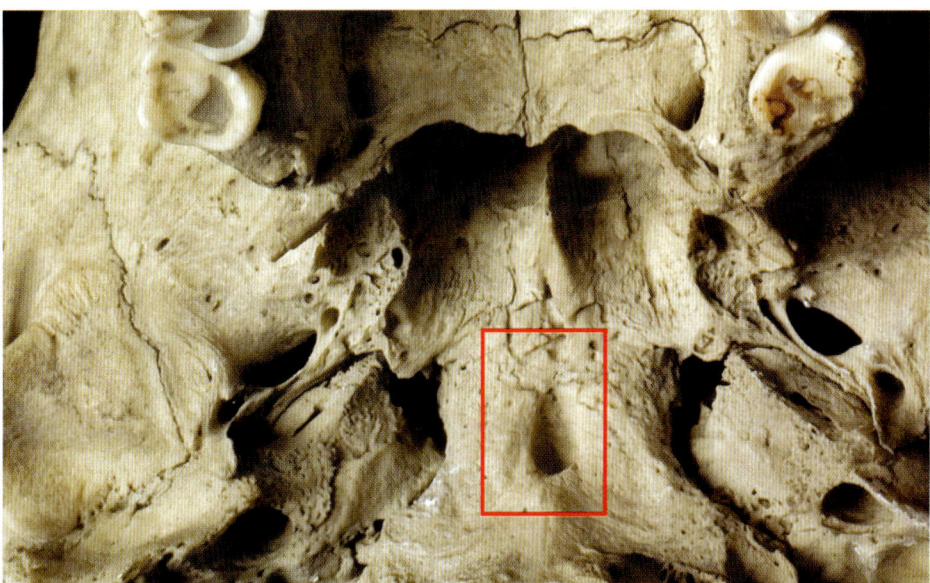

Figure 504. Large, teardrop shaped fossa navicularis in an adult Indian female skull (UPenn 413). Hauser and DeStefano (1989).

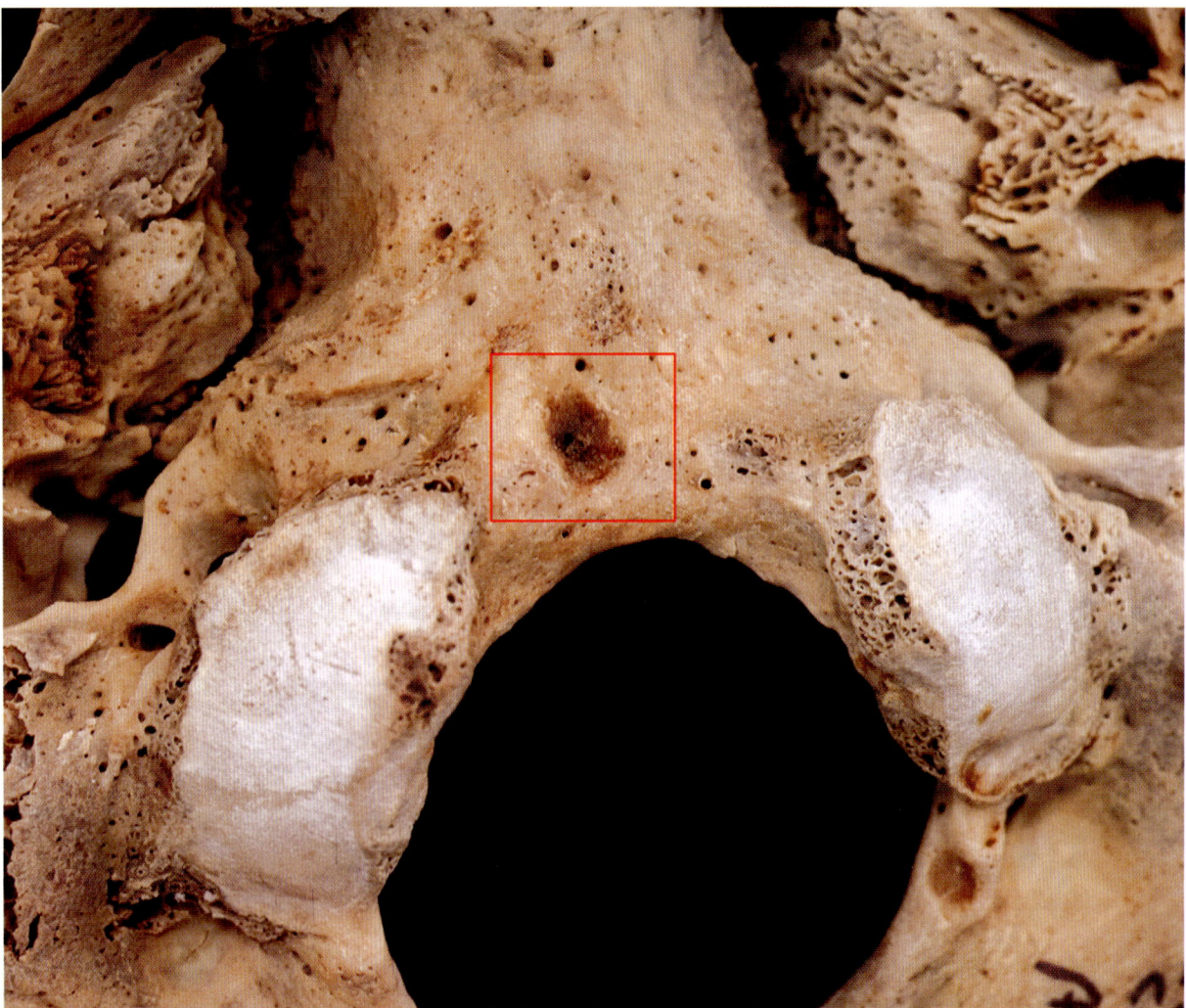

Figure 505. Posteriorly positioned fossa navicularis (square) near the margin of the foramen magnum in an elderly Asian female (CSC AC019). Cankal et al. (2004) found this pit in 26 of 492 skulls (5.3%). These researchers used CT to examine 525 patients and found 16 (3%) with fossa navicularis, none of which contained soft tissue lesions.

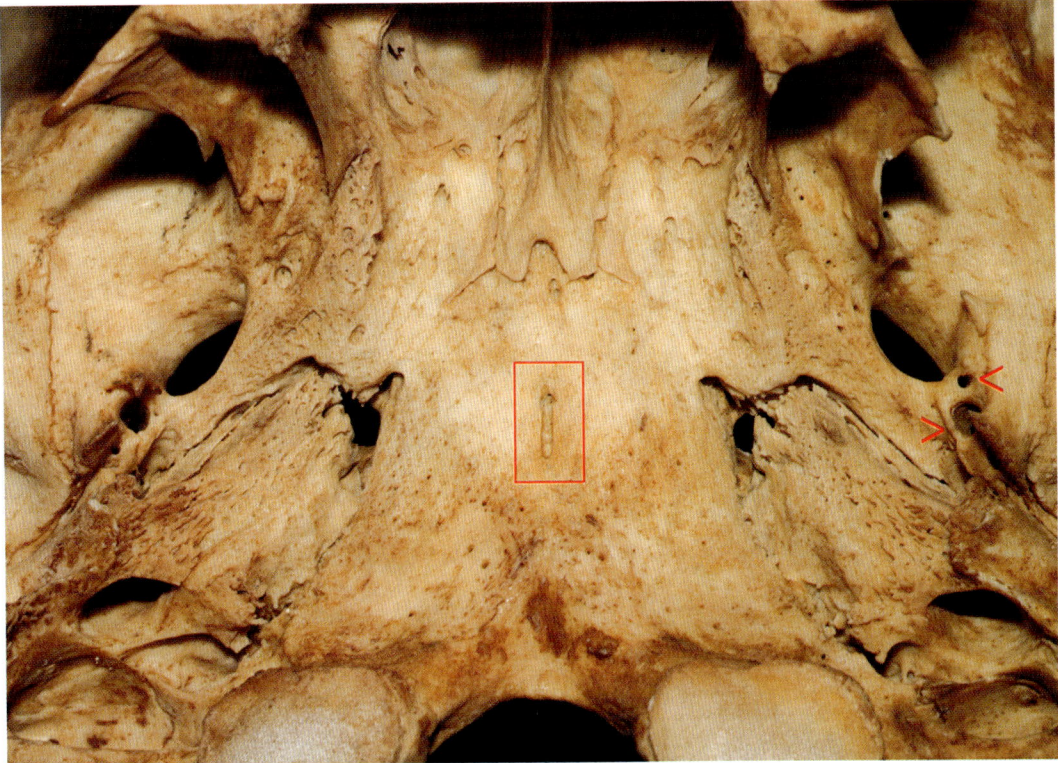

Figure 506. Slit-like fossa navicularis (rectangle) in a 30- to 50-year-old African, probable male (TM 20, Ditsong Museum). Slit-like fossae such as this are uncommon findings. Also present are a foramen of Arnold (<) and a thin bar of bone (>) spanning medial to the left foramen spinosum.

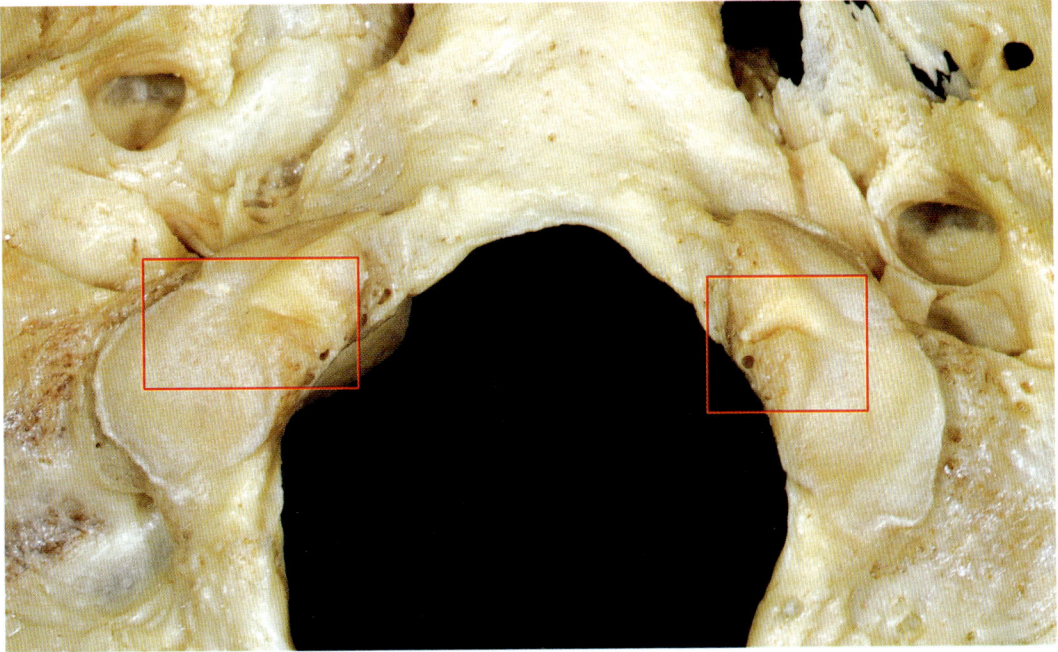

Figure 507. Partially divided occipital condyles (square and rectangle) in an adult (1134 JABSOM). The left condyle exhibits a small notch (small square) along its medial margin.

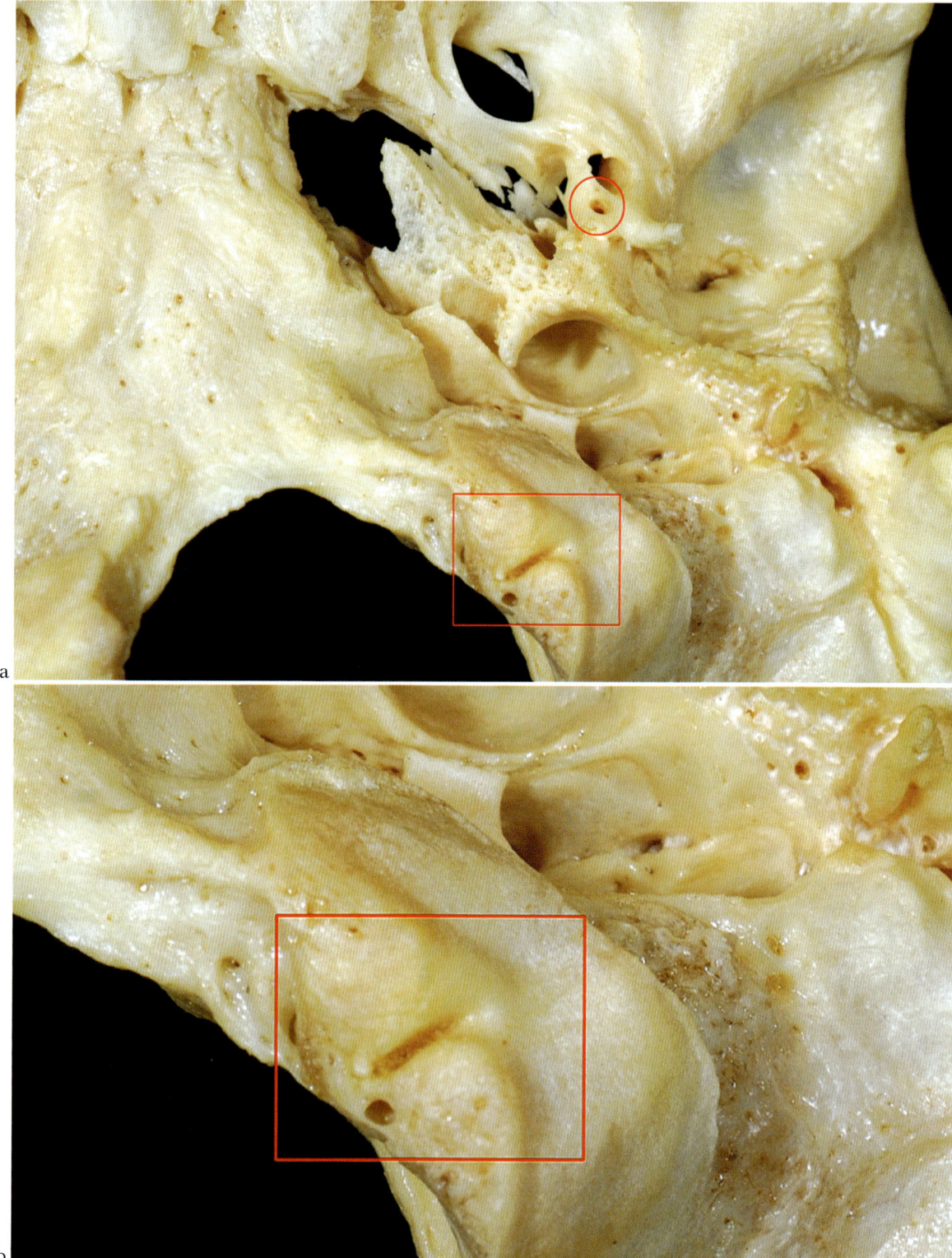

Figure 508a-b. Variant of the basioccipital synchondrosis and an accessory foramen. (a) Remnant of the basioccipital synchondrosis (rectangle) joining the lateral part of the left occipital to the basilar bone and a small accessory foramen (circle) medial to the left foramen spinosum (possibly the foramen of Arnold) (1134 JABSOM). (b) Higher magnification of the left occipital condyle (rectangle).

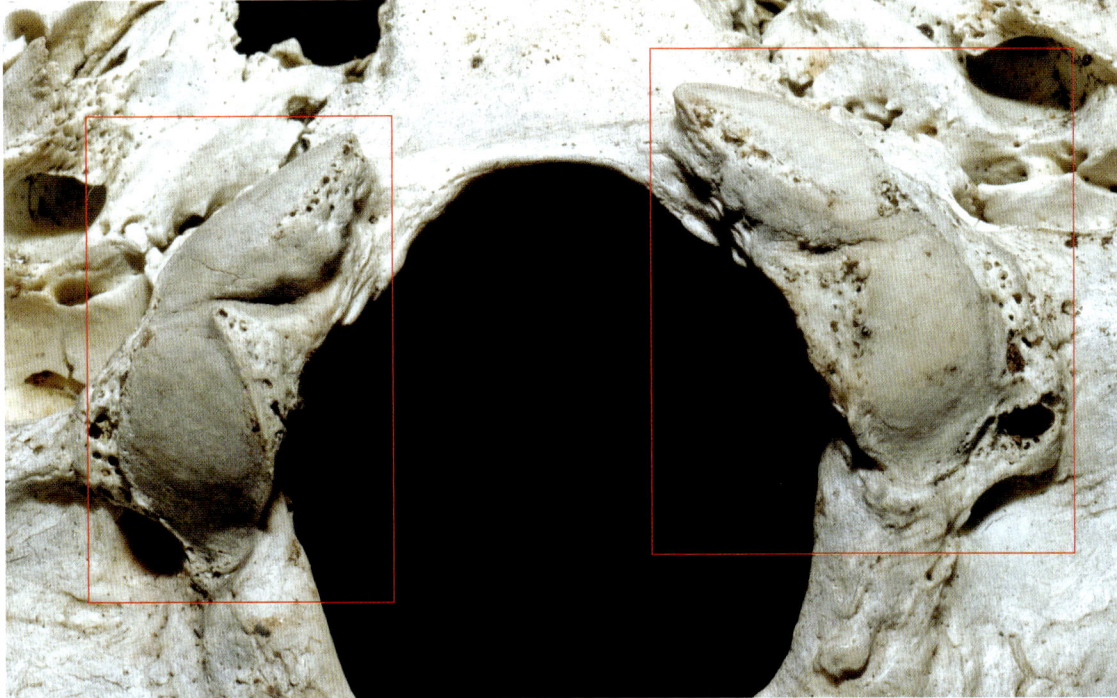

Figure 509. Variously divided occipital condyles (rectangles), reflecting a cranial shift, in an adult White female (SI Terry). Uncommon to common finding. See Tubbs et al. (2005) for a case described as an extremely rare variant where the condyles are spaced further apart.

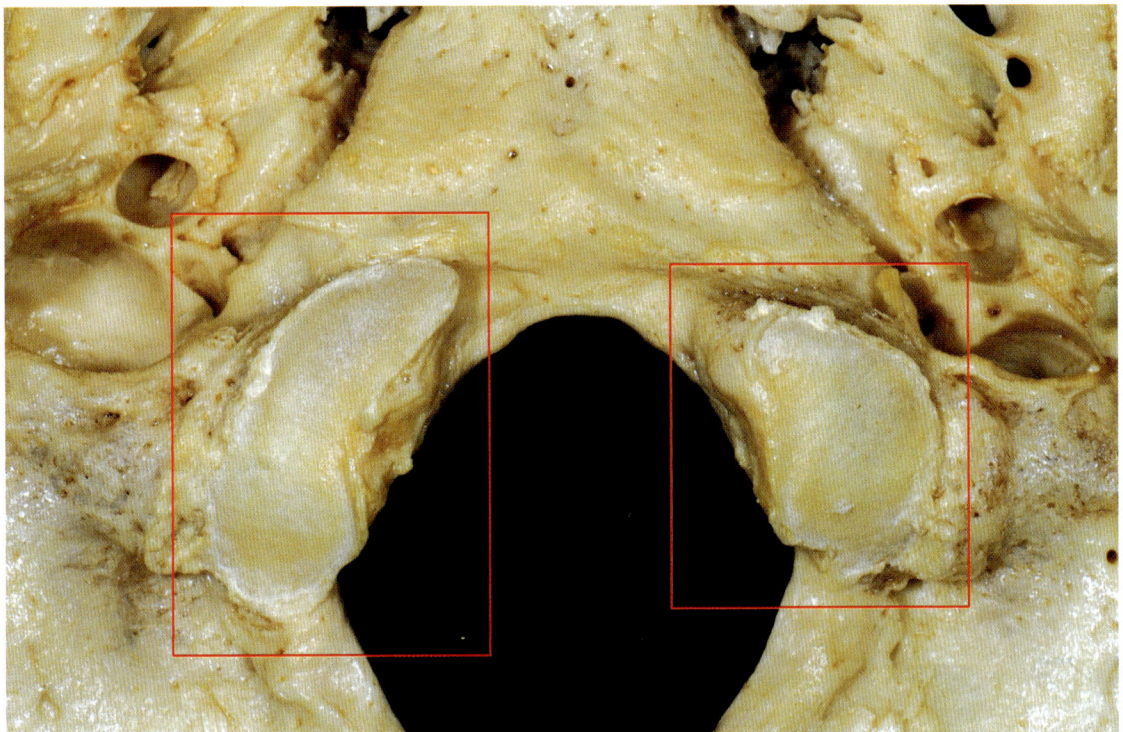

Figure 510. Asymmetrical occipital condyles (rectangle and square) in an adult (1040 JABSOM).

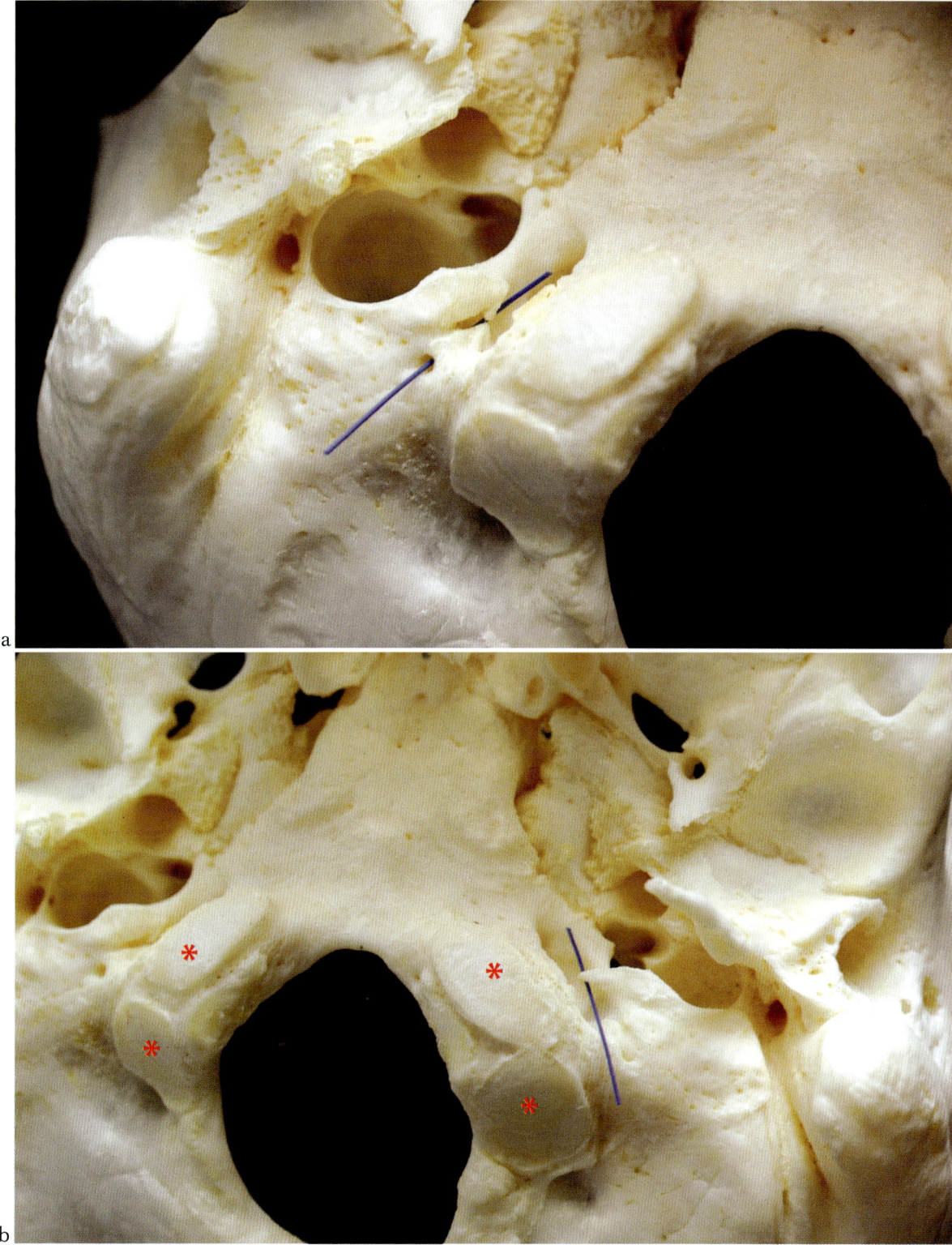

Figure 511a-b. Paracondylar foramen and divided occipital condyles. (a) Paracondylar foramen and canal (probe). (b) Divided right occipital condyles (*) and partial formation (probe) of a left paracondylar foramen/bridge in an elderly individual (FSA AC054).

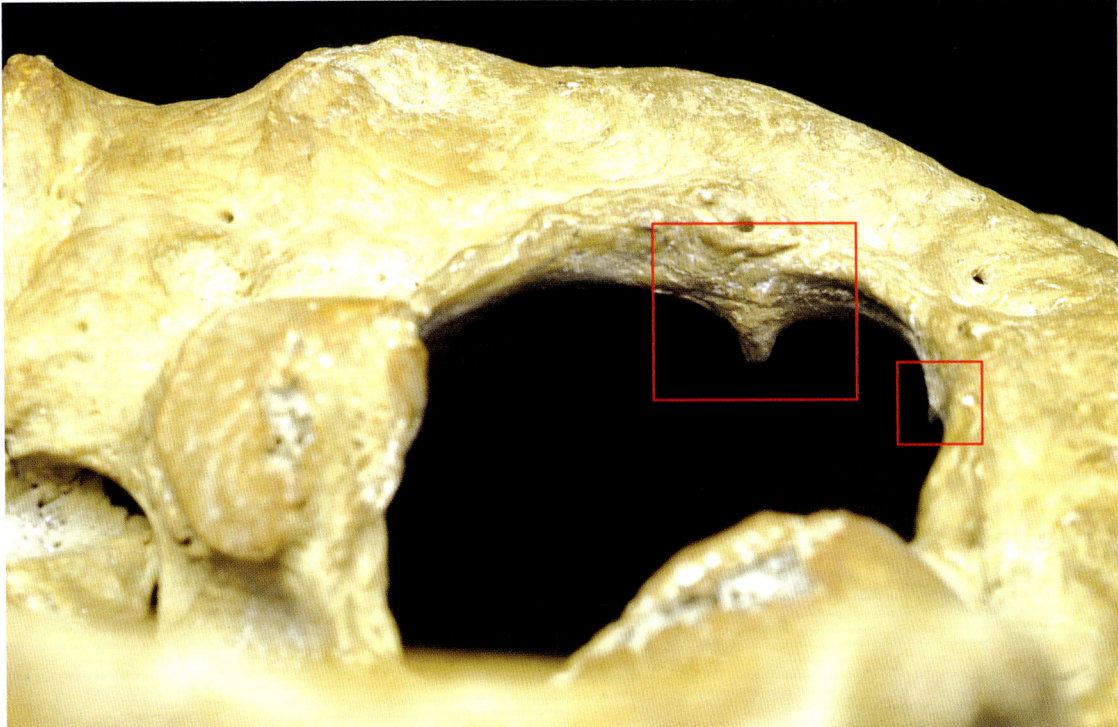

Figure 512. Two small spikes (rectangle and square) of unknown etiology along the posterior margin of the foramen magnum in an adult. Note small foramina opposite each spike (Mütter Museum). Rare finding.

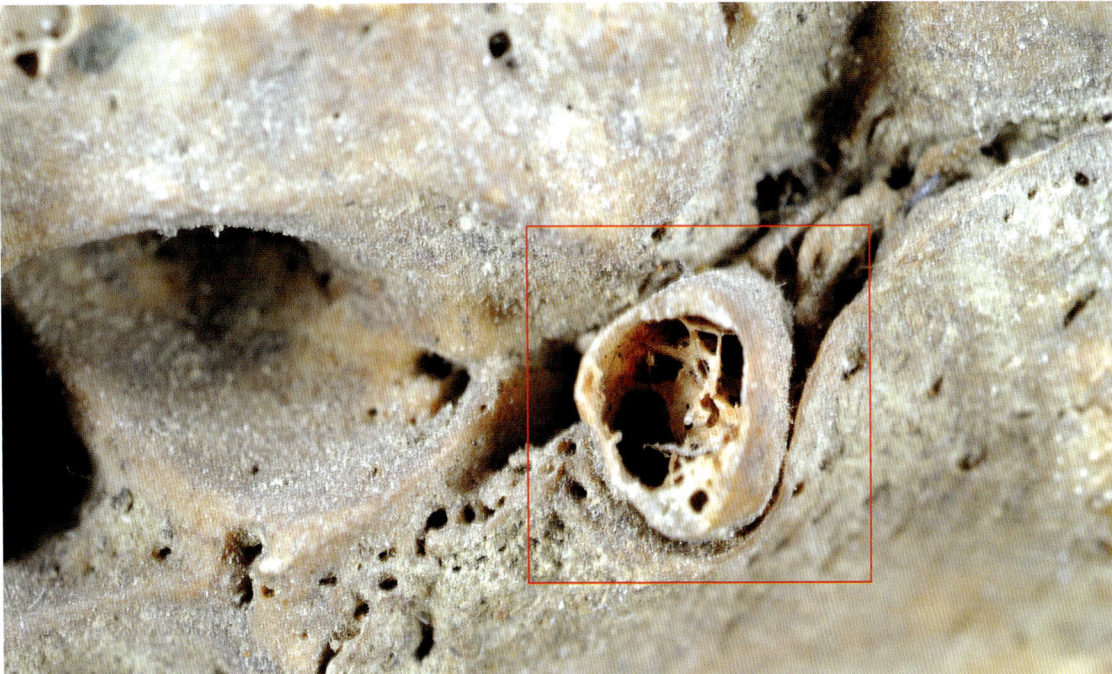

Figure 513. Typical internal morphology and architecture of the right styloid process (square) of the temporal bone in a middle-aged Thai male (KKU). Styloid processes may be solid or "hollow" and with a trabecular lattice pattern variously along its length.

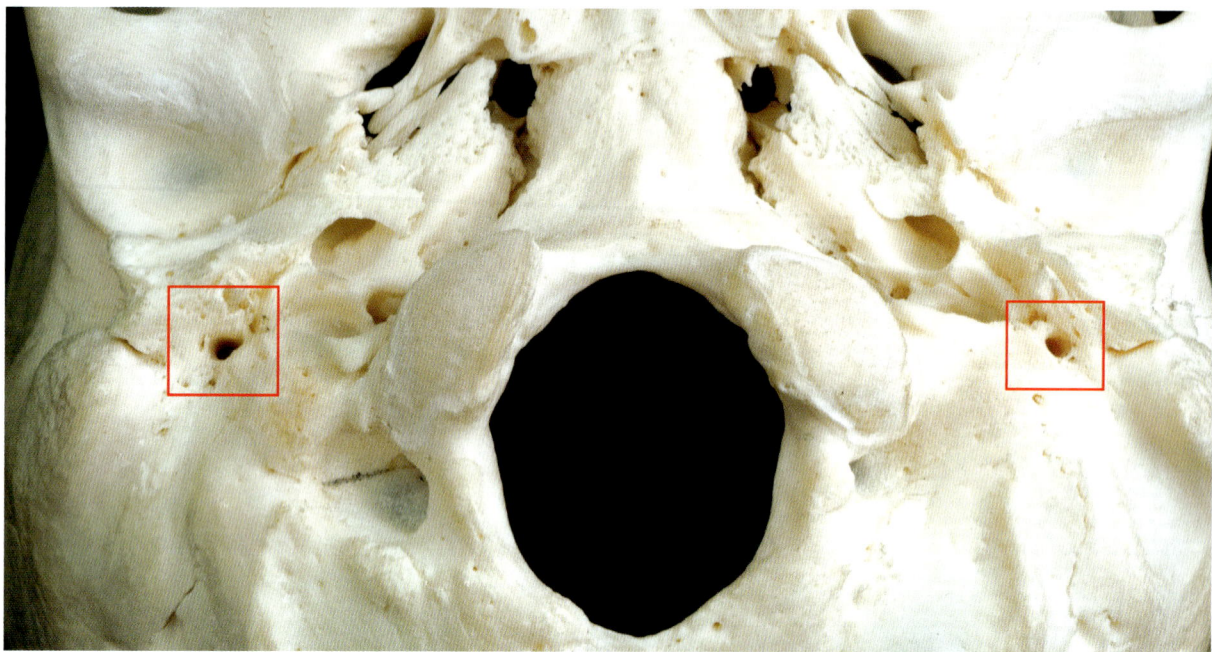

Figure 514. Stylomastoid foramen (squares) transmitting the motor branch of the facial nerve (cranial nerve VII) in an adult Asian (CSC AC27). Common finding and typical anatomy. Cf. Berge and Bergman (2001); Boyd (1930); Hauser and DeStefano (1989); Vázquez et al. (2001).

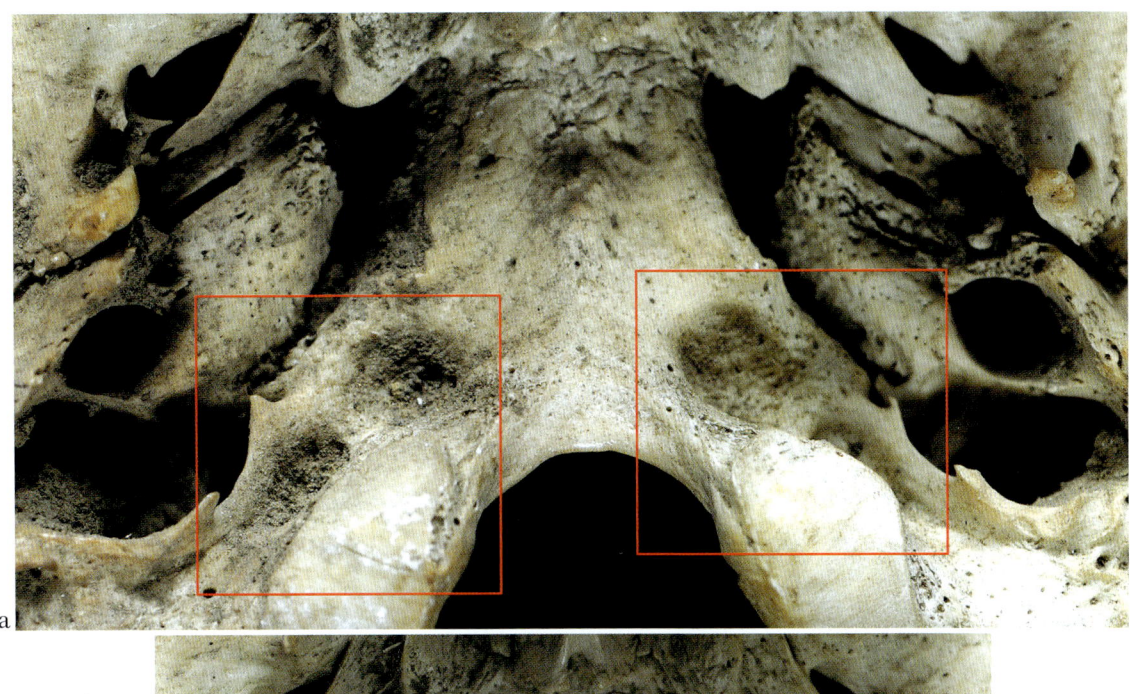

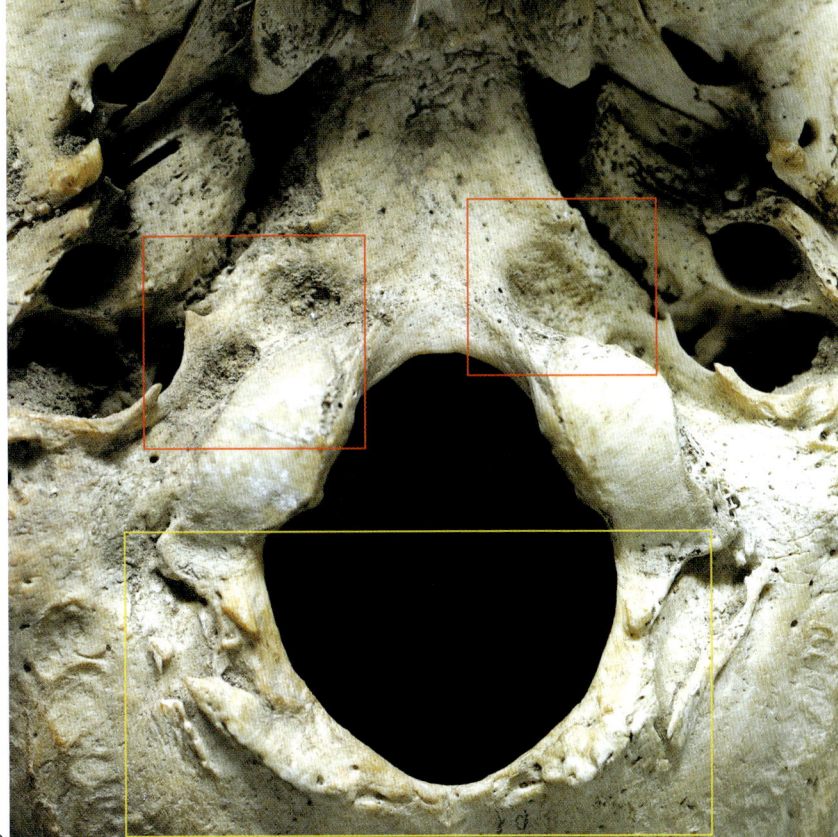

Figure 515a-b. Basilar depression (red squares) in an adult Thai (KKU). (a) Scooped-out depressions (rectangles) in the basilar bone that serve for attachment of the rectus capitis anterior muscles (typical anatomy, but uncommonly pronounced). (b) Basilar impressions (squares) with irregular rim of the foramen magnum (rectangle), a mild form of basilar impression due to contact with the posterior arch of the atlas (C1). Basilar impression is an uncommon finding (severe forms may reflect a pathological condition).

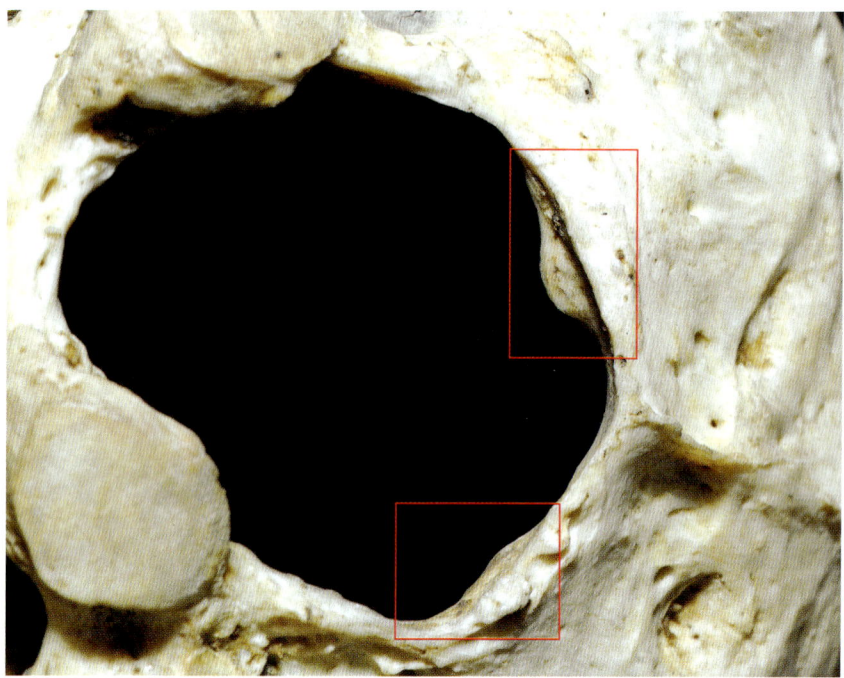

Figure 516. Endocranial tubercles (rectangles) along the posterior margin of the foramen magnum (Mütter Museum). These bony ledges are uncommon findings and their etiology is unknown.

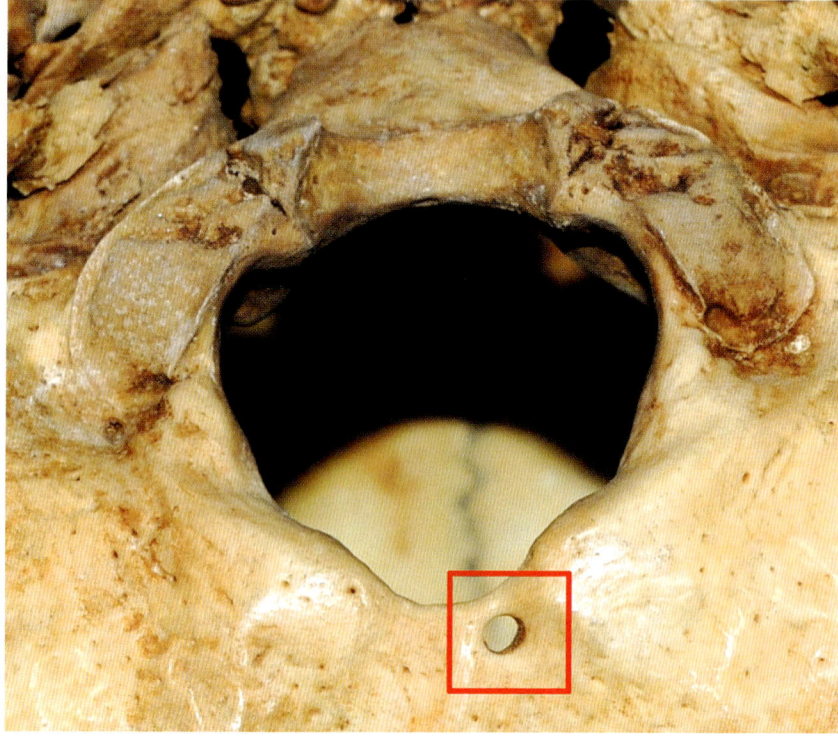

Figure 517. Large posterior foramen along the foramen magnum in a subadult Thai (KKU). While small foramina in this area are common, large foramina such as this are uncommon and of unknown frequency and etiology. Cf. Madeline and Elster (1995).

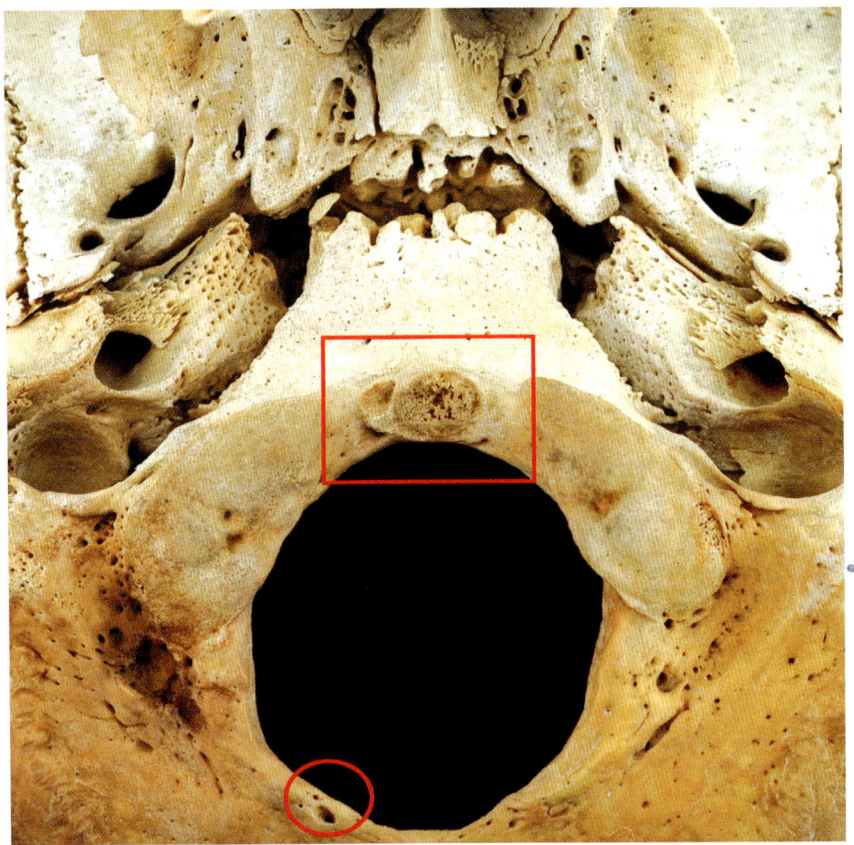

Figure 518. Tertiary condyle (rectangle) and accessory foramen (circle) in a Thai child (KKU). The tertiary condyle (condylus tertius) is an uncommon to rare finding. Cf. Allen (1880); Freyschmidt et al. (2002); von Ludinghausen et al. (2005); McCall et al. (2010); Taitz (2000).

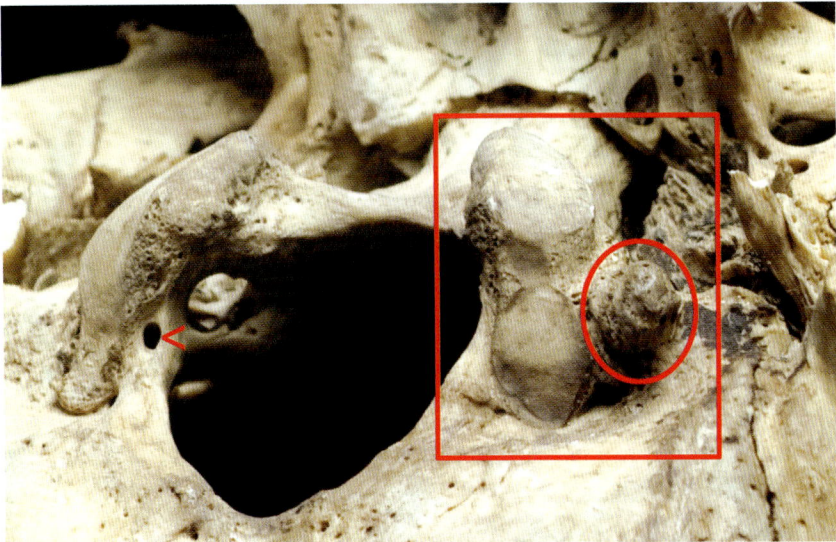

Figure 519. Unilateral paracondylar tubercle (circle), divided left occipital condyle (rectangle) and accessory canal and foramen (<) in an adult skull (UPenn, Wistar Collection). All are uncommon to rare features.

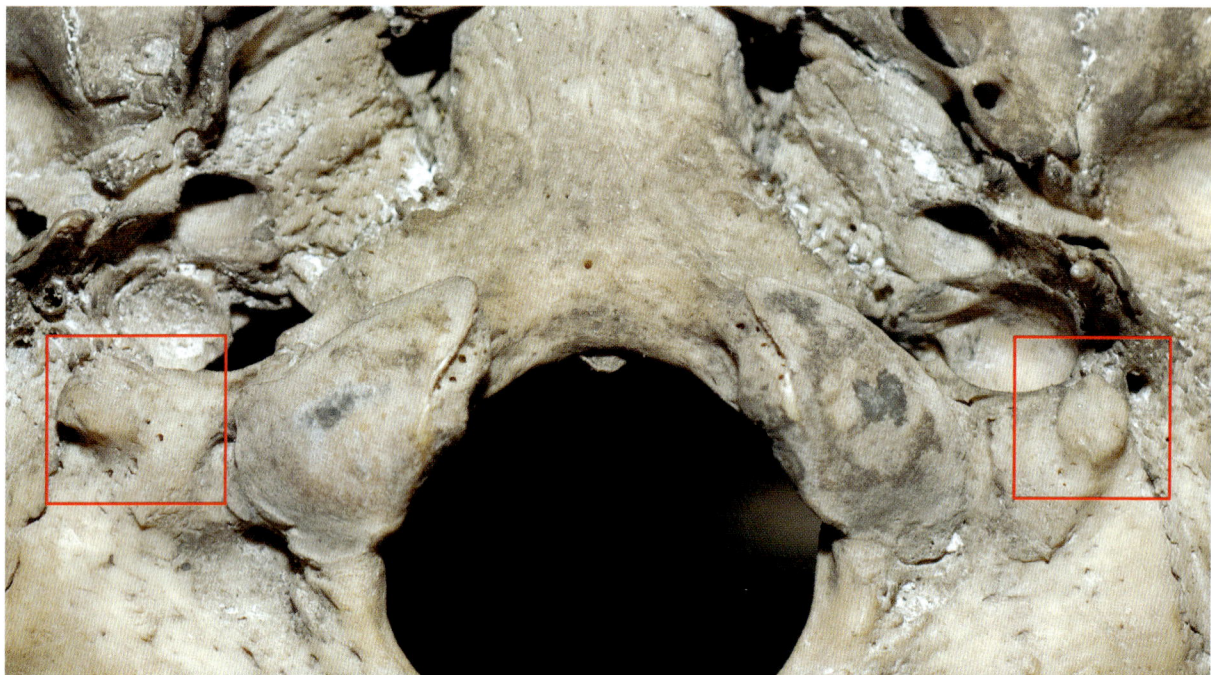

Figure 520. Bilateral paracondylar tubercles (squares) and ossified apical odontoid ligament (circle) in an adult ancient Peruvian (UPenn L-606 75). Uncommon to rare findings.

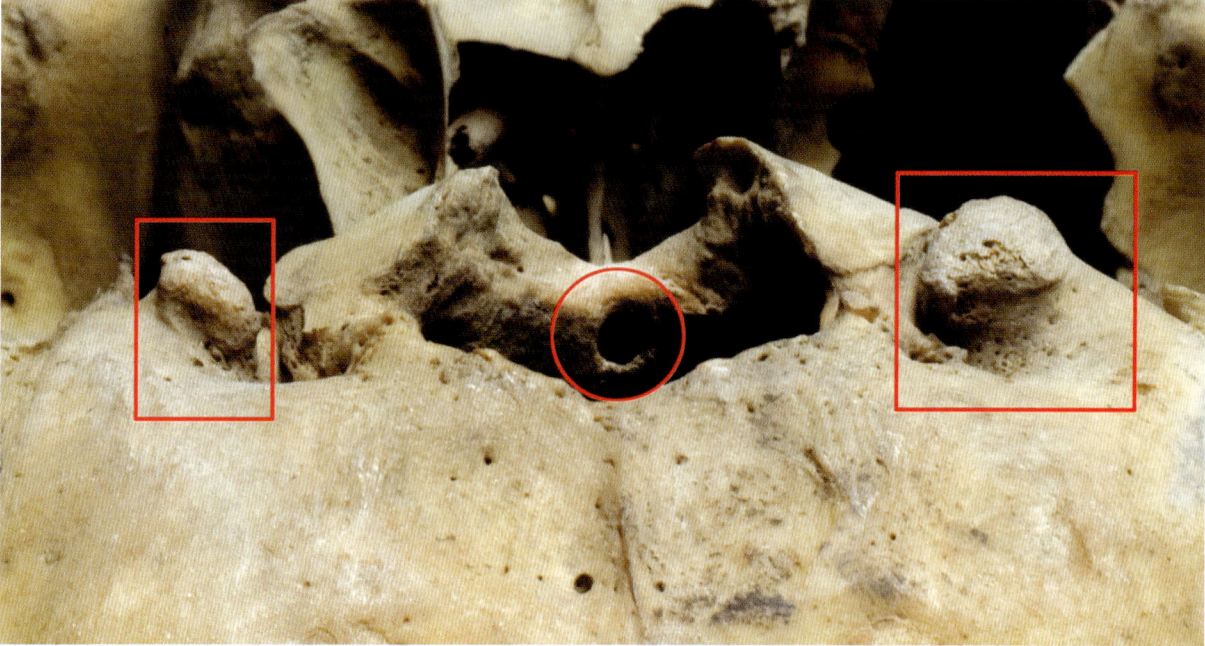

Figure 521. Bilateral paracondylar tubercles (rectangle and square) and an unusually large median canal (circle) in an ancient Peruvian adult female (UPenn L-606 409). Rare finding. Cf. Hauser and DeStefano (1989); McCall et al. (2010).

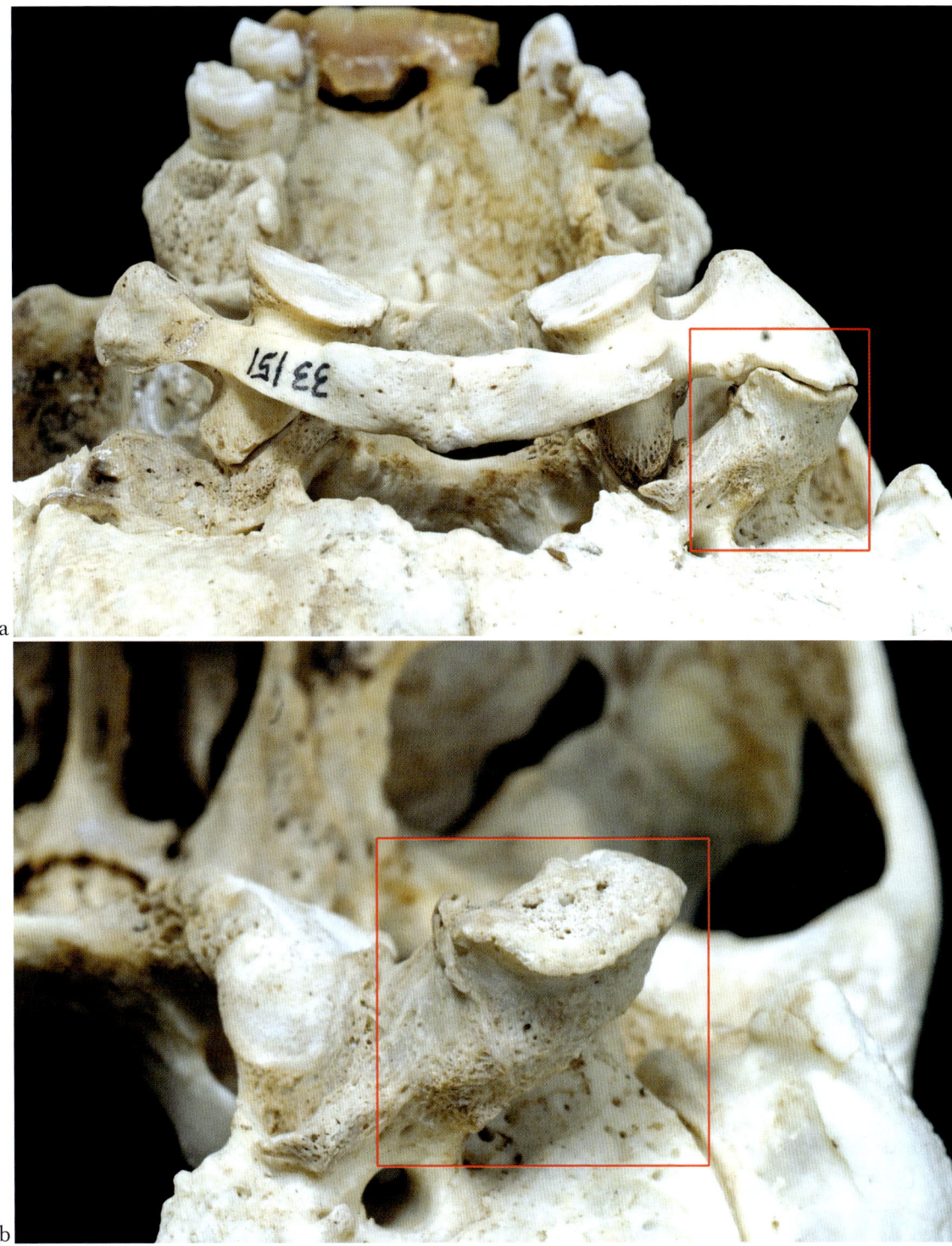

Figure 522a-b. Paracondylar process in an adult male (CMU 33 51). (a) Posterior view of a left paracondylar process or pedestal (rectangle) that articulates with the left transverse process of the atlas. This rare process is classified as an occipital vertebra and may result in partial (synovial joint) or complete fusion of the atlas to the cranial base. (b) Higher magnification showing the morphology of the articular surface of the pedestal (square). Cf. Hauser and DeStefano (1989); Nolet et al. (1999).

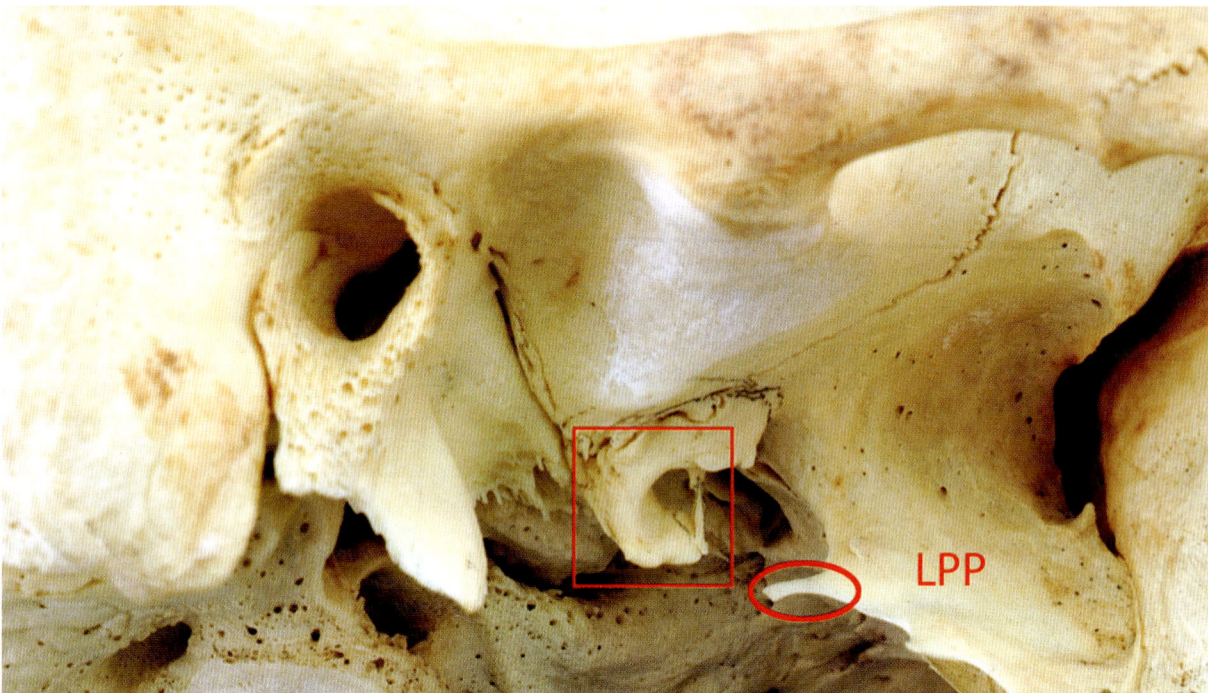

Figure 523. Bridged foramen spinosum (square; thin vertical bar of bone) and partial pterygospinous bridge (oval; lateral pterygoid plate, LPP) in an adult Thai skull (KKU). Uncommon to common finding. Cf. Nayak et al. (2007); Peker et al. (2002); Rossi et al. (2011); Skrzat et al. (2005, 2006).

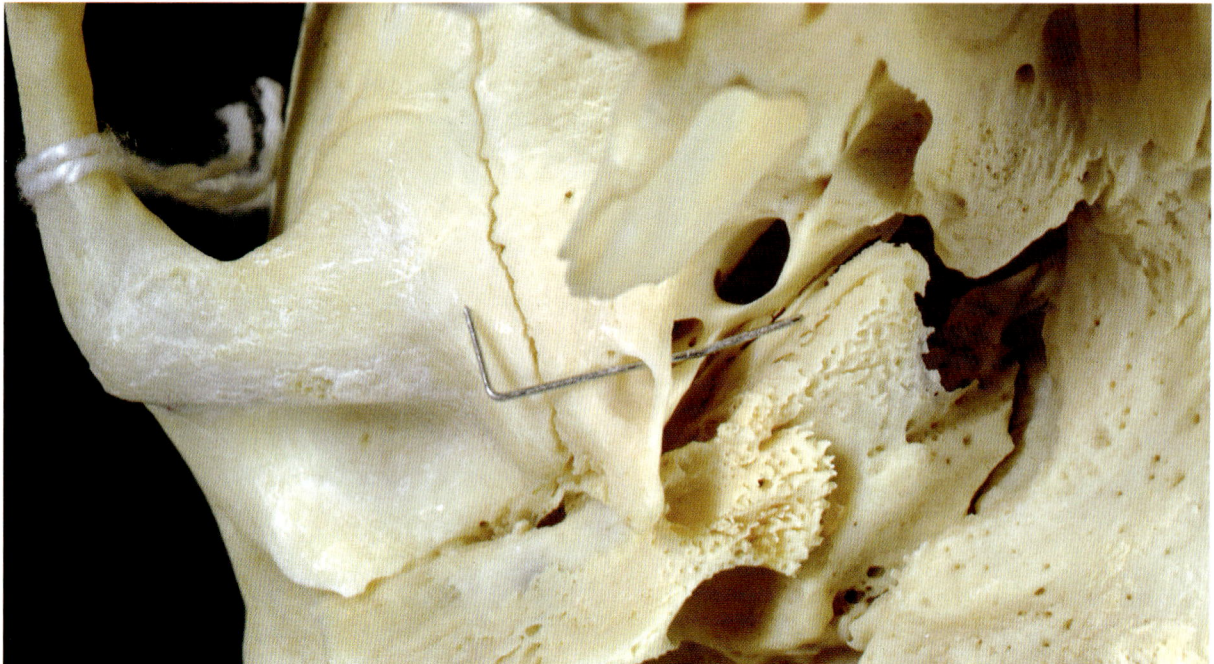

Figure 524. Bridged right foramen spinosum (probe) in an adult Thai skull (KKU). Common finding. Cf. Buikstra and Ubelaker (1994); Hauser and DeStefano (1989).

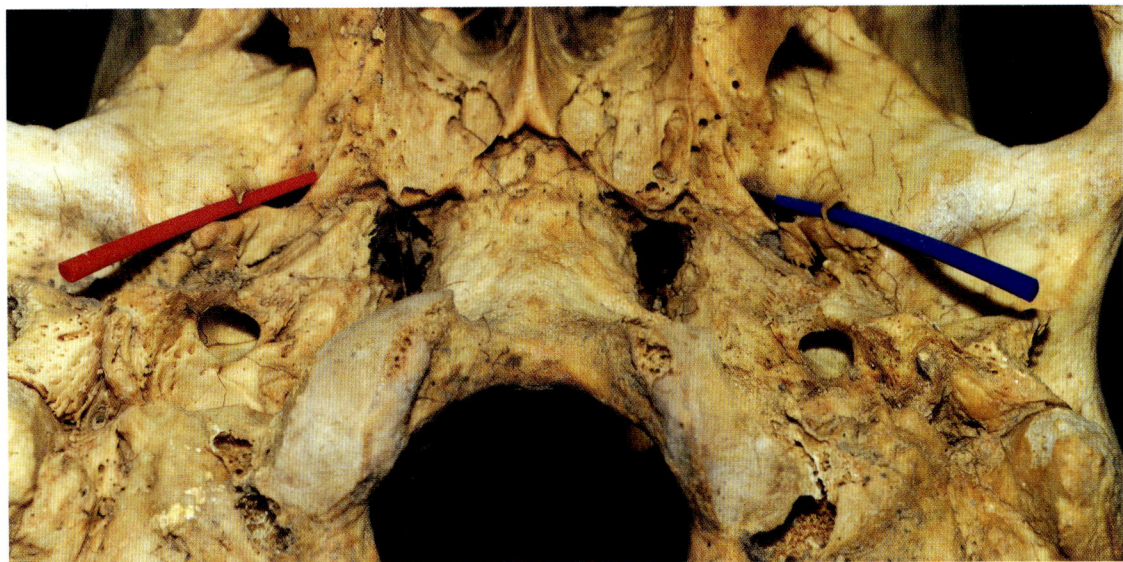

Figure 525. Bridged foramen spinosum in an adult Vietnamese skull (PAVN Forensic Institute). Complete bridging (blue probe) and incomplete bridging (red probe) are both common traits.

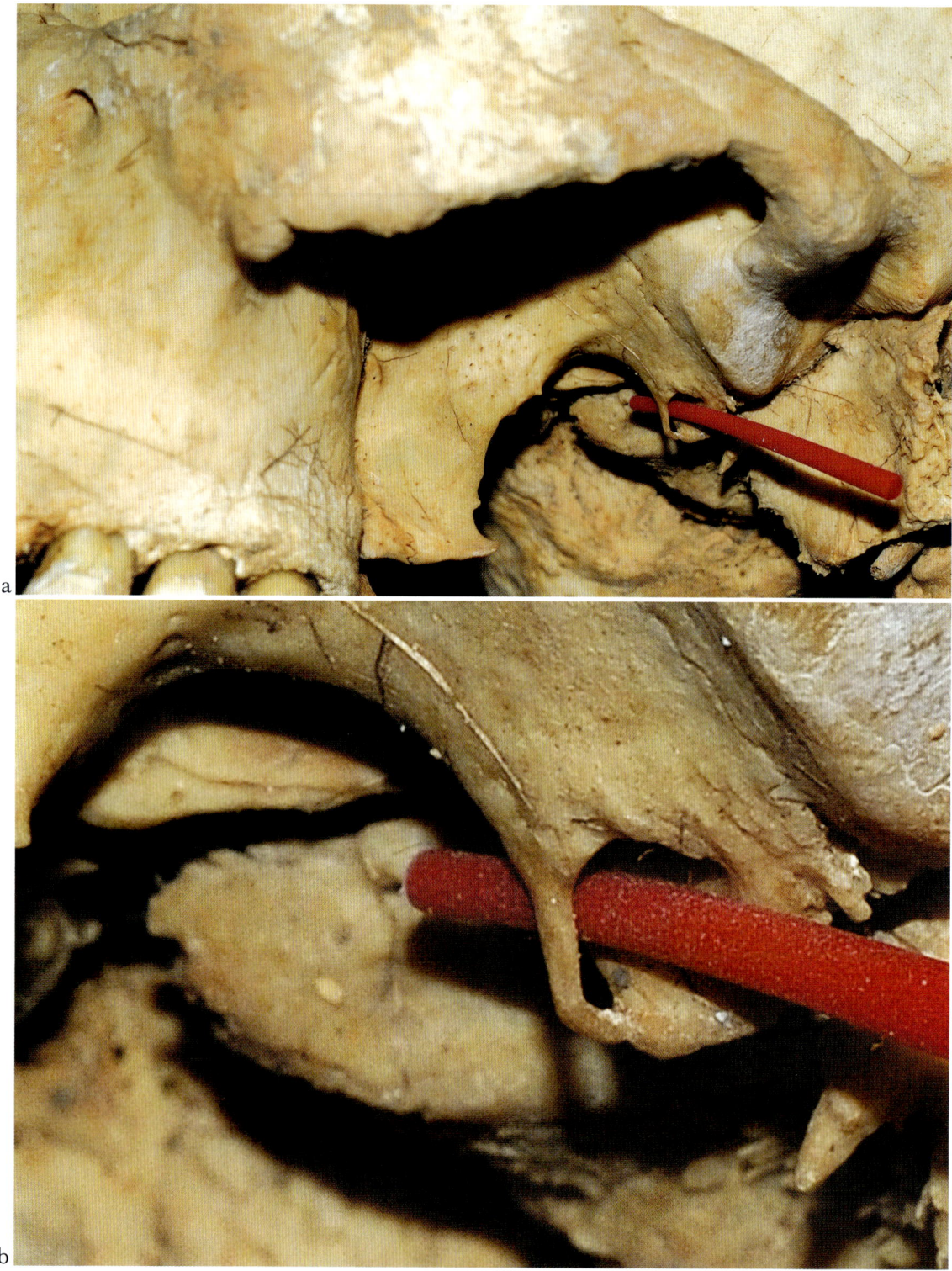

Figure 526a-b. Bridged foramen spinosum. (a) Left lateral and (b) higher magnification of a bridged left foramen spinosum in an adult Vietnamese skull (PAVN Forensic Institute). Common finding.

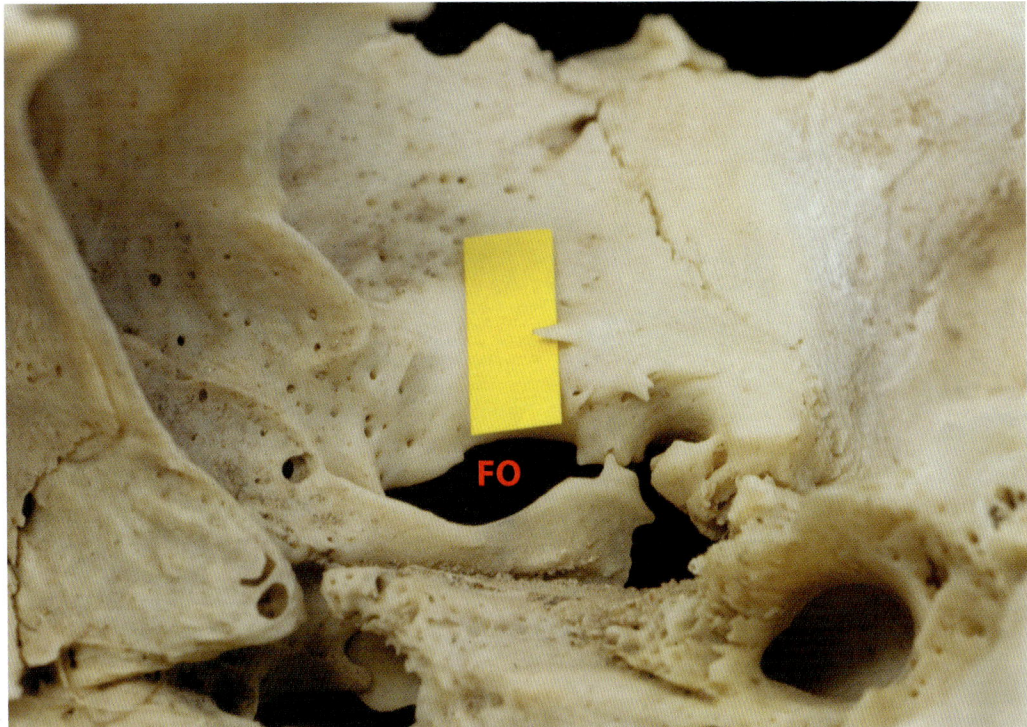

Figure 527. Trace (bony projection highlighted by yellow background) of a left pterygoalar bridge in an adult Asian male skull (CSC AC018). Note that the spine is positoned laterally to the foramen ovale (FO).

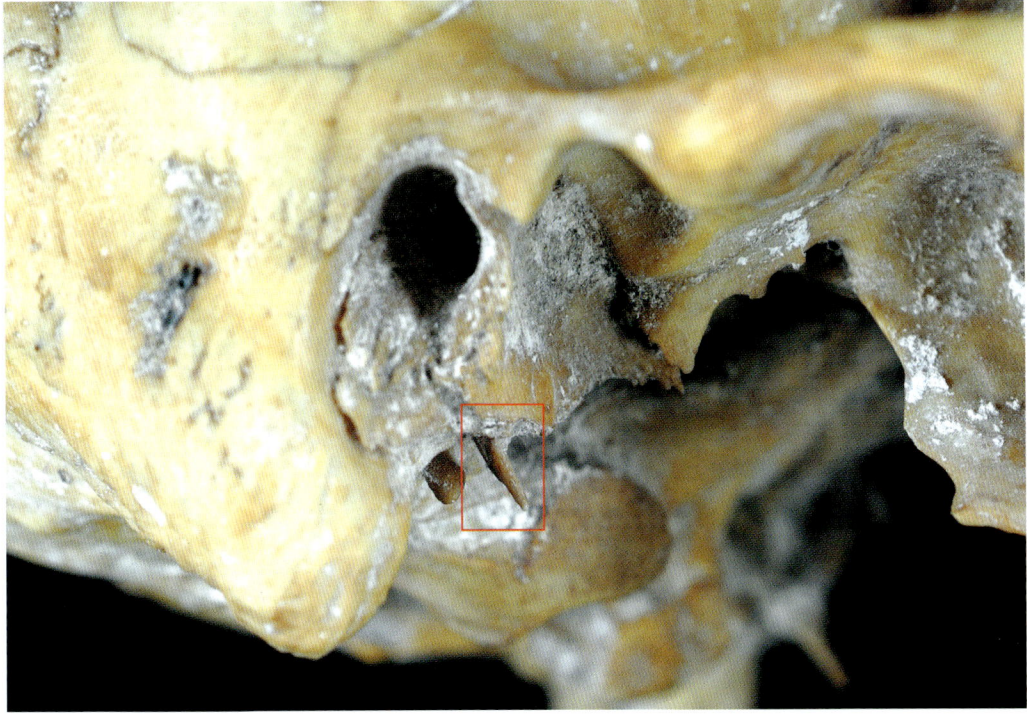

Figure 528. Short (5 mm) styloid process (rectangle) of the right temporal bone in an Asian adult skull (CIL historic). The styloid process may be absent or separate/unfused. Common finding.

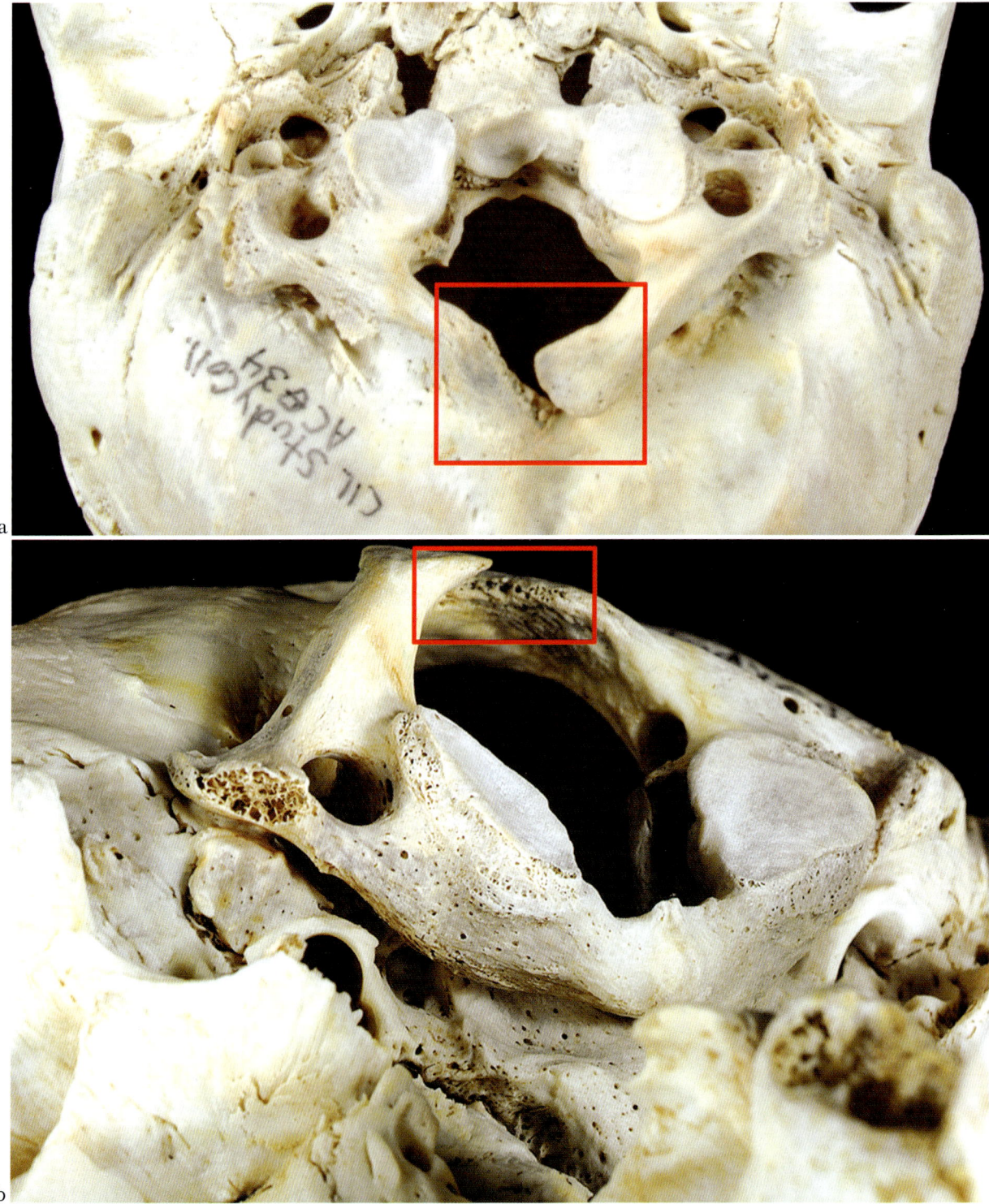

Figure 529a-b. Bifid atlas and atlanto-occipitalization. (a) Inferior view of a bifid atlas (rectangle) and atlanto-occipitalization, also known as atlano-occipital assimilation in an adult Asian skull (CSC). (b) Oblique view of the bifid atlas and assimilation of C1 into the cranial base. Uncommon findings. Cf. Allen (1879); Gladstone and Wakeley (1925); Kassim et al. (2010); Al-Motabagani and Surendra (2006); Sharma et al. (2008). Congenital fusion of the atlas to the cranial base may be partial or complete.

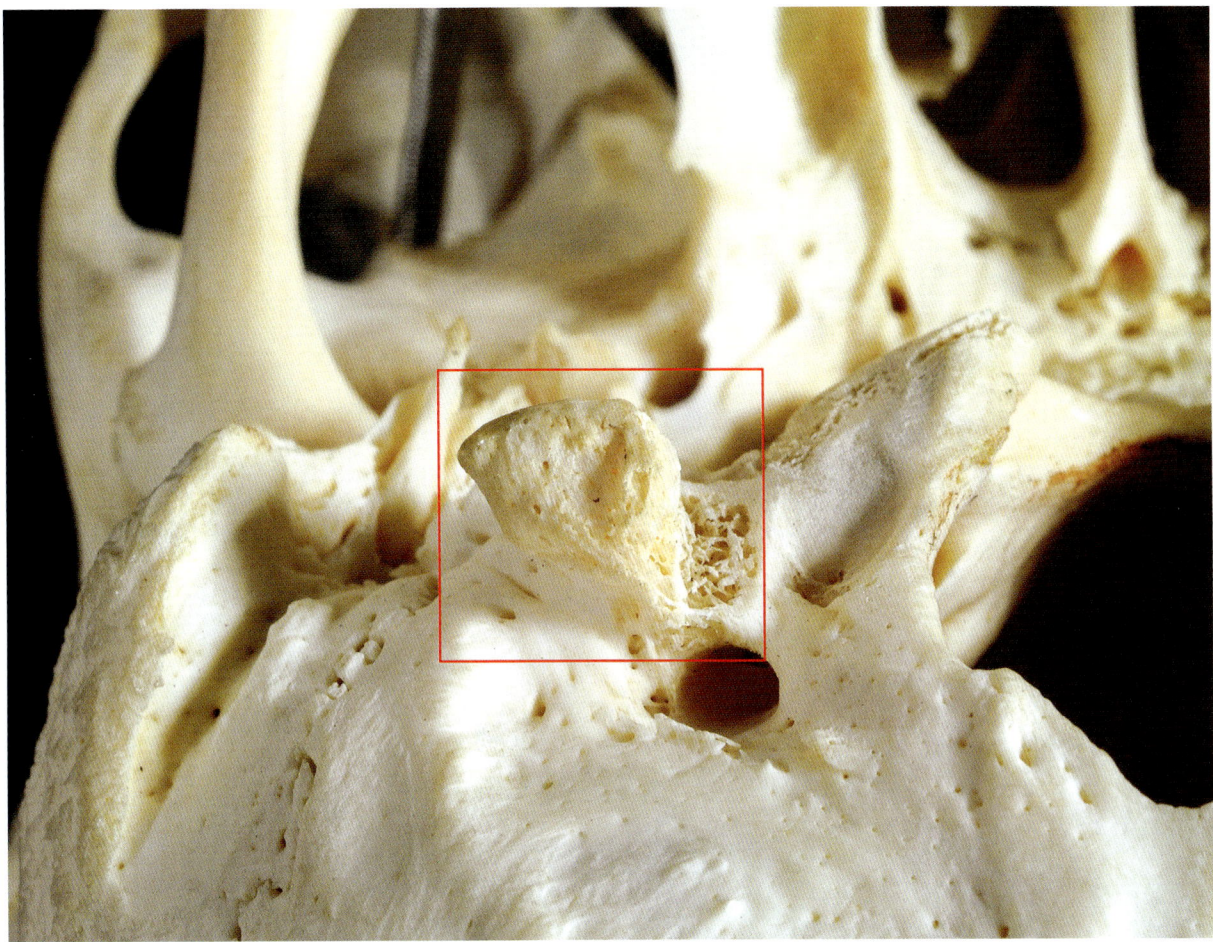

Figure 530. Large right paracondylar process (square) in an adolescent (late teens) Asian male (CSC AS005). This congenital condition of the craniovertebral junction may result in variously sized and shaped bony projections (exostoses), pedestals, masses, and platforms that may partially or completely fuse the atlas to the cranial base. Cf. de Graauw et al. (2008); Nolet et al. (1999).

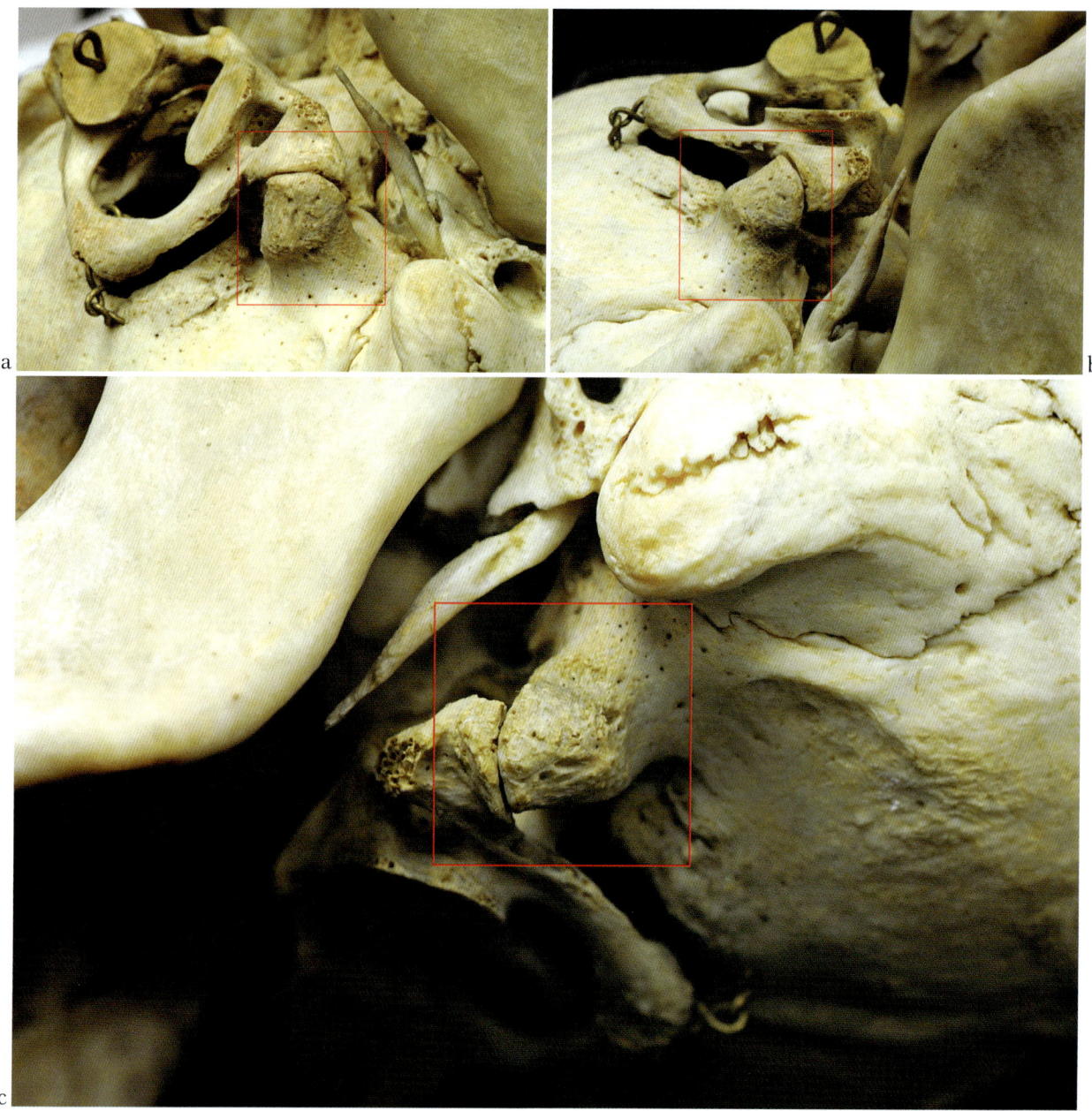

Figure 531a-c. Left paracondylar process and articulation and epitransverse process of the atlas. (a) Oblique and (b) lateral inferior views of a left paracondylar process (rectangle) with articulation and epitransverse process of the atlas (C1) (Mütter Museum 1183.00). (c) Left lateral view demonstrating the paracondylar process and articulation of the atlas (square). Rare finding. Cf. McCall et al. (2010); Prescher (1997).

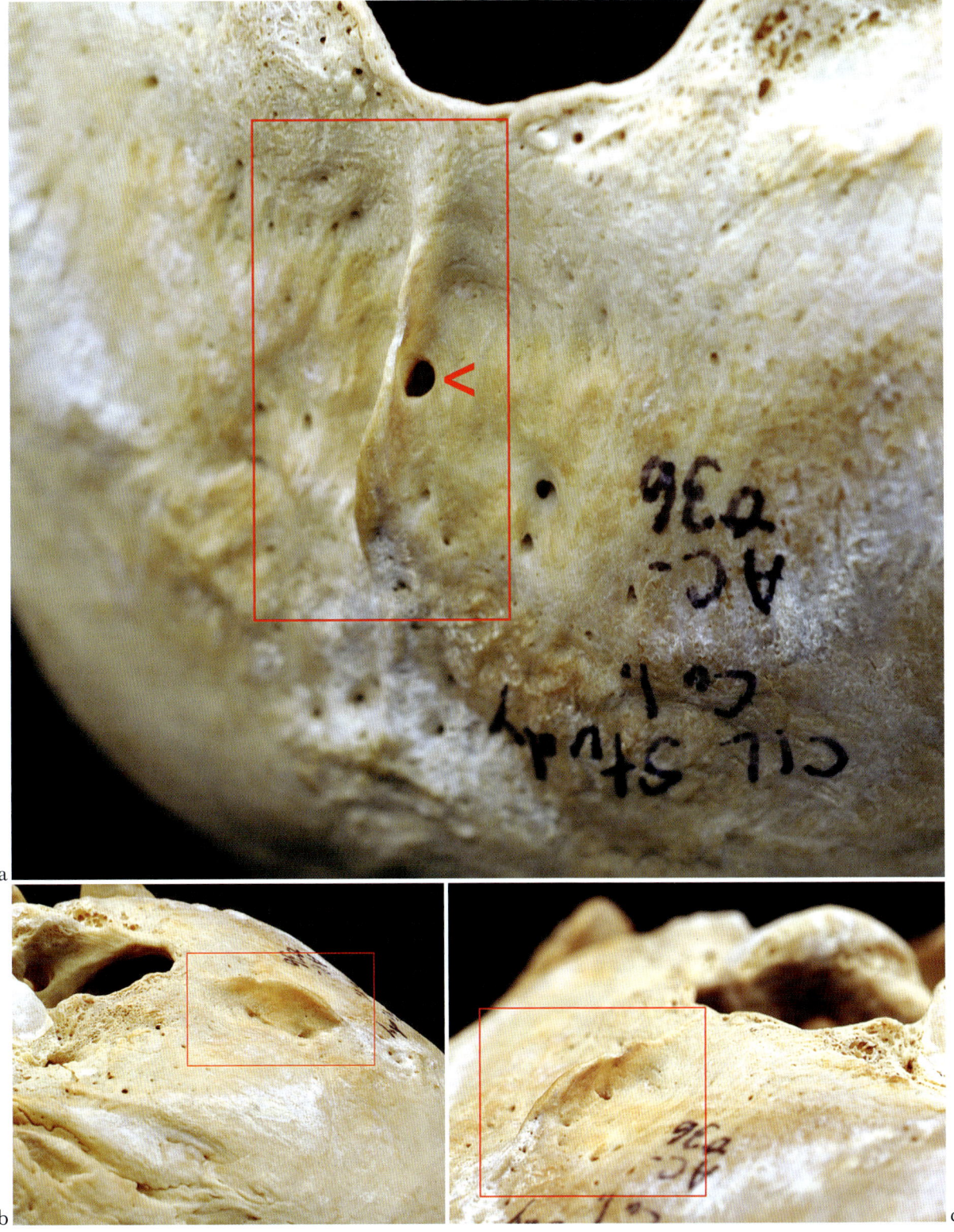

Figure 532a-c. External occipital crest and emissary occipital foramen. (a) Small external occipital crest (rectangle) and an emissary occipital foramen (<) in an adult Asian skull. (b and c) Oblique views of the occipital crest (rectangles). The crest serves for attachment of the nuchal ligament (ligamentum nuchae) (CSC AC036). Common findings. Cf. Boyd (1930); Hauser and DeStefano (1989).

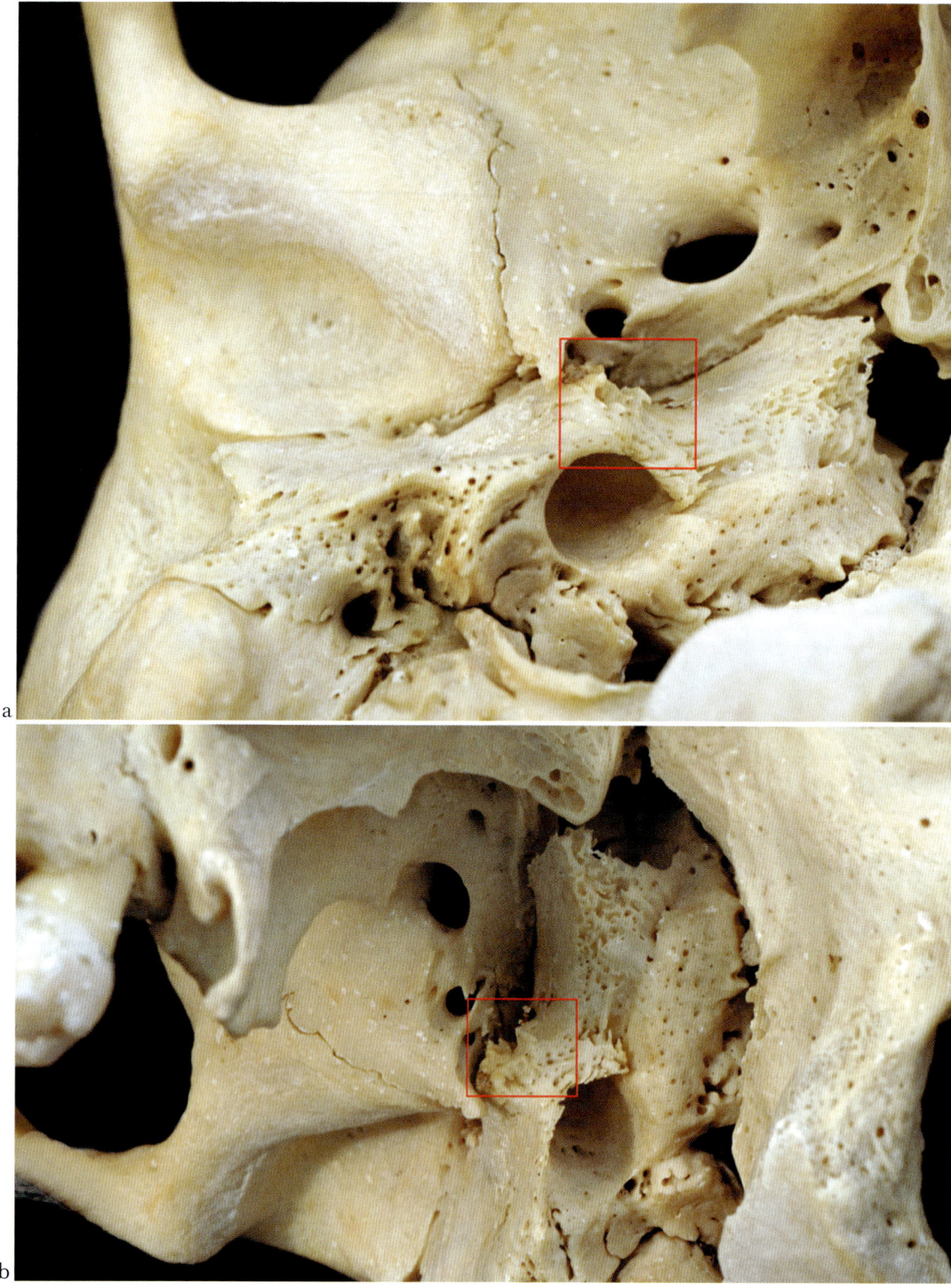

Figure 533a-b. Absence of the styloid process. (a) Congenital absence of the right styloid process (square). (b) Higher magnification of the temporal bone revealing absence of the styloid process and no evidence of breakage. Both styloid processes were absent in this Asian adult skull (CSC). Common to uncommon finding. Cf. Cousins et al. (2009).

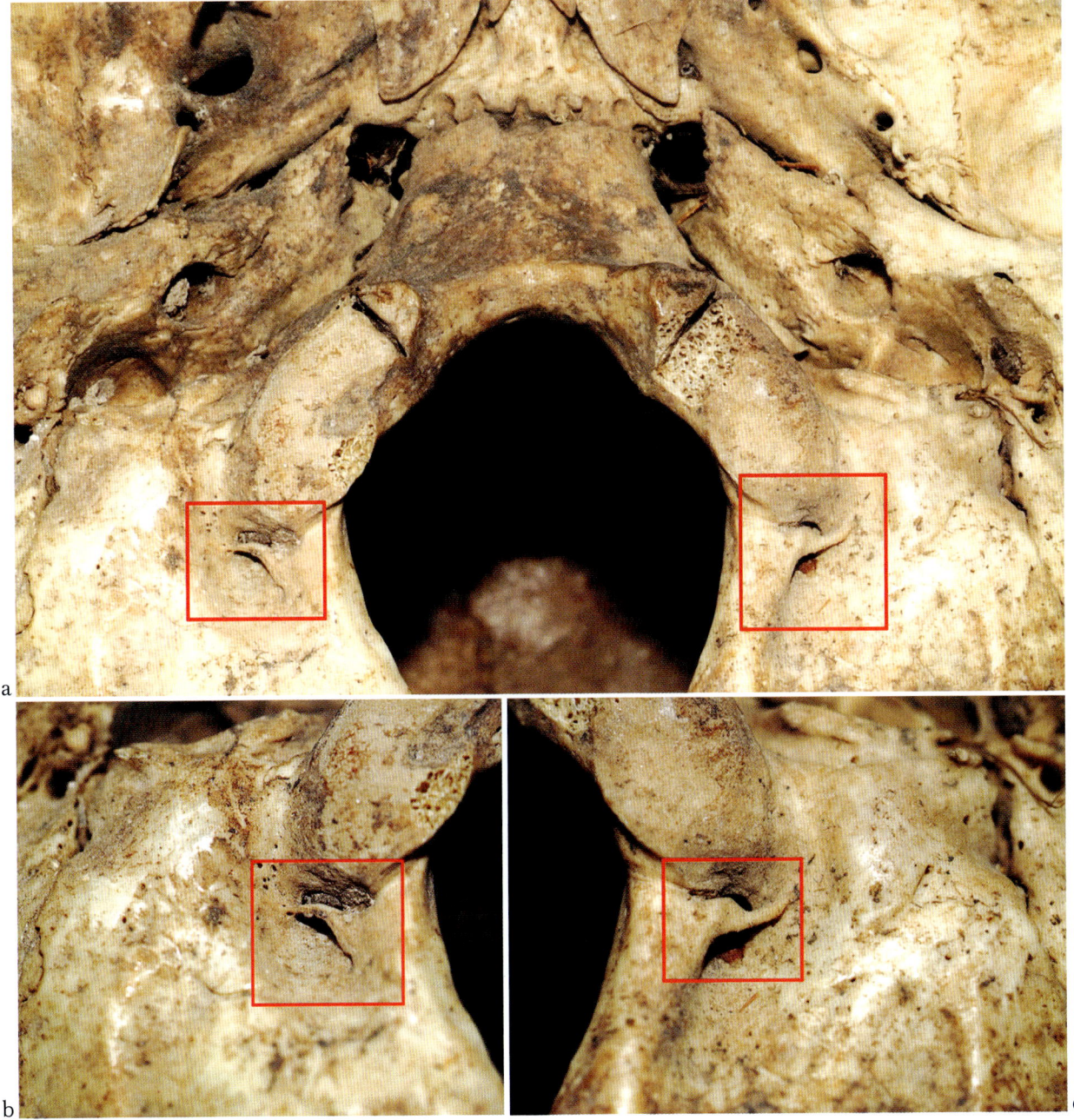

Figure 534a-c. Partially bridged postcondyloid foramina. (a) Small, tapered bone projections (squares) extending across the postcondyloid foramina in a subadult Thai skull (KKU). (b) Magnified view of the right and (c) left foramina demonstrating that the two curved projections (squares) originate along the external rim of the foramen magnum, not within them as in divided foramina, and are not fused to the cranial base. Uncommon to rare finding of unknown etiology.

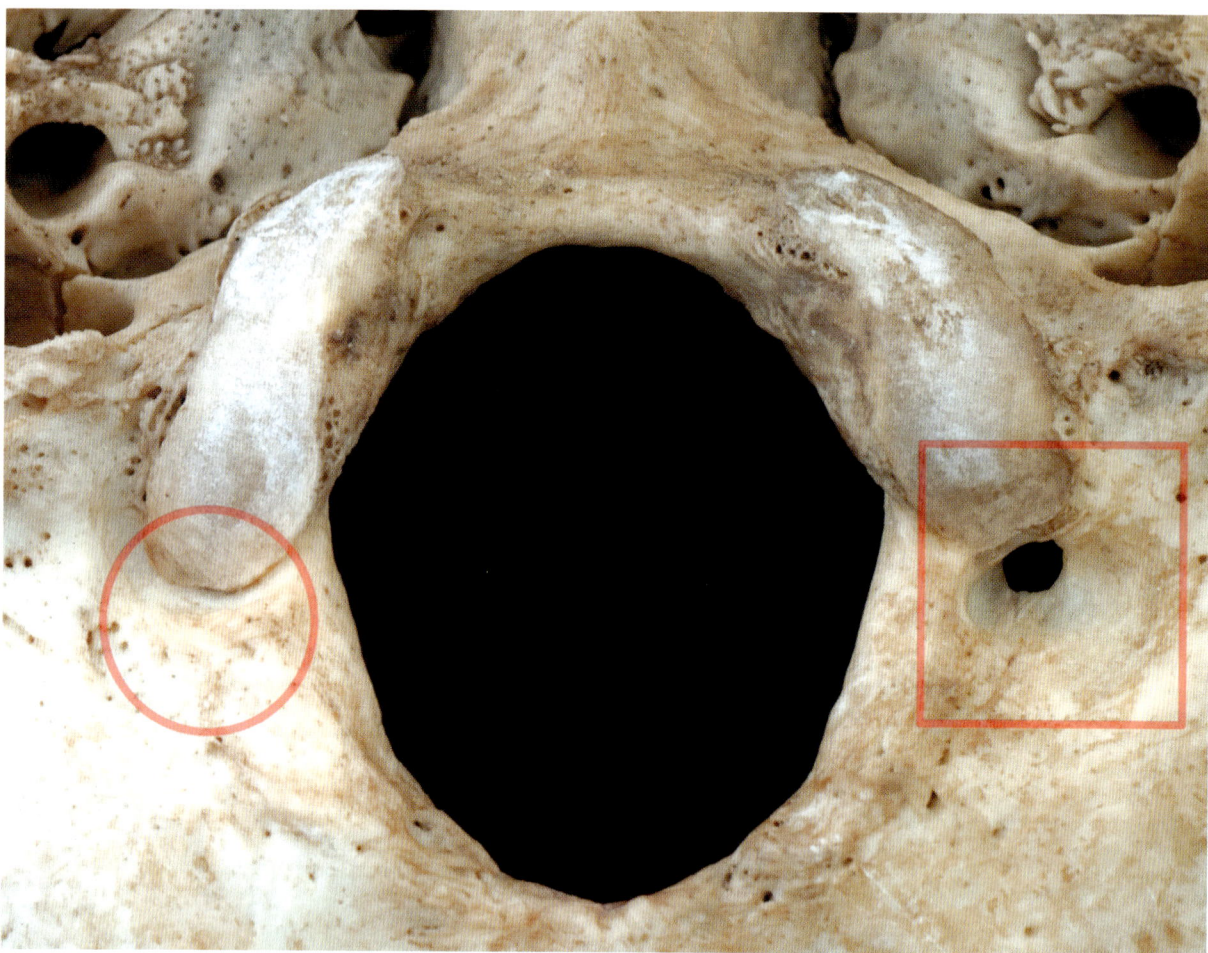

Figure 535. Absent right (circle) and patent left (square) postcondyloid canal in an adult Thai skull (KKU). This combination is a relatively common finding.

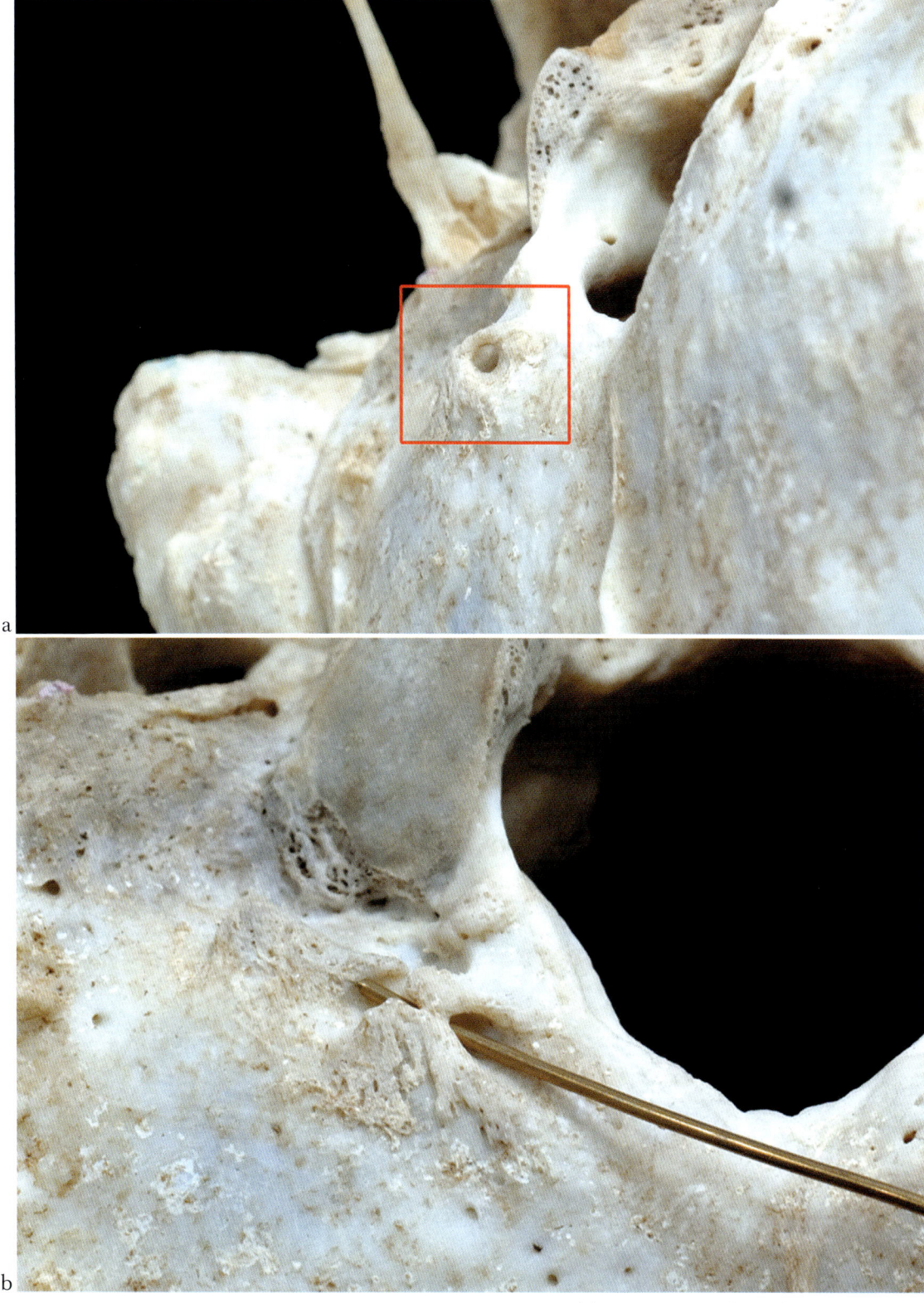

Figure 536a-b. Foramen along the margin of the foramen magnum. (a) Small foramen (square) formed by calcification, possibly along the right posterolateral border of the foramen magnum in a 57-year-old Thai skull (CMU 53 51). (b) Higher magnification of the foramen (probe) showing the roughened area of new bone. Uncommon to rare finding.

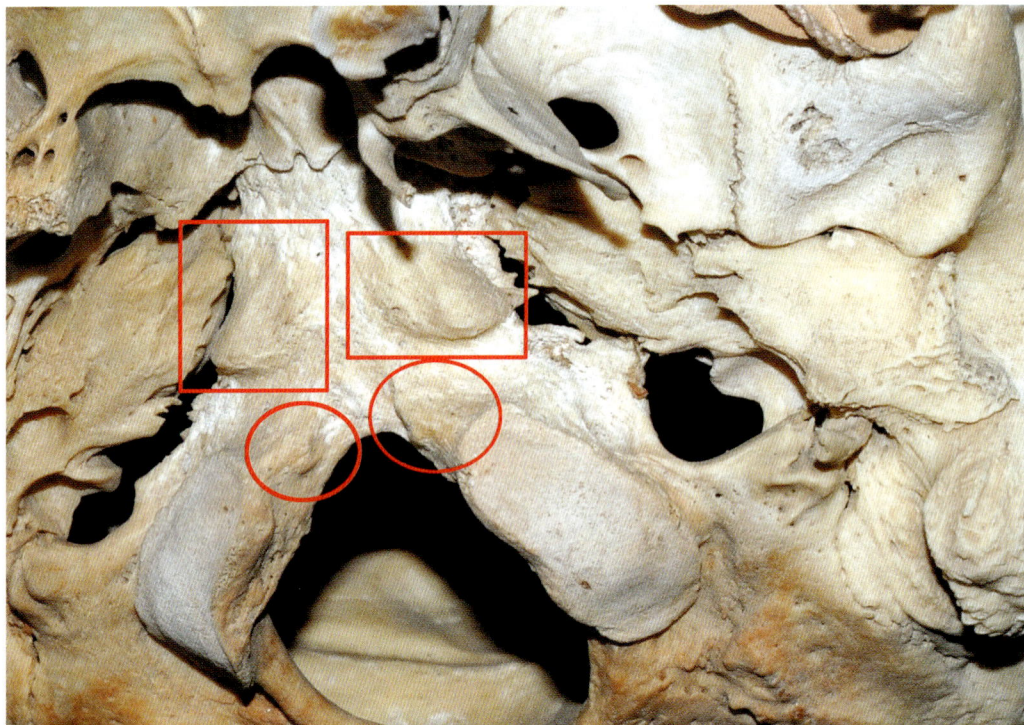

Figure 537. Basilar tubercles/wings (rectangles) and precondylar tubercles/processes (circles) in an adult ancient Peruvian (SI). Uncommon to common findings. Cf. Broman (1957); Oetteking (1923).

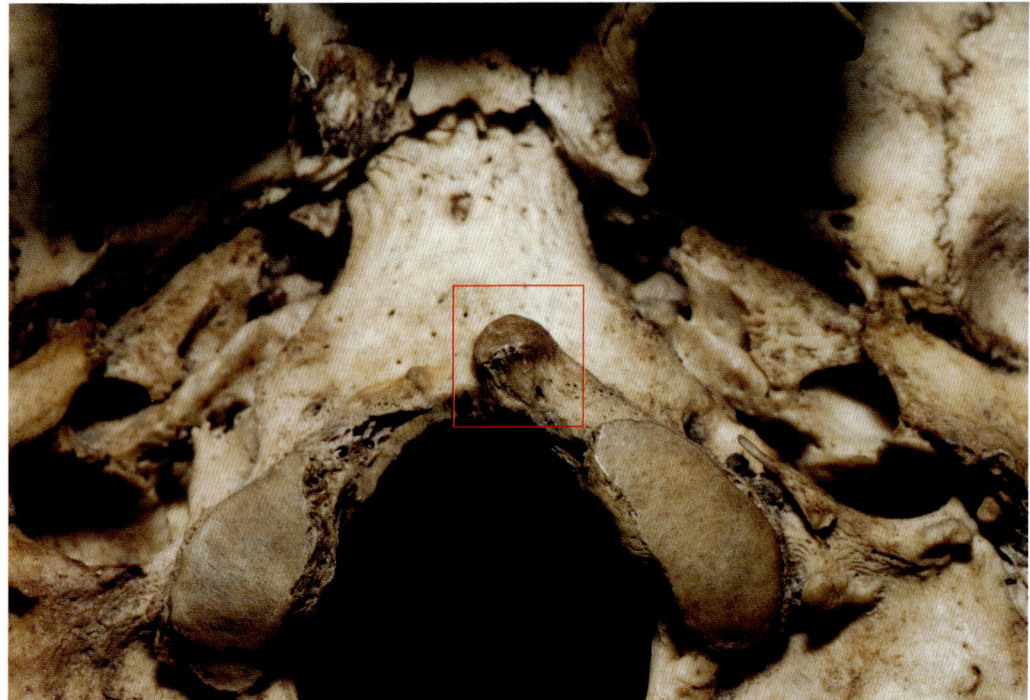

Figure 538. Unilateral left precondylar tubercle (square) (Mütter Museum). See Broman (1957); Hauser and DeStefano (1989); Oetteking (1923).

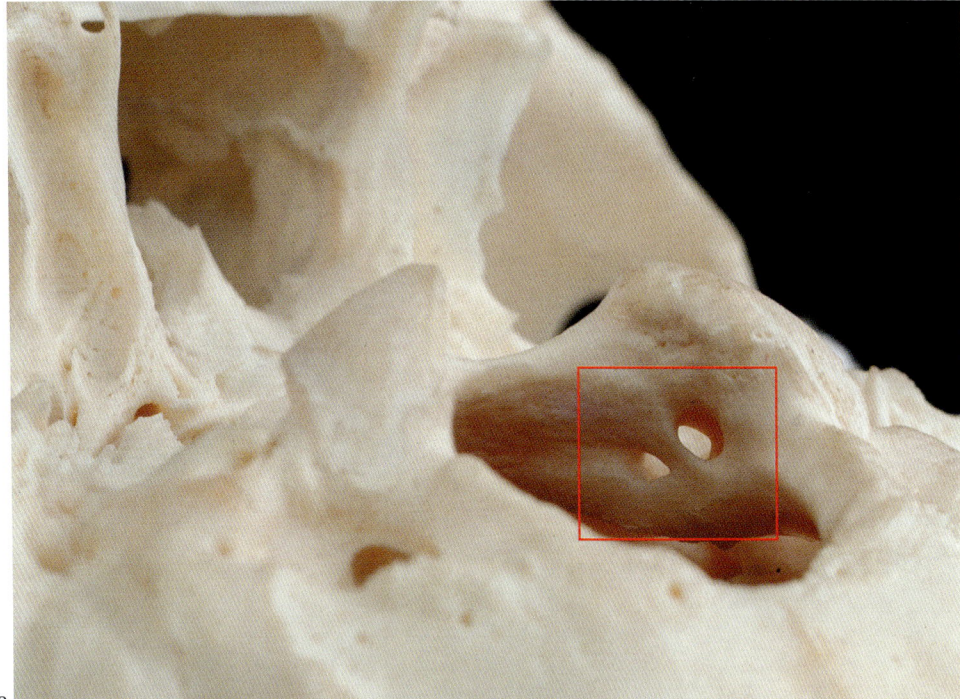

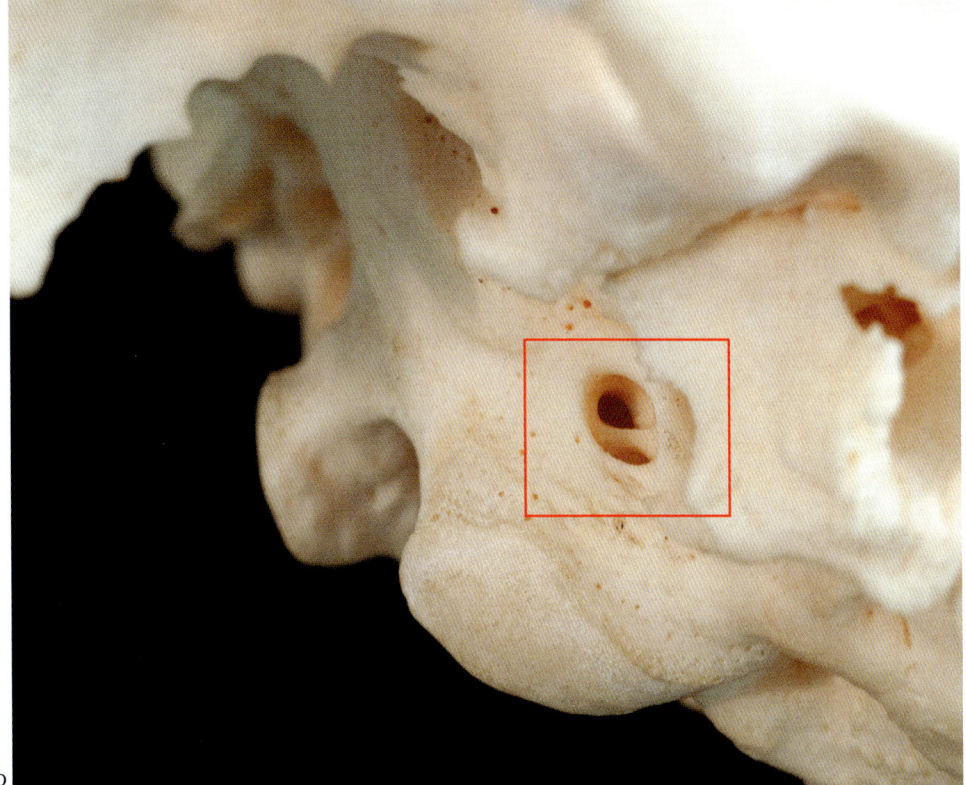

Figure 539a-b. Internally divided left hypoglossal canal. (a) Inferior and (b) left lateral views of an internally divided left hypoglossal canal (rectangles) in an adult Asian skull (CSC). Division of this canal has a genetic basis and may be present in fetuses. Cf. Berge and Bergman (2001); Hanihara and Ishida (2001b); Hauser and DeStefano (1989).

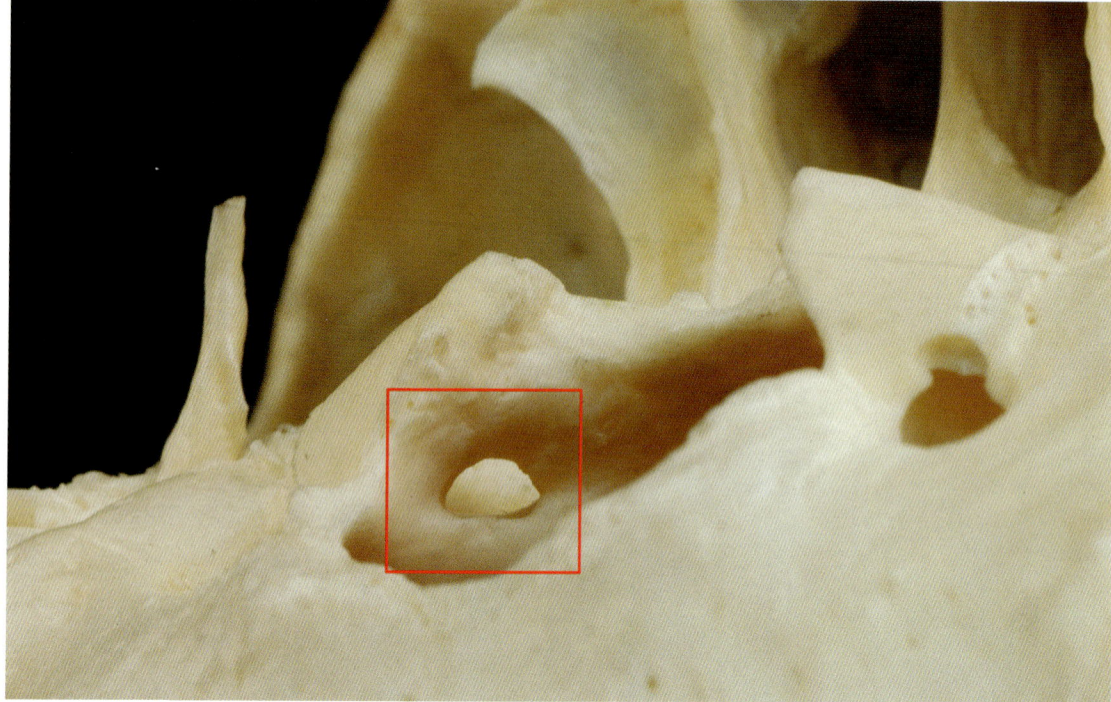

Figure 540. Non-divided, single hypoglossal canal (square) (CSC). Cf. Berge and Bergman (2001); Hanihara and Ishida (2001b); Hauser and DeStefano (1989). Common finding.

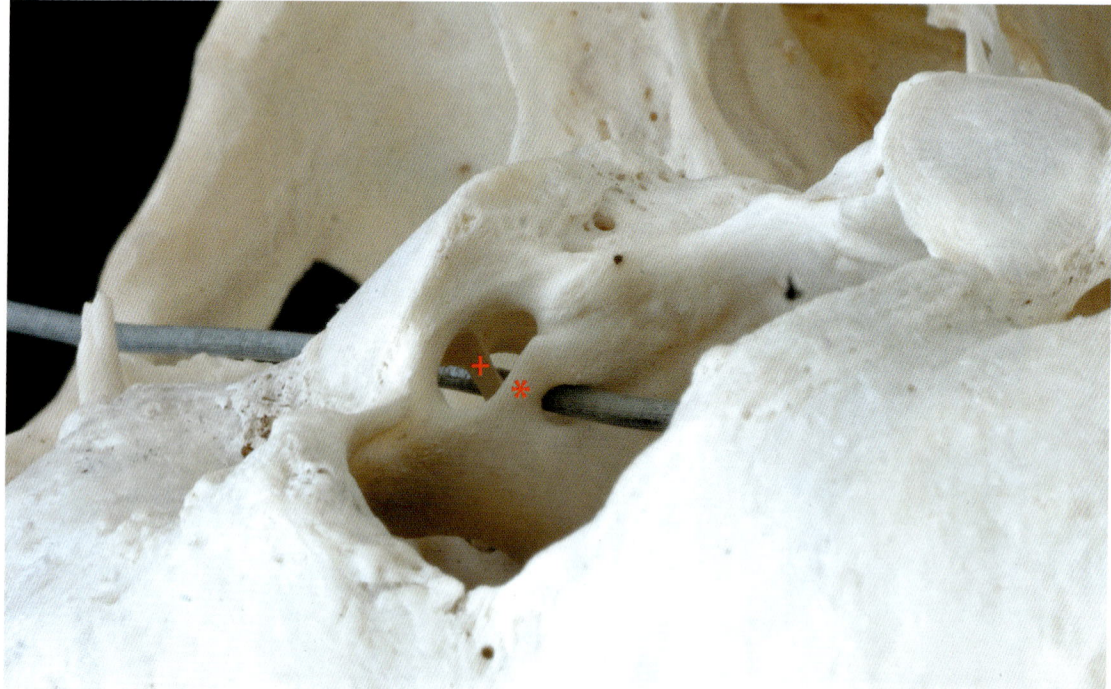

Figure 541. Oblique view of an interally (*) and externally (+) divided right hypoglossal canal (probe) resulting in one internal and two external foramina in a 57-year-old Thai male skull (CMU 143 50). Note that the calcified septa are oriented in different directions. Cf. Berge and Bergman (2001); Hanihara and Ishida (2001b); Hauser and DeStefano (1989).

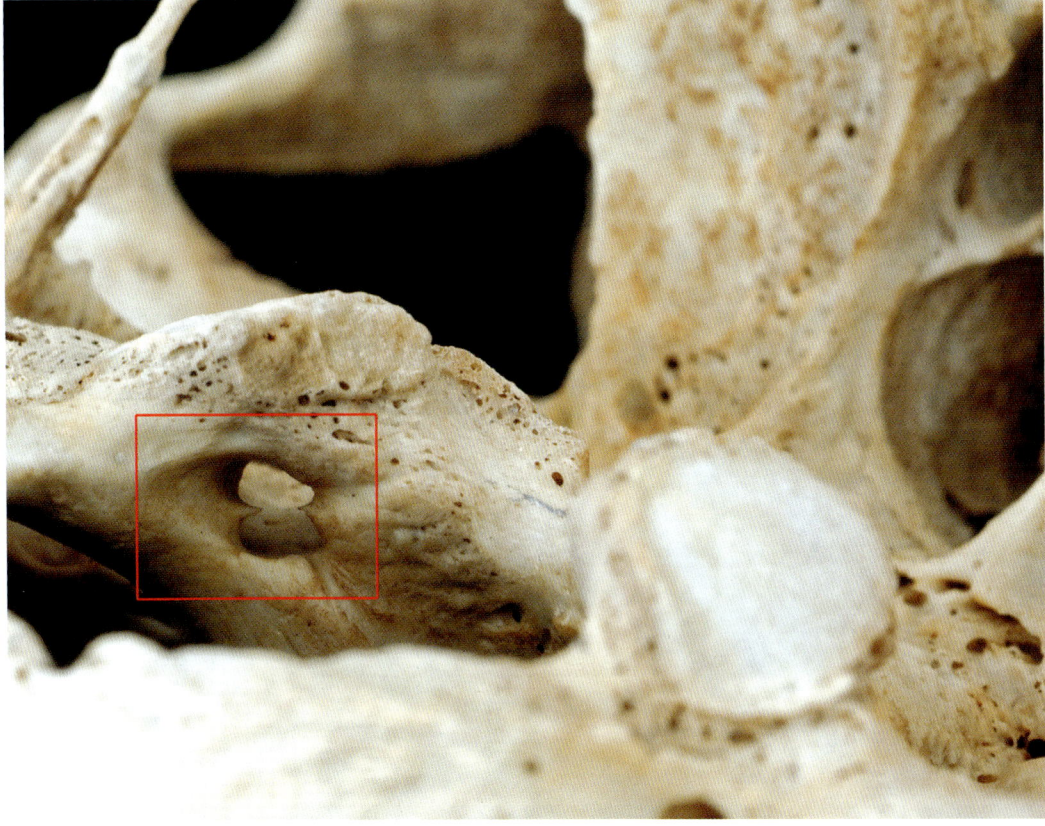

Figure 542. Small calcified spicules (rectangle) forming in the right hypoglossal canal of an adult Thai male (CMU). This specimen is unusual, as the spicules usually form from the superior and inferior borders of the canal, not the anterior and posterior borders as in the figure below.

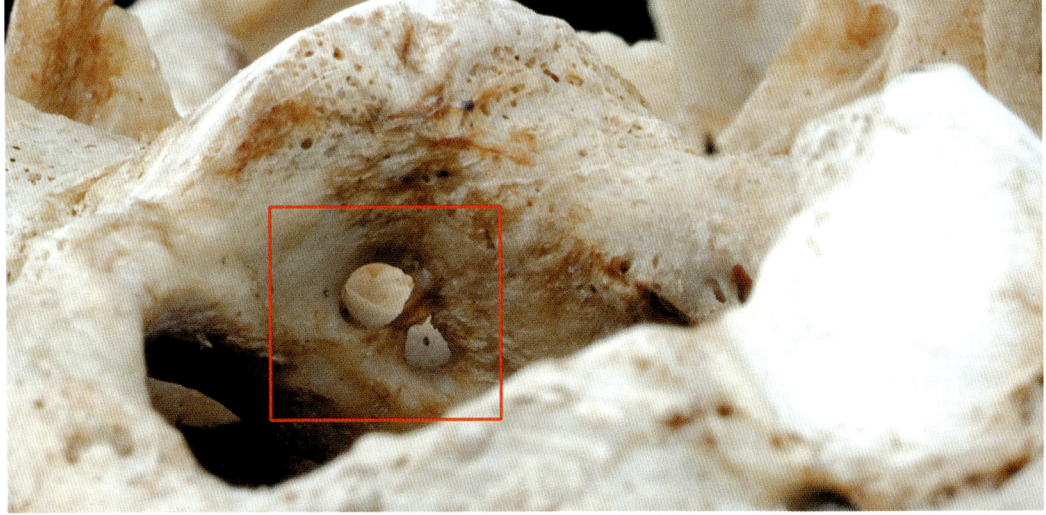

Figure 543. Nearly complete calcification of a fibrous bar/septum across the right hypoglossal canal (square) and approximately meeting at the middle in an 87-year-old Thai male (CMU 143 50). Formation of a calcified septum across this canal often begins as one or two triangular-shaped spicules that gradually grow in length towards one another. This septum divides the two roots of the hypoglossal nerve. Cf. Berge and Bergman (2001); Hanihara and Ishida (2001b); Hauser and DeStefano (1989).

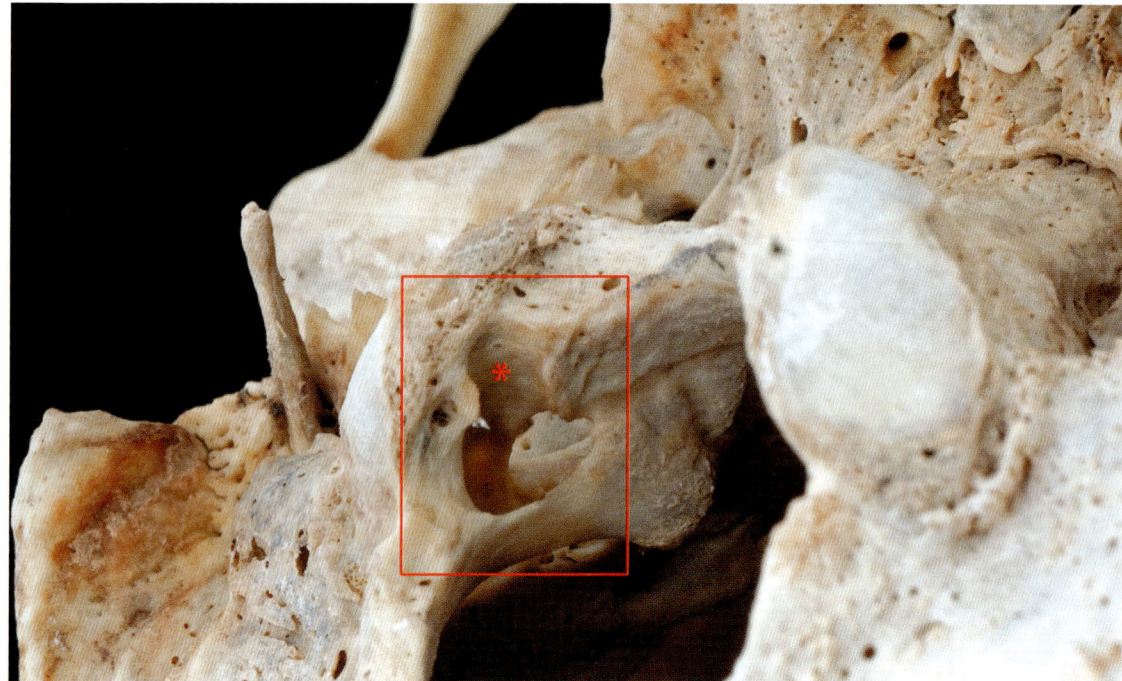

Figure 544. Vertically grooved right hypoglossal canal (rectangle and *) in a 67-year-old Thai male skull (CMU 83 51). Uncommon, but typical anatomy.

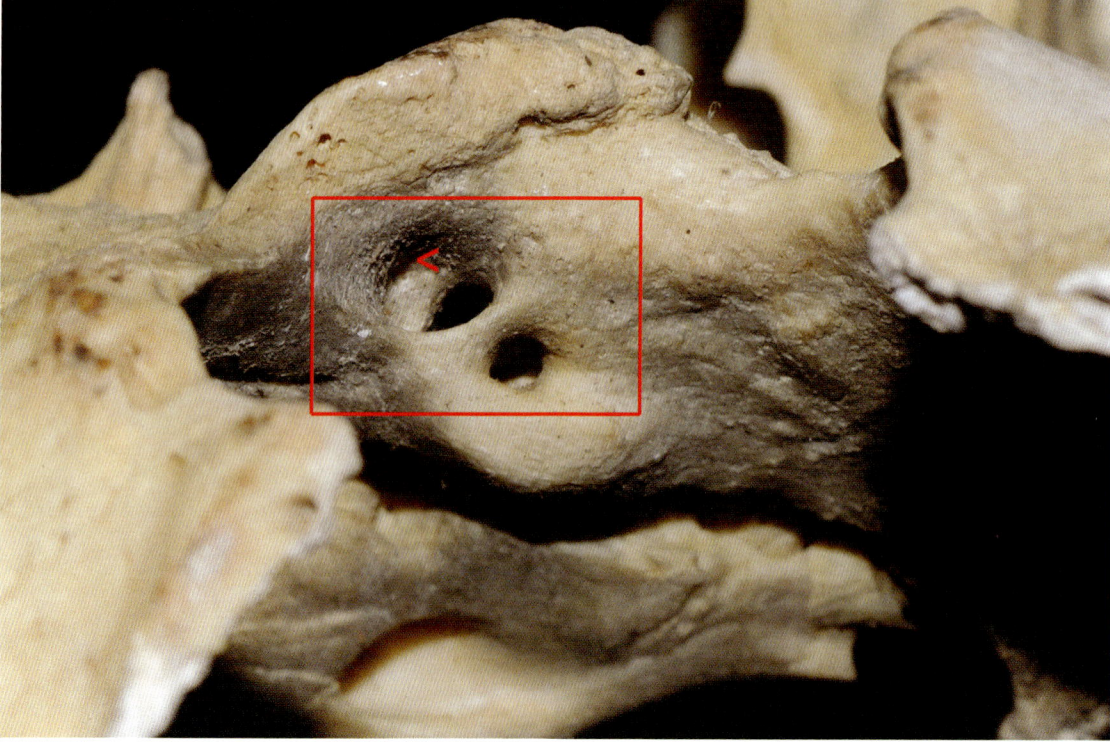

Figure 545. Rare triple right hypoglossal canal (rectangle with third canal), likely the result of calcified tissue spanning the canal (<) (RV69).

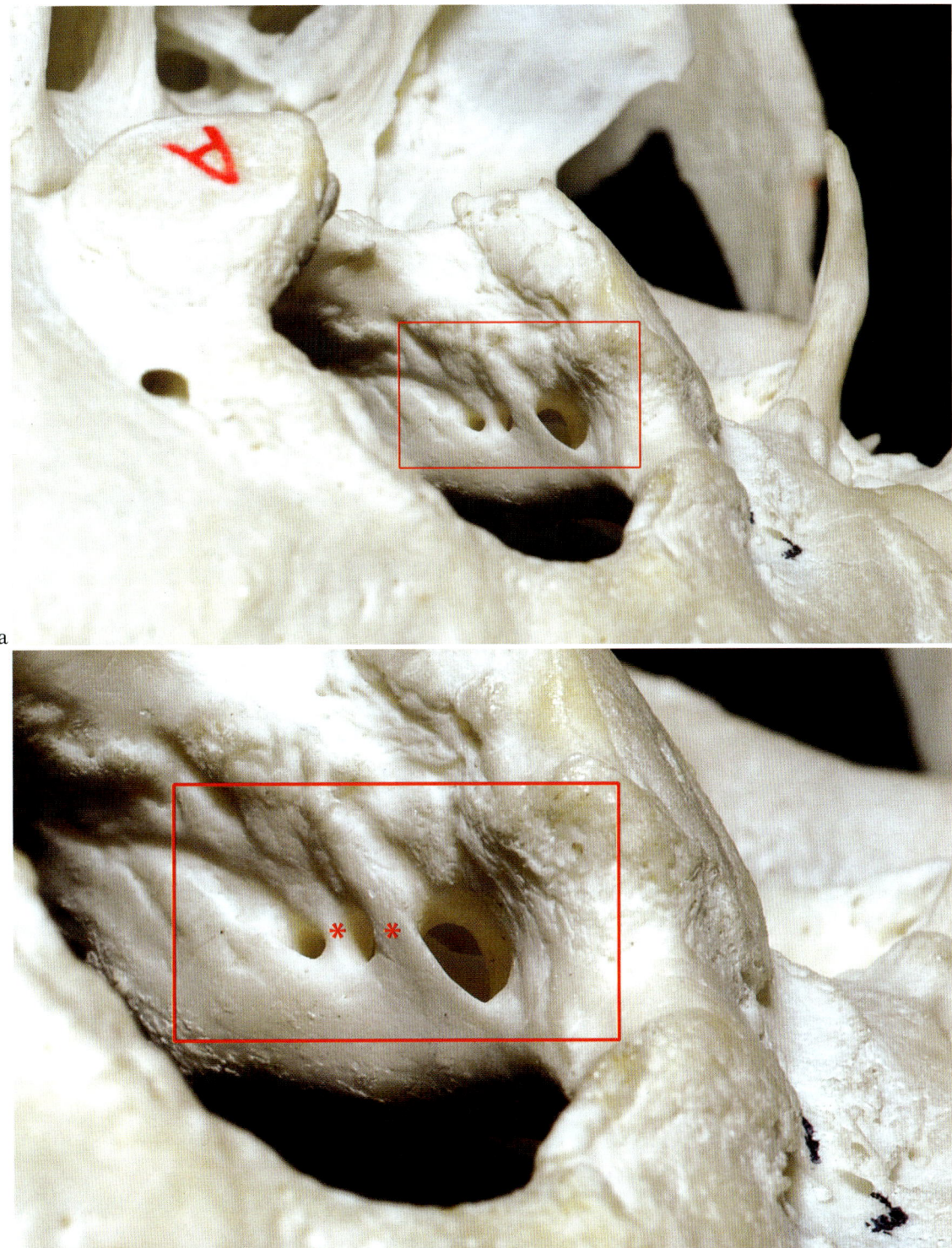

Figure 546a-b. Triple hypoglossal canal. (a) Rare triple left hypoglossal canal (rectangle) (JABSOM). (b) The three canals (rectangle), which increase in size from anterior to posterior, are formed by two calcified bridges (*) spanning the canal.

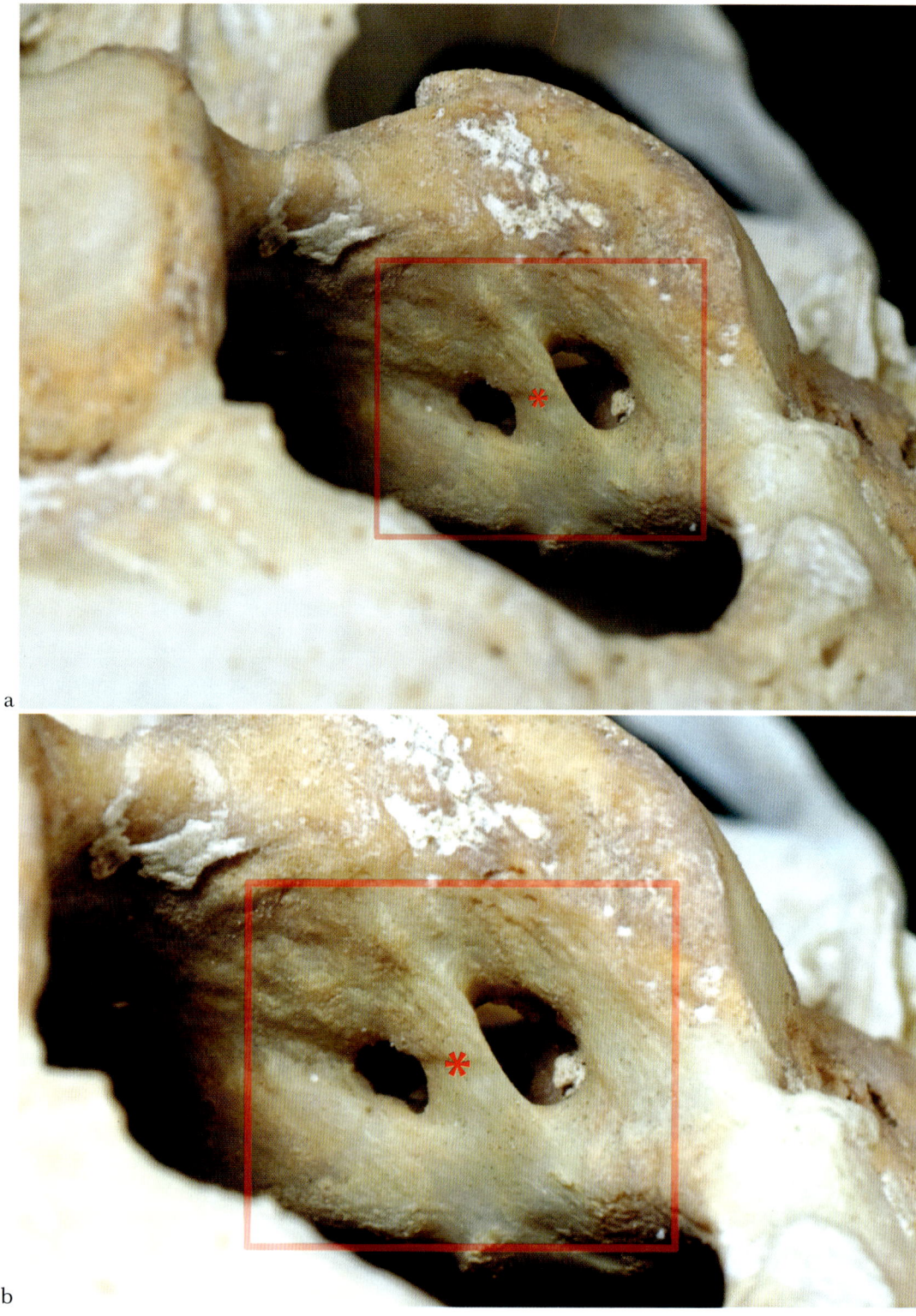

Figure 547a-b. Divided left hypoglossal canal. (a) Wide band of calcification (*) resulting in a divided left hypoglossal canal (rectangle) in a 51-year-old male skull (KKU 46-112). (b) Magnification showing detail of the calcified septum. Cf. Berge and Bergman (2001); Hanihara and Ishida (2001b); Hauser and DeStefano (1989); Naderi et al. (2005); Wysocki et al. (2004).

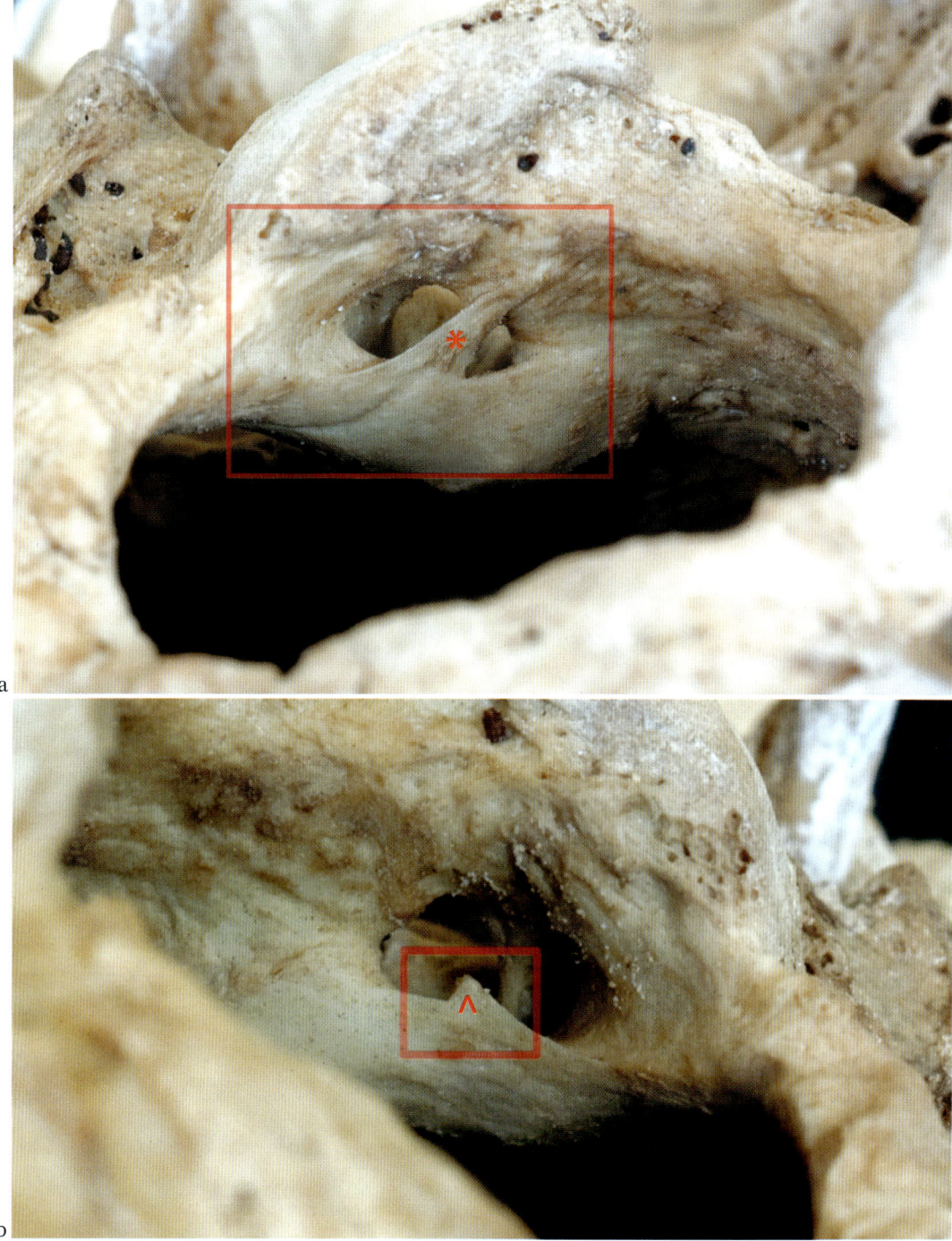

Figure 548a-b. Complete and partial bridging of the hypoglossal canal in an individual. (a) Complete bridging of the right canal due to the formation of a wave-like band of calcification (*) spanning the canal. (b) partial or trace bridging of the left hypoglossal canal in an adult male skull (KKU 4738-43). As in most individuals, calcification begins as a small triangular projection along the superior margin of the canal (∧) and grows towards a roughly similar small bony projection along the inferior margin of the canal. Cf. Berge and Bergman (2001); Hauser and DeStefano (1989); Hanihara and Ishida (2001b); Naderi et al. (2005); Wysocki et al. (2004).

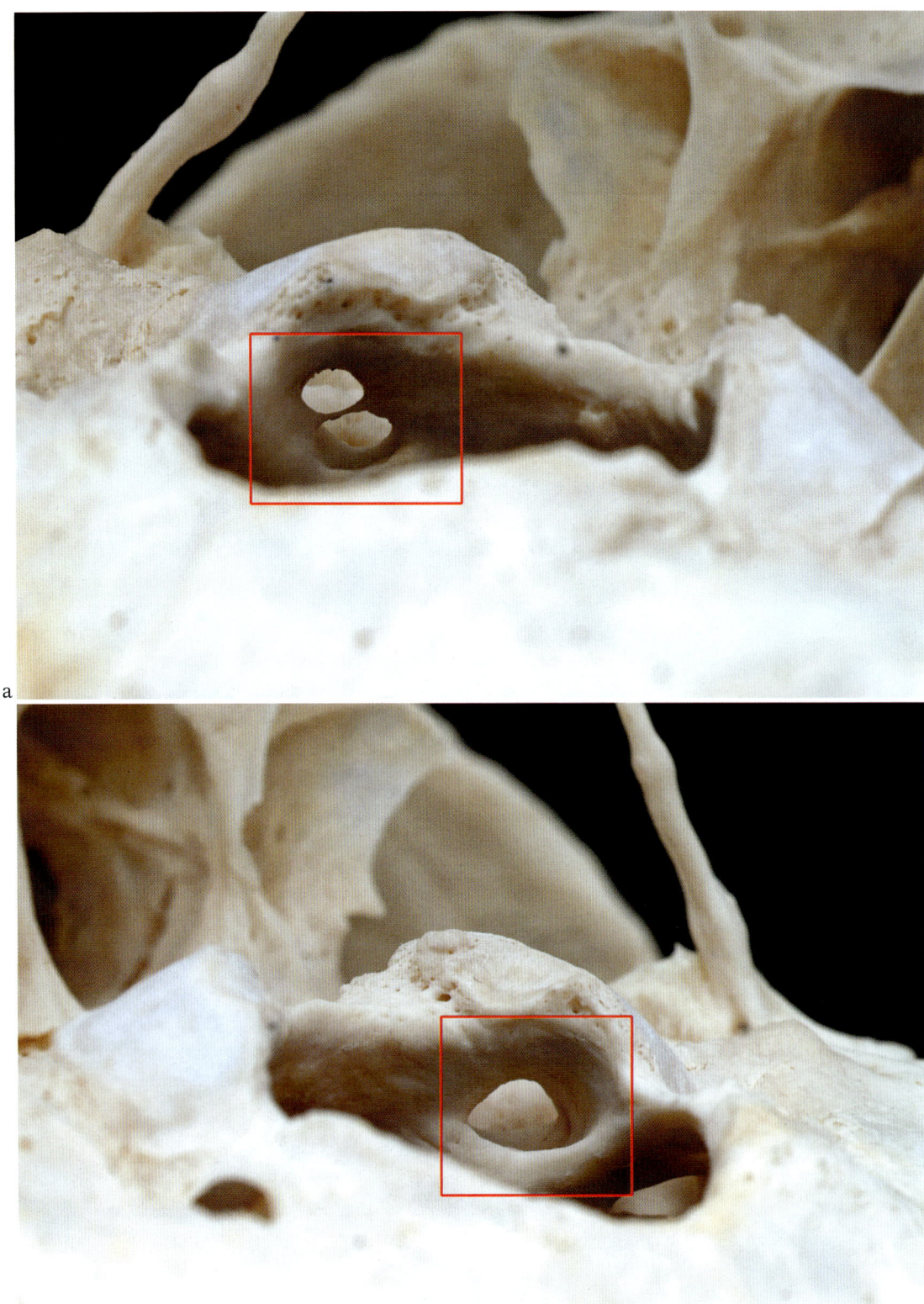

Figure 549a-b. Variants of the hypoglossal canal. (a) Divided right and (b) single left hypoglossal canal in a 60-year-old Thai male skull (CMU 13 51). Cf. Berge and Bergman (2001); Hauser and DeStefano (1989); Hanihara and Ishida (2001b); Naderi et al. (2005); Wysocki et al. (2004).

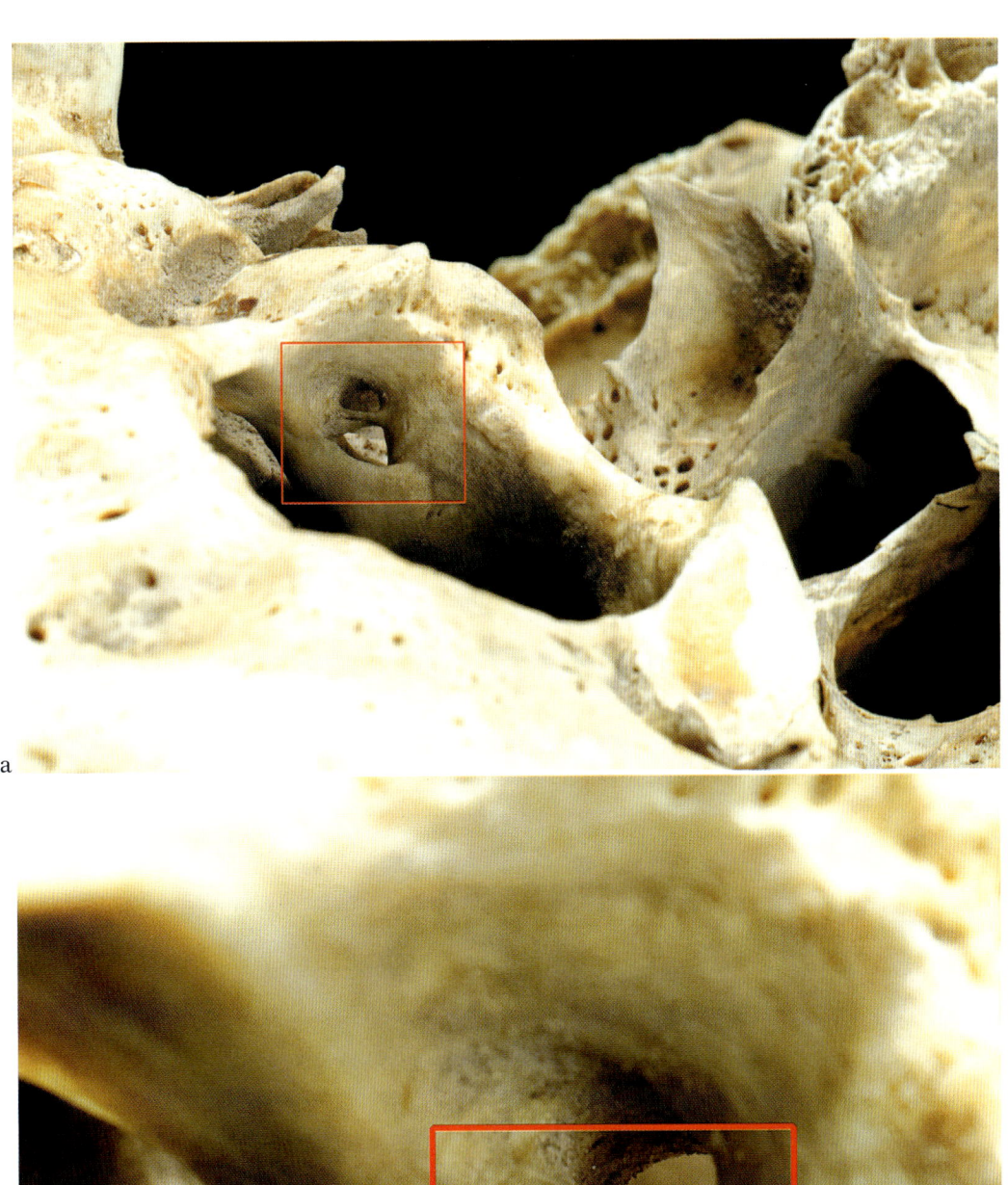

Figure 550a-b. Rare triple division of the right hypoglossal canal. (a) Right oblique view illustrating that the calcified bridge spanning the canal internally (rectangle), not along the outer rim as in most cases, actually consists of two separate bands of bone. (b) Higher magnification showing the double-bridges separating the right hypoglossal canal (UPenn). Cf. Berge and Bergman (2001); Hauser and DeStefano (1989); Hanihara and Ishida (2001b); Naderi et al. (2005); Wysocki et al. (2004).

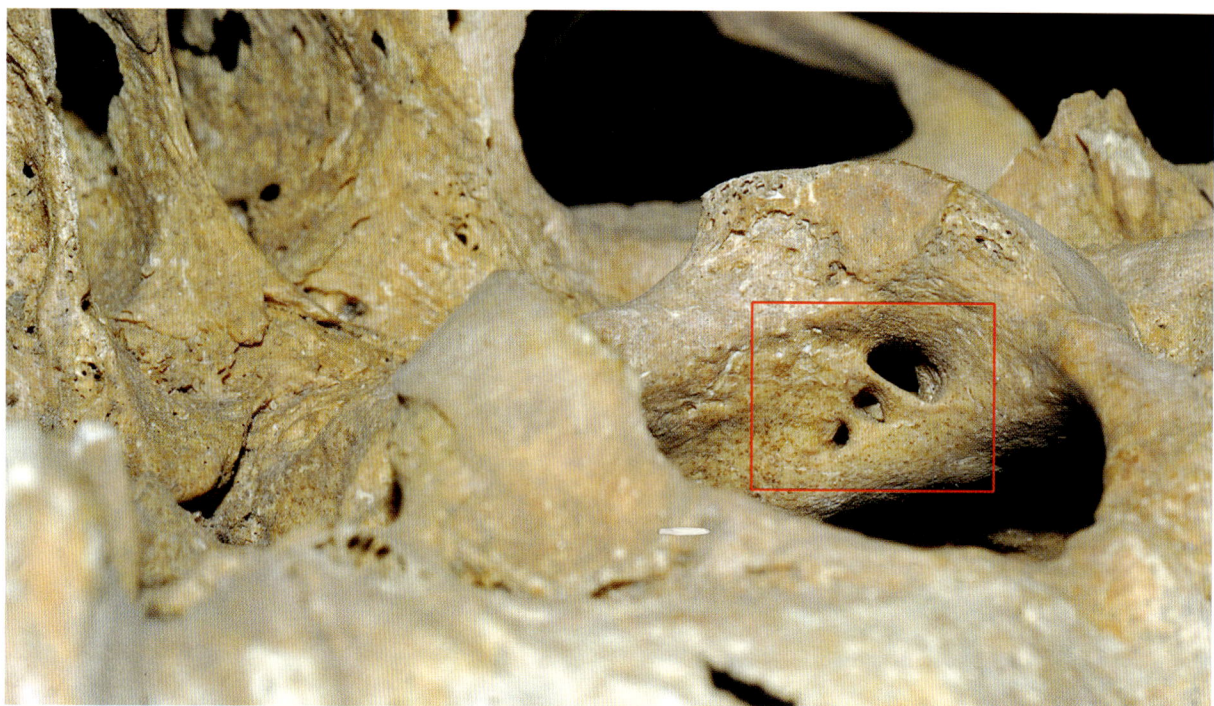

Figure 551. Rare double bridging (rectangle) of the left hypoglossal canal as the result of two bands forming three foramina in an elderly female (RV495). Division of the hypoglossal canal may be present in individuals of any age.

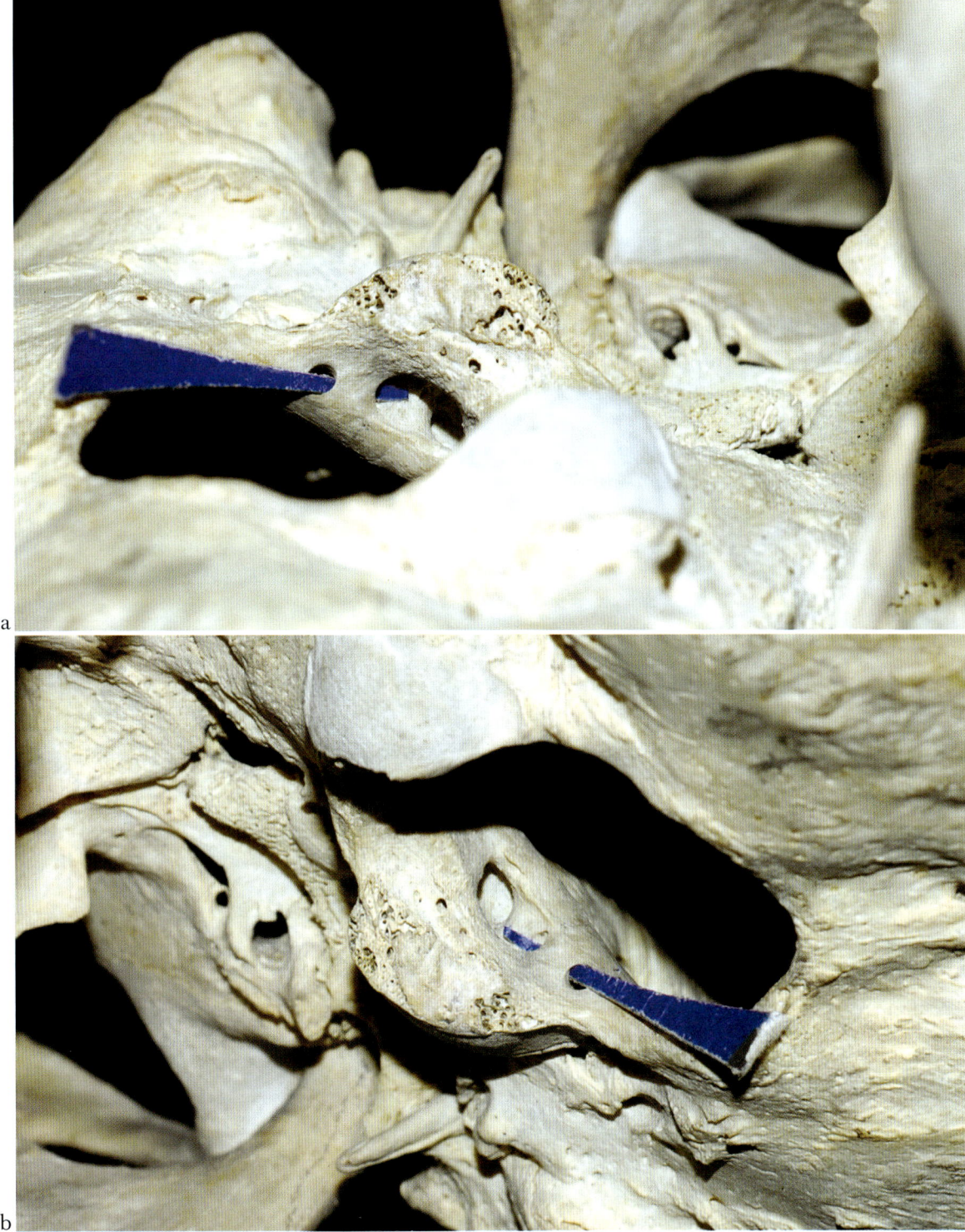

Figure 552a-b. Accessory foramen adjacent to the right hypoglossal canal viewed from the inferior view on an inverted skull. (a) Accessory foramen posterior and internal to the right hypoglossal canal (RV87, Celebes) with an entrance and exit posterior to the hypoglossal canal (trait is absent on the left side). (b) This foramen may have formed by calcification of a band of dura across the posterior-interior portion of the hypoglossal canal.

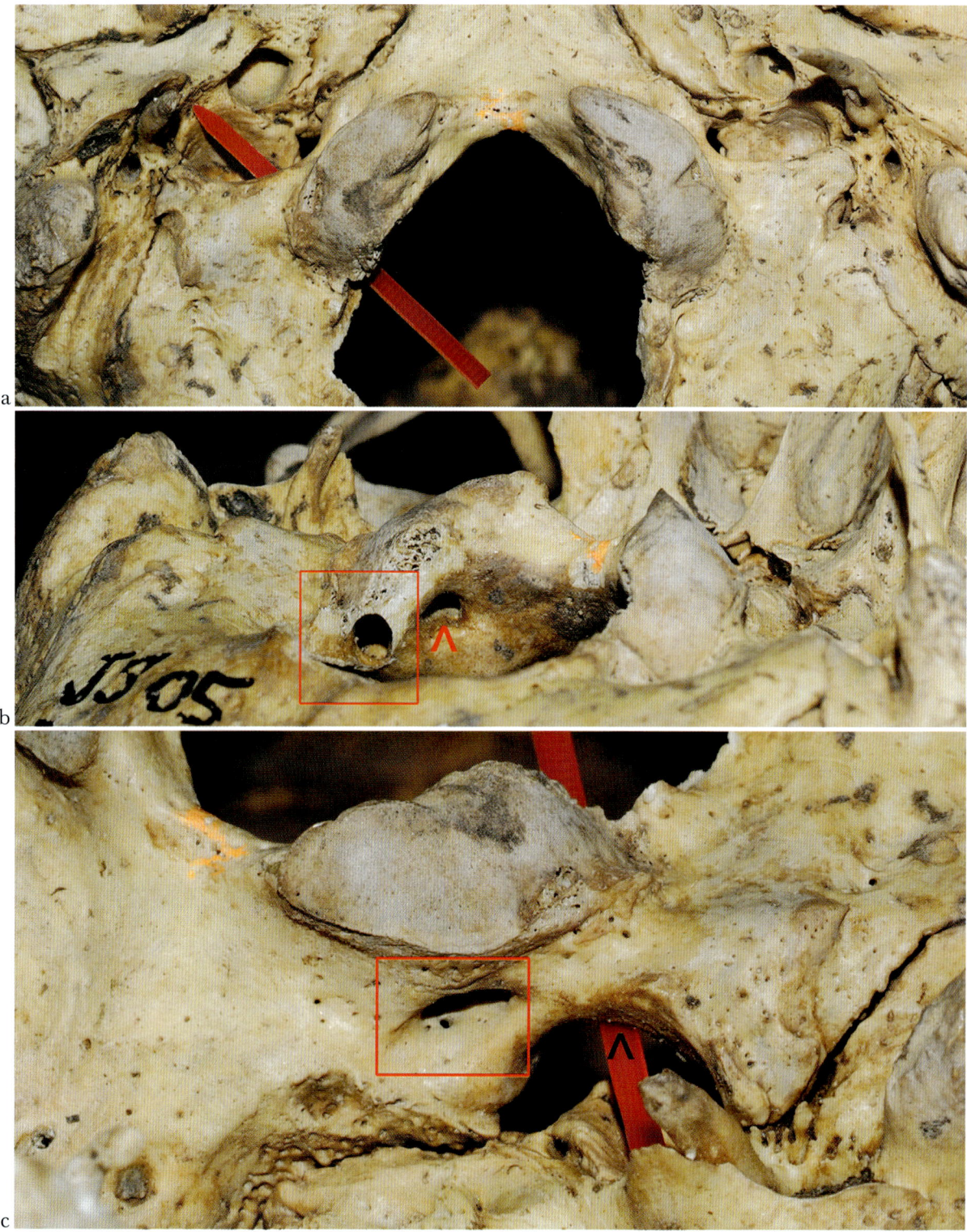

Figure 553a-c. Divided or accessory right hypoglossal canal. (a) Inferior view of a divided or accessory right hypoglossal canal that does not communicate with the primary canal in an adult Vietnamese skull (PAVN Forensic Institute). (b) Position of the accessory canal (square) posterior to the hypoglossal canal (∧). (c) Typical right hypoglossal canal (rectangle) and external opening (red probe and ∧) situated posterior to the hypoglossal canal.

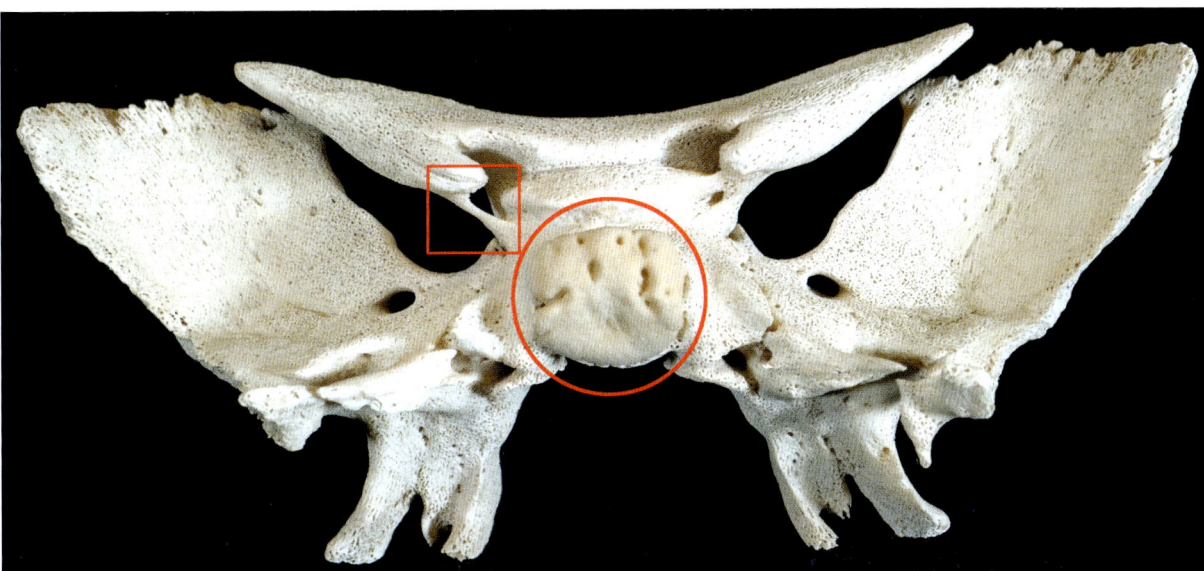

Figure 554. Sphenoid bone showing normal bridging (square) of the left anterior and posterior clinoid processes forming the optic foramen and normal morphology of the body, forming the basilar synchondrosis (circle) in an anatomical fetus (SI 249551). Typical anatomy.

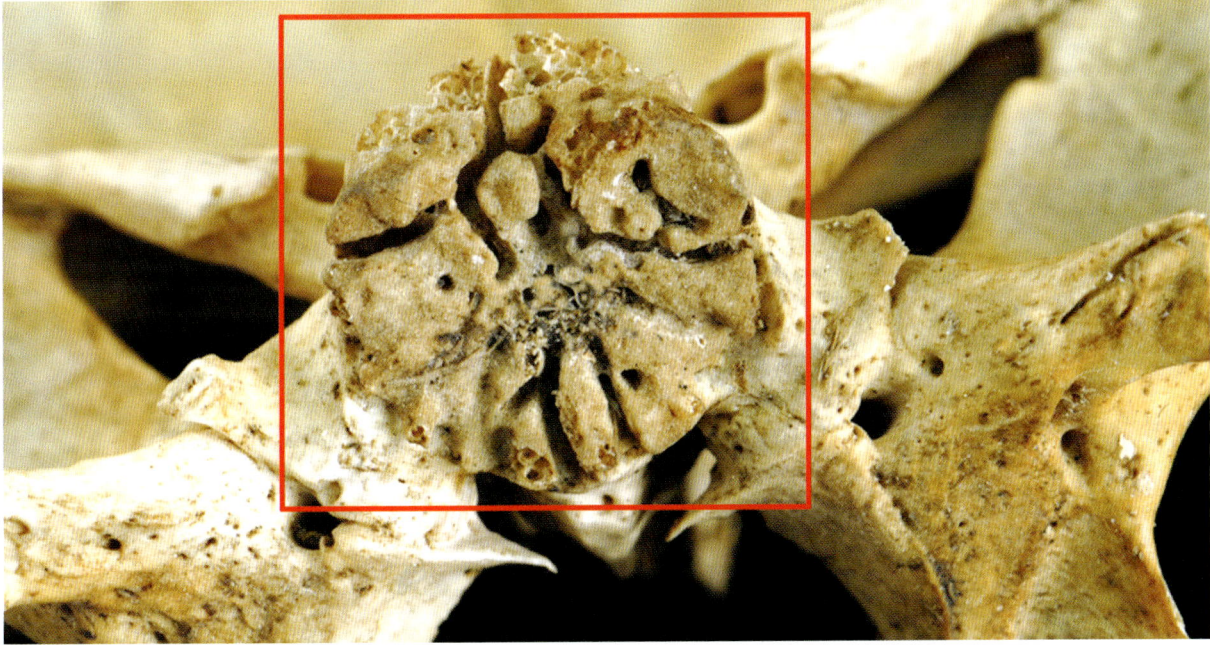

Figure 555. Basilar synchondrosis on the body of sphenoidal bone demonstrating its billowy surface (square) in a ancient Peruvian child (SI) – this individual has some burial debris adhering within the grooves. Note that the furrows have increased in number and depth compared to a younger individual in the image above. Typical anatomy.

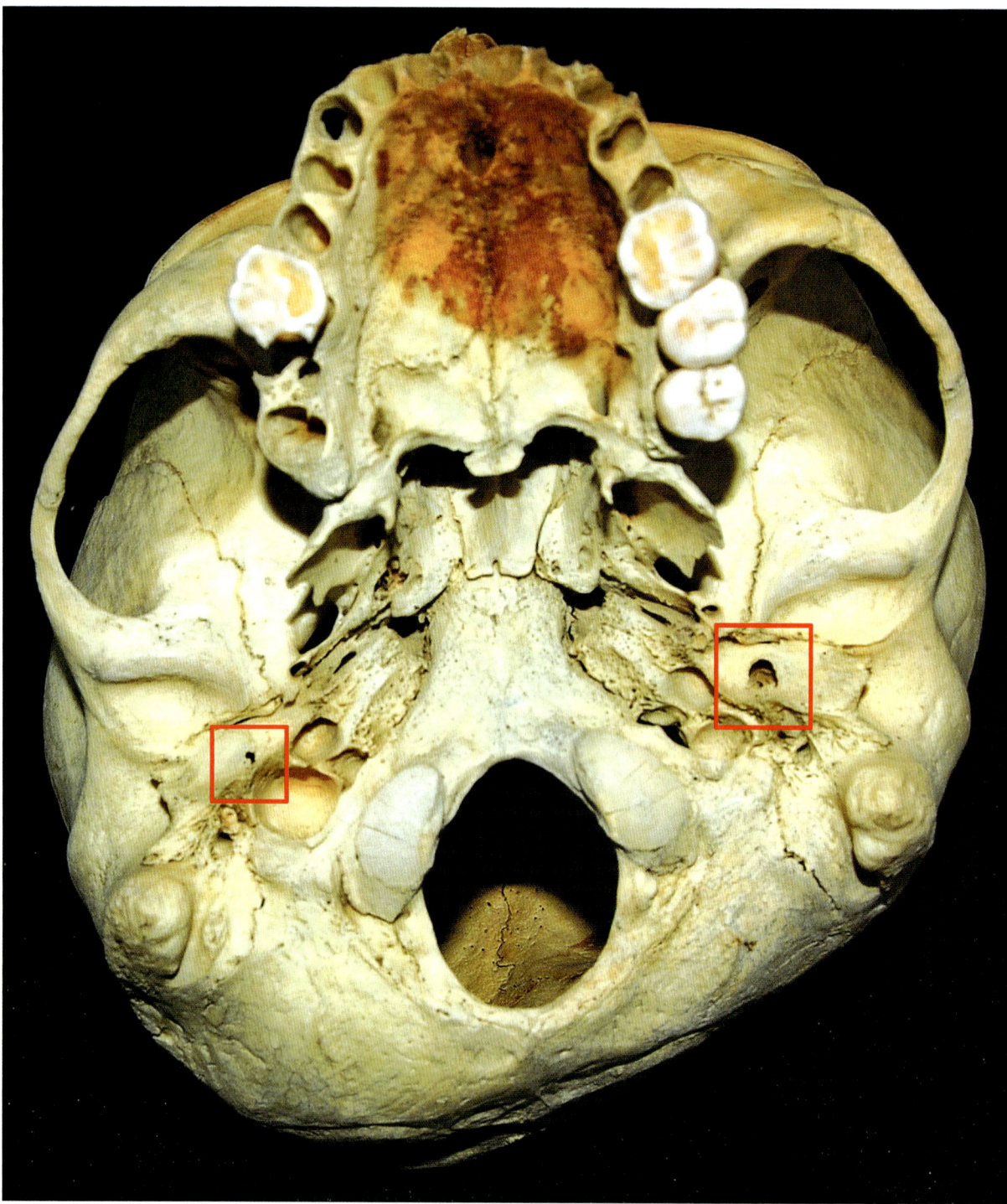

Figure 556. Cranial modification resulting in a flattened adult cranium with bilateral tympanic dehiscences (squares) in an adult ancient Peruvian cranium (SI). These openings are normal developmental features that typically close by about 5 years of age, but may persist into adulthood (Baker et al. 2005). Common finding. Cf. Hanihara and Ishida (2001); Hauser and DeStefano (1989).

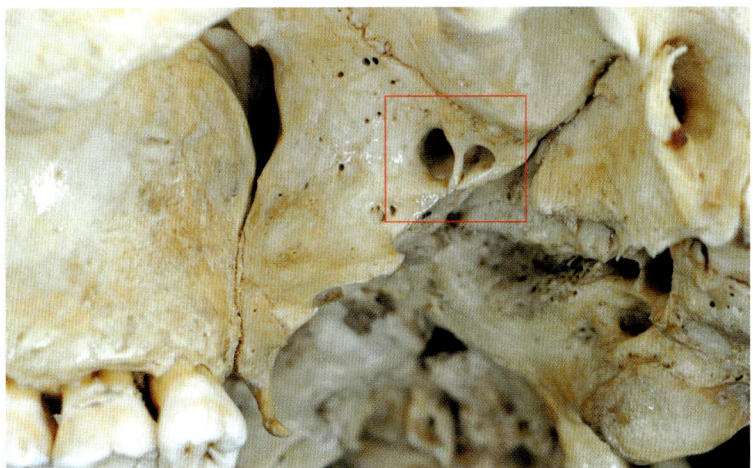

Figure 557. Pterygospinous foramen with bony bridging (square) in an adult Thai skull due to calcification of the spinous and alar ligaments (KKU). Common finding. Cf. Galdames et al. (2010); Nayak et al. (2007); Peker et al. (2002); Rossi et al. (2011); Skrzat et al. (2005, 2006).

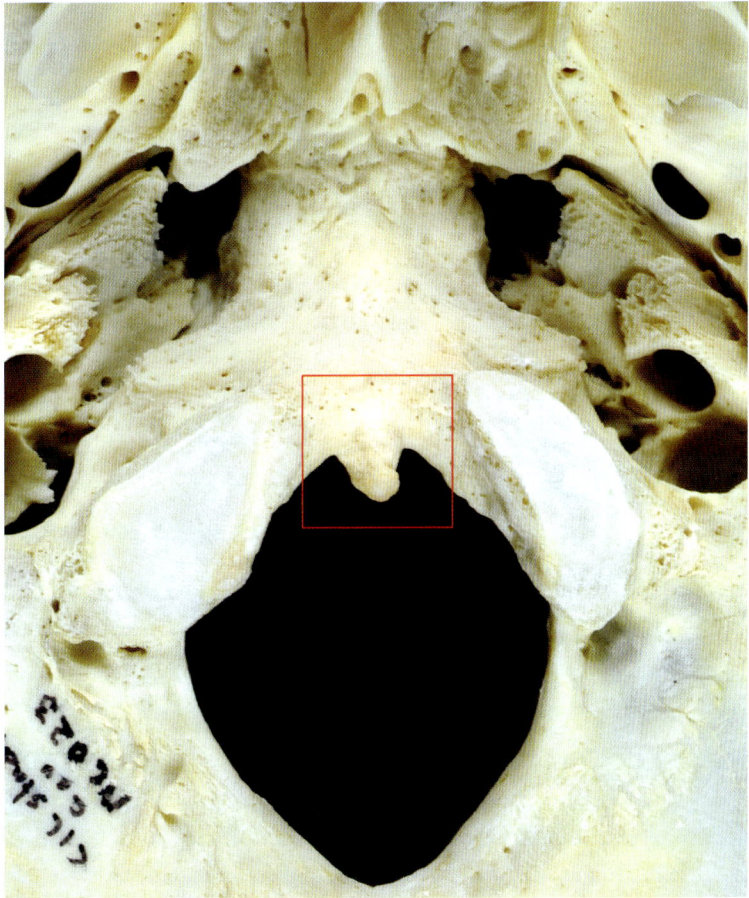

Figure 558. Probable calcification of the apical ligament (square) of the atlas resulting in a precondylar tubercle, in an adult Asian (CSC). Bony tubercles along the anterior rim of the foramen magnum vary greatly in size and shape while the tubercle in this example is conical and projects posteriorly. Common to uncommon finding. Cf. Oetteking (1923); Taitz (2000).

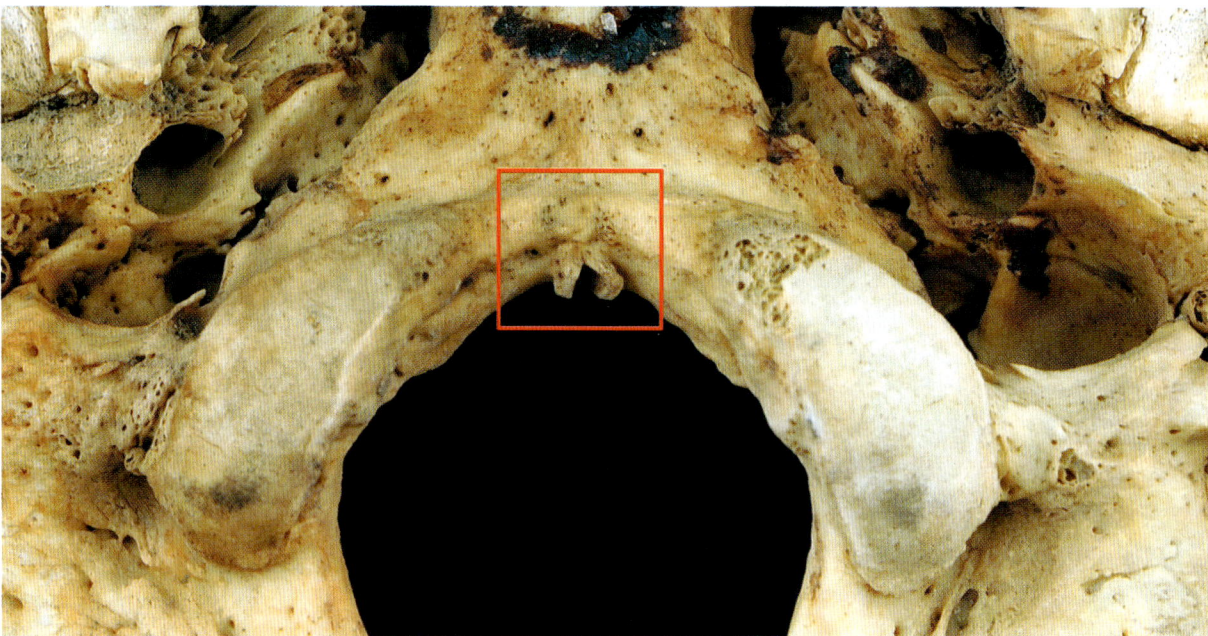

Figure 559. Bifurcated calcification of the apical ligament (square) of the atlas in an adult Thai skull (KKU). These horizontal tubercles are directed posteriorly. Uncommon to common finding. Cf. Oetteking (1923).

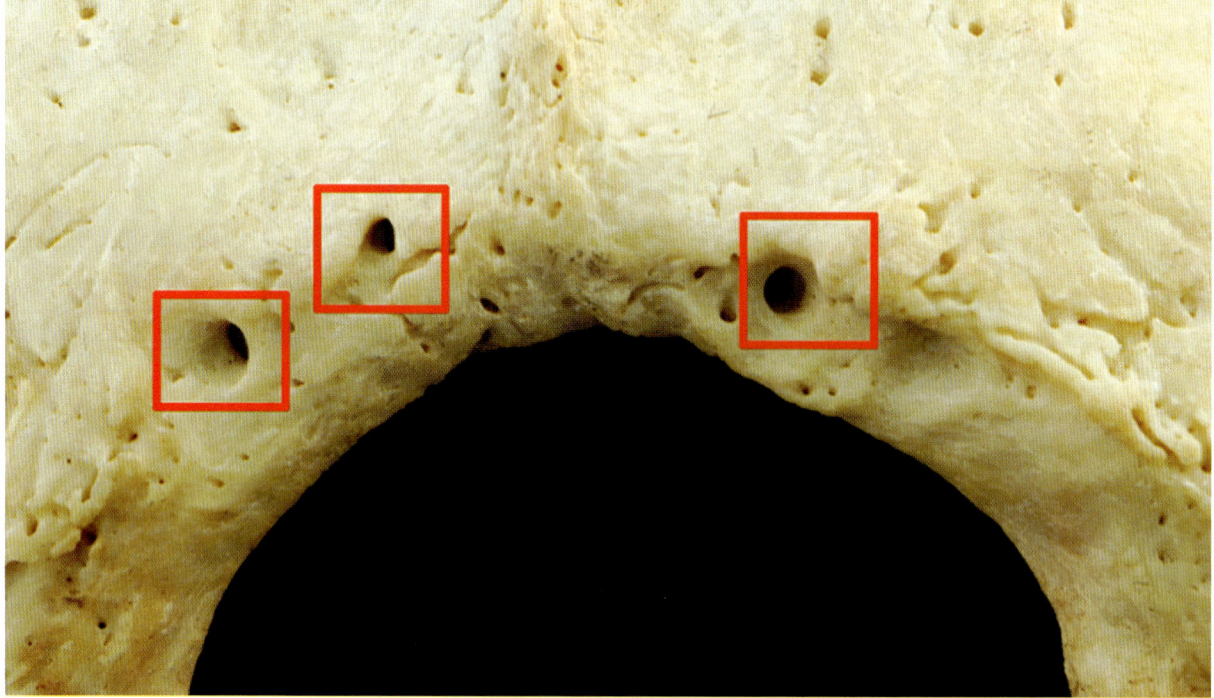

Figure 560. Unusually large occipital foramina (squares) along the posterior margin of the foramen magnum (ancient Peru, SI). Uncommon to common finding.

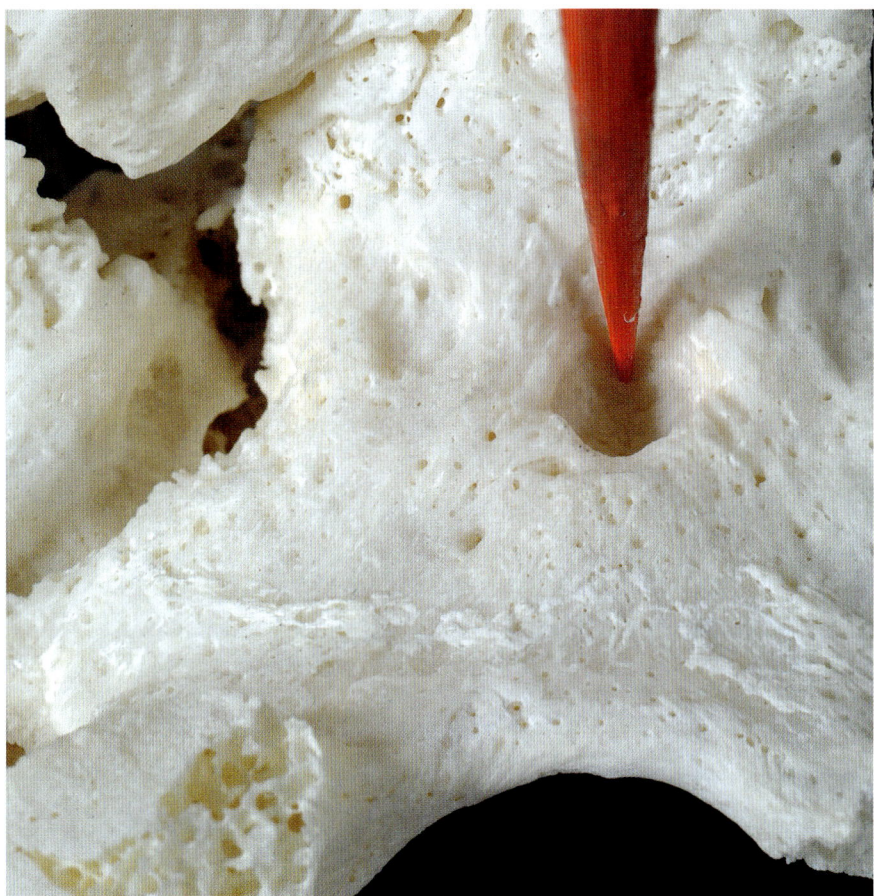

Figure 564. Deep pharyngeal foveola/fossa navicularis (probe tip). Common finding. Cf. Cankal et al. (2004).

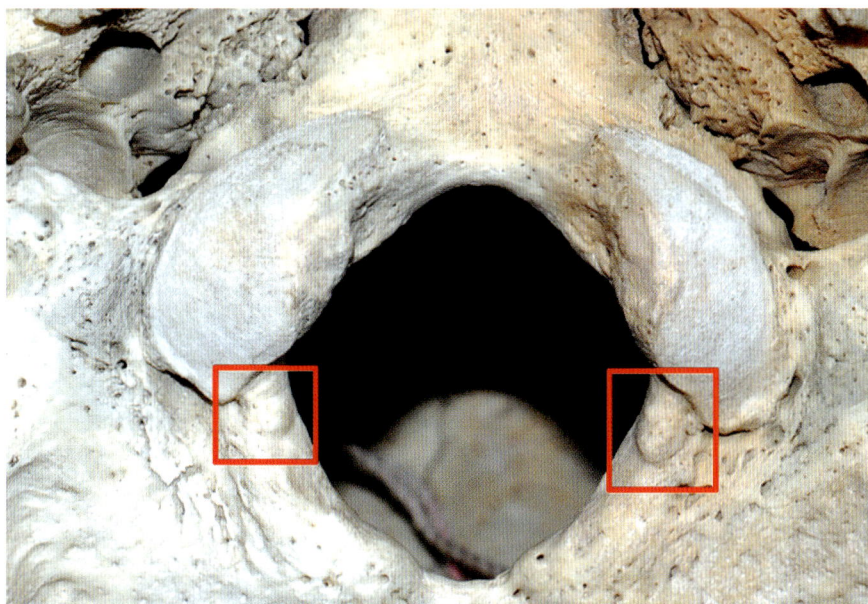

Figure 565. Postcondylar tubercles (squares), an uncommon to rare trait in an ancient Peruvian (SI). Uncommon finding depending on the group being studied.

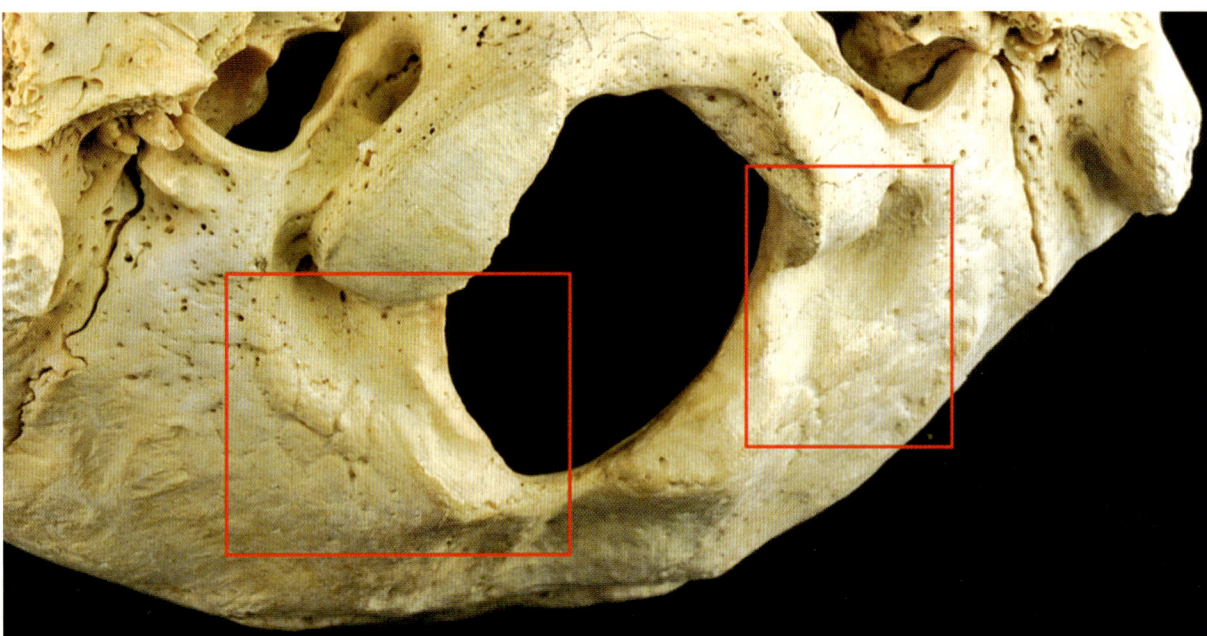

Figure 566. Postcondylar depressions or basilar invaginations (square and rectangle) in an Asian adult skull (CSC). Uncommon to common finding.

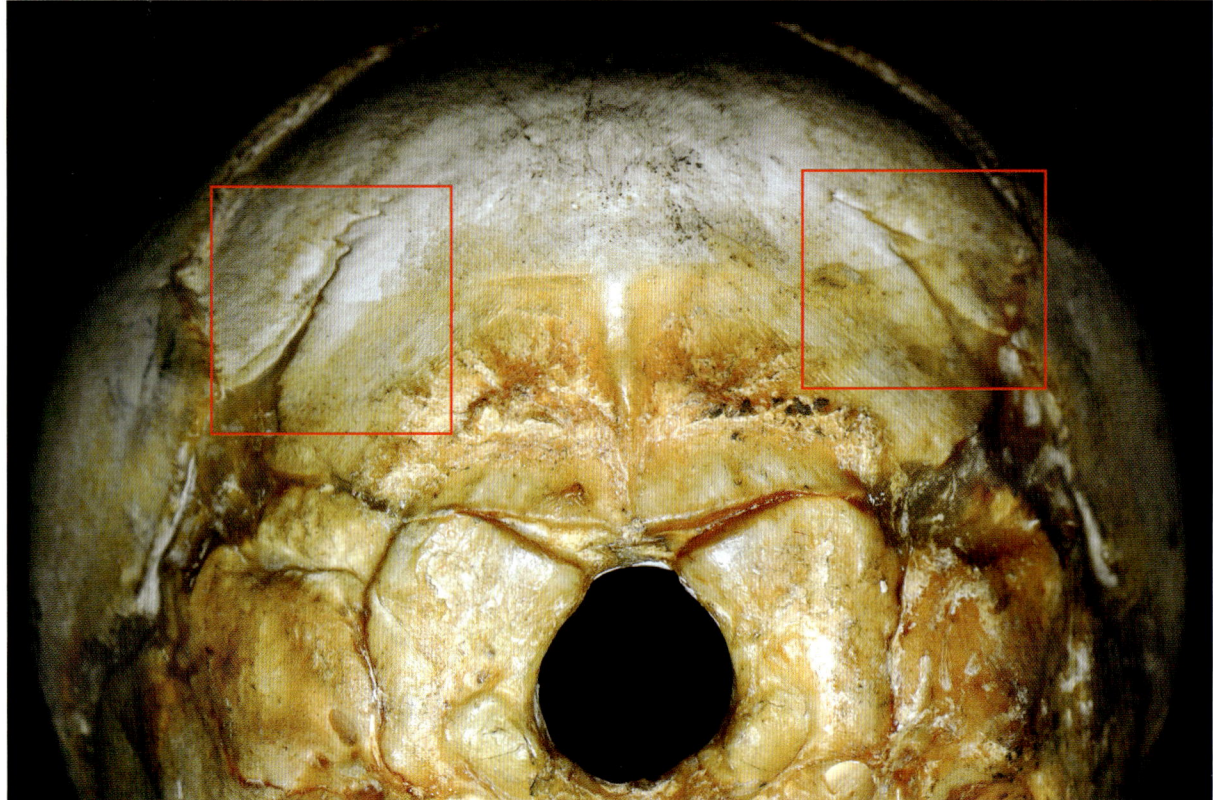

Figure 567. Remnant of Mendosal sutures (squares) in a child (anatomical, SI). Common finding.

Basilar (Inferior) View of the Skull

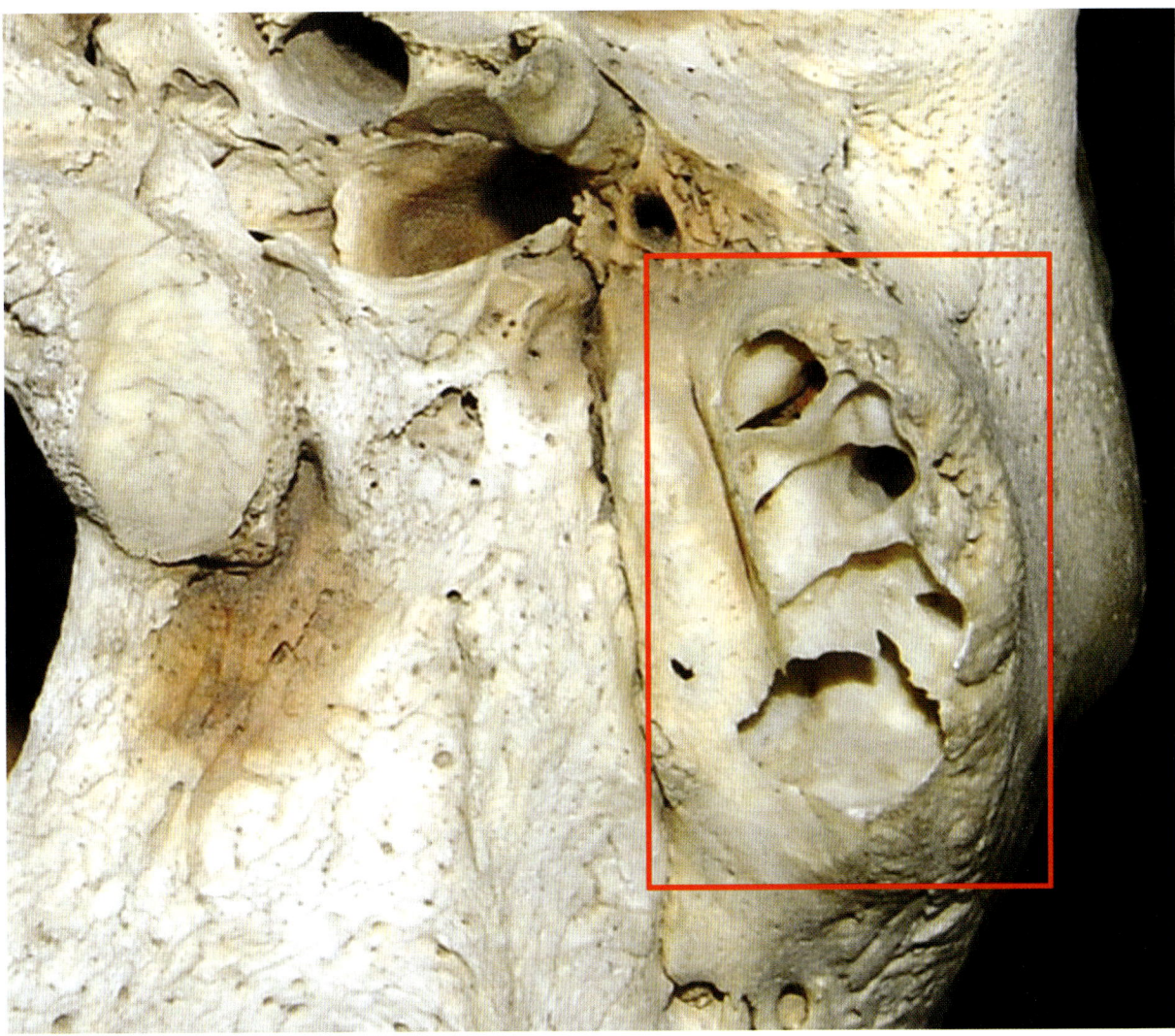

Figure 568. Typical internal anatomy and architecture of adult mastoid process (rectangle). Note the bony air cells and compartments as well as the "eggshell" thin bone forming the ectocranial border (KKU).

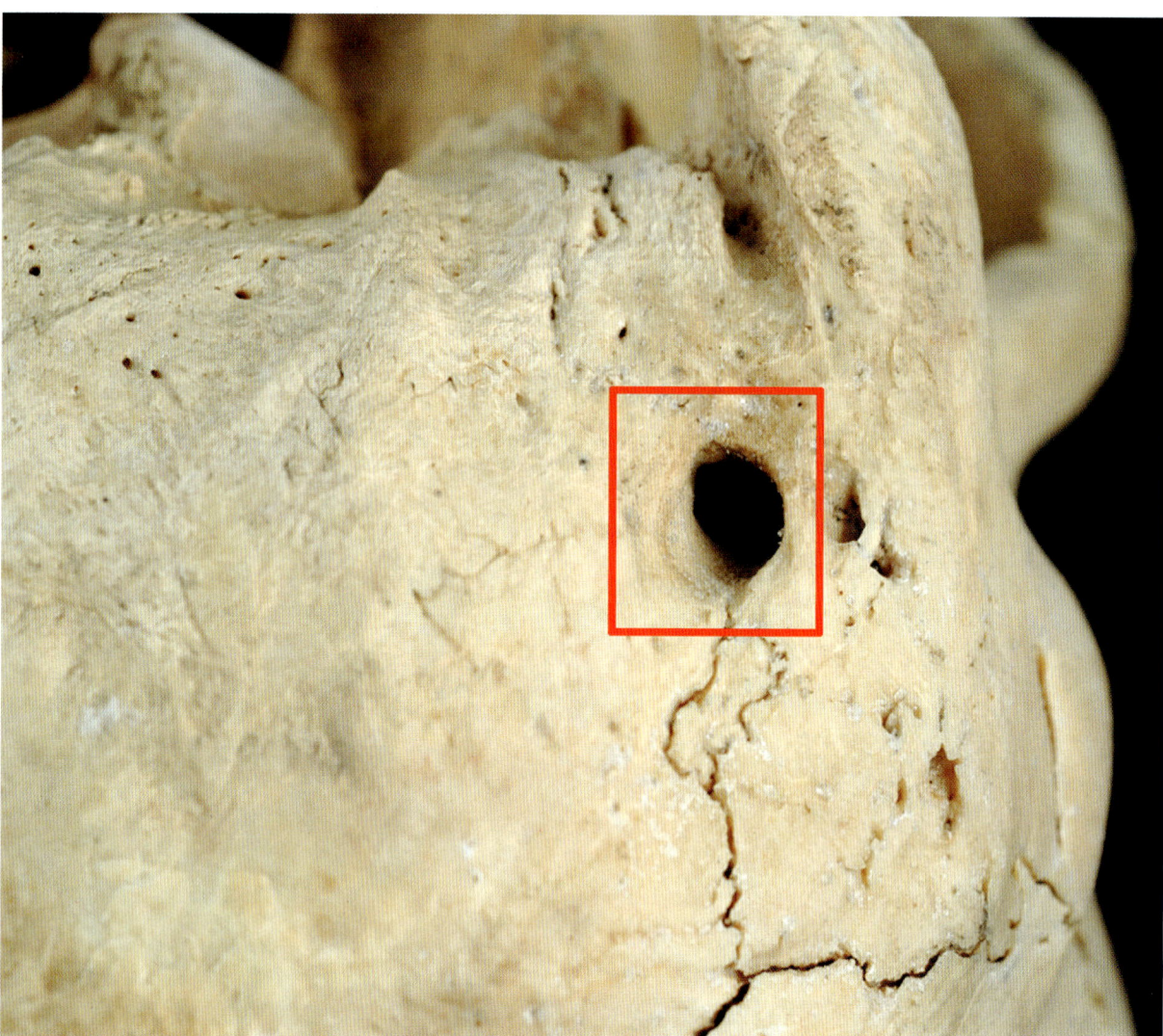

Figure 569. Unusually large mastoid foramen (square) along the suture and two smaller foramina (temporal) in an adult Thai male skull (KKU). Most mastoid foramina lie on (sutural) or beside (exsutural) the suture, with the latter form being less common. The endocranial opening of this foramen communicates with the sigmoid sinus. Large foramina such as shown here are uncommon. Cf. Berry and Berry (1967); Hauser and DeStefano (1989).

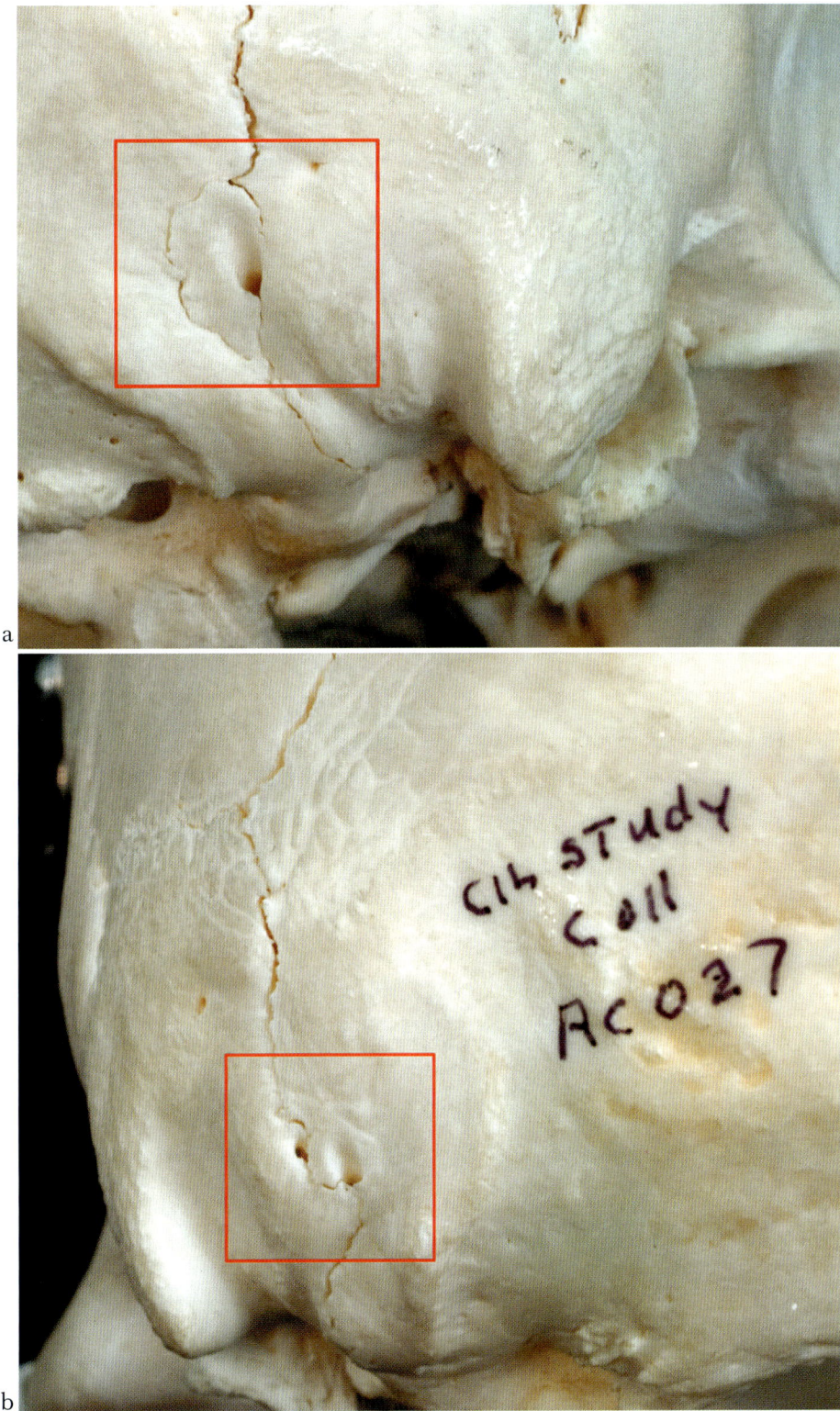

Figure 570a-b. Occipitomastoid ossicle and mastoid foramen. (a) Occipitomastoid ossicle (ossicle of Riolano; square) (Vázquez et al. 2001) and sutural foramen. (b) Two mastoid foramina (square) in the occipitomastoid suture of an adult Asian female skull (CSC AC 027). Note that one of the foramina is situated in the temporal bone and the other is in the occipital bone. Cf. Hauser and DeStefano (1989); Boyd (1930) for mastoid foramen.

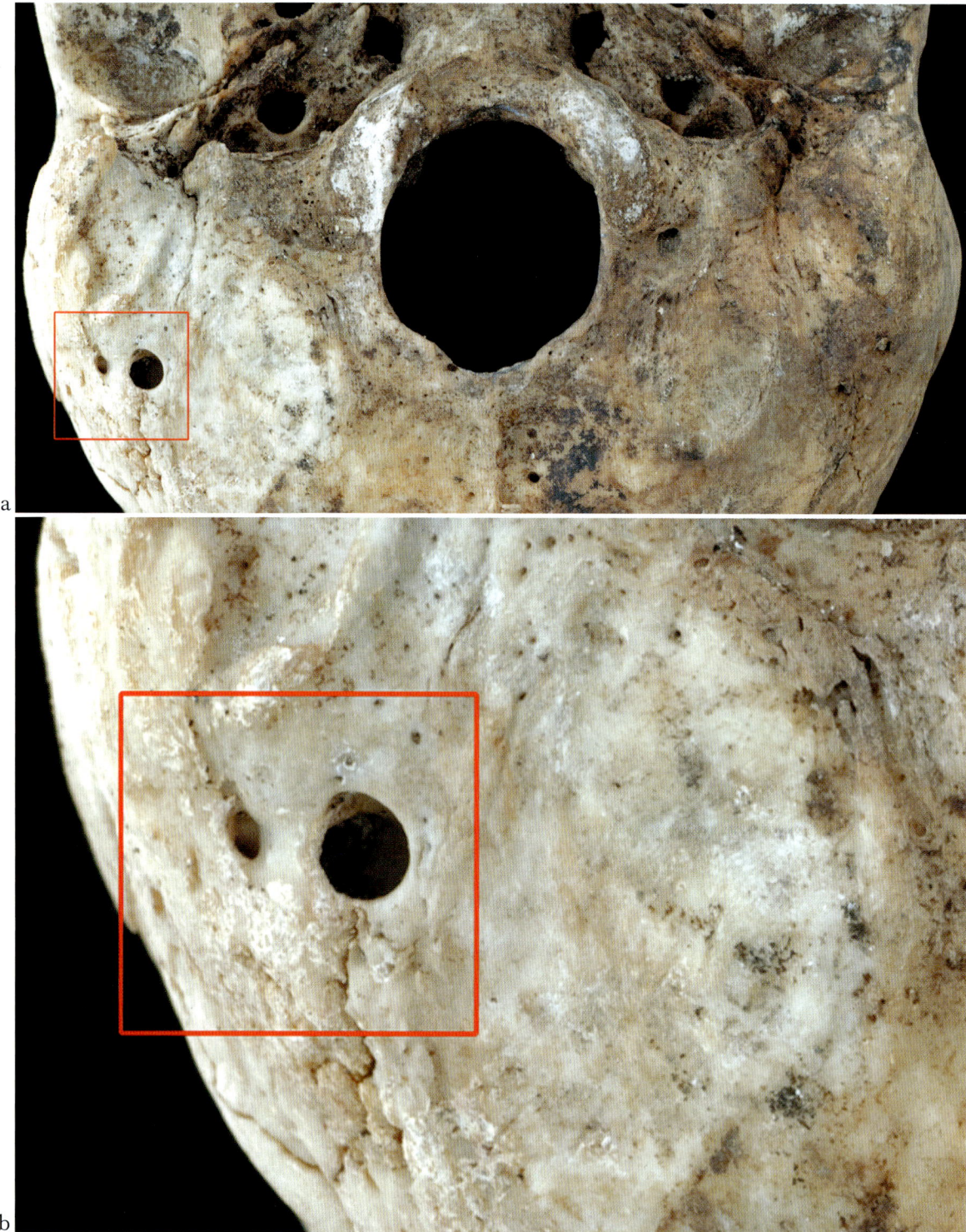

Figure 571a-b. Large and small mastoid foramina. (a) Inferior view of unusually large and small (typical) right mastoid foramina (square) in a 69-year-old Thai male skull (CMU 18 53). (b) Note the internal structure and "hollow" appearance of the large foramen (square). The large foramen lies on the suture ("sutural") and the small foramen lies distant to it ("exsutural").

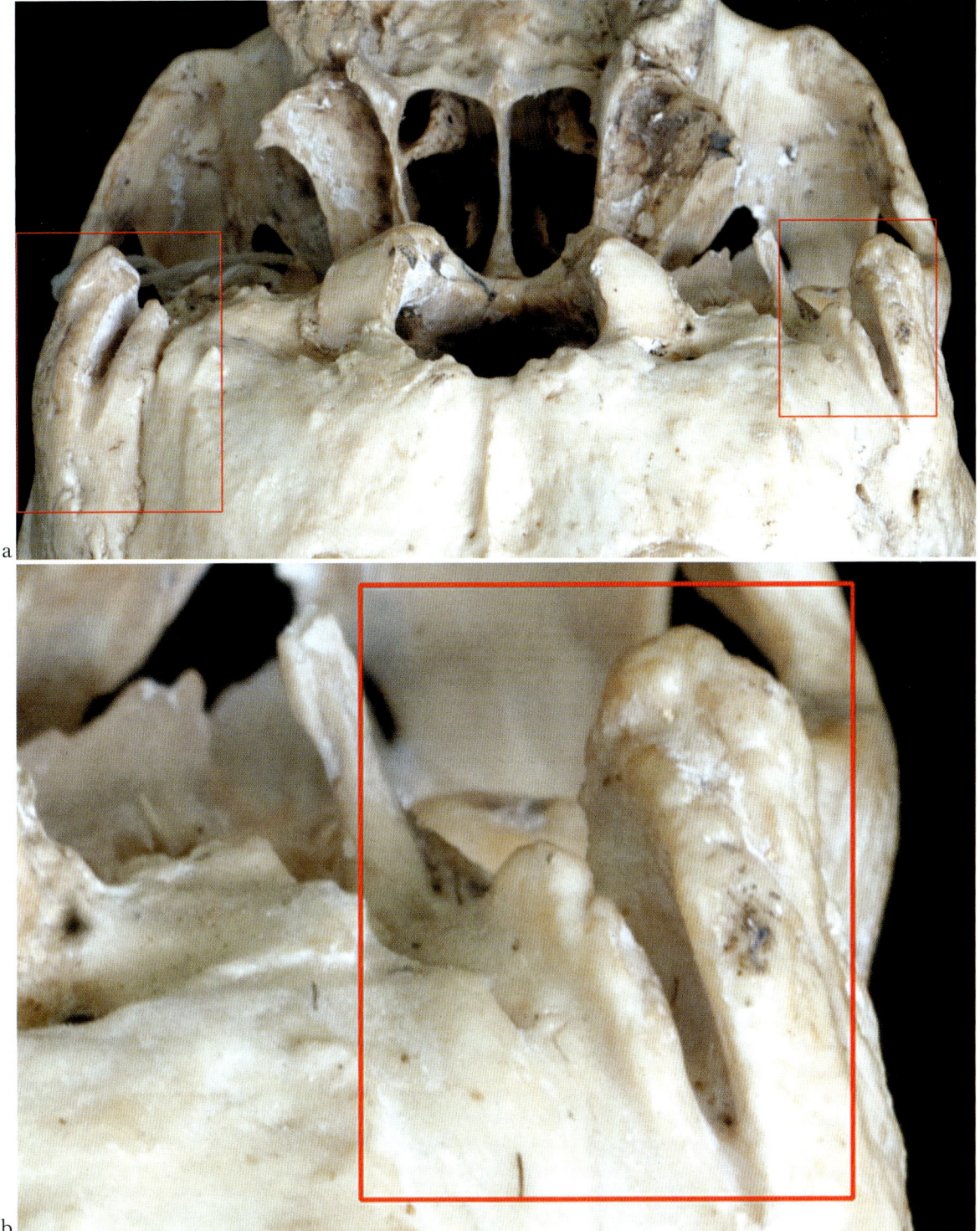

Figure 572a-b. Divided mastoid processes. (a) Posterior view of divided mastoid processes (rectangle and square) in an adult Thai male skull (KKU 275 36 A5 134). (b) Higher magnification of the left mastoid process (rectangle).

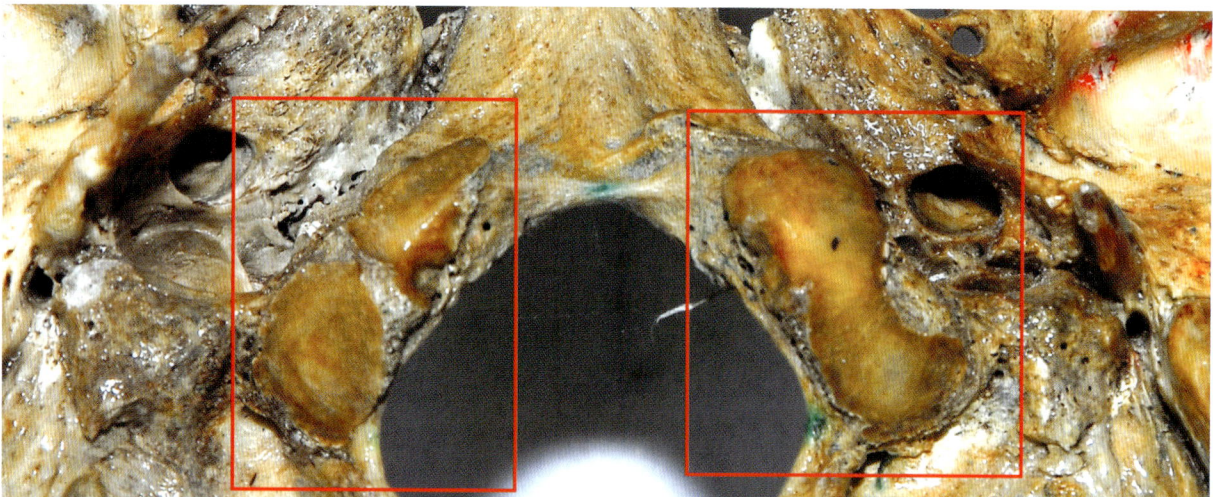

Figure 573. Asymmetrical occipital condyles (rectangle and square) – double on the right (uncommon) and single (common) facet on the left in an adult Thai skull (KKU).

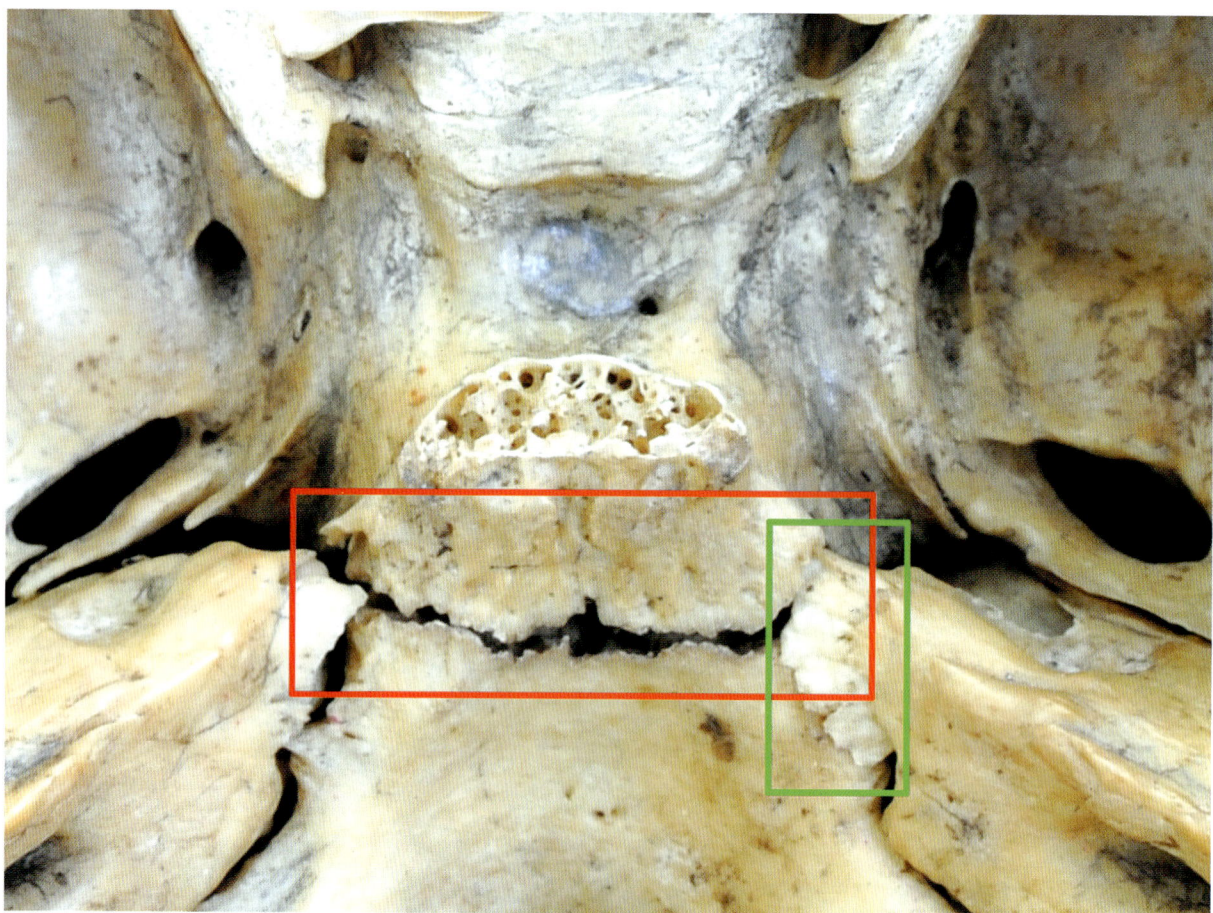

Figure 574. Fan-like ossification along the apex of the petrous bone (green rectangle) and an open basilar synchondrosis (red rectangle) in a subadult. Both are normal features in subadults.

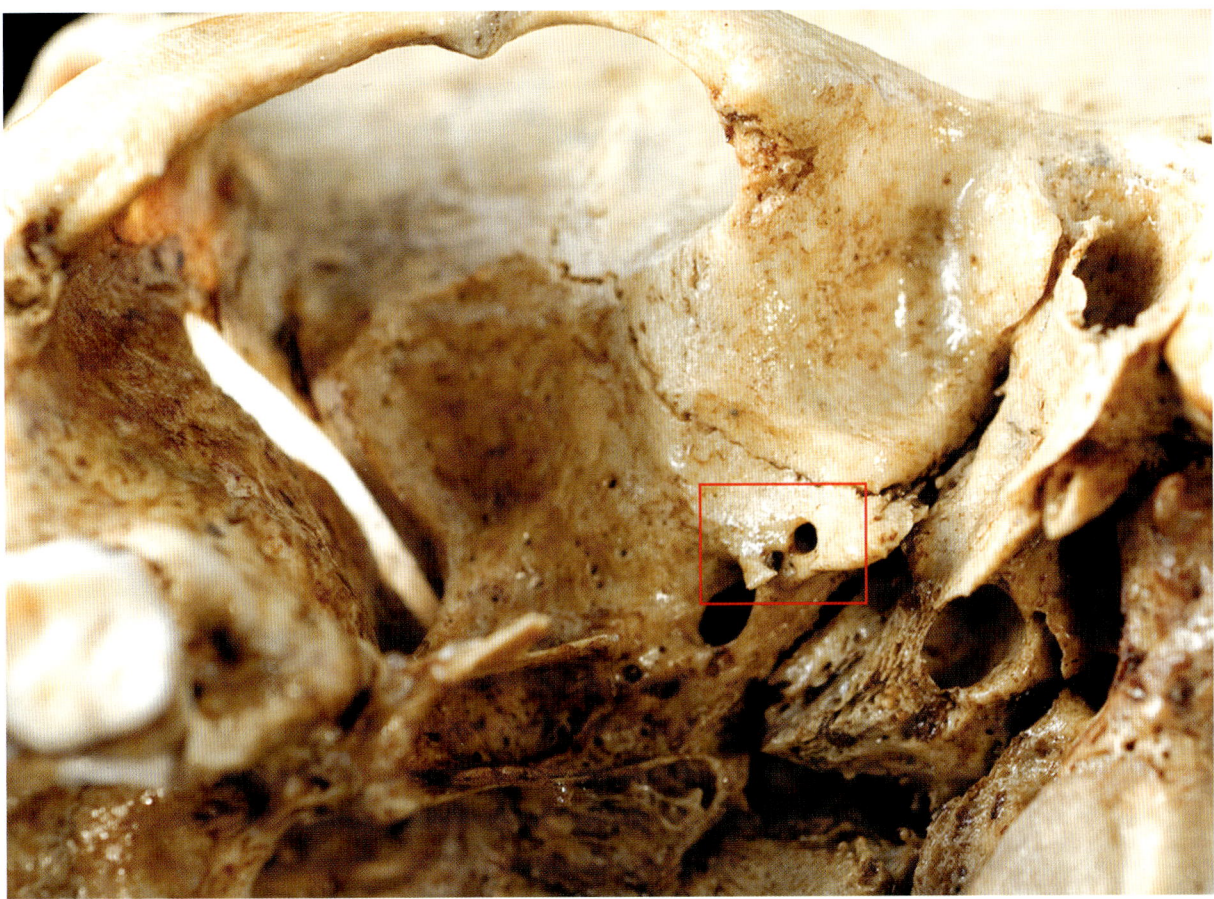

Figure 575. Double foramen spinosum (rectangle) in an Asian skull (CSC).

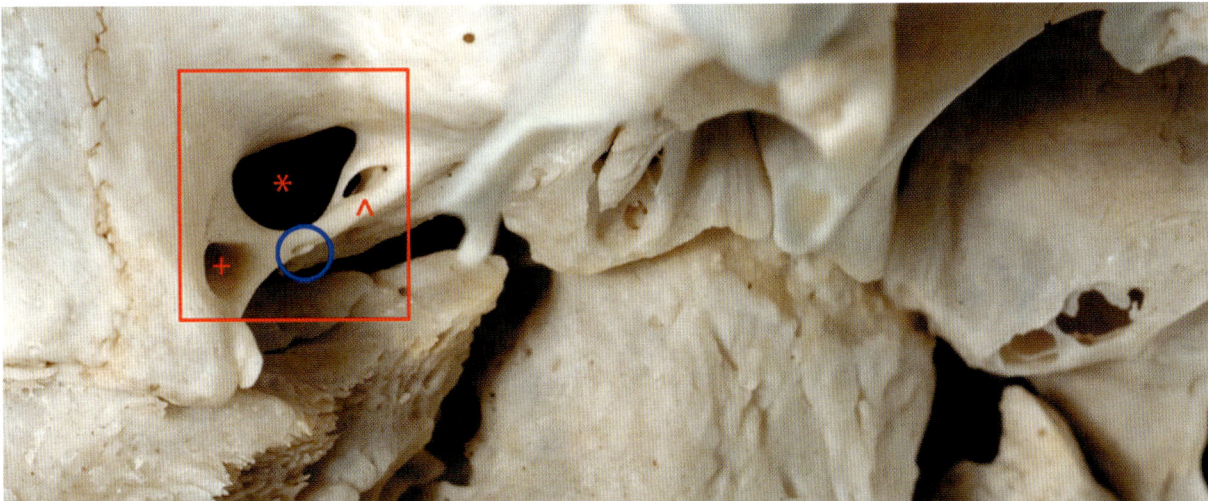

Figure 576. Foramen ovale (*), foramen of Vesalius (∧), canaliculus innominatus or foramen of Arnold (circle) and foramen spinosum (+) in an Asian adult (CSC AC026). Typical anatomy.

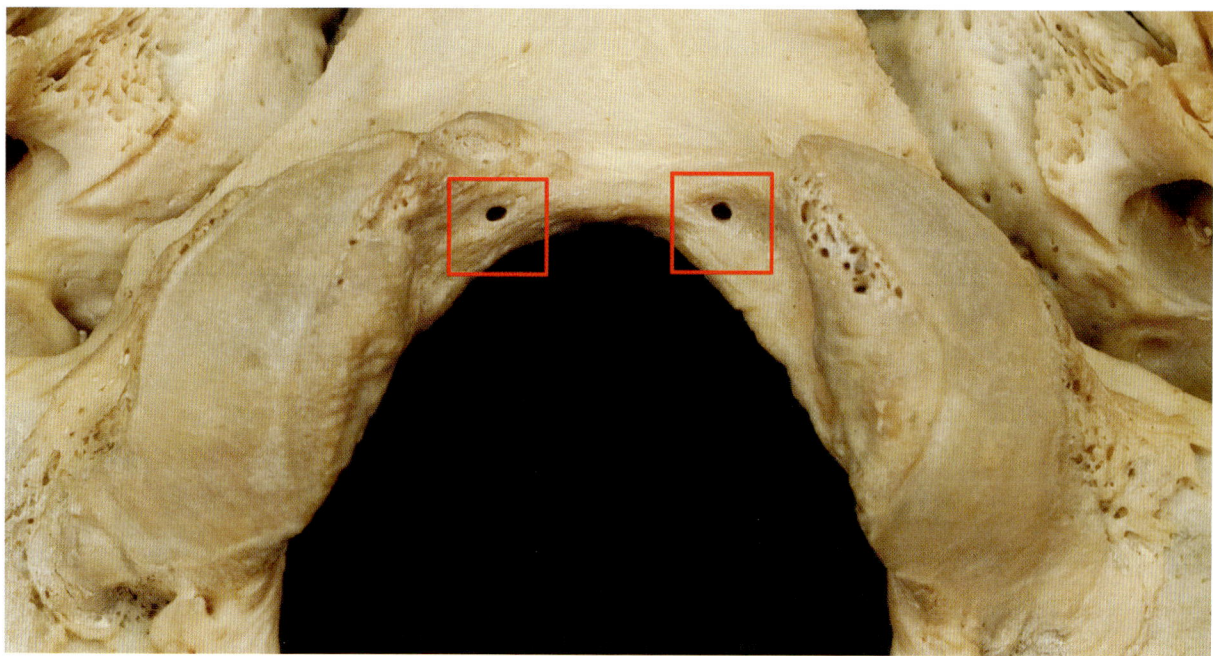

Figure 577. Bilateral median foramina (squares) medial to the occipital condyles in an adult (SI Terry106R).

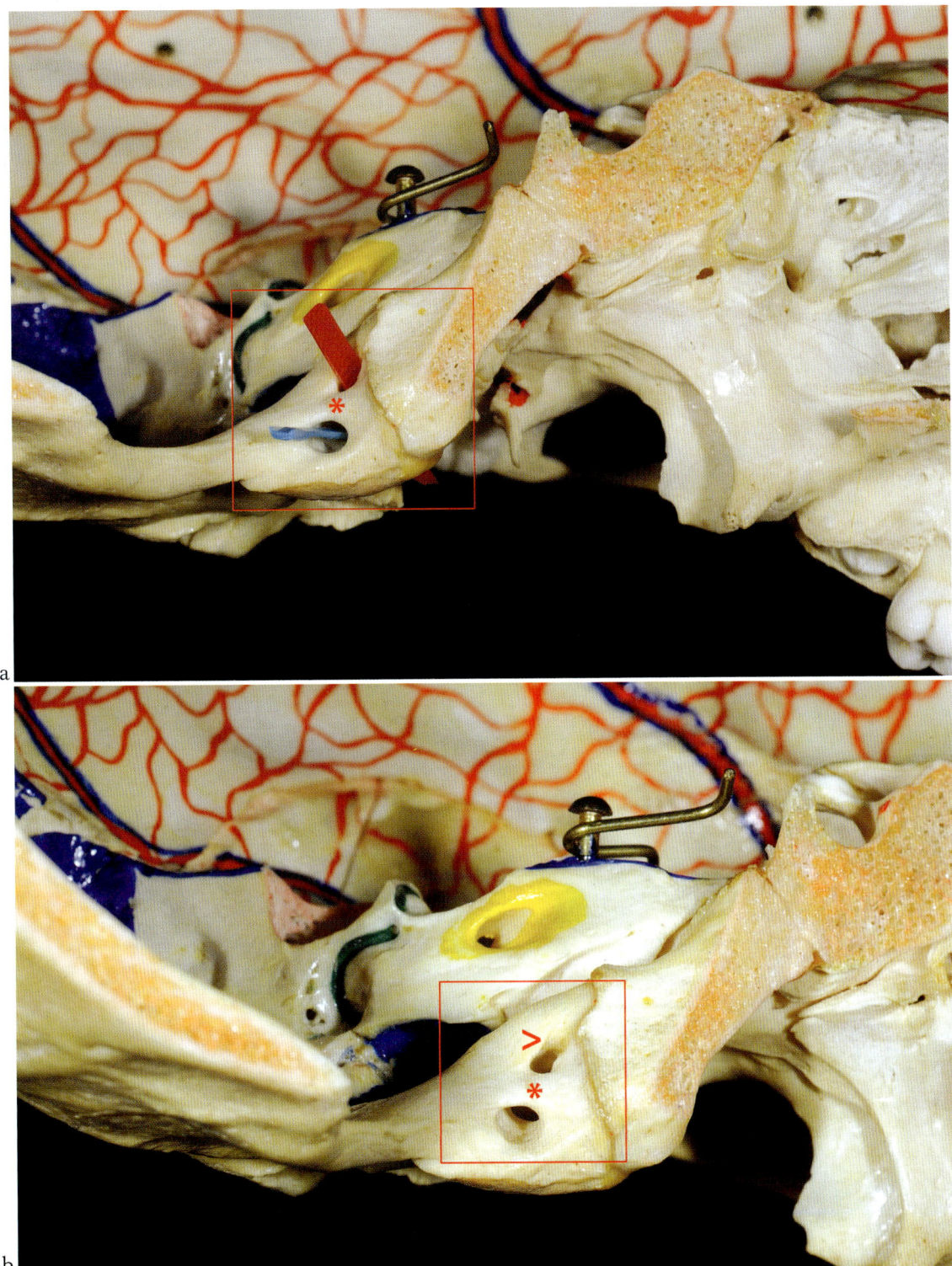

Figure 578a-b. Demonstration of hypoglossal canals in a teaching specimen (JABSOM) viewed on an inverted skull. (a) Unusual left hypoglossal canal (square) resulting in horizontal division of the canal by a wide bar of bone (*). (b) Vertical groove (>) and divided left hypoglossal canal (square) by a bar of bone (*). Most hypoglossal canals are divided by one or more bars of bone, many of which resemble a "wave" or inverted pyramid that is oriented superior-inferiorly.

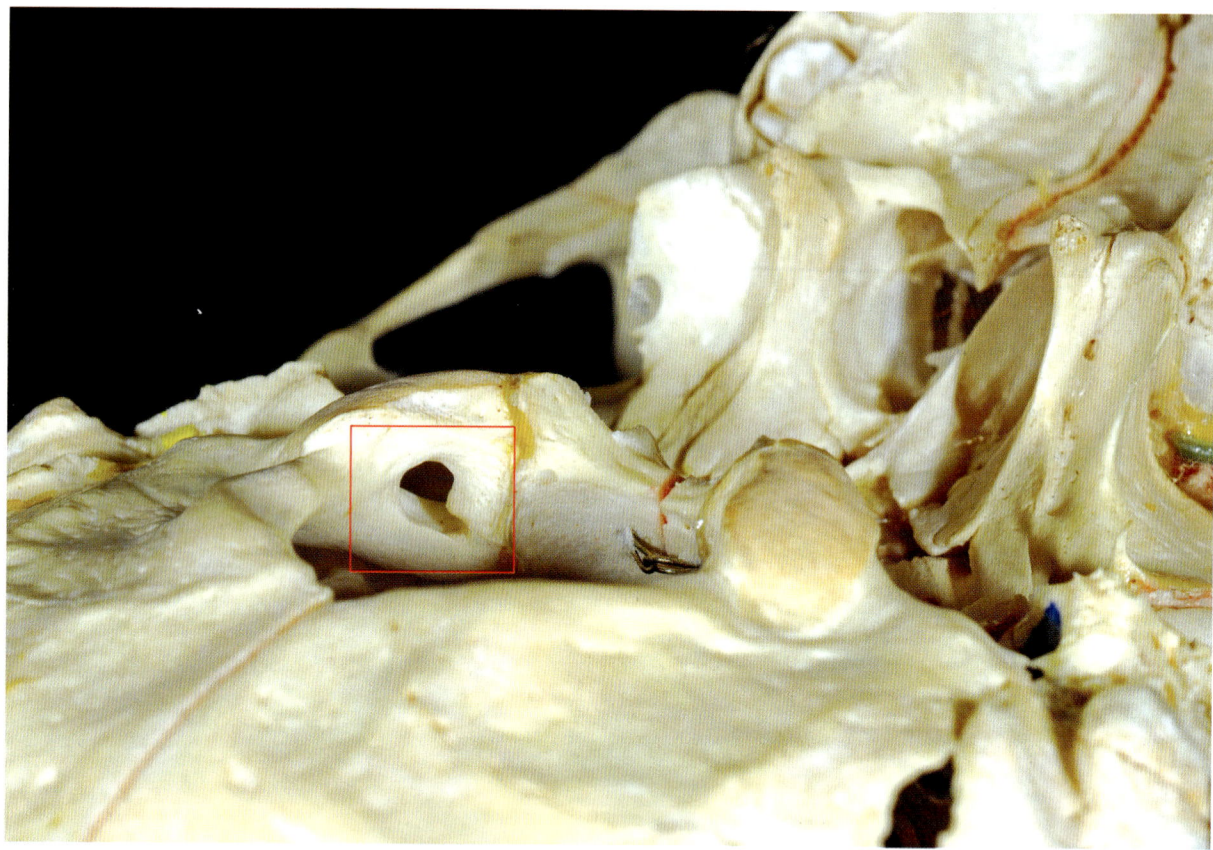

Figure 579. A single (non-divided) right hypoglossal canal (rectangle) showing its teardrop or "comma-like" shape (JABSOM teaching specimen).

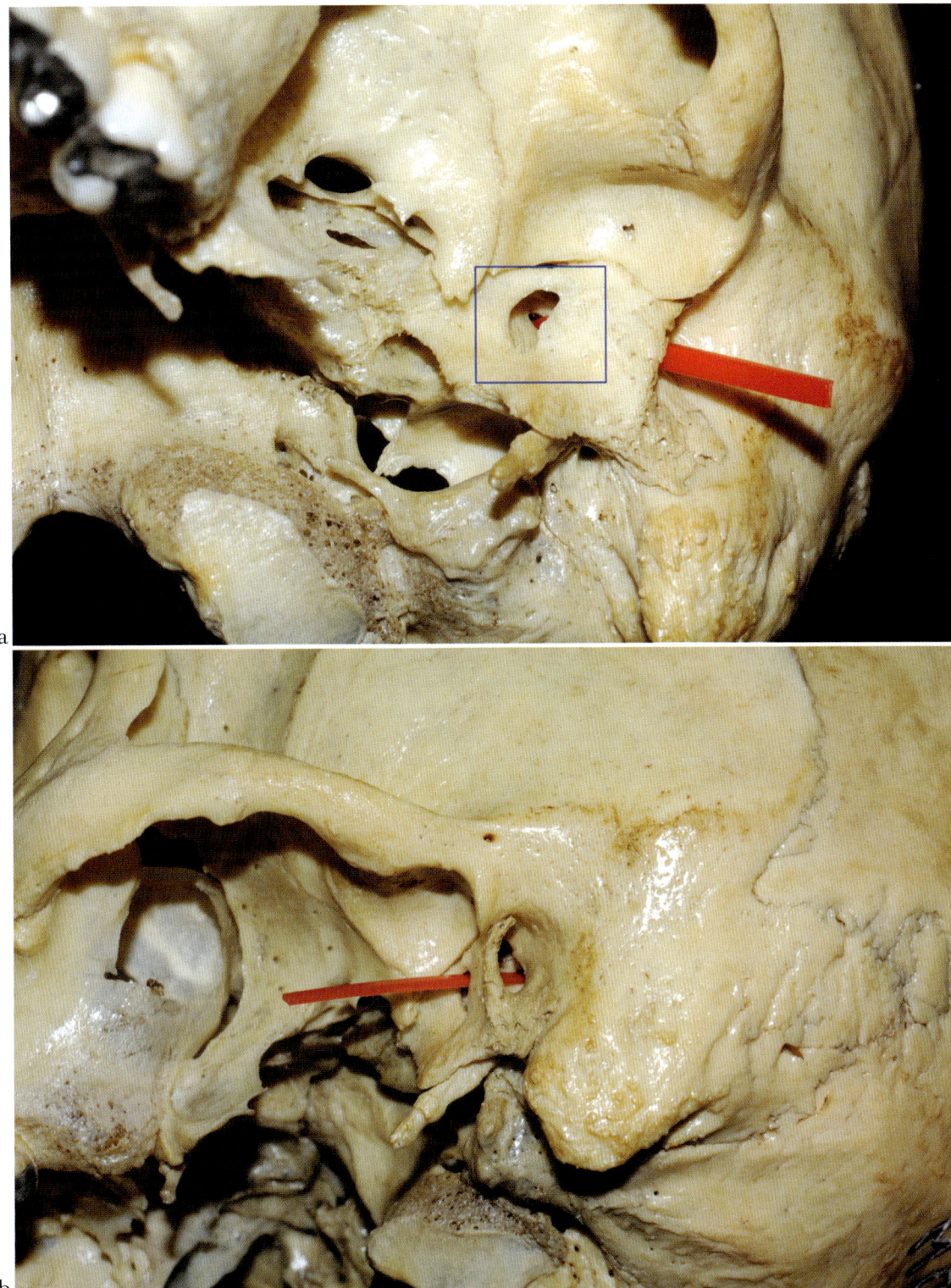

Figure 580a-b. Demonstration of a tympanic dehiscence and oval window. (a) Red probe inserted into the left external auditory meatus and pointing to the oval window through a small tympanic dehiscence (square), also known as a foramen of Huschke. (b) Left lateral view showing a red probe inserted through a dehiscence in the left tympanic plate and entering the oval window (JABSOM M02).

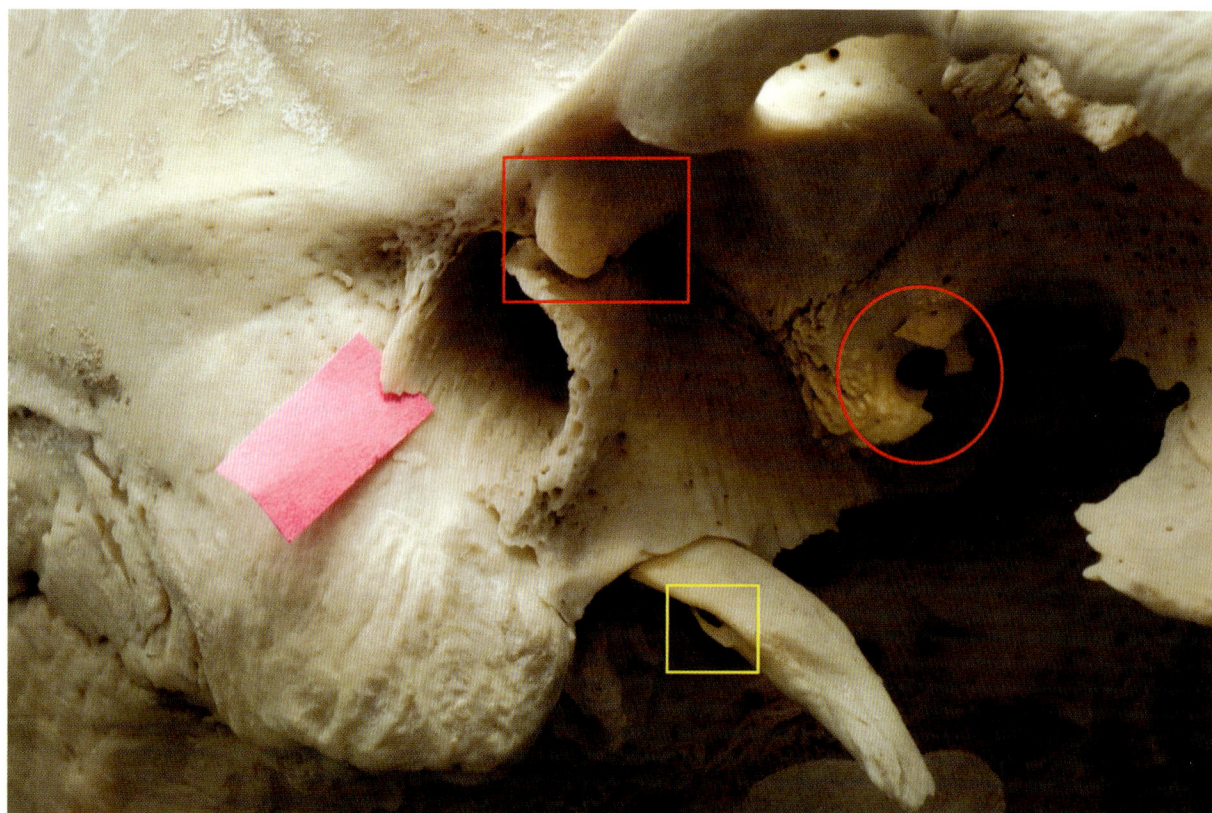

Figure 581. Small osseous projection along the posterior surface of the right styloid process (yellow square), partial bridging above the foramen spinosum (circle), a projecting spine of Henle (pink paper) and postglenoid process (red rectangle) (CSC018). While all are typical features in many older individuals, the postglenoid tubercle and spine of Henle are more developed in this individual than usual.

Basilar (Inferior) View of the Skull

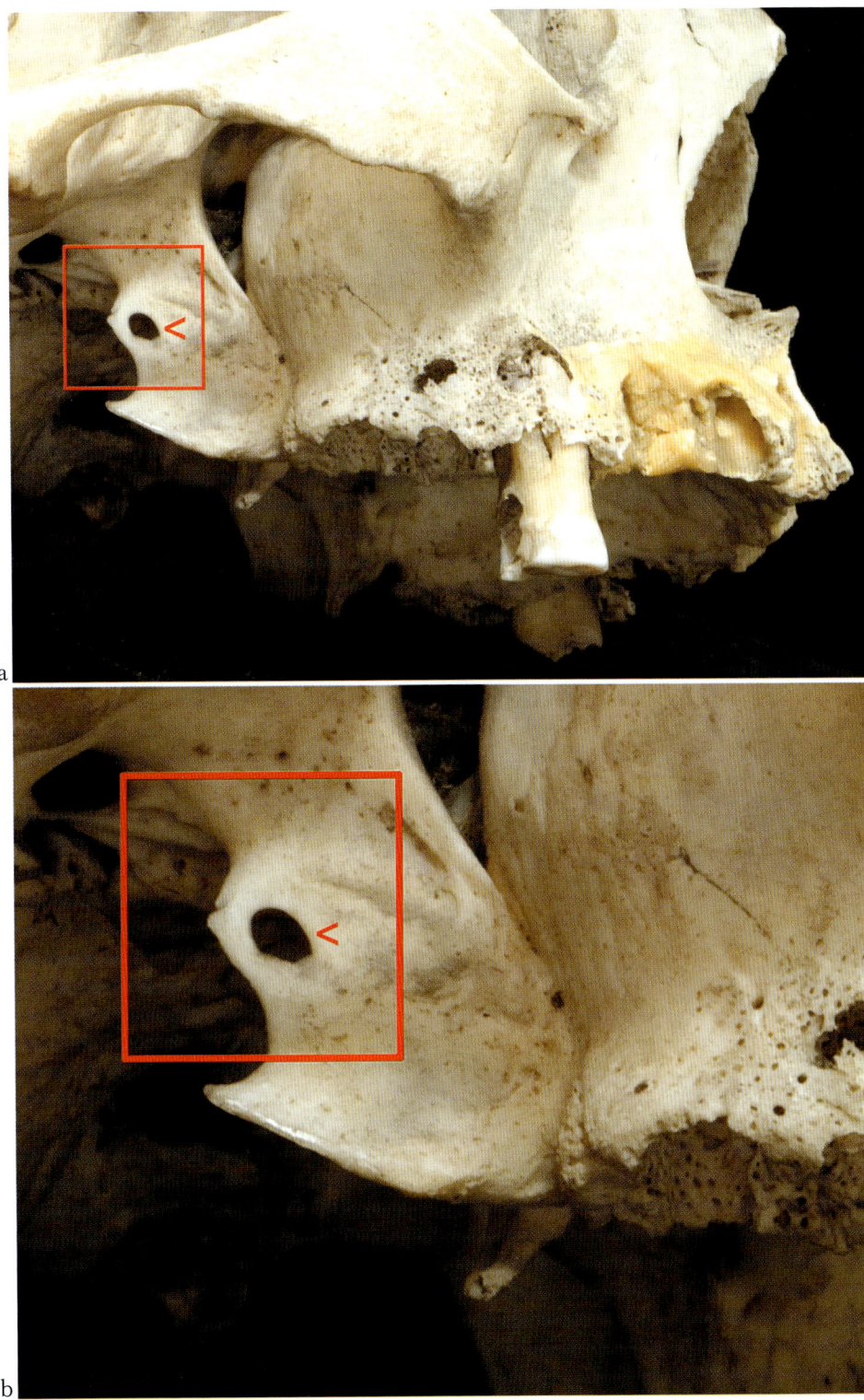

Figure 582a-b. Pterygoalar bar and foramen of Hyrtl in an adult skull (UPenn L606). (a) Lateral view of a right pterygoalar bar (square) and foramen of Hyrtl (<), in some of the literature also known as porus crotaphiticobuccinatorius (Hyrtl 1862) and foramen masticatorium. (b) Higher magnification of the pterygoalar bar of bone and right foramen of Hyrtl (<).

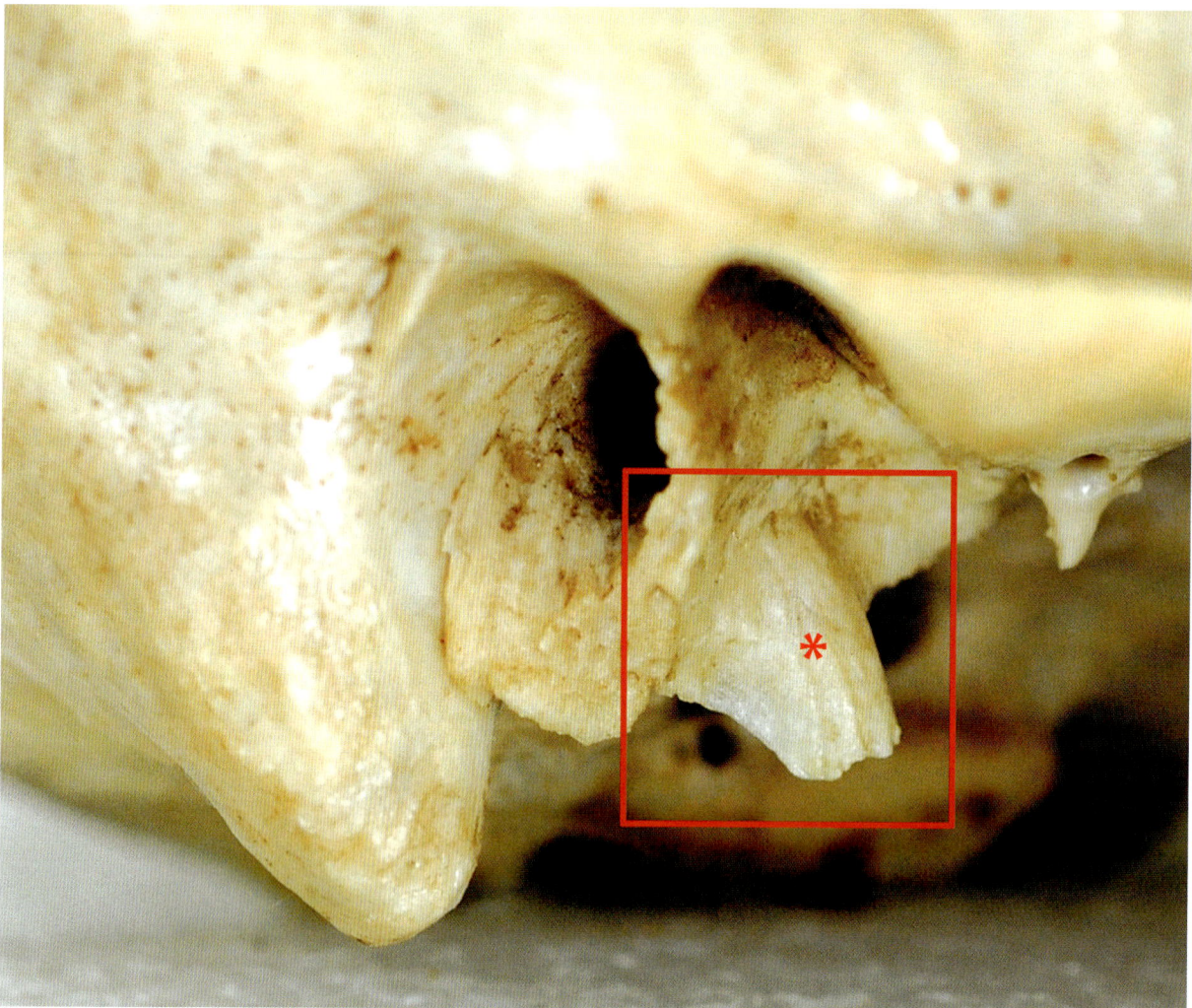

Figure 583. Large right vaginal process of the temporal bone (square and *) in an adult. The temporal styloid process is posterior and medial and usually in contact with the vaginal process. This process is a typical variant, but differs in size.

Chapter 8

MANDIBLE AND TEETH, HYOID, MAXILLA AND TEETH

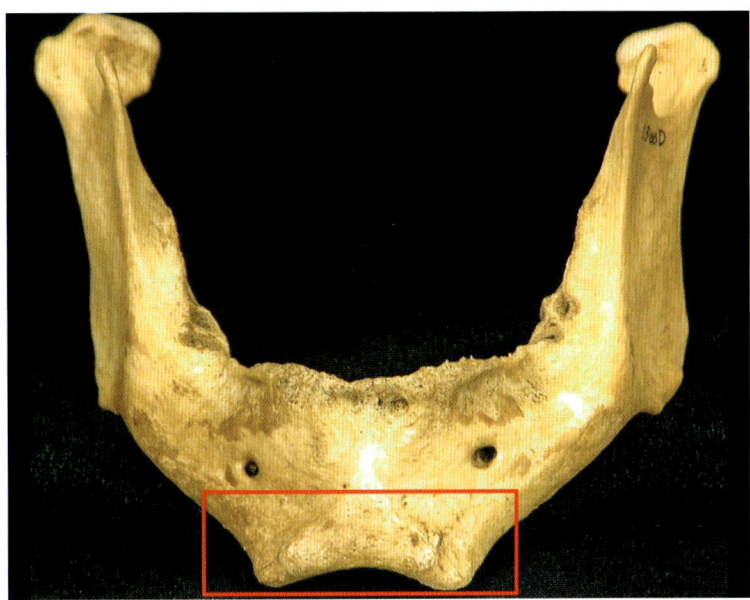

Figure 584. Prominent bilobate mandible resulting in a very square chin (rectangle) in an ancient Peruvian male (UTK, Hefner). A male trait and common to uncommon finding in most groups.

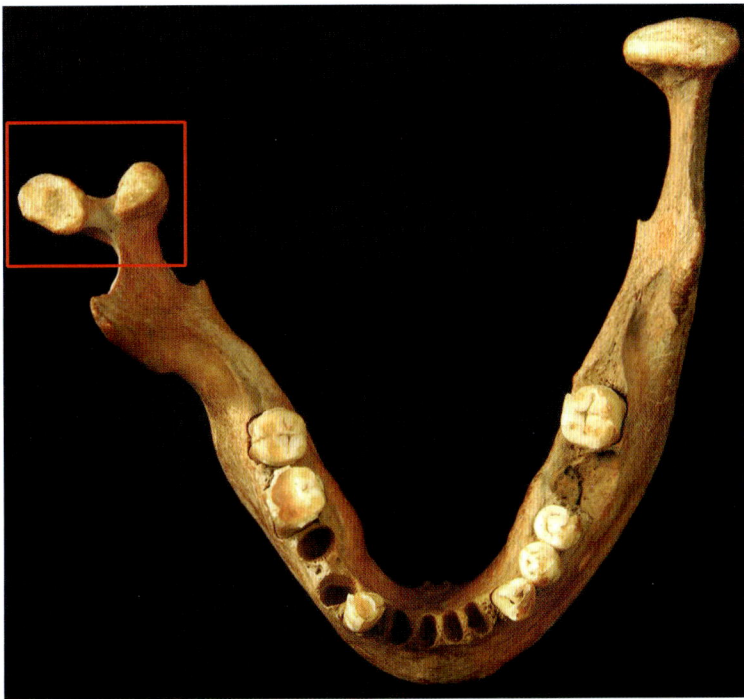

Figure 585. Divided/bifurcated right mandibular condyle (rectangle) (SI).

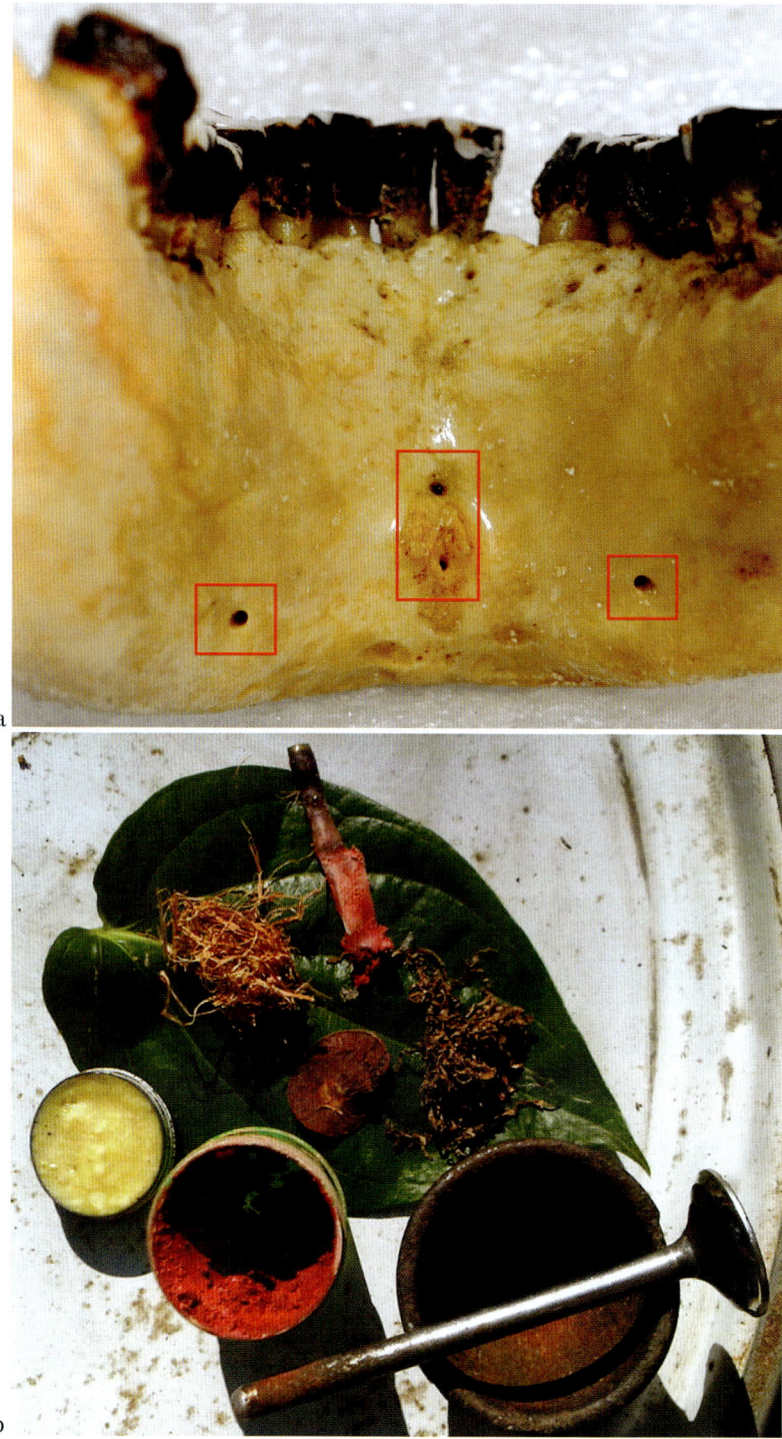

Figure 586a-b. Lingual foramina and betel nut kit. (a) Multiple lingual foramina (squares and rectangle) in the anterior mandible of an adult Thai skull (KKU). Multiple pits is a common finding (Singh et al. 2000). Black staining of the teeth is due to chewing betel nut. McDonnell et al. (1994) found lingual foramen in 311 of 314 mandibles (all transmitted branch of the lingual artery). Cf. Liang et al. (2007) and Nagar et al. (2001) for midline foramina. (b) Thai betel nut "kit" consisting (clockwise) of petroleum jelly to soothe the lips, shredded betel nut husk for cleaning the teeth, spatula to spread the lime on the leaf, tobacco, ceramic mortar and pestle (motorcycle cylinder valve), red lime and two slices of dried betel nut (center) on a betel nut leaf. Most mortar and pestles used for betel nut are made of stone, wood, terra cotta or other materials to grind the mixture by older individuals who can no longer masticate effectively.

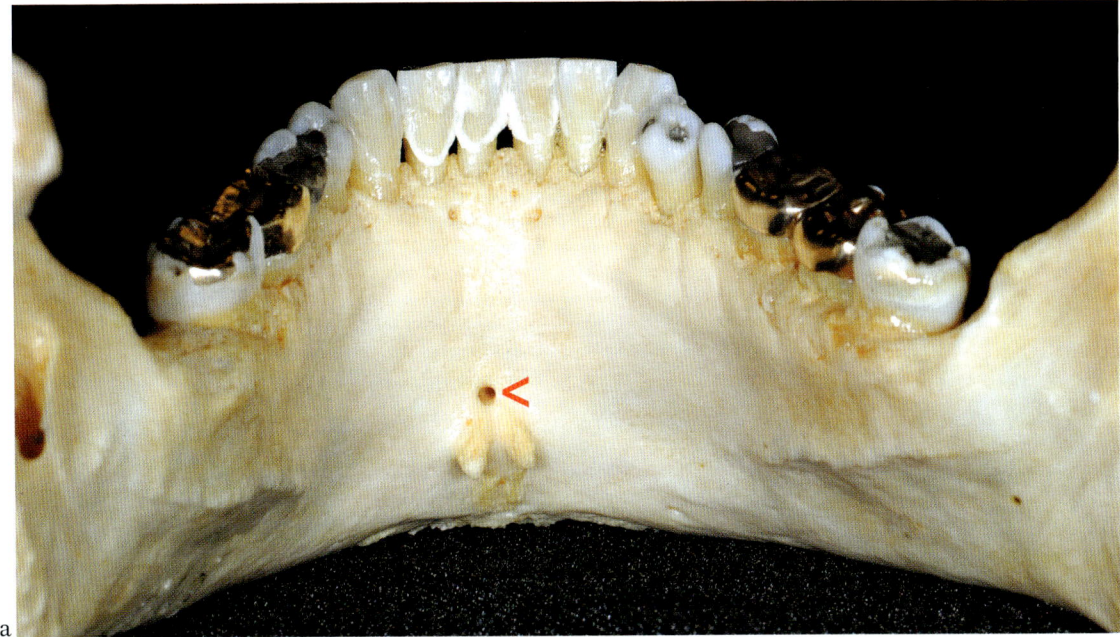
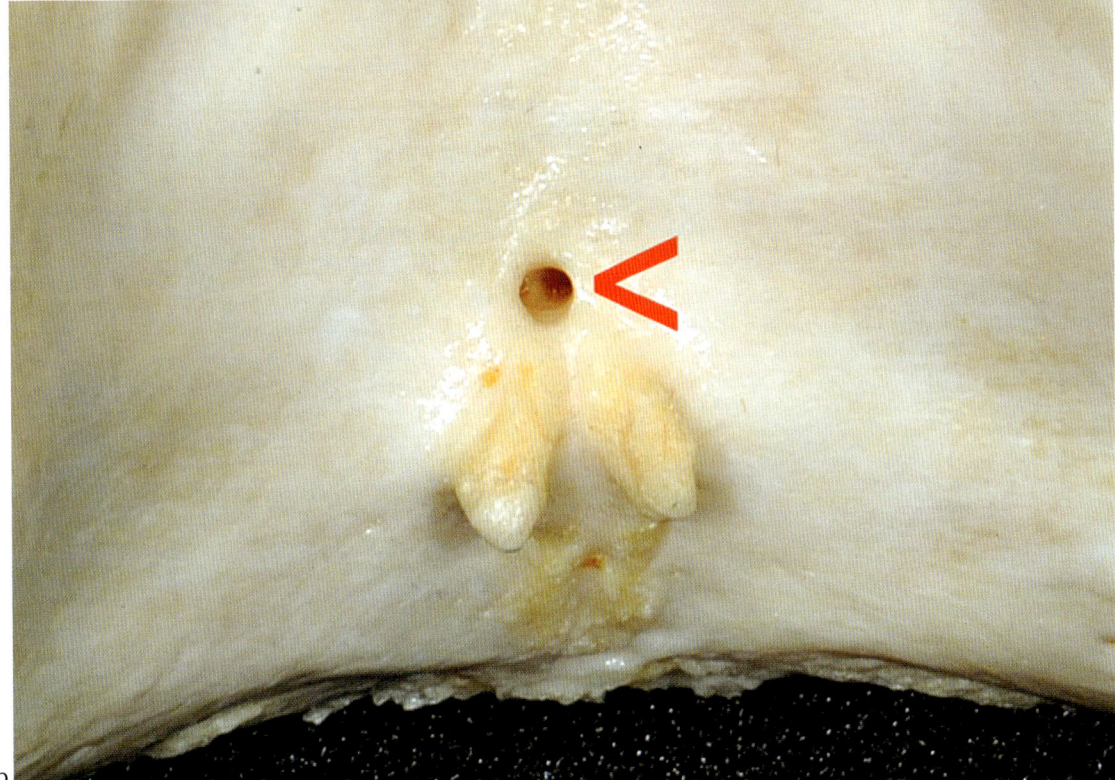

Figure 587a-b. Lingual foramen. (a) Normally occurring, single lingual foramen (<) above the genial tubercles in an elderly adult (JABSOM 1163). (b) Higher magnification of the lingual foramen (<). Nagar et al. (2001) found that 72.45% (sample size not stated) of dried adult Indian mandibles had a midline foramen that carried a single branch of the left sublingual artery (no accompanying vein or nerve).

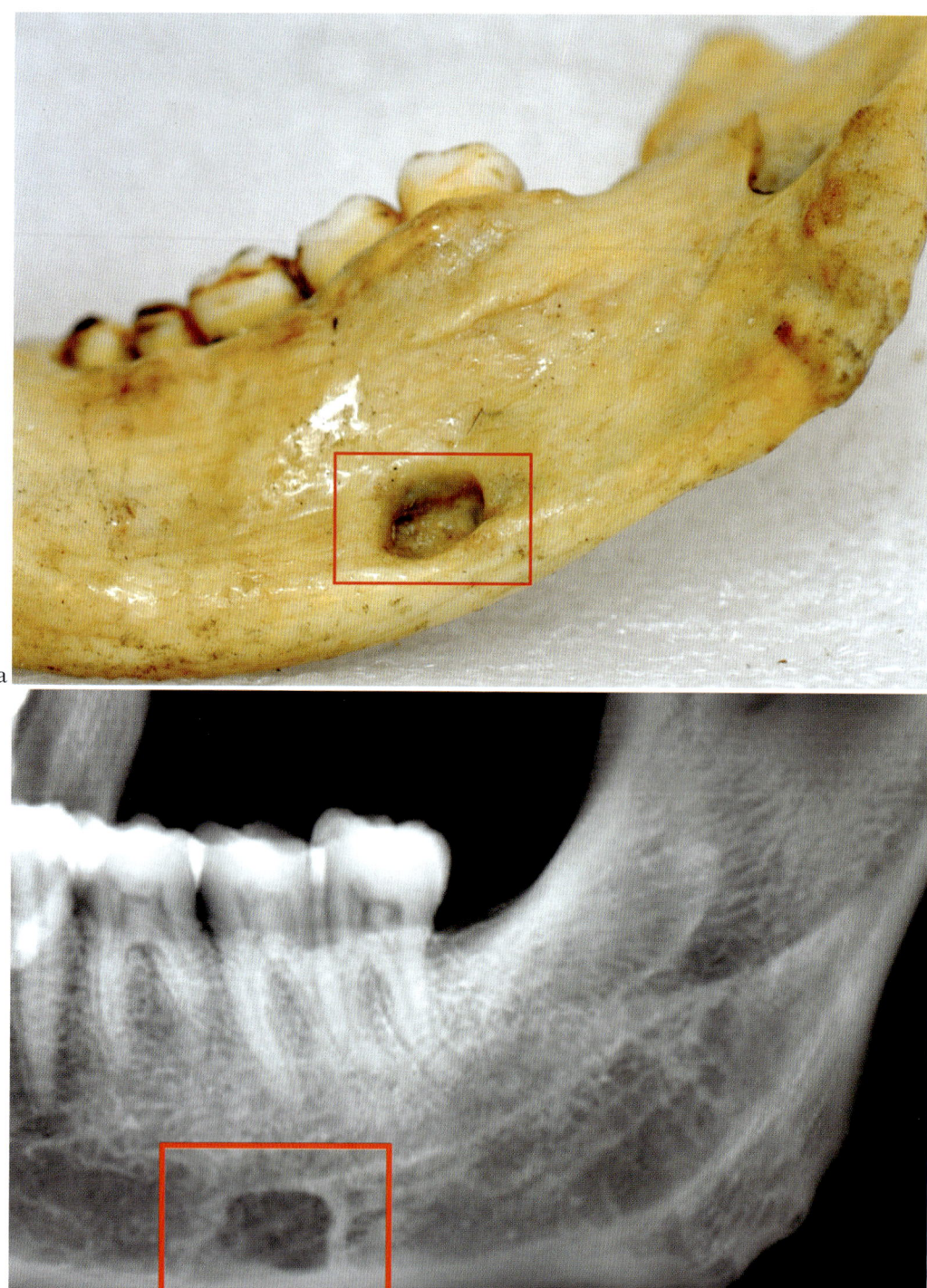

Figure 588a-b. Photograph of a Stafne's defect. (a) Stafne's defect (rectangle), also known as static bone cavity, idiopathic bone cavity, and salivary gland depression, among others, in the left corpus of an adult Thai male mandible (KKU). (b) X-ray showing resorption of the lingual cortical plate and "sclerotic" margin (rectangle) around the defect. Uncommon to common finding. Cf. Mann (2001); Finnegan and Marcsik (1980, 1981); Stafne (1942); Vodanovic et al. (2011); Wasterlain and Silva (2012).

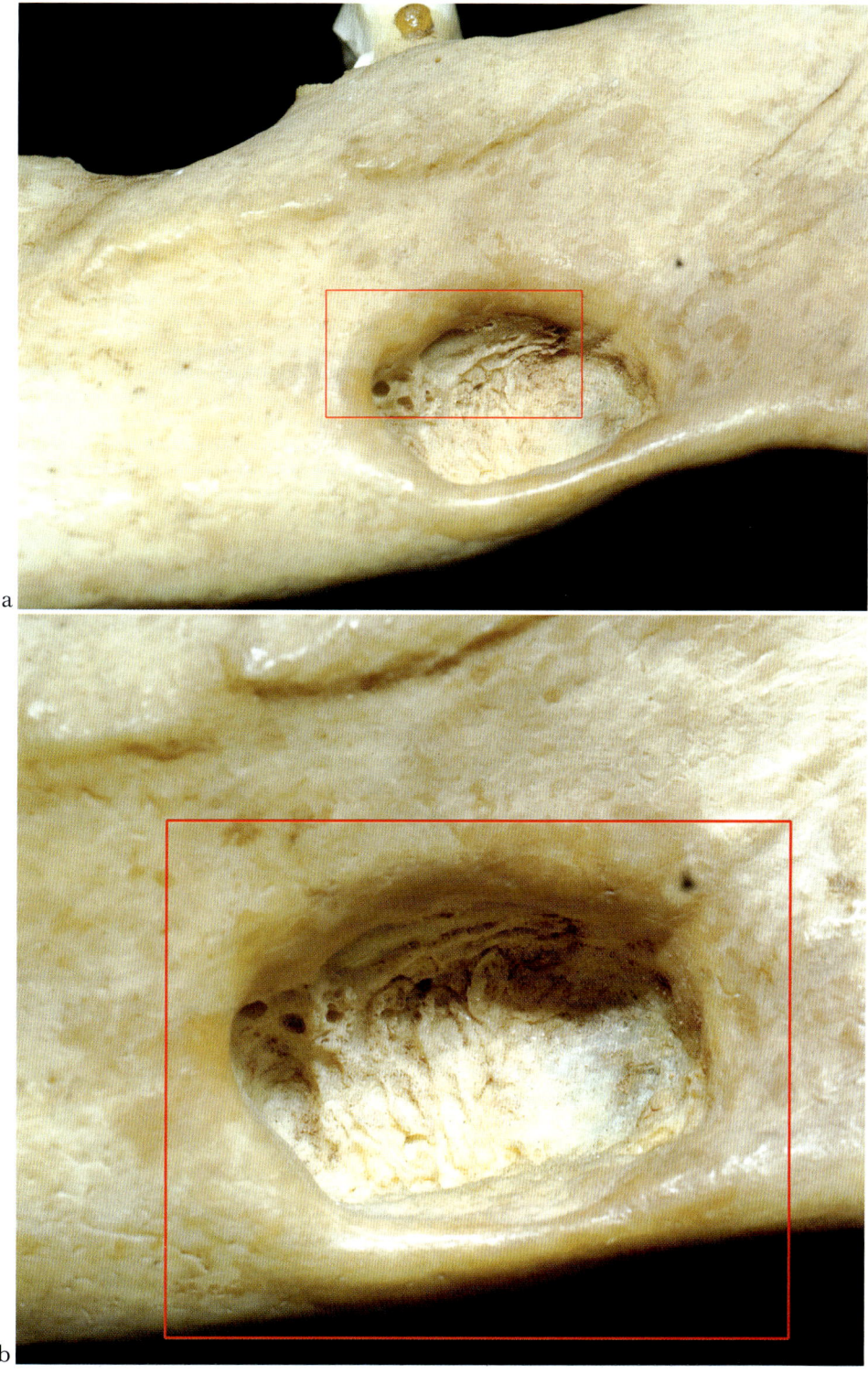

Figure 589a-b. Stafne's defect. (a) Stafne's defect (rectangle) in the right lingual plate of the mandible showing an irregular and corrugated floor (UPenn). Note that the mandibular canal is visible along the superior border of the defect. (b) Higher magnification showing the rugged appearance of the floor (rectangle) of the defect.

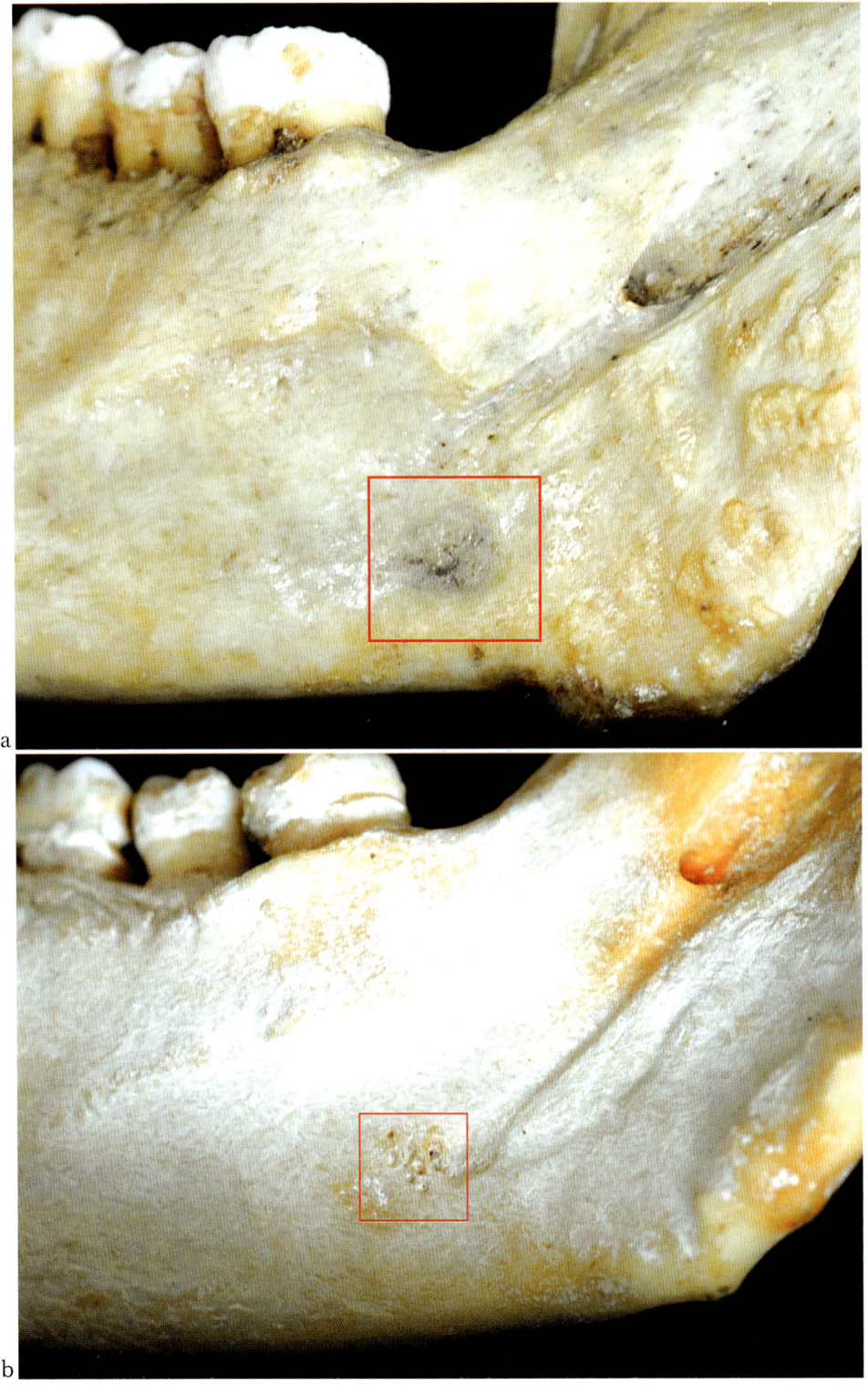

Figure 590a-b. Early-stage Stafne's defects. (a and b) Rare examples (rectangles) of early-stage Stafne's defects in the right hemi-mandibles of two adult Thai male mandibles (KKU). These defects likely would have developed into deep concavities and would have been classic Stafne's defects. Early-stage defect is an uncommon finding.

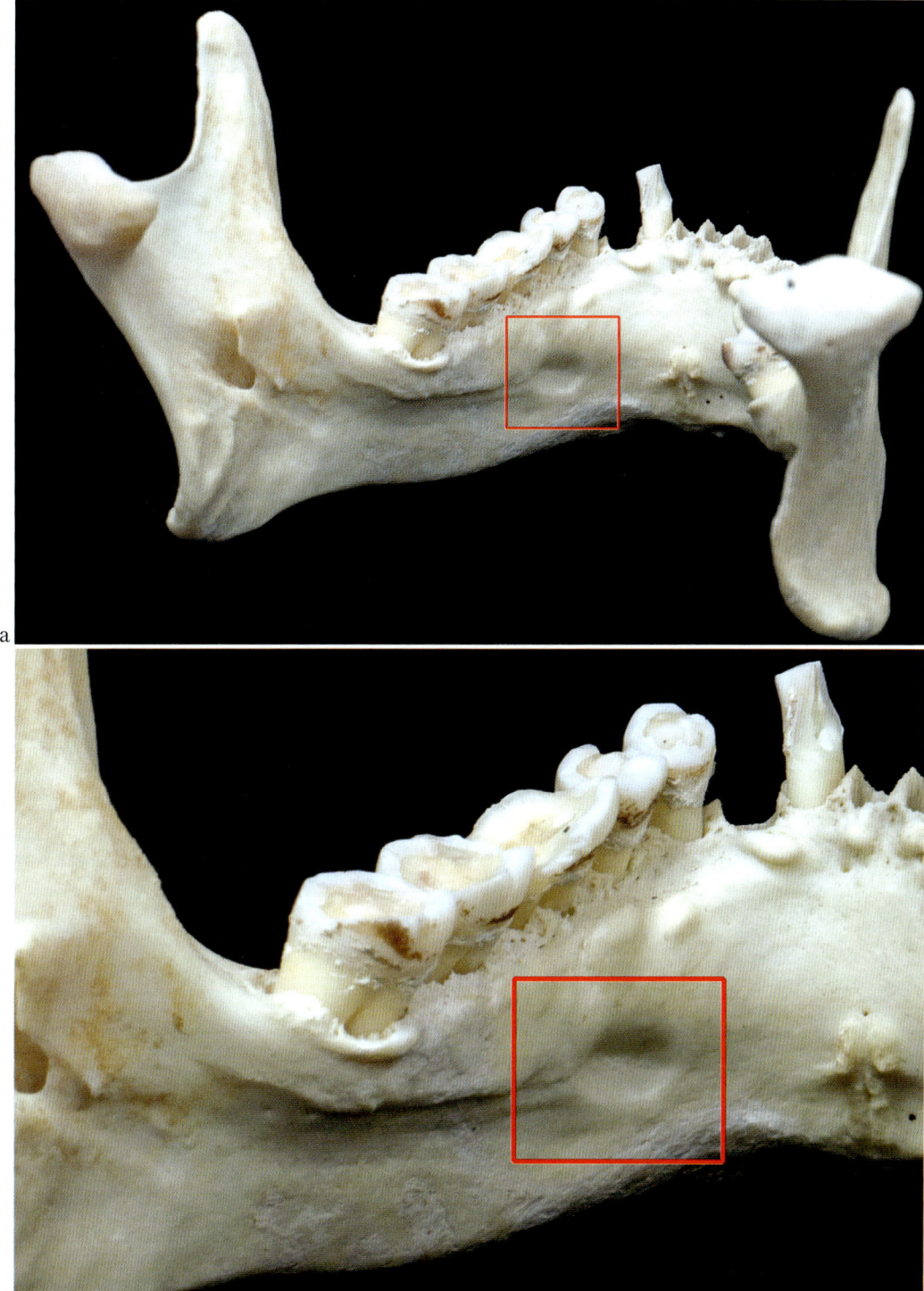

Figure 591a-b. Anterior Stafne's defect. (a) High (b) and low magnifications of a rare anterior Stafne's defect (sublingual gland) located inferior to the left second premolar and in line with the mylohyoid groove in a 55-year-old Thai male mandible (MCU 65 52). Classsic Stafne's defects, in comparison, are situated inferior to the molars in the region of the submandibular salivary gland, while anterior defects are inferior to the premolars and canines. Cf. Dereci and Duran (2012); Mann (2001).

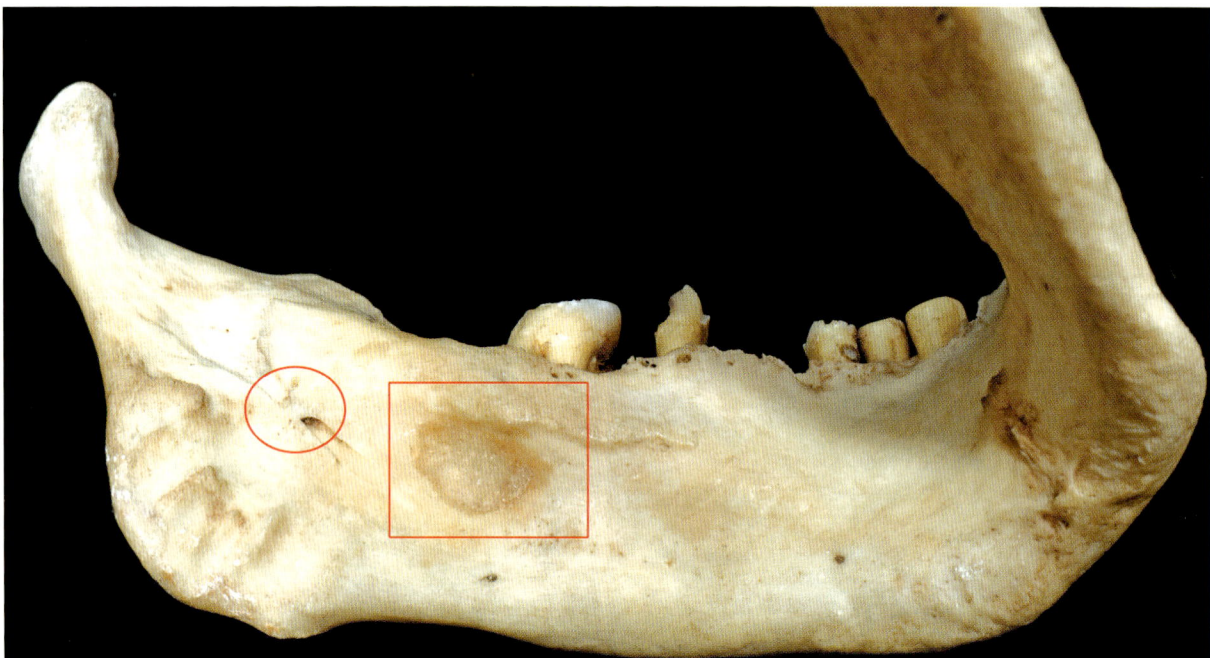

Figure 592. Large Stafne's defect (rectangle) and small mylohyoid bridge (circle) in the left lingual plate of the mandible (UPenn). Cf. Mann (2001); Stafne (1942); Vodanovic et al. (2011); Wasterlain and Silva (2012).

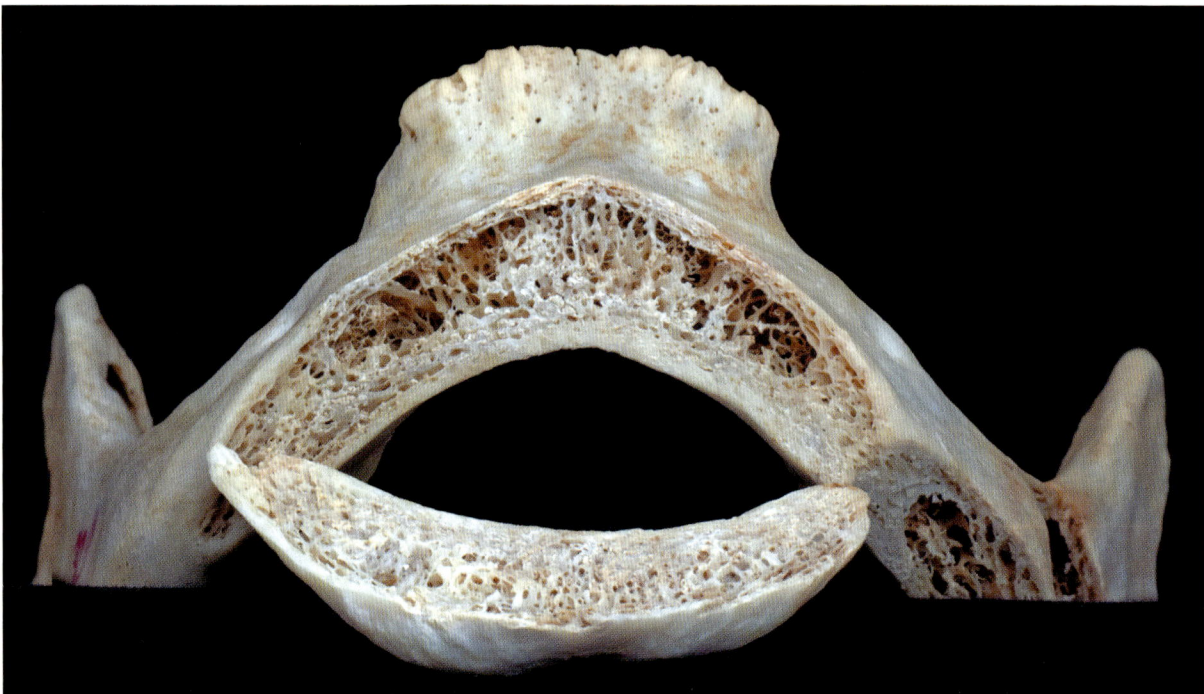

Figure 593. Sectioned mandible showing its normal architecture consisting of cancellous bone in an 88-year-old Thai female (CMU 32 51).

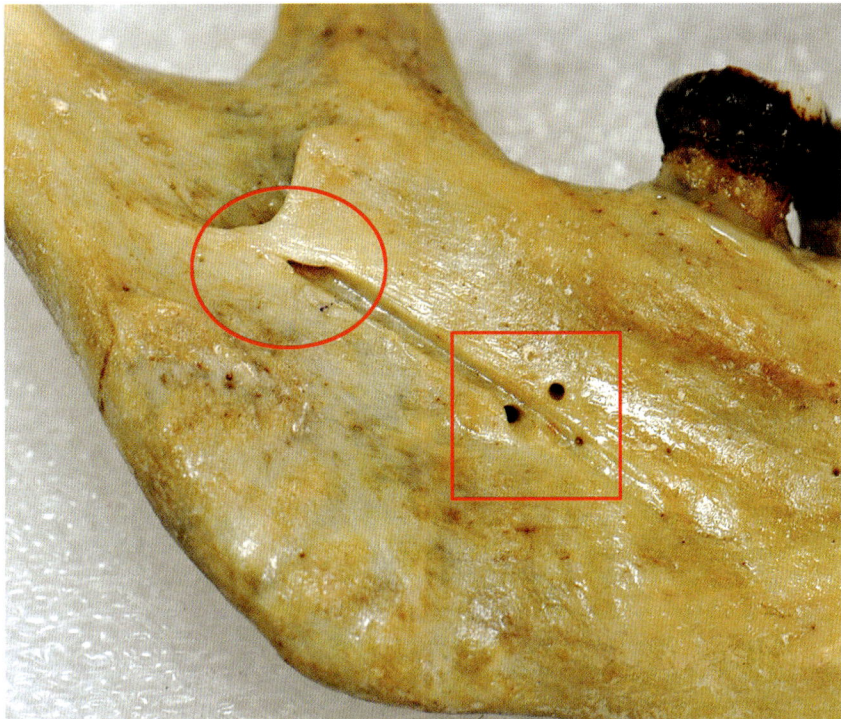

Figure 594. Mylohyoid bridge (circle) and multiple perforations (square) along the mylohyoid canal in an adult Thai (KKU). Common to uncommon findings. Cf. Hauser and DeStefano (1989).

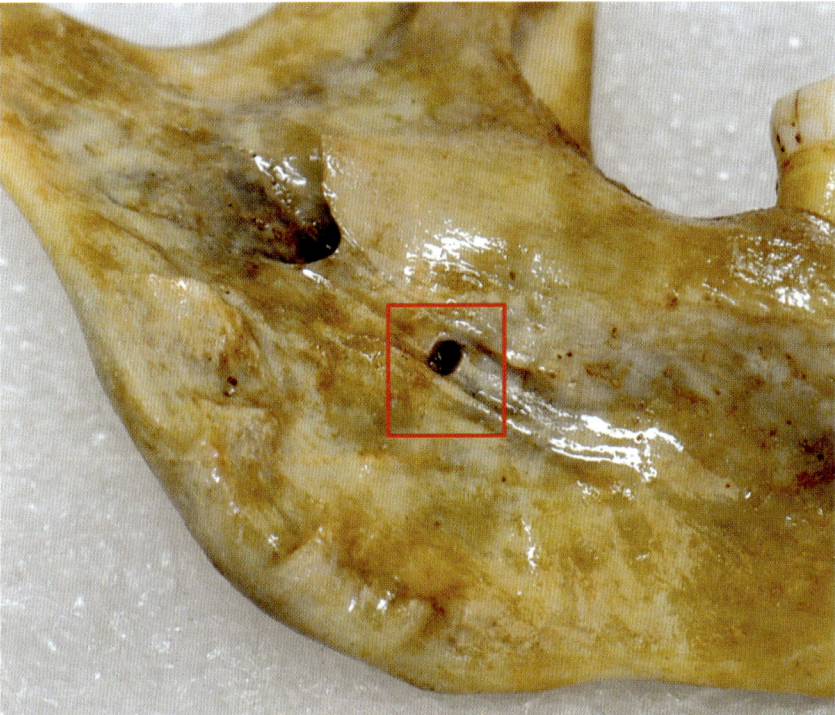

Figure 595. Perforation of the mylohyoid canal (rectangle) in an adult Thai mandible (KKU). While subject to interpretation, some researchers might identify this as mylohyoid bridging. Uncommon to common finding.

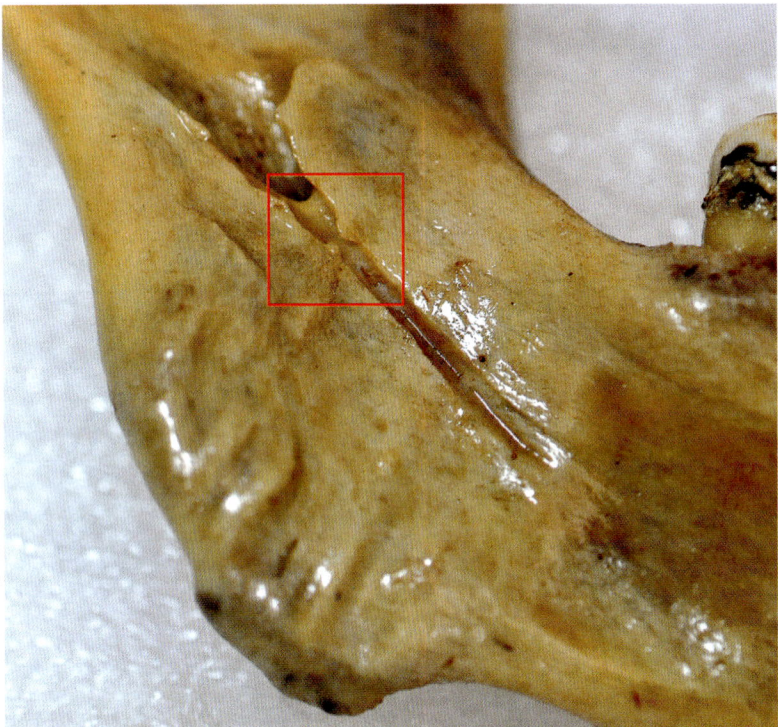

Figure 596. Partial bridging (square) of the left mylohyoid canal in an adult Thai mandible (KKU). Common finding. Cf. Hanihara and Ishida (2001b); Hauser and DeStefano (1989).

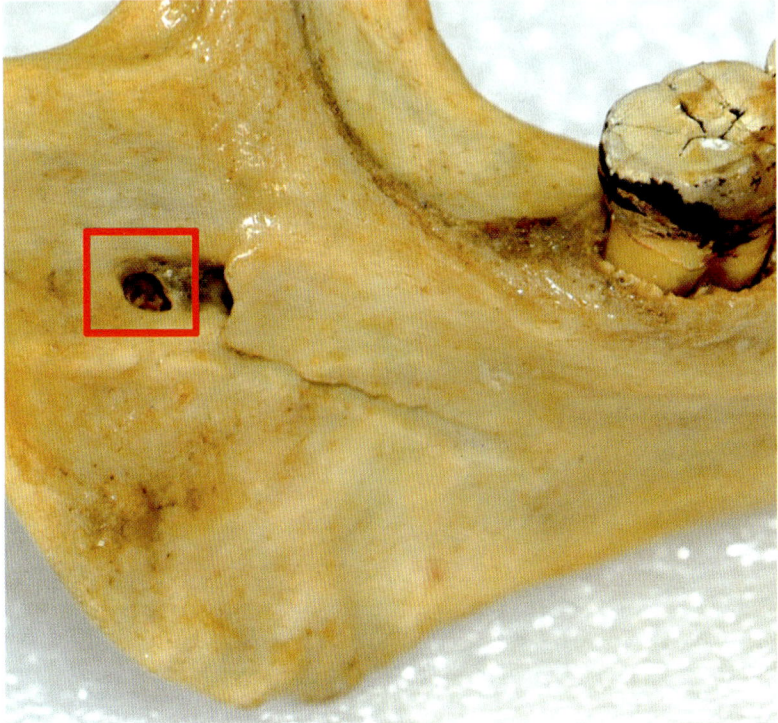

Figure 597. Double perforation (square) referred to as an accessory mandibular foramen in the left mylohyoid canal in an adult (KKU). Uncommon finding. Murlimanju et al. (2011b).

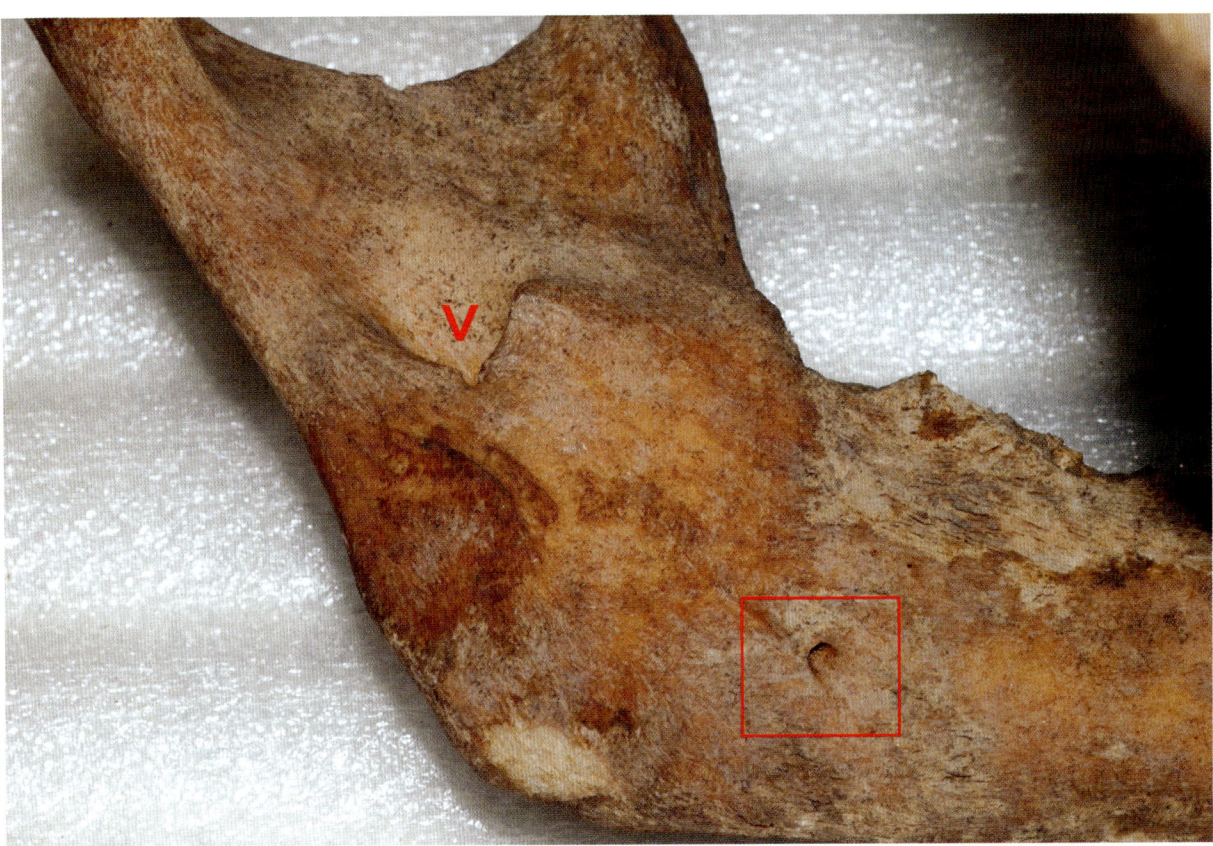

Figure 598. Unusually long mylohyoid bridge with an entrance (∨) located far posterosuperior to a foramen (square) in an adult White female (TM 91, Ditsong Museum). It could not be discerned whether the entrance and foramen were connected, as the foramen was too small to explore with a probe. The unusually wide "bridge" and presence of a foramen at this location are uncommon findings.

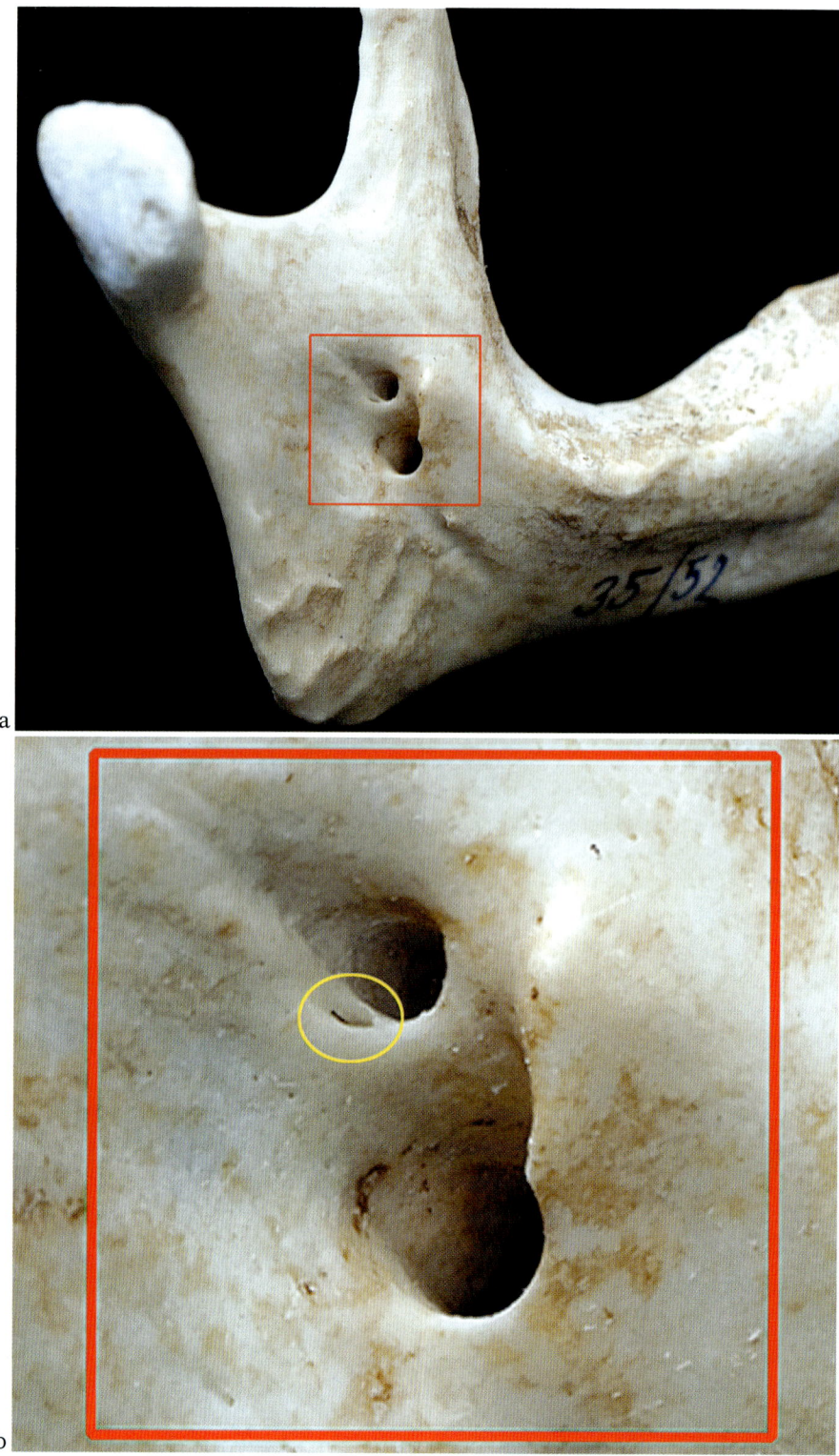

Figure 599a-b. Triple mandibular foramen. (a) Uncommon triple left mandibular foramen (square) in the ramus of an adult Thai male (CMU 35 52). Only one foramen occurred on the right side. (b) Note the small third foramen (oval) between the two larger foramina (square). Murlimanju et al. (2011 a & b) found accessory foramina in 16.4% of 67 mandibles studied. Cf. Barner and Lockett (1972).

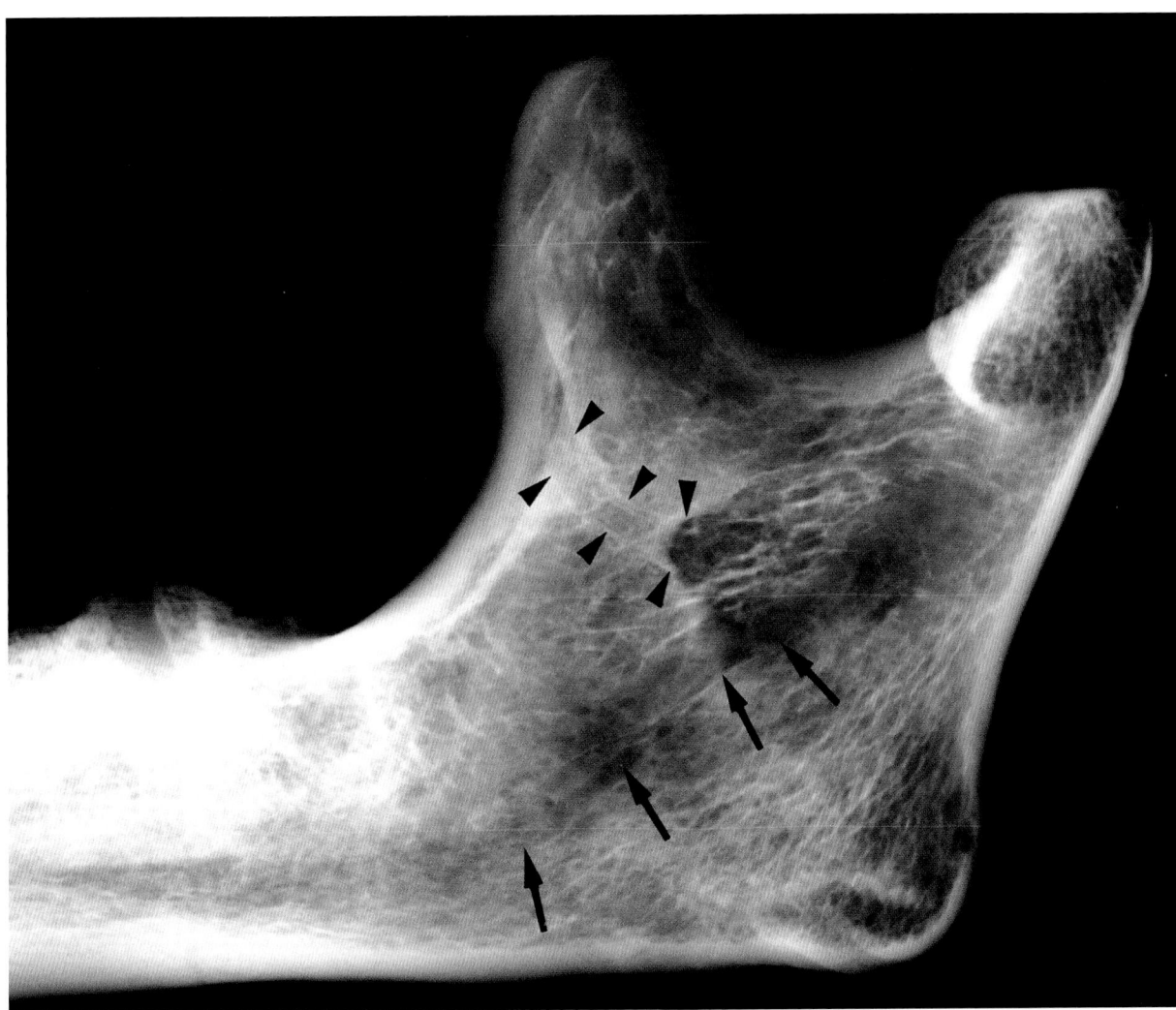

Figure 600. Vertically-oriented accessory (arrowheads) bifid/bifurcated mandibular canal in an Asian adult (SI). The arrows indicate the path of the normally occurring mandibular canal as it courses downward and anteriorly through the inferior one-third of the mandible to the mental foramen. Bifid mandibular canals are rare findings in most populations with a reported frequency of 0.35% in 2012 patients in Spain and may be more prevalent in women (Sanchis et al. 2003). Uncommon finding. Ramadhan et al. (2010) found triple foramina each transmitting a nerve in 1.2% of dry skulls and radiographs. See Sahin et al. (2010) for an example of two mental nerves from two mental foramina; and see Singh et al. (2010); Rouas et al. (2007) for radiographic study of the mandibular canal. Cf. Mardini and Gohel (2008); von Arx et al. (2011).

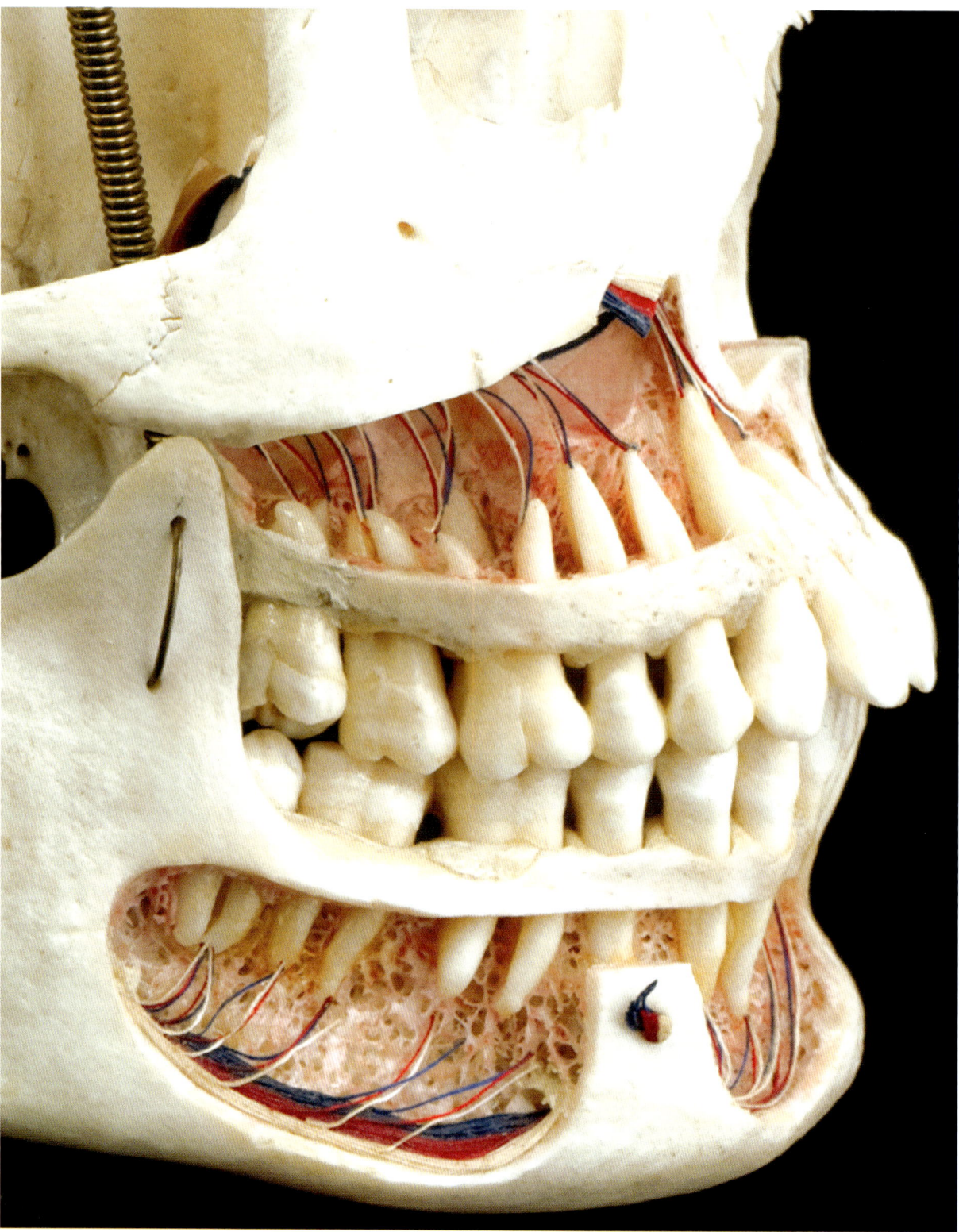

Figure 601. Sectioned maxilla and mandible simulating the superior and inferior alveolar neurovascular bundles supplying the teeth in a young adult (CSC AC 039). A terminal branch of the inferior alveolar nerve passes through the mental foramen and provides sensory innervation to the mental eminence.

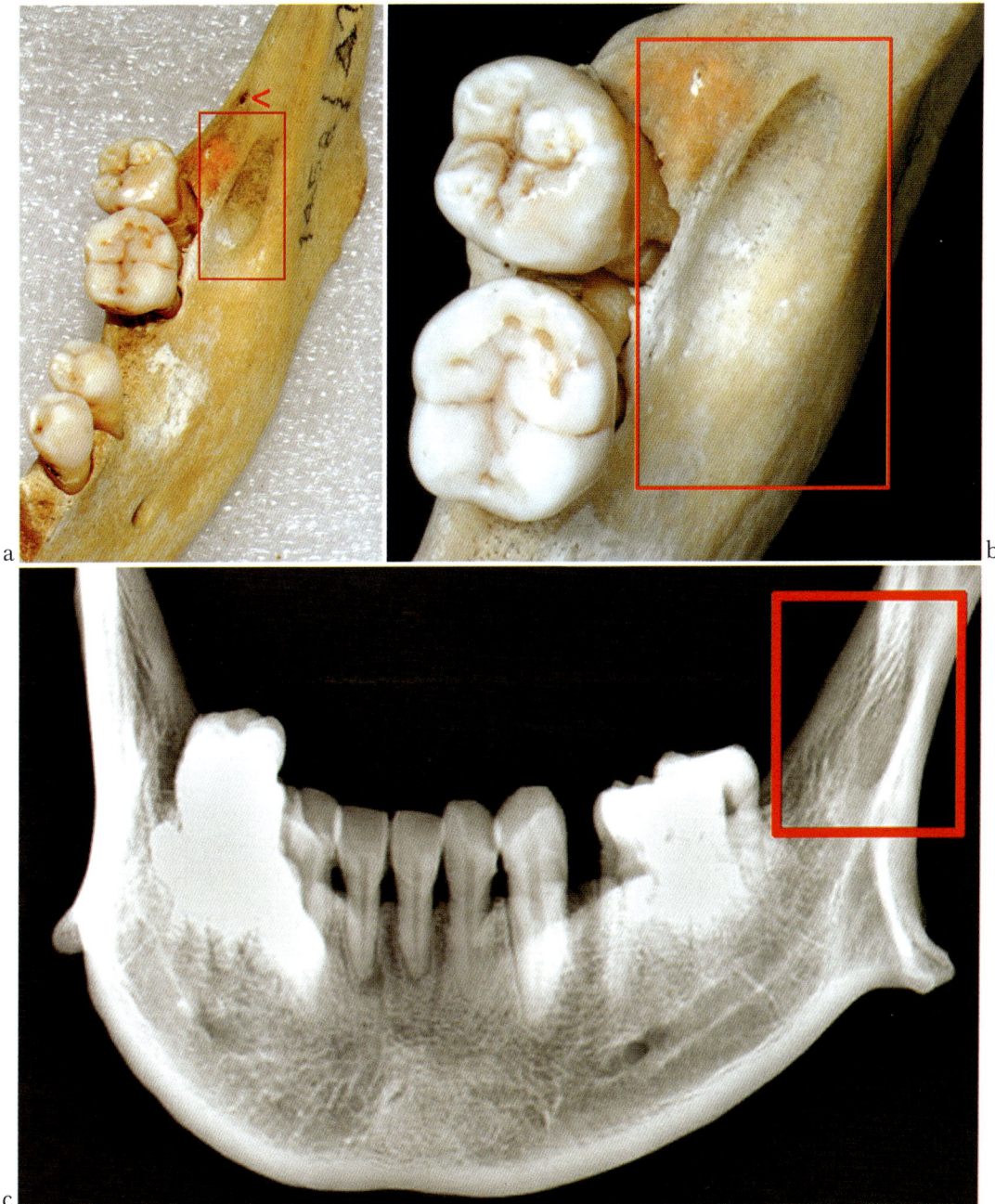

Figure 602a-c. Rare defect in the left mandibular sulcus. (a and b) Rare defect in the left mandibular sulcus (rectangles) in an adult Thai skull (KKU). Note the small retromolar foramen (<), possibly innervating the mandibular molars or carrying an accessory or aberrant buccal nerve (von Arx et al. 2011). (c) X-ray of the resorptive defect in the left ramus (rectangle). While the gross and radiographic appearance of this feature resembles a Stafne's defect, it is located in the retromolar region and its etiology and possible relationship to the parotid gland and other soft tissues is unknown (Mann and Tsaknis 1991). (a) Cf. Ossenberg (1987) and Rossi (2012) for more on the retromolar foramen, found to be present in approximately 25% of individuals.

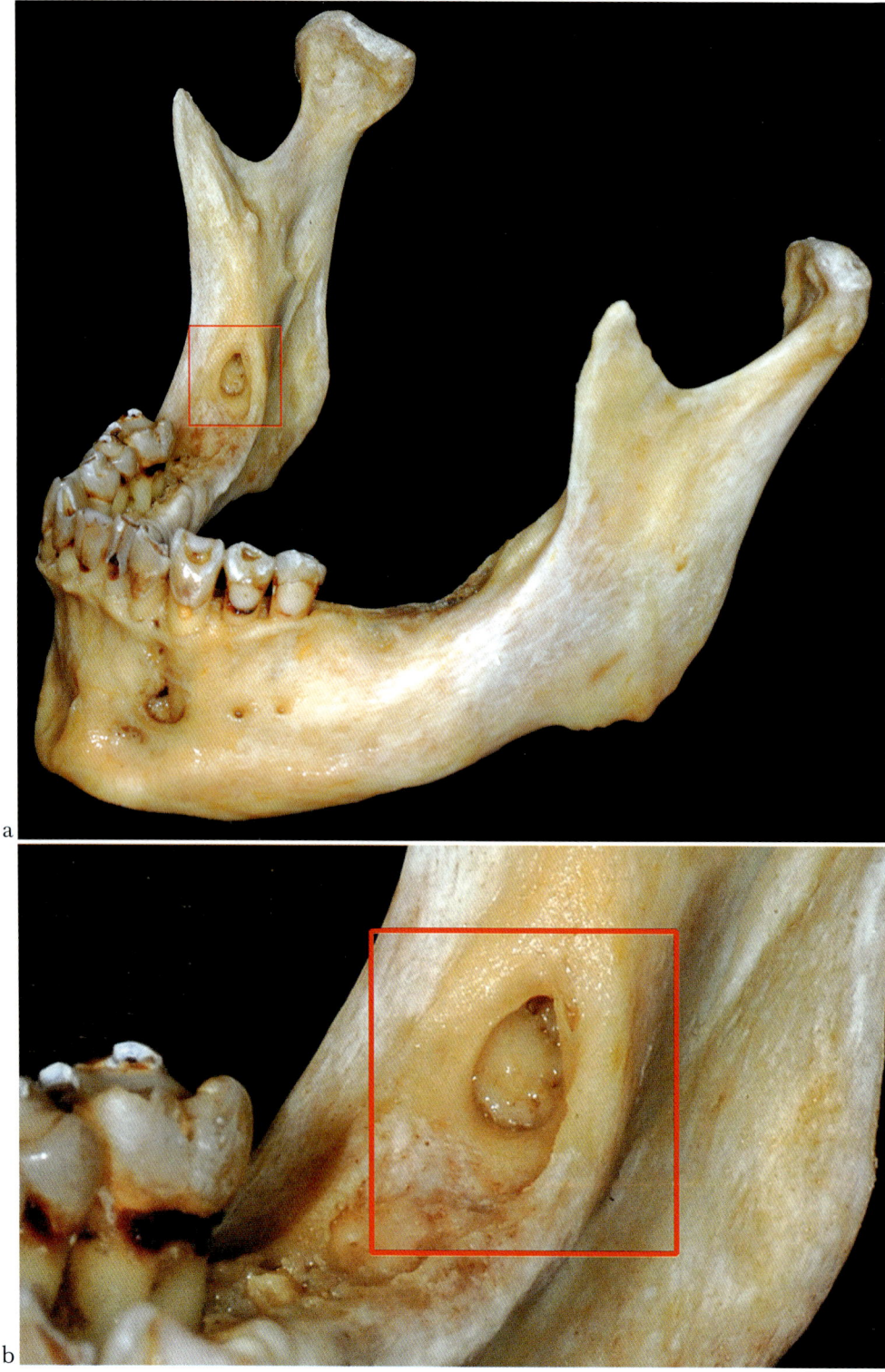

Figure 603a-b. (a) Uncommon to rare cavitation defect in the retromolar fossa in an elderly male (JABSOM 1232). (b) Higher magnification showing the smooth margins and internal morphology of the defect (square). While the etiology and frequency of this unilateral defect is unknown, its position and smooth, rounded margin contraindicates a third molar defect.

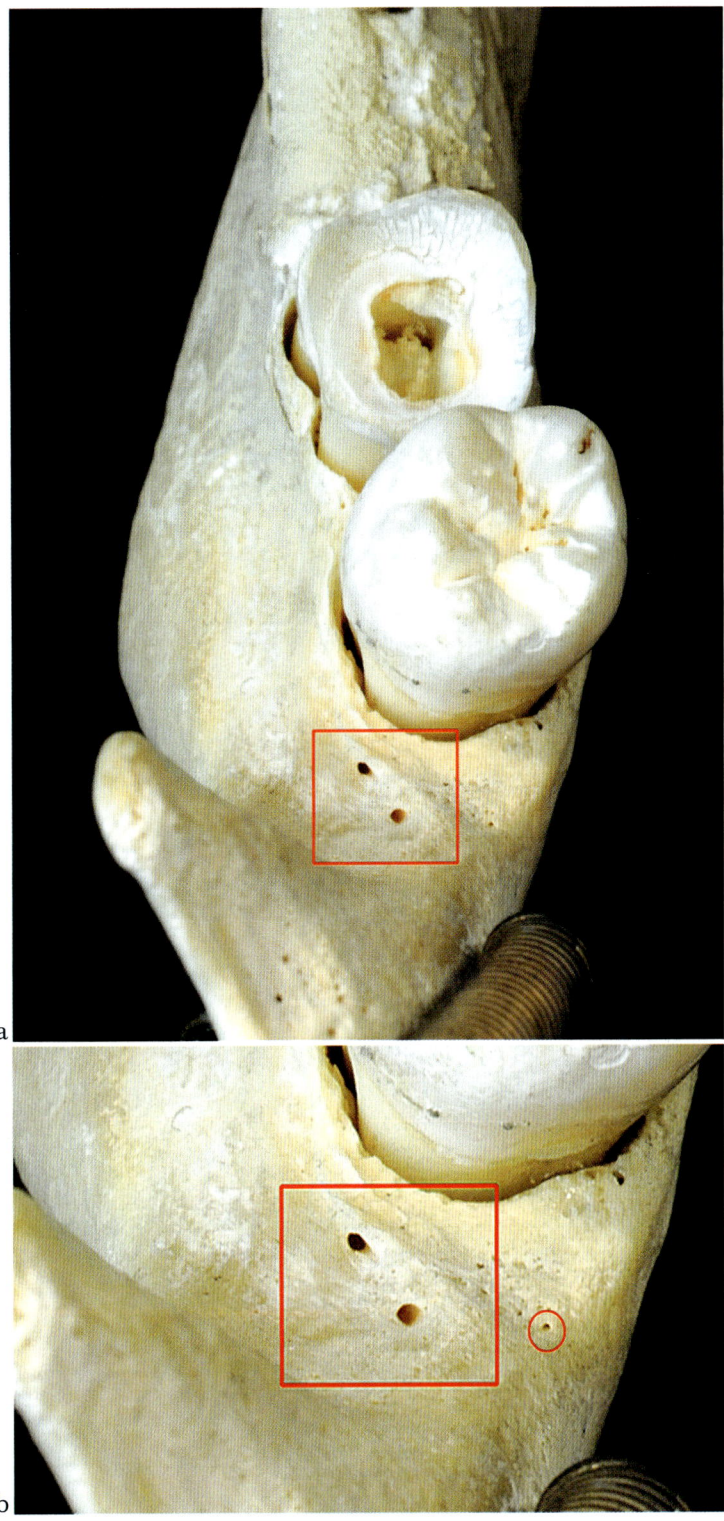

Figure 604a-b. Double left retromolar canals. (a) Double left retromolar canals (square) and (b) a small foramen (circle) that likely does not communicate with the molar or mandibular canal. Note that this tiny foramen would not be scored as a retromolar foramen due to its diminutive appearance (FSA DS-041). Cf von Arx et al. (2011); Ossenberg (1987).

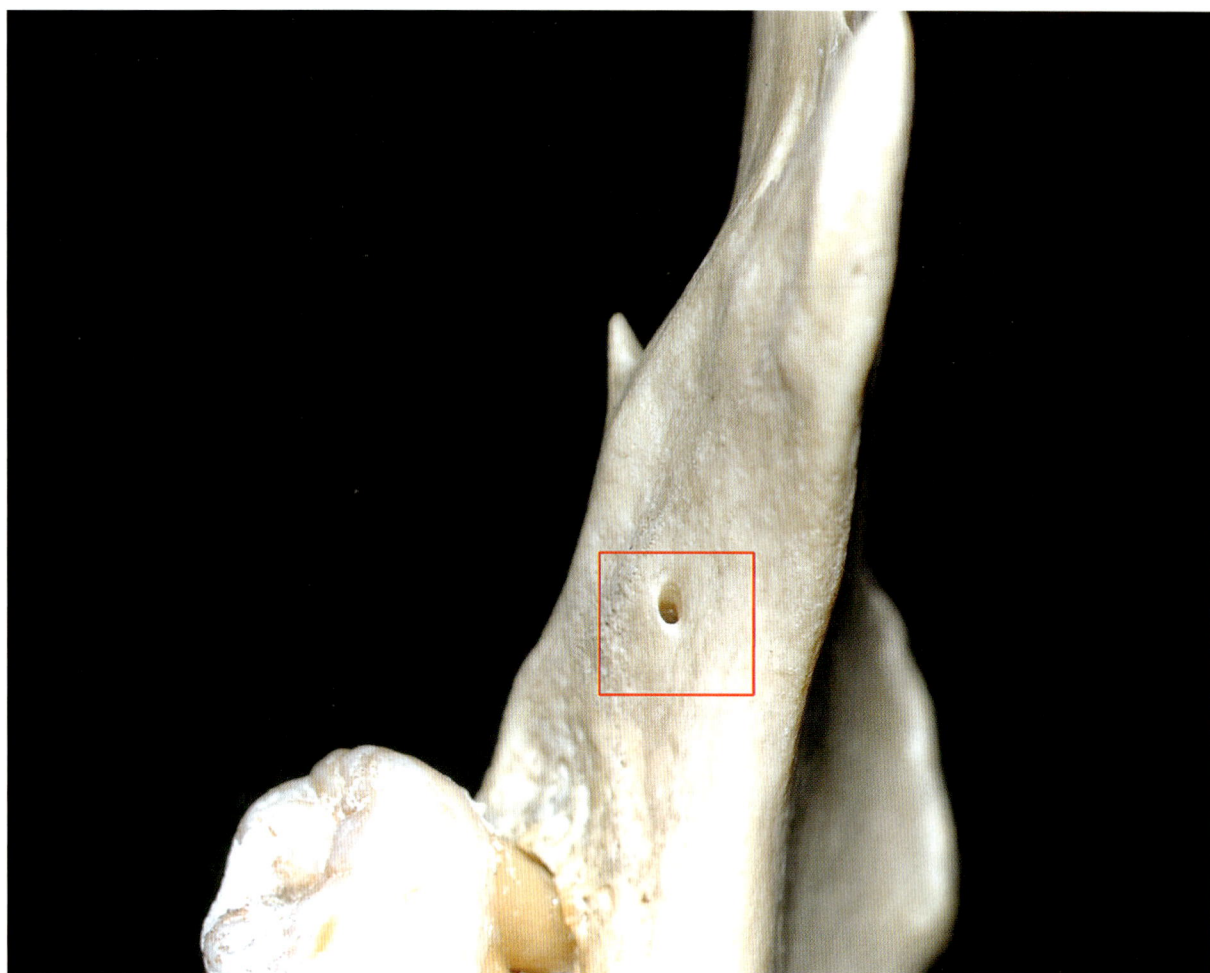

Figure 605. Large, but typical single left retromolar canal (square) (FSA AC-030). Although researchers report differing frequencies of this canal in ancestral groups, possibly due to scoring techniques and confusion with osteoporosis and remnants of molar crypts, it appears to be present in approximately 25% of individuals.

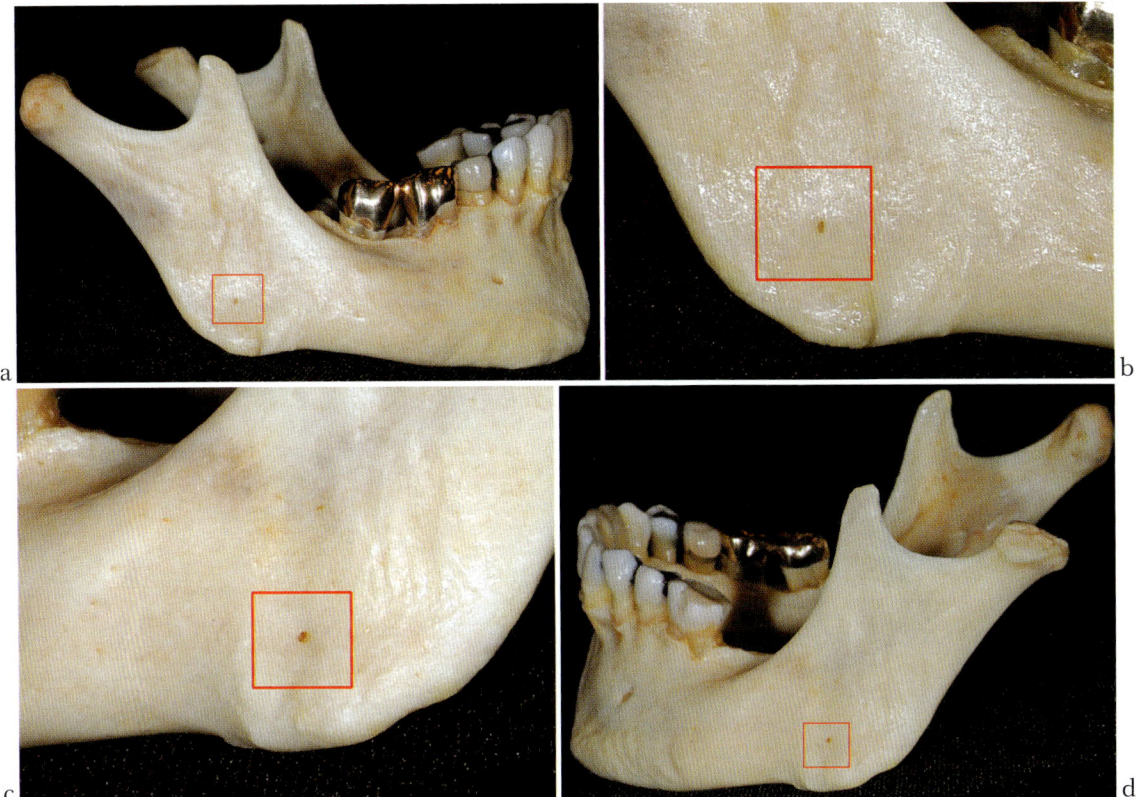

Figure 606a-d. Bilateral buccal foramina. (a and b) Bilateral buccal foramina superior to the gonial angle in the right ramus. (c and d) Bilateral foramina in the left ramus in a 58-year-old female (JABSOM 1206).

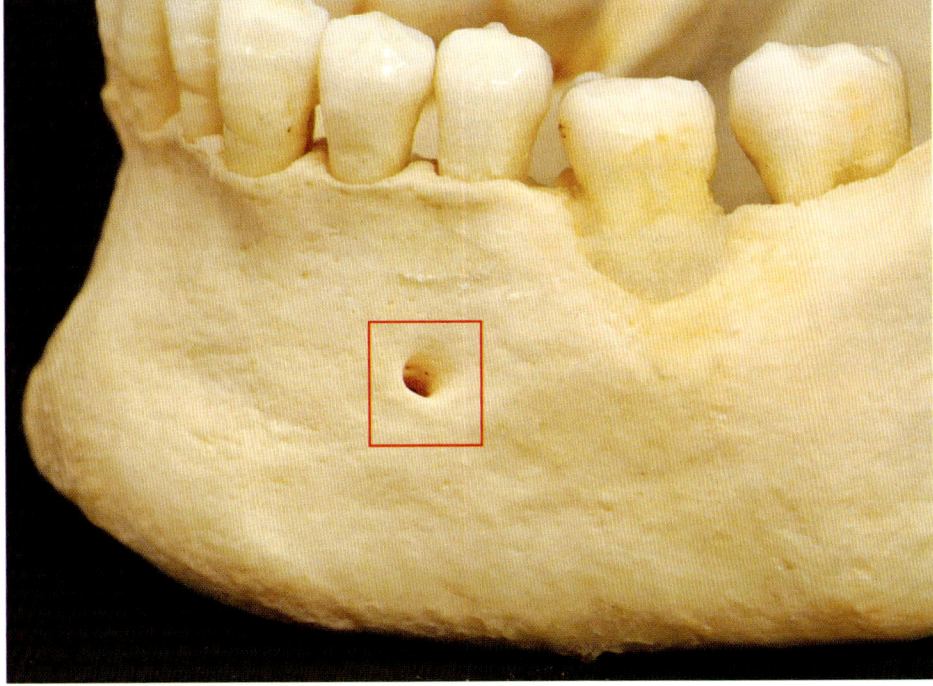

Figure 607. Single left mental foramen (square) in an adult Thai (KKU). Typical anatomy and common finding.

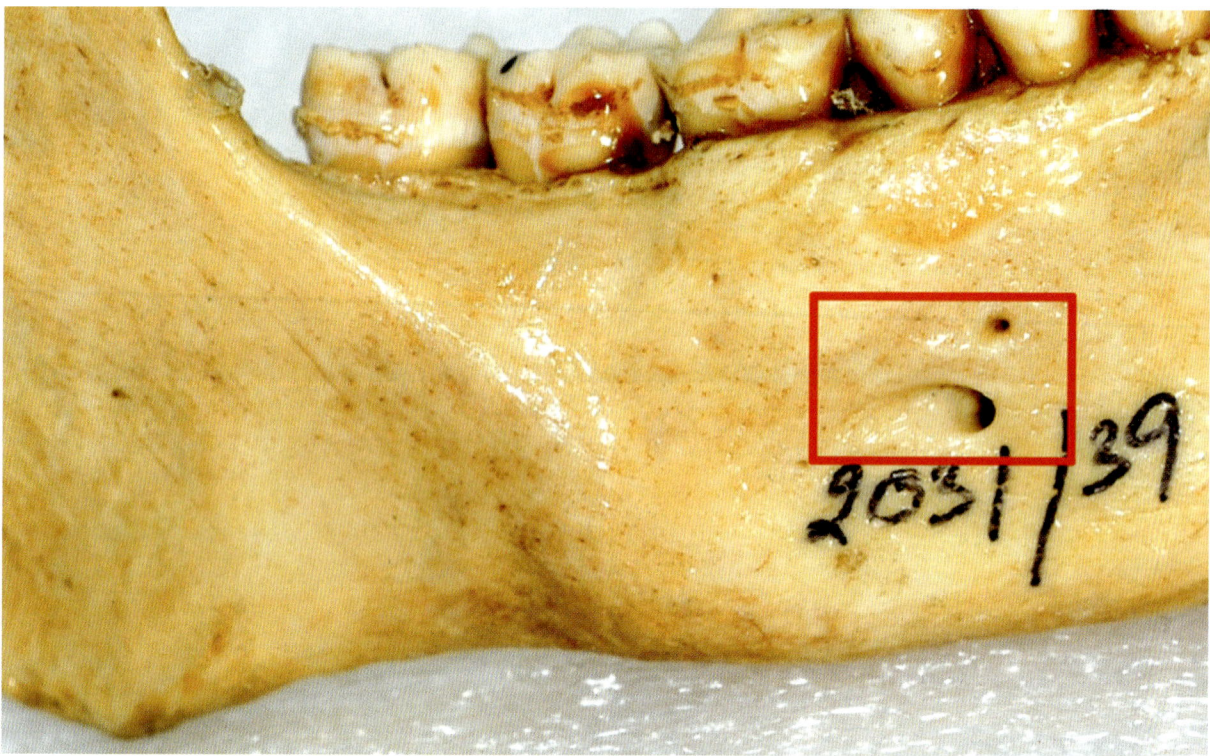

Figure 608. Double right (accessory) mental foramina (rectangle) in a young adult Thai (KKU 2031/39) – common finding. Note that the primary foramen is much larger than the accessory foramen – both probably transmitted cutaneous nerves to the lips and chin. See Serman (1989) for a clinical example of double foramina; see Vayvada et al. (2006) for anatomy.

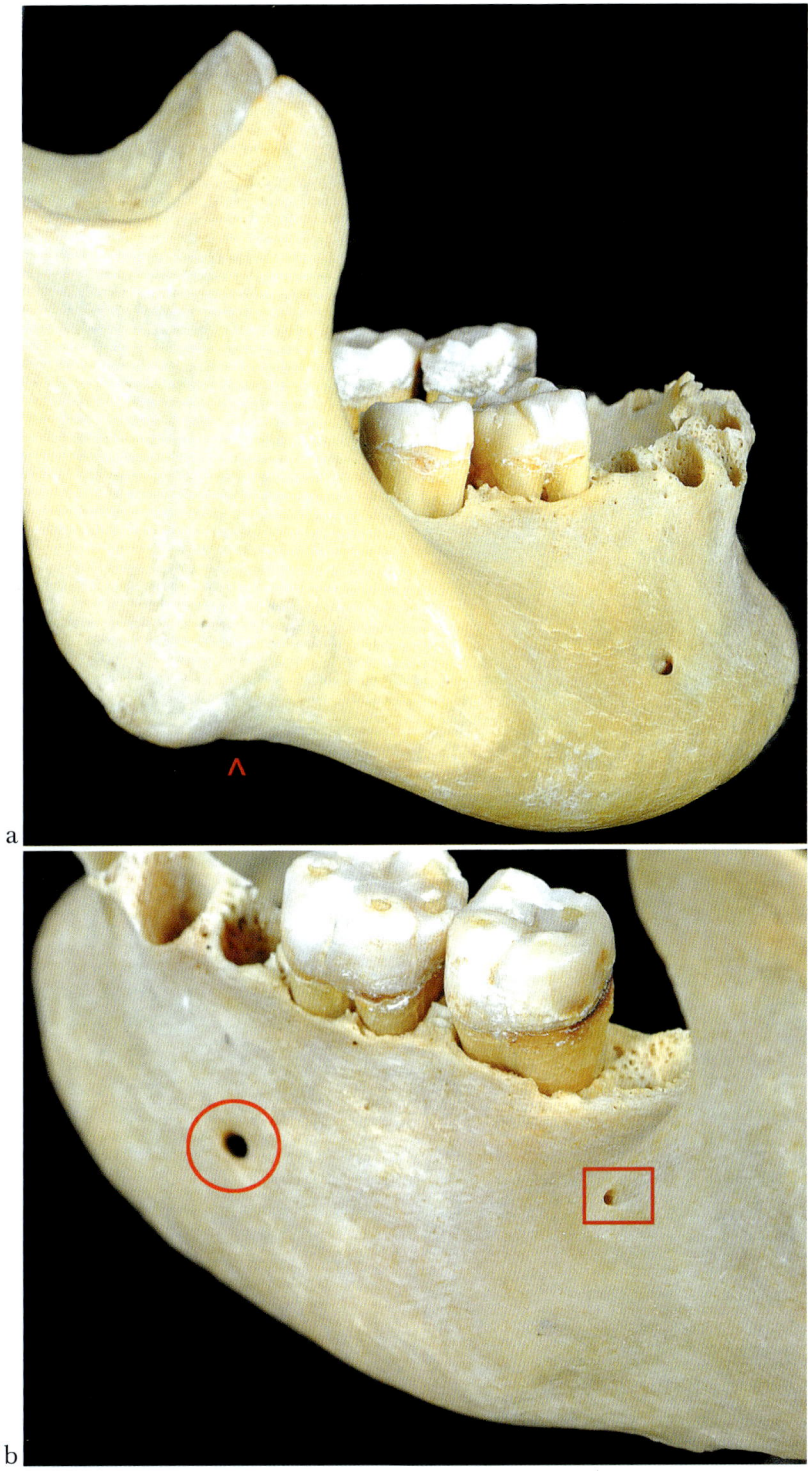

Figure 609a-b. Unusually short mandible (a) with a rounded mental eminence and a deep antegonial notch (∧) in an adult Thai (KKU). (b) Note the normal mental foramen (circle) and a small accessory foramen (rectangle) on the left side. An accessory foramen in this region is uncommon to rare. Neves et al. (2010) reported on an extremely rare case of an accessory mental foramen in the lingual surface of the mandible associated with a duplicate mandibular canal. Cf. Ramadhan et al. (2010) for an example of triple mental foramina and nerves on one side of the mandible.

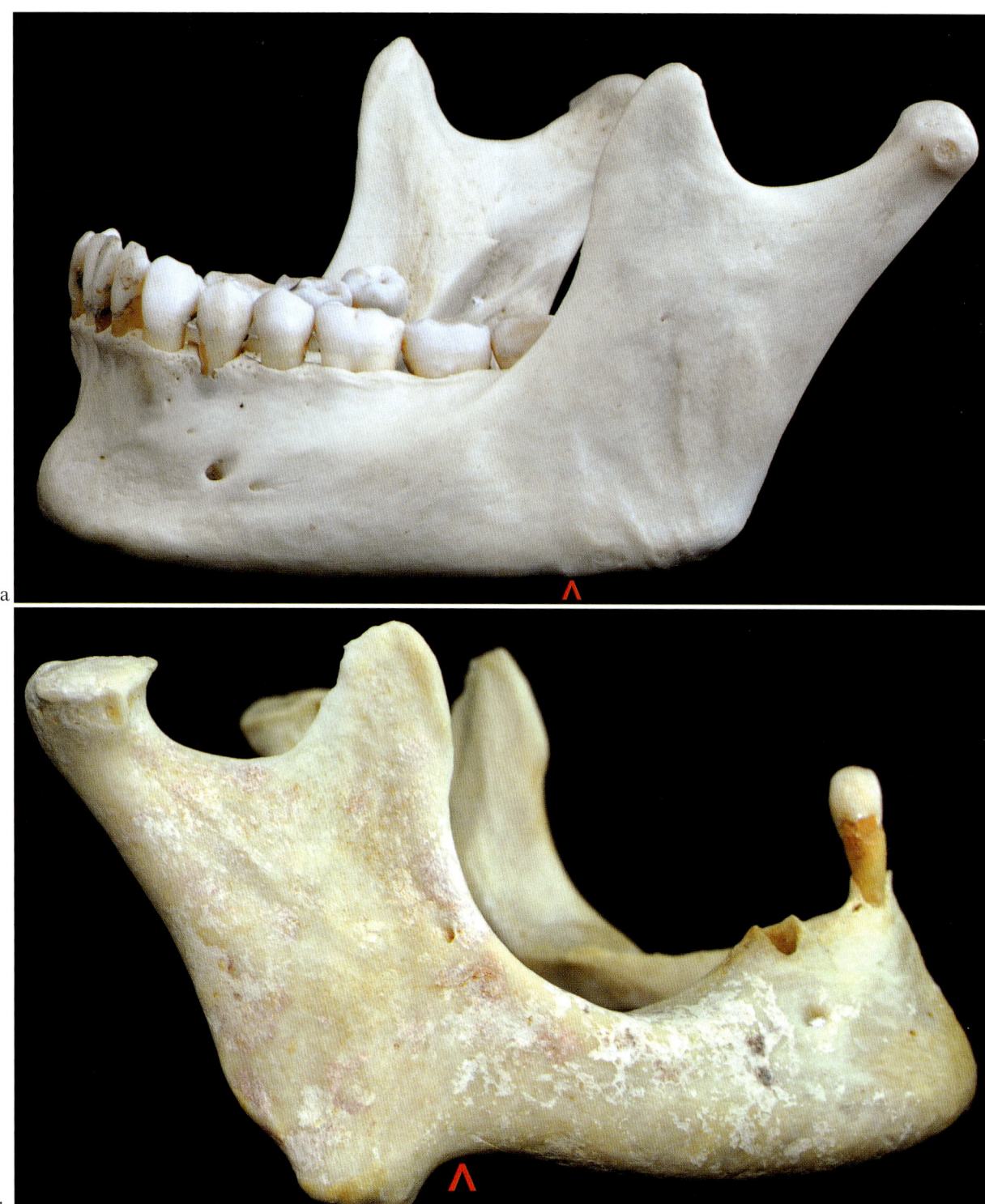

Figure 610a-b. Antegonial notch. (a) Absence of an antegonial notch (∧) resulting in a straight lower border in an adult Asian female (CMU FO 804 56 043) and (b) a deep antegonial notch (∧) in an adult Asian male (CMU FO 804 56 035). The presence and depth of the antegonial notch is often used as an indicator of sex (present and deepest in males). See Mangla et al. (2011) on depth of the notch, and Ongkana and Sudwan (2010) for a study of Thai mandibles.

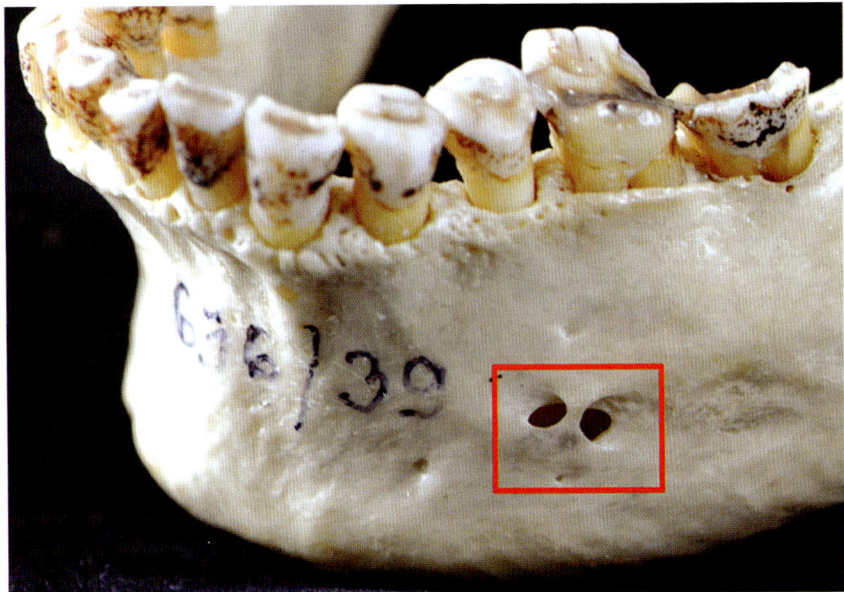

Figure 611. Vertically-divided mental foramen (rectangle) in an adult Thai mandible (KKU). Note that the external bony bridge, which has divided the foramen, is thin and translucent; both openings, however, likely transmitted neurovascular bundles. Although there are two external openings, in this specimen, there is only one internal canal. A study of 464 dry Greek mandibles revealed 6% with double foramina (Zografos and Mutzuri 1989). Balcioglu and Kocaelli (2009) report accessory mental foramina are rare. Cf. Ramadhan et al. (2010); von Arx (2013).

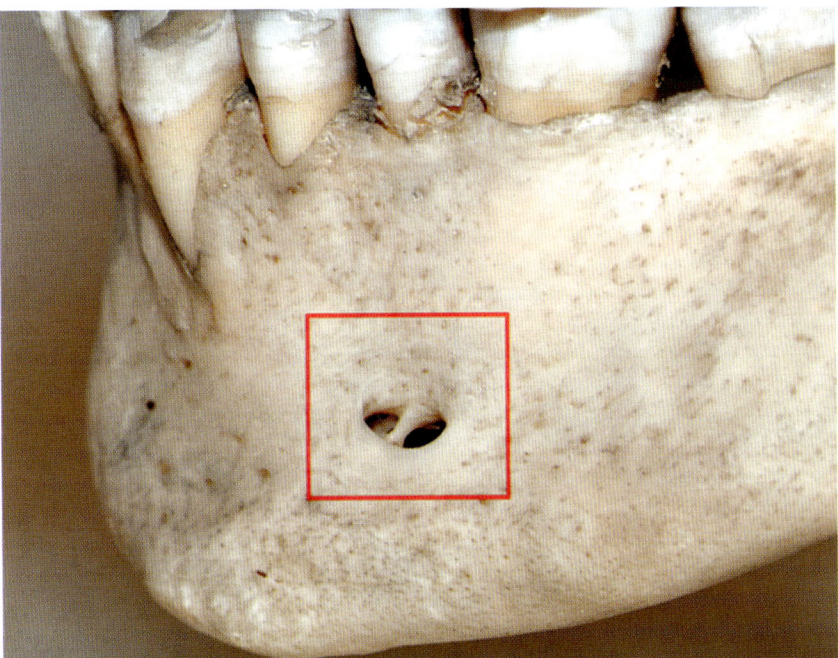

Figure 612. Internally-divided left mental foramen (square) in an 18-year-old male (Mütter Museum 1006-110). Examination of 1,435 mandibles revealed absence of a mental foramen twice on the right side and once on the left side (de Freitas et al. 1979). Rarely, a mental foramen may communicate/perforate the lingual mandible (Cf. Neves et al. 2010). Cf. Hasan et al. (2010).

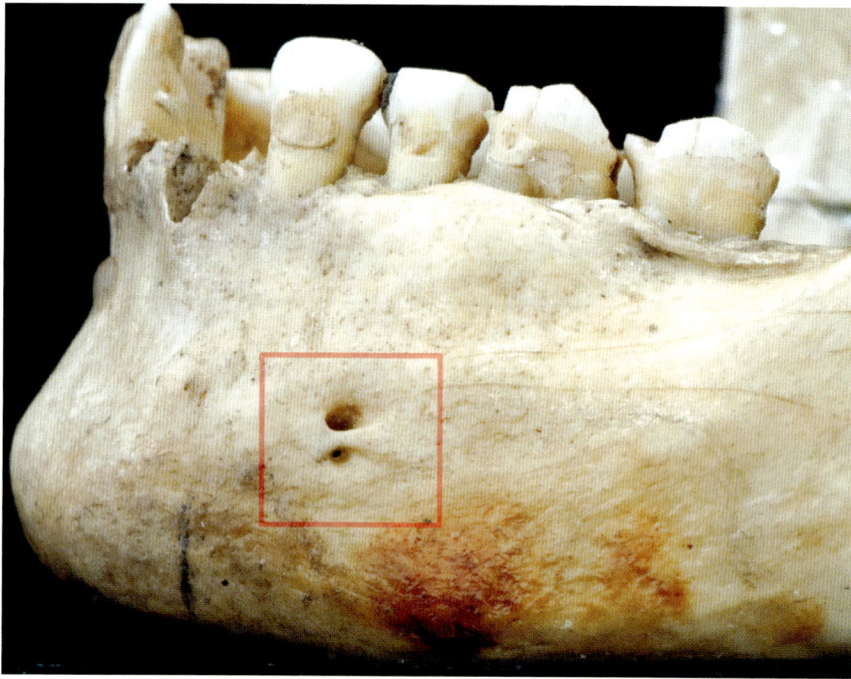

Figure 613. Horizontally-divided left mental foramen (square) that probably transmitted separate neurovascular bundles (KKU 329-32).

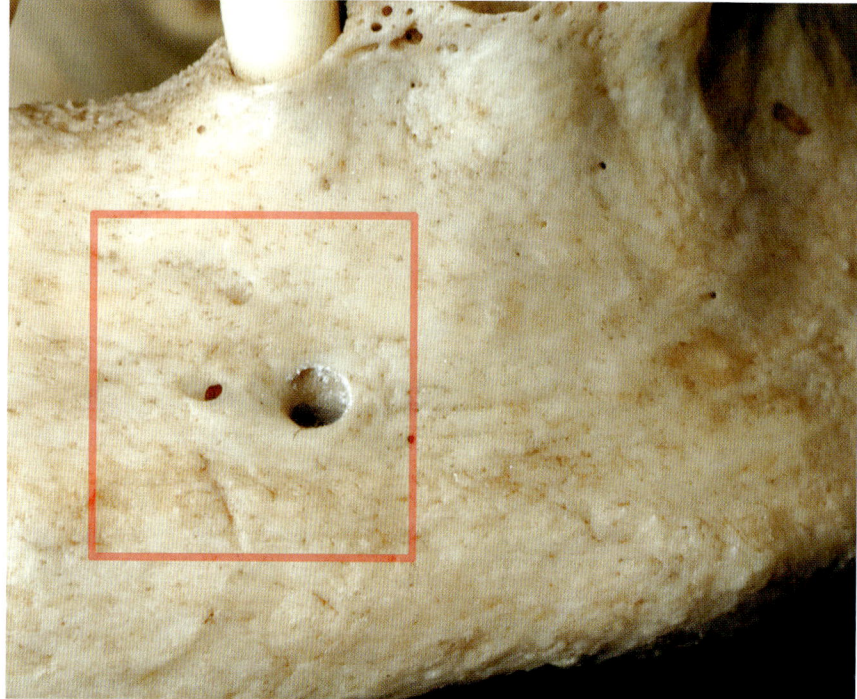

Figure 614. Vertically-divided or double left mental foramen. Two buccal foramina (square) leading into a single mandibular canal (KKU E6 672). While the smaller foramen is an accessory foramen, both probably transmitted neurovascular bundles to supply superficial structures of the mandible. See Ramadhan et al. (2010) for an example of triple foramina. See von Arx (2013) for detailed information on multiple foramina and the vessels and nerves that pass through them.

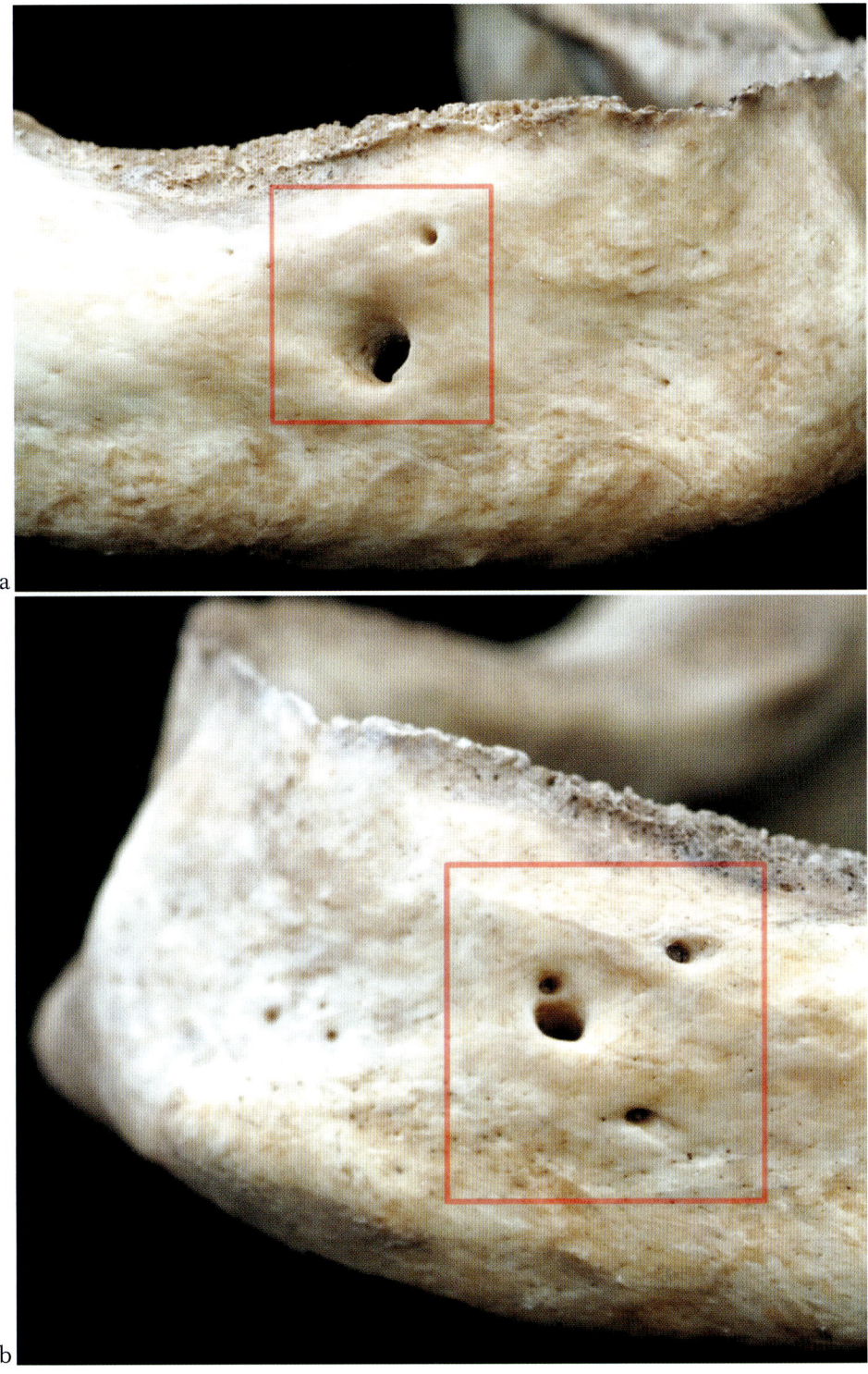

Figure 615a-b. Double right mental foramina and rare four left mandibular foramina. (a) Double right (square) mental foramina and (b) rare four left mandibular foramina (square) in an elderly Thai mandible (KKU C2 395). See Neves et al. (2010) for a rare lingual accessory mental foramen associated with a duplicate mandibular canal and Ramadhan et al. (2010) for triple mental foramina and corresponding nerves. Murphy (1957) classified divided foramina as a minor variant and totally separate accessory foramina as a major trait. DeVilliers (1968); von Arx (2013).

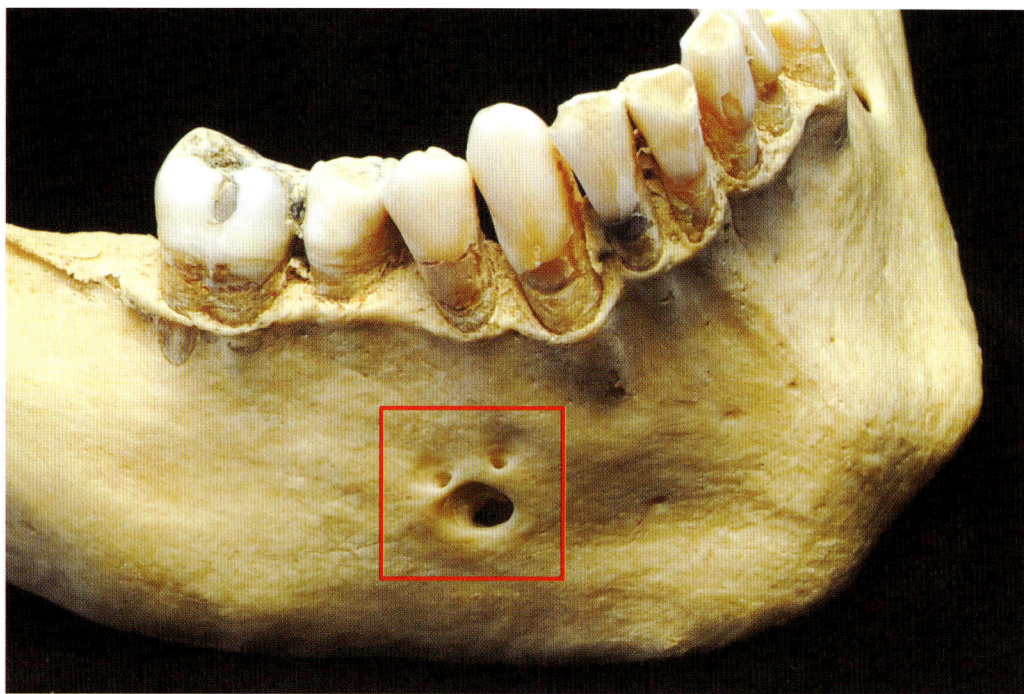

Figure 616. Triple right mental foramina (square) in an adult African (University of Pretoria). The two small foramina communicate with the large foramen and probably transmitted small neurovascular bundles. Cf. von Arx (2013).

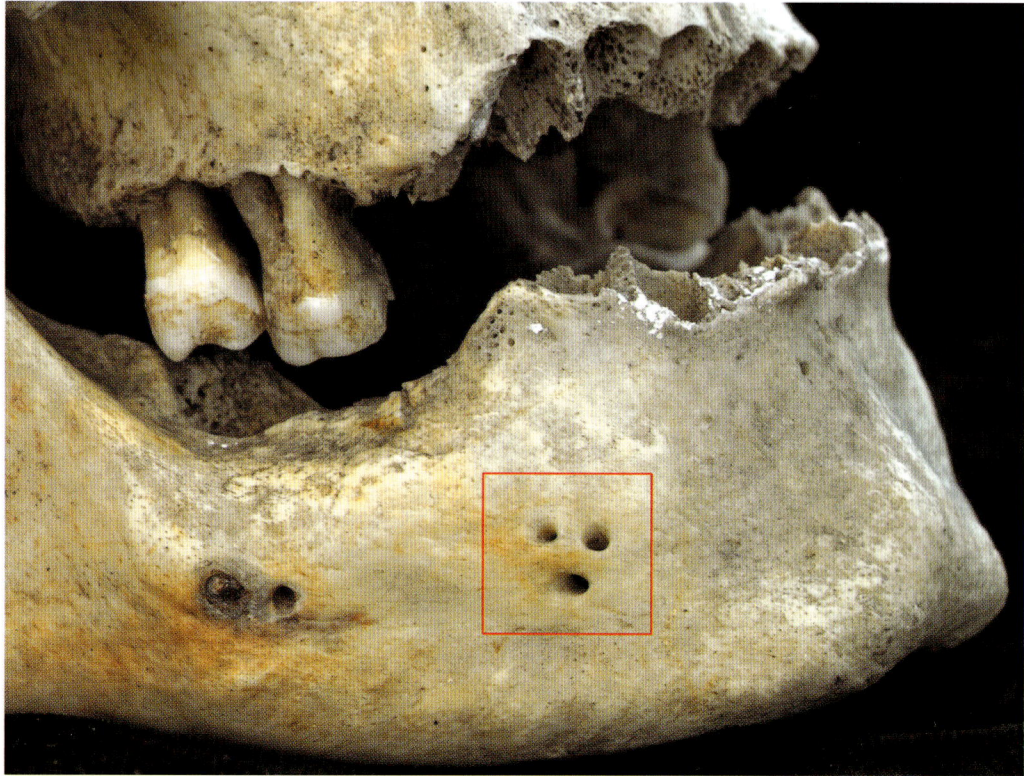

Figure 617. Triple right mental foramina (square) in an adult male (RV 1069).

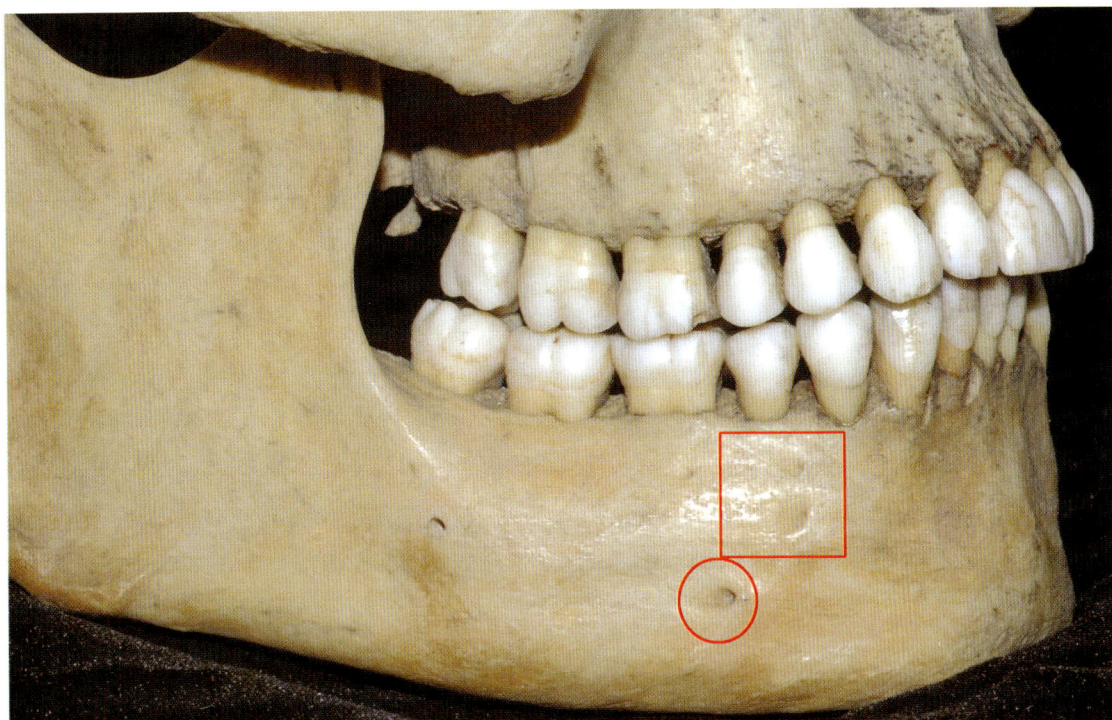

Figure 618. Three right mental foramina consisting of a double superior foramen (square) and single inferior foramen (circle) (RV1472), all of which likely carried neurovascular bundles.

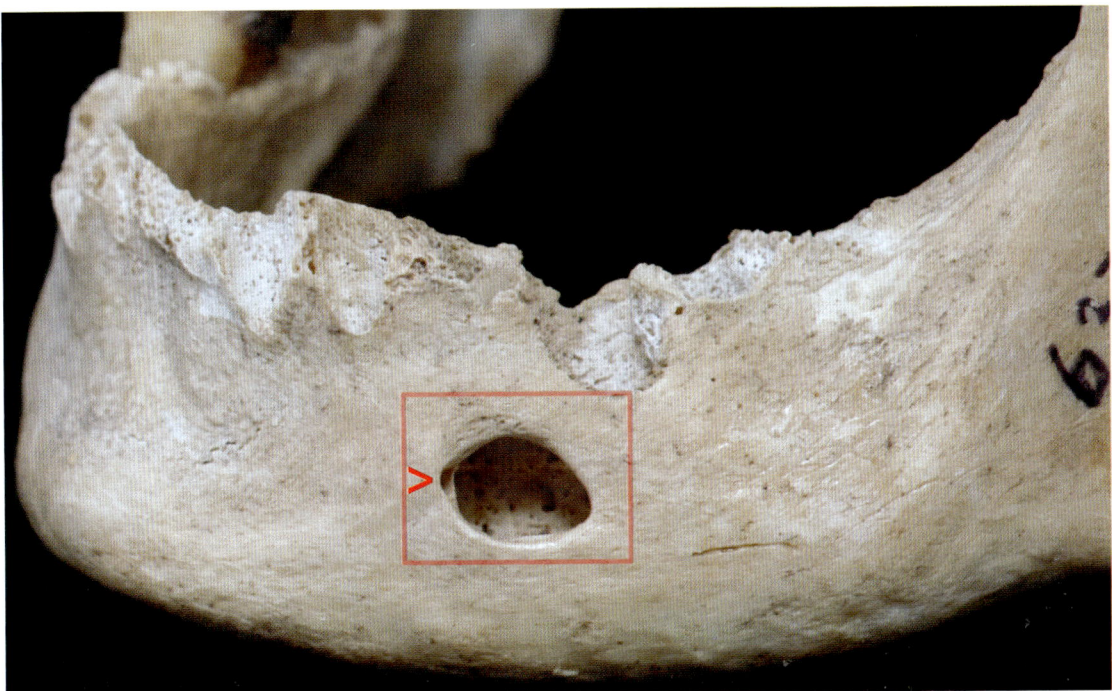

Figure 619. Unusually large left mental foramen with a small foramen (>) along its medial margin in an elderly female. The right mental foramen is also larger than usual, but neither foramen appears to communicate with or be enlarged due to age, dental abscess or localized disease (KKU 637-32). See von Arx (2013) for more on the mental foramen.

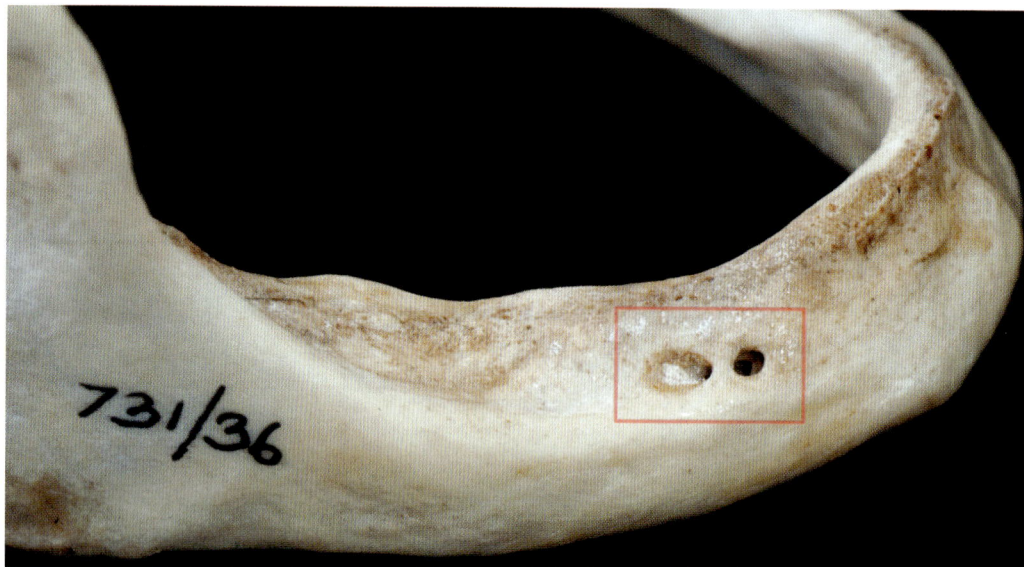

Figure 620. Vertically-divided right mental foramen (rectangle) in an elderly Thai female (KKU 731-36). Loss of the teeth resulted in severe resorption and posterior angulation of the corpus and foramina, that appear lower in the mandible compared to the dentulous condition. Cf. Amorim et al. (2008) and von Arx (2013).

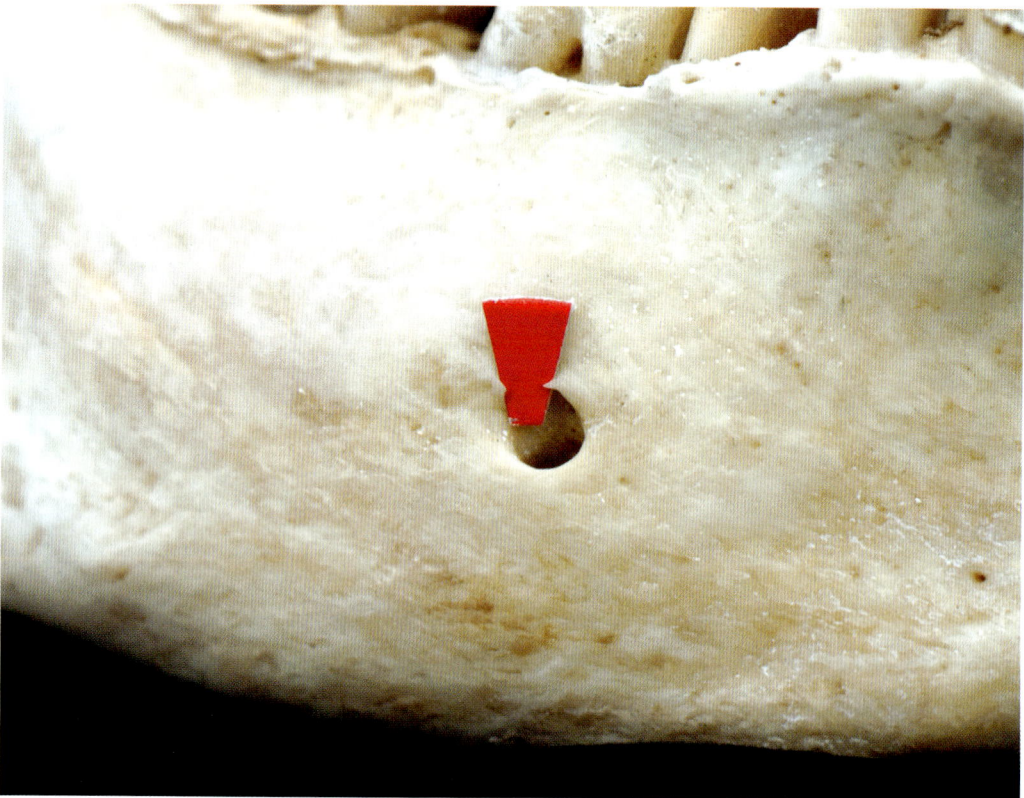

Figure 621. Partial bridging of the right mental foramen in an adult Thai mandible (KKU 43-725). Note the two small bony spicules (red arrowhead) projecting towards one another.

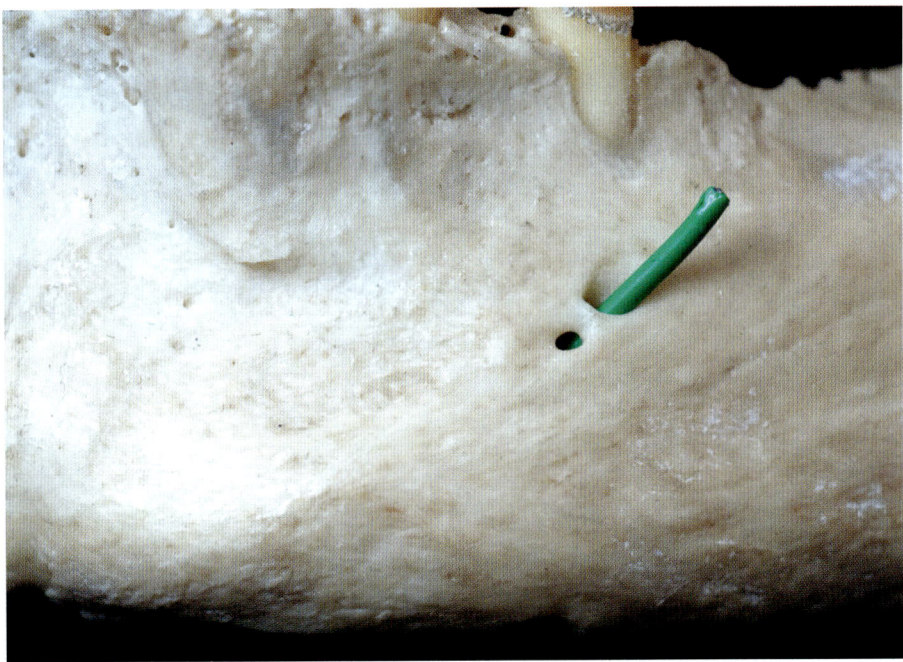

Figure 622. Diagonal bridging resulting in a double mental foramen (green wire) in an adult Thai mandible (KKU E3 0662).

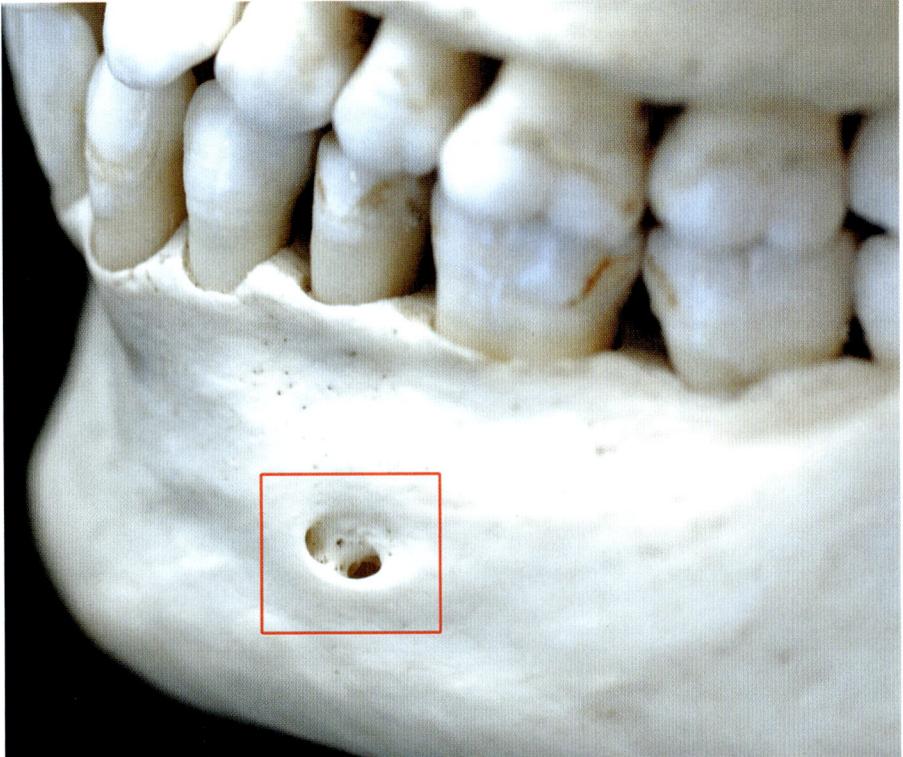

Figure 623. Single external foramen and double internal foramina (square) (FSA CSC AC043). Rarely a mandible will exhibit absence of one or both mental foramina (de Freitas et al. 1979).

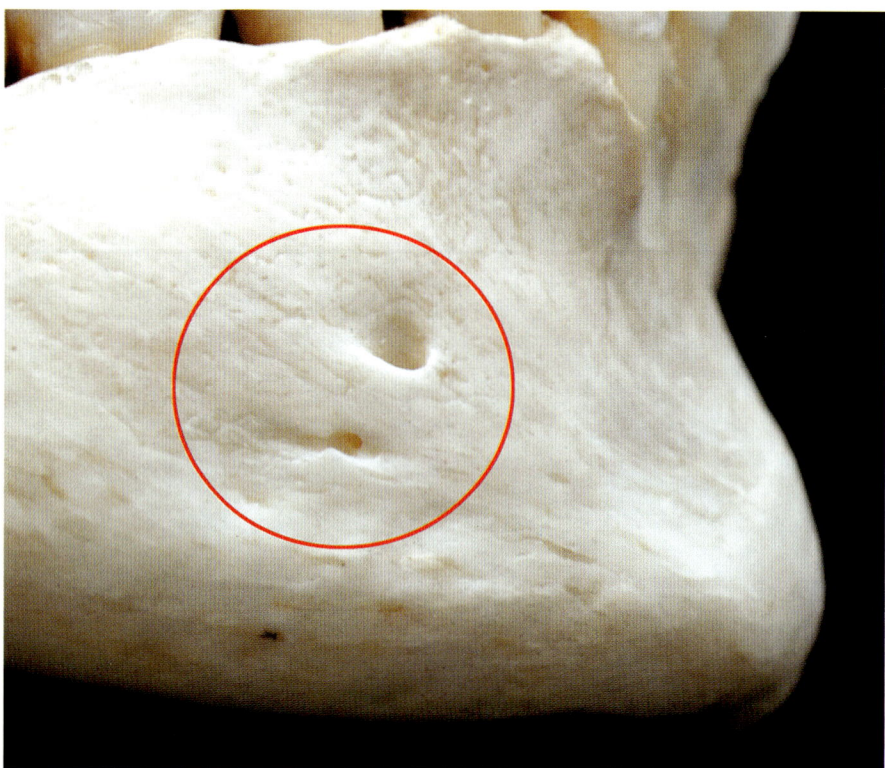

Figure 624. Separate large superior and small inferior mental foramina (circle) in an adult (FSA CSC AS008). Note the small foramen has a shallow horizontal groove that transmitted vessels and nerves.

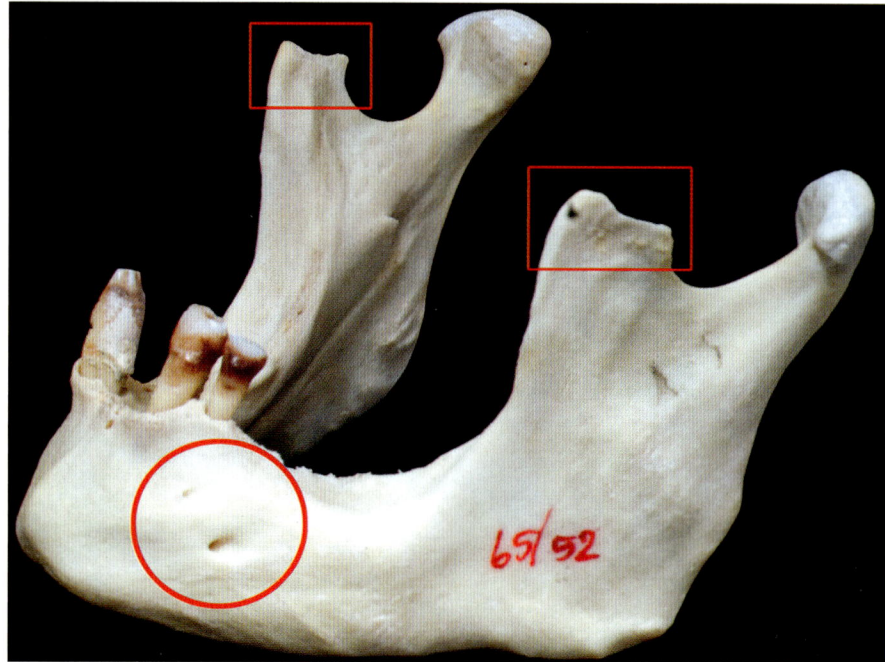

Figure 625. Double left mental foramina (circle) and flattened coronoid processes (rectangles) in a 69-year-old Thai male mandible (CMU 65 52). The coronoid process is usually hook shaped, triangular or rounded (Isaac and Holla 2001; Priya et al. 2004).

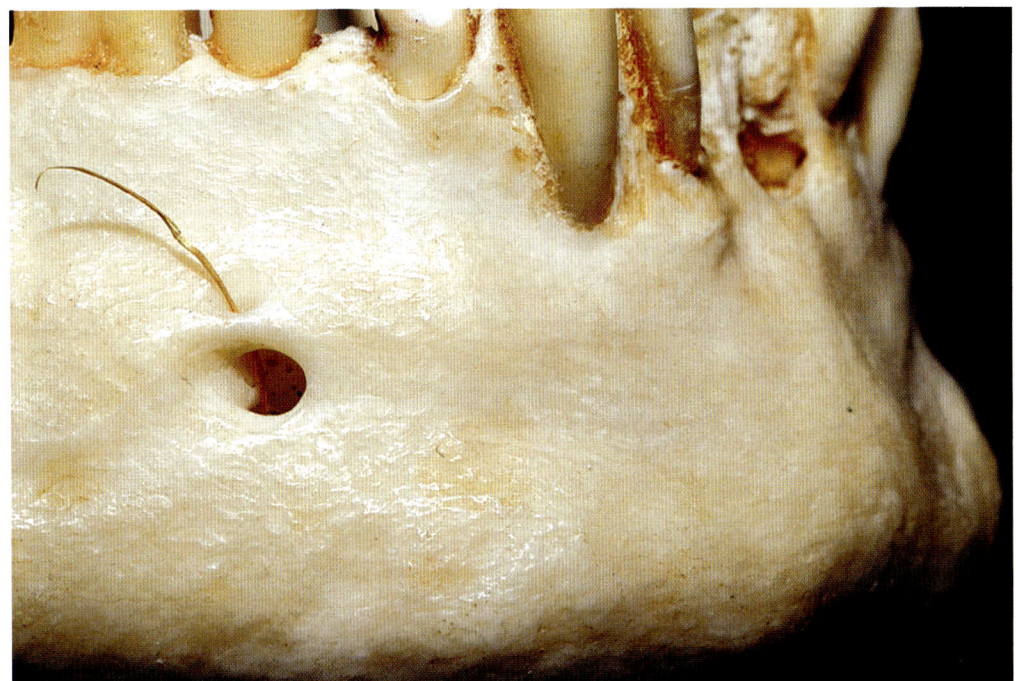

Figure 626. Horizontally divided/double right mental foramen. In this specimen a small superior foramen communicates (straw probe) with a large inferior foramen, both of which likely carried neurovascular bundles (JABSOM). The left mental foramen is single.

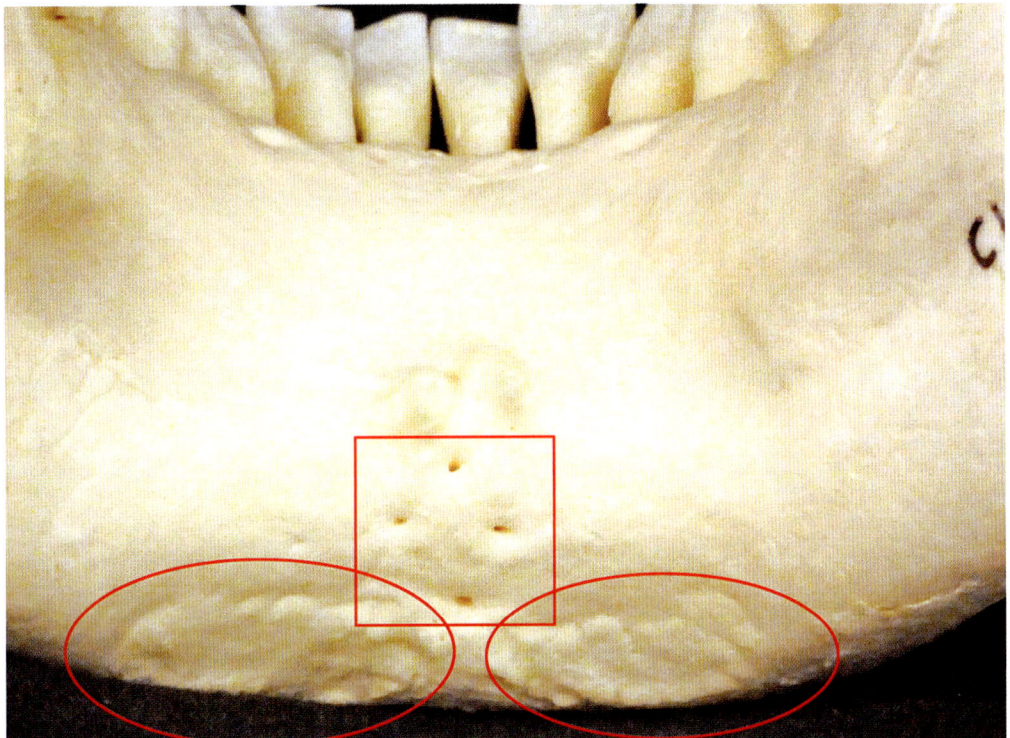

Figure 627. Accessory foramina (square) and roughened areas for the anterior digastric muscles (ovals) in an Asian adult (CSC). Both are common findings. Cf. Singh et al. (2000).

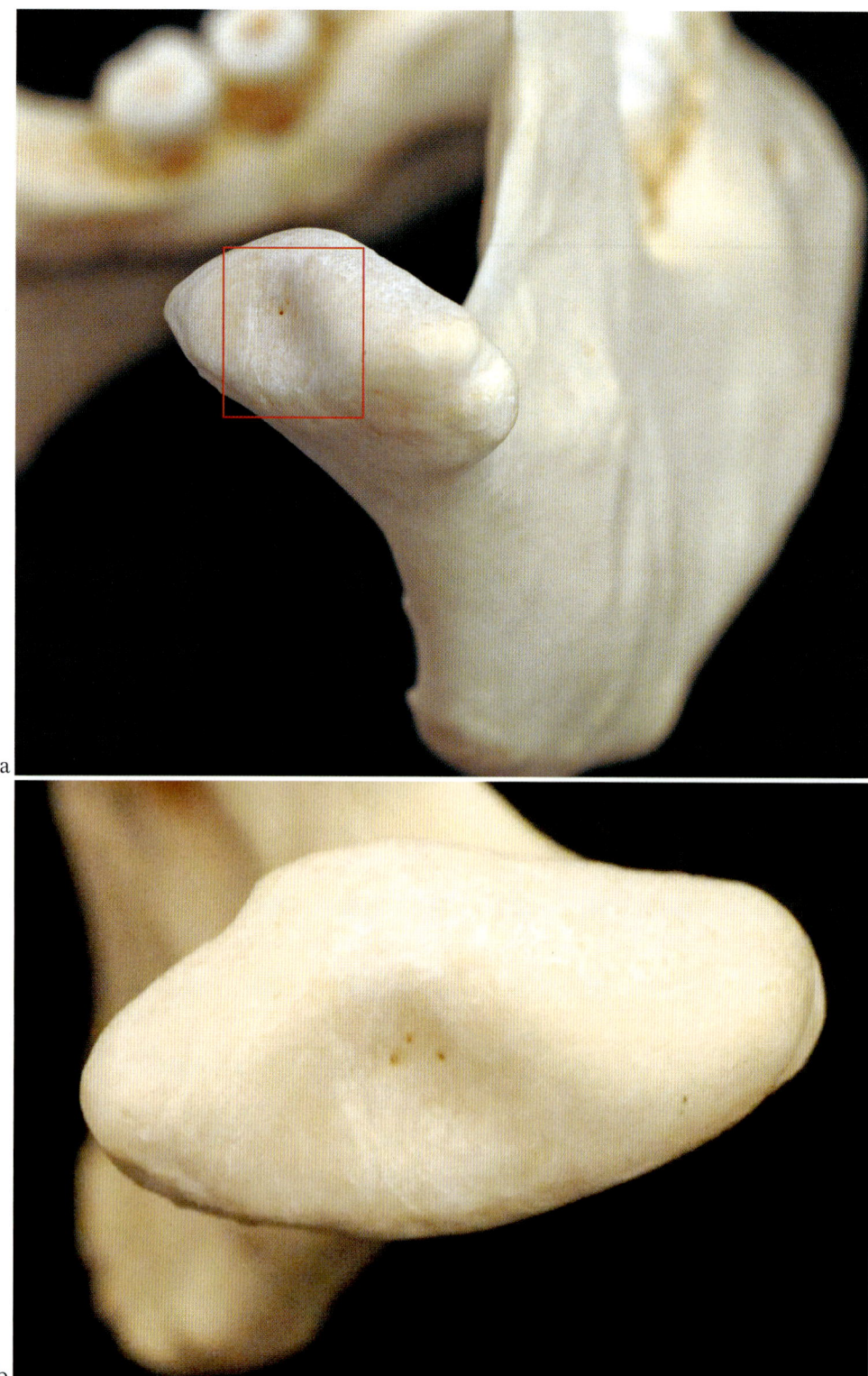

Figure 628a-b. Shallow fossa of the right mandibular condyle with perforations. (a) Oblique view of fossa with perforated (square) right mandibular condyle while the corresponding left condyle was not affected. (b) Superior view of tiny foramina inside the fossa. Such "dimpling" is an unusual finding of unknown etiology and may reflect disease of the craniomandibular joint, i.e., osteoarthritis.

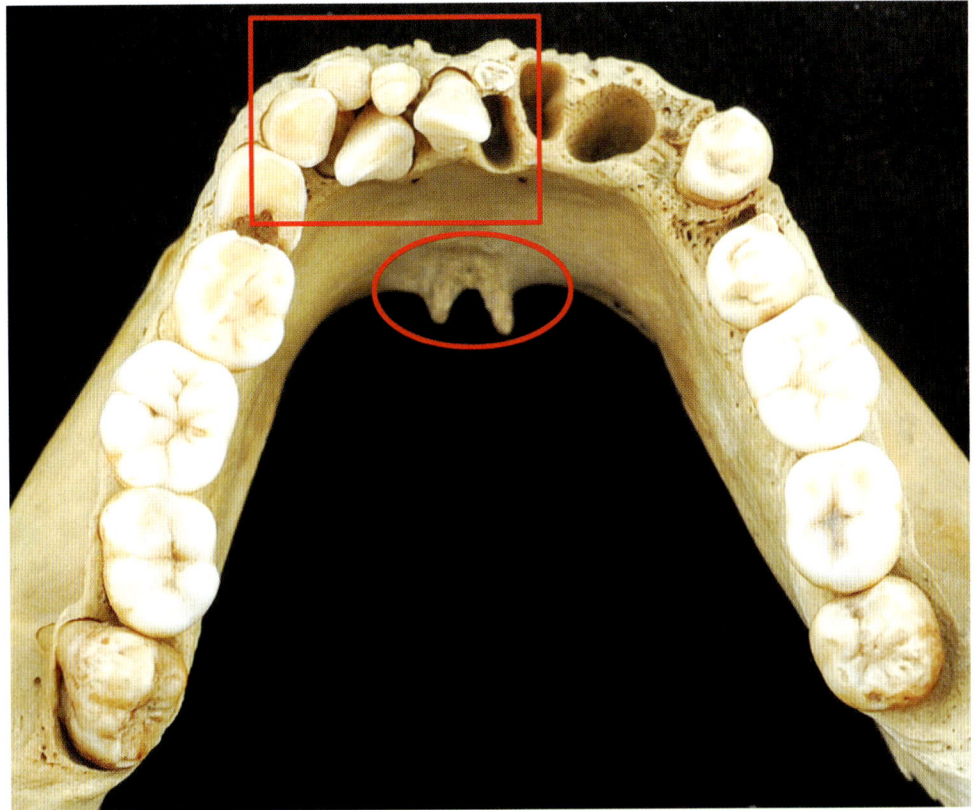

Figure 629. Dental crowding (rectangle), four left molars and long genial tubercles (oval) in an ancient Peruvian mandible (SI). Common findings. Cf. Greyling et al. (1997); Singh et al. (2000).

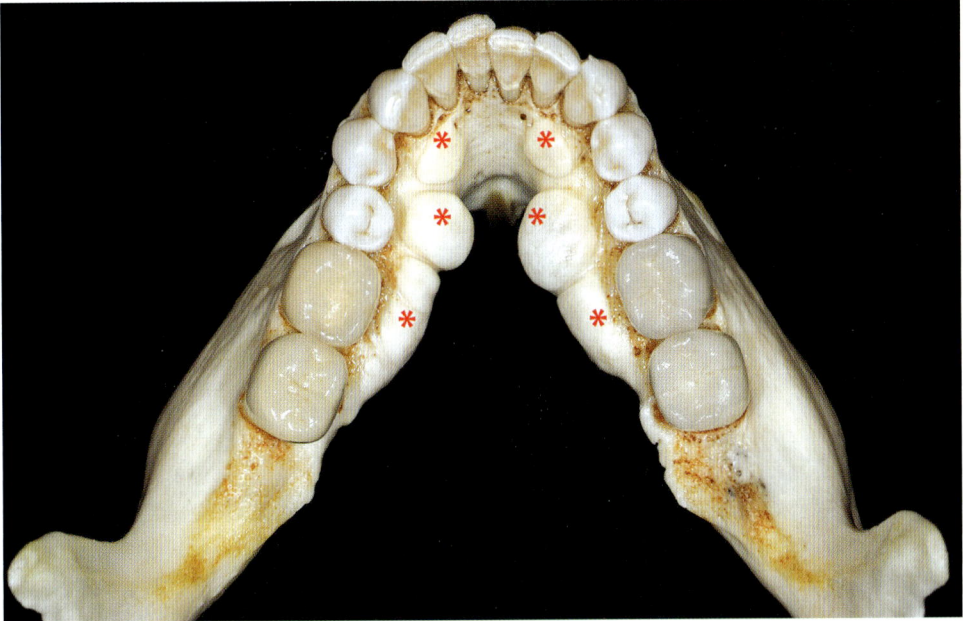

Figure 630. Lingual exostoses (*) in an adult. The exostoses are separate anteriorly, but coalesce posteriorly into elongated bars of bone (JABSOM 1170). These bony growths may form in response to mechanical stresses associated with mastication.

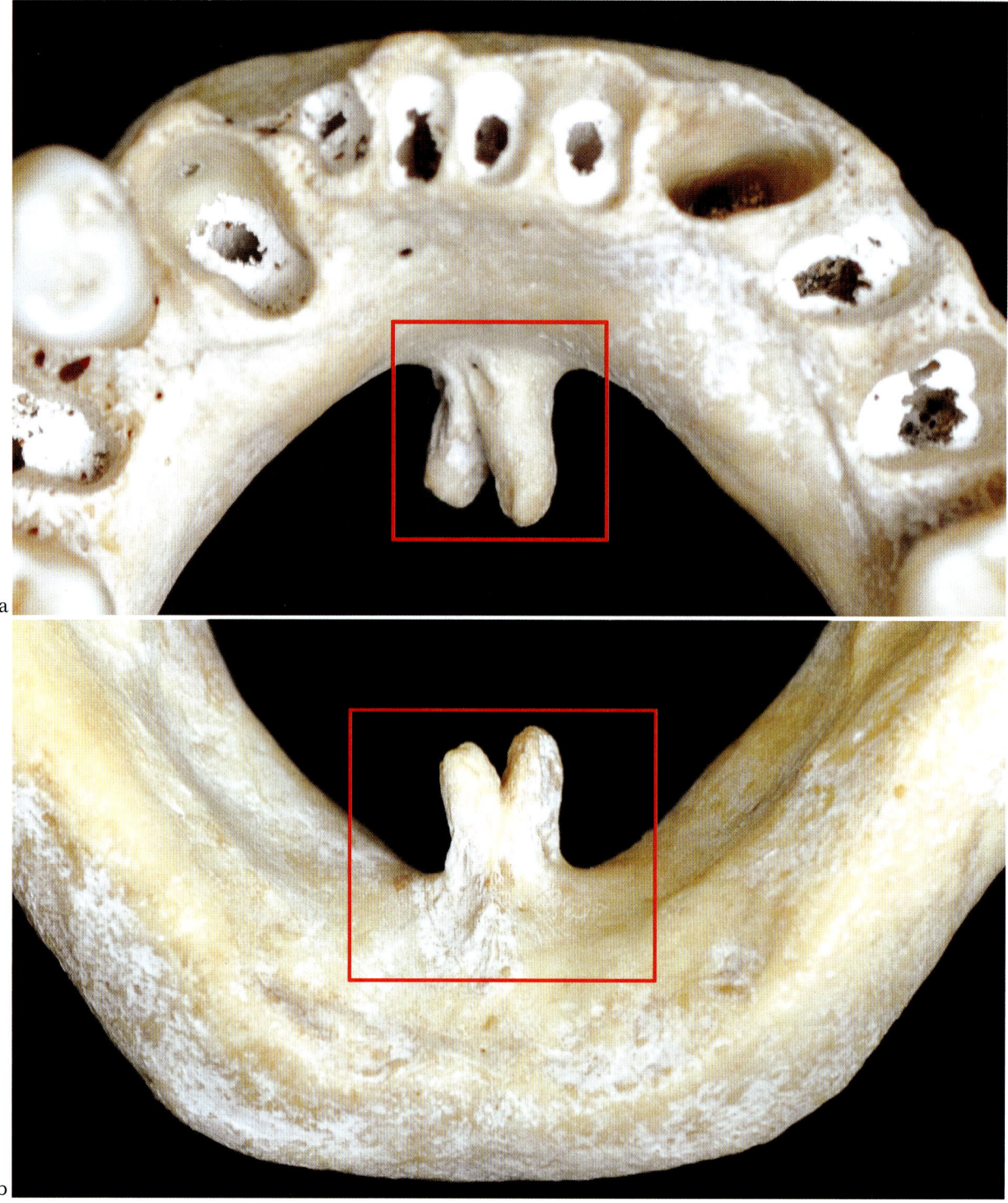

Figure 631a-b. Unusually large and fused genial tubercles viewed from superior (a) and (b) inferior perspectives These tubercles are typically separate but many elongate with age (KKU). Uncommon finding. Cf. Singh et al. (2000).

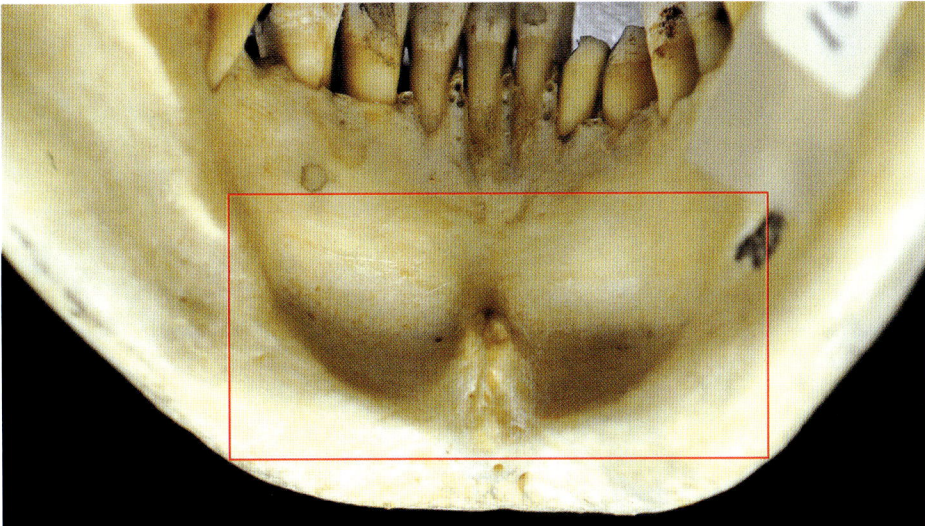

Figure 632. Bilateral anterior depressions called sublingual fovea of the anterior and internal aspect of the mandible (rectangle) that are sometimes misidentified as "anterior" Stafne's defects (Mütter Museum 1008.48). Anterior Stafne's defects will have the same characteristics of those found inferior to the molars, but will be in the region of the canines or anterior to the premolars. Typical anatomy, but uncommon to be so deep.

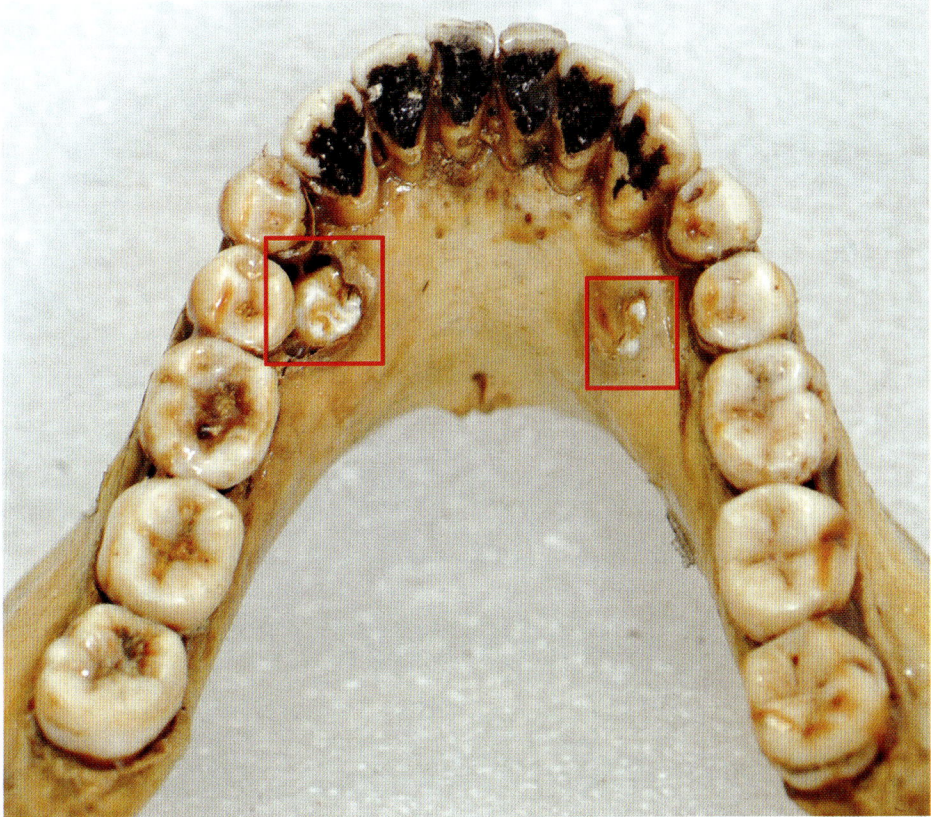

Figure 633. Bilateral accessory premolars (square and rectangle) in an adult Thai mandible. Note the black lingual staining often attributed to smoking, but may also occur in children or individuals who have never smoked (KKU) due to diet and betel nut chewing in middle-age and older individuals. Uncommon finding.

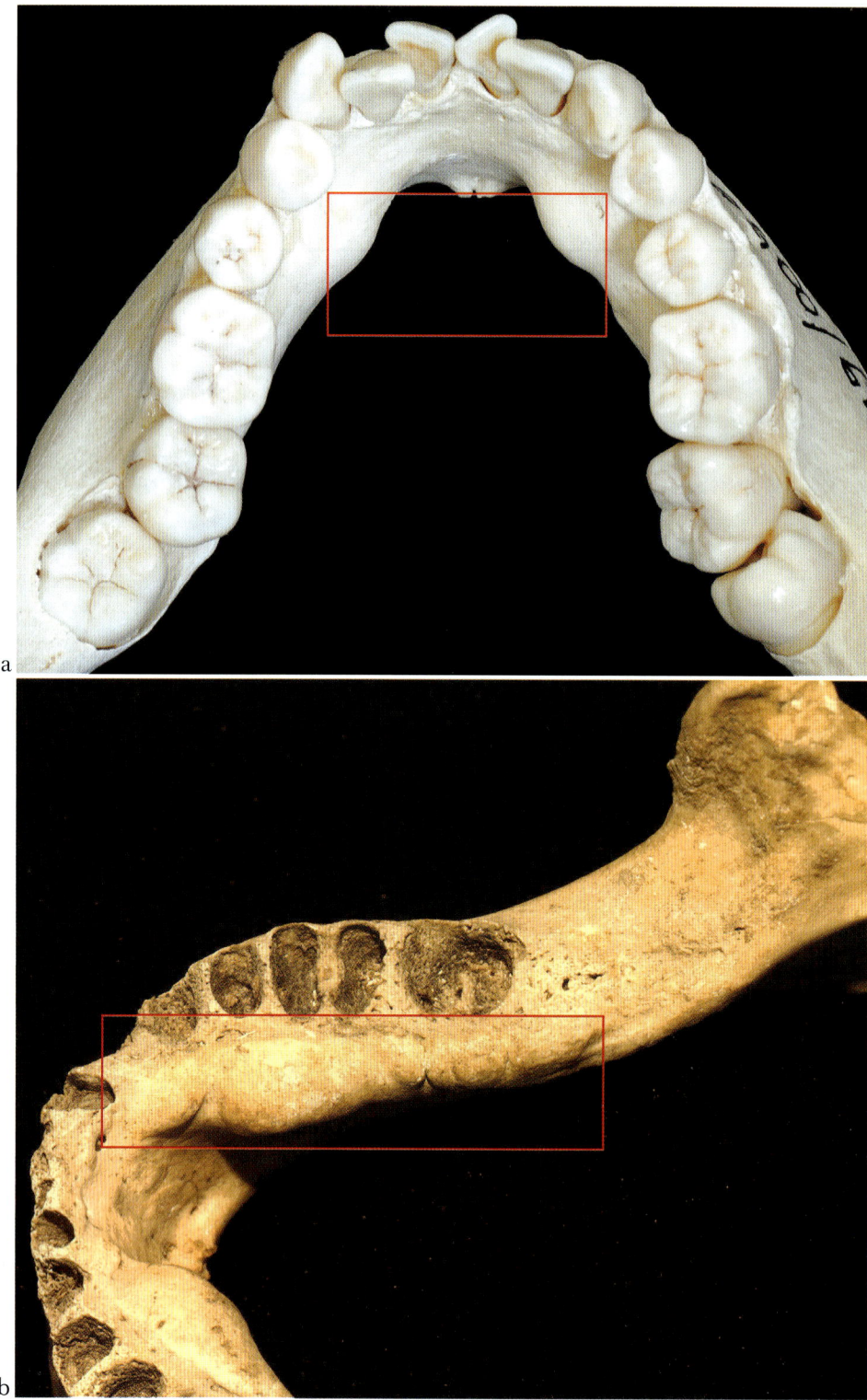

Figure 634a-b. Photographs of mandibular tori. (a) Mandibular tori (rectangle) with small localized tori (KKU) compared to (b) large tori (rectangle) that extend along the entire length of the dental alveolar ridge (SI). Mandibular tori are uncommon to common findings, depending on the group, increase in size with age (Moorrees et al. 1952) and may regrow if surgically removed. Cf. Hassett (2006).

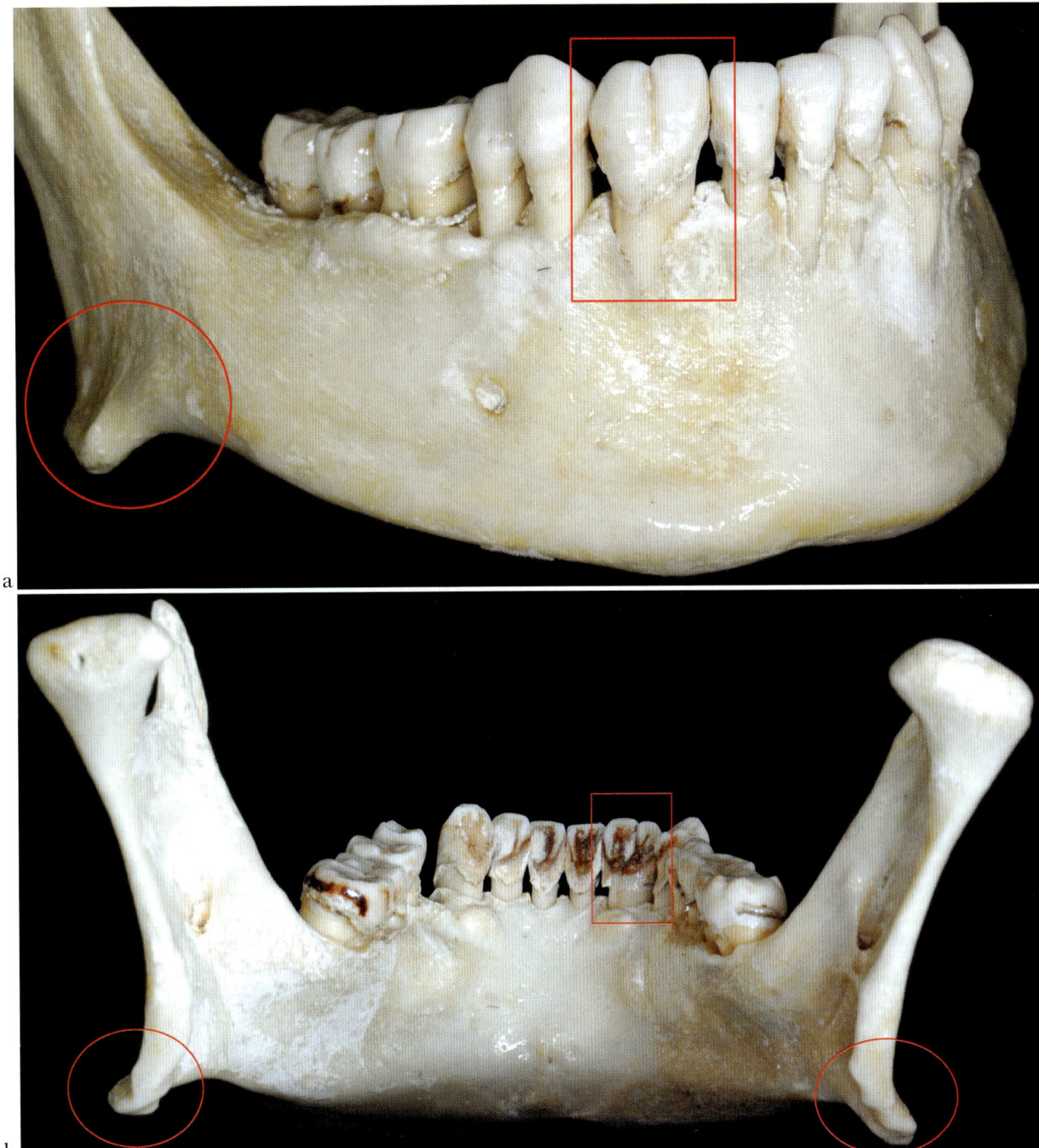

Figure 635a-b. Synodontia of the right lateral mandibular incisor. (a) Oblique view of geminated teeth (rectangle) with two crowns, but only one root, and marked gonial eversion (circle) in an adult Thai male mandible (KKU). (b) Posterior view of the geminated tooth (rectangle) and bilateral gonial eversion (circles). A radiographic study by Altug-Atac and Erdem (2007) reported that of 3,043 Turkish children only two cases of synodontia were observed (0.07%). Mild expression of synodontia is a common male trait, while severe forms are uncommon to rare. Deep unilateral or bilateral indentations such as these anterior to the angle of the mandible have been attributed to insertion of the masseter muscle and not necessarily age (Apofisis Lemuriana de Albrecht or the Angle of Sandifort – Vázquez et al. 2001). See Figure 636a-b for more images of this specimen.

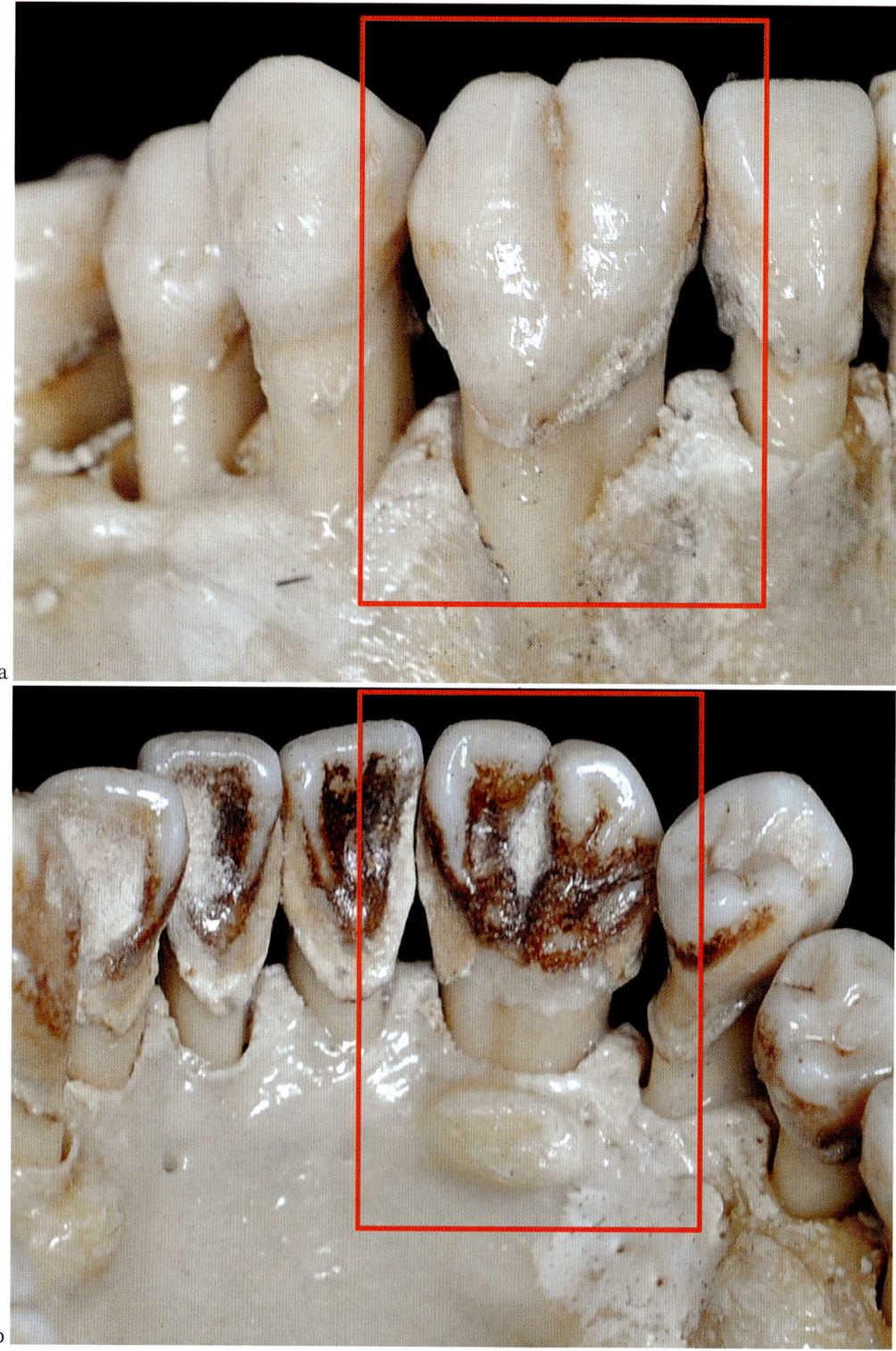

Figure 636a-b. Higher magnification of synodontia. (a) Buccal and (b) lingual views of the geminated mandibular lateral incisor (rectangles) in an adult Thai mandible (see Figure 635a-b for more images) (KKU). Rare finding.

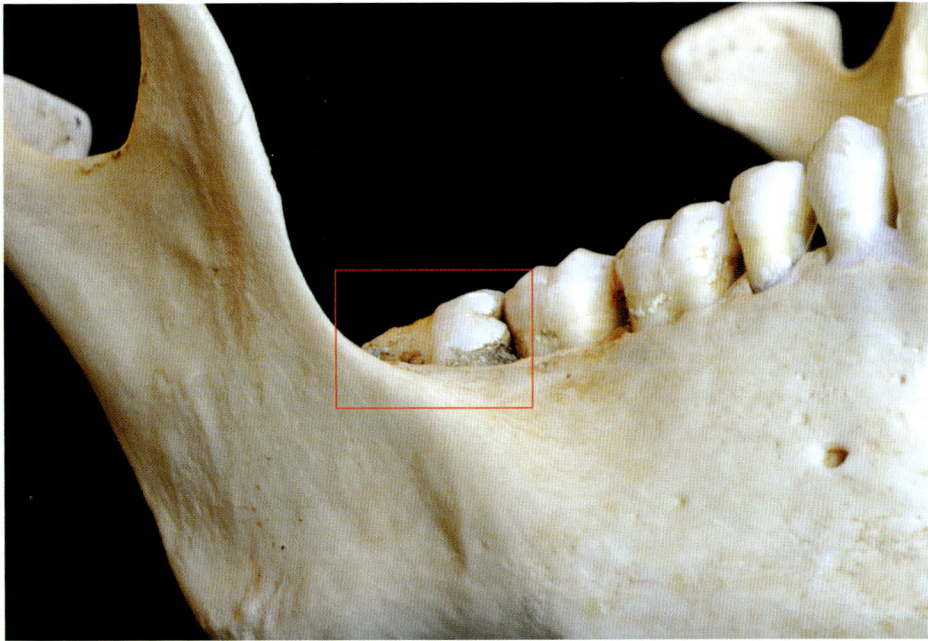

Figure 637. Horizontally-impacted right third molar (rectangle) in an adult Thai mandible (UHWO). Uncommon archaeological finding, but common clinical finding.

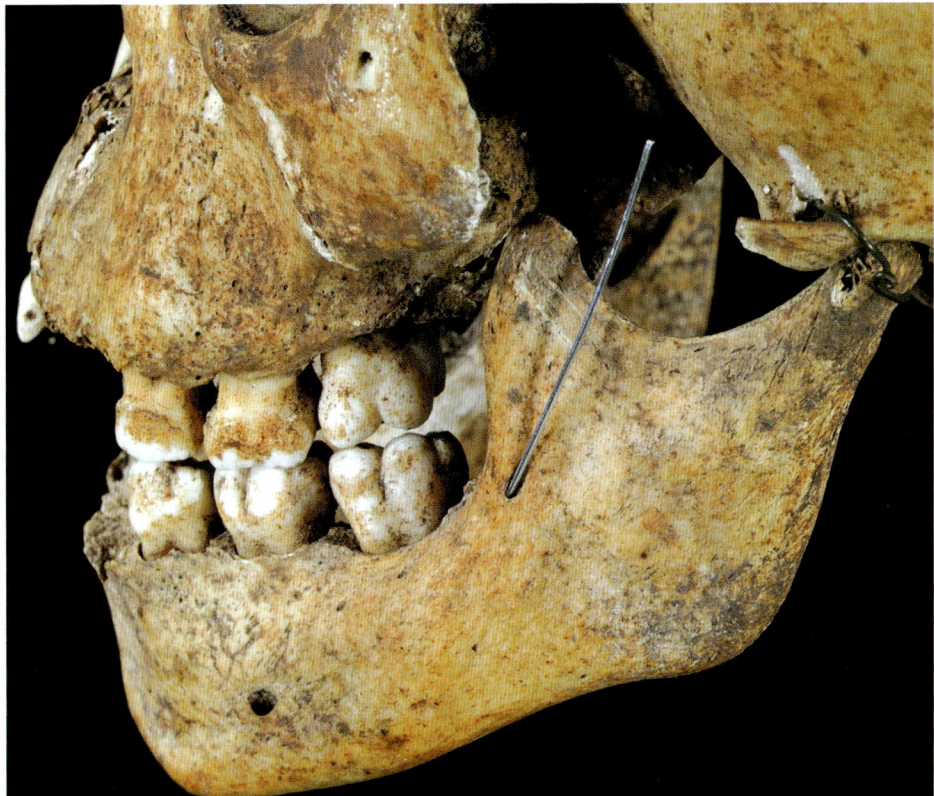

Figure 638. Small accessory foramen (metal probe) in the left ramus of an Asian child (CSC AC 003). Uncommon to rare finding.

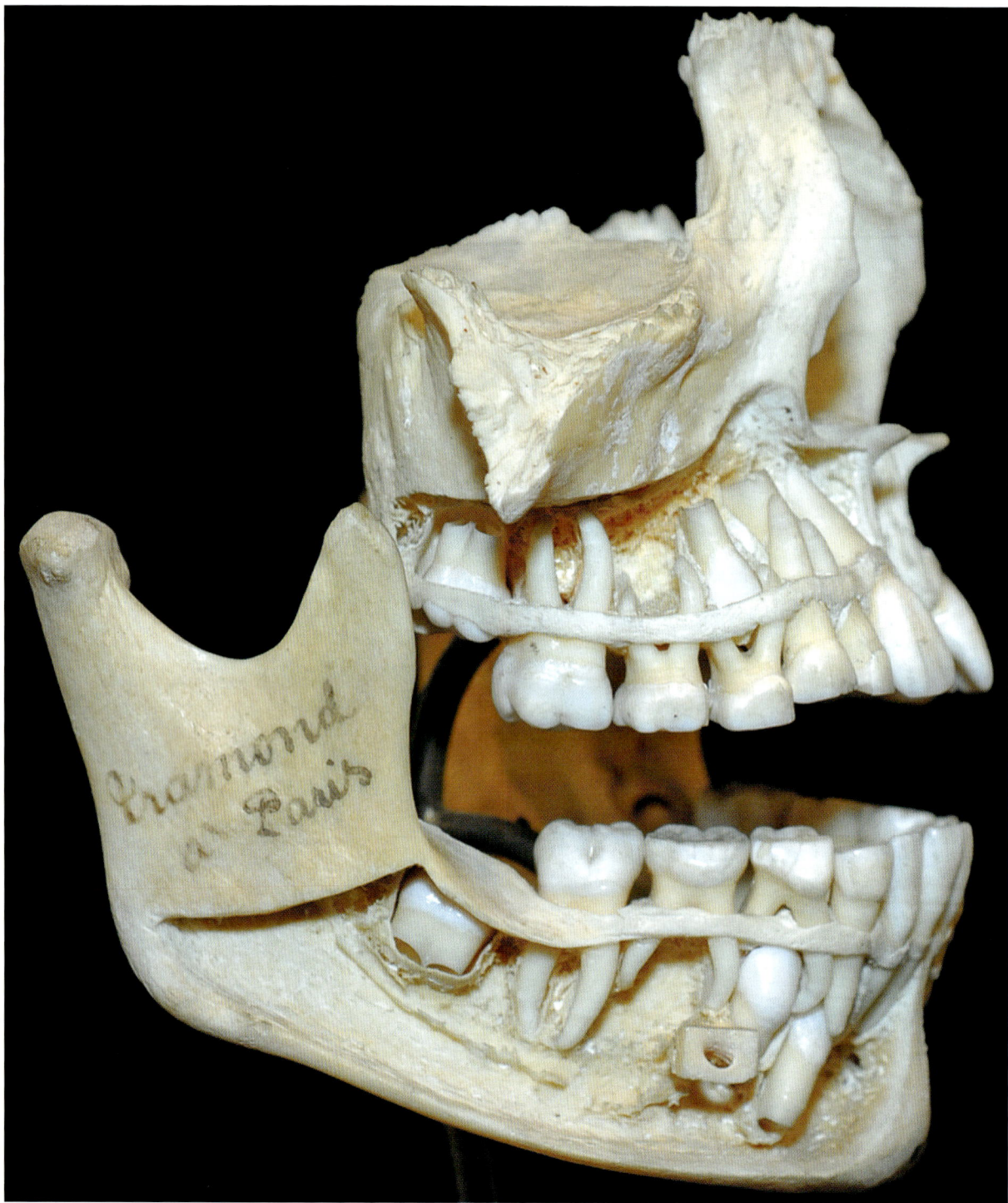

Figure 639. Beautifully sectioned and well-preserved teeth and jaws showing the normal anatomy and location of the mandibular canal, right mental foramen, which is sometimes doubled, and developmental stages of the tooth roots in a child (Mütter Museum 1098.10). Cf. Berge and Bergman (2001); Serman (1989).

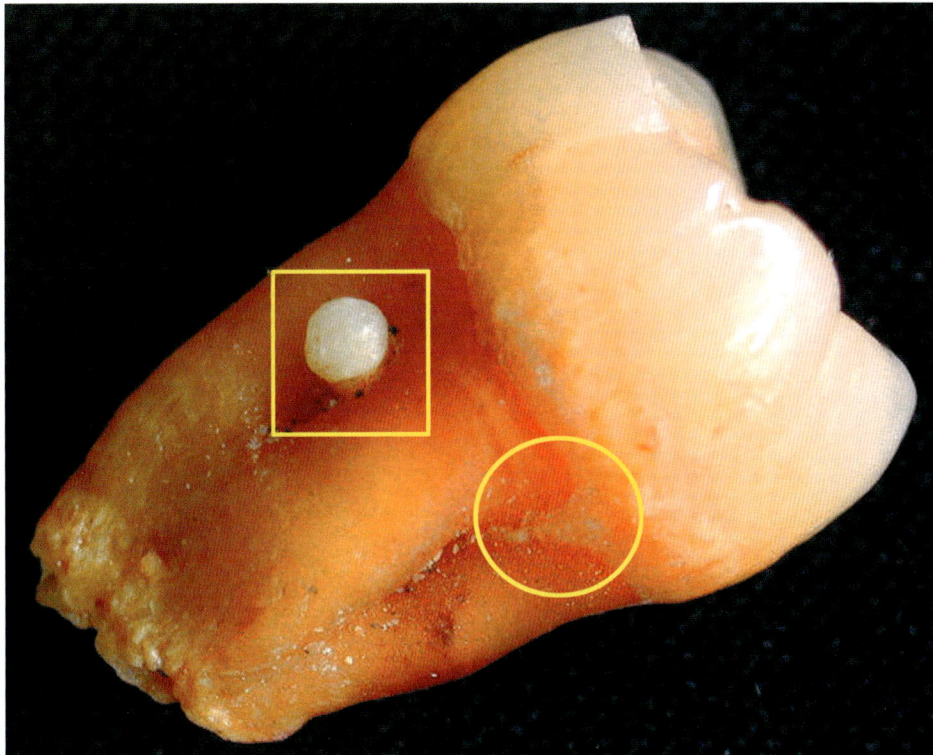

Figure 640. Enamel pearl (square) and extension (circle) in a mandibular molar (VES, Rhode). Enamel pearls and extensions form along the bifurcation of the roots. Common (especially in deciduous molars) to uncommon findings depending on the group studied.

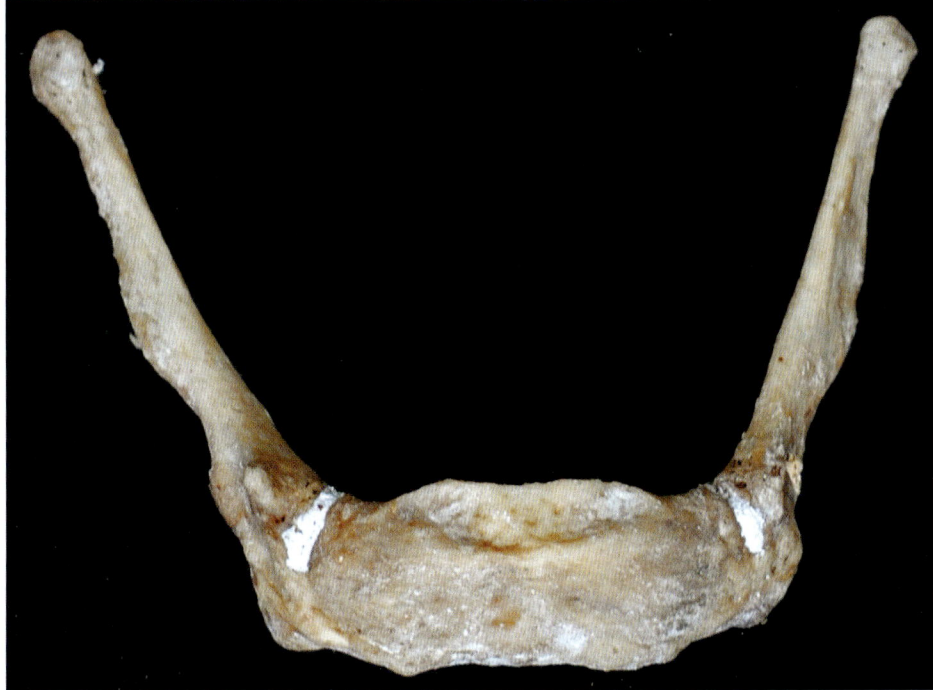

Figure 641. Adult hyoid bone (KKU). Normal anatomy. Cf. Parsons (1909) for a detailed report on the hyoid.

MAXILLA (HARD PALATE) AND TEETH

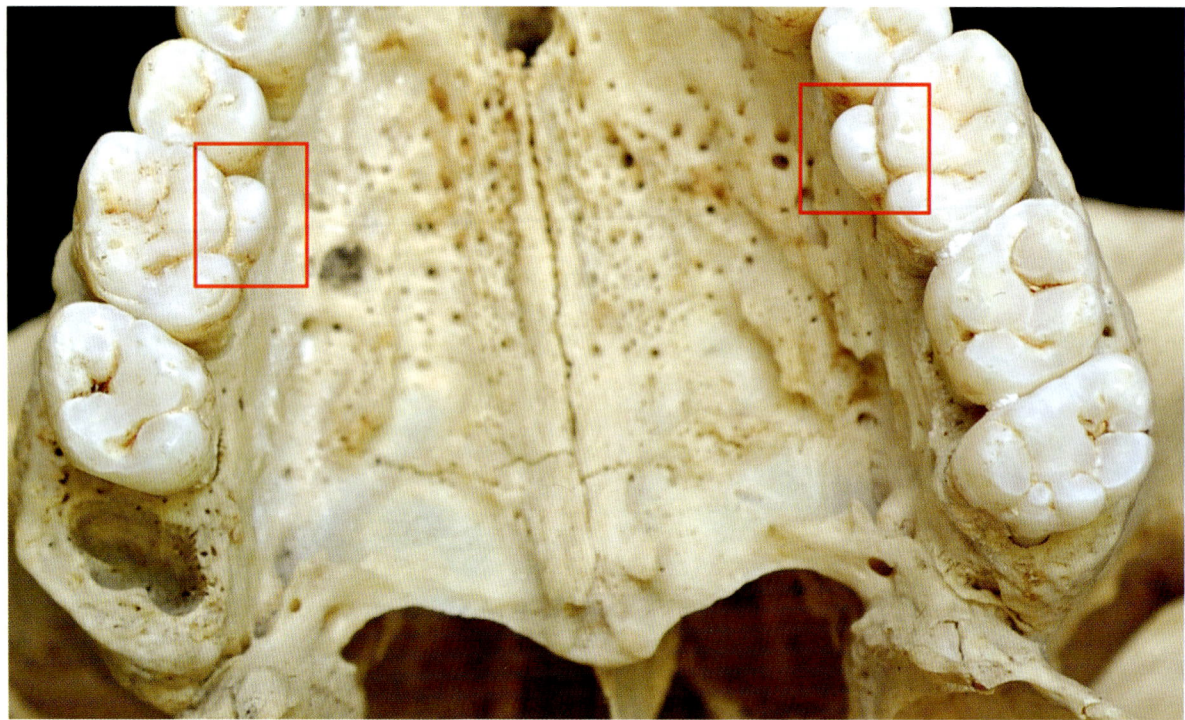

Figure 642. Large bilateral Carabelli's trait ("cusp") (square and rectangle) in an Asian adult maxilla (UHWO). Common finding. Cf. Scott (2008).

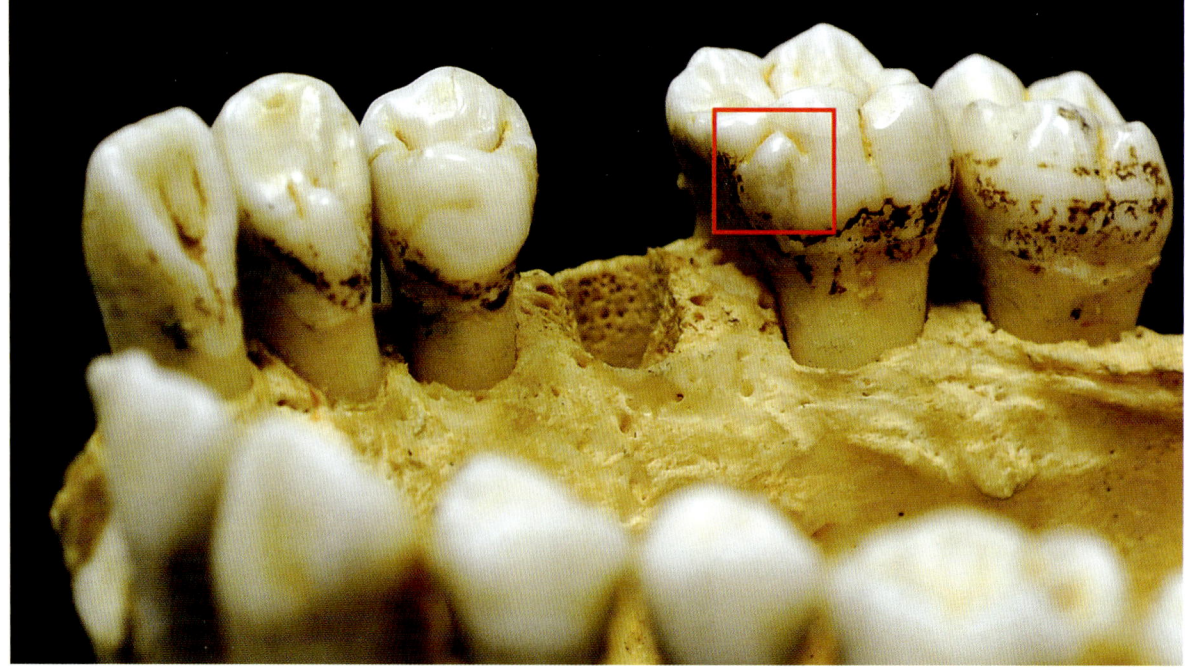

Figure 643. Small Carabelli's trait (square) (Mütter Museum). Common finding. Cf. Scott (2008).

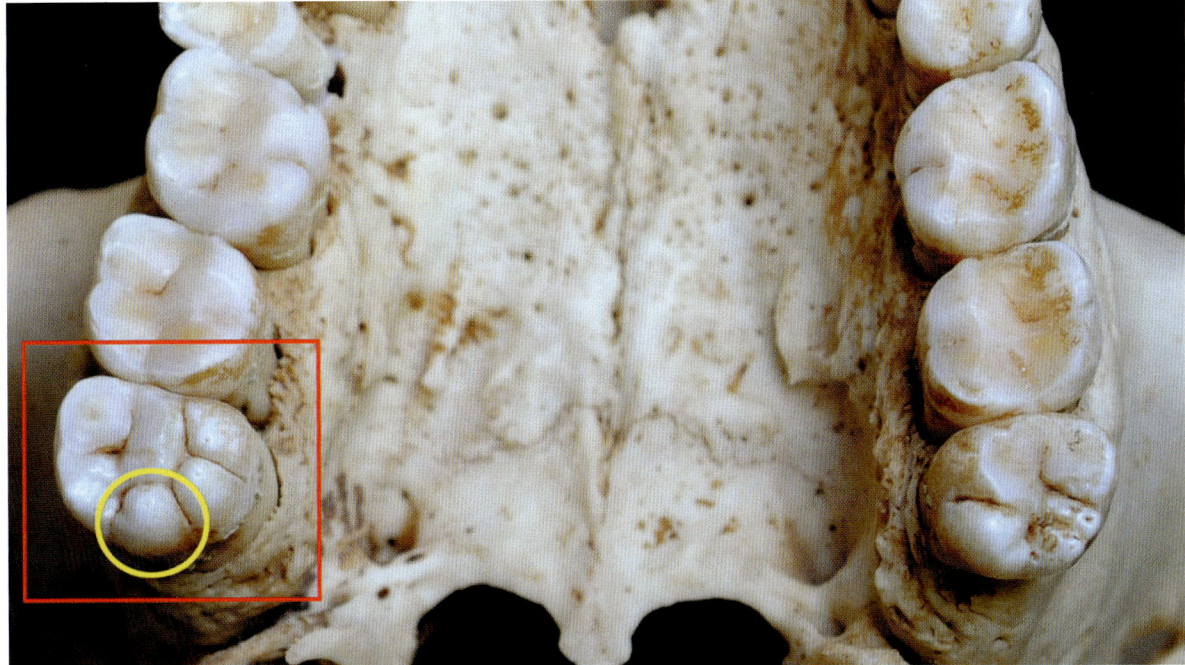

Figure 644. The right maxillary third molar (square) exhibits a well-developed hypocone and metacone, with an intervening cusp 5 (metaconule = yellow circle). It is likely that the mesial lingual cusp is a Carabelli's cusp and distal to that is a second, accessory lingual cusp that developed on the protocone between the Carabelli's cusp and the large hypocone (UHWO) (personal communication, Dr. Marin Pilloud). Uncommon to rare trait. Cf. Scott (2008) for more on dental morphology.

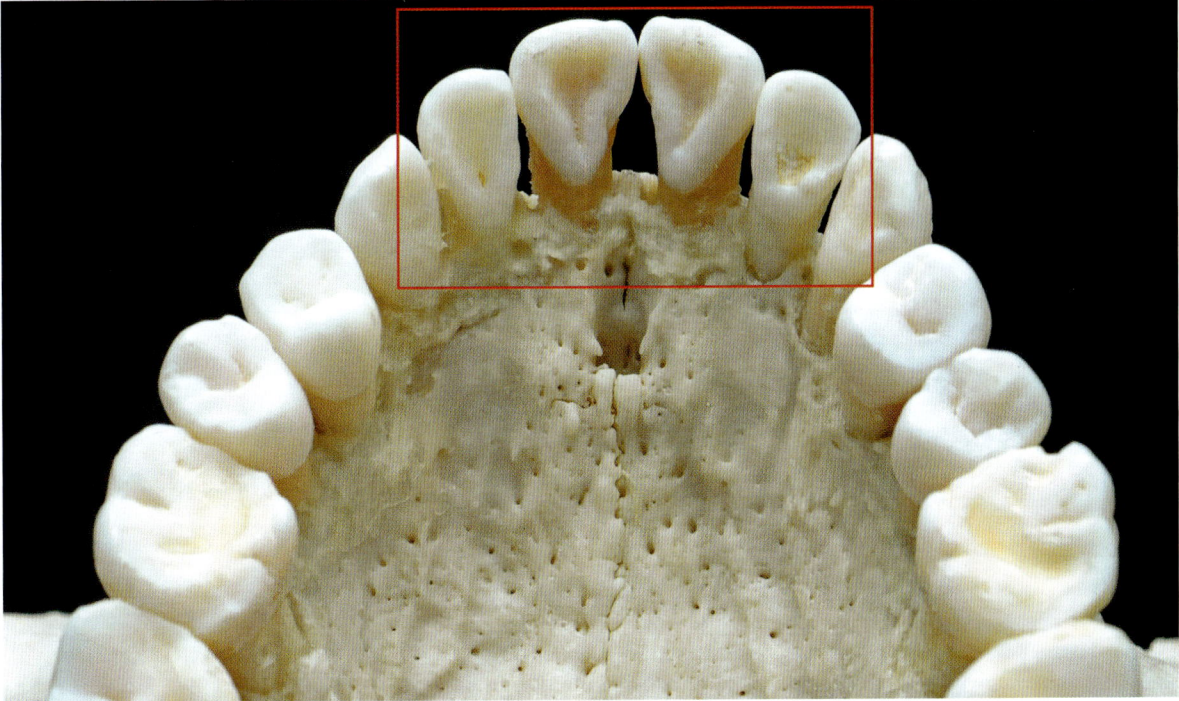

Figure 645. Shovel-shaped maxillary incisors (rectangle) in an adult Asian (CSC). Common finding.

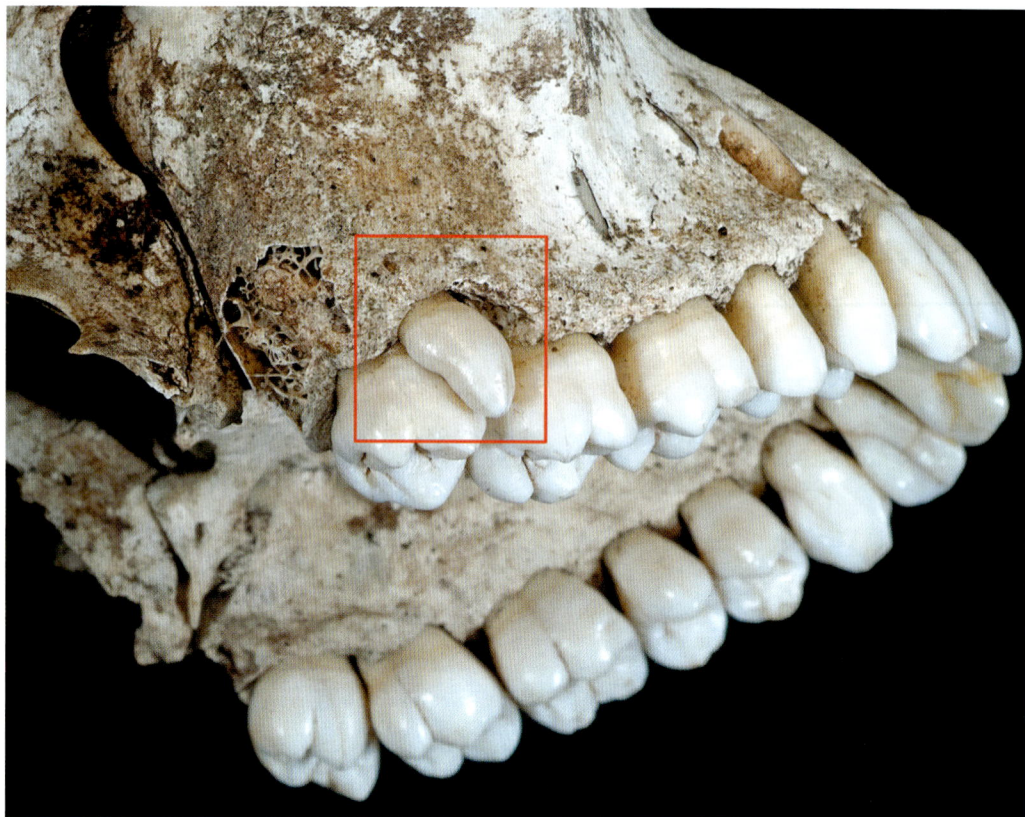

Figure 646. Supernumerary tooth, also known as hyperdontia (square) in a teenage Black female (SI 257579). Uncommon to common finding.

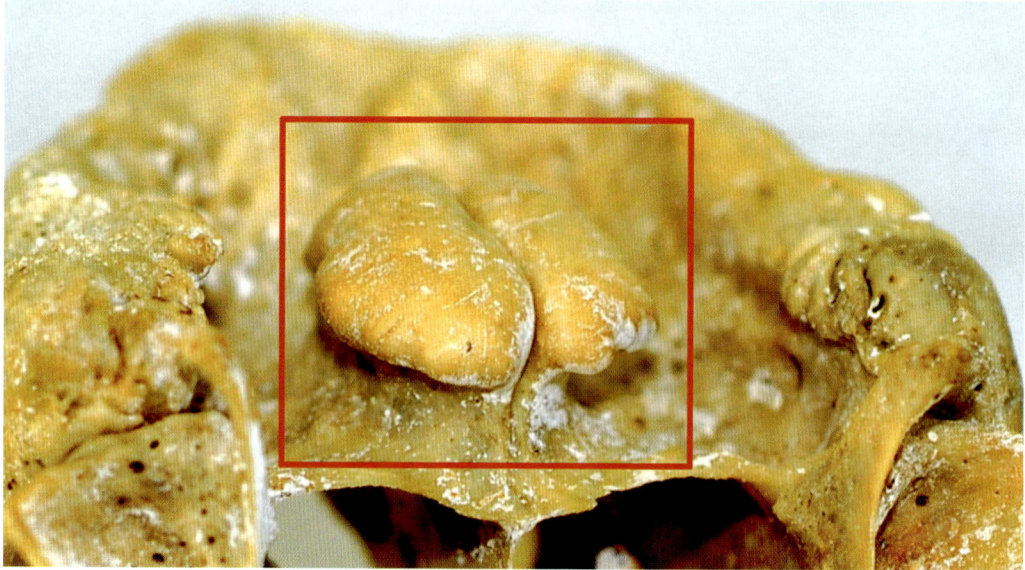

Figure 647. Large maxillary tori (torus palatinus) (rectangle) in a 54-year-old Thai maxilla (KKU). These tori are slowly developing tumor-like growths along the midline of the palate (Belsky et al. 2003). Common finding in some groups, particularly Asians. Cf. Garcia-Garcia (2010); Hauser and DeStefano (1989); Jainkittivong et al. (2007).

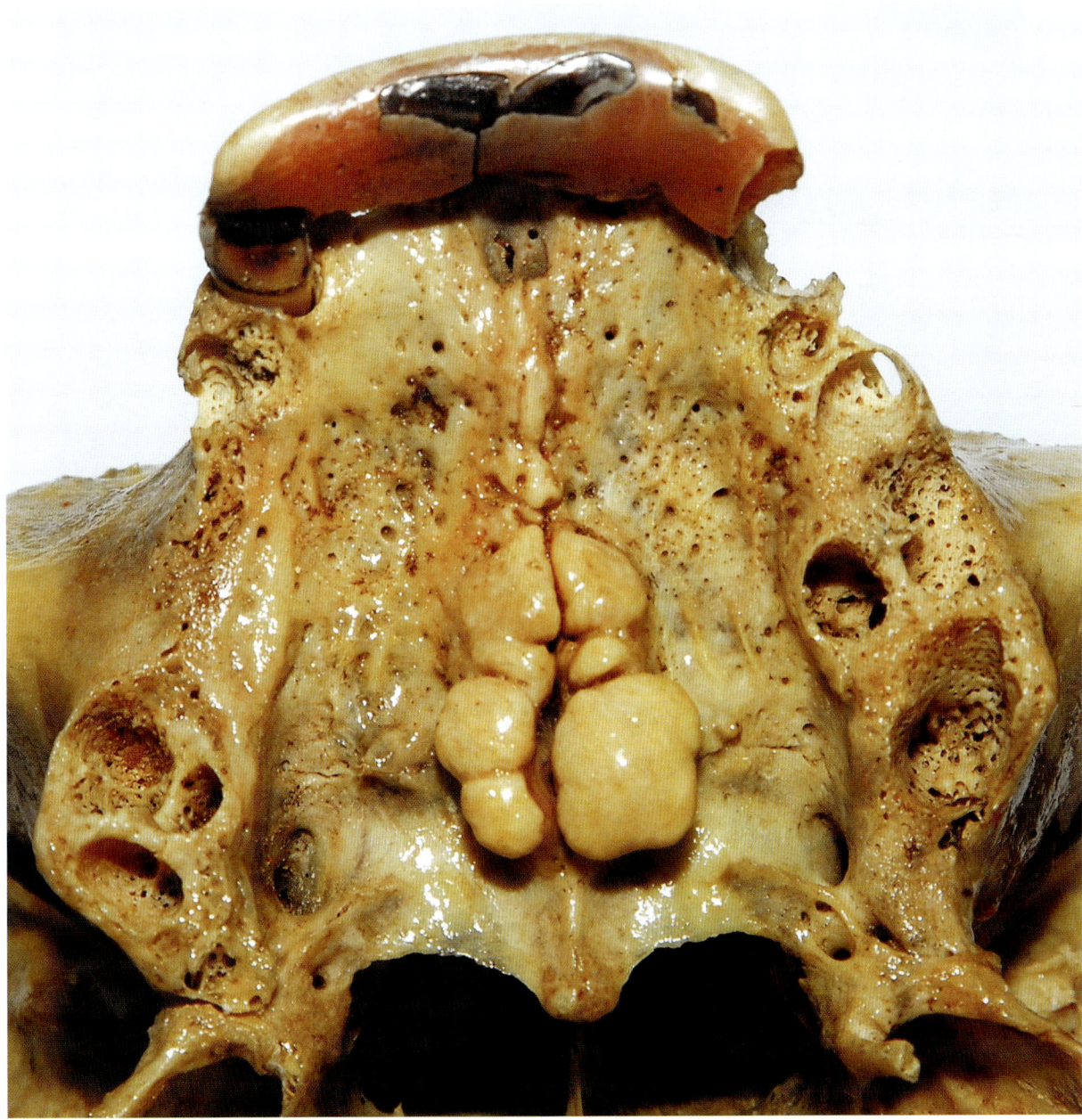

Figure 648. Cauliflower-like torus palatinus (palatal torus, palatine torusm maxillary torus) along the midline of the palate and an anterior dental appliance in an elderly Thai (KKU). Tori are common findings in some groups. Jainkittivong et al. (2007).

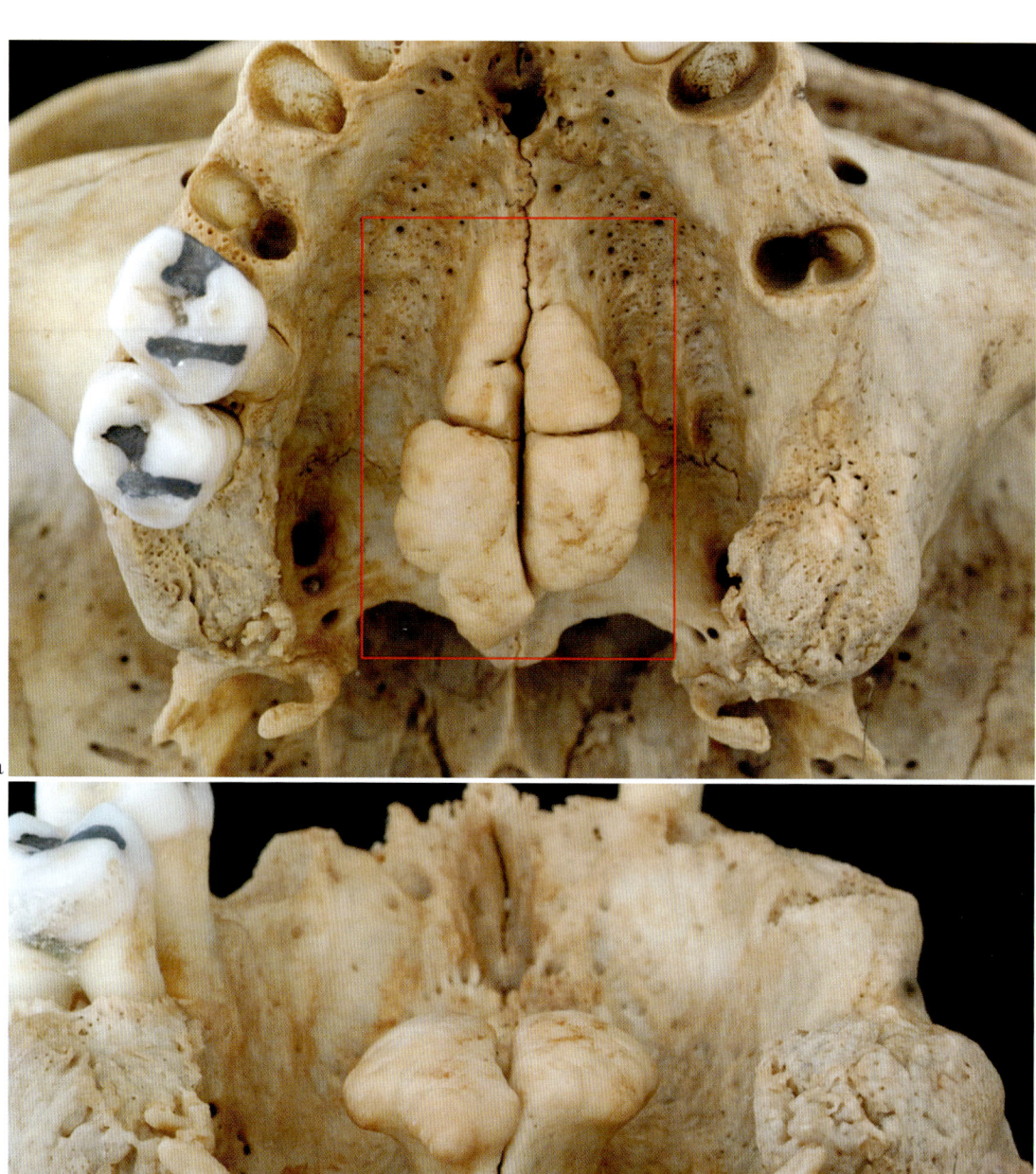

Figure 649a-b. Large torus palatinus (maxillary torus) in a 58-year-old Thai female (CMU 114 50). (a) A torus (rectangle) that consists of two lobules along the anterior median palatine suture and two smaller posterior lobules along the posterior median palatine suture. Also note that the corresponding sutures are open. Whether a torus palatinus alters the rate of closure and obliteration of the maxillary sutures warrants further research. (b) Posterior view showing the "mushroom" shape of the torus along the midline. See Jainkittivong et al. (2007) for frequencies in a Thai population.

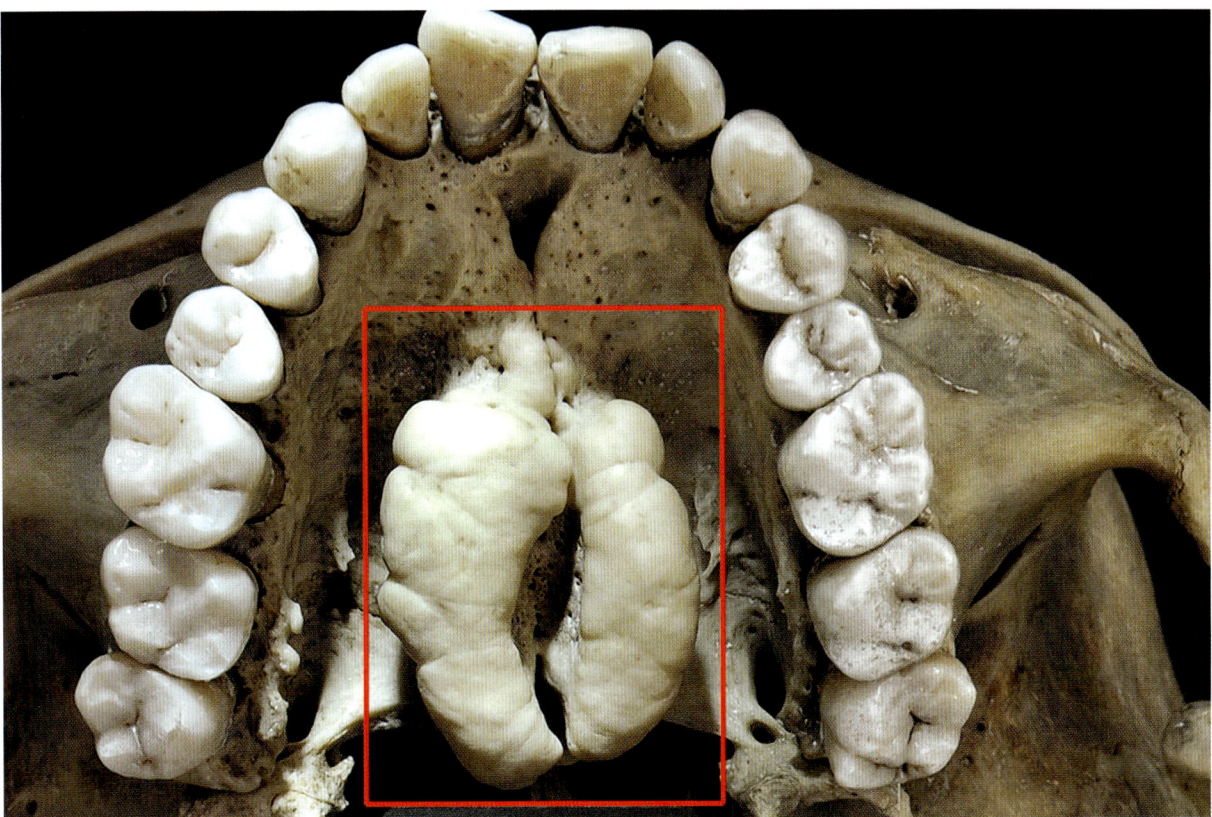

Figure 650. Unusually long and divided torus palatinus (rectangle) in an adult (MPIC, photo courtesy Nunto Sartprasit). Note that the suture between the two tori has obliterated.

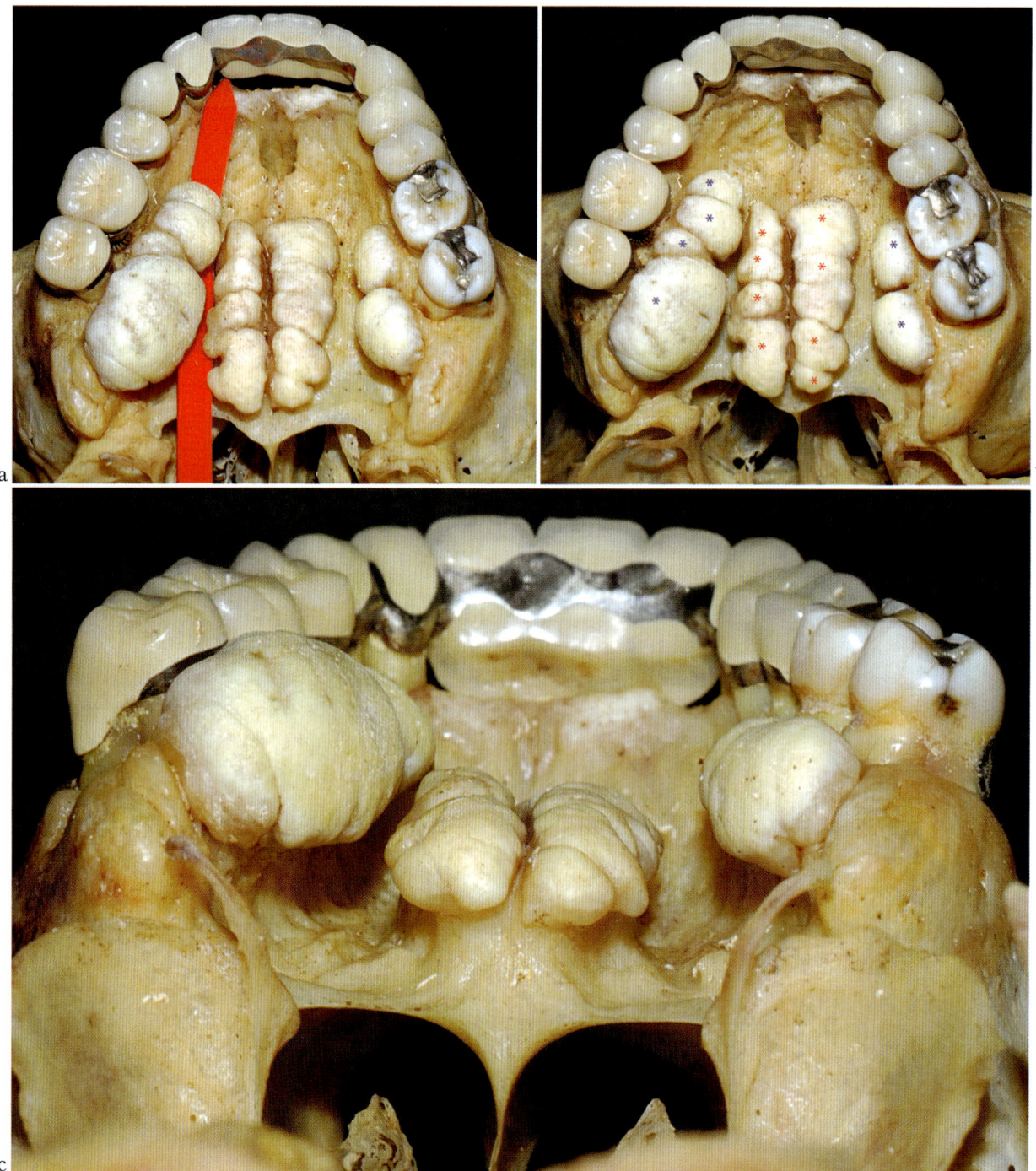

Figure 651a-c. Large maxillary tori or exostoses and torus palatinus. (a) Large torus palatinus (red asterisks) arising from the midline and lingual alveolar exostoses (blue asterisks) in an elderly Asian female (JABSOM 1367). (b and c) Note that the alveolar exostoses arise from beneath the dental crown and project, toward the midline (red probe), but do not fuse with the torus palatinus. The etiology of tori and exostoses is still debated, but appears to be multifactorial (genetics and environment), may begin to develop in children, are more common in Asians, and they typically increase in size with age. See Hassett (2006); Jainkittivong et al. (2007); Lee et al. (2013); Sisman et al. (2008).

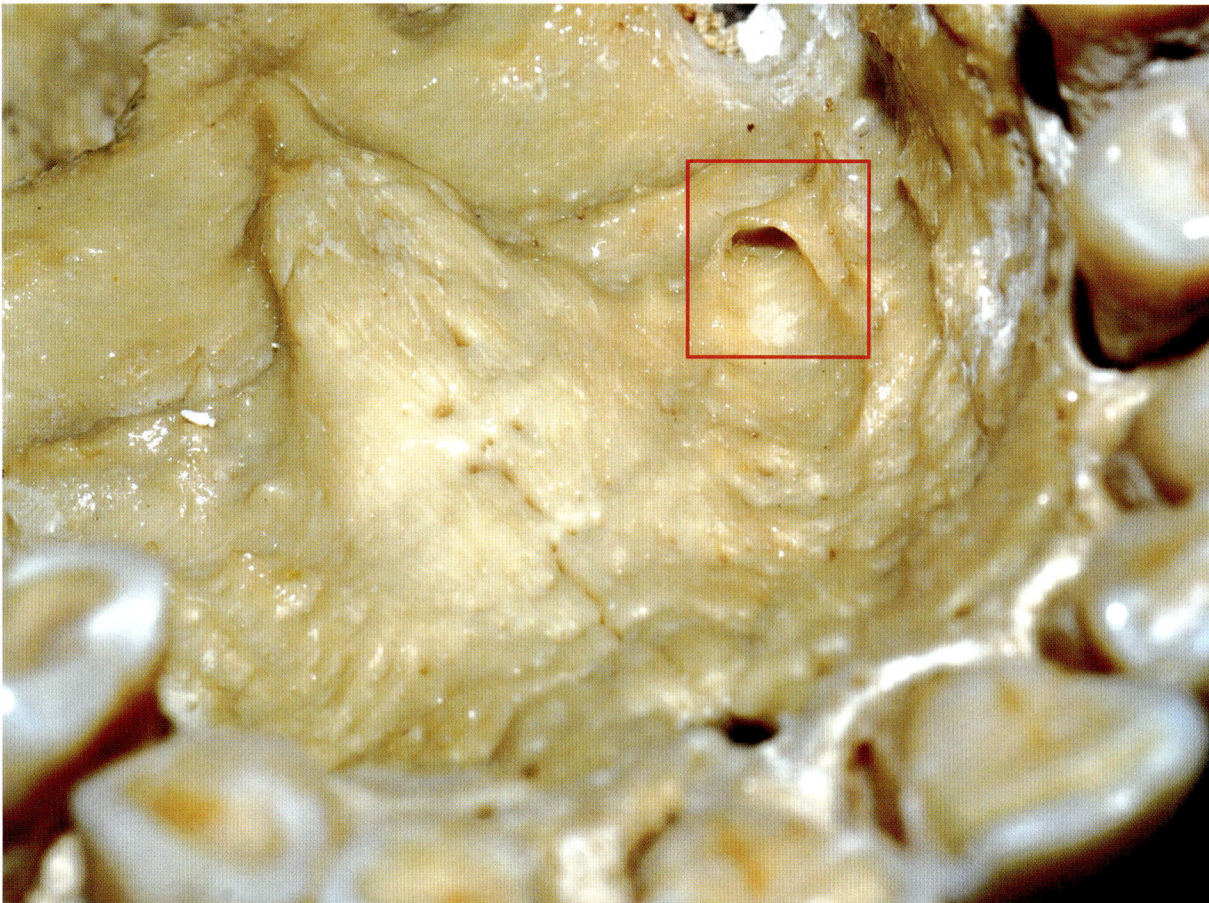

Figure 652. Palatal bridge (square) in an adult Thai maxilla (KKU). This common trait may consist of partial or complete bridging unilaterally, bilaterally, or absent (most common).

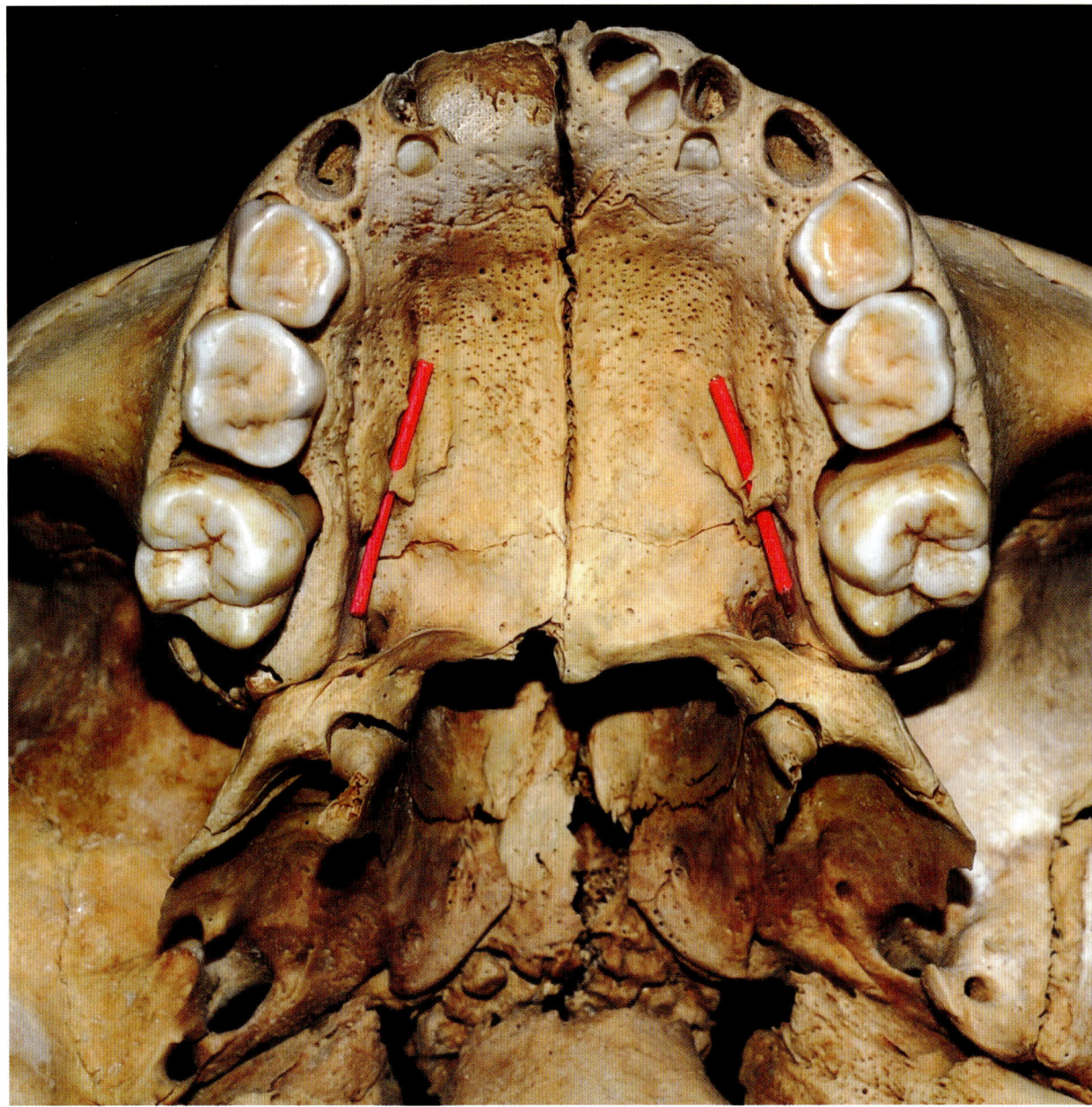

Figure 653. Bilateral palatal bridging (red probes) in an ancient Peruvian child (SI). Note the extreme degree of dental wear exposing the dentine in some teeth, open basilar synchondrosis, erupted first permanent molars (6-year molars) and gubernacular or "guiding" canals (eruption pathways) that will help guide the anterior adult teeth. Lee et al. (2001) noted palatal bridges in 2.2% of 320 palate halves (160 adult Korean skulls). Common finding. Cf. Jamieson (1937); Morris (1907); Orban (1986).

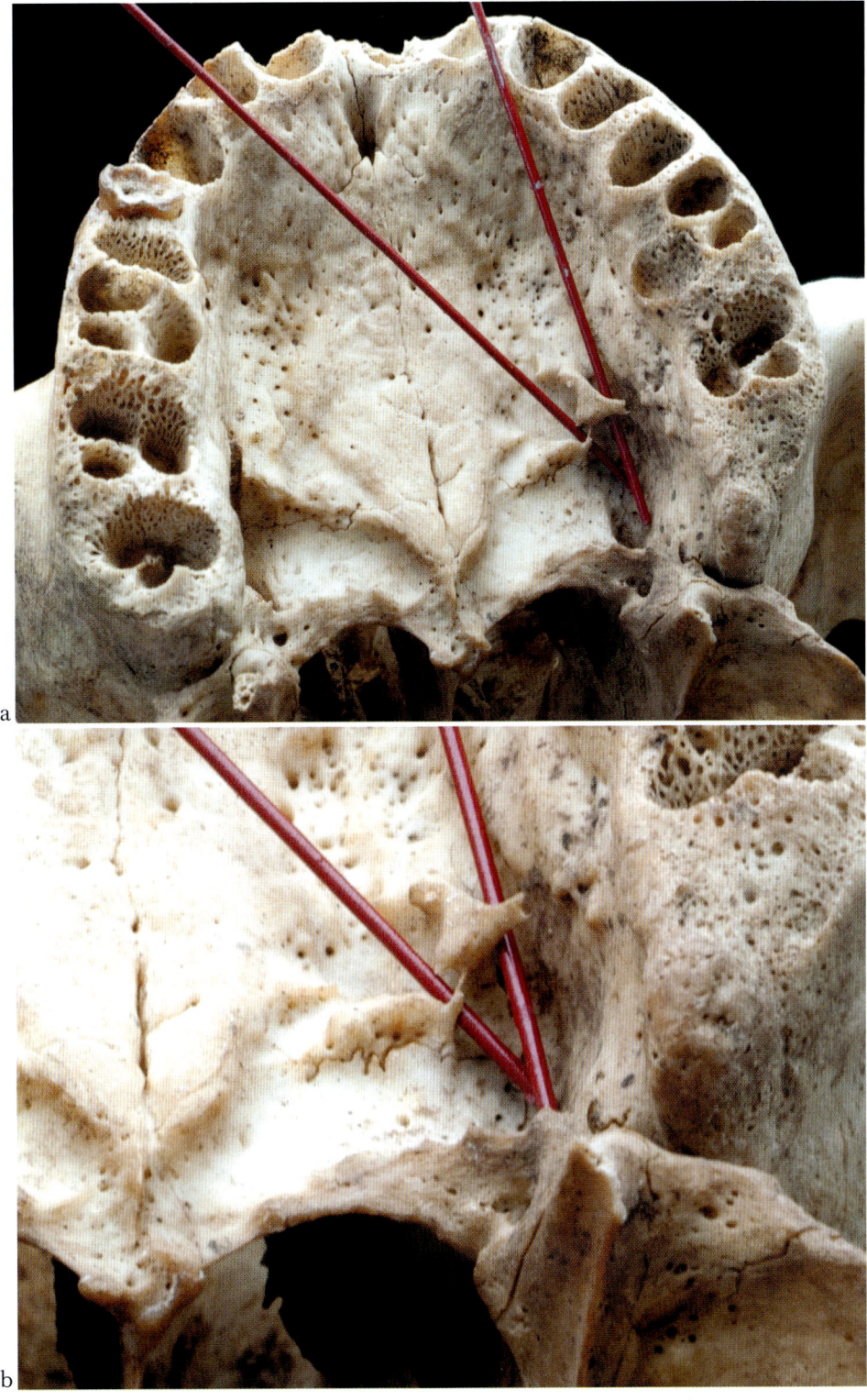

Figure 654a-b. Complete and partial greater palatine groove bridging (probes) in an adult Asian male (CSC AC029). (b) Higher magnification of the morphology of the small spikes (probes) of bone forming a partial bridge over the groove.

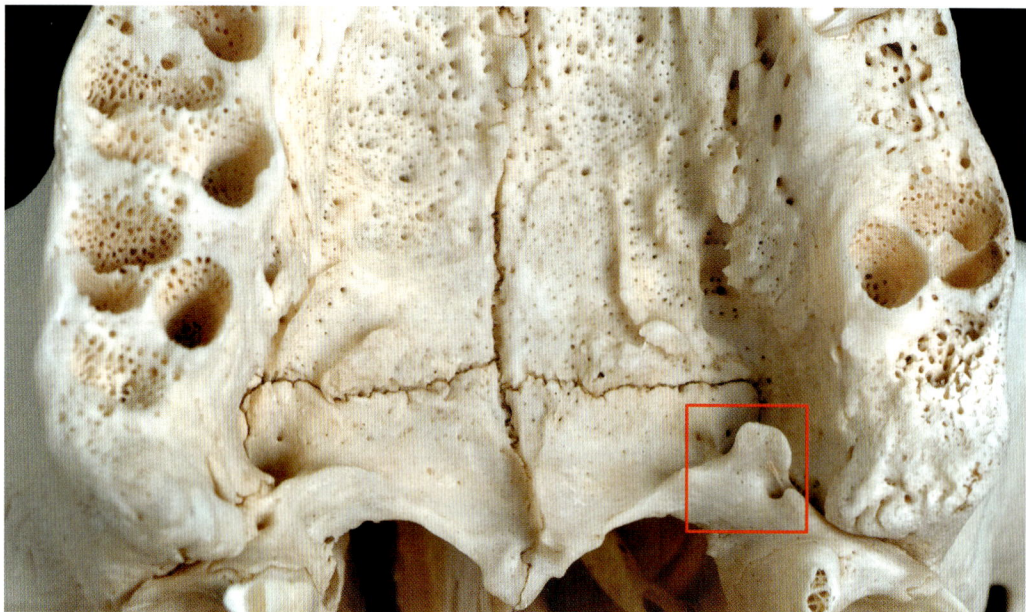

Figure 655. "Tag" (square) along the palatine crest in an adult Asian, probable male (CSC AC 026). Common finding.

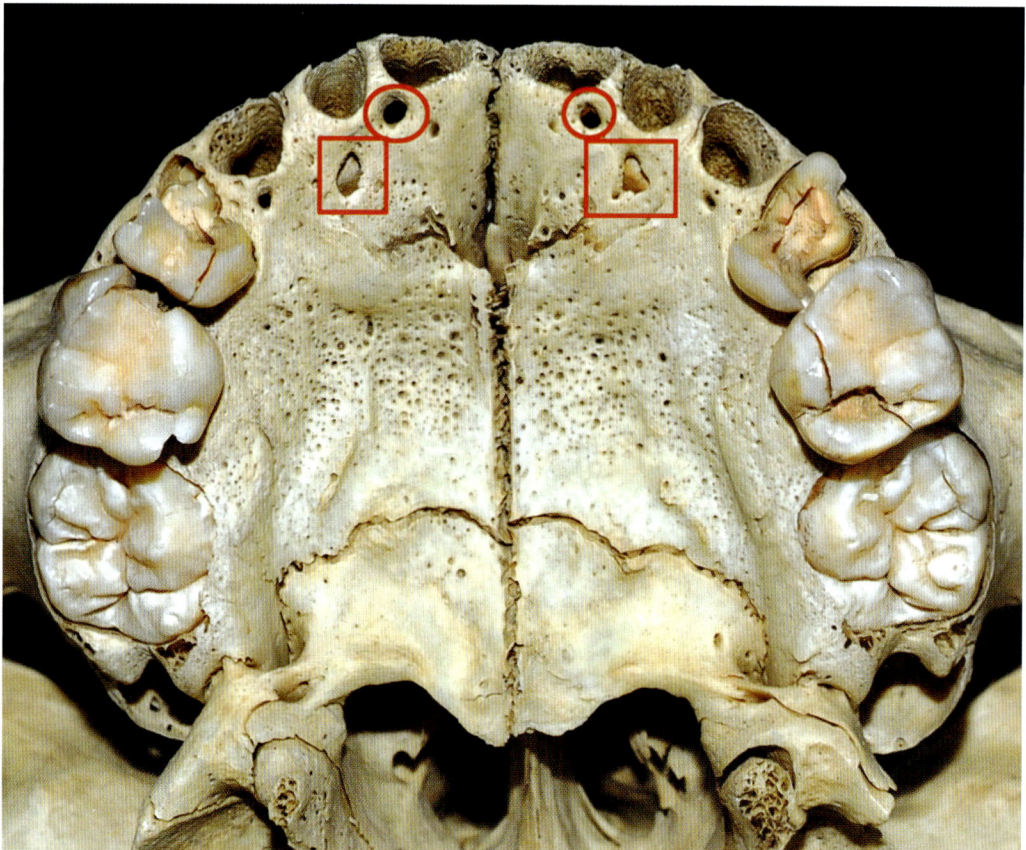

Figure 656. Gubernacular canals (circles and squares) in a Thai child (KKU). Note that the six-year molars are erupting. Typical anatomy. Cf. Morris (1907); Jamieson (1937); Orban (1986).

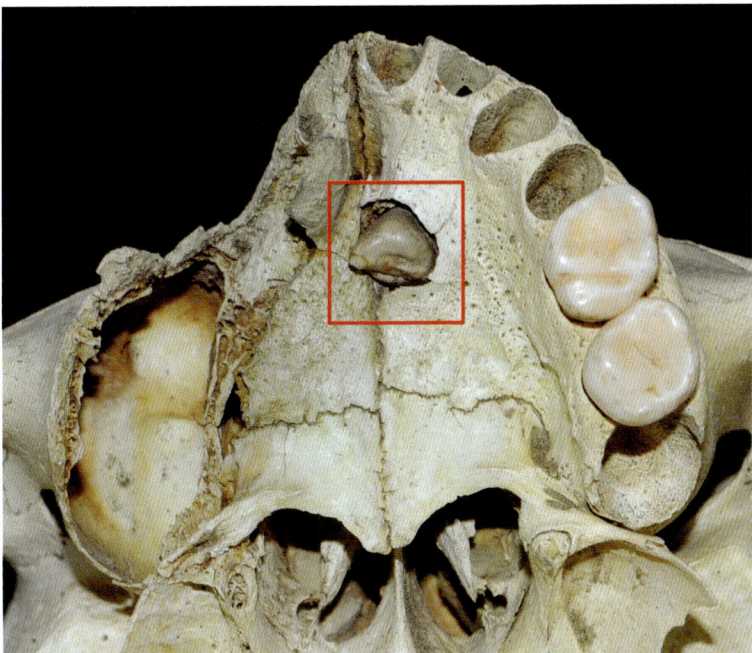

Figure 657. Child's palate with an ectopic canine, also known as mesiodens and odontoma (square) along the anterior median palatine suture in an ancient Peruvian (SI). Common to uncommon finding. Mesiodens are the most common (0.15 to 1.9%) accessory tooth (van Buggenhout, 2008).

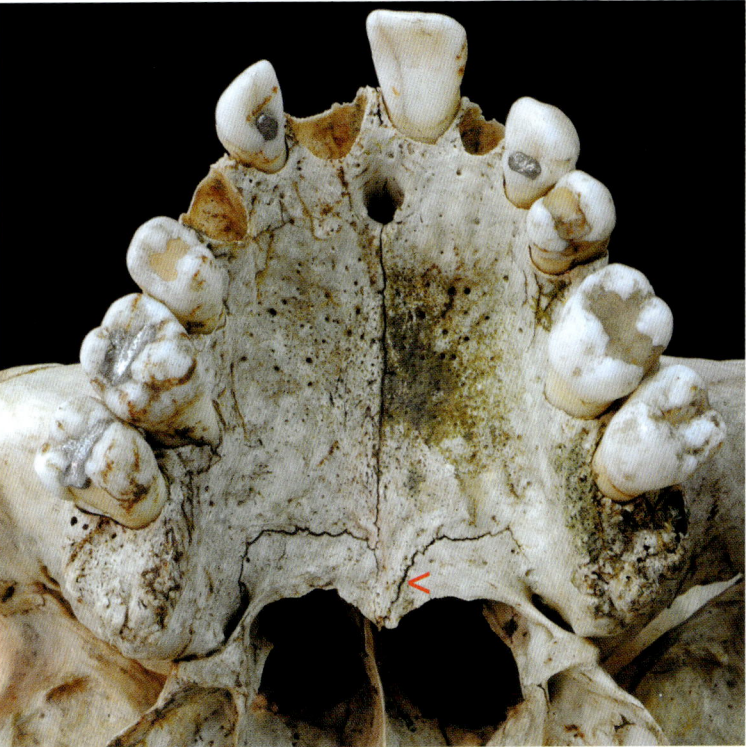

Figure 658. Rare deviation of the medial portion of the transverse palatine suture (<) in an elderly White male that terminates at the posterior nasal spine (University of Milan). Magnified examination revealed that this is not a fracture. This individual also exhibits what appears to be bilateral absence of the pterygoid hamulus.

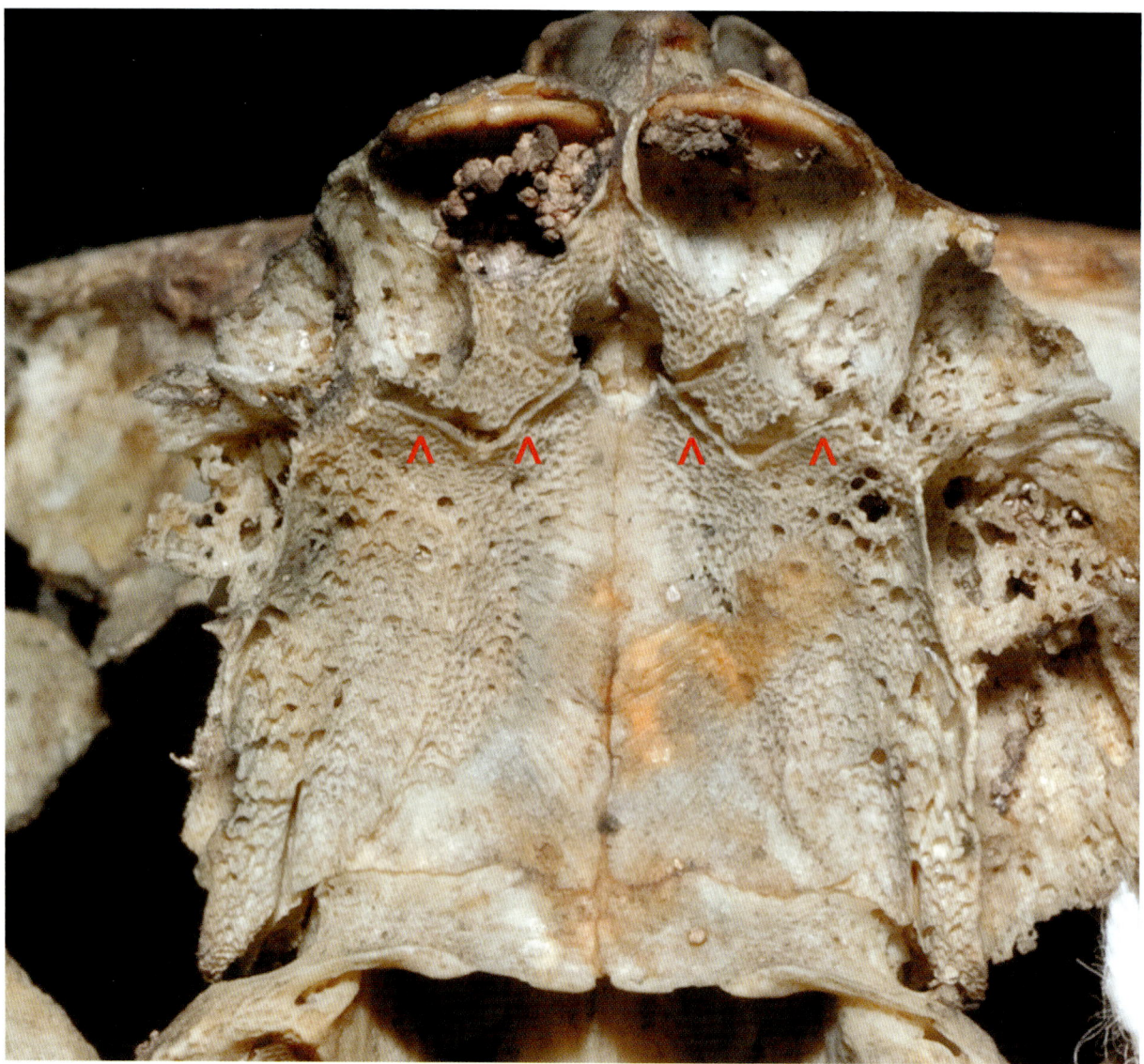

Figure 659. Maxillary sutures in a child – note the W-shaped incisive suture (∧) posterior to the central incisors and incisive fossa (Mütter Museum). Typical anatomy.

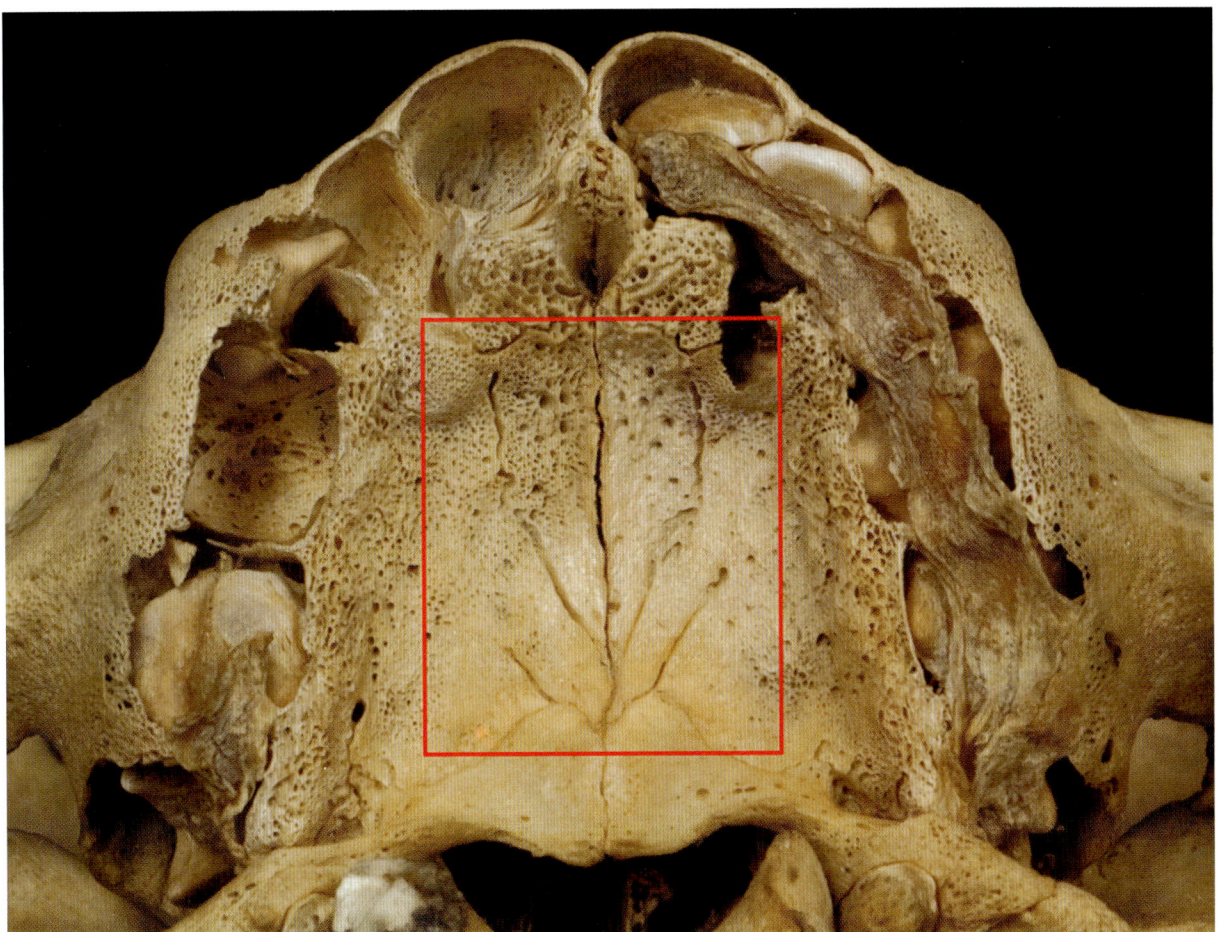

Figure 660. Accessory palatal sutures, also known as anterior medio-palatine bones (rectangle) in a child (Mütter Museum 1008.84). These sutures are uncommon findings at any age and are among the rarest of the cranial anomalies (Ashley-Montagu 1940). See Brothwell (1981) for drawings of anterior and posterior medio-palatine bones. Cf. Woo (1948). Rauber-Kopsch (1914) refer to this feature as Calorische Naht ("caloric seam") stating that it extends from the transverse palatine suture to the incisive suture and that it may fade, suggesting to the present authors that it is a suture and not a vessel marking. Rauber-Kopsch present an example (similar to Fig. 660) of "Calorische Naht" showing it as bilateral and symmetrical, but they do not provide information on how this feature develops or its frequency, other than it is rare. Although the age of Rauber-Kopsch's example in their Fig. 166 is not given, it appears to be a composite of an adult (developed third molar sockets) and a very young child (incisive suture has not begun to obliterate.)

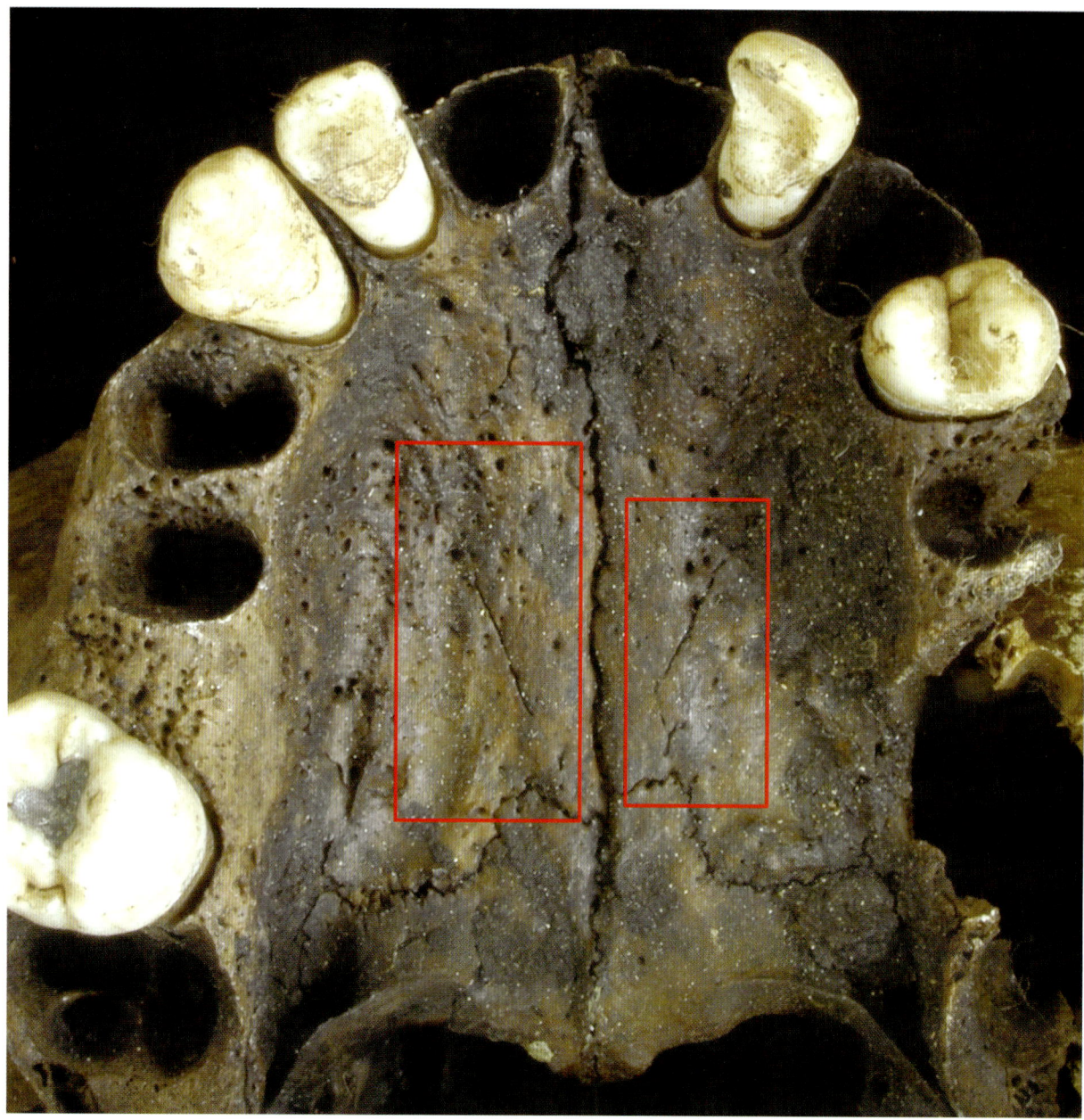

Figure 661. Anterior medio-palatine bones (rectangles) that have partially obliterated in an adult White male (CIL, Mann). See description by Ashley-Montagu (1940) and Zona (1935) and drawings by Brothwell (1981). Cf. Woo (1948). See Rauber-Kopsch (1914) for Calorischen Naht.

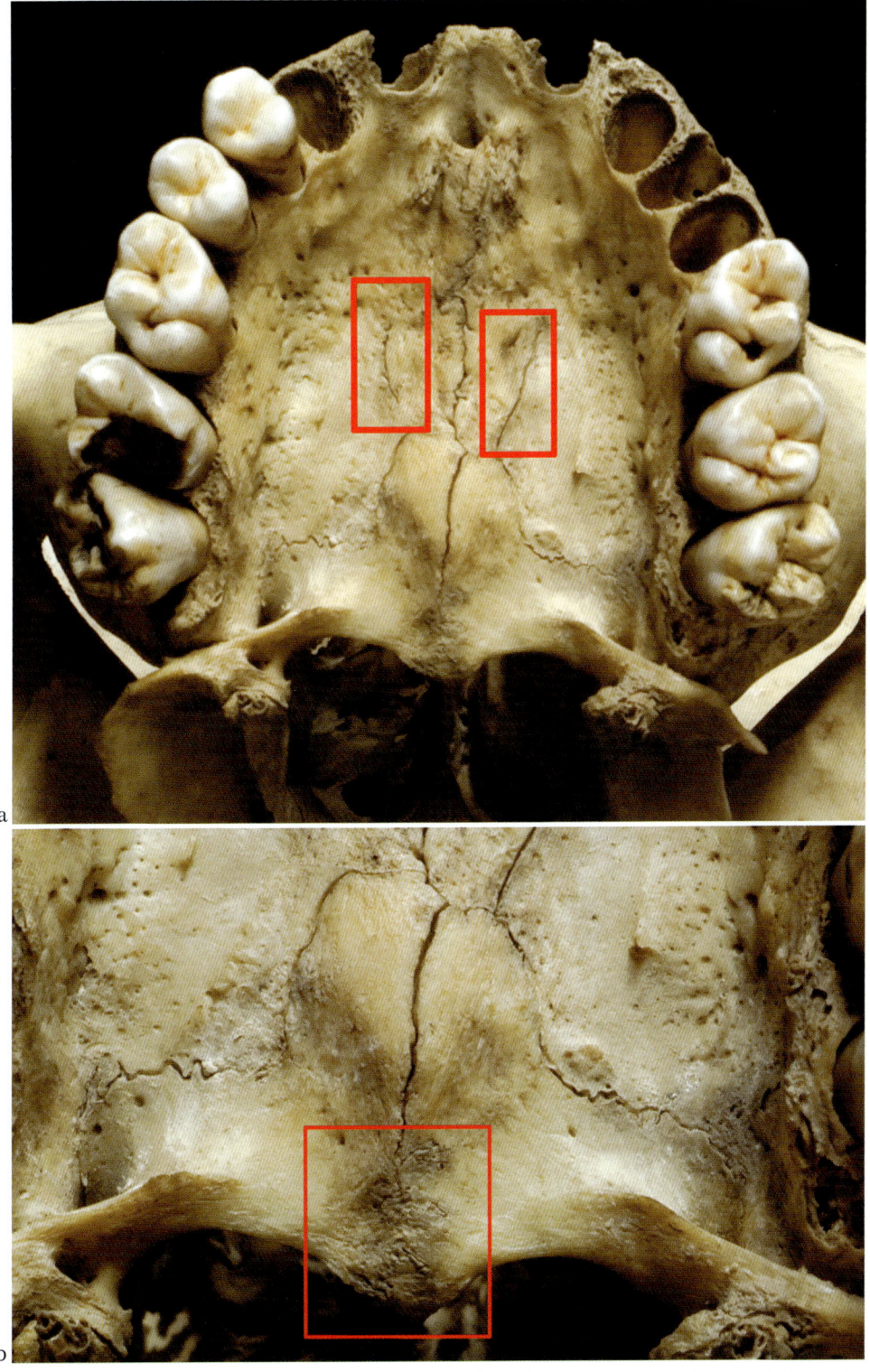

Figure 662a-b. Rare anterior medio-palatine bones. (a) Medio-palatine bones (rectangles) and (b) an unusually complex posterior median palatine suture (square) in an approximately 30-year-old adult with a developmental anomaly of the cranial base (UPenn L-606 98). See Ashley-Montagu (1940); Brothwell (1981); Woo (1948); Zona (1935). See Rauber-Kopsch (1914) for Calorischen Naht.

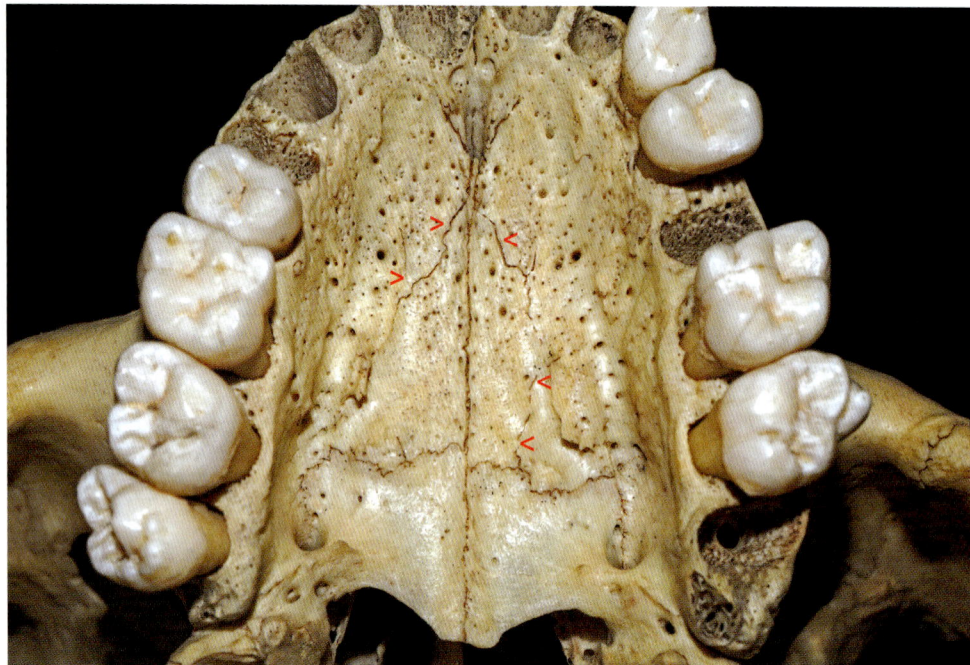

Figure 663. Rare anterior medio-palatine bones (< and >) in a young adult African (RV220). See Ashley-Montagu (1940) for early description of this trait and Brothwell (1981) for drawings. Cf. Woo (1948); Zona (1935). See Rauber-Kopsch (1914) for Calorischen Naht.

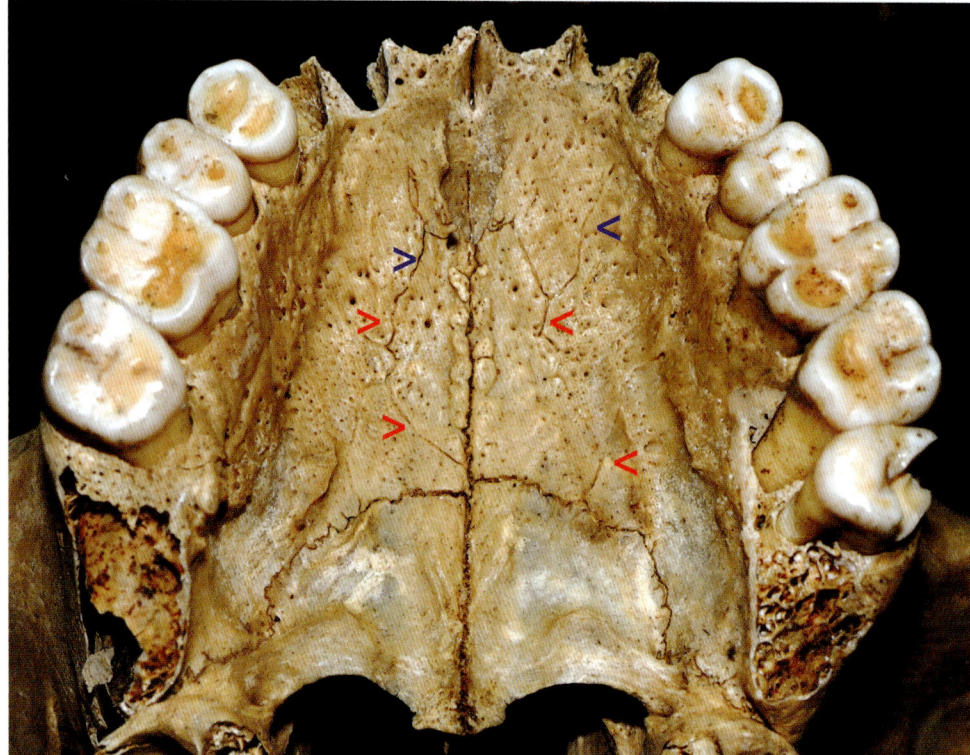

Figure 664. Accessory palatal sutures (red arrowheads) in a young adult female (RV1066). The blue arrowheads indicate the normally occurring incisive suture. Uncommon to rare trait. See Rauber-Kopsch (1914) for Calorischen Naht.

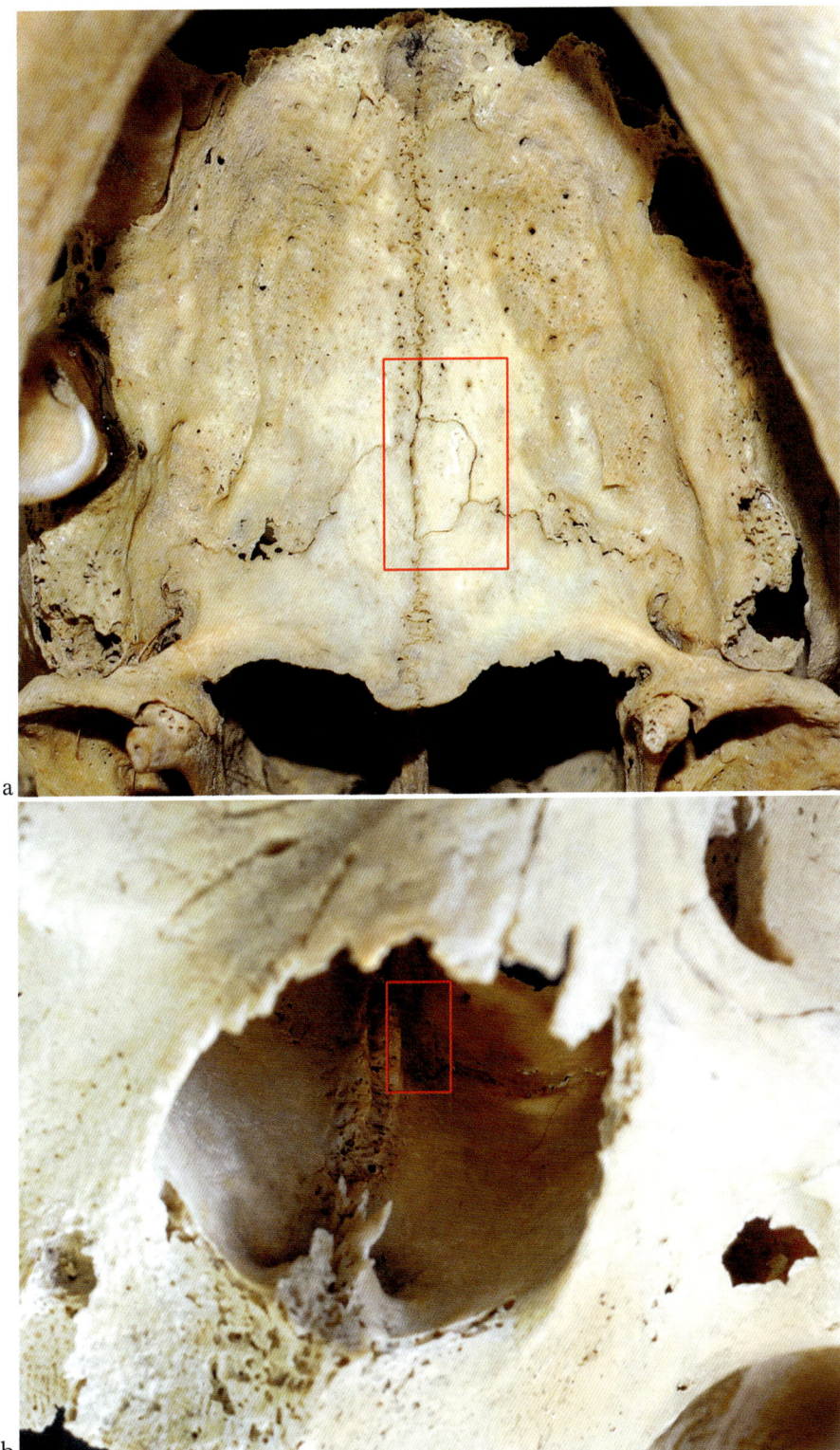

Figure 665a-b. Posterior medio-palatine bone. (a) Rare posterior medio-palatine bone (rectangle) showing its size and shape in the hard palate. (b) Partial obliteration of the suture (rectangle) along the nasal floor revealing that obliteration of the margin of this ossicle, at least in this individual, begins in the nasal aperture and not the lingual surface of the palate (M0001 0138 Freiburg University Archives). Rare trait.

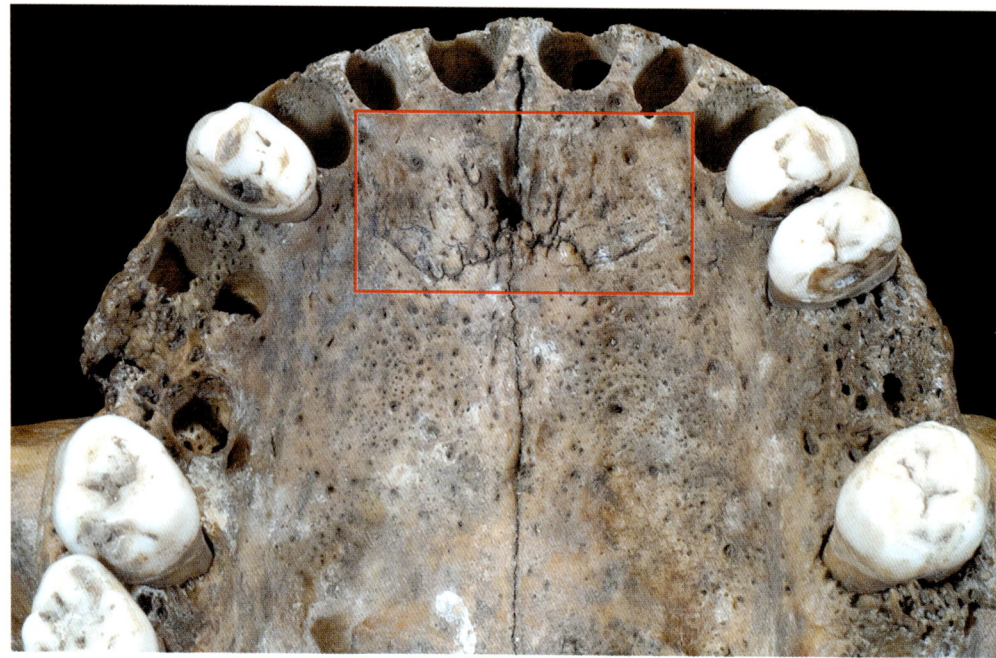

Figure 666. Unusually complex incisive suture (rectangle) in an adult Black (SI 244083). Uncommon finding. The incisive suture is W-shaped in children and obliterates by about 20 years of age.

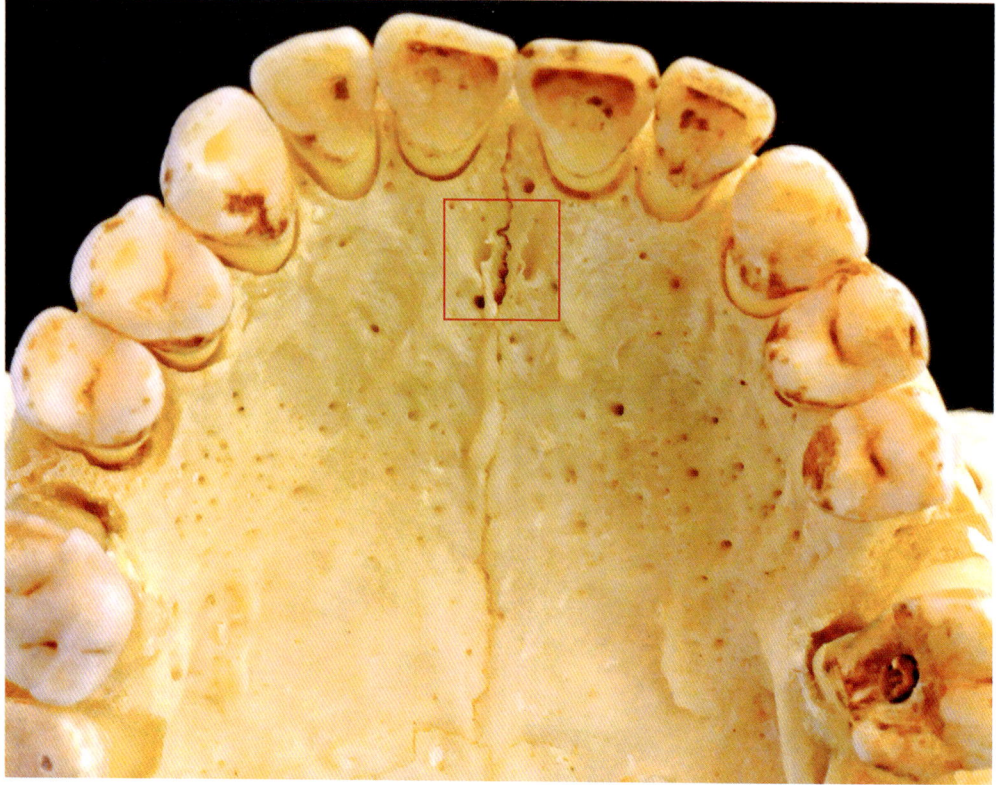

Figure 667. Possible atresia or congenital absence or an extremely shallow incisive fossa (square) and premature closure of the entire incisive suture in an adult (CSC). Rare findings.

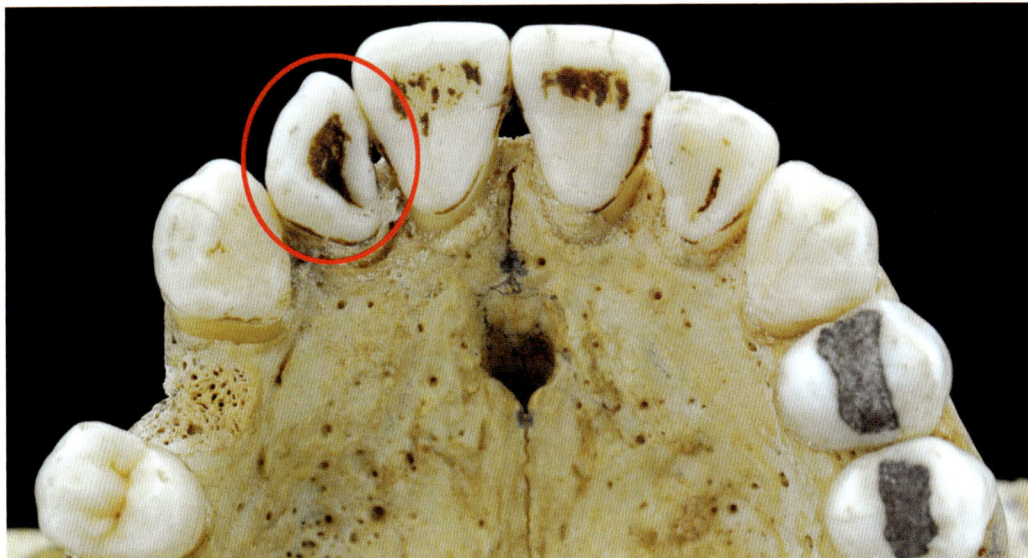

Figure 668. Shovel-shaped (nearly barrel-shaped, circle) right lateral incisor in an adult Thai dental arcade (KKU). Note the dental fillings in the left premolars, loss and remodeled right first premolaralveolus. Typical anatomical variant. Cf. Hrdlička (1920).

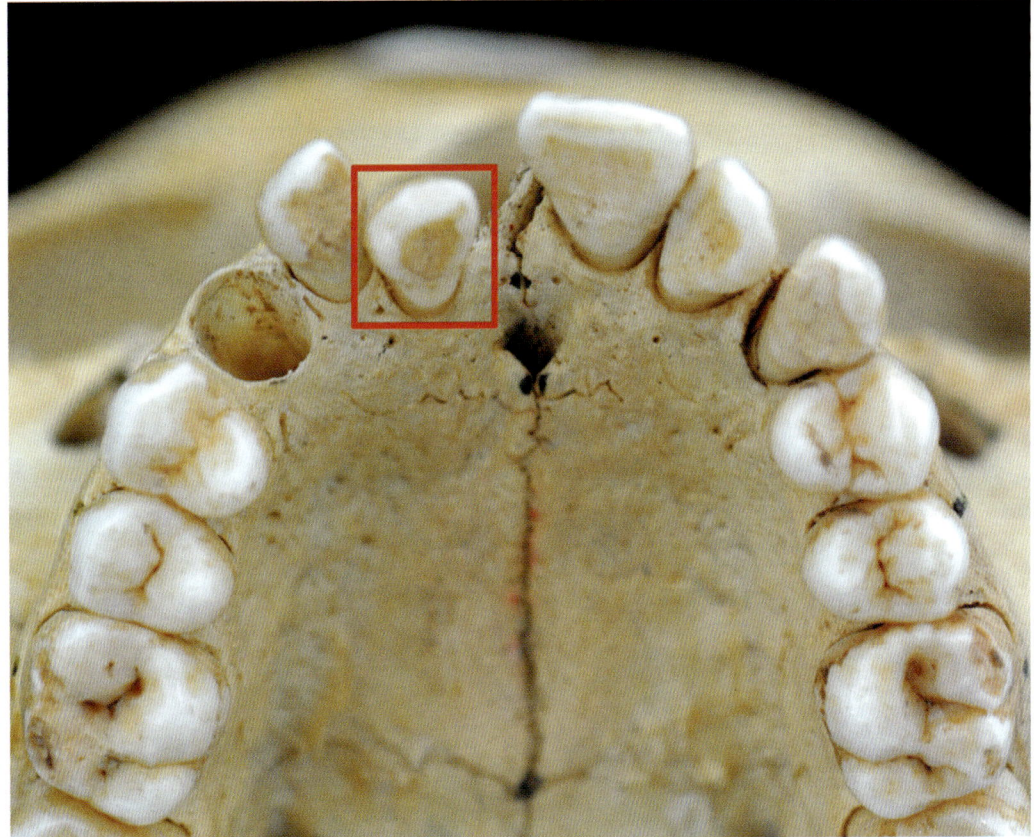

Figure 669. Accessory/supernumerary and misplaced maxillary right lateral incisor (square) in a subadult Thai dental arcade (KKU). Uncommon finding archaeologically, but common clinically.

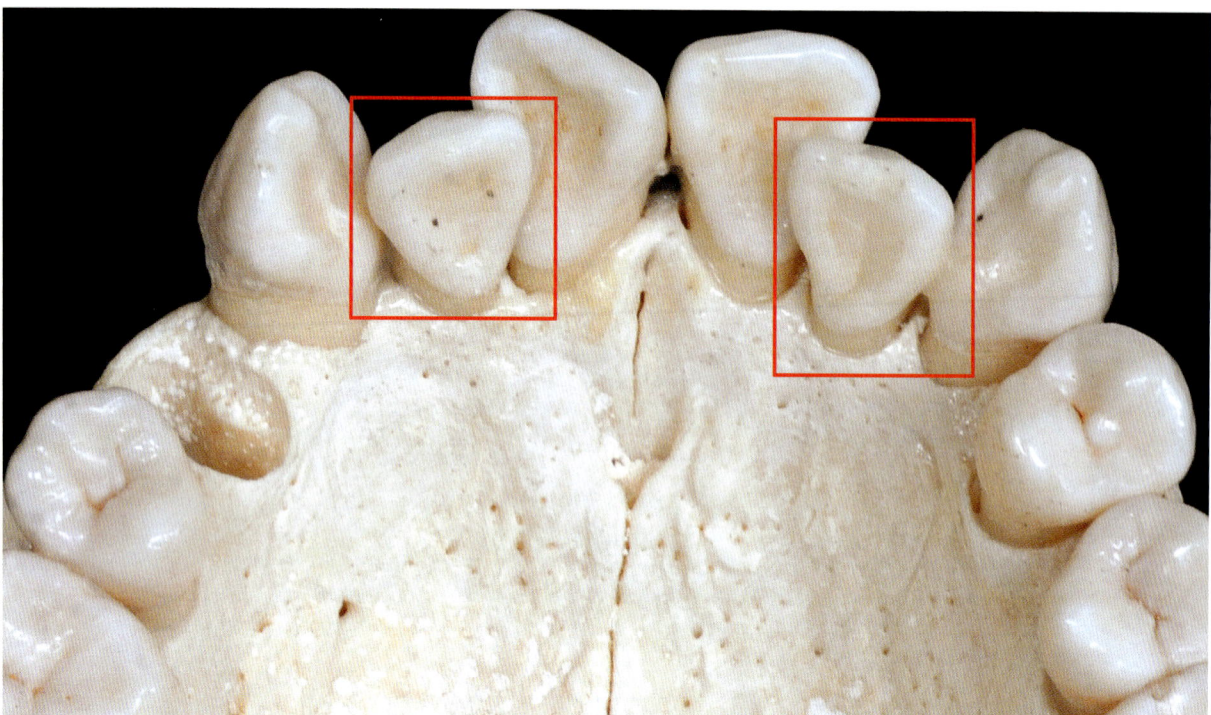

Figure 670. Bilaterally malpositioned maxillary lateral incisors (squares) in an adult Thai dental arcade (KKU). Uncommon finding in archaeological, but not clinical samples.

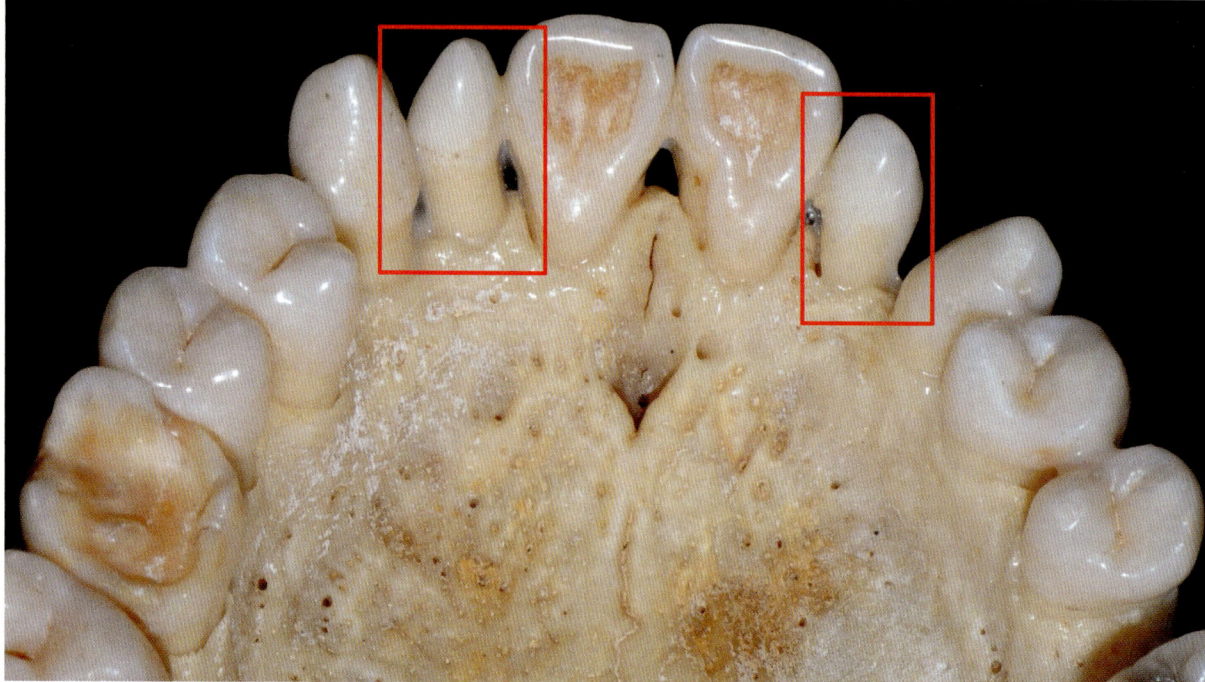

Figure 671. Pegged lateral incisors (rectangles) in an adult Thai dental arcade (KKU) (the White substance is a glue used to preserve the teeth). Uncommon finding.

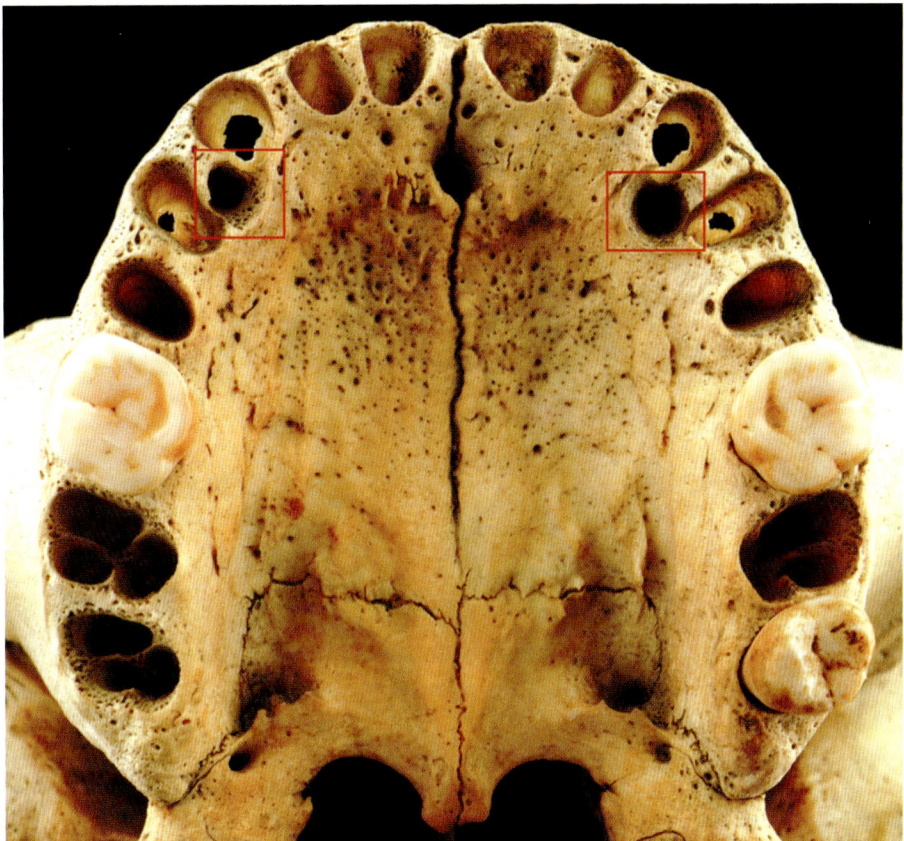

Figure 672. Alveoli (squares) for accessory canines or premolars in an adult Thai (KKU). Uncommon finding.

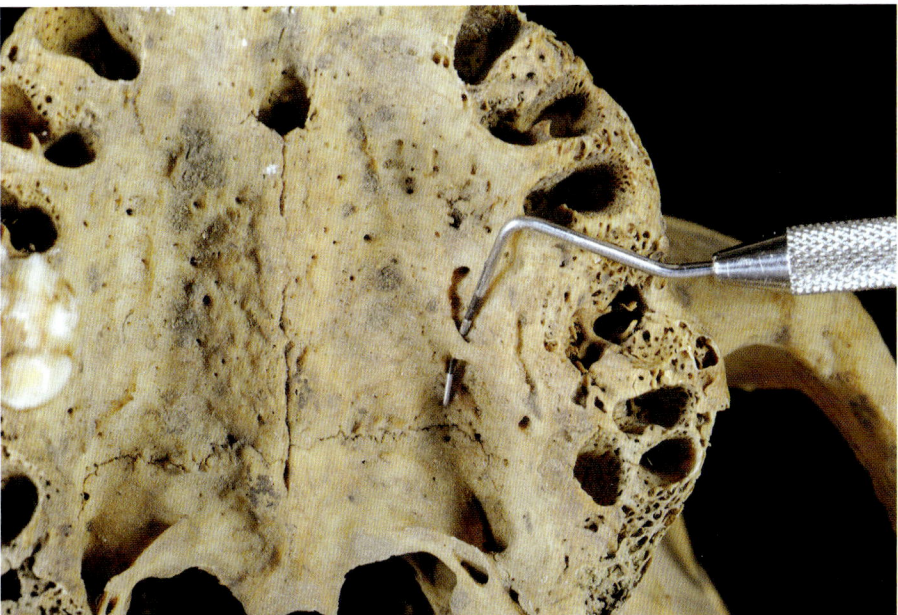

Figure 673. Maxillary/palatal bridging (probe) in an adult Thai (KKU). Common finding.

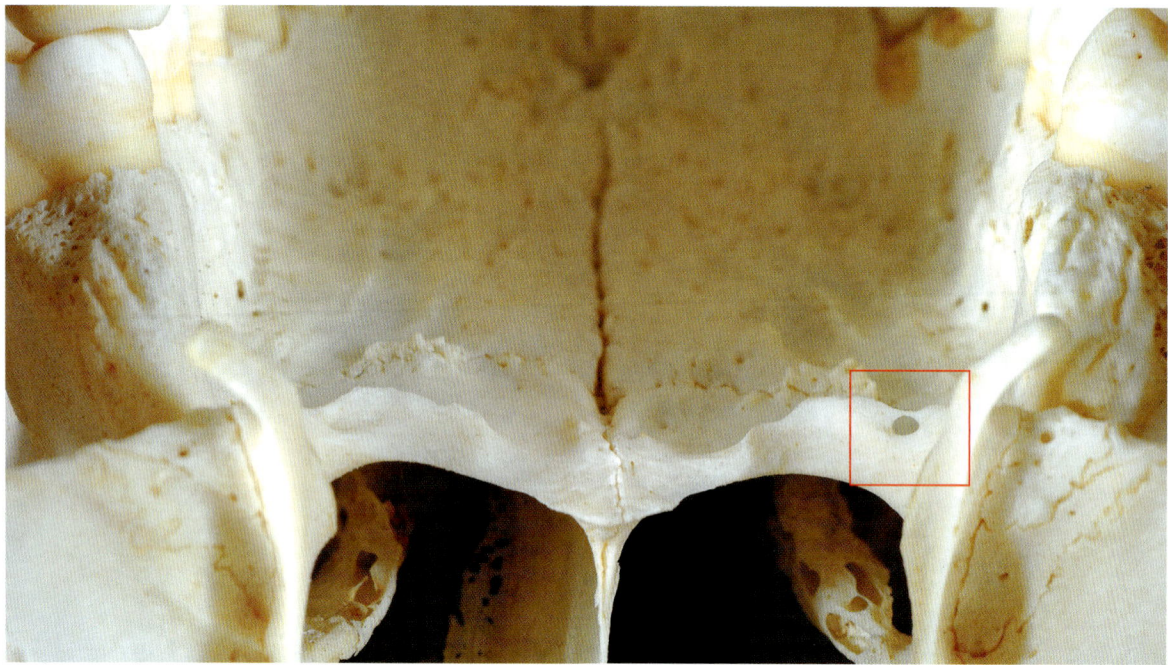

Figure 674. Unilateral lesser palatine foramen (square) transmitting the lesser palatine nerve, artery and vein in the left palatine bone of a young adult Asian male (CSC AS 005). Common finding.

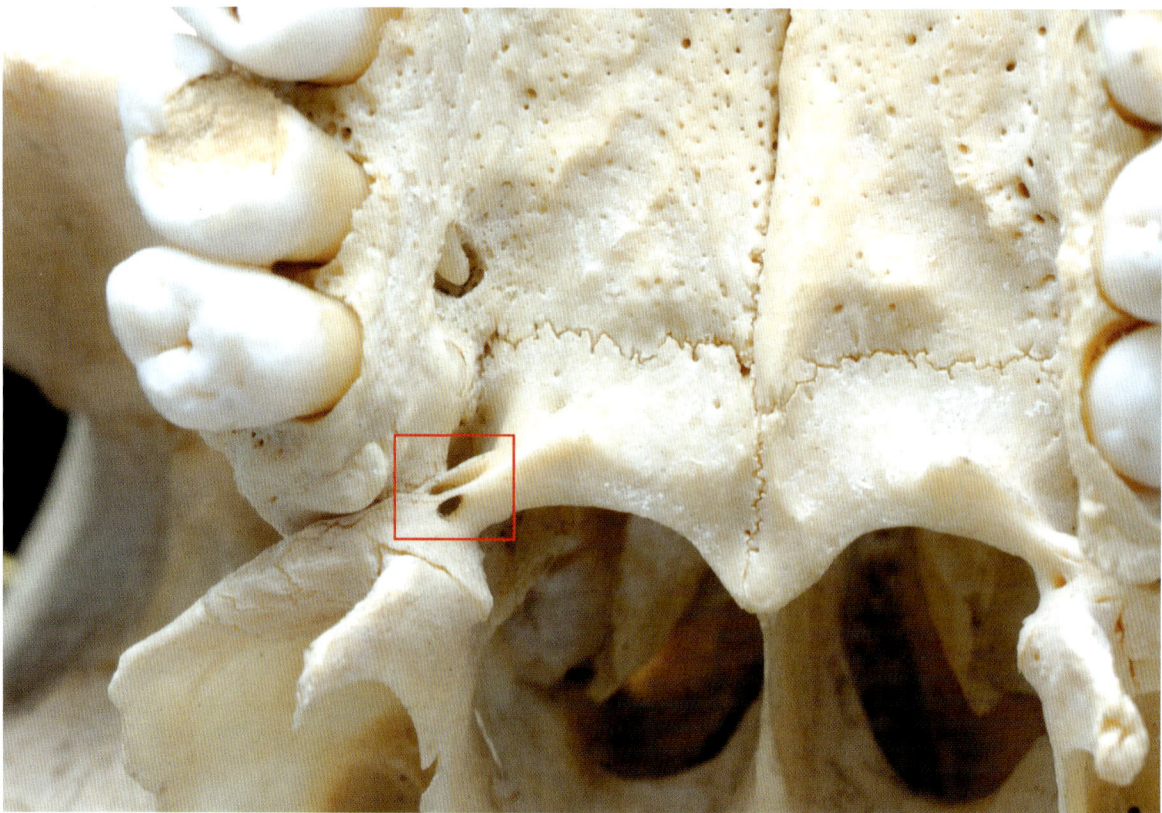

Figure 675. Double lesser palatine foramina (rectangle) in an adult male (FSA DS043).

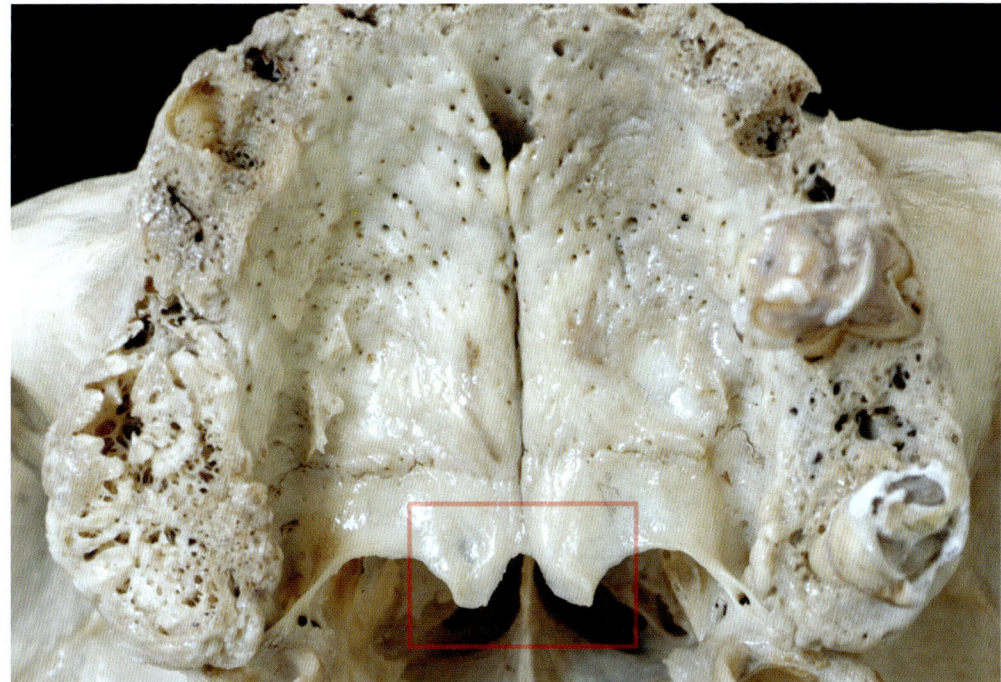

Figure 676. Uncommon but typical anatomy (usually single and pointed or blunt) showing bifurcated/divided posterior nasal spine (rectangle) of the palate (KKU 37-1587).

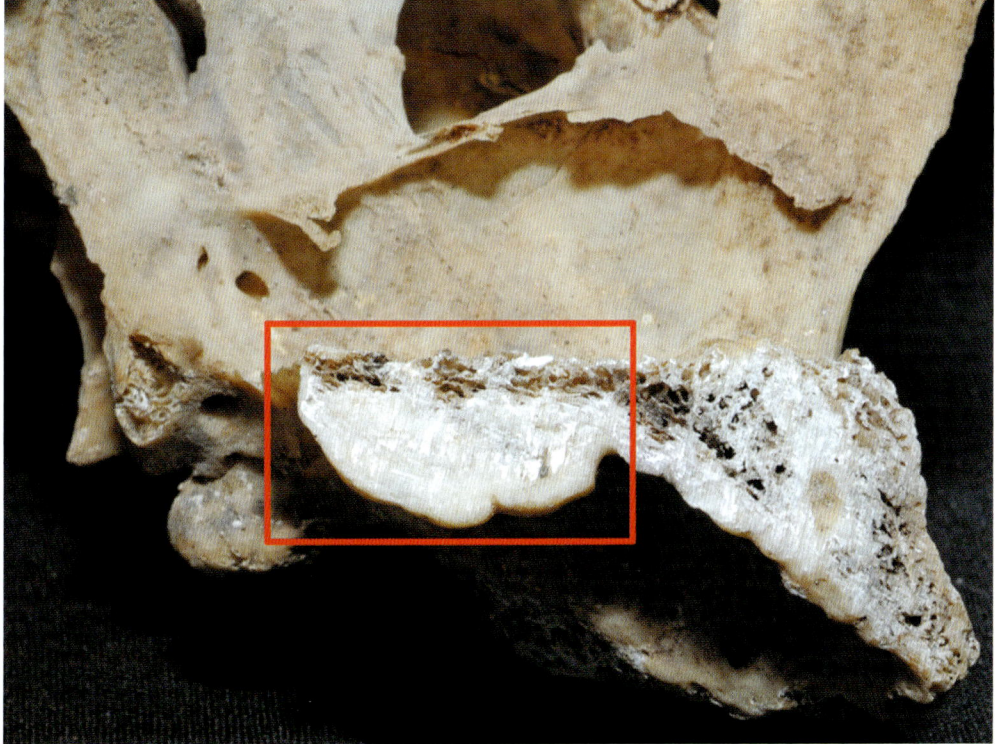

Figure 677. Cross-section through torus palatinus (maxillary torus, rectangle) in an adult Thai (KKU). Common finding in some groups. See Lee et al. (2001) for frequencies in Korean skulls.

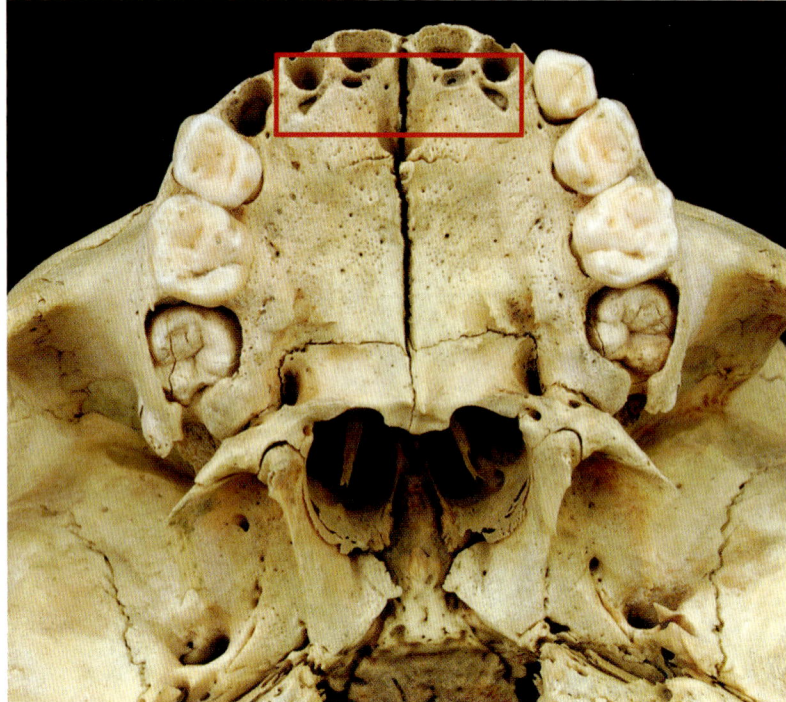

Figure 678. Gubernacular or "guiding" canals (rectangle) for the permanent anterior teeth in a Thai child of about 5 to 6 years (KKU). Normal anatomy. Morris (1907); Orban (1986).

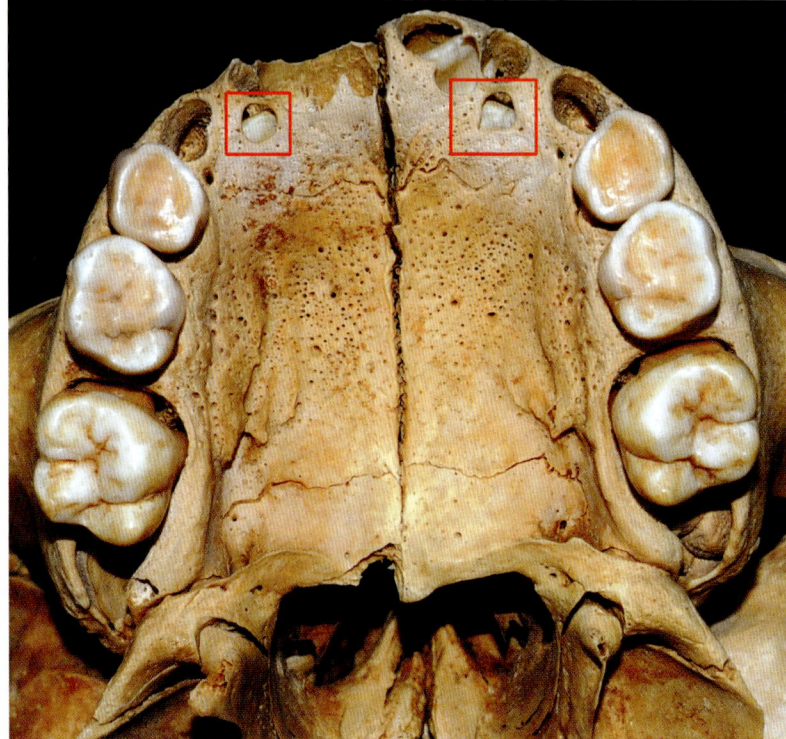

Figure 679. Gubernacular (guiding) canals (squares) in a child. Note the occlusal attrition on the deciduous at this early age.

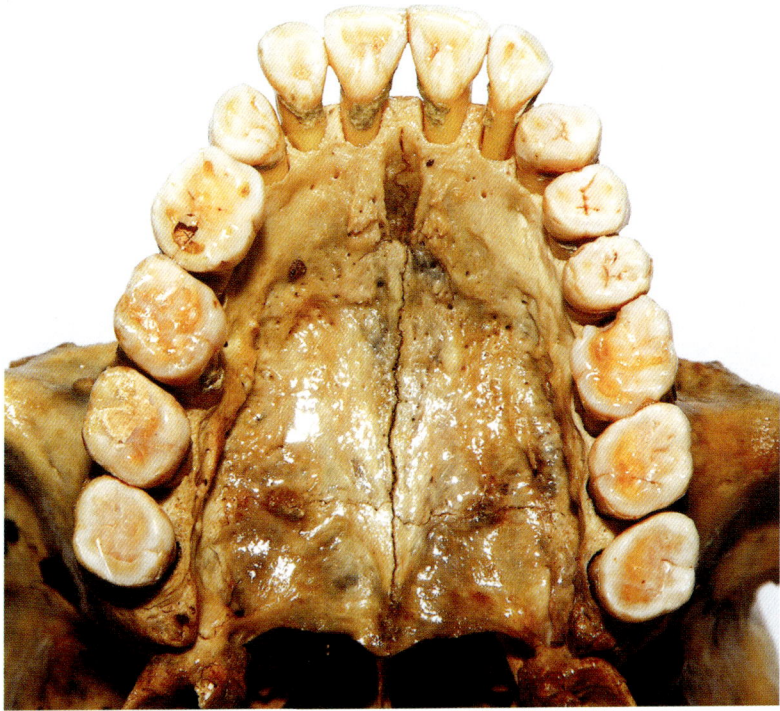

Figure 680. Congenital agenesis of the maxillary canines, the retention of the right second deciduous molar, and a supernumerary left premolar with a molarized crown pattern in an adult Thai dental arcade (KKU). Uncommon to rare findings.

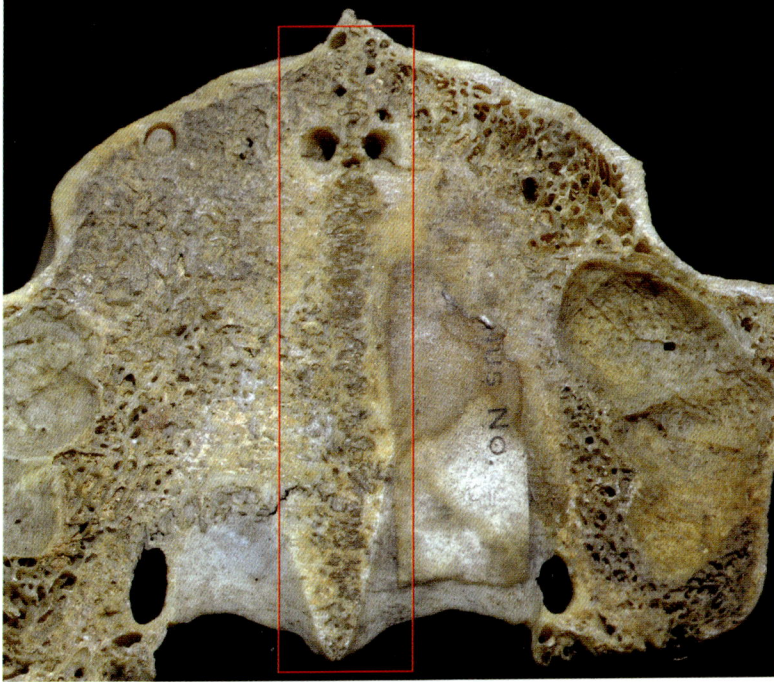

Figure 681. Transverse section through the nasal region of an adult showing the superior aspects of the incisive canal and palatal sutures. The anterior median palatine and posterior median palatine sutures (red rectangle) are faintly visible (Mütter Museum). Normal anatomy.

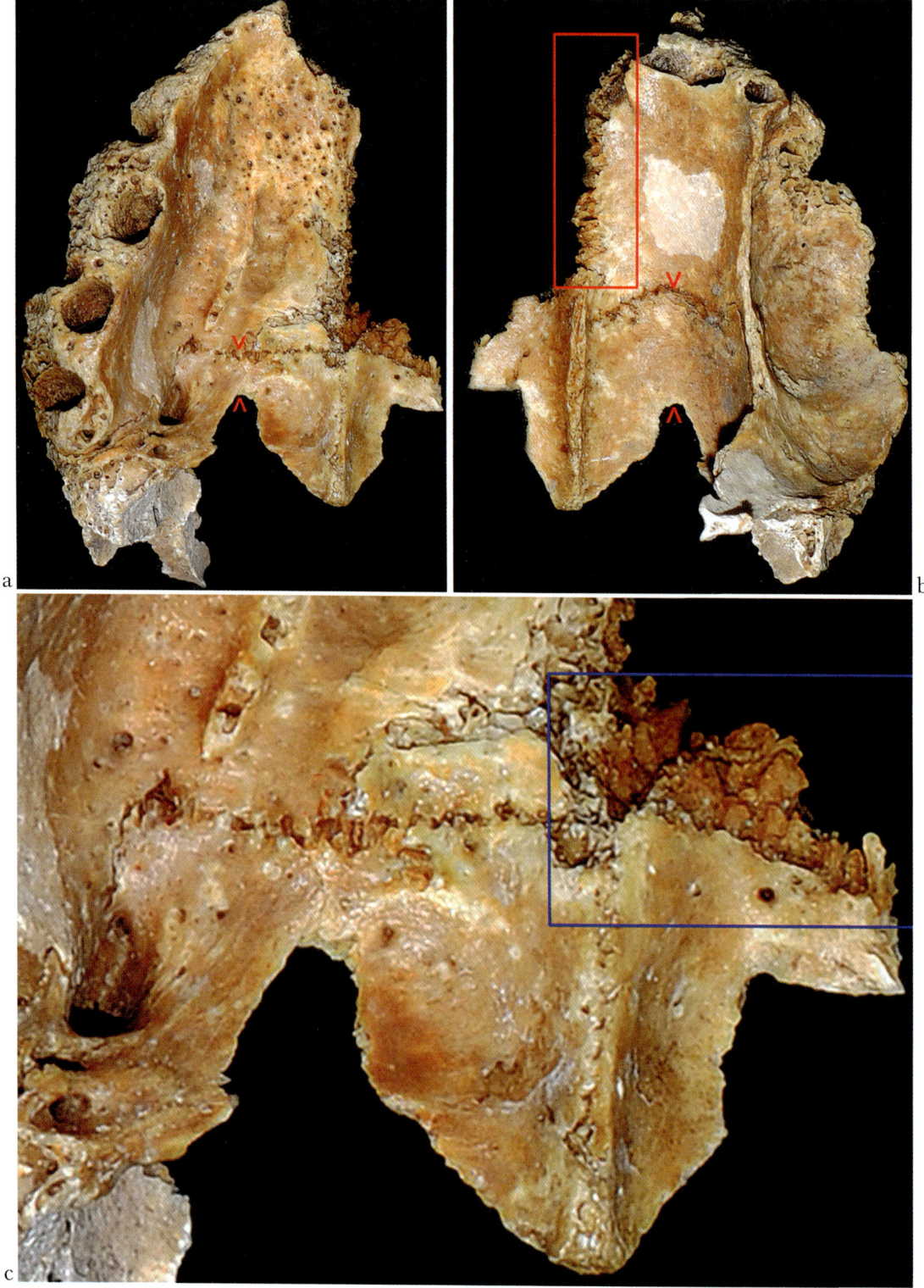

Figure 682a-c. Morphology of the maxillary sutures. (a) Lingual view of the transverse palatine suture showing that its distance from the posterior border (broken postmortem) is shorter on the lingual side than the nasal side (b) reflecting the approximately 45-degree angle (rectangle) of this suture (bottom). The distance between the arrowheads (a) is 3.18 mm and the distance between the same points on the nasal side (b) is 10.11 mm. (c) The rectangle is the median palatine suture in this teaching specimen. Typical anatomy.

Mandible and Teeth, Hyoid, Maxilla and Teeth 519

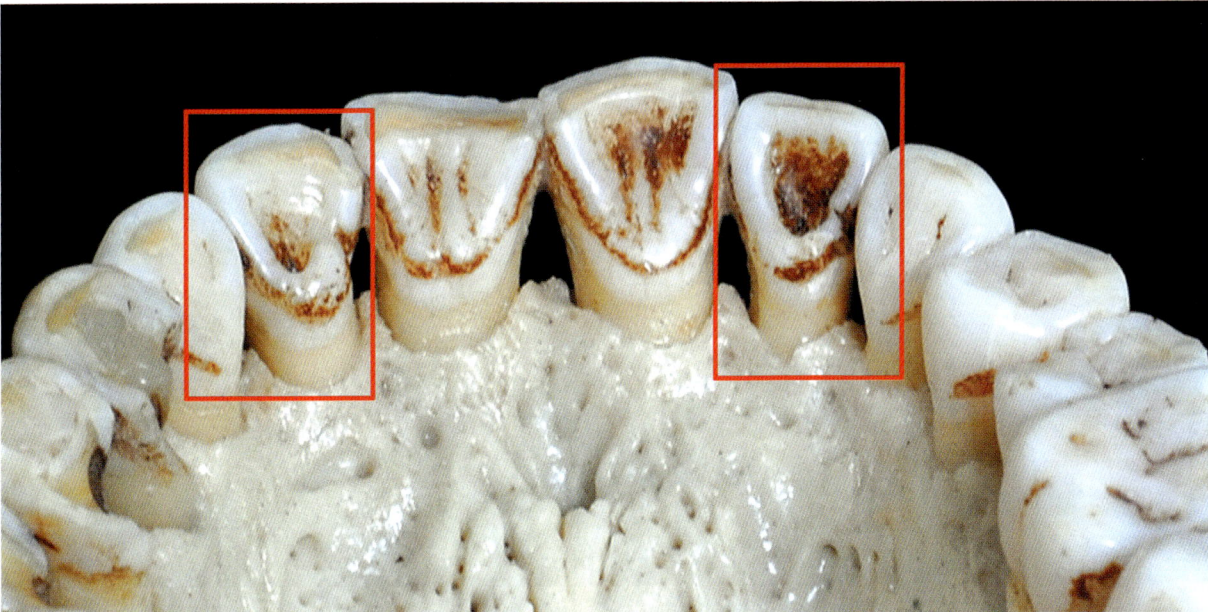

Figure 683. Shovel-shaped lateral maxillary incisors (rectangles). Note the vertical ridge in the central incisors in an adult Thai (KKU). Uncommon finding in most groups. Cf. Hrdlička (1920).

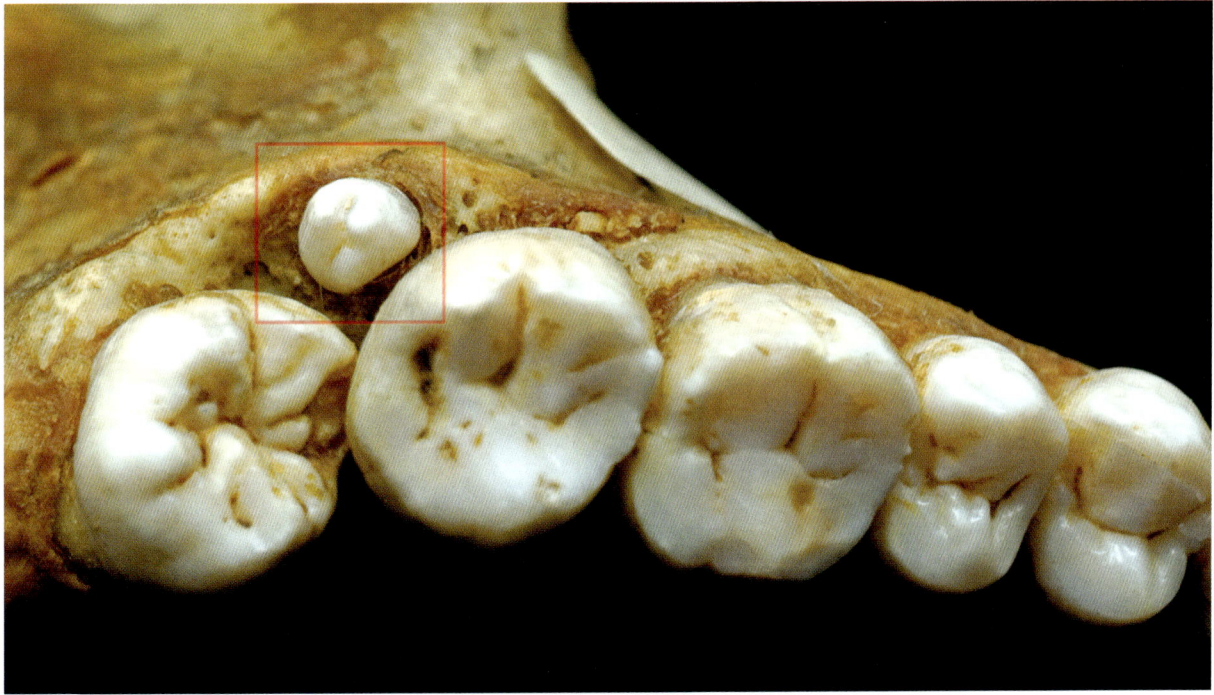

Figure 684. Supernumerary (hyperdontia) pegged tooth between the right second and third maxillary molars in an adult male (Mütter Museum).

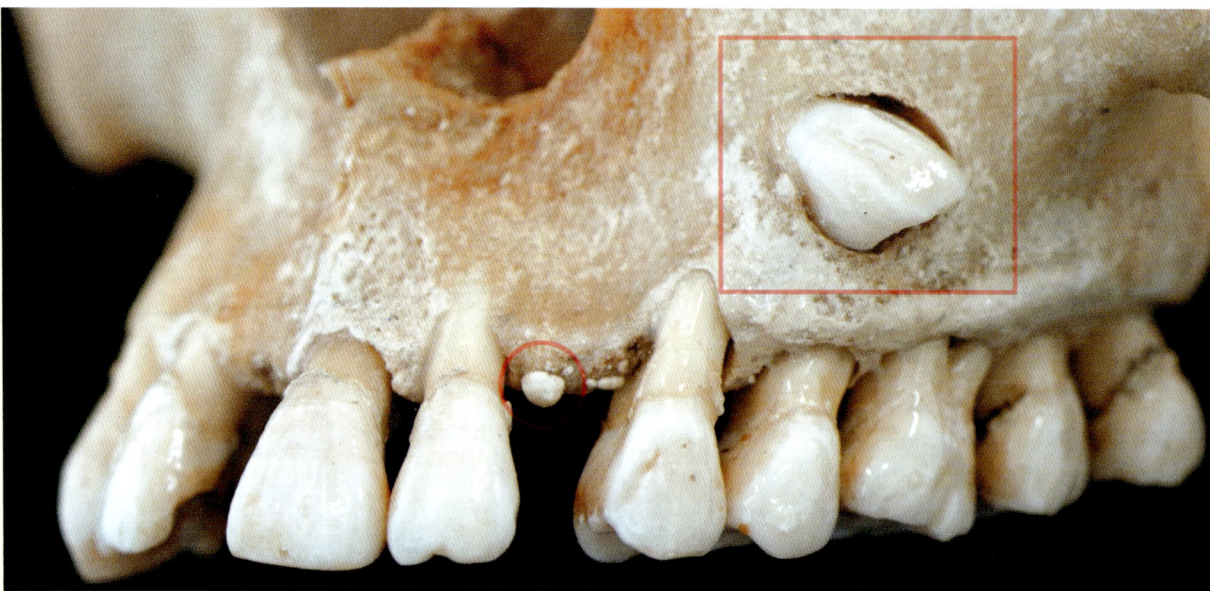

Figure 685. Malpositioned/ectopic left canine tooth (rectangle) and several enamel remnants (possible odontoma) (circle) in the diastema/space created by the repositioned left canine (KKU 42-3734). Note the wide diastema between the central incisors and the grooved incisal edge of the left lateral incisor. Odontomas are uncommon findings in most osteological collections.

Chapter 9

SHOULDER, ARM AND HAND
(CLAVICLE, SCAPULA, HUMERUS, RADIUS, ULNA, CARPAL)

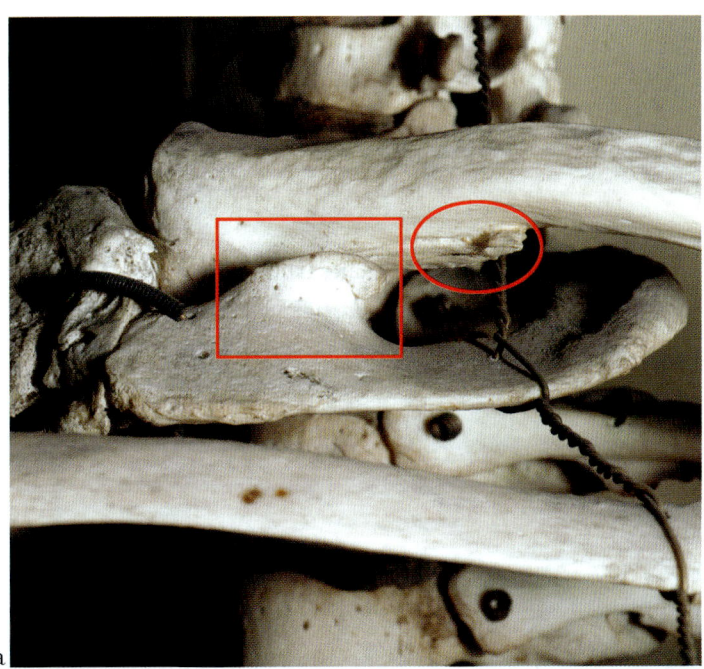

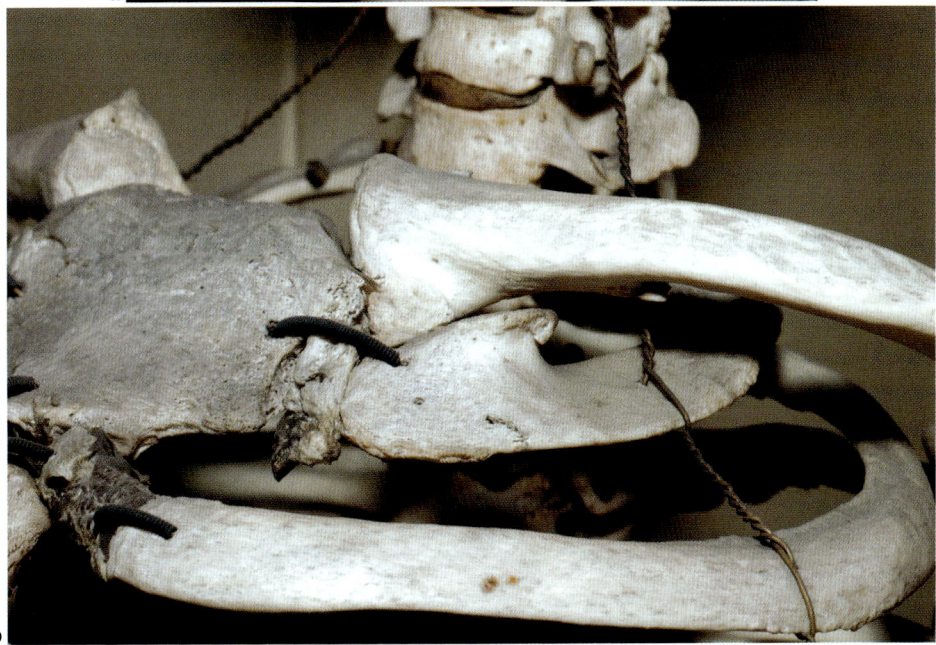

Figure 686a-b. Rare congenital unilateral costoclavicular joint. (a) Raised plateau (rectangle) along the superior surface of the left first rib (b) where it articulates (forming a false or artificial joint called a nearthrosis) with the inferior surface of the clavicle (oval) in a 47-year-old German male (Mütter Museum). Note the roughened and ridge-like area lateral to this joint that replaces the usual ligamentous connection. Cf. Cave (1961); Rani et al. (2009, 2011); Redlund-Johnell (1986).

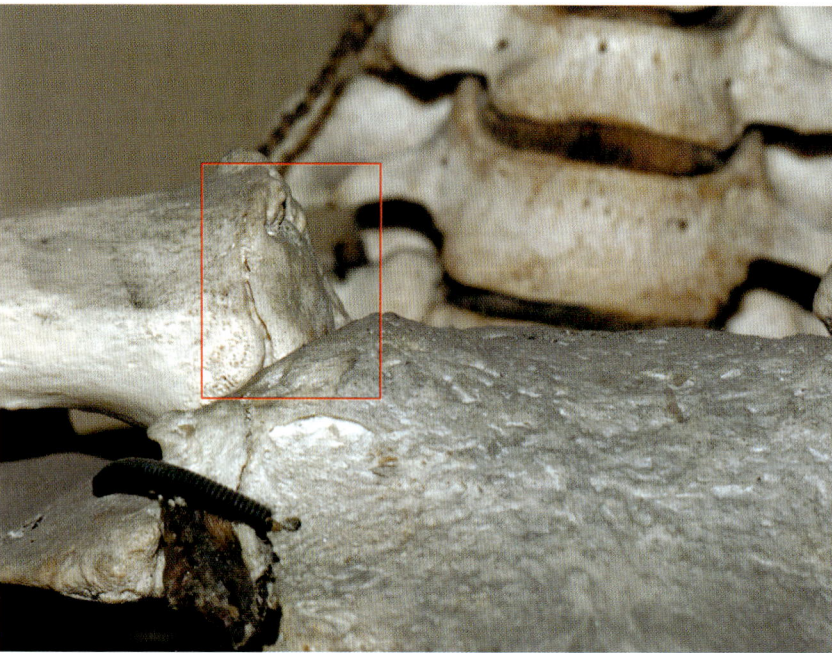

Figure 687. Incompletely fused medial epiphysis of the right clavicle (rectangle) in a 47-year-old German male (Mütter Museum). The medial epiphysis, which usually fuses by 32 years of age (Singh and Chavali 2011), is usually the last epiphysis to unite/fuse/obliterate in the human skeleton.

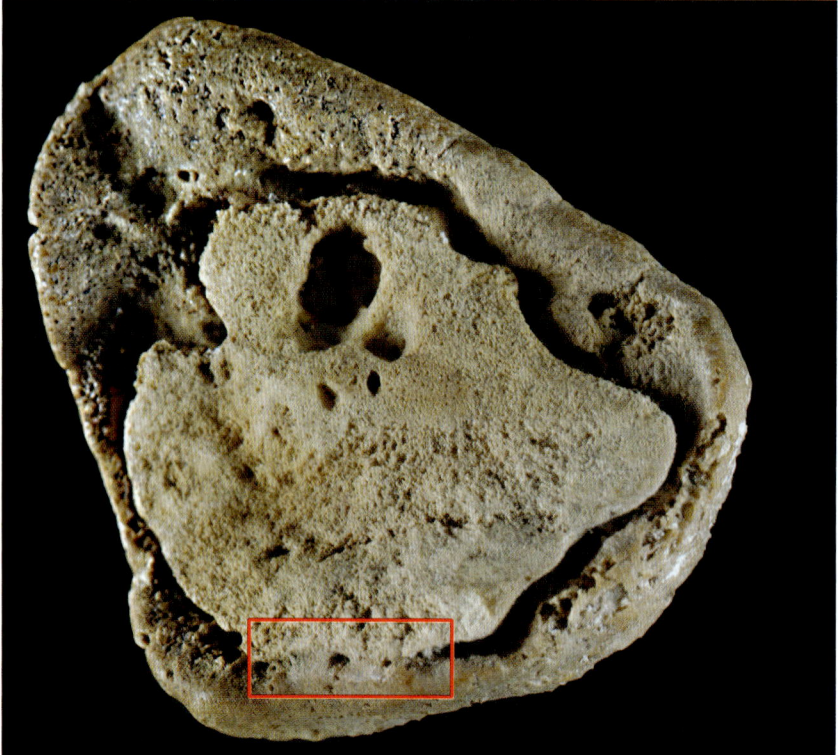

Figure 688. Early-stage fusion (rectangle) of the medial epiphysis of the clavicle in a young adult male (CIL). Note that this epiphysis often forms as a central island that slowly enlarges laterally and asymmetrically (graphics correction by Christopher Sciotto.)

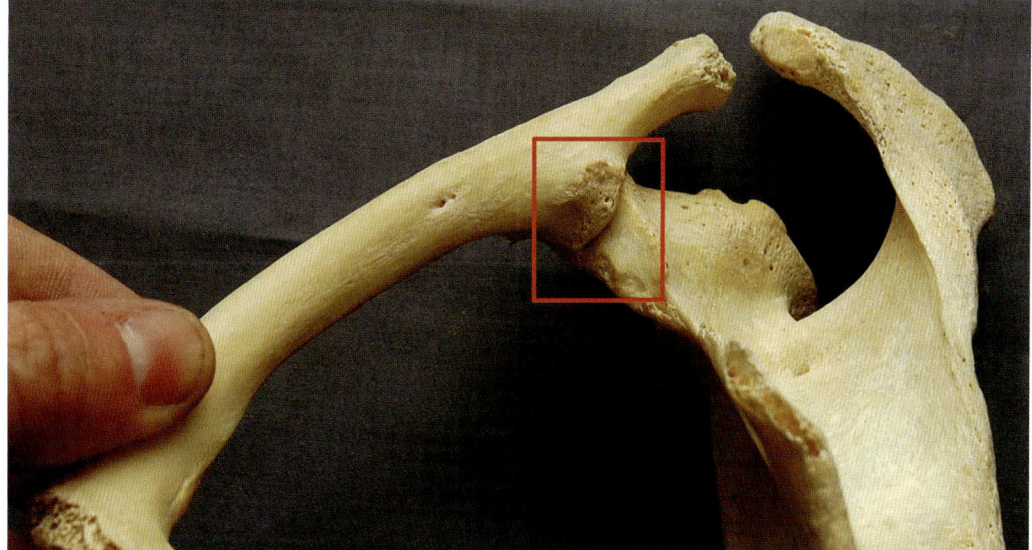

Figure 689. Coracoclavicular/conoid joint or facet (rectangle) in a right clavicle and scapula (Chiba University, Hugh Tuller). Research by Kaur and Jit (1991) of 1,000 adult northwest Indians revealed this joint in 10% of males and 8% of females, but absent in 85 fetuses, neonates and young children, showing it is not a congenital anomaly. Pillay (1976) reported the conoid joint as an inherited simple Mendelian trait. A radiographic study of 1,020 human clavicles (Gumina et al. 2002) revealed 8 (8%) of these joints in 6 males and 2 females. Uncommon finding in most groups.

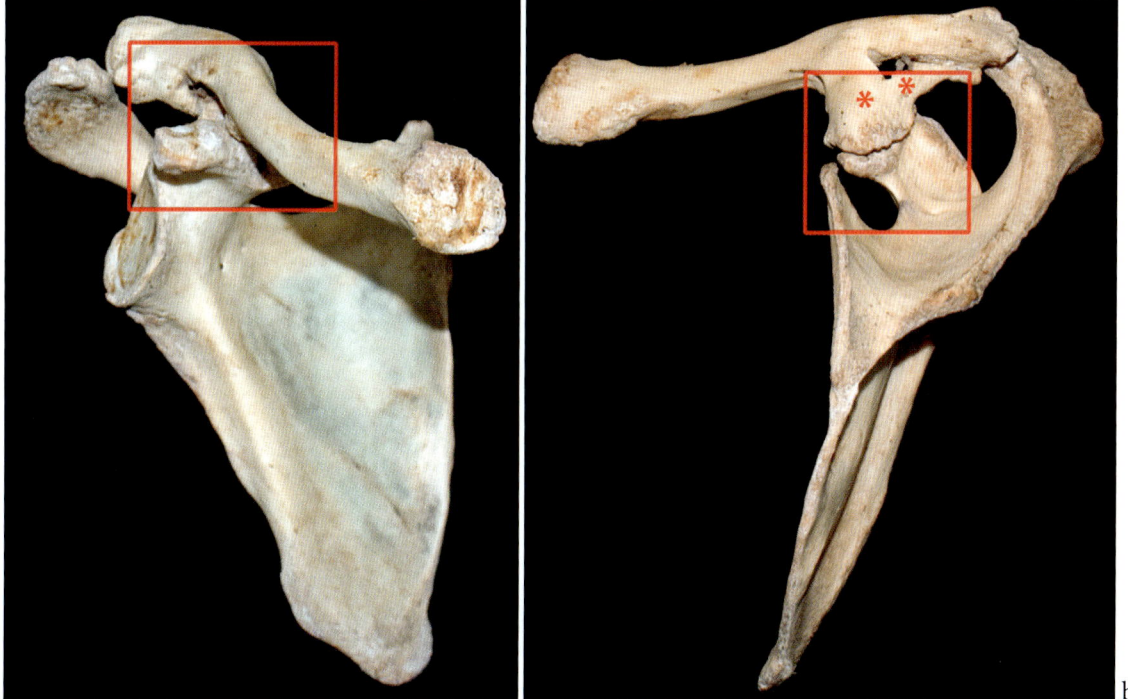

Figure 690a-b. Calcification and formation of an articular facet/pseudoarthrosis of the right scapula and clavicle in an adult, probably due to acute trauma to the shoulder (KKU 0674). (a) The surface where the two bones meet to form a pseudoarthrosis (rectangle) is rough and irregular and not smooth like a normal cartilage-covered joint. (b) Note that the two bars of bone (*) forming the pseudoarthrosis are the result of trauma and calcification of the muscles reflecting myositis ossificans traumatica (not to be confused with a normal variant).

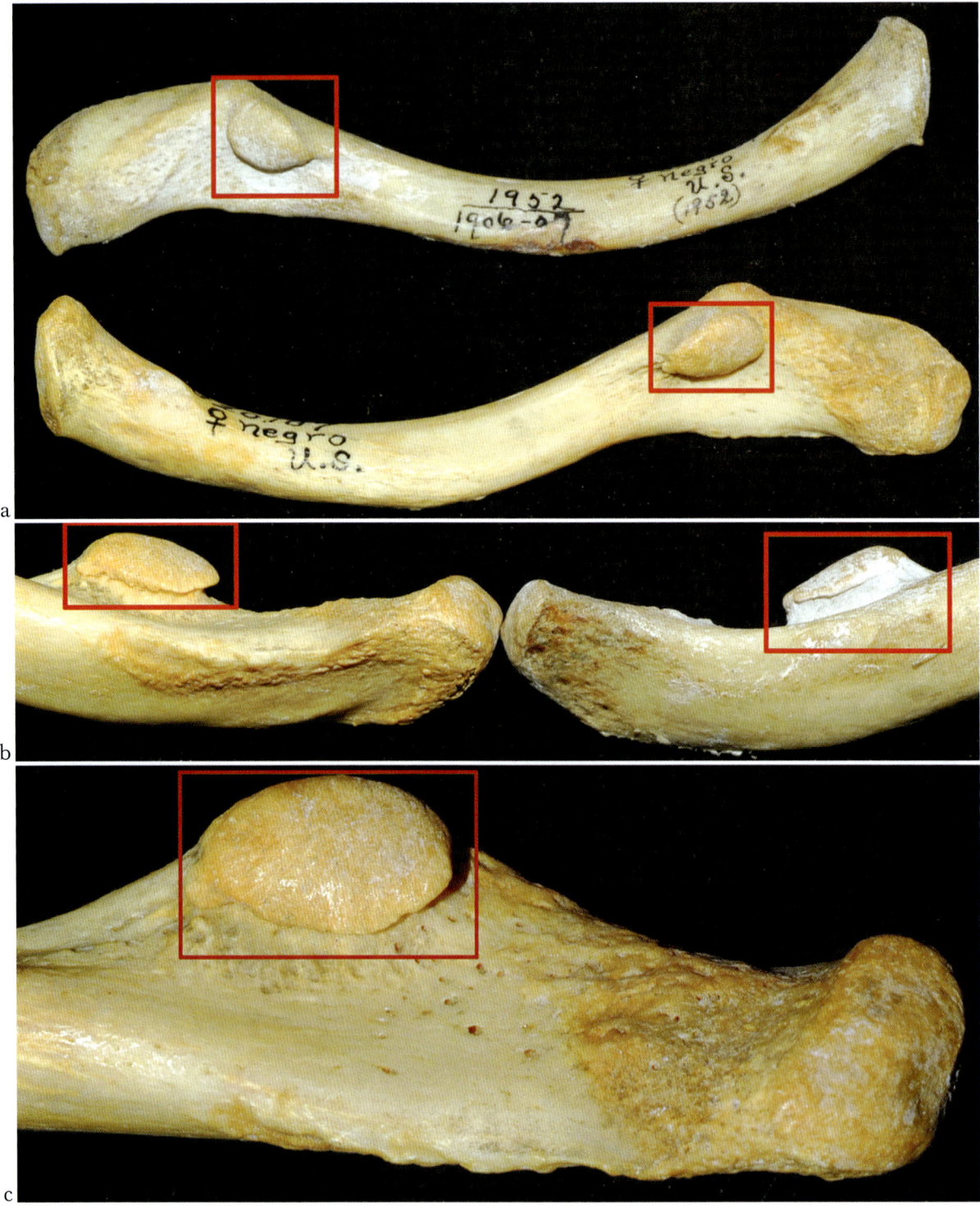

Figure 691a-c. Clavicular facets of the coracoclavicular joint (conoid) joint in an adult female (SI). (a) Inferior, (b) posterior and (c) inferior views of the oval-shaped platform forming the conoid joint (rectangles). The frequency of this joint varies among groups from 0.55% (Olotu et al. 2008) to 9.8% (Cho and Kang 1998) or higher, is associated with increased frequencies of OA in neighboring joints (Gumina et al. 2002) and may have a genetic component (Nehme et al. 2004). Cf. Cockshott (1979, 1992); Kaur and Jit (1991); Lewis (1959); Nalla and Asvat (1995); Rani et al. (2009). See Piyawinijwong et al. (2006) for gross anatomy dissections in a Thai sample.

Shoulder, Arm and Hand (Clavicle, Scapula, Humerus, Radius, Ulna, Carpal)

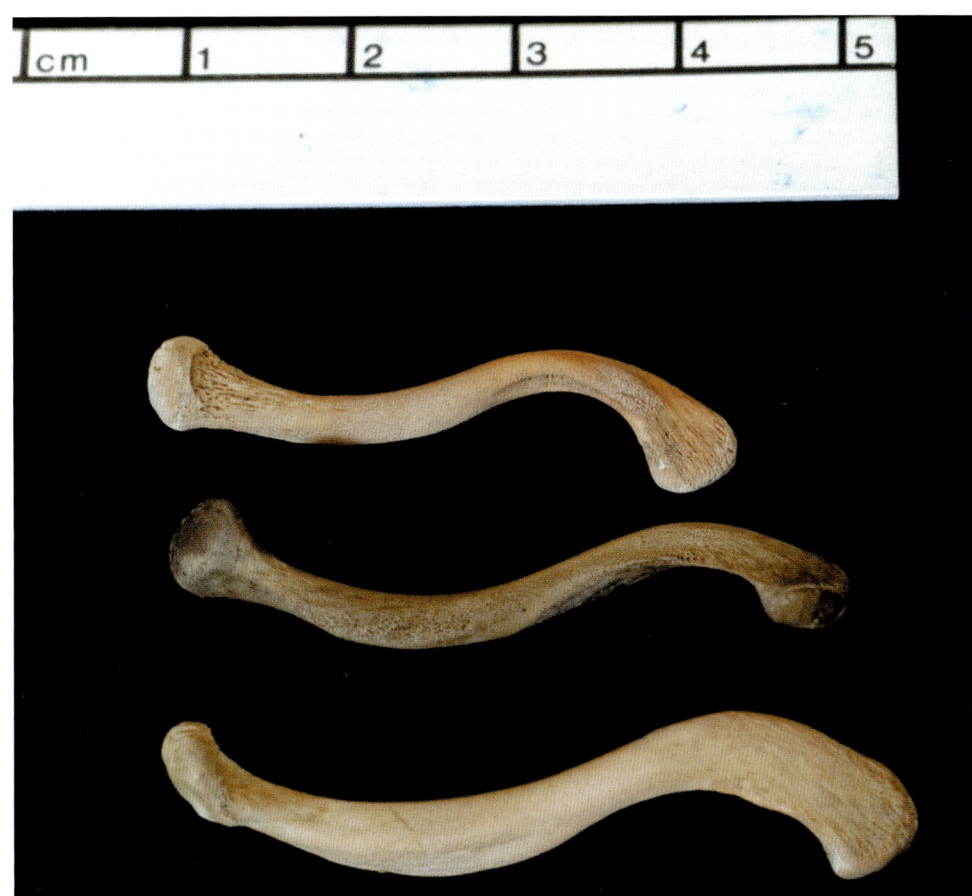

Figure 692. Left fetal clavicles showing an increase in their size with age (SI).

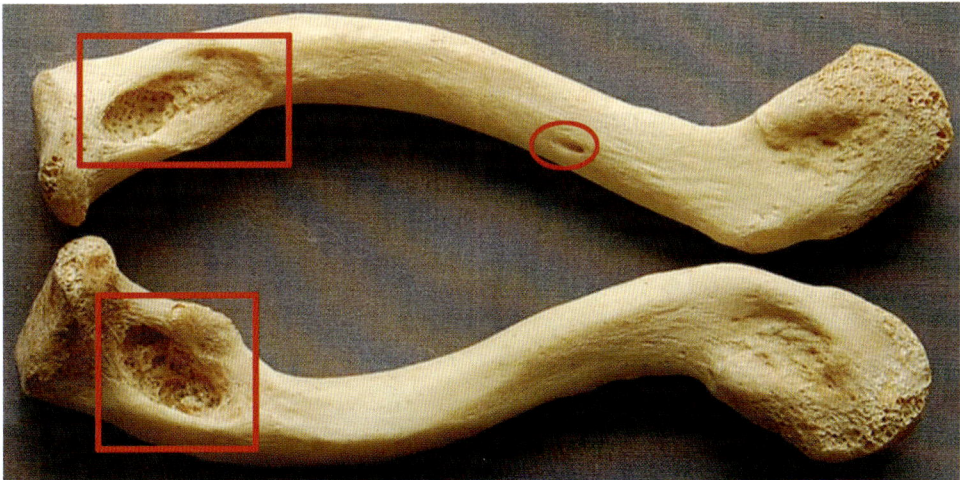

Figure 693. Rhomboid fossae (squares) and nutrient foramen (circle) in an adult Japanese (Chiba University, Hugh Tuller). The rhomboid fossa serves for attachment of the costoclavicular ligament and its site of attachment may be a concavity as in this individual, flat, raised, or any combination thereof – both are normal variants. The rhomboid fossa is so named because of its rhomboid shape. Cf. Rani et al. (2011). Cf. Natsis et al. (2007b) for a rare example of an intermediate supraclavicular nerve that perforated the clavicle; Rogers et al. (2000) for age and sex variation.

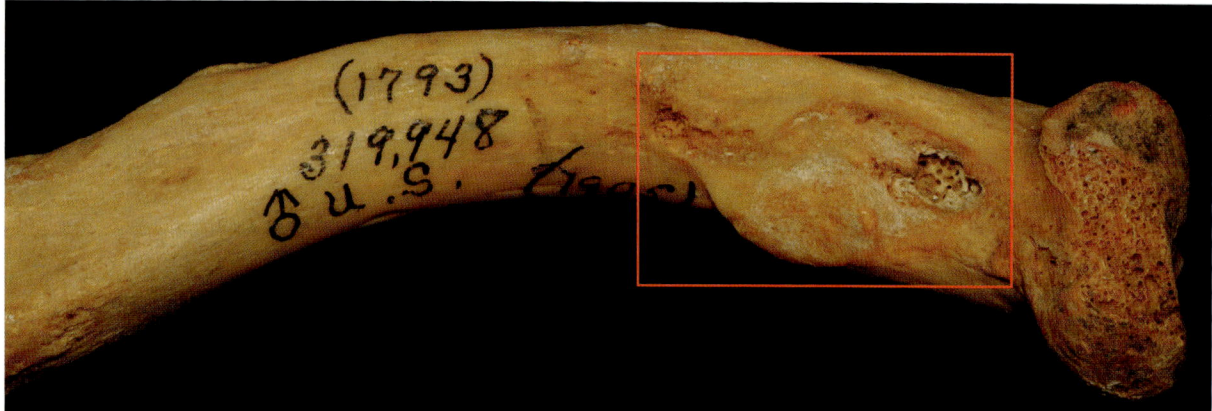

Figure 694. Combination of a pit/fossa and lipped ridge (rectangle) at the site of attachment of the costoclavicular ligament in an adult male (SI 319948). Normal variant and common finding. For sex and age determination from the Rhomboid fossa see Rogers et al. (2000).

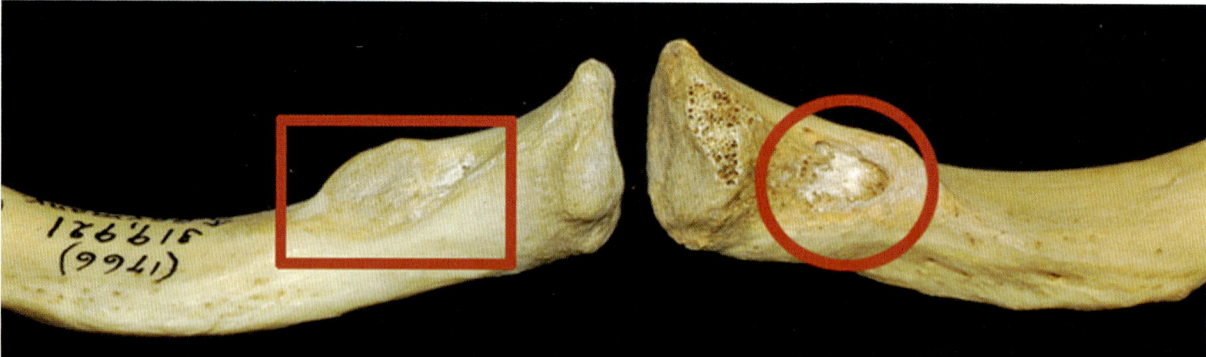

Figure 695. Asymmetry of the rhomboid fossae in the form of a pit (circle) and groove/ridge (rectangle) in an individual (SI 319921) – the left and right rhomboid fossae/facets/joints are often very asymmetrical in the same individual. Cf. Rani et al. (2011).

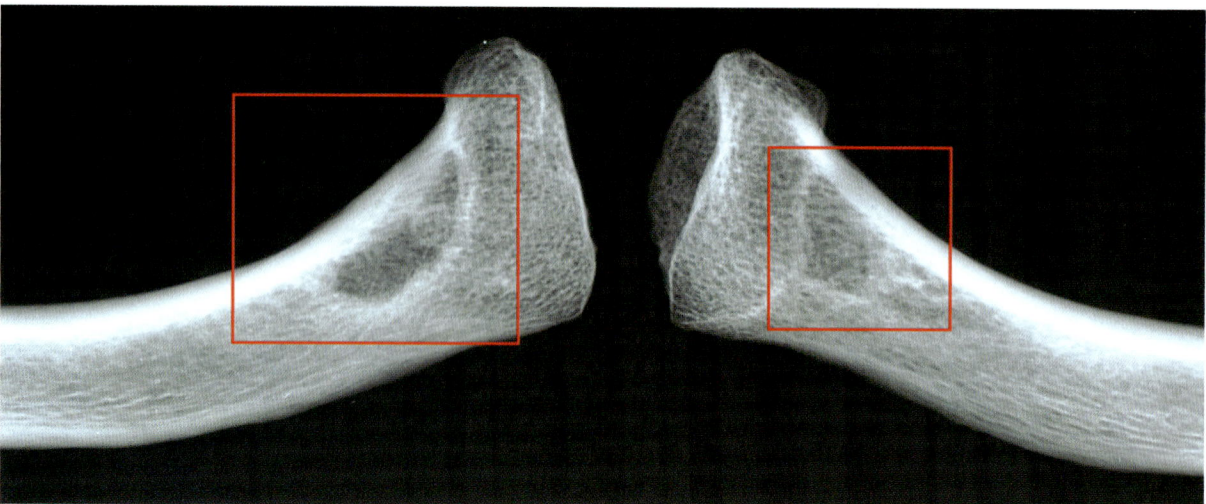

Figure 696. Radiographic appearance of rhomboid fossae (square and rectangle) in an adult (SI).

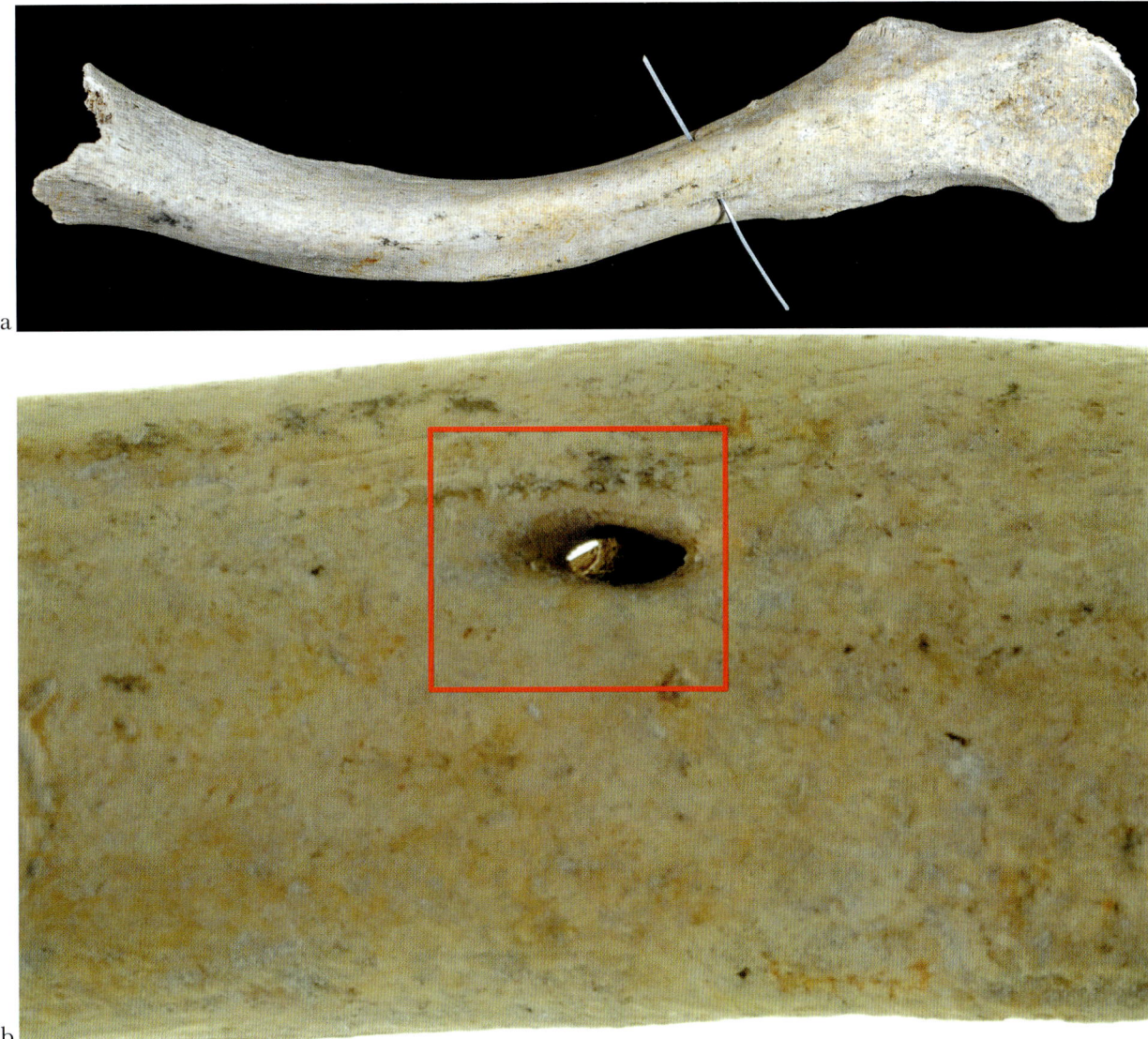

Figure 697a-b. Nutrient foramen (canalis intracavicularis) in an adult left clavicle. (a) Superior view of the left clavicular foramen (probe) that transmits a nutrient artery and sometimes a nerve. (b) Close-up of the foramen (rectangle) illustrating its oval shape and rounded margin. Common finding.

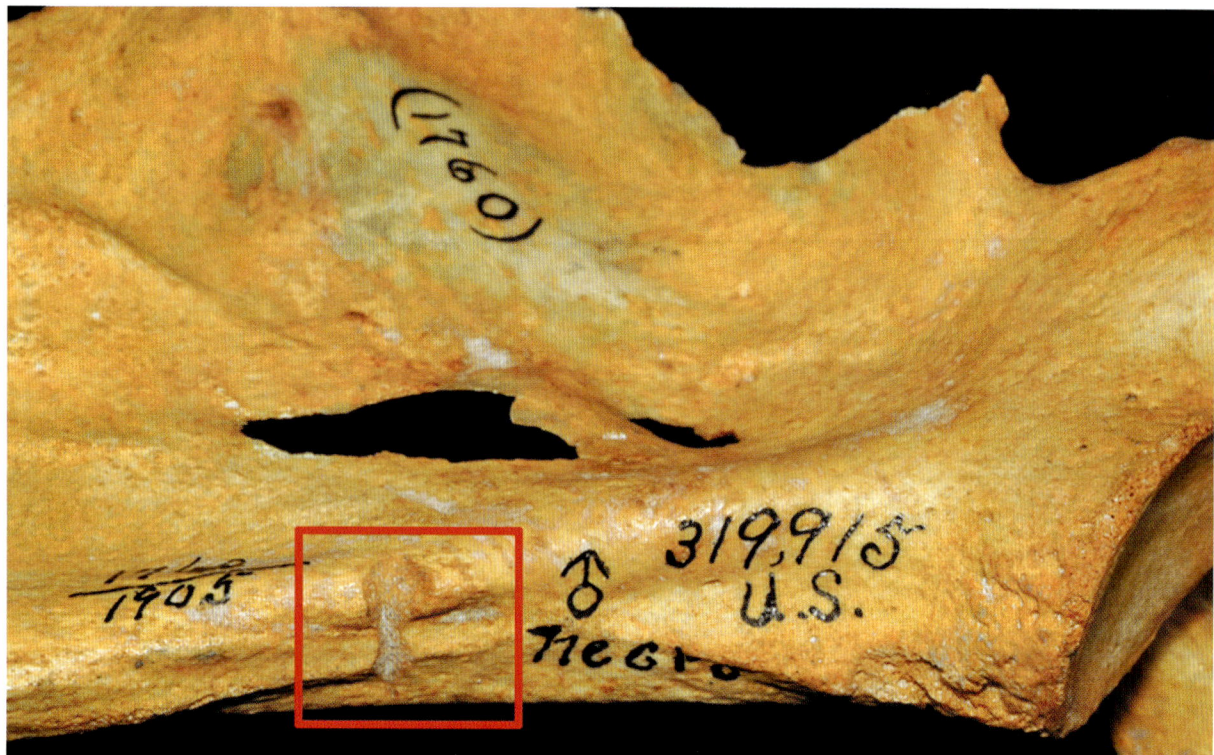

Figure 698. Circumflex sulcus (rectangle) for the circumflex artery in the left scapula of an adult (SI 319915) (some bone breakage occurred postmortem). Common finding.

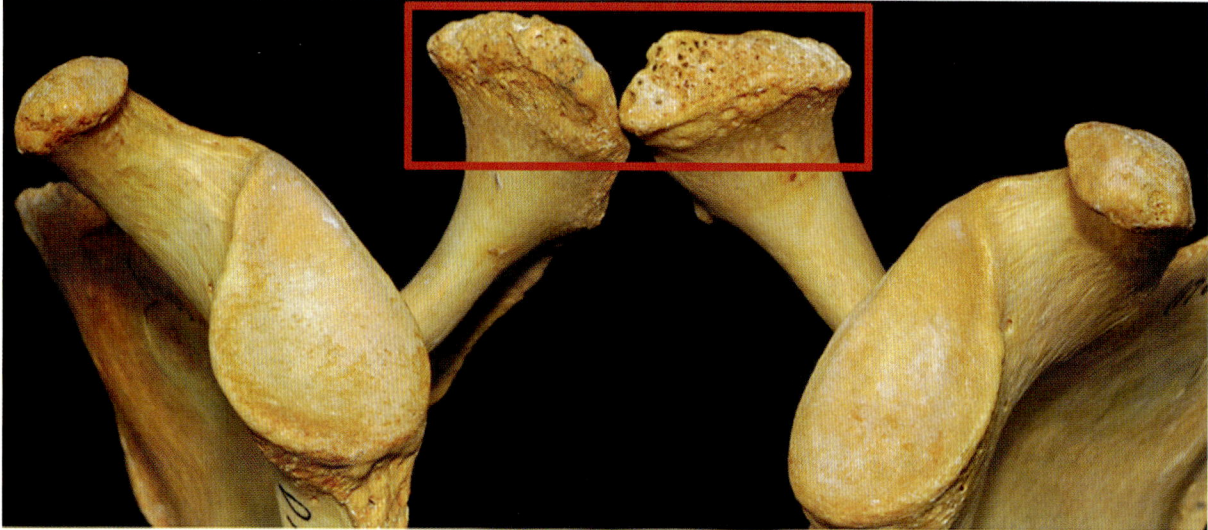

Figure 699. Bilateral os acromiale (rectangle) in an adult (SI Huntington). Common to uncommon finding, often the result of a developmental anomaly (failure of fusion) rather than pulling/functional/activity stresses to the shoulder (Hunt and Bullen 2007; Case et al. 2006). Cf. Sammarco (2000) for more on the frequency, anatomy and clinical implications of this feature.

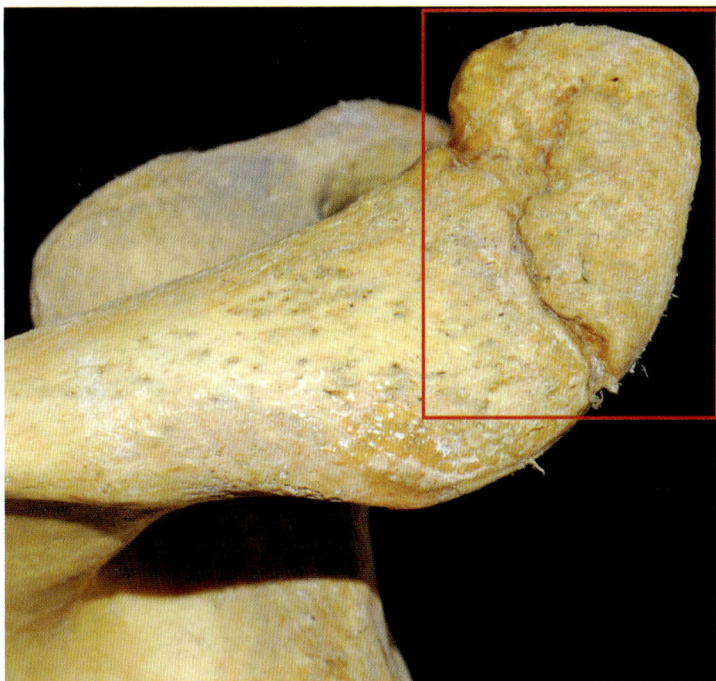

Figure 700. Os acromiale (rectangle) in the right scapula of an adult (SI Huntington). Uncommon to common finding.

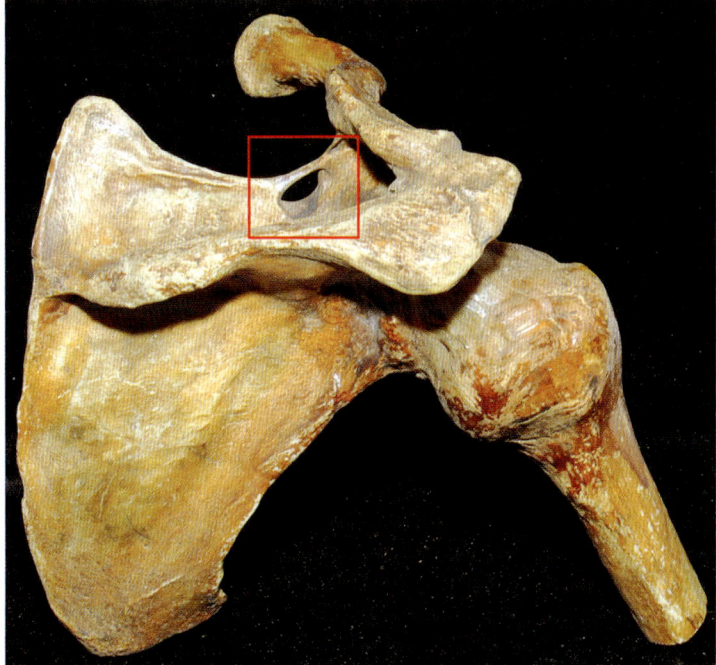

Figure 701. Calcified suprascapular (transverse) ligament resulting in a suprascapular foramen (square) in an adult right scapula (Mütter Museum). The shape of the suprascapular border in this region varies from straight, to indented (suprascapular notch), to a partial or complete foramen (suprascapular foramen). Foramina in this area are due to calcification of the ligament spanning the notch and not perforation of the scapular body. Common finding. Cf. Freyschmidt et al. (2002); Natsis et al. (2007); Sinkeet (2010); Tubbs et al. (2013b); Wang et al. (2011).

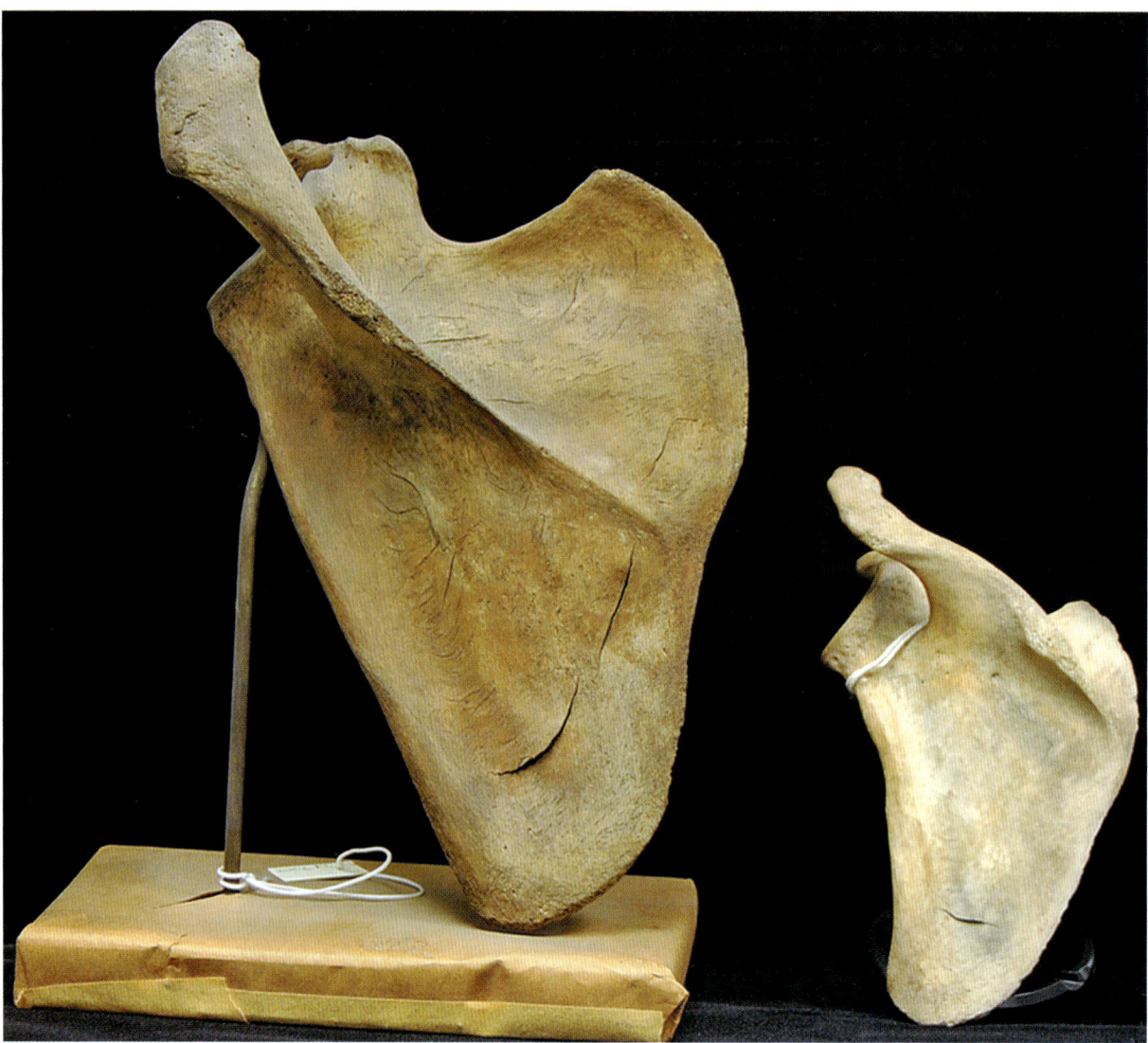

Figure 702. Unusually large ("giant") left scapula compared to an average-sized adult scapula (Mütter Museum) – the scapula on the left originated from someone who was almost certainly more than 7 feet tall. The cracks in the two bones are postmortem drying cracks. Rare finding.

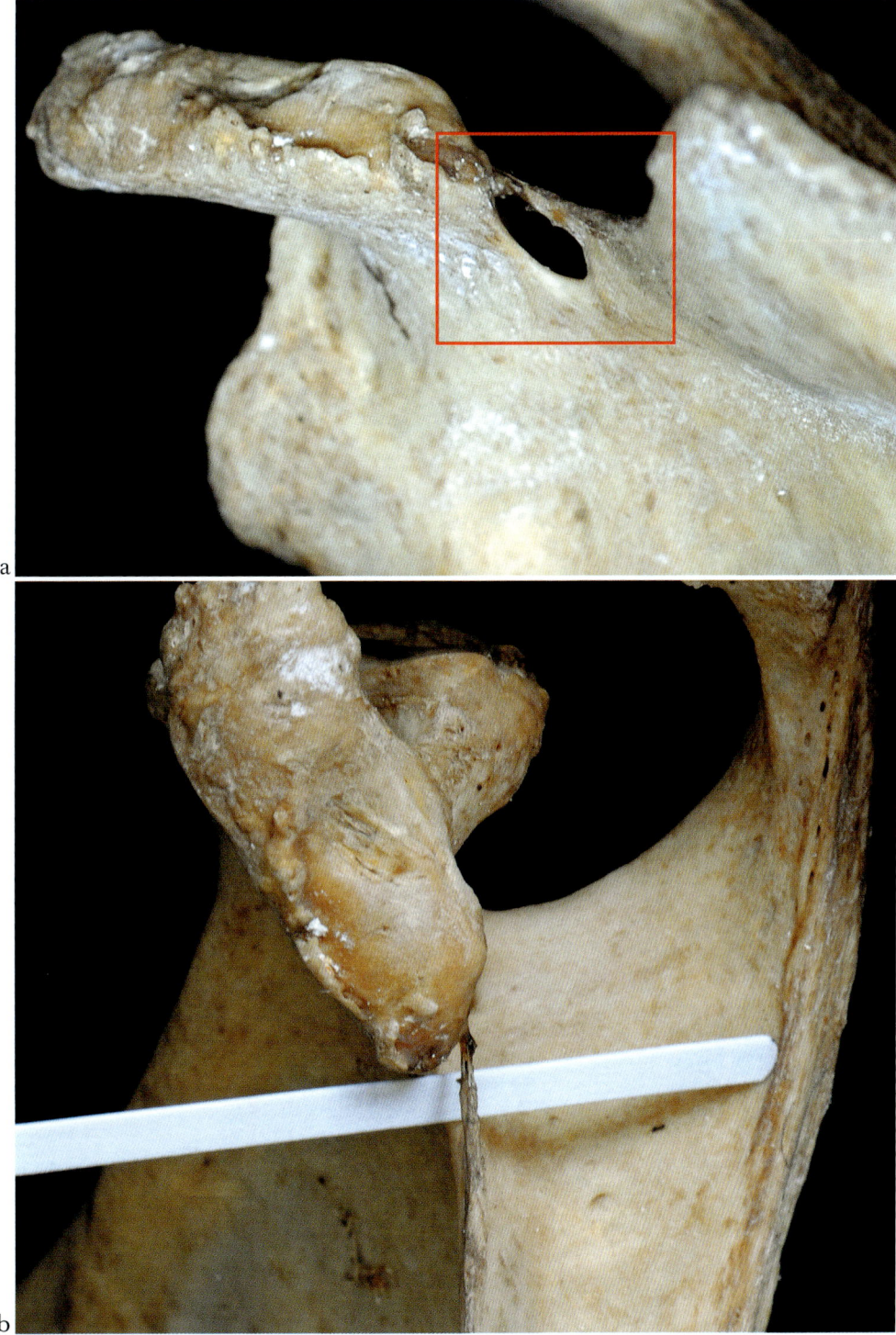

Figure 703a-b. Suprascapular foramen in the process of forming – the suprascapular transverse ligament in this adult right scapula is still calcifying (KKU). (a) Posterior view of the foramen and ligament (square) spanning the suprascapular notch. (b) Probe passing beneath the ligament. Polguj et al. (2011) examined 86 Polish scapulae and found complete and partial ossification of this ligament in 7% and 23% of scapulae, respectively. A study of 138 Kenyan scapulae revealed 2.9% of scapulae with a suprascapular foramen (Sinkeet 2010). Common finding. Cf. Natsis et al. (2007b); Wang et al. (2011).

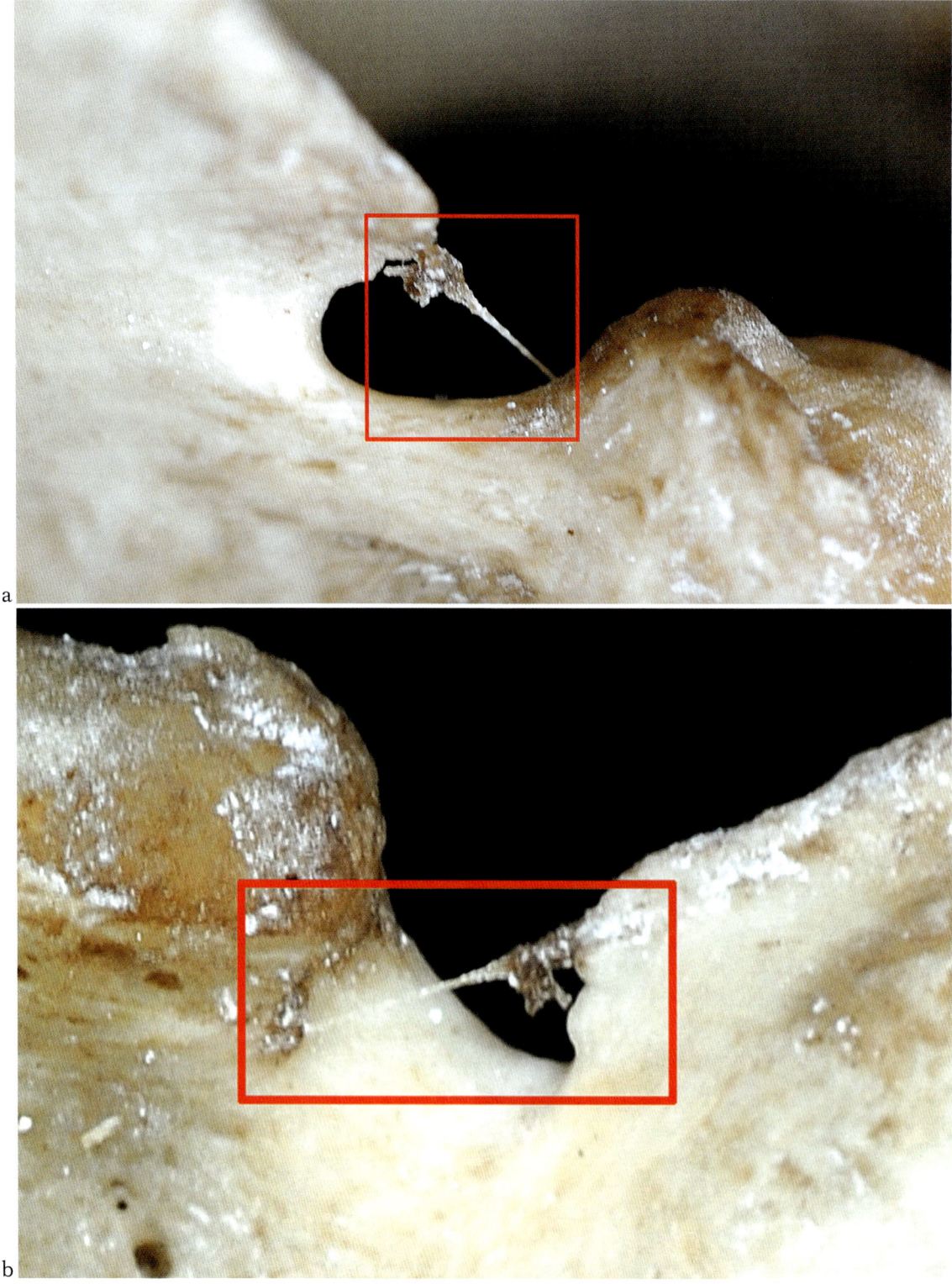

Figure 704a-b. Partially calcified suprascapular ligament in an adult Thai (KKU). (a) Ventral and (b) dorsal views of the suprascapular ligament extending across the U-shaped suprascapular notch. Uncommon to common finding (these fragile bridges often break postmortem or may be consumed by necrophagus insects).

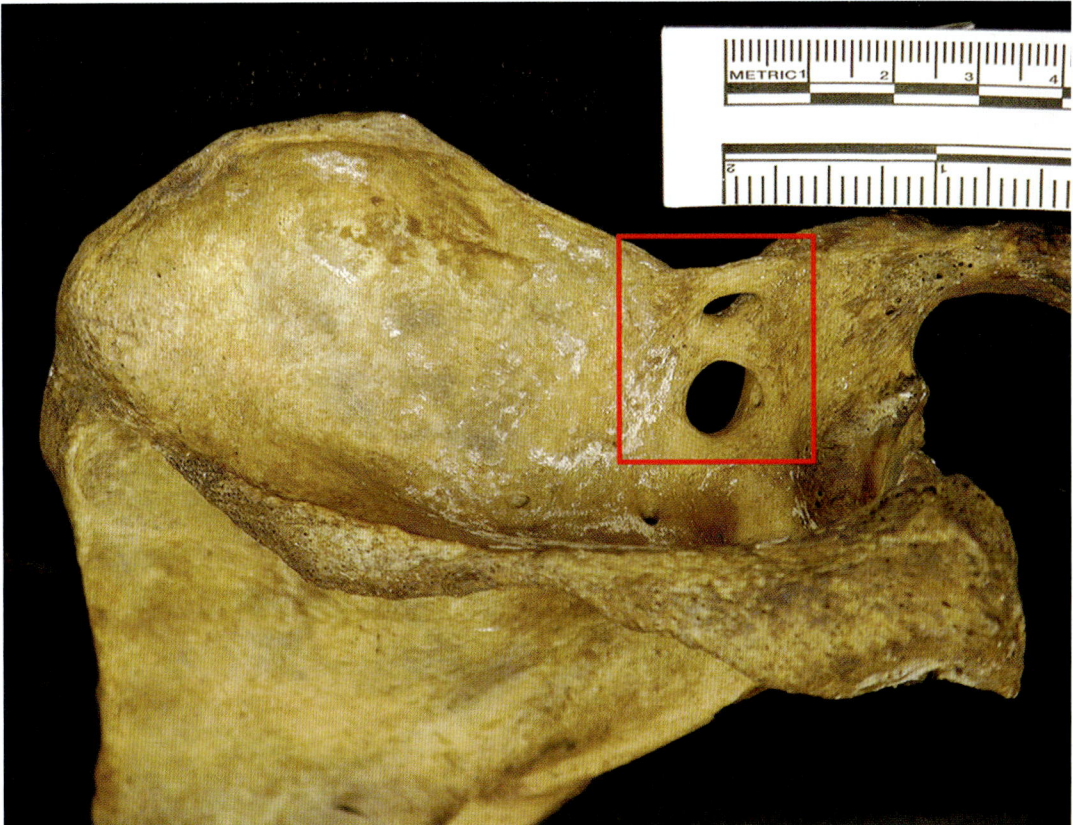

Figure 705. Rare double suprascapular foramen (square) joining the scapular body and coronoid process (UTK, Joe Hefner). These foramina formed due to ossification of the suprascapular transverse ligament, not perforation of the scapular body. Wang et al. (2011) found one example of double suprascapular foramen in 295 Chinese scapulas. Cf. Rengachary et al. (1979) and Natsis et al. (2007a) for the scapula. See Hrdlička (1942) for another example of double foramina.

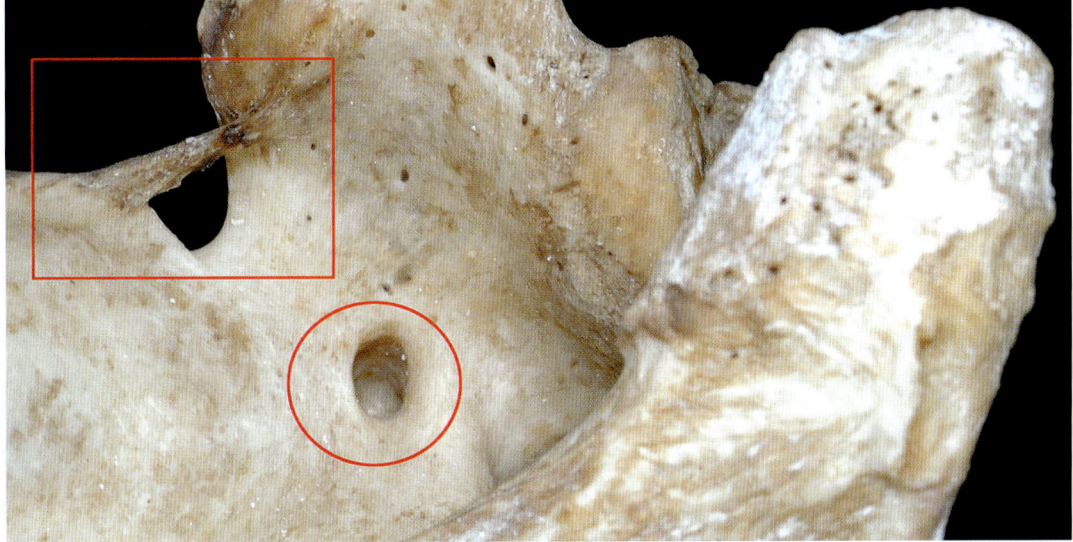

Figure 706. Actively forming (calcifying) suprascapular foramen (rectangle) and unusually large vessel foramen (circle) (KKU). A foramen in this location is common but one of this size is uncommon.

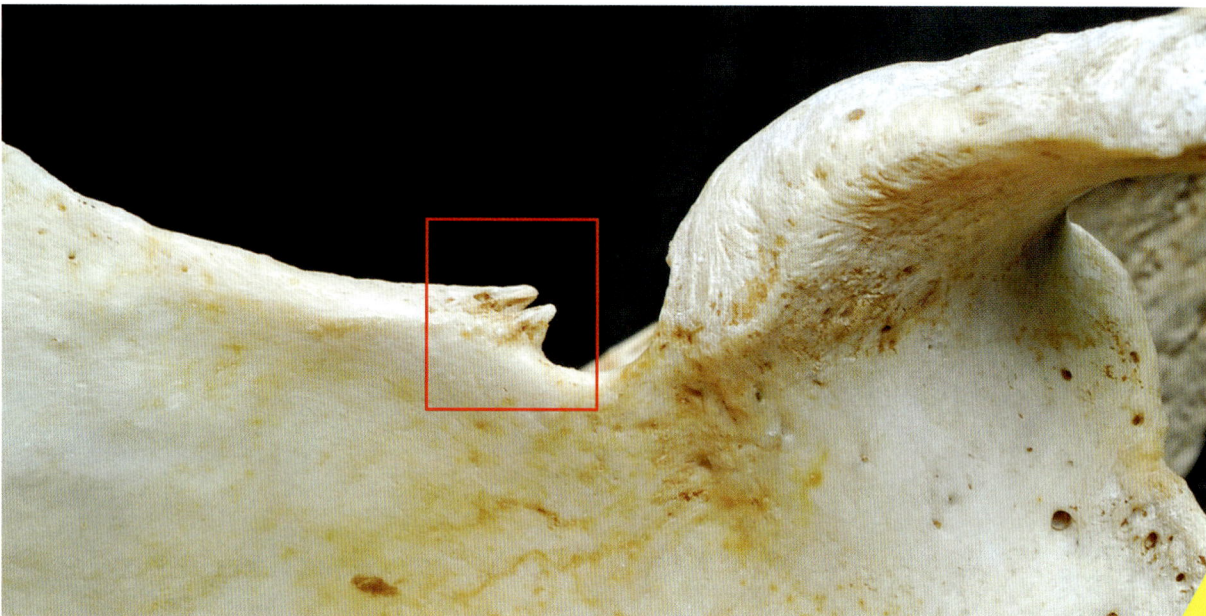

Figure 707. Spike-like projections (square) reflecting early-stage calcification of the suprascapular ligament in an adult (UHWO). Uncommon to common finding at this stage of development. Cf. Natsis et al. (2007a) for classification of the suprascapular notch.

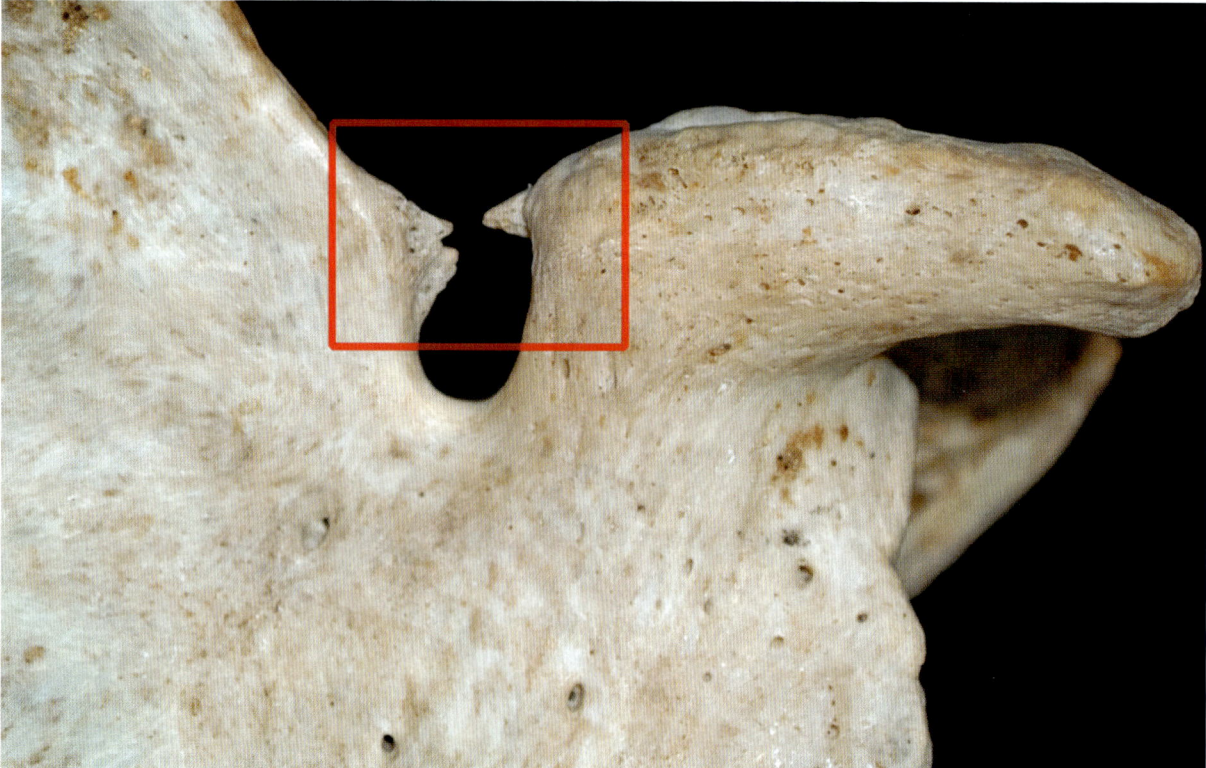

Figure 708. U-shaped suprascapular notch and early-stage suprascapular bridging (rectangle) resulting in small bony projections growing towards one another in the left scapula (KKU 51/076). The superior border of the scapula may be straight (without a notch), have a J-shaped or U–shaped suprascapular notch, a foramen (suprascapular foramen), or a complete or partial foramen formed by calcification of the suprascapular ligament.

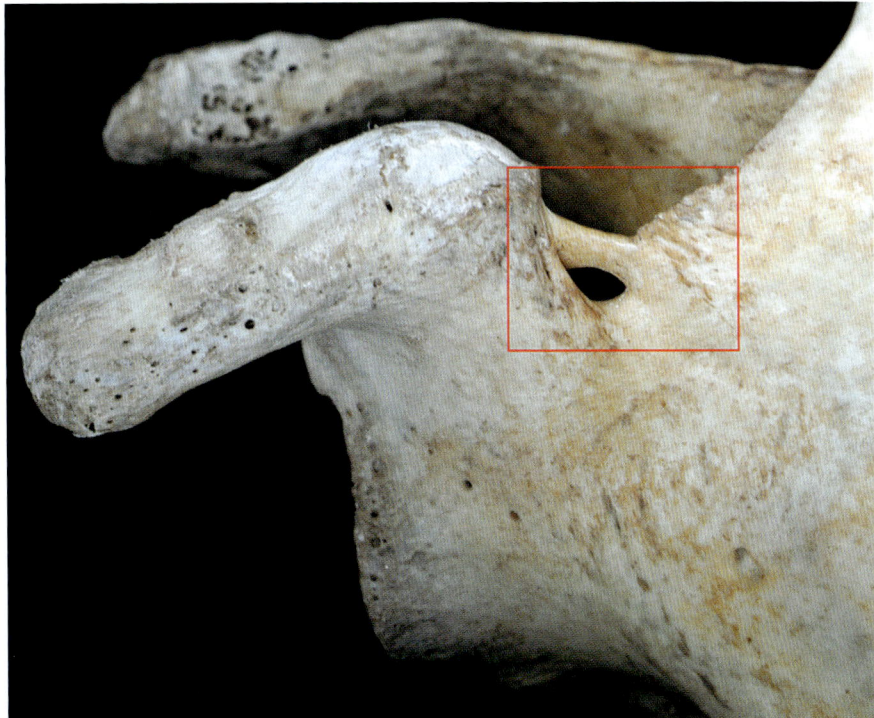

Figure 709. Calcified suprascapular ligament (rectangle) in an adult Thai (KKU).

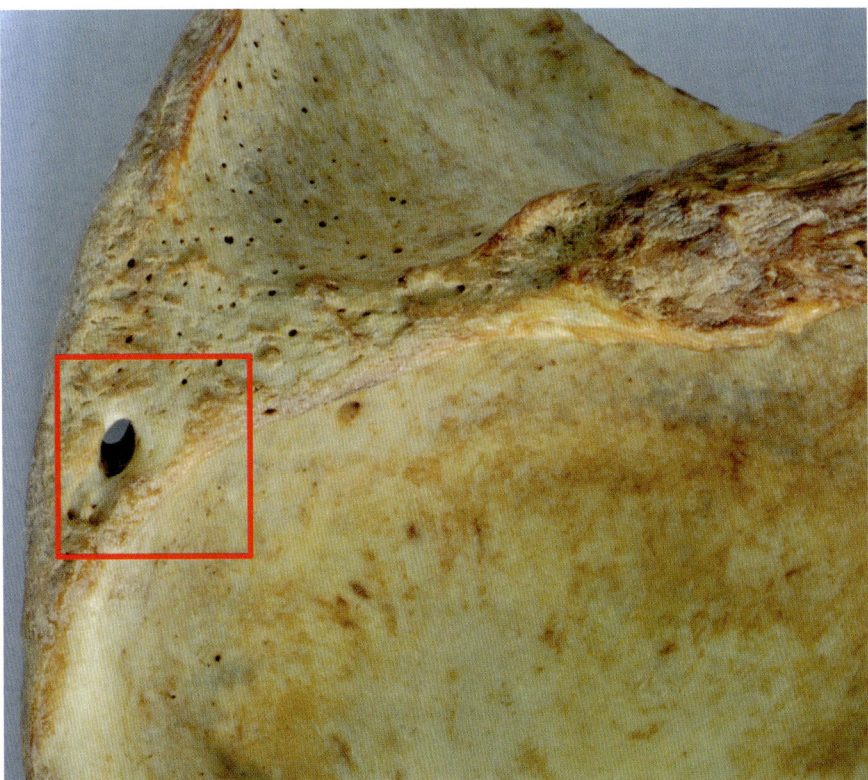

Figure 710. Uncommon to rare foramen, likely housing a vessel, along the vertebral border of the right scapula (KKU).

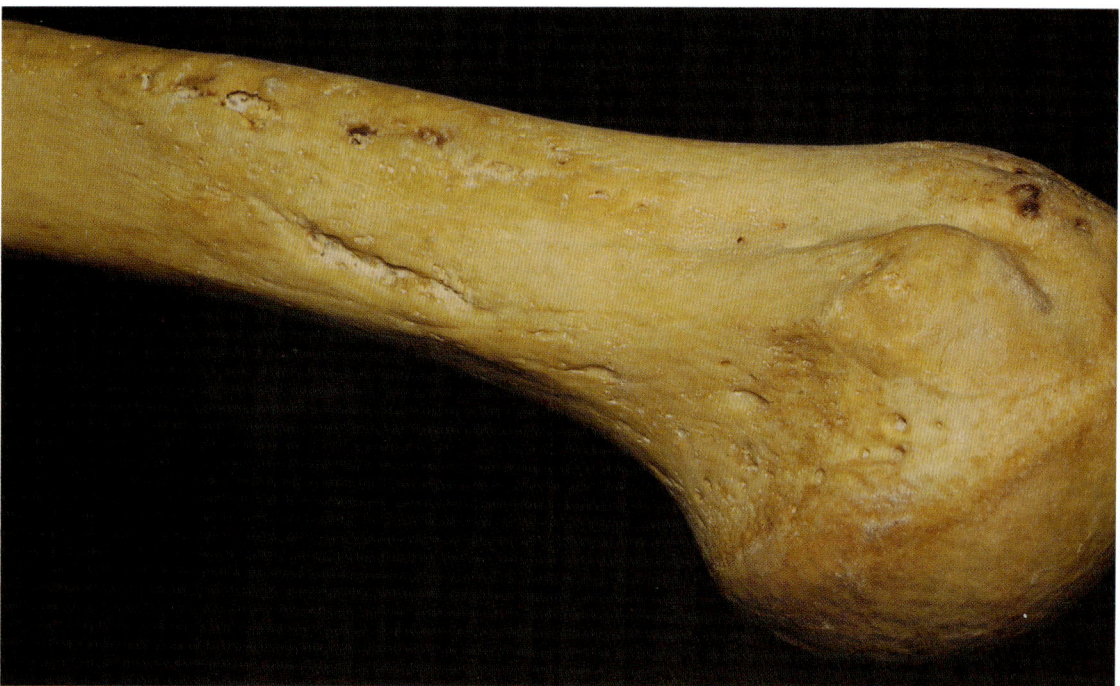

Figure 711. Cortical grooves (rectangle) in the right humerus of an adult (SI). Common finding in subadults and young adults. These grooves are sometimes attributed to heavy exercise and strenuous lifting and may be associated with the pectoralis, latissimus, and teres muscles. (Mann and Hunt 2012).

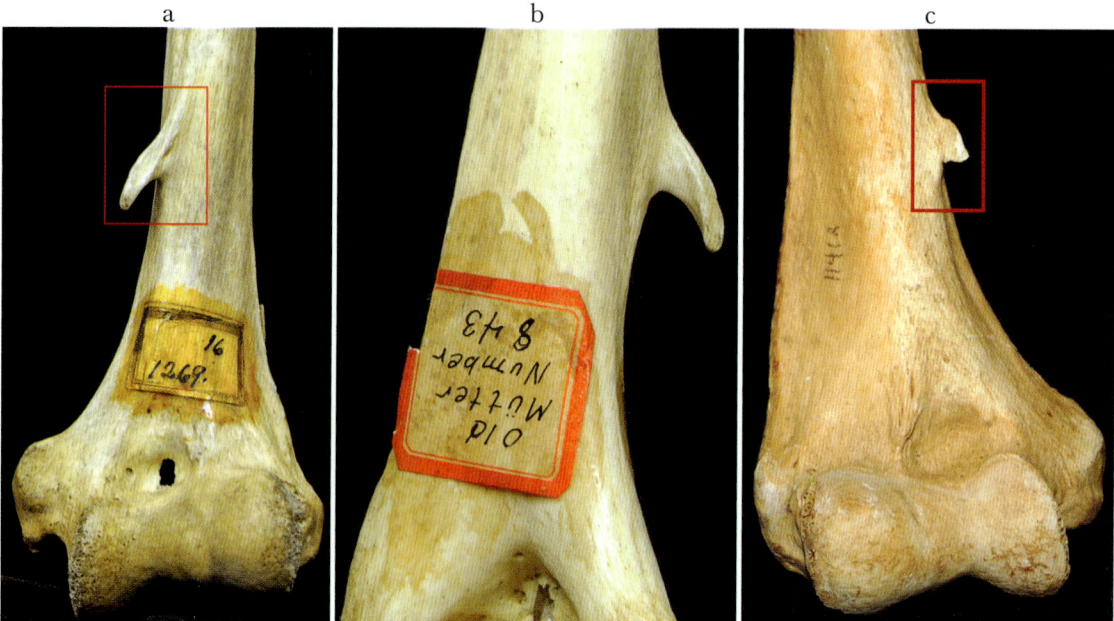

Figure 712a-c. Illustrations of a supratrochlear/supracondylar spur/supracondyloid process for attachment of the ligament of Struthers in three adults. (a) A large downwardly-projecting spur (rectangle) in a left humerus (Mütter Museum). (b) Dorsal view of a large spur in a left humerus (Mütter Museum). (c) Anterior view of a right humerus with a small supratrochlear spur (rectangle) from 12th Dynasty Egypt (SI). The ligament of Struthers, which sometimes calcifies, extends from this bony "hook" along the medial border to the medial epicondyle. Uncommon finding. Cf. Freyschmidt et al. (2002); Lordan et al. (2005); Natsis (2008); Singhal and Rao (2007); Rau (1931); Yazar and Acar (2006).

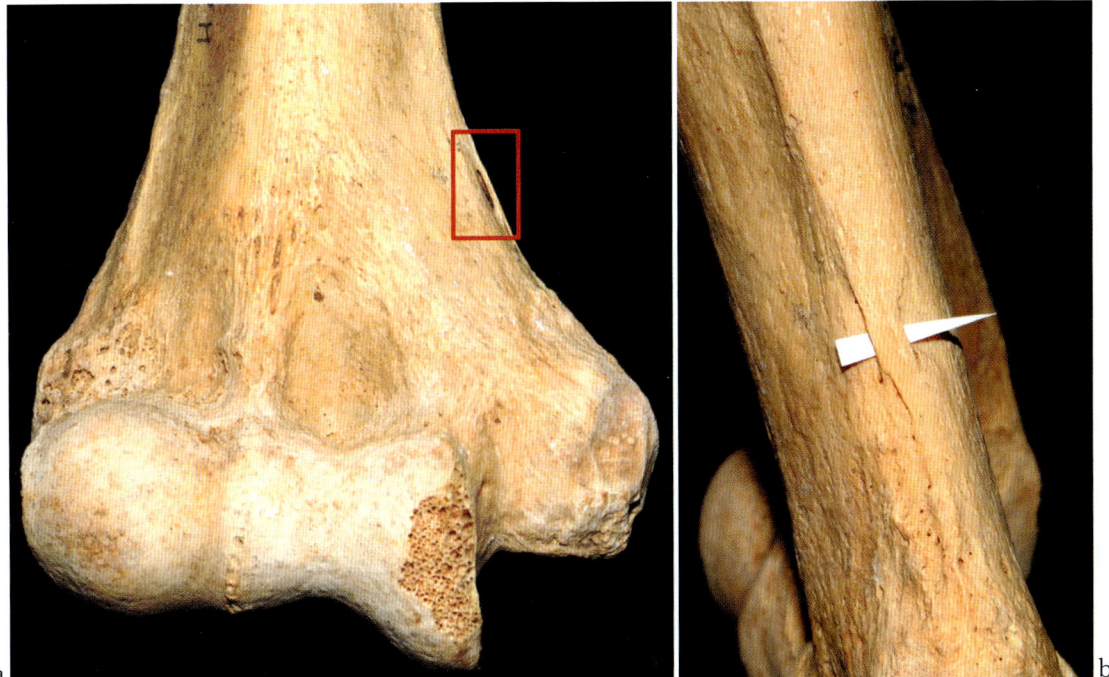

Figure 713a-b. Right humerus showing a variant of the supracondyloid foramen (Dwight 1904), tunnel (Verna 2014) and physiological notch (Freyschmidt et al. 2002). (a) Anterior and (b) medial views of the slit-like foramen or aperture (rectangle and paper arrowhead) along the medial border in a 12th Dynastic Egyptian (SI). Uncommon to rare finding.

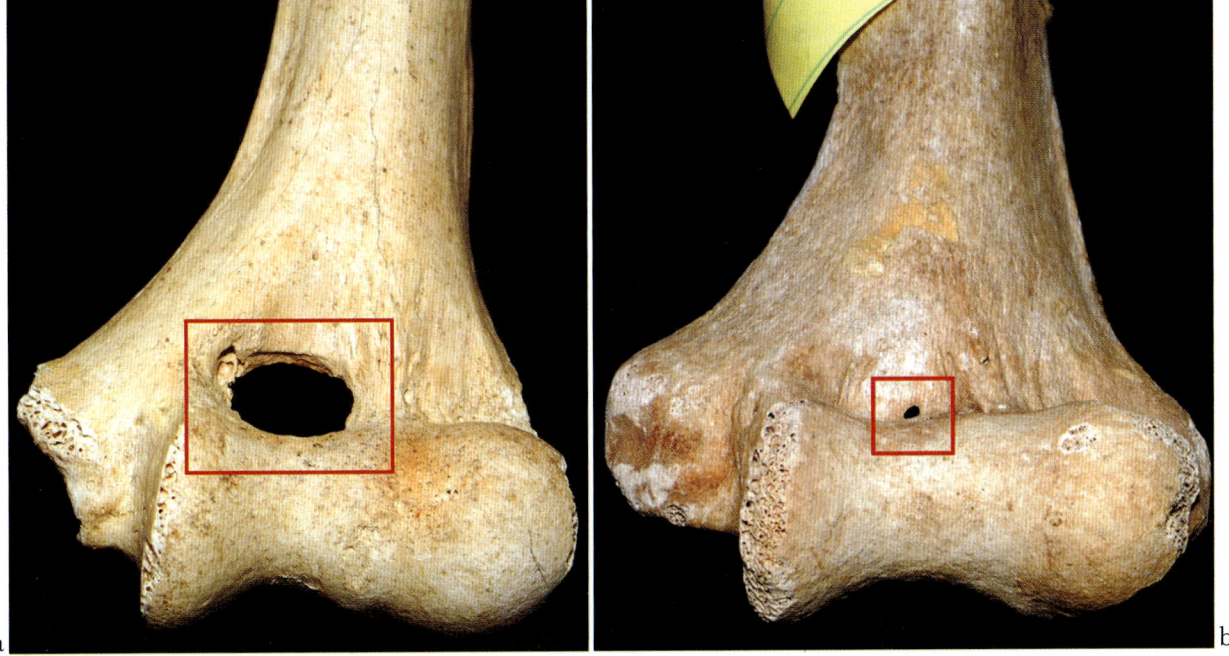

Figure 714a-b. Septal apertures. Illustration of (a) large and (b) small septal apertures (rectangle and square) in two 12th Dynastic Egyptian adults (SI). Both variants are common findings and may vary (asymmetrical) in size and shape in the same individual. Cf. France, 1983; Freyschmidt et al. (2002); Singhal and Rao (2007) noted apertures in 42 of 150 (28%) adult Indian humeri; Trotter (1934) for American Blacks and Whites.

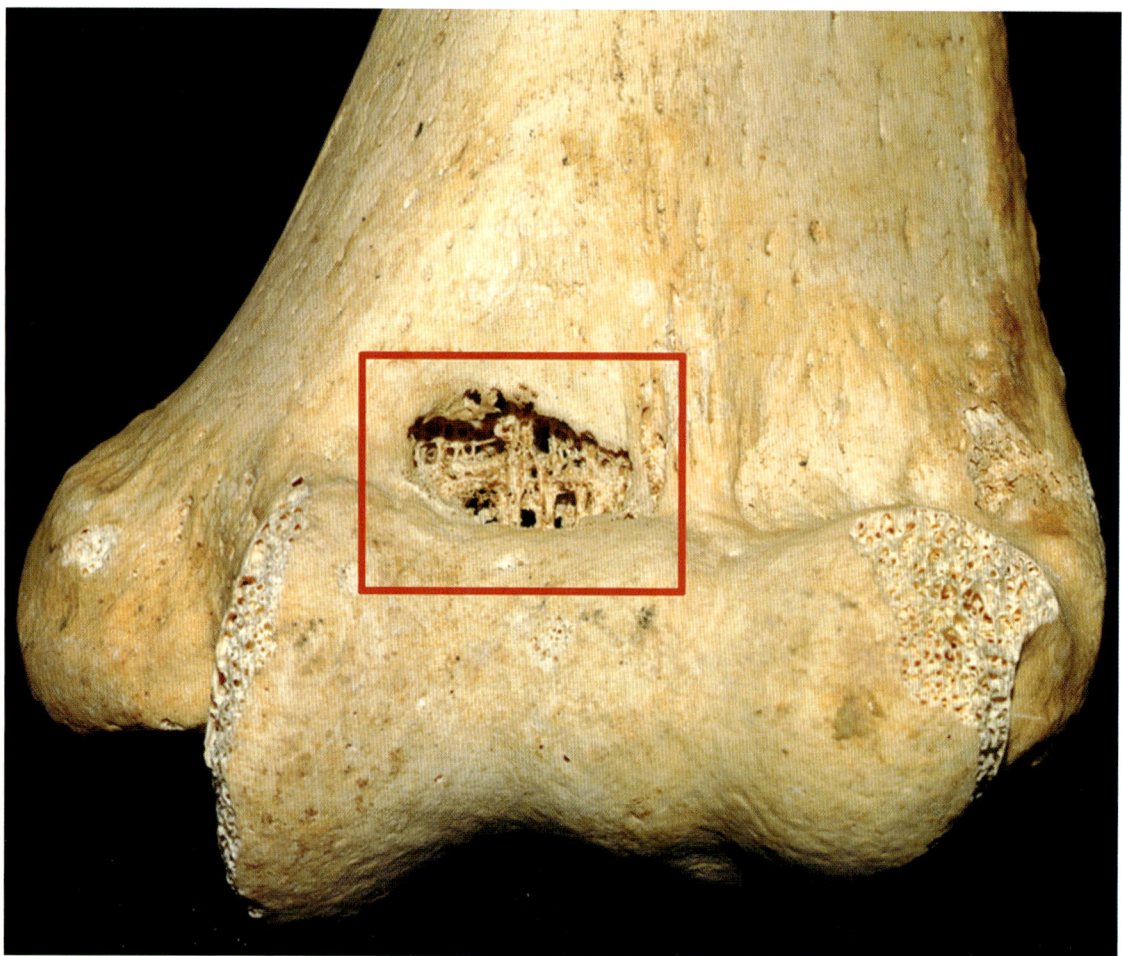

Figure 715. Possible early-stage septal aperture (rectangle) in the left humerus of an adult (SI). This is one of only a few examples of its kind the authors have encountered where the coronoid fossa/depression exhibits a "woven" and fibrous floor suggesting active remodeling.

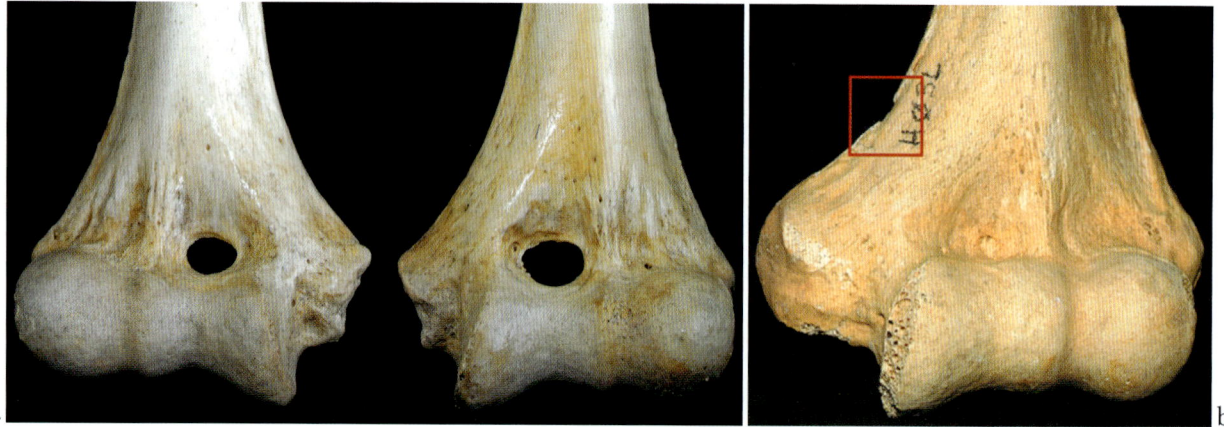

Figure 716a-b. Septal apertures and physiological notch. (a) Bilateral septal apertures in a subadult (KKU). (b) A physiological notch (square) in the medial margin of the left humerus in an (SI). Common (septal aperture) and uncommon (notch) findings. Trotter (1934) noted 4.3% of 960 White paired humeri and 12.6% of 784 Black paired humeri with septal apertures. Cf. Freyschmidt et al. (2002); Meier (2006); Meier and Hunt (2006); Singhal and Rao (2007); Trotter (1934).

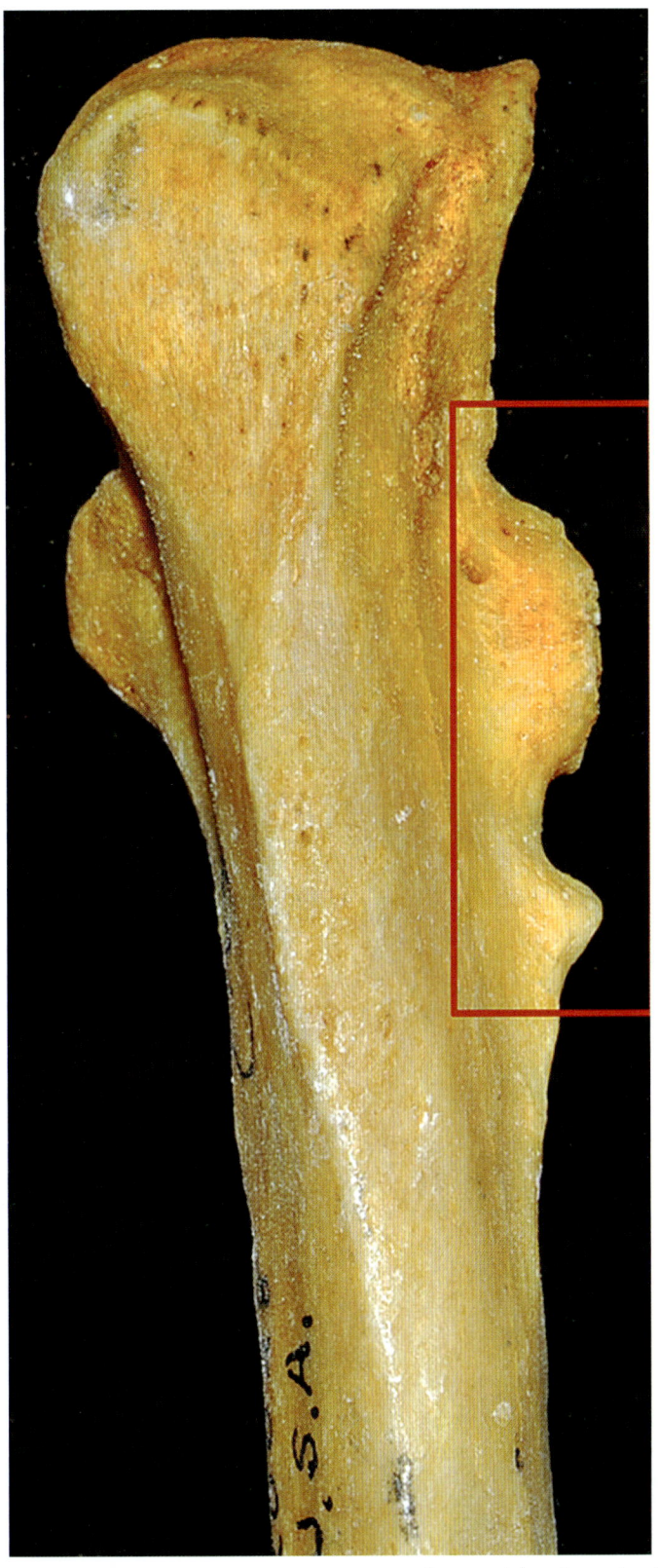

Figure 717. Highly developed and "doubled" supinator crest (rectangle) in the right ulna of an adult (SI Huntington). Uncommon finding. For discussion on occupational stress markers see Kennedy (1983).

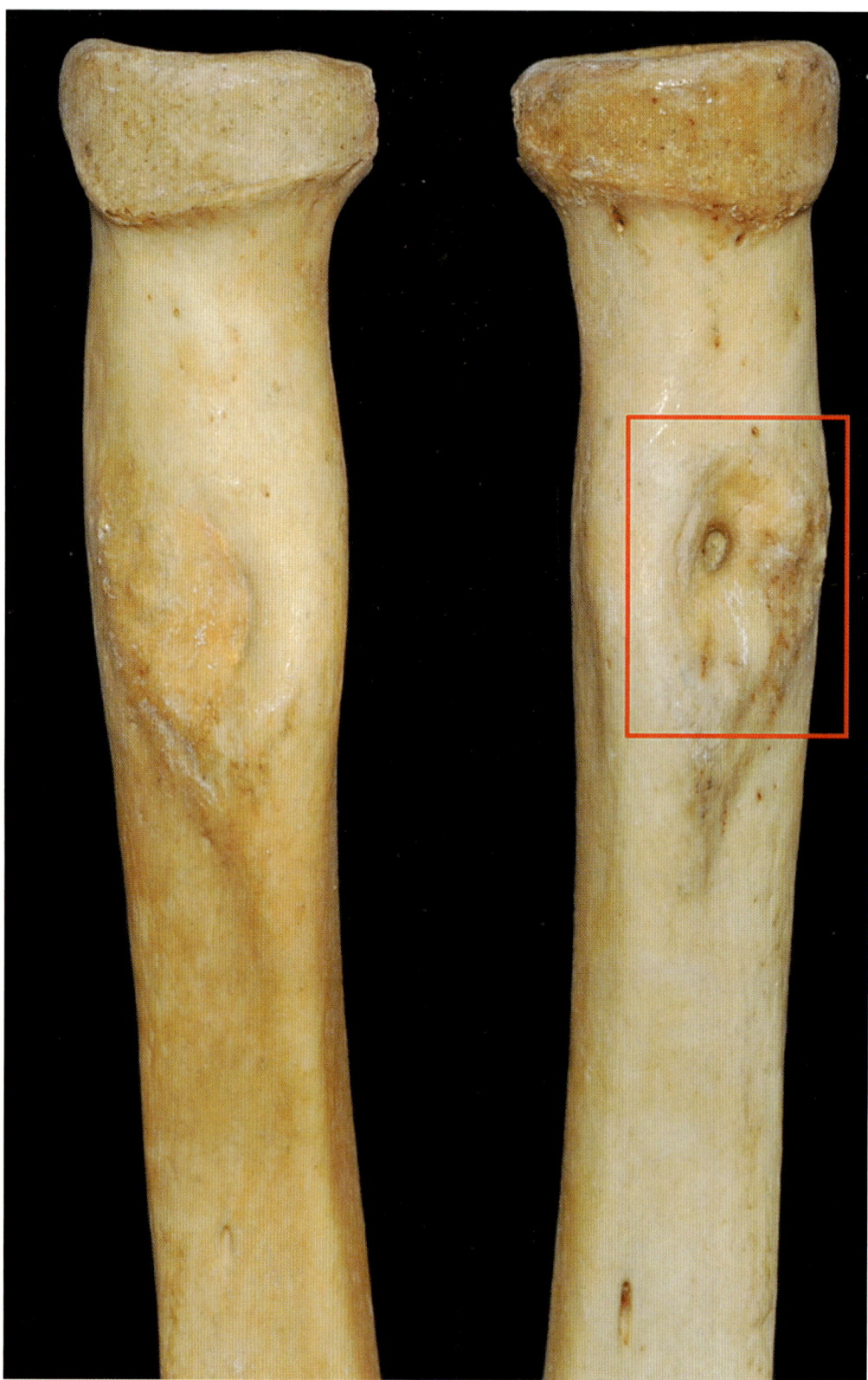

Figure 718. Dimpled radial tuberosity (rectangle) with a raised margin (SI). Uncommon to common finding of unknown etiology.

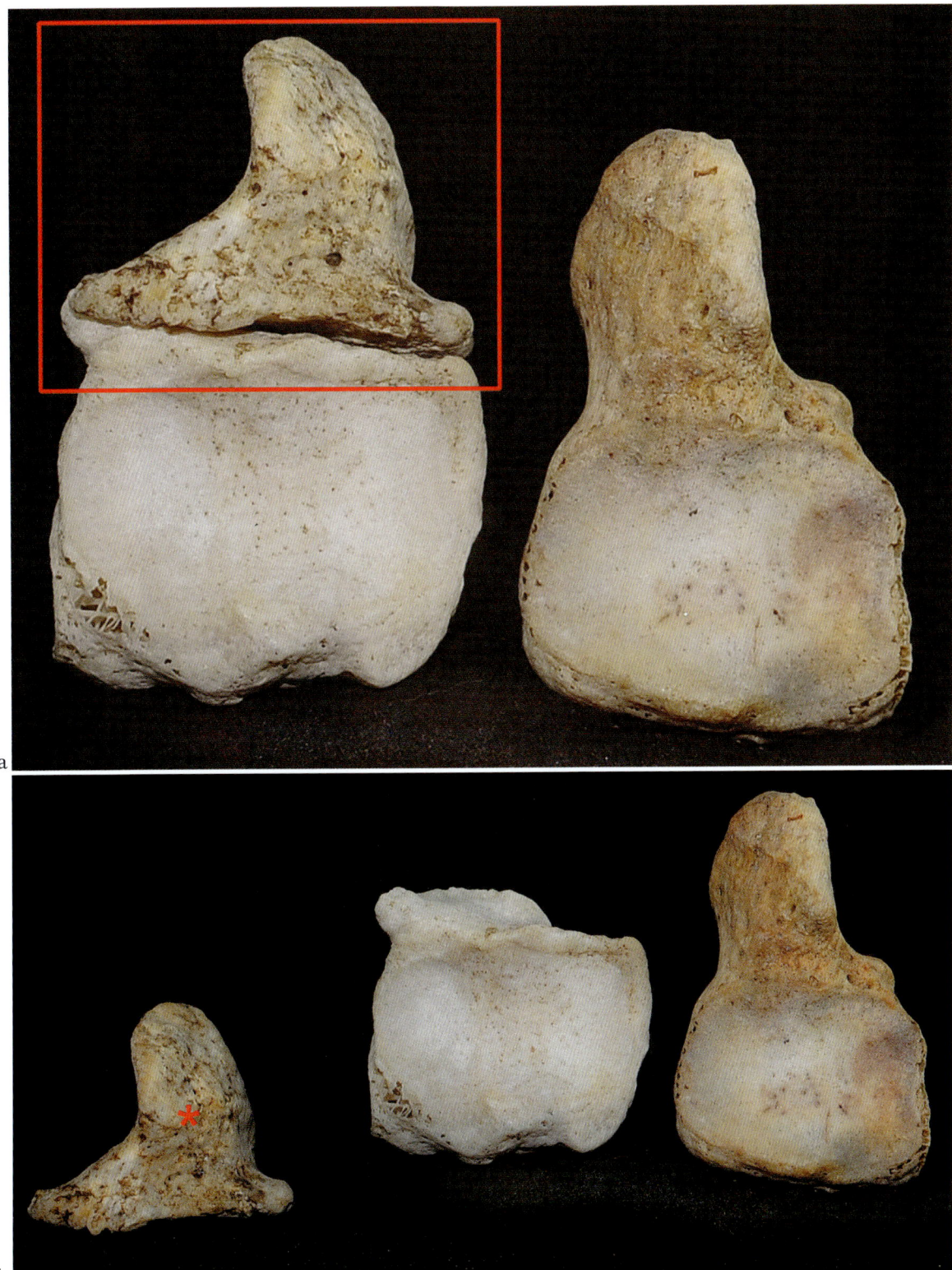

Figure 719a-b. Bipartite hamulus. (a) Bipartite right hamulus with the accessory bone attached (a – rectangle) and (b) unattached (*) in a 78-year-old male (CMU FO80456015). The individual's left hamulus (b) was not bipartite. Cf. Chow et al. (2005); Greene and Hadied (1981).

Chapter 10

STERNUM, SPINE AND PELVIS
(STERNUM, VERTEBRA, HIP AND SACRUM)

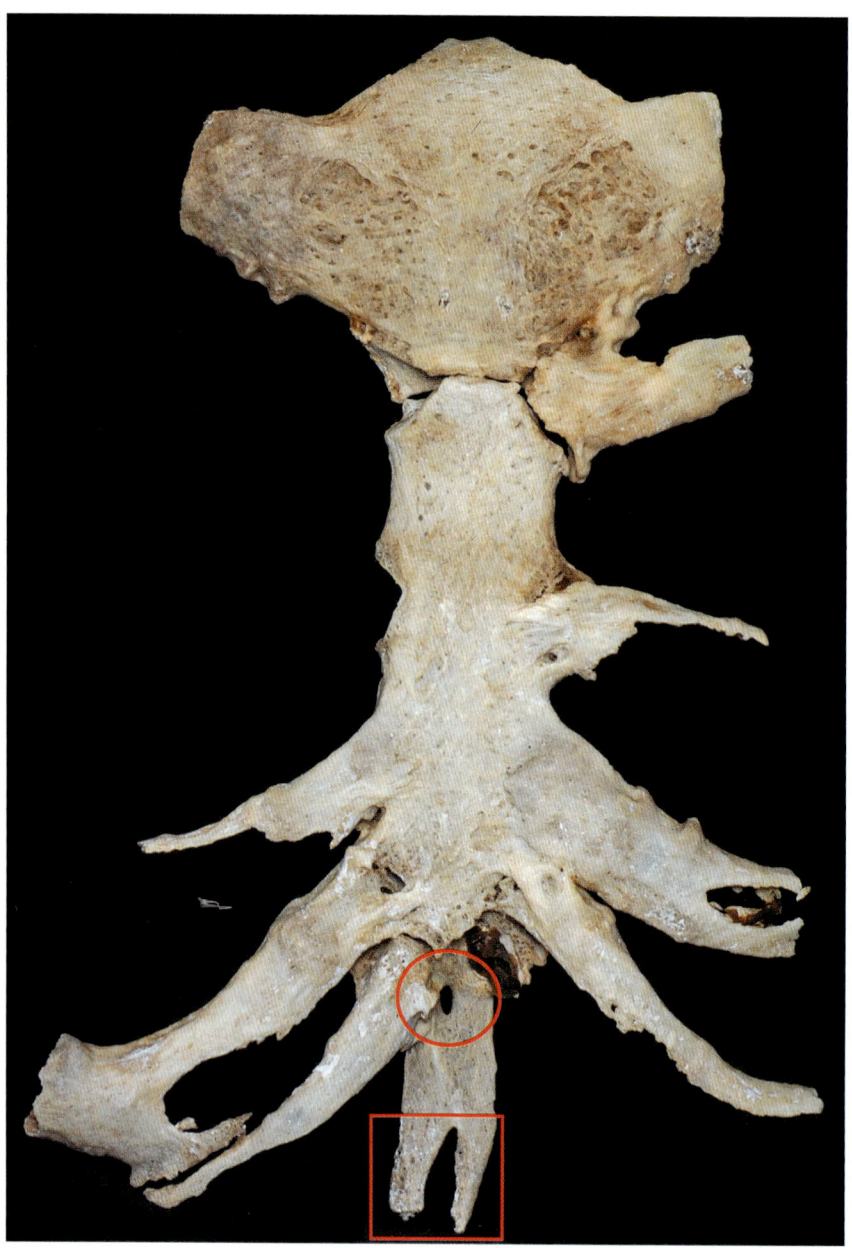

Figure 720. Normal calcification (resembling a crab claw) of the costal cartilage in an elderly Thai male (KKU). Note the small xiphoid foramen (circle) and bifid xiphoid process (square). Common findings. Cf. McCormick et al. (1985); Navani et al. (1970); Rejtarova et al. (2009); Sanders (1966); Verna et al. (1980) for sex determination from the cartilages. See Jit et al. (1980); Bongiovanni and Spradley (2012) for sex determination from the sternum. See Yekeler et al. (2006) for sternal variants and Scheuer (2002) for a radiographic example. For discussion on age-related feature of costal cartilage calcification see Inoi (1997); McCormick and Stewart (1988); Stewart and McCormick (1984); Vaziri et al. (2015).

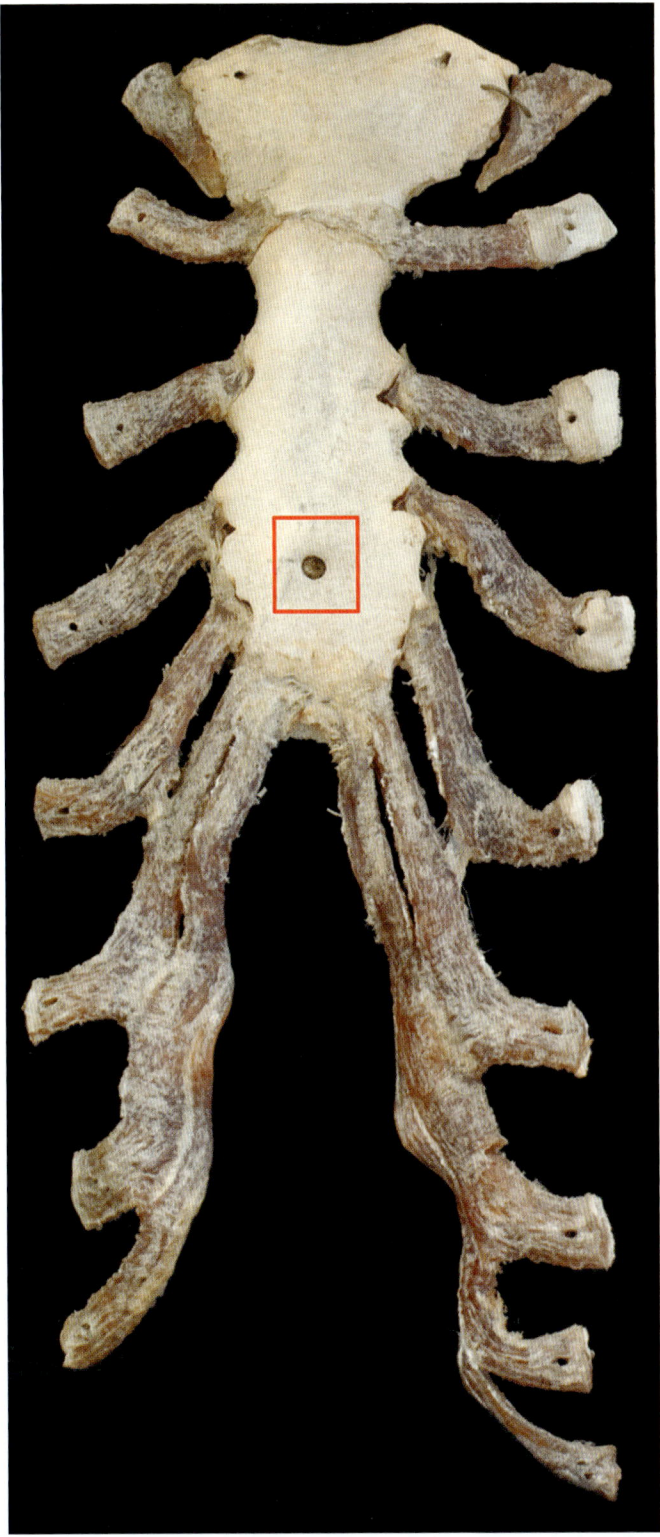

Figure 721. Normal anatomy of the chest plate (ventral view) showing attachment sites of the costal cartilage (ribs 1–10) and a small sternal foramen (square) in a 17- to 20-year-old Asian female (CSC AS 7). This chest plate was previously wired to the ribs. Cf. Yekeler et al. (2006). For discussion on sexing from the sternum see Bongiovanni and Spradley (2012).

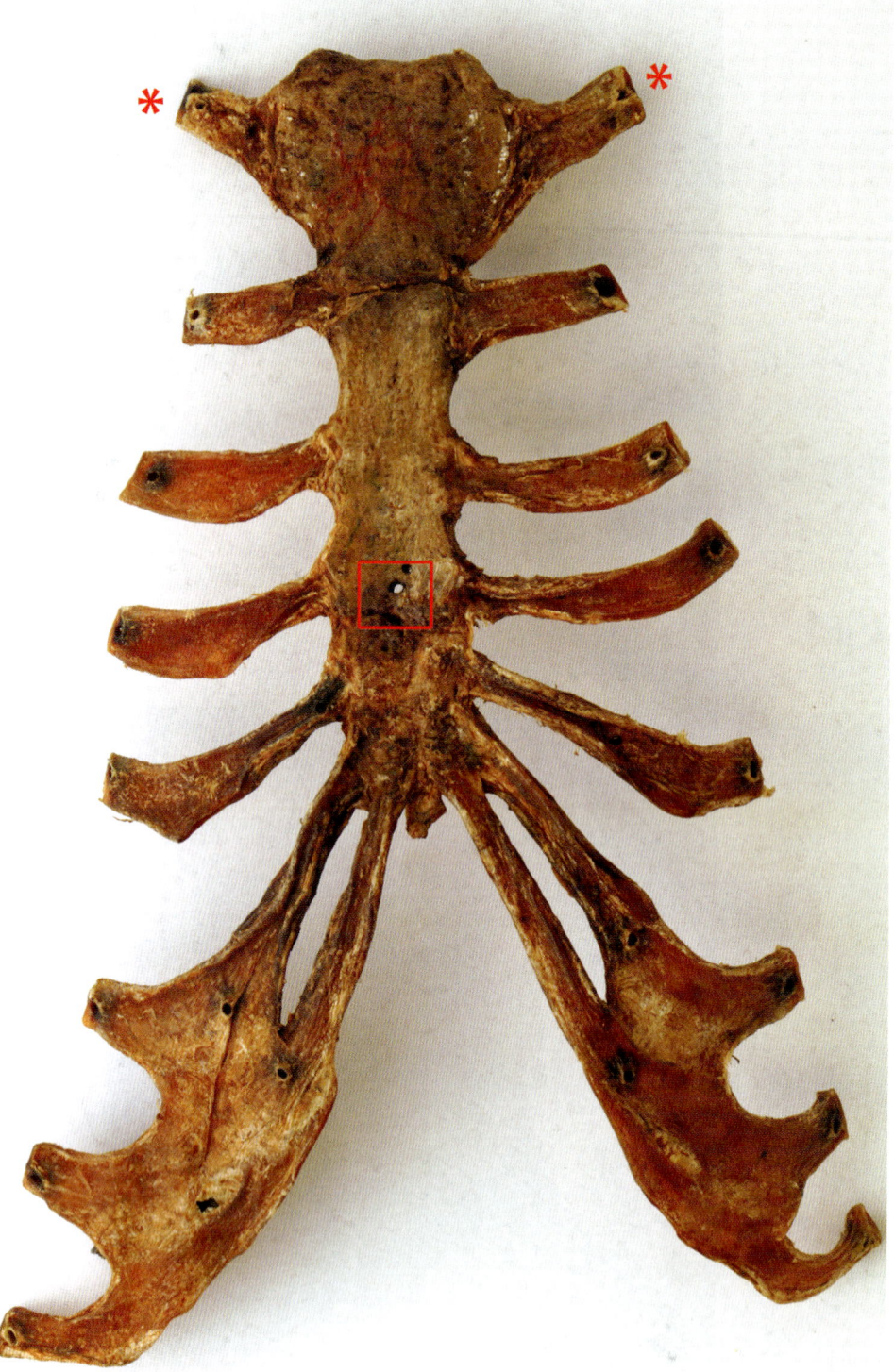

Figure 722. Chest plate consisting of the manubrium, body of sternum and costal cartilages in a teaching skeleton (FSA). The chest plate usually consists of seven sternocostal joints (ribs 1–7) that attach directly to the sternum (true ribs), three pairs of false ribs (8, 9 and 10) that join the sternum indirectly through the 7th costal cartilage, and two pairs of "floating" ribs (11 and 12) lacking bony attachment anteriorly. Ribs 1(*), 6 and 7 attach to the manubrium as synchondroses, whereas the other sternocostal joints are symphyseal joints. Cf. Gilroy et al. (2012). Note the small sternal aperture (square).

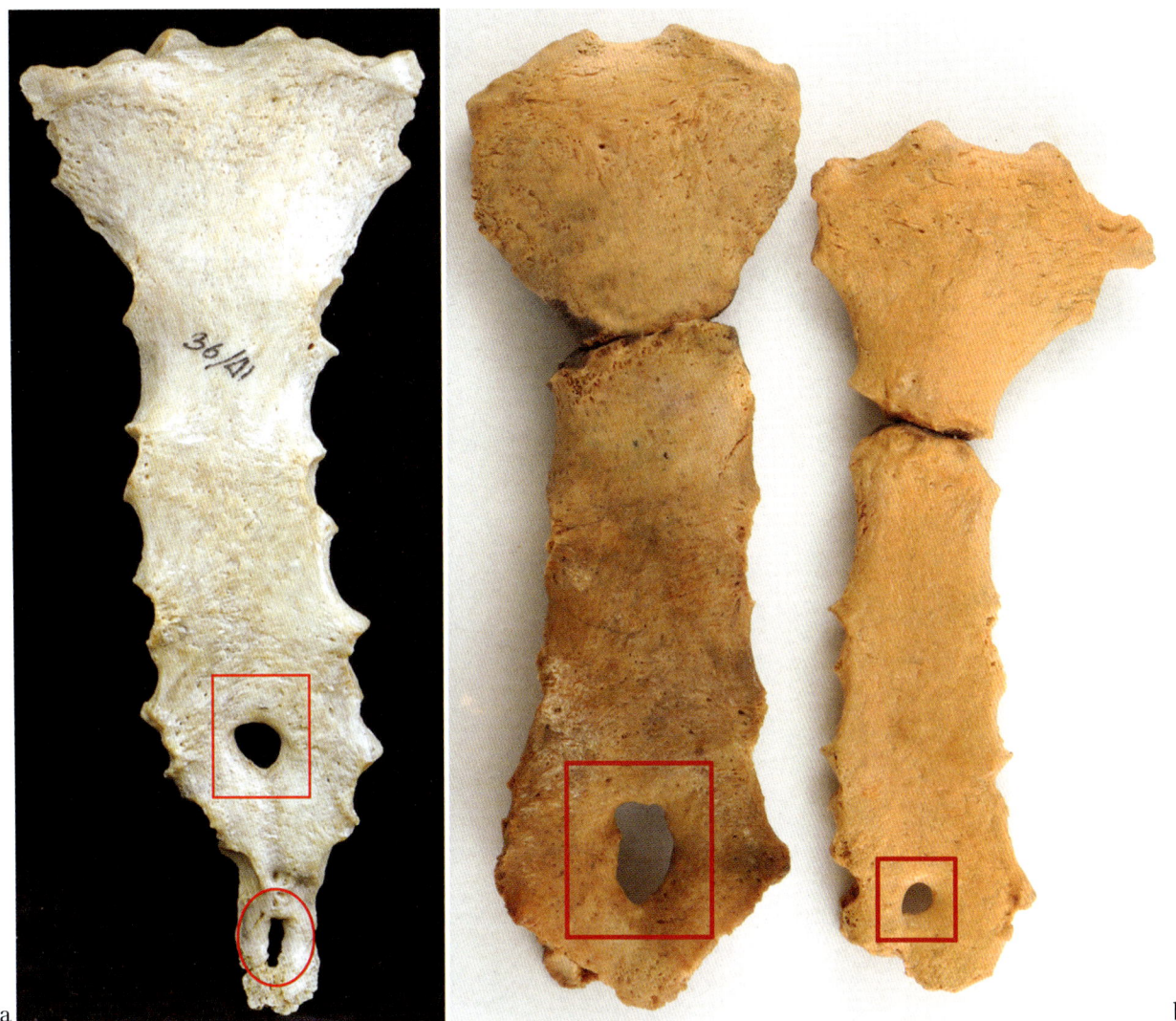

Figure 723a-b. Sternal aperture and xiphoid aperture. (a) Sternal foramen or aperture (rectangle) and xiphoid foramen (oval) in an adult (KKU). (b) Large and small sternal foramina in two young adults. These foramina are the result of incomplete fusion of multiple ossification centers. Yekeler et al. (2006) found xiphoidal foramen in 27.4% and sternal foramina in 4.5% of 1,000 patients. McCormick (1981) found 25 of 324 foramina (7.7%) in radiographs of decedents, were more common in men, were always single, round or oval and ranged in diameter from 3–18 mm. Common findings. Cf. Cooper et al. (1988).

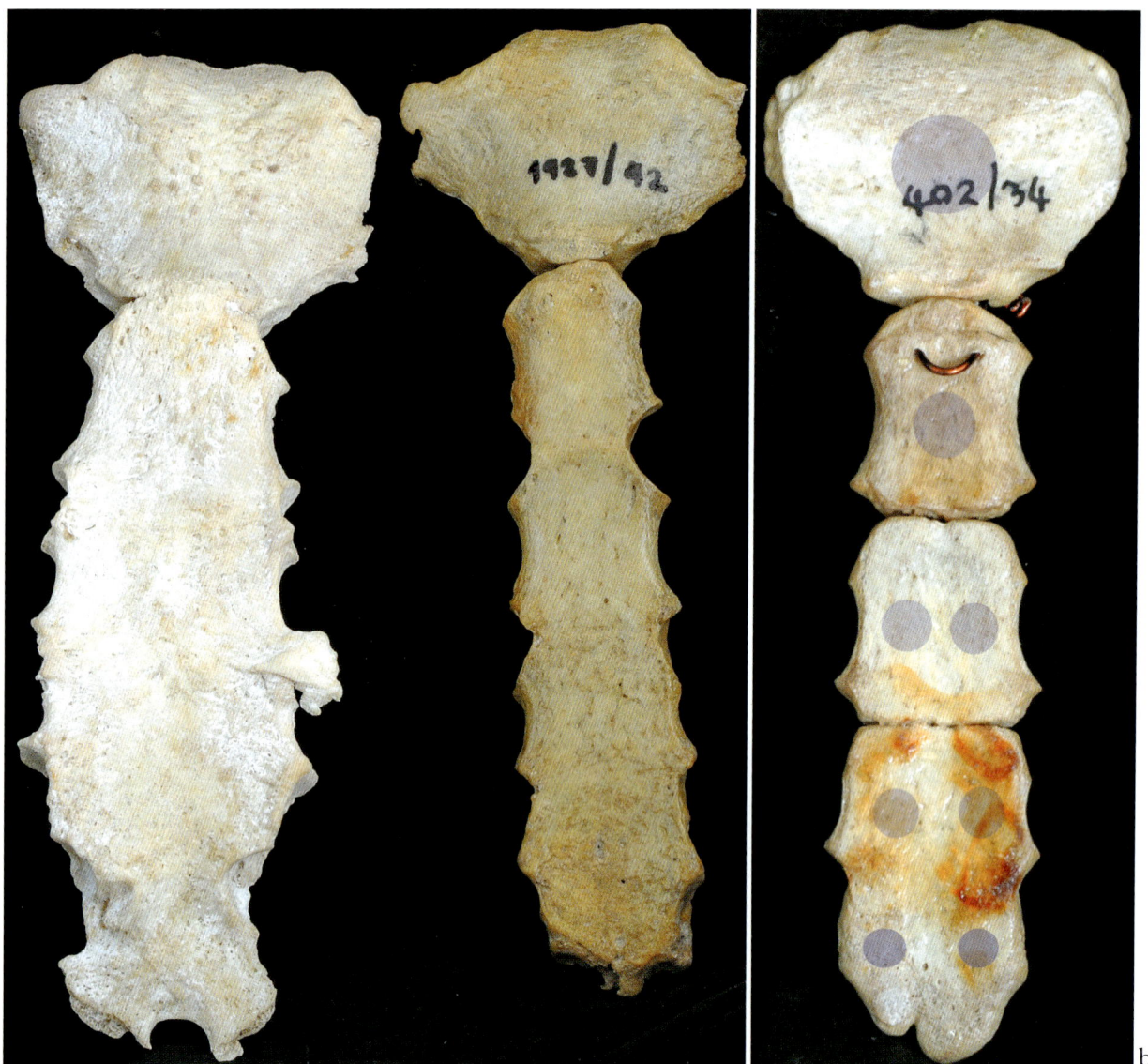

Figure 724a-b. Variation of the sternum. (a) Two adult sternums without sternal apertures. (b) Typical subadult sternum with its five segments, their lines of fusion and centers of ossification are illustrated in light purple (KKU). Ashley (1956) examined 581 human sterna from eight months fetal to four years of age and classified them into three types, based on the pattern of their centers of ossification: Type I displayed a single midline ossification in the center of the first three segments of the mesosternum; Type II with a single midline ossification in the center in the first segment and two bilateral or obliquely positioned centers in the third segment; Type III exhibited two bilaterally or obliquely positioned centers in each of the first three segments. Type II was the most common pattern (60%), followed by Type I (22%) and Type III (18%). Wong and Carter (1988) found that mechanical stress played a signficant role in the morphogenesis, growth and development of the sternum. Typical anatomy and common findings. Cf. Freyschmidt et al. (2002); Barnes (1994).

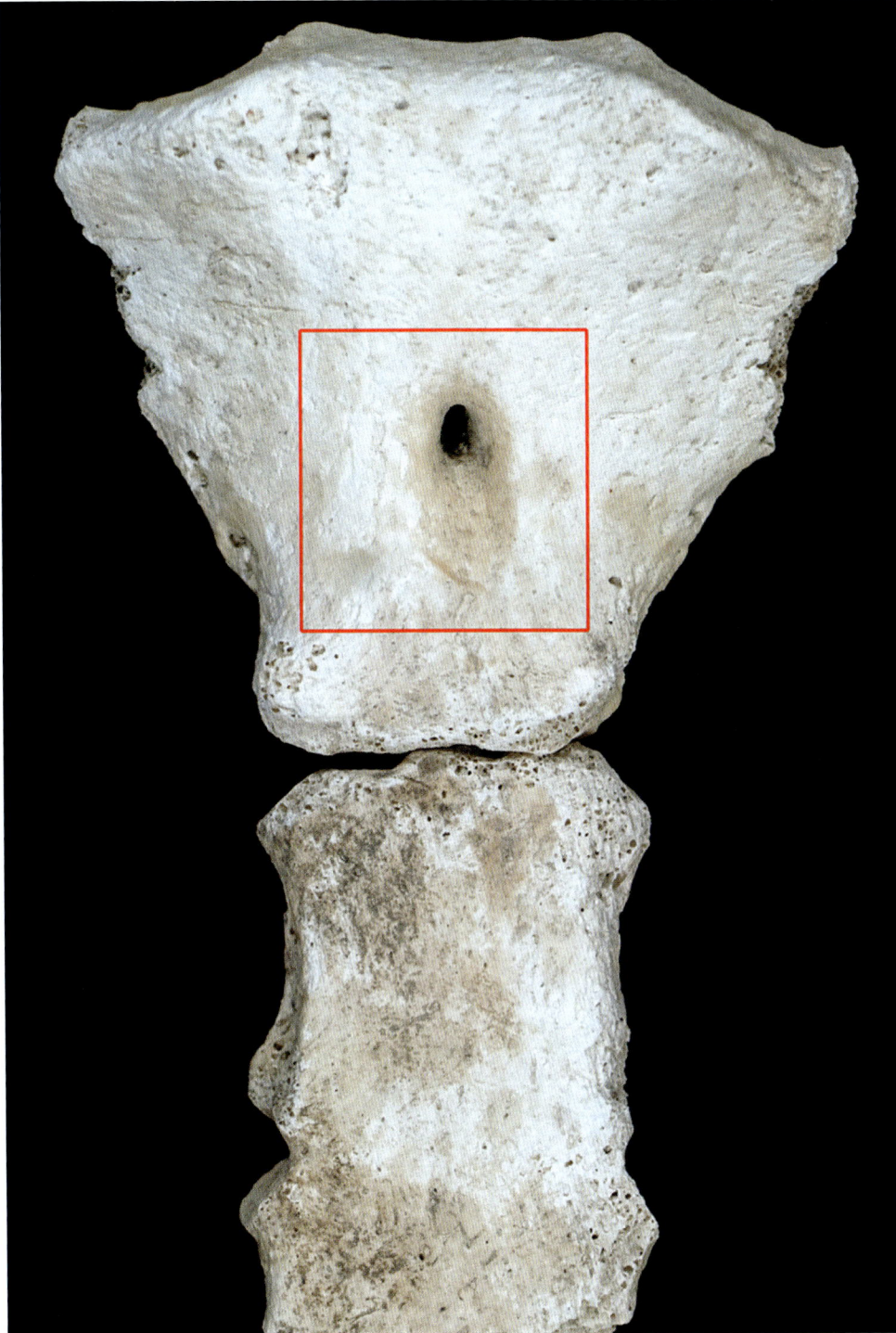

Figure 725. Manubrial aperture (square) in a probable adult (CIL). While the manubrium usually forms from one center of ossification, approximately 10% develops from two centers that form in a craniocaudal direction. A double center of ossification is often found in trisomy 21 and monosomy X (Clavelli et al. ND). CT (MDCT) examination of 1,000 manubria failed to reveal a foramen (Yekeler et al. 2006). Cooper et al. (1988) found one manubrial foramen in an elderly female in 236 autopsied chest plates and 580 infant cadavers. This trait may also be referred to as a manubrial foramen or perforation. Rare finding; this is the only example of this trait that the authors have seen.

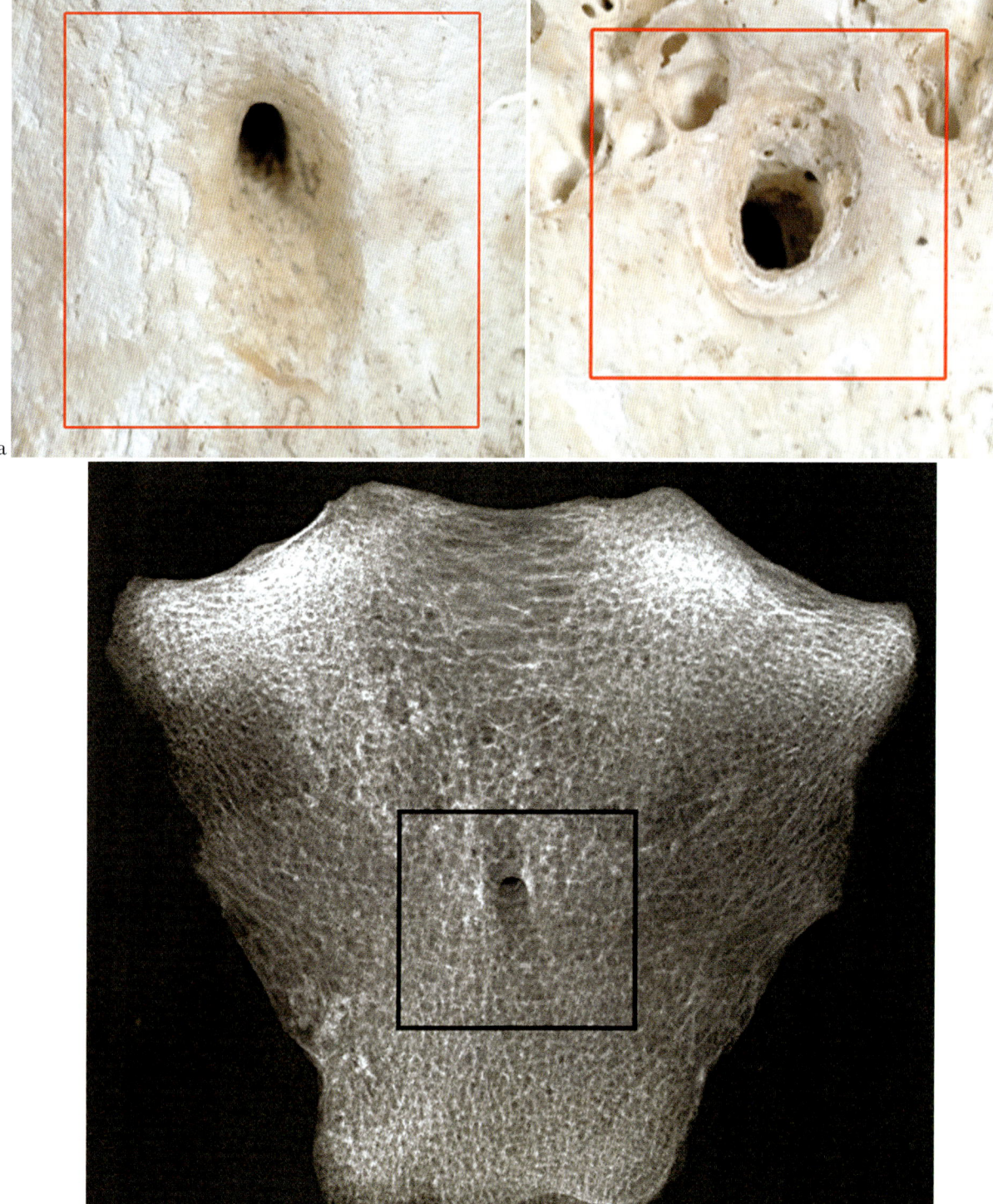

Figure 726a-c. Higher magnification and x-ray of manubrial aperture (CIL). (a) Ventral and (b) dorsal views (squares) (see Figure 725). When viewed ventrally, note the sloping inferior margin of the feature as it enters the aperture at an angle from inferior to superior. (c) AP x-ray of the manubrial aperture (square).

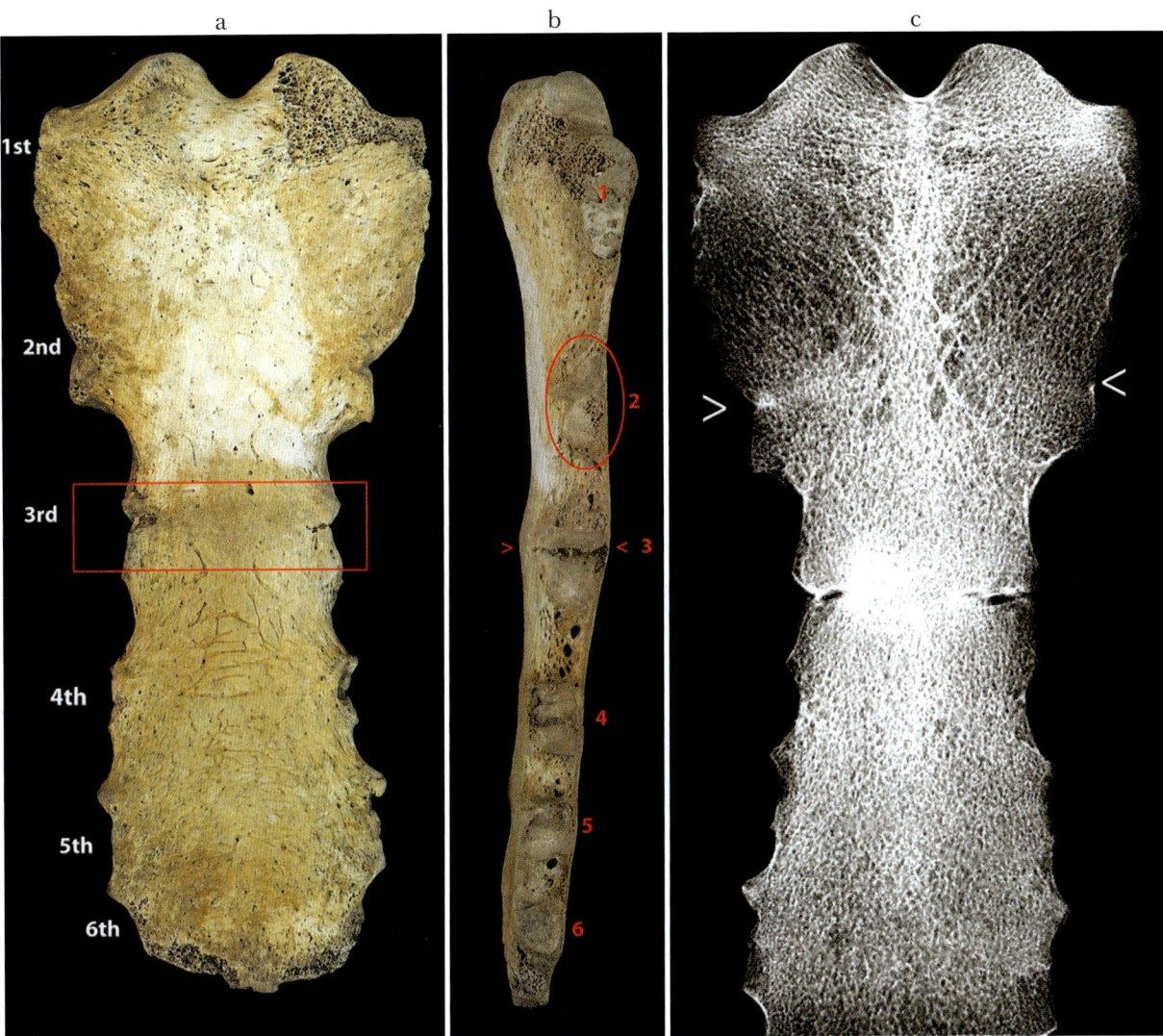

Figure 727a-c. Sternum with the second costal facet in the manubrium. (a) Anterior view shows the position of the sterno-manubrial junction that in this individual is located at the third costal facet (rectangle) in an adult male (CIL). (b) Lateral view of the costal facets demonstrating the morphology of the second (oval) and third facets (> and <). (c) X-ray illustrating the morphology of the 2nd costal facet (> and <) showing that the manubrium is unusually elongated from superior to inferior. Rare trait. See Bayaroğulları et al. (2014) for variation of the sternum using multidetector CT; and Jurik (2007) for radiographic imaging of the sternocostoclavicular region.

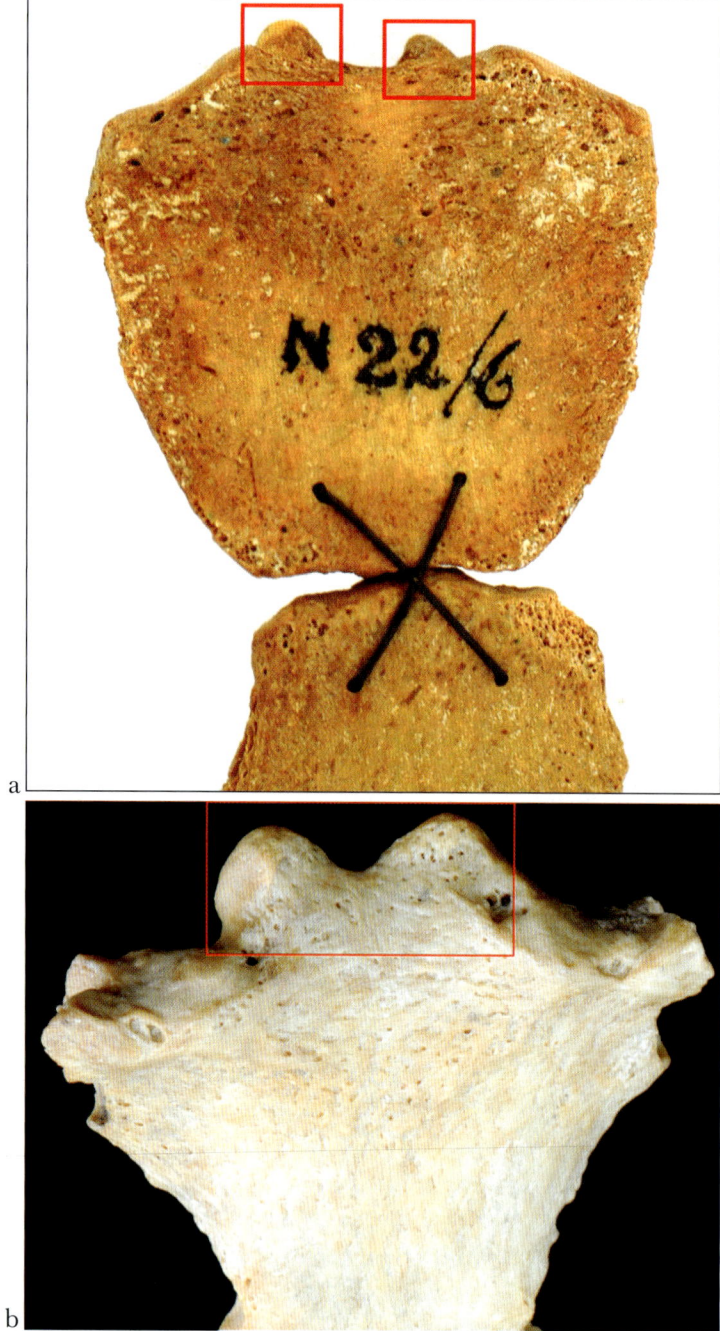

Figure 728a-b. Suprasternal or episternal bones in two adult Thais (KKU). (a) Small, bilateral suprasternal bones (squares). (b) Large, widely separate ossicles (rectangle) situated in the jugular notch. Episternal bones consist of cartilage that fail to attach to the manubrium (Arey 1946) and were found in 4% of 1,000 patients (Yekeler et al. 2006). Ogawa et al. (1979) reported 6.9% of 562 living Japanese subjects had suprasternal bones and 1.4% (8 of 562) had suprasternal tubercles, of which three individuals were bilateral. See Carwardine (1893) for drawings of these tubercles and their ligamentous attachment between the clavicle and jugular notch. This variant may appear as an attached (fused) tubercle or a separate pea-shaped bone that may easily be overlooked or misidentified. Freyschmidt et al. (2002) report about 1% to 7% of patients have these asymptomatic ossicles. Cf. Restrepo et al. (2009) for x-ray examples; Stark et al. (1987) for drawings of eight variants of these ossicles; Cobb (1937); Dixon (1914).

Sternum, Spine and Pelvis (Sternum, Vertebra, Hip and Sacrum) 551

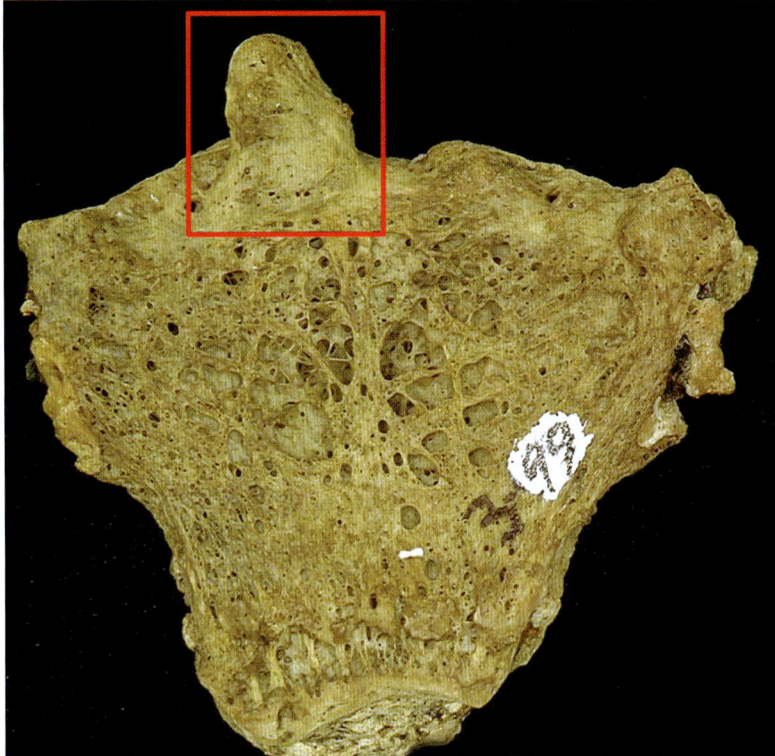

Figure 729. Unilateral suprasternal tubercle (rectangle) in an adult (UTK, Joe Hefner). Bilateral suprasternal tubercles are twice as common as the unilateral type (Yekeler et al. 2006). Cf. Freyschmidt et al. (2002). Stark et al. (1987) found 12 examples of episternal ossicles in 800 individuals. Eight cases were bilateral, 4 were unilateral, 7 were in men and 5 were in women. Cf. Cobb (1937); Dixon (1914).

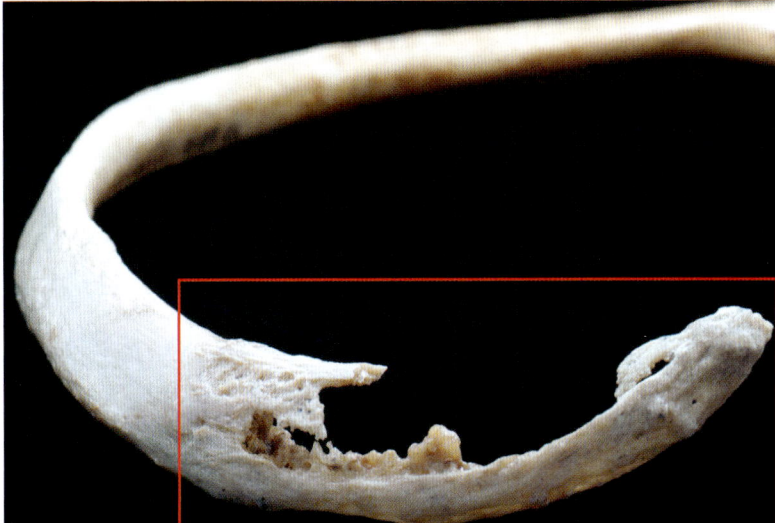

Figure 730. Calcification of the costal cartilage in a right rib (CSC DS007). Common finding in the elderly. Cf. McCormick (1983); Vastine et al. (1948). For sex determination: McCormick et al. (1985); Navani et al. (1970); Rejtarova et al. (2009); Sanders (1966); Verna et al. (1980). For discussion on costal cartilage calcification and association with age see: Inoi (1997); McCormick and Stewart (1988); Stewart and McCormick (1984); Vaziri et al. (2015).

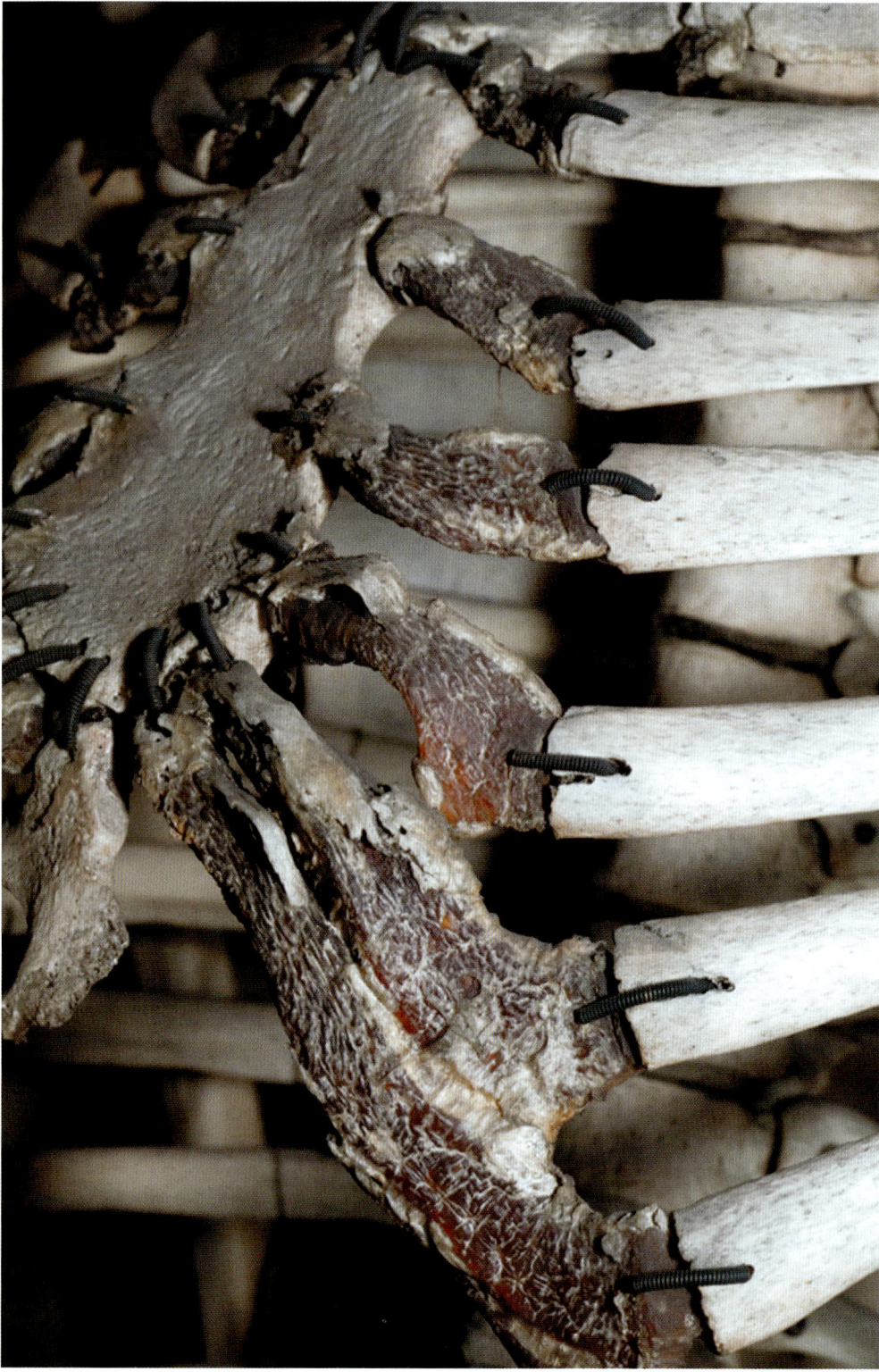

Figure 731. Normal calcification pattern of the (hyaline) costal cartilage in males (Mütter Museum). The covering of the costal cartilage, the perichondrium, shows numerous surface cracks, but no "vertical plates" as in Figures 732 and 733. Note bone formation along the upper and lower surfaces of the costal cartilage giving a "crab claw" appearance. Cf. McCormick et al. (1985); Scheuer (2002).

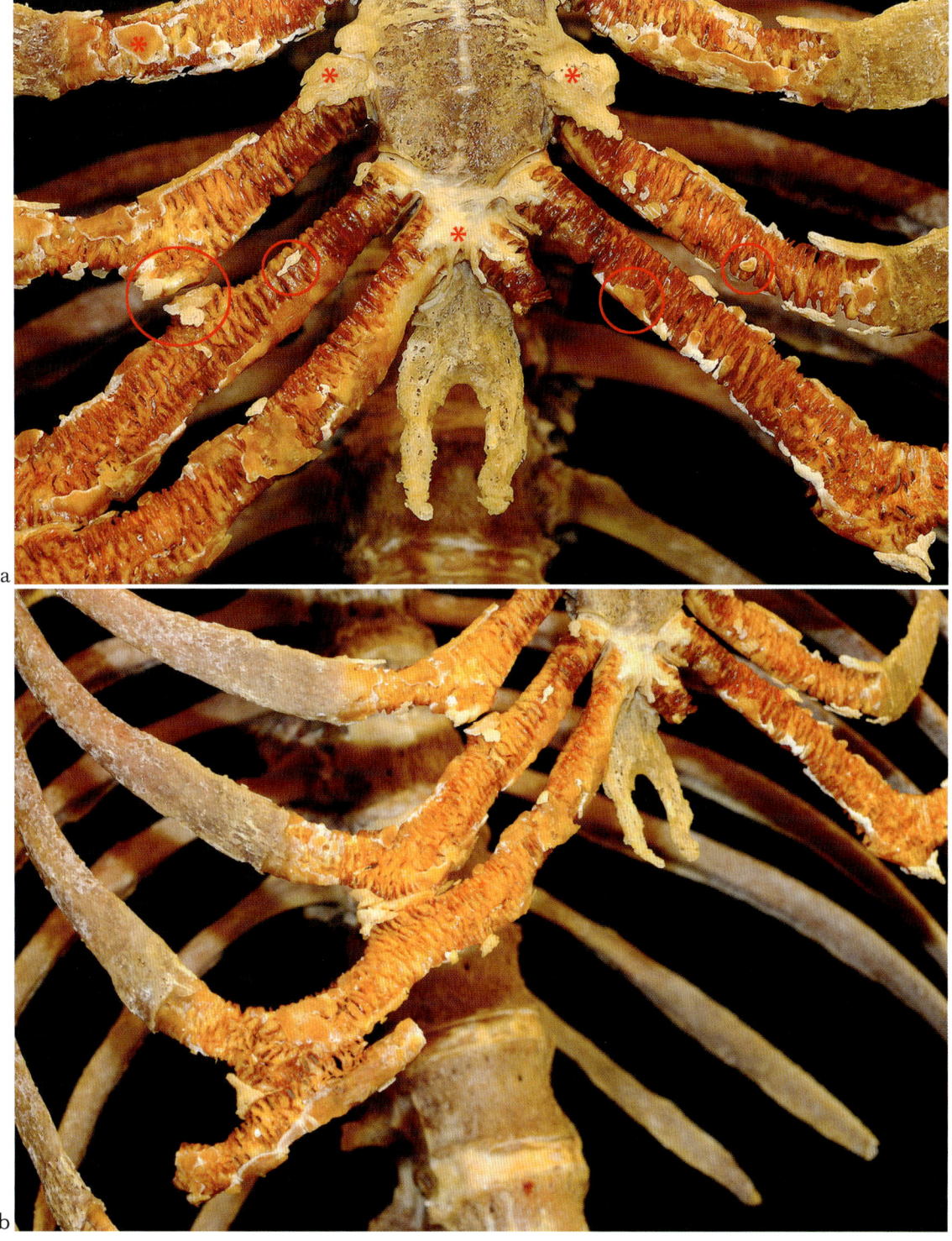

Figure 732a-b. Costal cartilage in a 72-year-old female (JABSOM). (a) Ventral view of the chest plate illustrating what the authors call "vertical plates" of costal cartilage (Type II collagen) and areas of calcification (circles and *) after immersion in bleach for 20 minutes. (b) Right oblique view showing numerous small areas of calcification and vertical plates after removal of the perichondrium and costal matrix with bleach. It is not known if these vertical plates reflect a normal underlying pattern of costal cartilage in all individuals or a pattern that accompanies elderly age. The authors are conducting additional research on this topic. See Figure 733 for an enlargement of vertical plates.

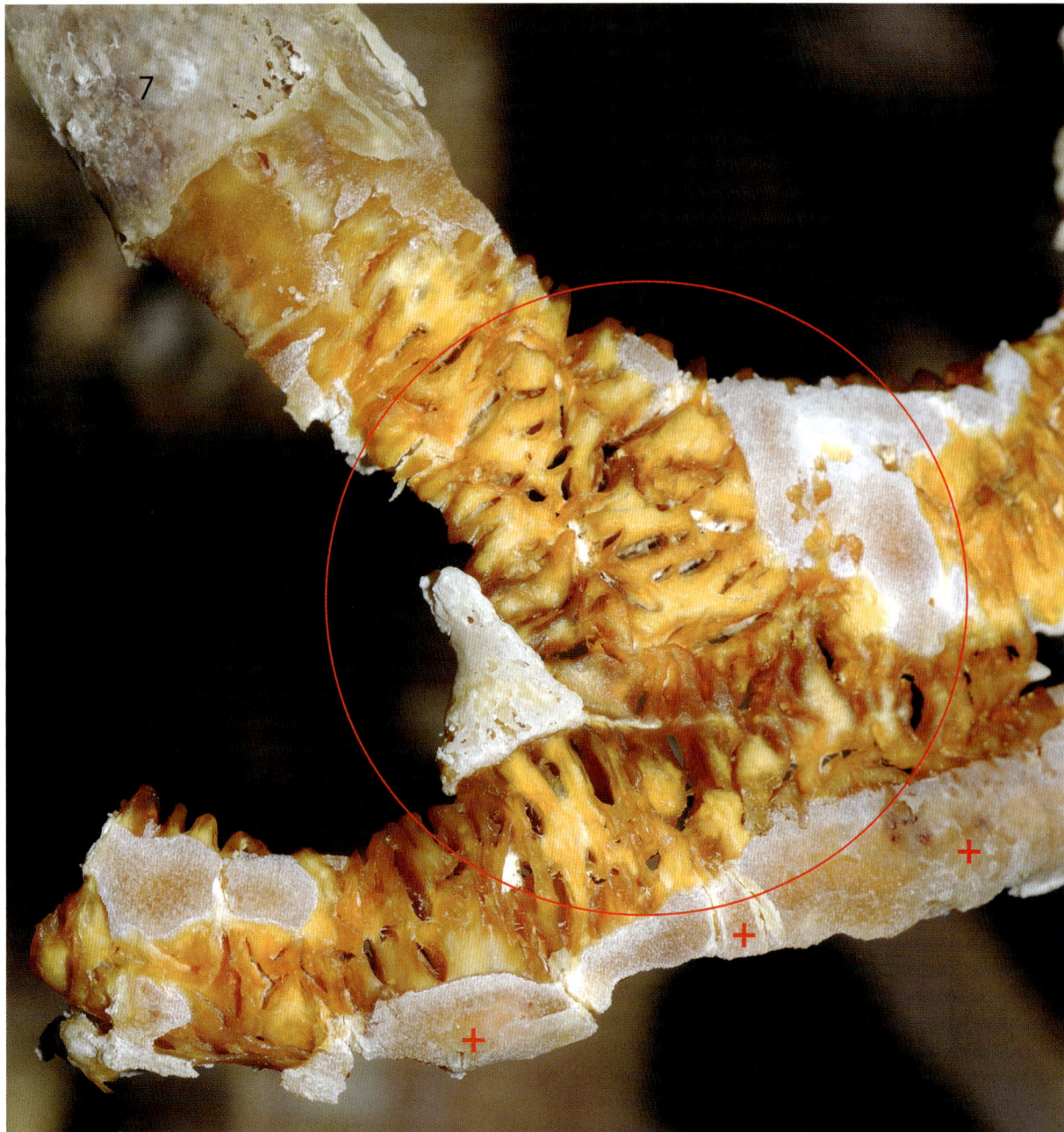

Figure 733. Oblique view illustrating translucent (whitish) areas of what appears to be calcification, especially noticeable along the inferior surface of the 8th costal cartilage (+) and a "disorganized" pattern of vertical plates joining the right 7th and 8th costal cartilages in a 72-year-old female (JABSOM). See Figure 732 for more images of this chest plate. Calcification is typically most developed along the dorsal surfaces of the costal cartilages. (Overlying perichondrium has been removed by immersion in bleach. The authors are researching whether this pattern is an artifact of the bleaching process or a previously unreported biological structure.)

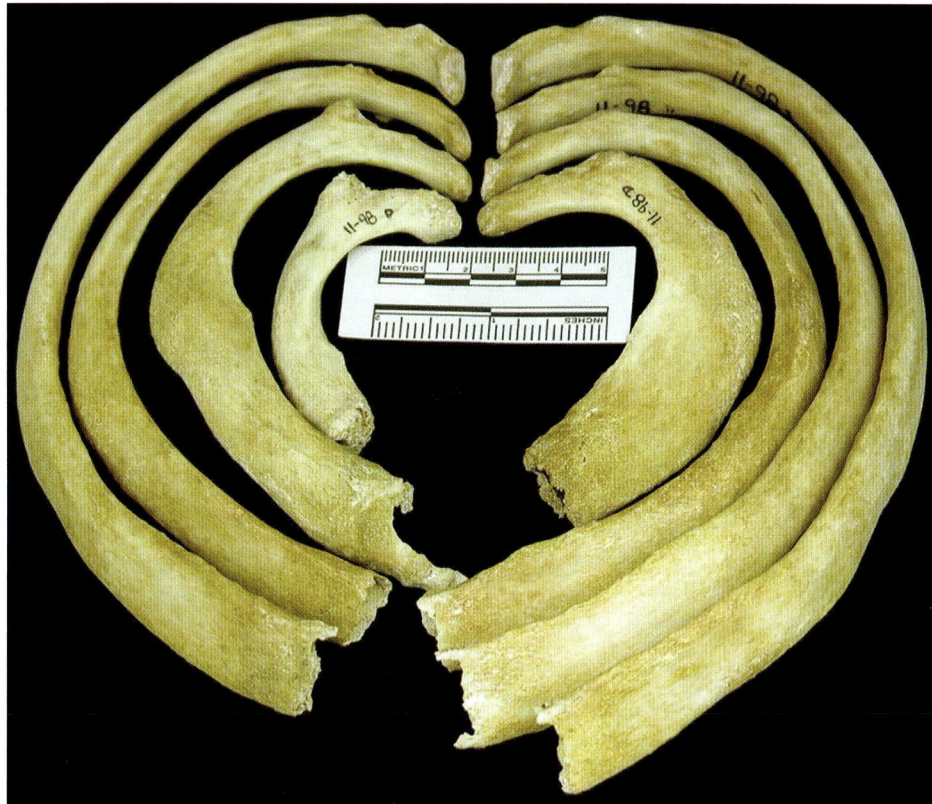

Figure 734. Asymmetrical and hypoplastic right ribs, possibly reflecting Klippel-Feil or scoliosis (Hefner, UTK 1998 11–98D). Uncommon finding.

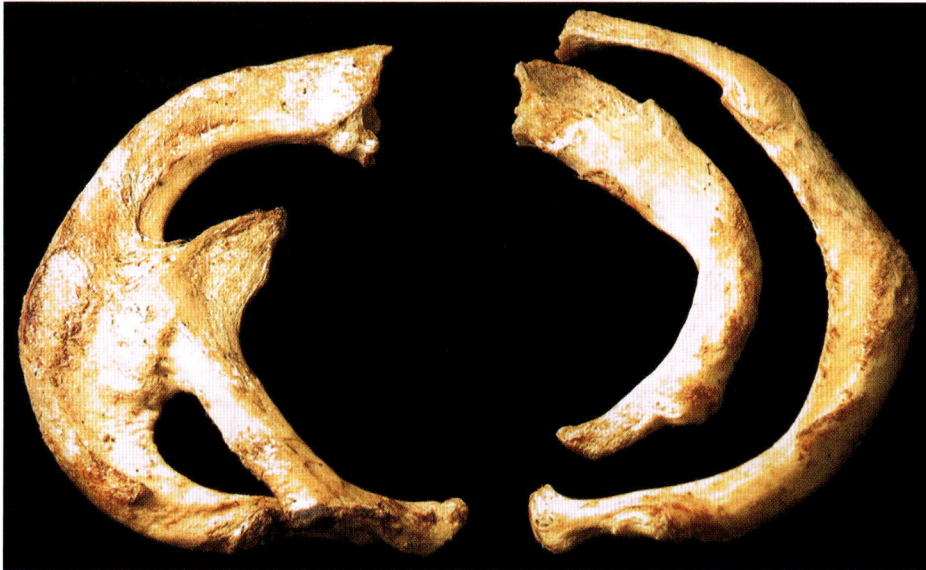

Figure 735. Lateral union, also referred to as synostosis, fusion, bridging or bifid rib, of the left first and second ribs. Srb's anomaly is also used to characterize this feature, but is broader in definition since it includes the partial or complete fusion of the first and second ribs (Yochum and Rowe 2005) (Joe Hefner, UTK). The right and left second ribs are approximately the same size. Uncommon to rare finding. Srb's anomaly cf. Barnes (1994, 2012); Campbell (1870); Gershon-Cohen and Delbridge (1945); Köhler and Zimmer (1968).

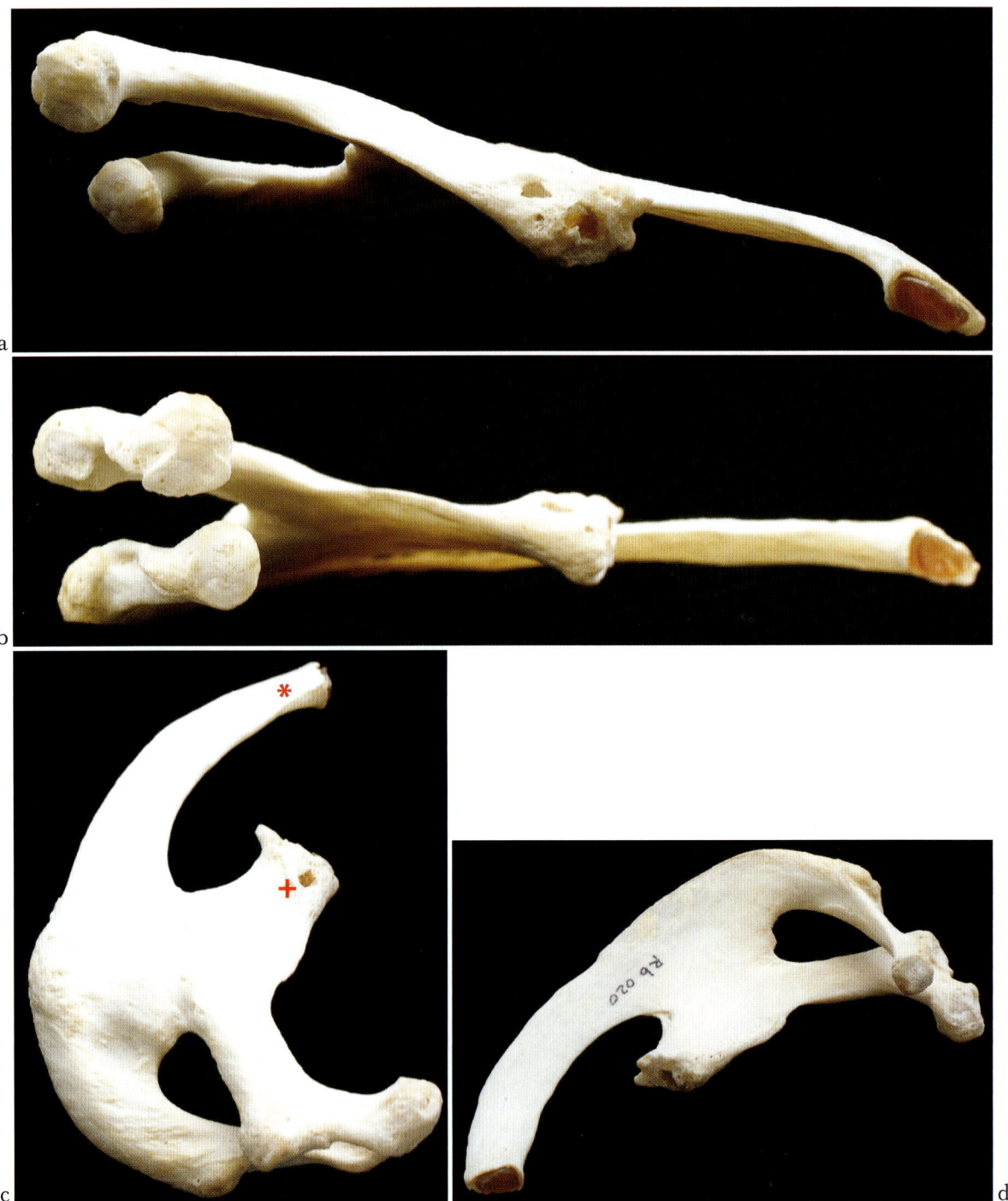

Figure 736a-d. Srb's anomaly (FSA Rb020). (a and b) Medial-lateral views of the ribs showing their overall morphology and area of fusion. (c) Superior view demonstrating the altered shape of the first rib and costal end (+) and second rib (*). (c and d) View from beneath showing the area of fusion of the two ribs and the altered shapes of both ribs. Cf. Barnes (1994, 2012) and Gershon-Cohen and Delbridge (1945) for anomalies of the first rib. A cervical rib, in contrast, is generally considered to originate from the seventh cervical vertebrae and does not contact the manubrium. However, some researchers believe that a cervical ridge may attach to the manubrium (Turner 1870). Note that the present authors were unable to discern the origin or meaning of "Srb," other than it probably refers to "J. Srb," a German anatomist from the 1800s.

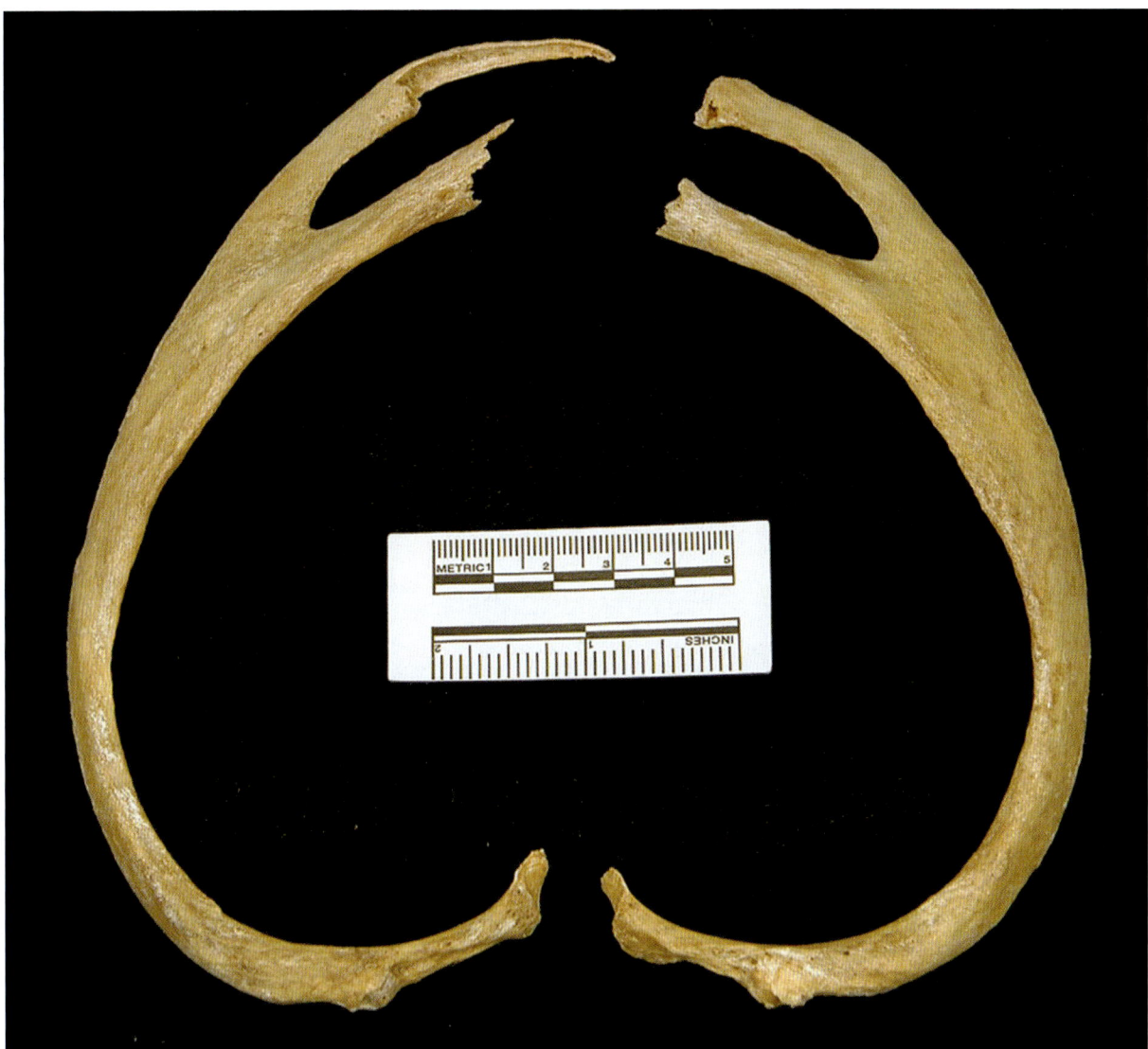

Figure 737. Bilateral Luschka's bifurcated ("forked") rib with perichondral calcification of the costal cartilage of the left rib (Hefner, UTK). Luschka's bifurcated rib, forking of the terminal, anterior portion of a rib is the most common of all rib anomalies, occurring in approximately 0.6% of chest radiographs (Yochum & Rowe 2005). Cf. Arey (1942); Barnes (1994, 2012); MacDonnell (1886).

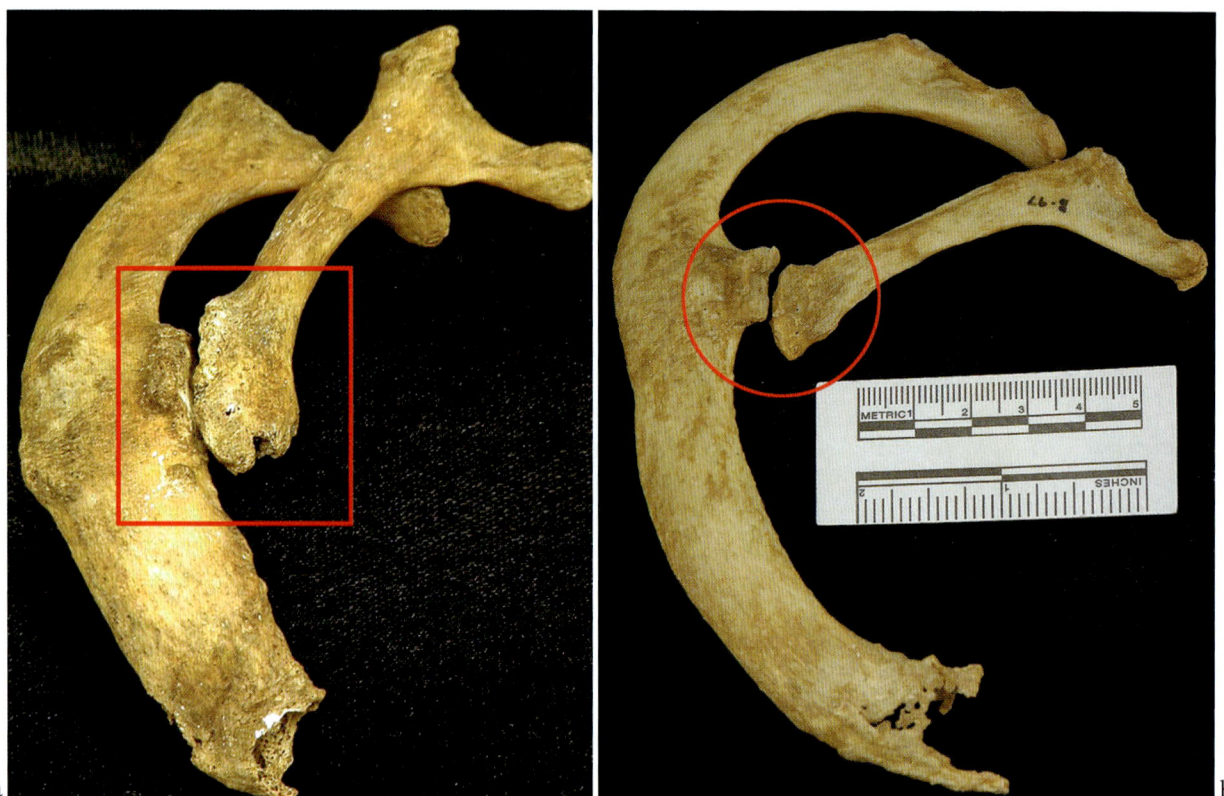

Figure 738a-b. Variation of two right cervical ribs with pseudoarthroses. (a) Cervical rib articulating through a pseudoarthrosis with the first thoracic rib (square) (Hefner, UTK 2001 16-01). (b) A cervical rib with pseudoarthrosis (circle) to the first rib in an adult (UTK 1997 08-97). Note the size and shape differences between the two first ribs. Etter (1944) found 68 cervical ribs in 40,000 consecutive chest x-rays films of men. Erken et al. (2002) found a significant correlation between the presence of cervical ribs and sacralization and scored "non-articulating" (attached) and elongated transverse processes of cervical vertebrae (C7) as cervical ribs if greater than 30 mm. Brewin et al. (2009) noted 10 individuals with cervical ribs of 1,352 chest radiographs. Cf. Todd (1912); Lucas (1915).

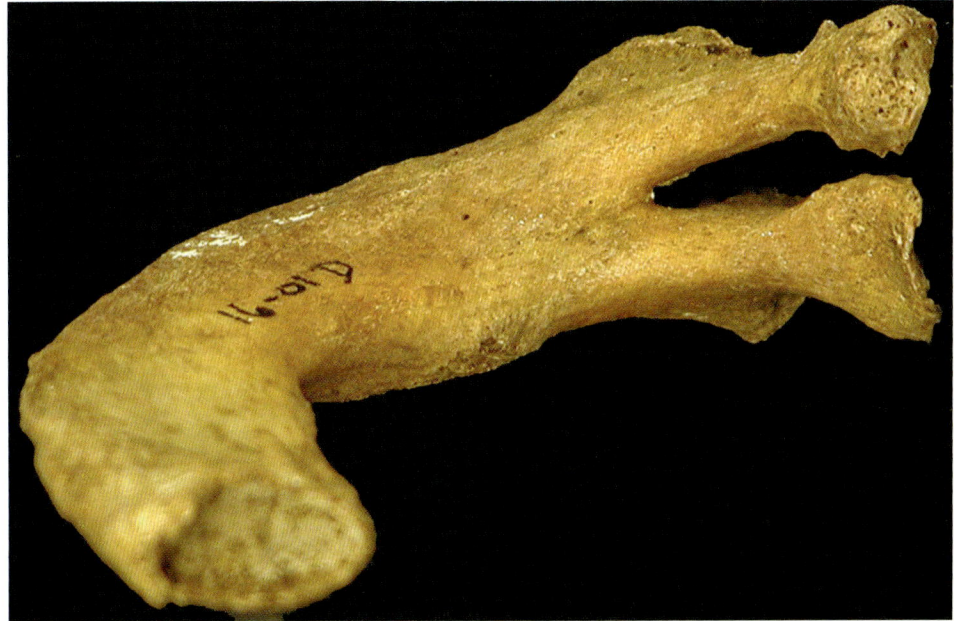

Figure 739. Synostosed first and second ribs, possibly Srb's anomaly, resulting in two articular vertebral facets and one body (Hefner, UTK). Turner (1883) referred to this as a bicipital rib (see MacDonnell 1886). Uncommon to rare finding in most osteology collections. Cf. Yochum and Rowe (2005) for radiographic example and description of Srb's anomaly.

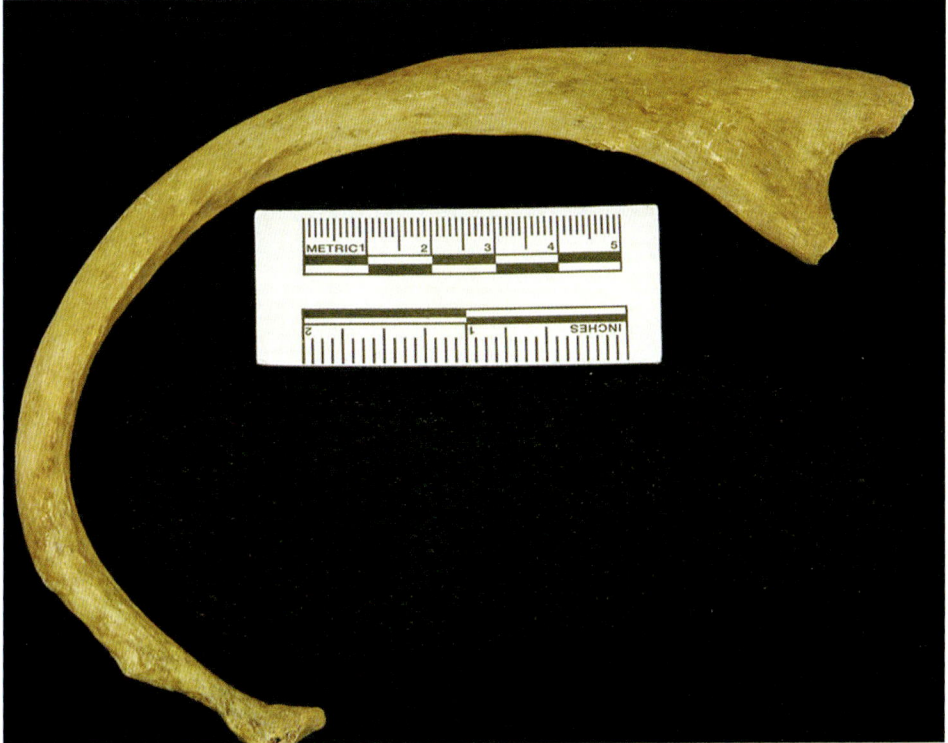

Figure 740. Luschka's (bifid, bifurcated) left rib with mild separation and bifurcation of the sternal end (Hefner, UTK 1999 22-99D). Although Luschka's rib was originally used only for the fourth rib, some researchers use this term for any upper rib that bifurcates anteriorly (Cf. Yochum and Rowe 2005).

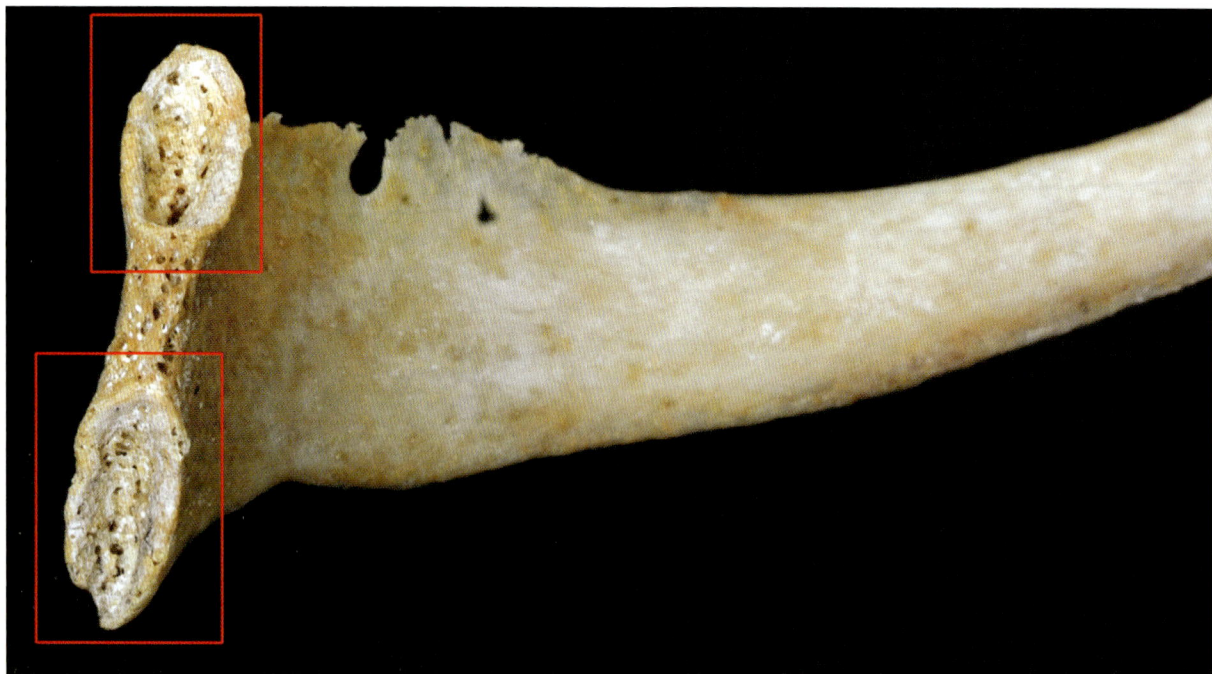

Figure 741. Anterior and internal view of a Lushka's bifid right fourth rib for attachment of the 4th and 5th costal joints (rectangles) of the sternum in an adult Thai male (KKU). Note that while sternal end of the right rib is mildly bifurcated the left rib is normal (KKU).

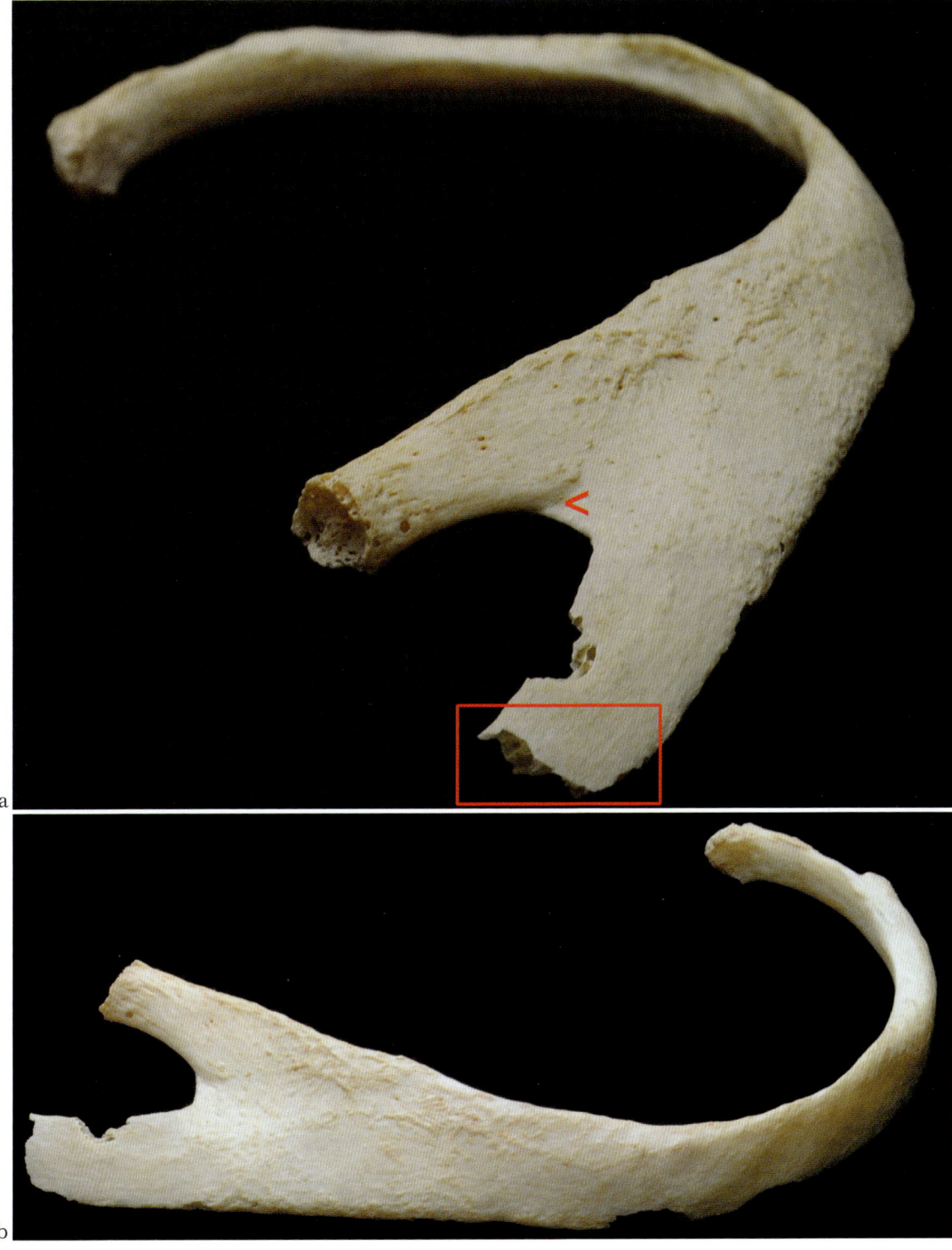

Figure 742a-b. Luschka's bifurcated left fourth rib (courtesy Vince Sava). (a) Mediolateral view demonstrating that the two sternal facets are widely divergent, the anterior portion of the rib becomes wider and thinner as it approaches the sternum and that there is a thin "web" of bone (<) that connects the two sternal facets with the single fourth rib. The inferior facet (red rectangle) was damaged postmortem. The two sternal facets would have articulated with the left 4th and 5th costal facets on the sternum. (b) Lateral view of the rib showing its anterior bifurcation.

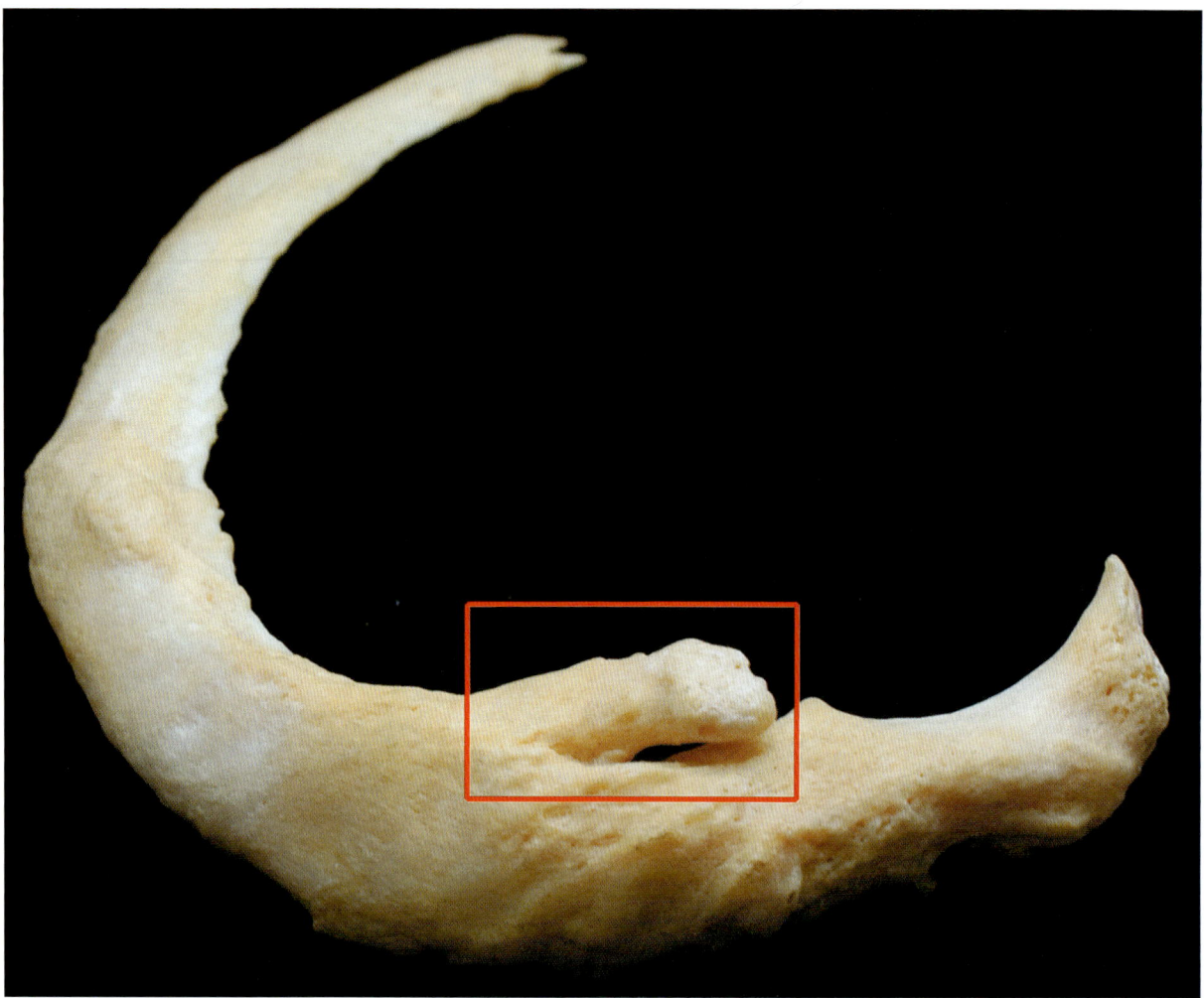

Figure 743. Rudimentary left first rib (rectangle) synostosed to the second rib (FSA Rb019).

VERTEBRAE AND PELVIS

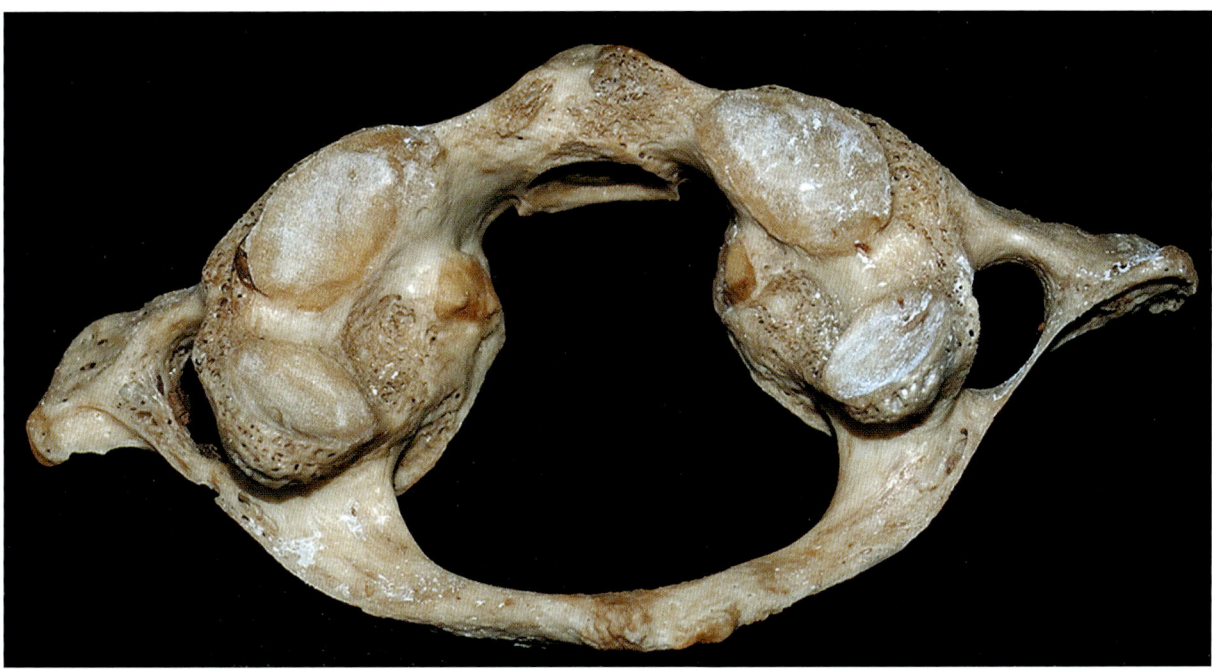

Figure 744. Divided or double superior articular facets of the atlas for articulation with the occipital condyles in an adult male (KKU 0684).

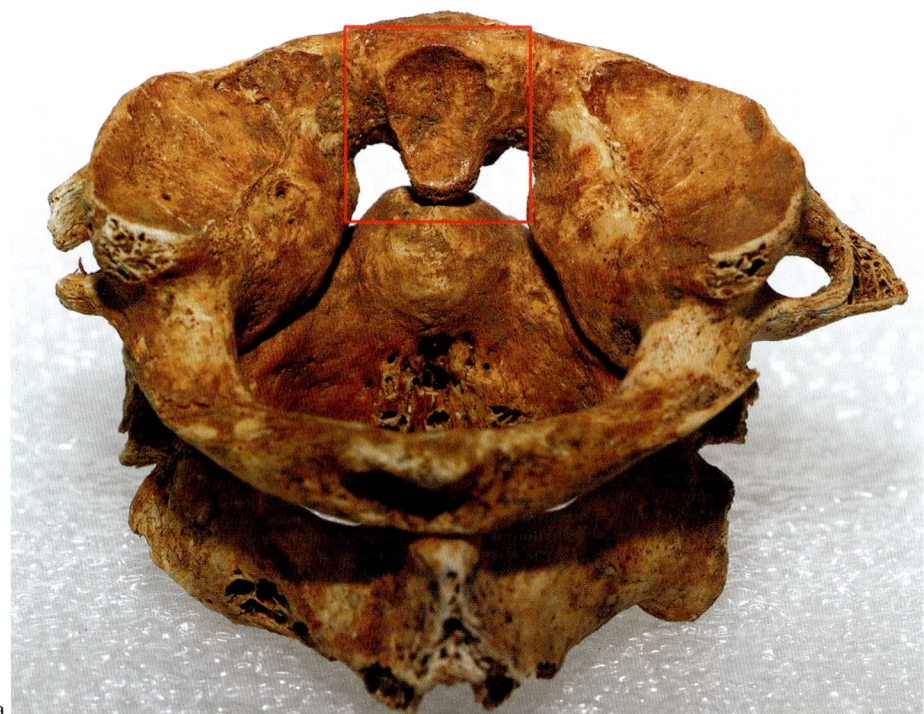

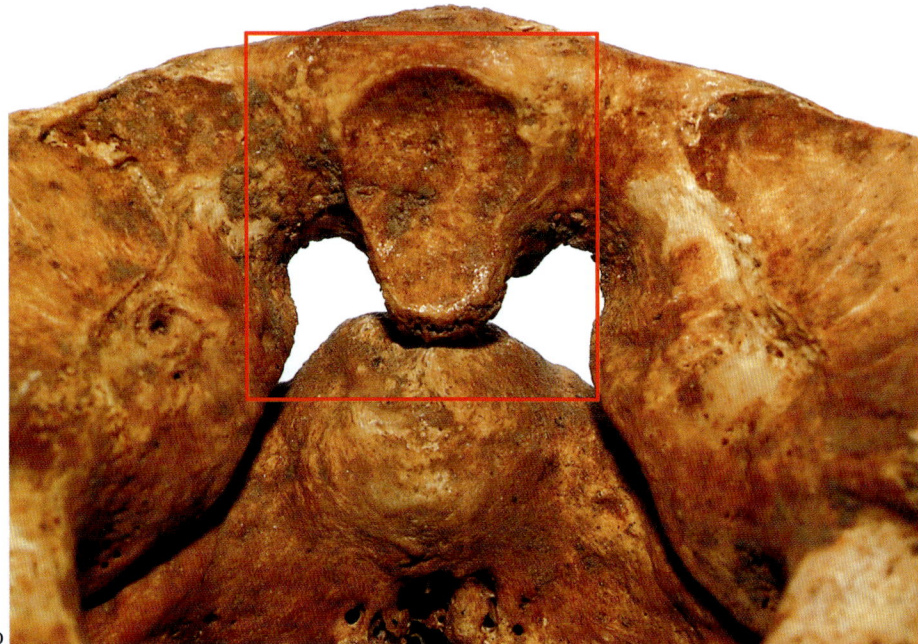

Figure 745a-b. Os odontoideum or congenital separation of the dens of the axis (C-2). (a) Note the well-developed articular facet on the atlas (square), indicating that the dens was present in this individual, although the dens was not recovered with this case (CIL). (b) Higher magnification of the articular facet (square) on the atlas. While subject to considerable debate, prior trauma may be associated with this condition. Cf. Barnes (1994, 2012); Leng et al. (2009); Pang and Thompson (2011); Prescher (1997); Smoker (1994); Turner (1890); Truumees (2010). Hunter (1924) reported on an atlas with a separate odontoid process fusing with the anterior face of the axis. See Cunningham (1886) for a discussion of the dens joining with the body of the axis. Rare finding.

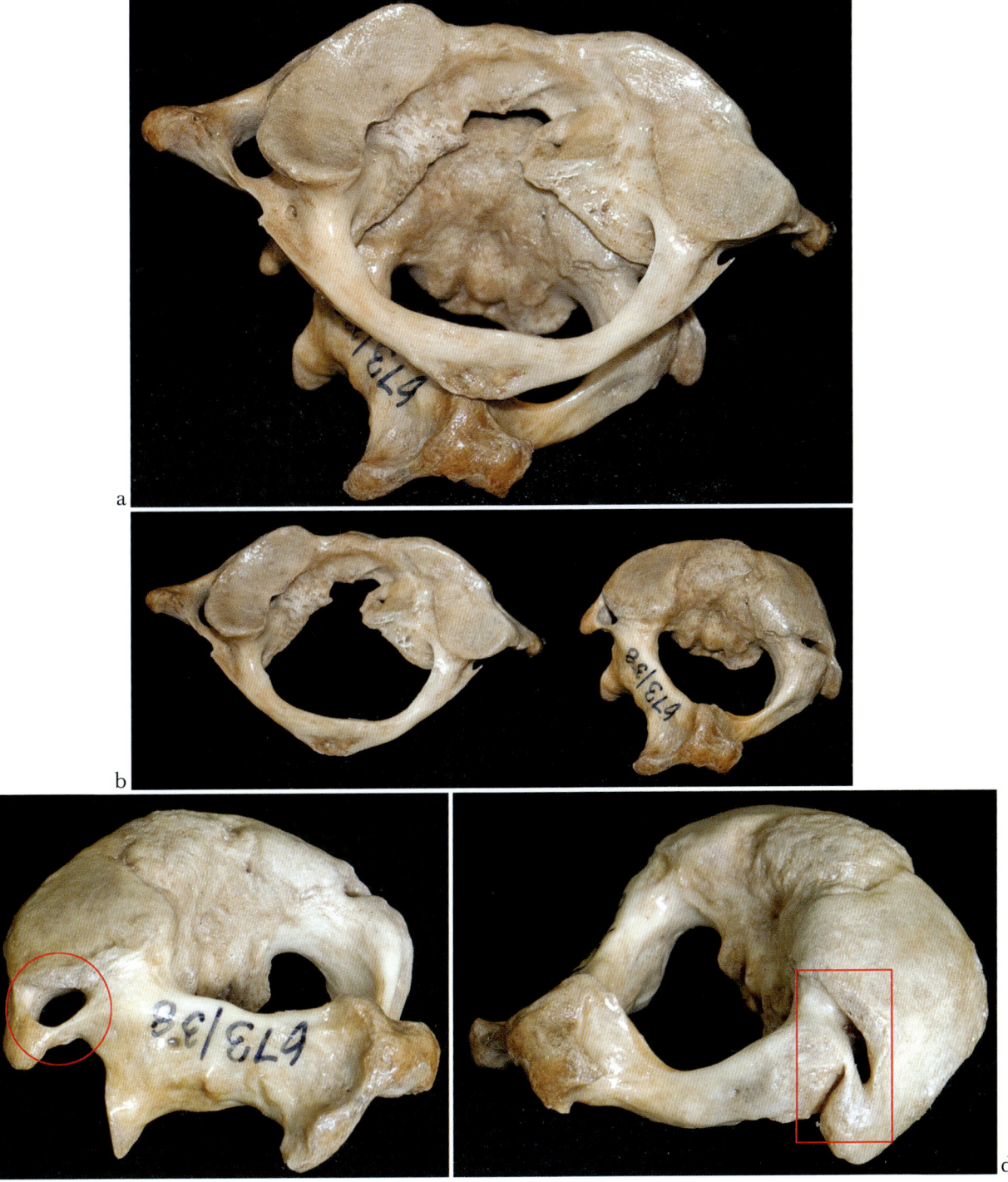

Figure 746a-d. Os odontoideum in a 25-year-old Thai male (KKU 0202). (a) C1 and C2 depicting morphology when articulated. (b) C1 and C2 disarticulated demonstrating the asymmetry and overall morphology of the articular facets. This specimen likely reflects congenital absence of the odontoid process or dens, although hypoplasia of the dens cannot be ruled out. Cf. Anderson (1987); Bajaj et al. (2010); Barnes (1994, 2012); Pang and Thompson (2011); Smoker (1994); Truumees (2010). (c) Note the normal left transverse foramen (circle) compared to the (d) stenotic and slit-like right transverse foramen (rectangle). This individual reportedly walked with assistance and could move his head with some difficulty until bedridden the last few years of his life, dying of pneumonia or cardiac arrest.

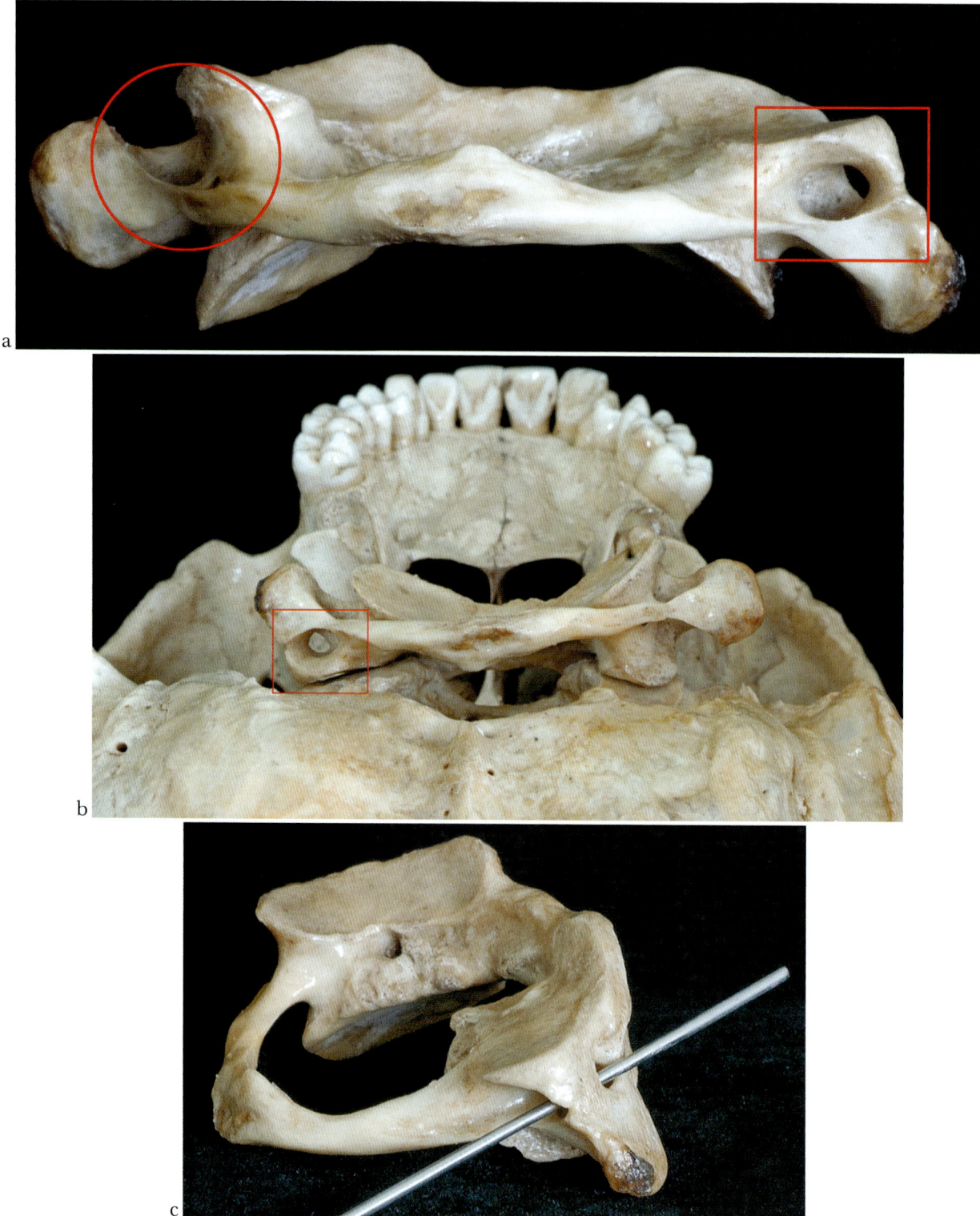

Figure 747a-c. Unbridged left transverse foramen (a, circle) and laterally bridged right transverse foramen (square) in the atlas of a 25-year-old Thai male with os odontoideum (KKU 0202). (b) C1 articulated with the cranial base showing the right foramen (rectangle). (c) Probe through the foramen. This is not Kimmerle's anomaly since the foramen in this specimen is bridged laterally, not posteriorly. See Macalister (1893) for variation of the atlas.

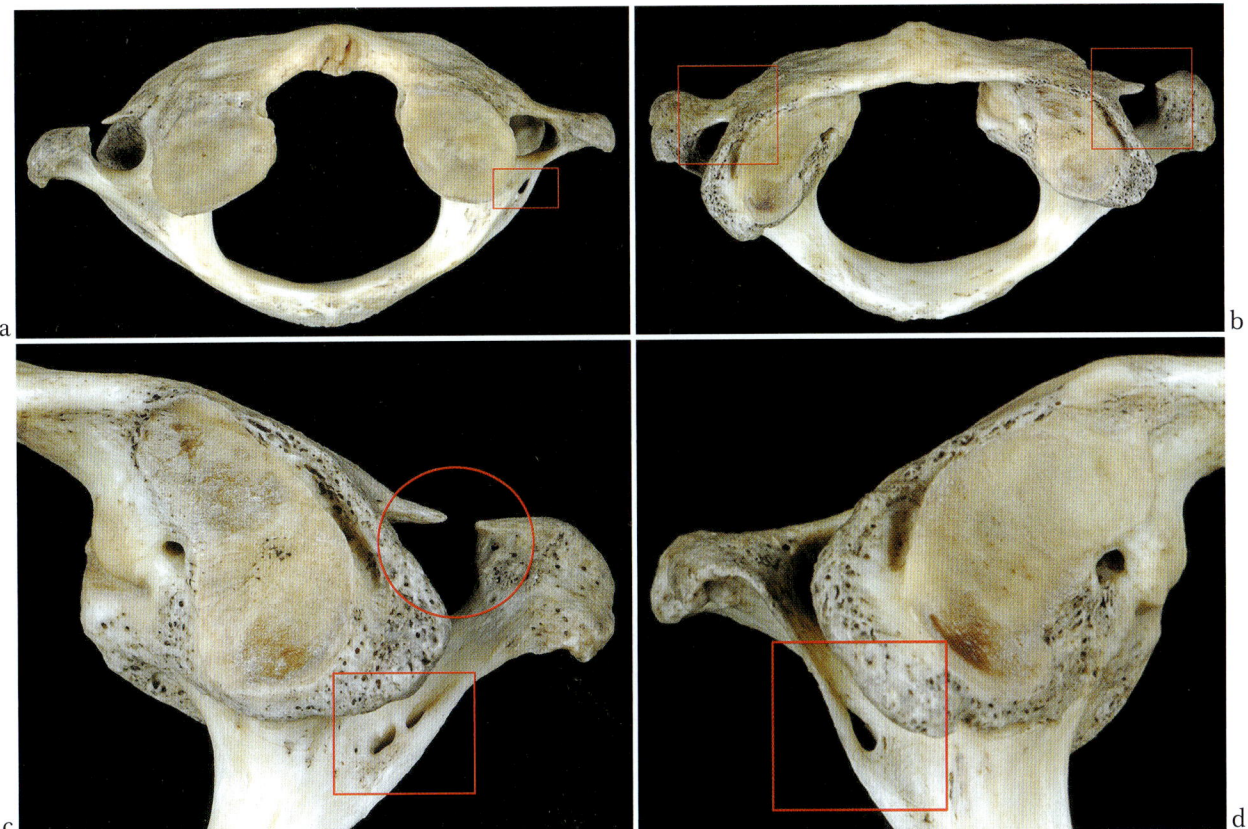

Figure 748a-d. Variation of partial and complete bridging in the atlas (CIL). (a and d) A small accessory foramen (rectangle and square). (b) Complete and partial bridging of the atlas (squares). (c) Partial bridging (circle) and accessory foramina (rectangle) in the atlas/C-1. (a and d) Differing views of a small, slit-like accessory foramina (square). All are common findings. Agrawal et al. (2012); Hauser and DeStefano (1989); Macalister (1893).

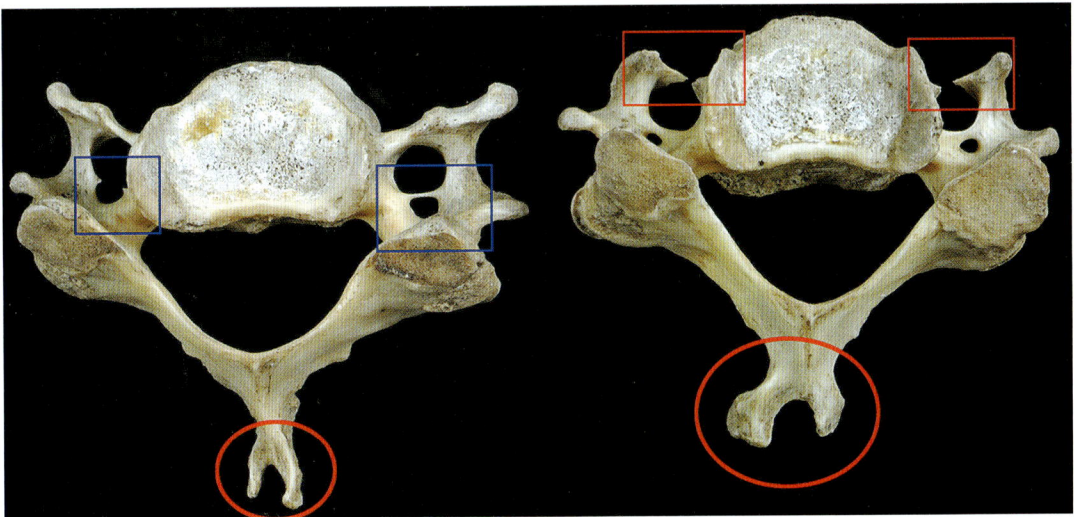

Figure 749. Partial and complete division (double foramina transversaria) (blue), partial bridging of the foramen for the vertebral artery (red squares) and bifid spinous processes (circles) in two cervical vertebrae (CIL). Common findings. Murlimanju et al. (2011a) noted in 363 cervical vertebrae studied that 1.6% had accessory foramina, 1.4% had double foramina and 0.3% had three foramina; no vertebra showed absence of the foramen transversarium.

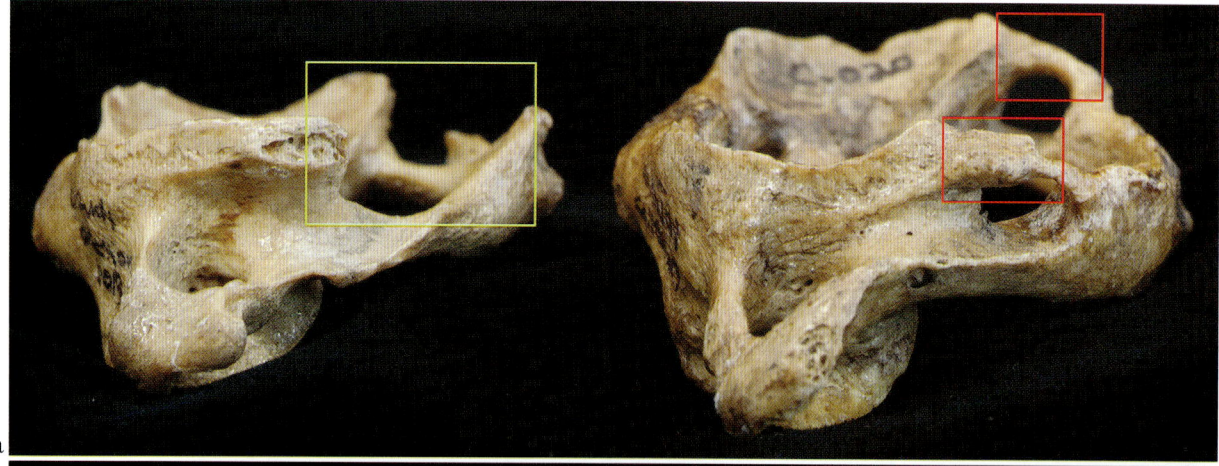

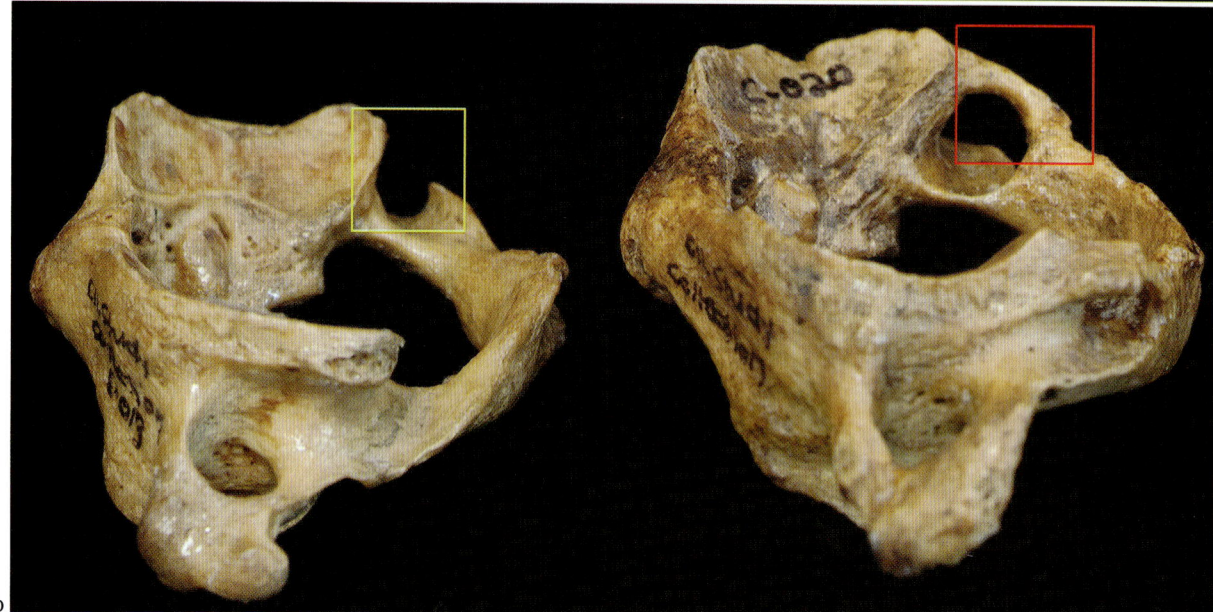

Figure 750a-b. Posterior osseous bridging of C1. (a) Osseous bridging (red rectangles), also known as Kimmerle's variant or anomaly, arcuate foramen and ponticulus posticus, among others, compared to a non-bridged (yellow rectangle) C1. (b) More superior view of osseous bridging (red square) and a non-bridged (yellow square) C1. This foramen, for which bridging can range from none, partial and complete bridging, houses the vertebral artery and first cervical nerve (Cf. Simsek et al. 2008) and forms by calcification of the atlanto-occipital membrane (Burgenen and Kormano 1997). Simsek et al. (2008) noted 6 of 158 C1 vertebrae (3.8%) with complete bridging. Cf. Prakash et al. (2010). See Leonardi et al. (2009) for more on the relationship between ponticulus posticus and posterior arch defects of the atlas, sella turcica bridging, interclinoid bridging and palatally displaced canine teeth.

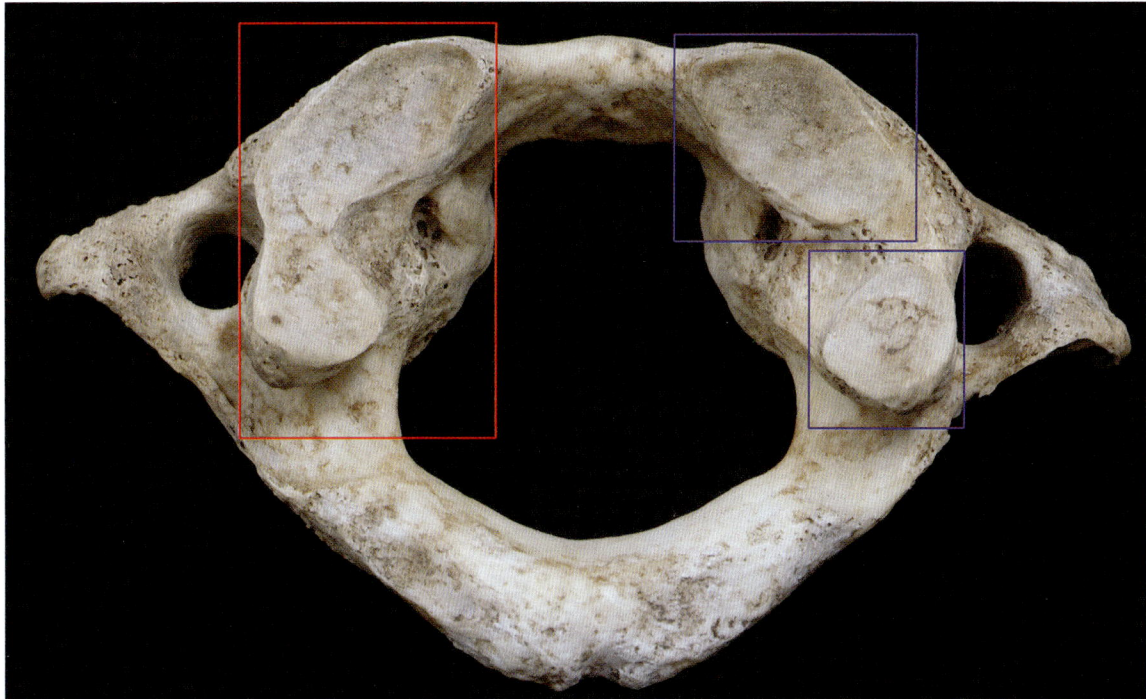

Figure 751. Single left (red rectangle) and double right (blue square and rectangle) superior articular facets for articulation with the occipital condyles in a 26-year old Thai female (CMU 3 50). The right occipital condyle is single in this individual.

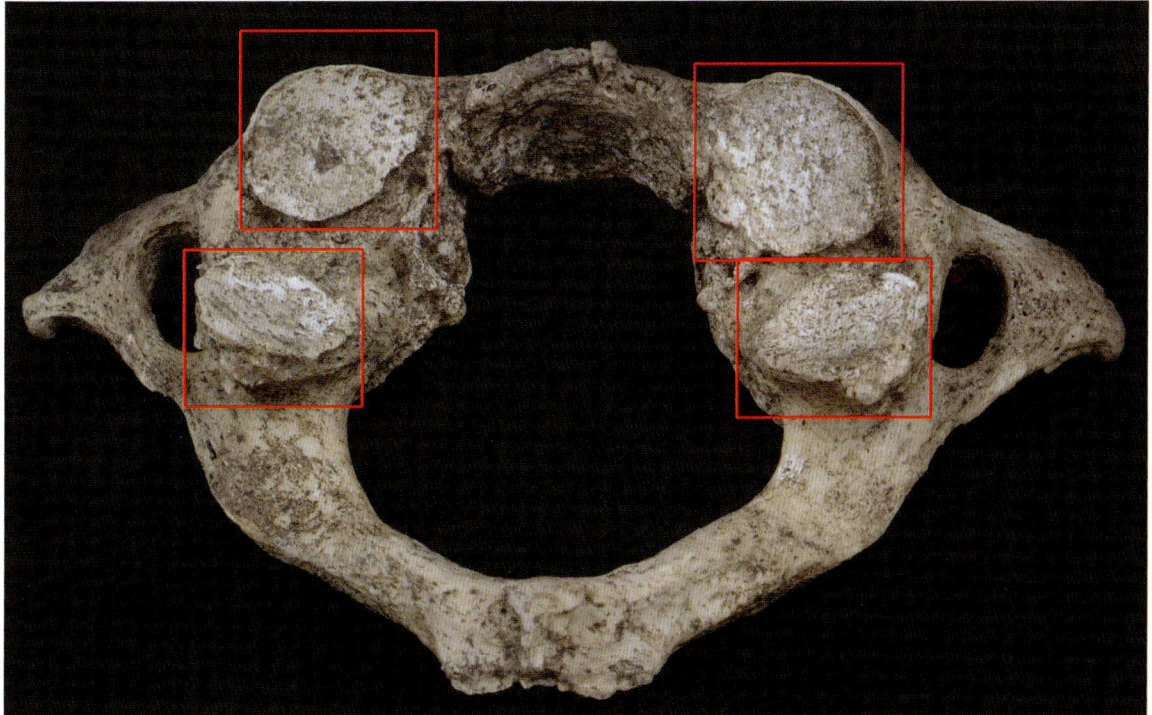

Figure 752. Divided/double superior condyles (squares) in an atlas in a 74-year-old male (CMU 75 53). Cf. Barnes (1994); Billmann et al. (2007).

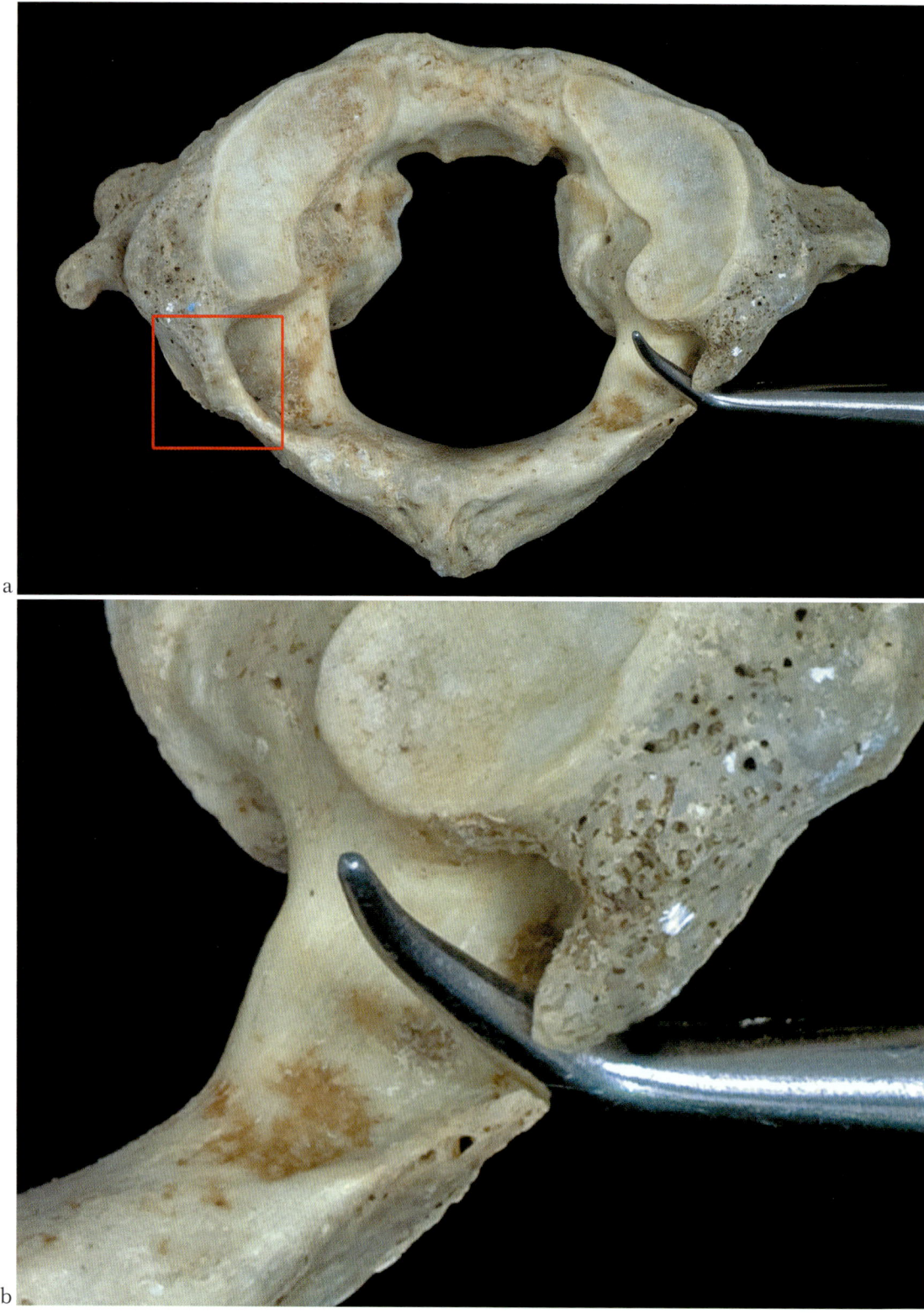

Figure 753a-b. (a) Complete left (square) and partial right (probe) bridging of the border of the posterior articular facets resulting in Kimmerle's anomaly in an adult (CMU). (b) Higher magnification of the partial bridging (probe) on the right side.

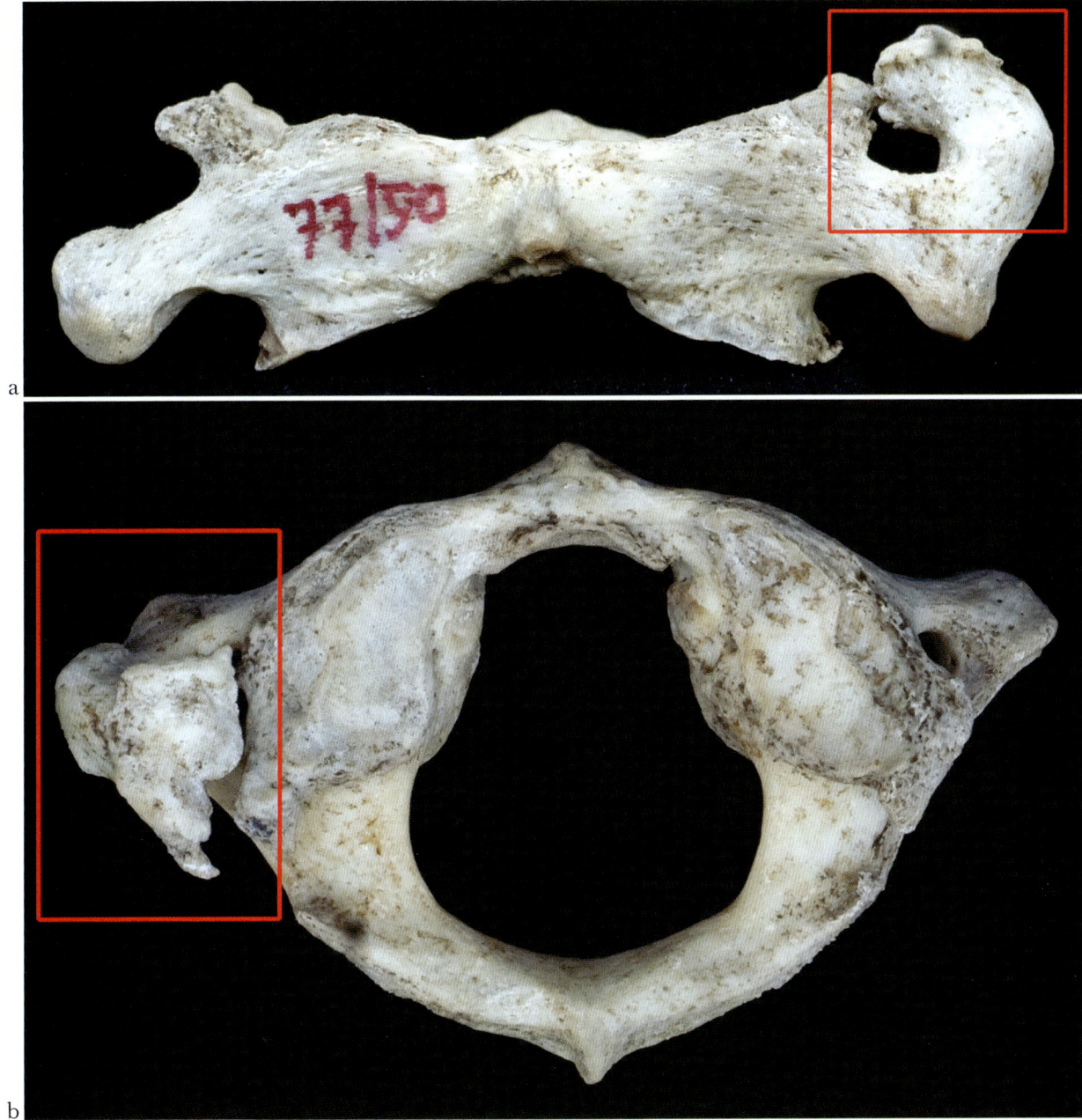

Figure 754a-b. Developed left paracondylar process or pedestal (red square and rectangle) resulting in an anteroposterior directed foramen in an elderly Thai female (CMU 77 50). (a) Anterior and (b) superior views of the paracondylar process.

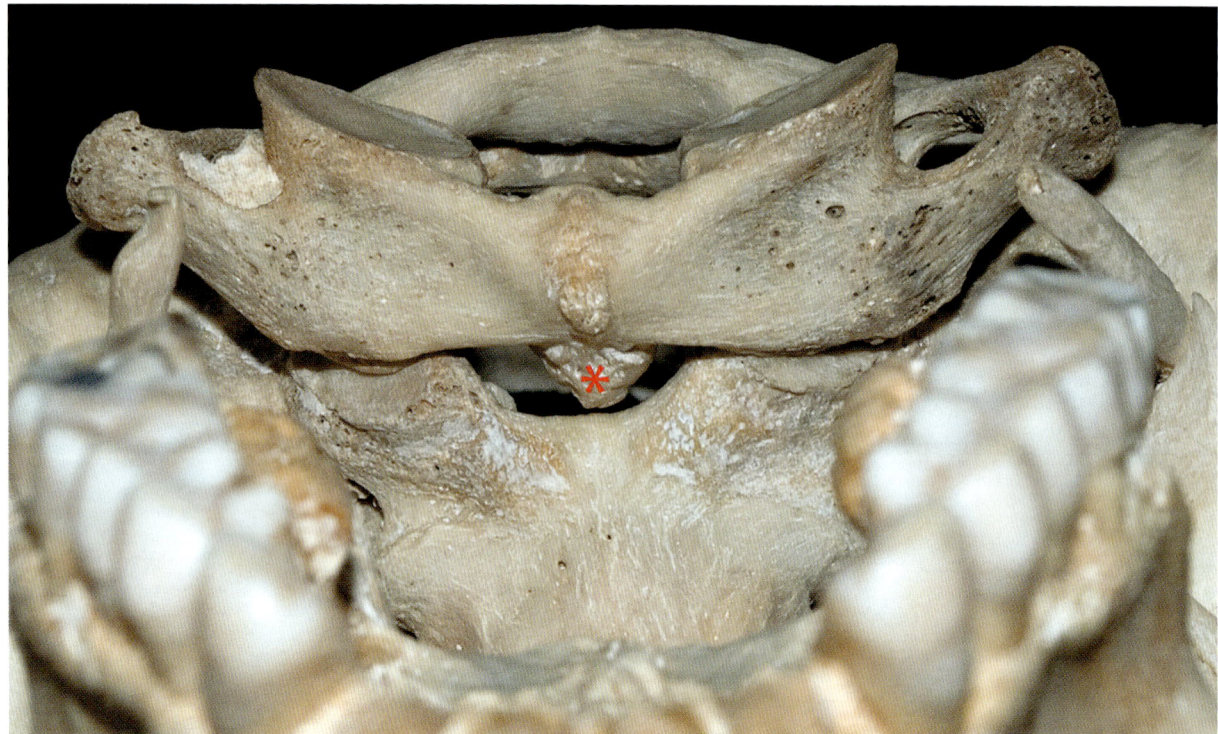

Figure 755. Unusually long extension (asterisk) of the odontoid facet in the atlas viewed from the anterior perspective with an inverted specimen. The extension did not articulate with the cranial base in this elderly male (KKU 0670).

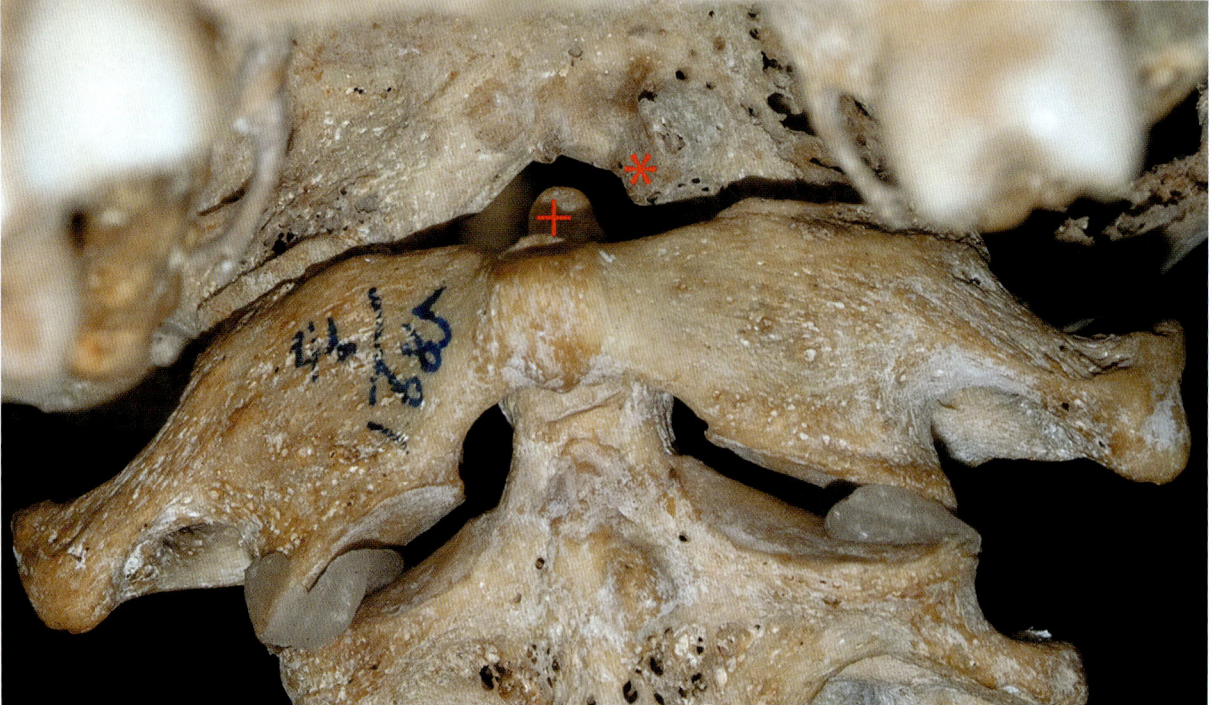

Figure 756. Unusually long odontoid process (+) of the axis that appears to have articulated with a faceted precondylar tubercle (*) on the cranial base in an adult female (KKU 643).

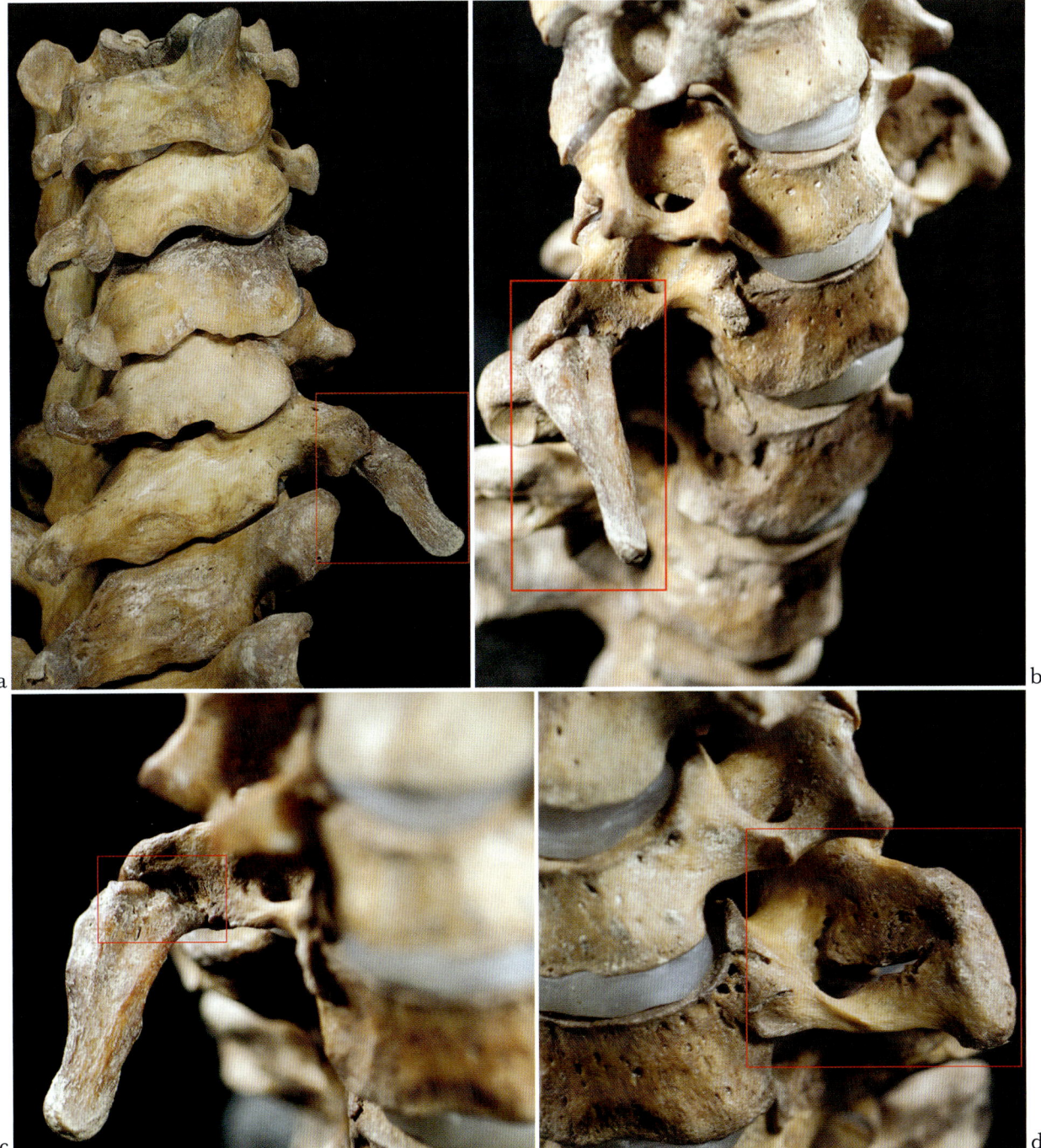

Figure 757a-d. Right cervical rib (rectangle) on the 7th cervical vertebra in a young adult male (CIL). (a) Posterior oblique view showing the cervical rib (square). (b) Anterior and right oblique view of the rib demonstrating the absence of an attachment site (facet) for the rib on the centrum of C7. (c) Anterior view showing the site of attachment (rectangle) of the rib to the transverse process. This unilateral rib, which in the living was attached by soft tissue to the transverse process and not through bony union, was oriented downward in the typical "angel wing" fashion. (d) The left cervical rib (rectangle) was attached to the centrum and the transverse process, was shorter and projected more horizontally compared with the right side. Both types of ribs are uncommon to rare in most groups (0.5% of the population – Fisher 1981). Incidence of cervical ribs and the complete absence or presence of rudimentary 12th ribs appears to correlate with a high frequency of stillbirths and malformations (Bots et al. 2011). Cf. Brewin et al. (2009); Shore (1930); Turner (1869, 1883).

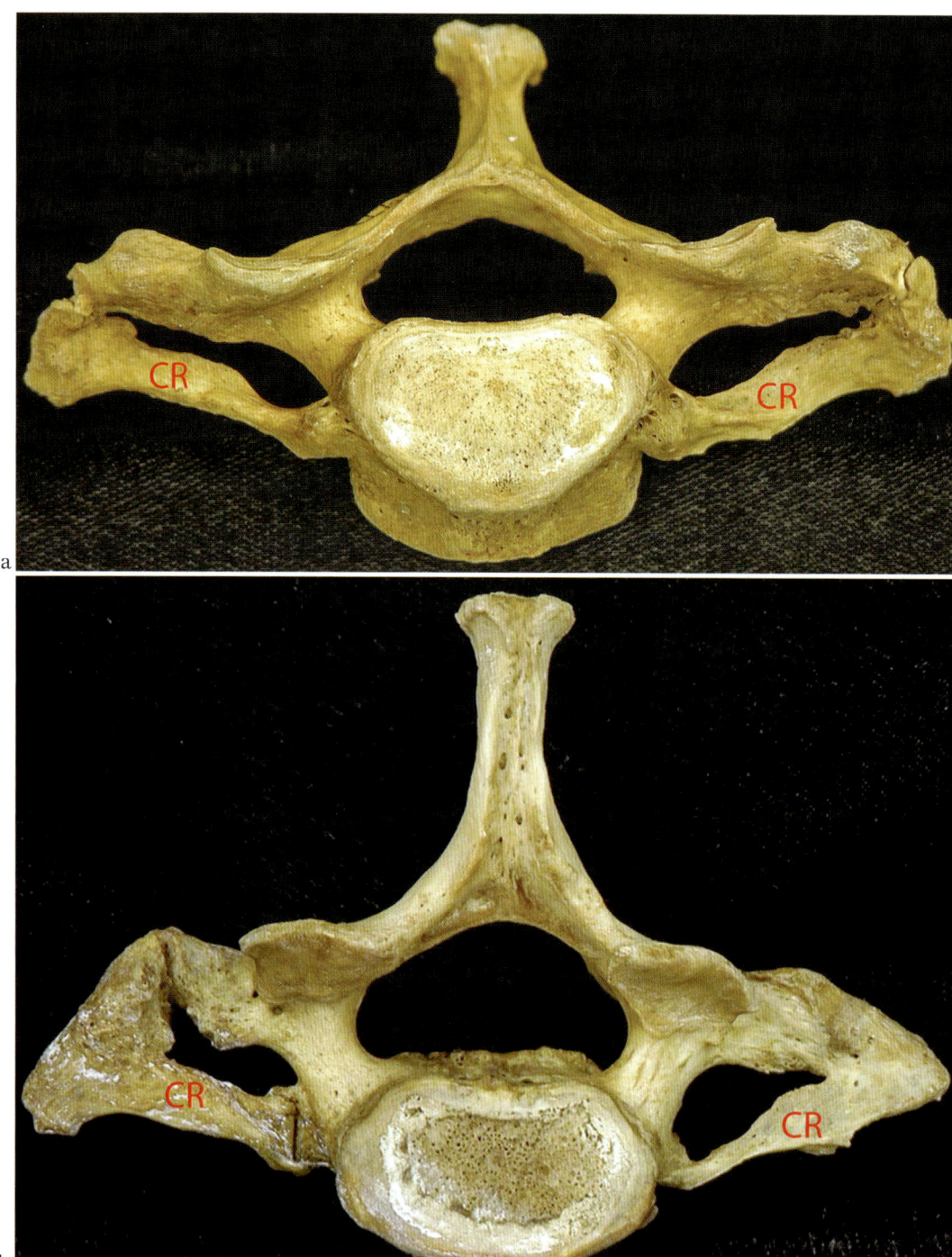

Figure 758a-b. Variation of the cervical rib. (a) Superior view of bilateral cervical ribs (CR) in a 7th cervical vertebra (Joe Hefner; UTK). (b) Inferior view of the cervical ribs (CR). Note the asymmetry in size and shape of these ribs and their sites of attachment. Cervical ribs are typically found in less than 1% of individuals and can appear as finger-like projections on the seventh, sixth, fifth or fourth vertebrae, in descending order of frequency (Church 1919). Overdevelopment of a costal process may lead to the formation of a cervical rib (Arey 1942). Brewin et al. (2009) examined 1,352 chest radiographs of London patients and found an overall prevalence of 0.74% (7 females and 3 males). These researchers noted a total of 12 cervical ribs in 10 individuals. Cf. Cave (1975); Etter (1944) examined x-ray images of 40,000 soldiers; Turner (1883). This is usually considered a minor variant (personal communication, Barnes 2012).

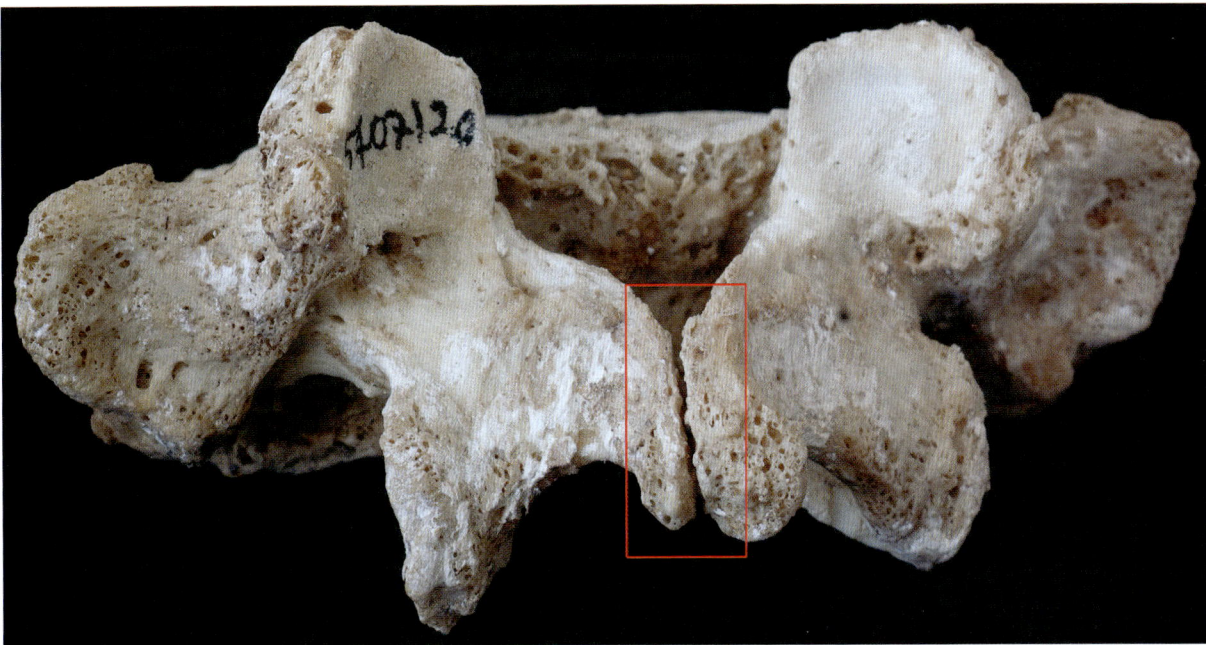

Figure 759. Bifid spinous process (rectangle) also referred to as cleft in an L5 vertebra in a 70-year-old Thai male (CMU 5407120). Cf. Barnes (1994, 2012). This individual also had six lumbar vertebrae, a left lumbar rib (L1) and complete clefting of the sacrum.

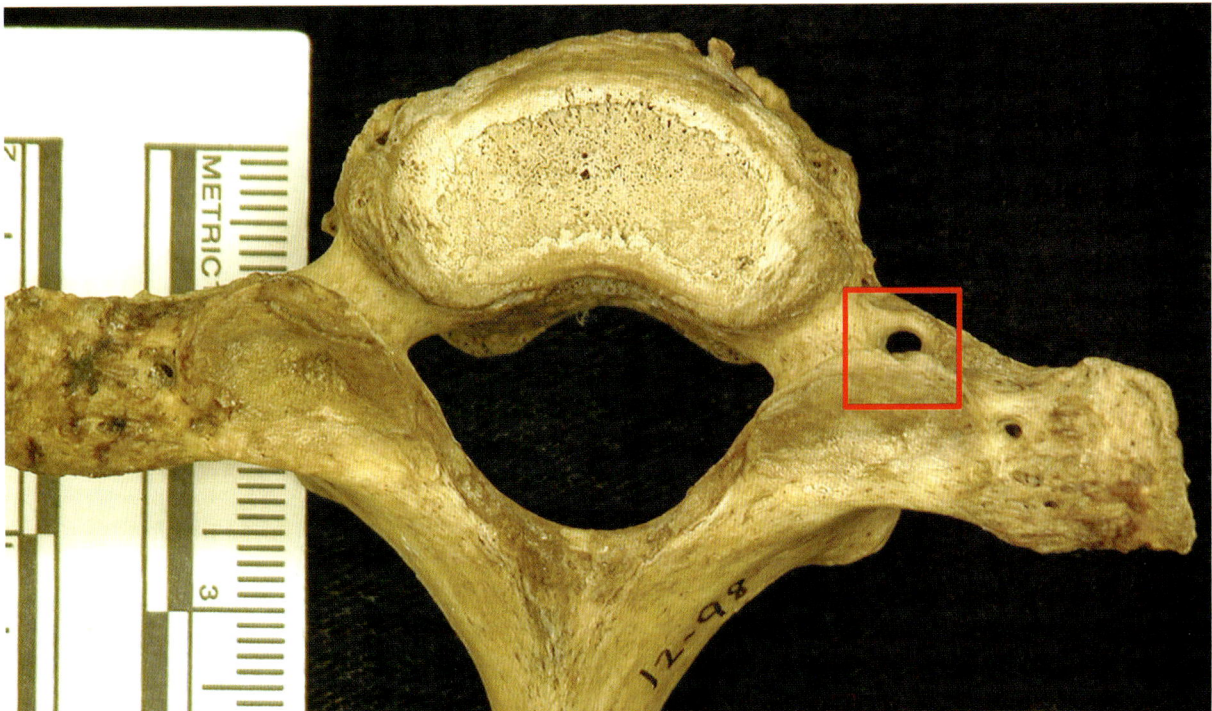

Figure 760. Foramen (square) in the right pedicle of a thoracic vertebra (UTK, Joe Hefner). Uncommon finding.

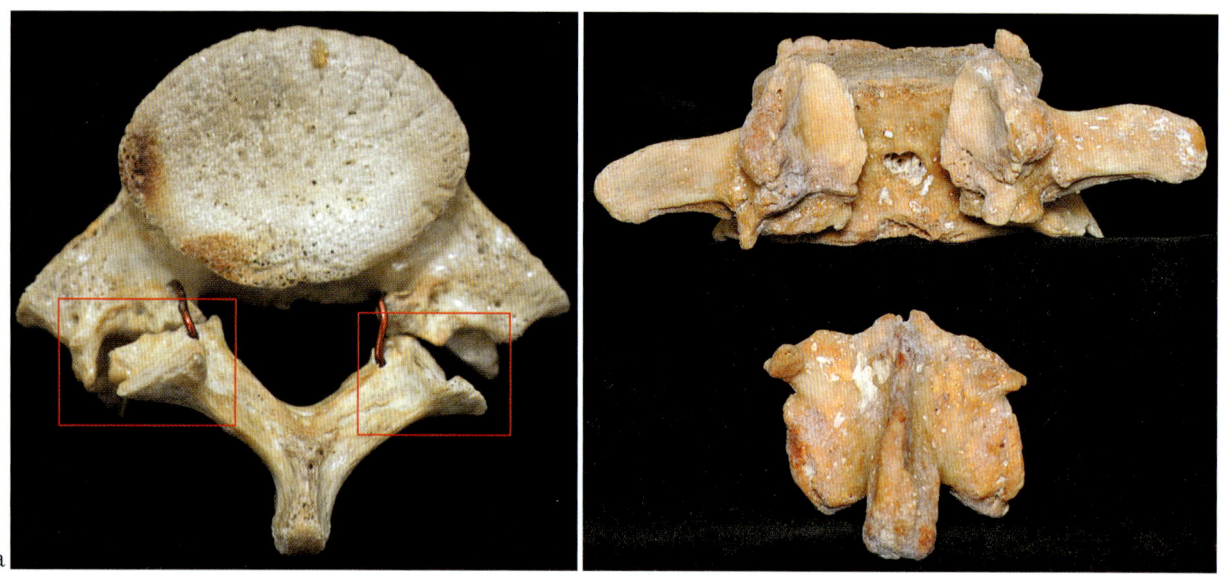

Figure 761a-b. Bilateral lumbar spondylolysis. (a) Bilateral spondylolysis (rectangles) through the pars interarticularis in a subadult (KKU). (b) Spondylolysis in an adult (KKU) with the separate neural arch removed from its articulation just beneath the superior articular facets. Spondylolysis is a repetitive stress fracture leading to joint instability and it occurs through the L5 pars interarticularis in 85%–95% of cases (Bono 2004). Willis (1931) attributed it to "imperfect ossification" (p. 721), regardless of the causative event. There are numerous reports of both healing (Morita et al. 1995; Wiltse et al. 1975) and non-healing with no evidence of callus in unilateral and bilateral specimens (Willis 1931). This condition is found more often in teenage boys than girls and in adolescents than in adults. Spondylolysis is seen in high frequencies in divers (43%), wrestlers (30%) and weight lifters (23%) (Bono 2004). While spondylolysis is most commonly seen in the lower lumbar vertebrae, it can occur in the cervical spine, especially C7. Cf. Barnes (1994, 2012); Beutler et al. (2003); Gunzburg and Szpalski (2005); Manners-Smith (1910); Mellado et al. (2011a, b); Roche and Rowe (1952); Shore (1932); Saifuddin et al. (1998). See Beutler et al. (2003) for a discussion of the developmental history of spondylolysis and spondylolisthesis spanning 45 years. Beutler et al. (2003) found healing of the pars in only three people with unilateral defects (none with bilateral defects) and none of the individuals with unilateral defects progressed to bilateral defects. The present authors have not seen any examples of healing in uni- or bilateral spondylolysis in dry bone specimens. Common finding with high frequencies in some groups (e.g., Thai).

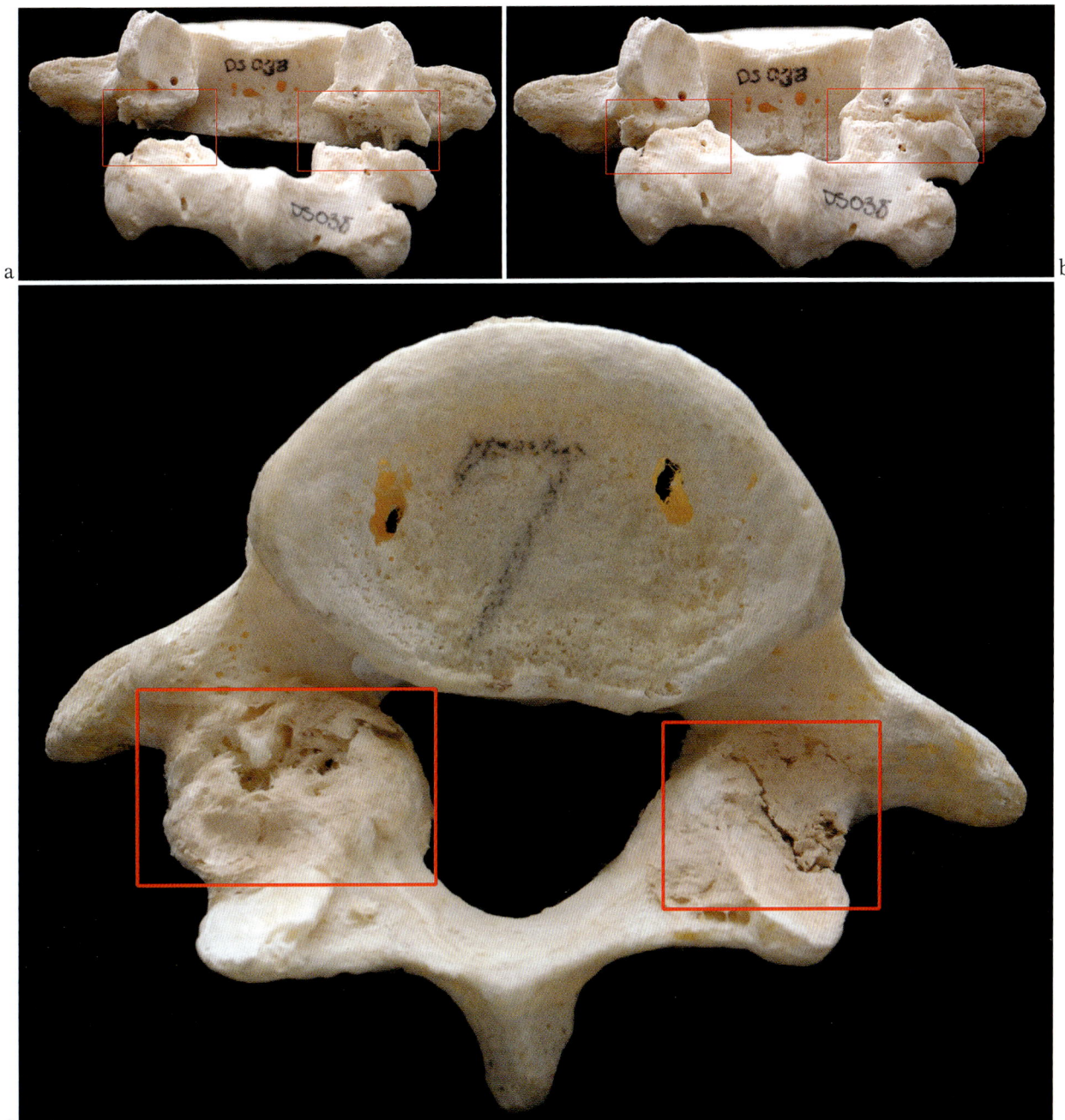

Figure 762a-c. Separate neural arch. (a) Dorsal view of a bilateral separate neural arch, also known as spondylolysis, in the L5 of an adult. (b) Dorsal view of the neural arch rearticulated in its approximate *in vivo* position using clear dental wax. (c) Inferior view showing the lines of separation of the separate neural arch through the pars interarticularis (rectangle and square) (FSA CIL DS038, Christopher Sciotto). Note that separation of the neural arch occurs inferior to and not through the articular facets. The bony separation is bridged by fibrous tissue in patients. Examination of 4,200 human skeletons revealed 178 individuals (4.2%) with neural arch separations; 94.6% were in L4 or L5 (Roche and Rowe 1952). Willis (1931) found 79 of 1,520 (5.2%) human skeletons with a separate neural arch. Cf. Mellado et al. (2011a, b) and Eisenstein (1978) for more on neural arch defects. Cf. Beutler et al. (2003) for a 45-year prospective study of these defects.

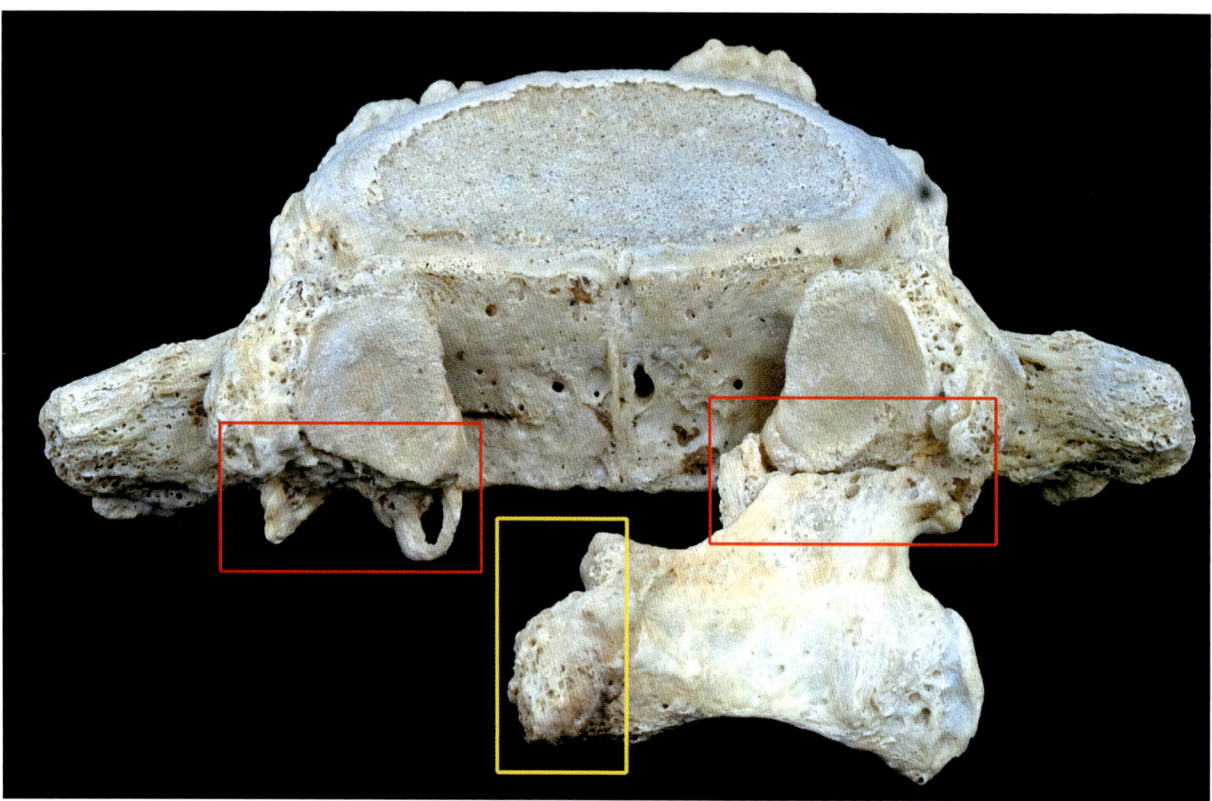

Figure 763. Bilateral spondylolysis through the pars interarticularis (red rectangles) and cleft spinous process (left half of the neural arch is missing postmortem) (CMU). Cf. Barnes (1994, 2012); LeDouble (1912).

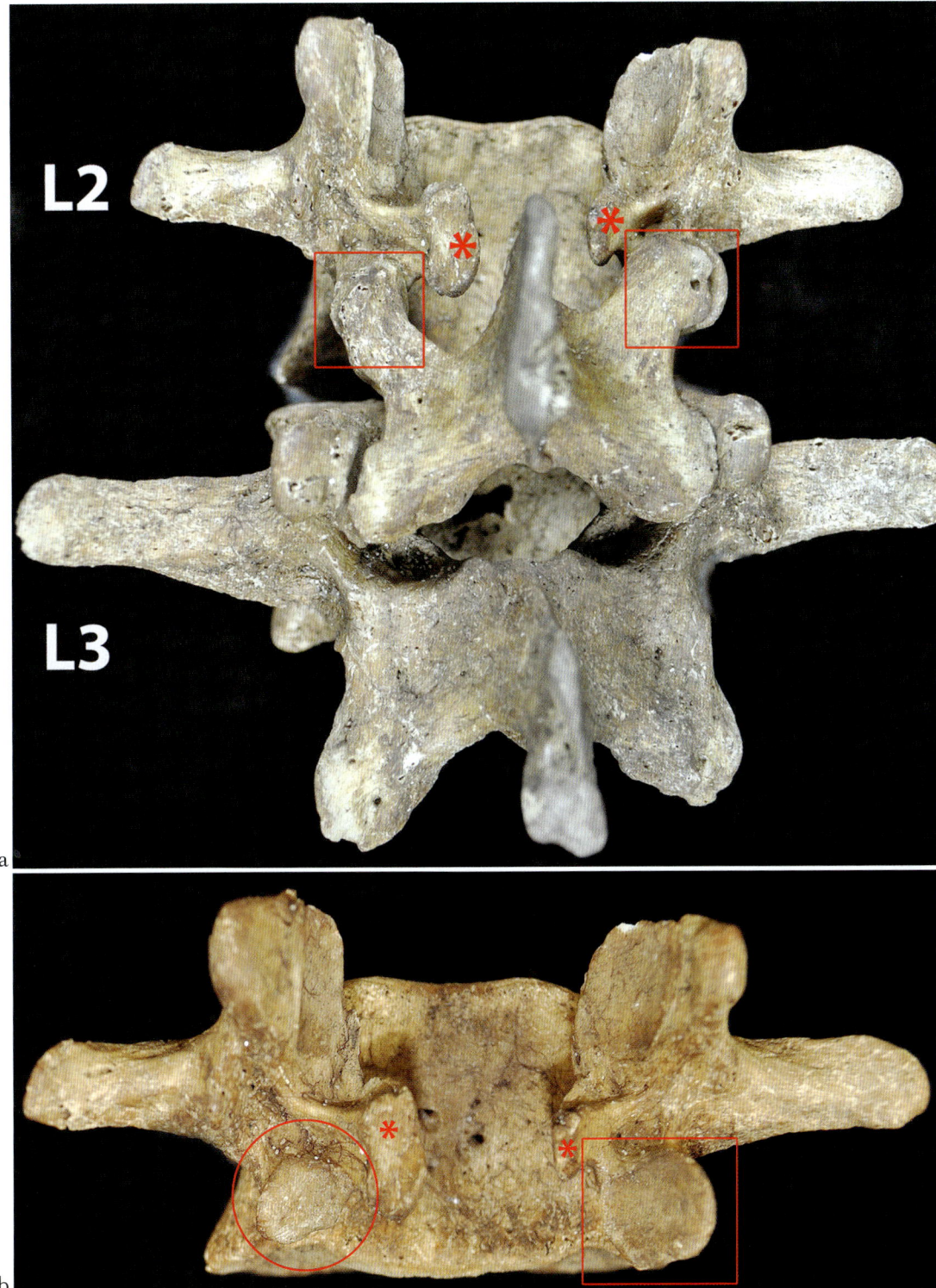

Figure 764a-b. Congenital articulating neural arch (ANA). (a) This extremely rare condition consists of bilateral accessory facets (red squares) and cleft (*) of the laminae in L2 of a young adult male (CIL and Ashley Burch). (b) L2 showing the wide cleft (*), with the small left and larger right superior facets (circle and square, respectively). This condition is likely a congenital developmental defect and not traumatic separation resulting from fracture as seen in spondylolysis. L3 is normal in size and shape. Cf. Mellado et al. (2011a, b) and Eisenstein (1978) for more on neural arch defects.

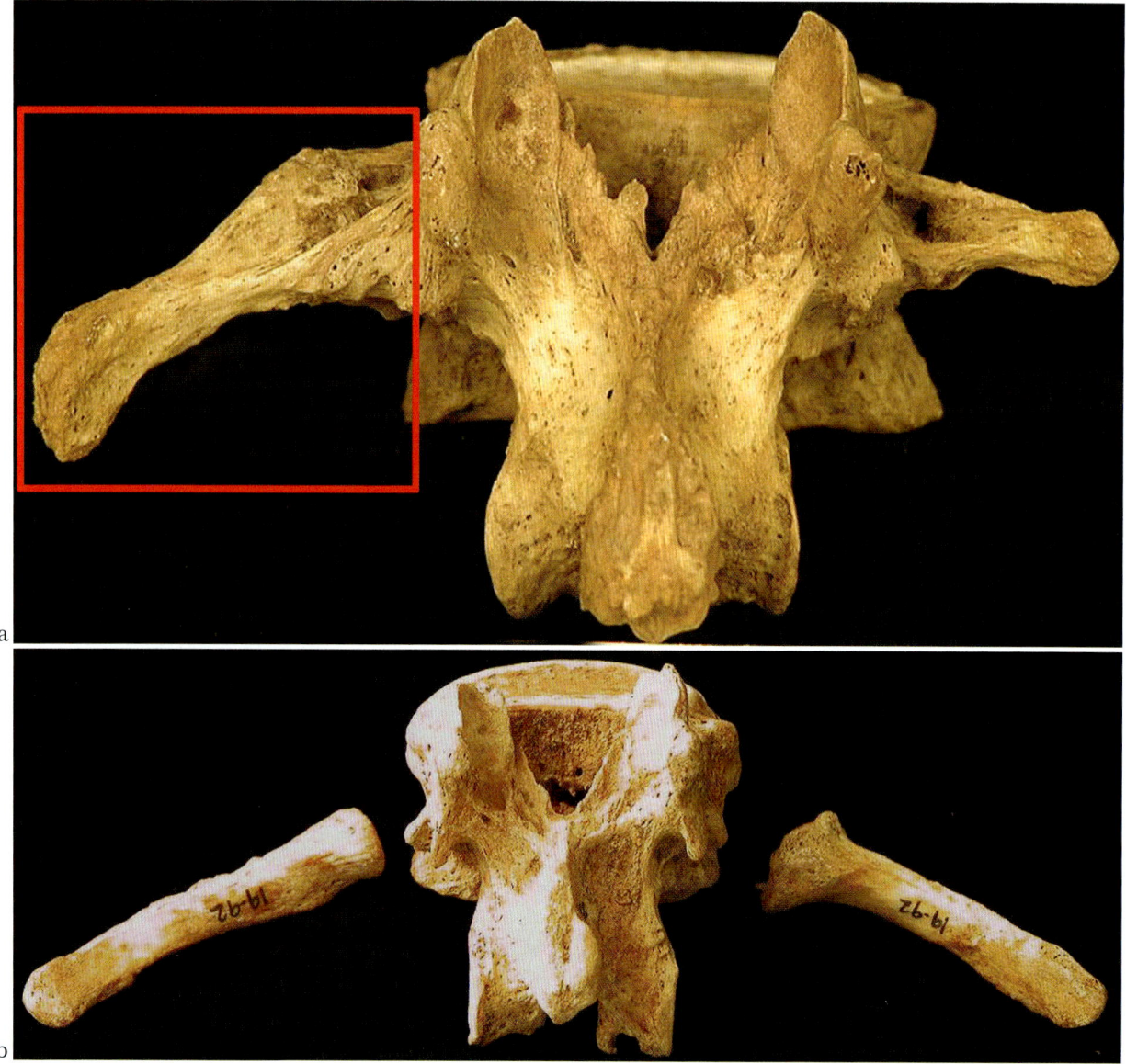

Figure 765a-b. Fused and unfused lumbar ribs. (a) Fused lumbar ribs in an adult demonstrating asymmetry with a left rib (rectangle) larger than the right. (b) Bilateral non-fused and asymmetrical lumbar ribs in an adult (Hefner, UTK 19-92). Uncommon to rare finding.

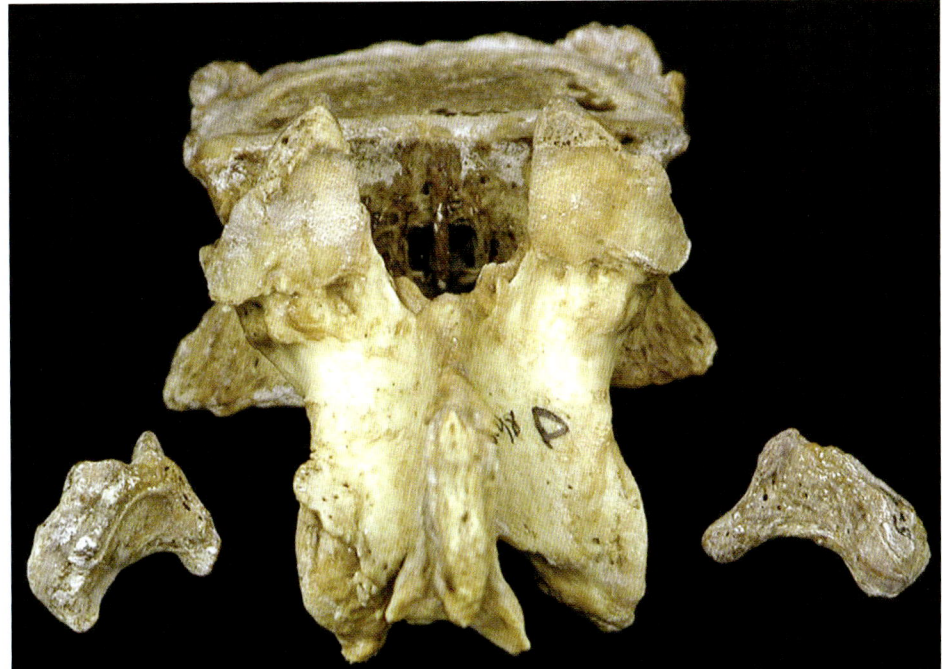

Figure 766. Separate transverse processes in a lumbar vertebra, sometimes referred to as lumbar ribs (Gray 1901) (Hefner, UTK). Rare finding.

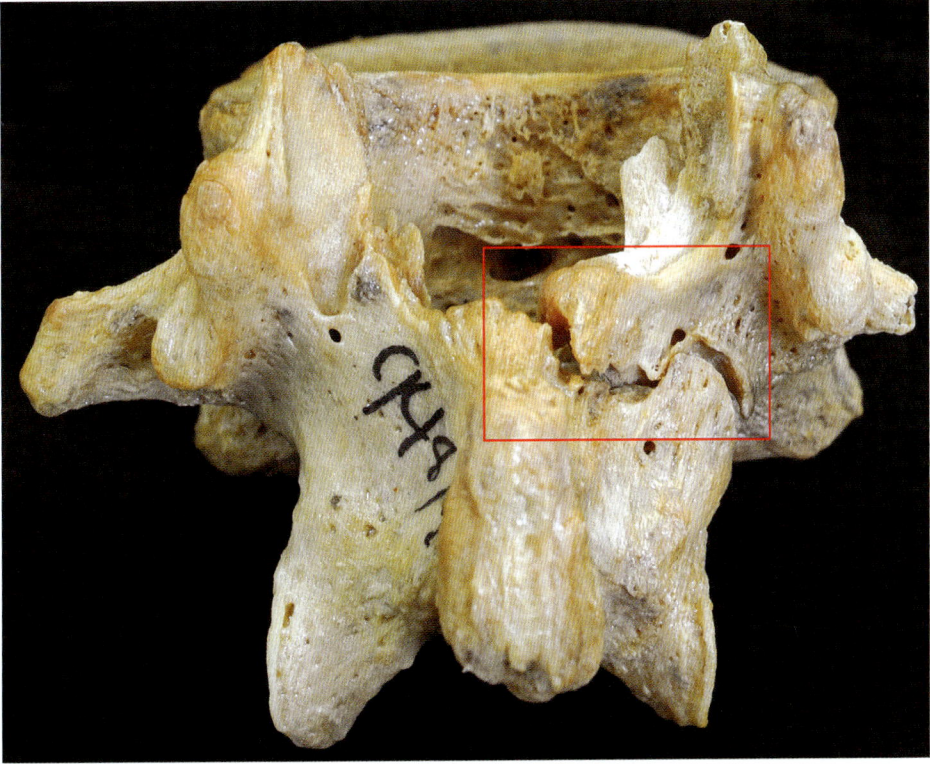

Figure 767. Unilateral spondylolysis (rectangle) through the right pars interarticularis in a lumbar vertebra of an adult (KKU). Uncommon finding. Cf. Roche and Rowe (1952).

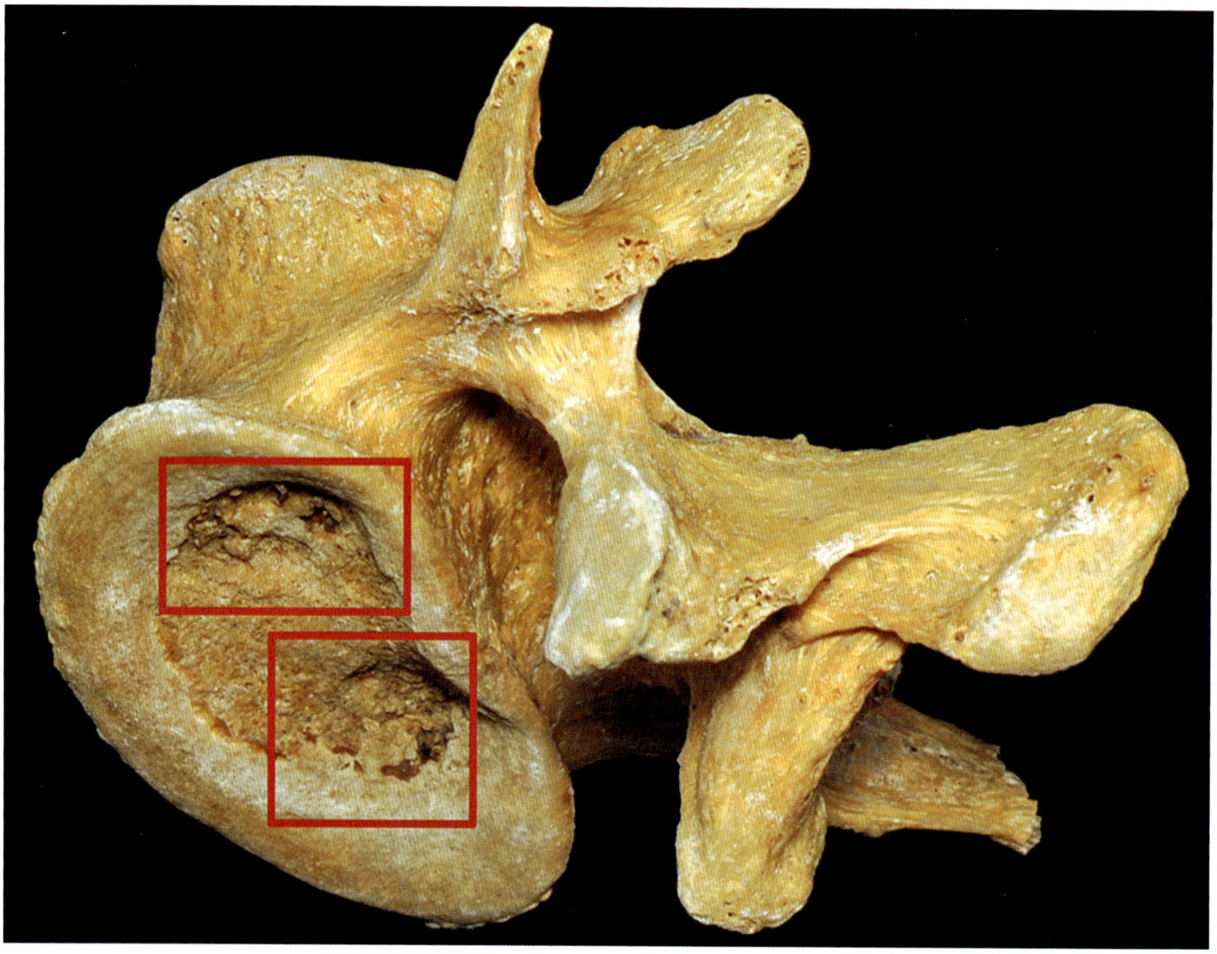

Figure 768. Normal "double concavities" in the inferior endplate of L5 that can also occur in other lumbar vertebrae. These concavities are not the result of osteoporosis, herniation, or acute trauma. Cf. Wang et al. (2012) for information on distinguishing four types of endplate lesions, including Schmorl's nodes.

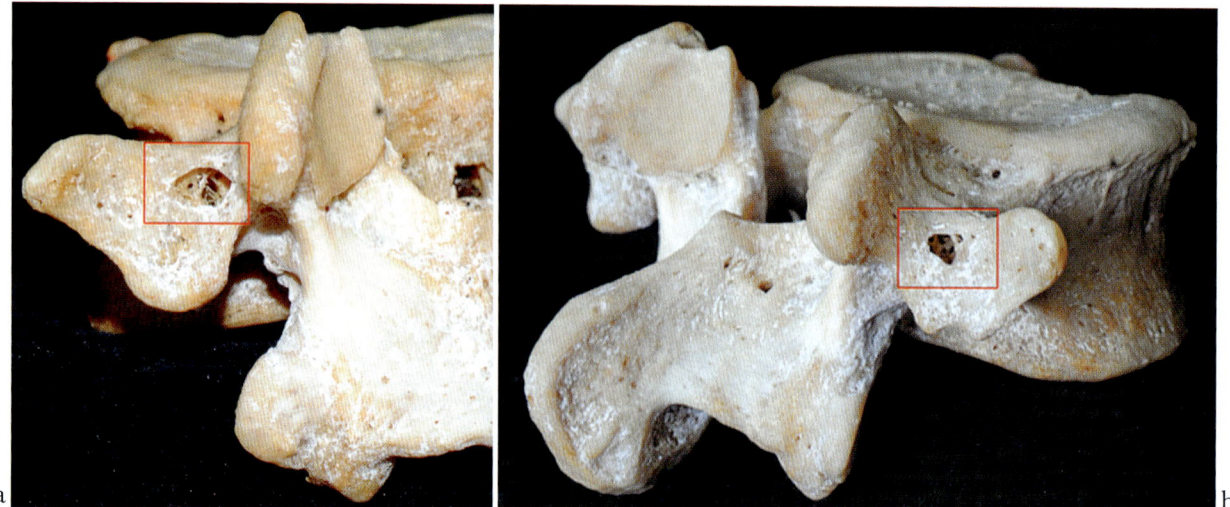

Figure 769a-b. Bilateral accessory foramina (rectangles) in a lumbar vertebra. (a) Large left foramen and (b) smaller right foramen of unknown etiology in an adult Asian (KKU). Smaller foramina in this area are uncommon to common findings.

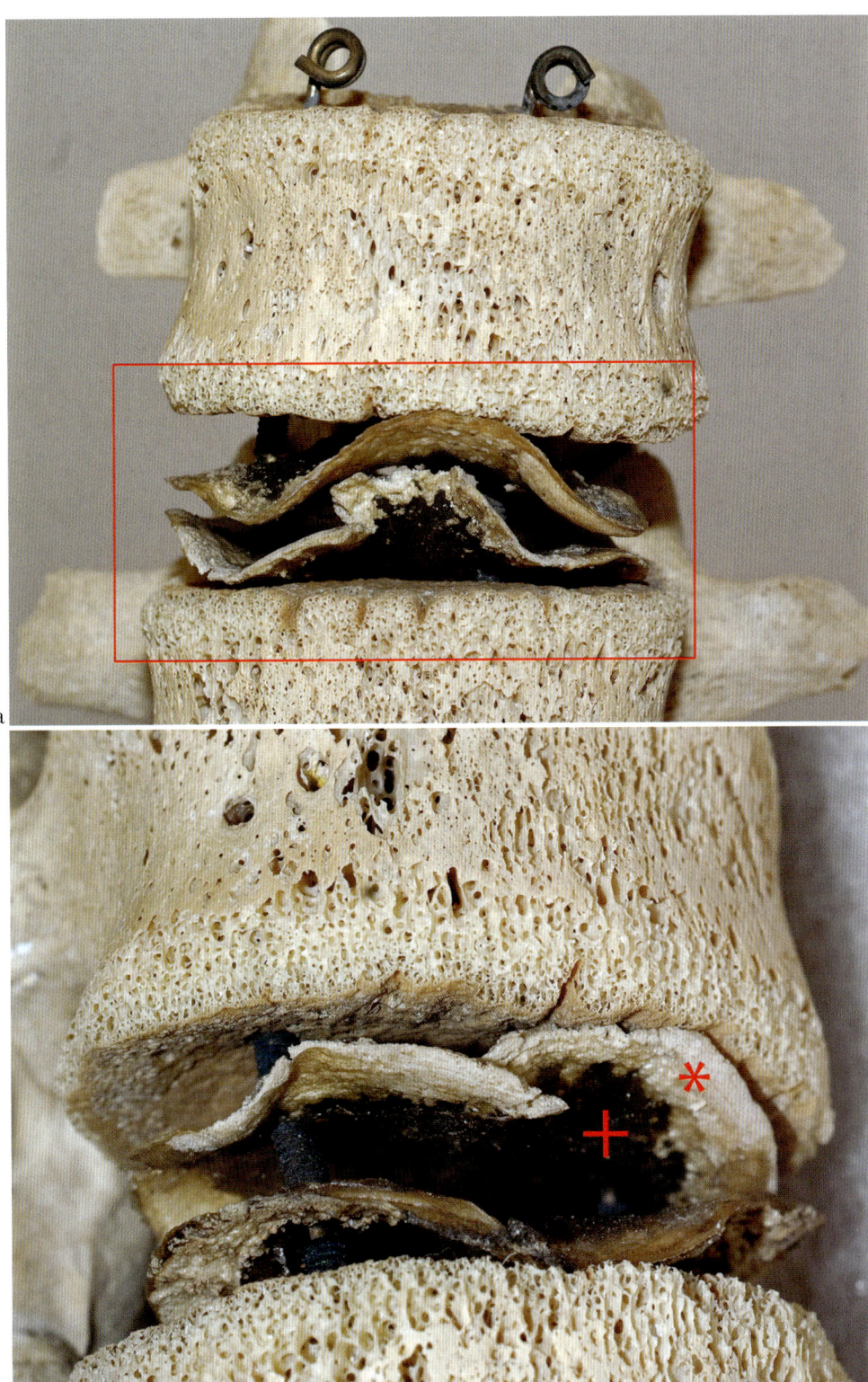

Figure 770a-b. Ossification, but not united superior and inferior endplates (rectangle) of two lumbar vertebrae in a subadult. (a) Ventral view demonstrating inferior and superior apophyseal endplates (rectangle) between two vertebrae. (b) Apophysis (*) and cartilaginous portion of the intervertebral disc (+) (Mütter Musuem).

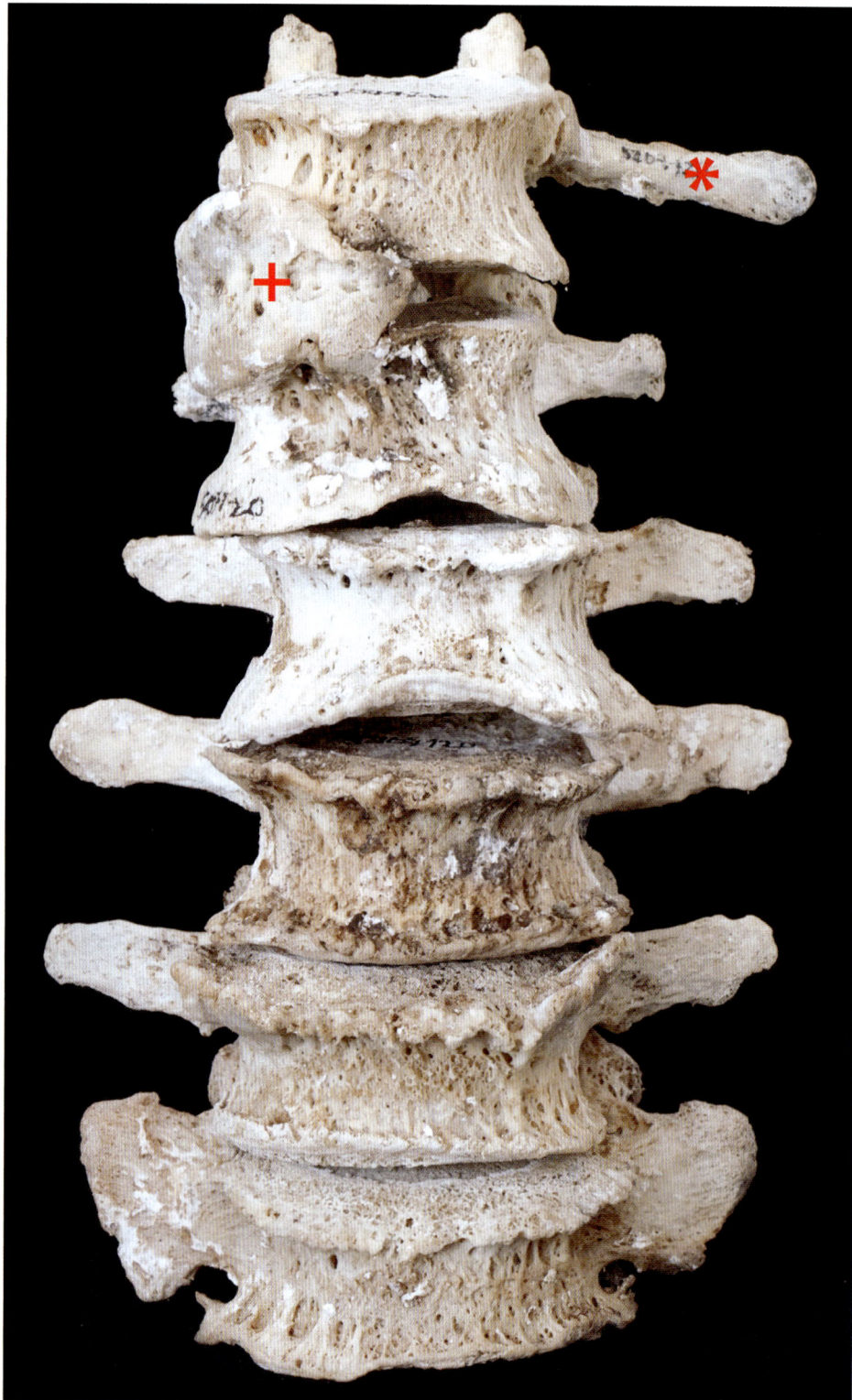

Figure 771. Six lumbar vertebrae from a spinal column with 24 total pre-sacral vertebrae and a left lumbar rib (*) in a 70-year-old Thai male (CMU 5407120) who also had a cleft spinous process of L1 and a rudimentary right transverse process. Luboga (2000) noted 20 of 591 (4%) African skeletons with six lumbar vertebrae. Cf. Barnes (1994, 2012) for six vertebrae and lumbar ribs. Also note the large bridging osteophyte (+) between L1 and L2.

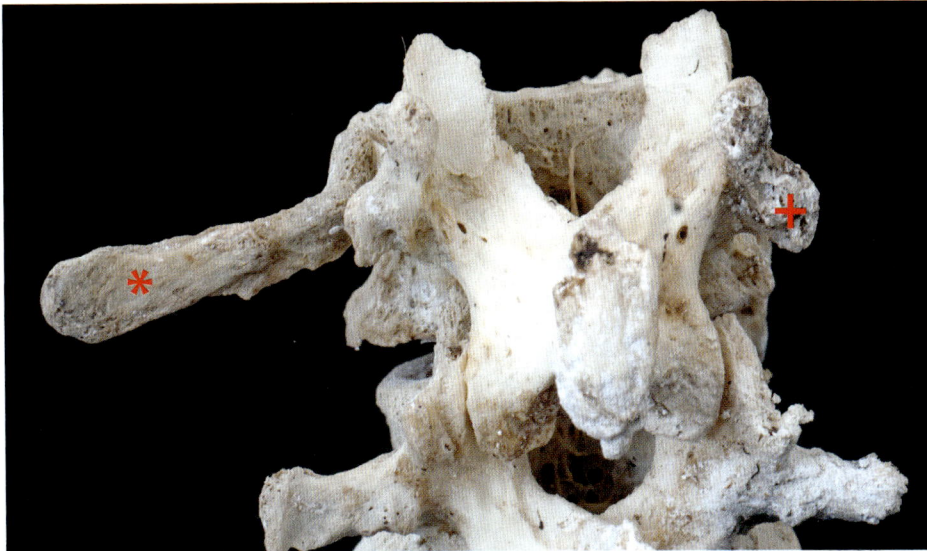

Figure 772. Left lumbar rib (*) and a small right transverse process (+) in a 70-year-old Thai male with six lumbar vertebrae (CMU 5407120).

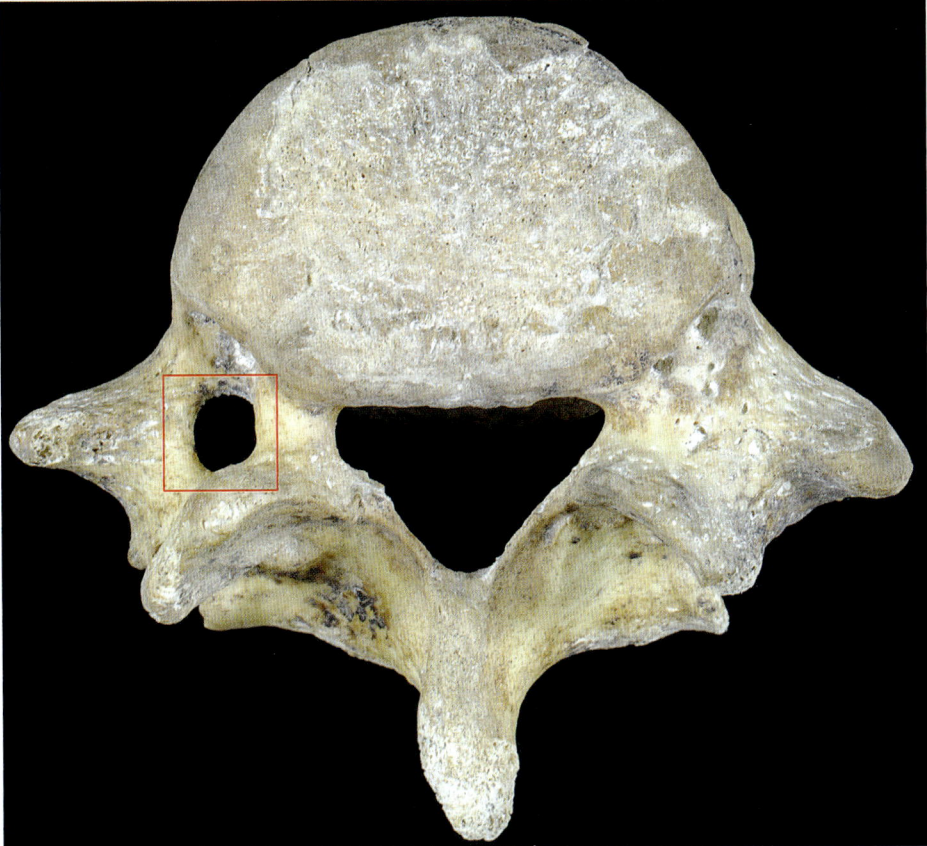

Figure 773. Superior view of a fifth lumbar vertebra exhibiting a foramen (square) in the left pedicle of a young adult male (CIL). Note that the right pedicle is more robust than the left. The structure that traversed the foramen is unknown. Rare trait, possibly the result of faulty development of the left pedicle. See Beers et al. (1984); Dwight (1902); Mahato (2014); Szawlowski (1901).

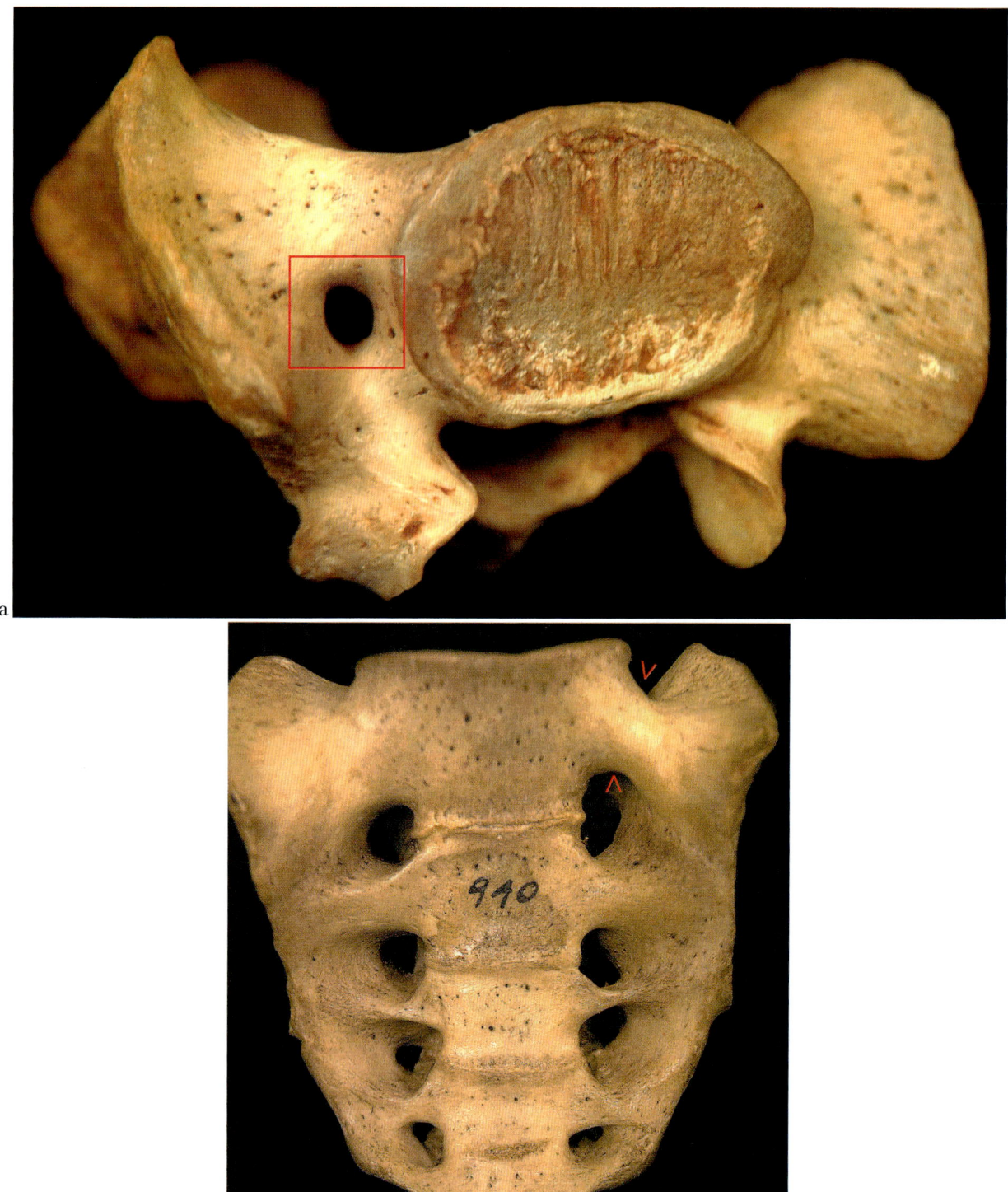

Figure 774a-b. Rare accessory foramen in the sacrum in an adult (SI Terry 940). (a) In this specimen, the foramen (square) communicated with the (b) left first sacral foramen (and ∨). Singh (2012).

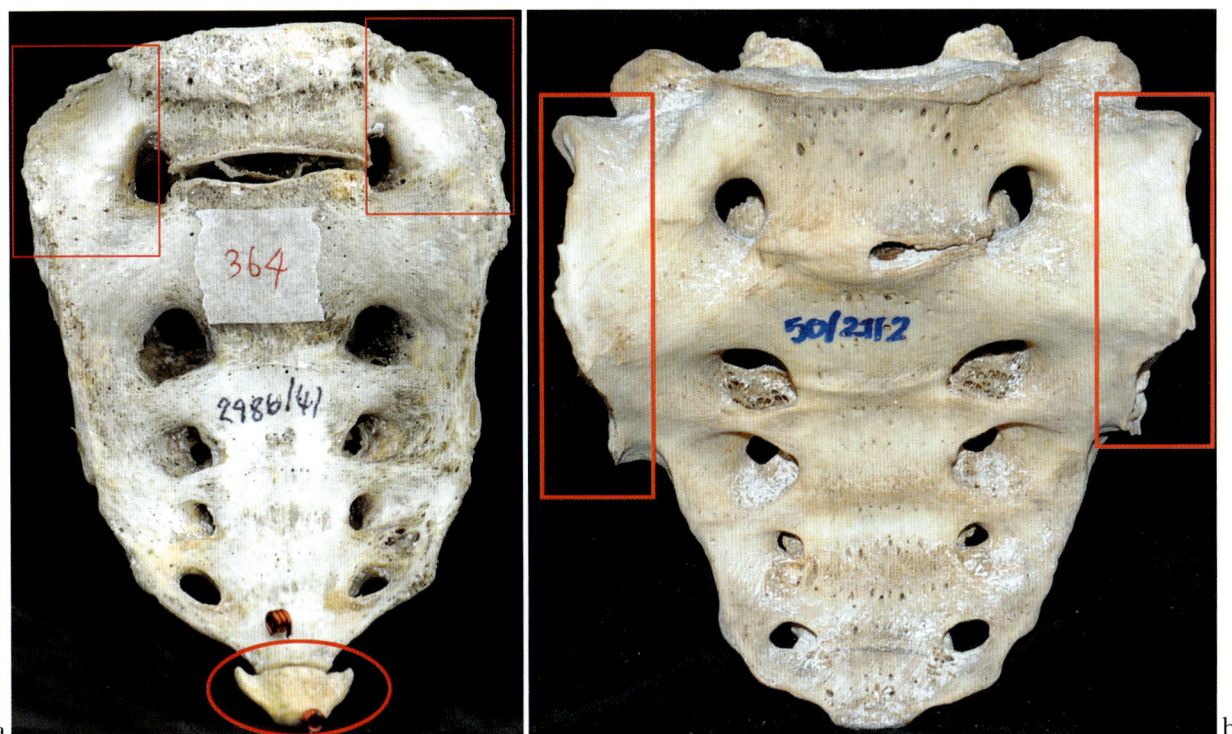

Figure 775a-b. Sacralization and variation in the size and shape of two adult sacra. (a) A narrow, long sacrum with sacralized L5 vertebra squares (personal communication, Ethne Barnes 8 June 2011) and unfused coccyx (oval). (b) Short and triangular sacrum with wide and protruding alae (rectangles) (KKU). Sacralization of L5 is more common than lumbarization of S1. Erken et al. (2002) found a significant correlation between sacralization and the presence of cervical ribs. Common finding. Cf. Barnes (1994, 2012); Mahato (2010); Savage (2005); Shore (1930).

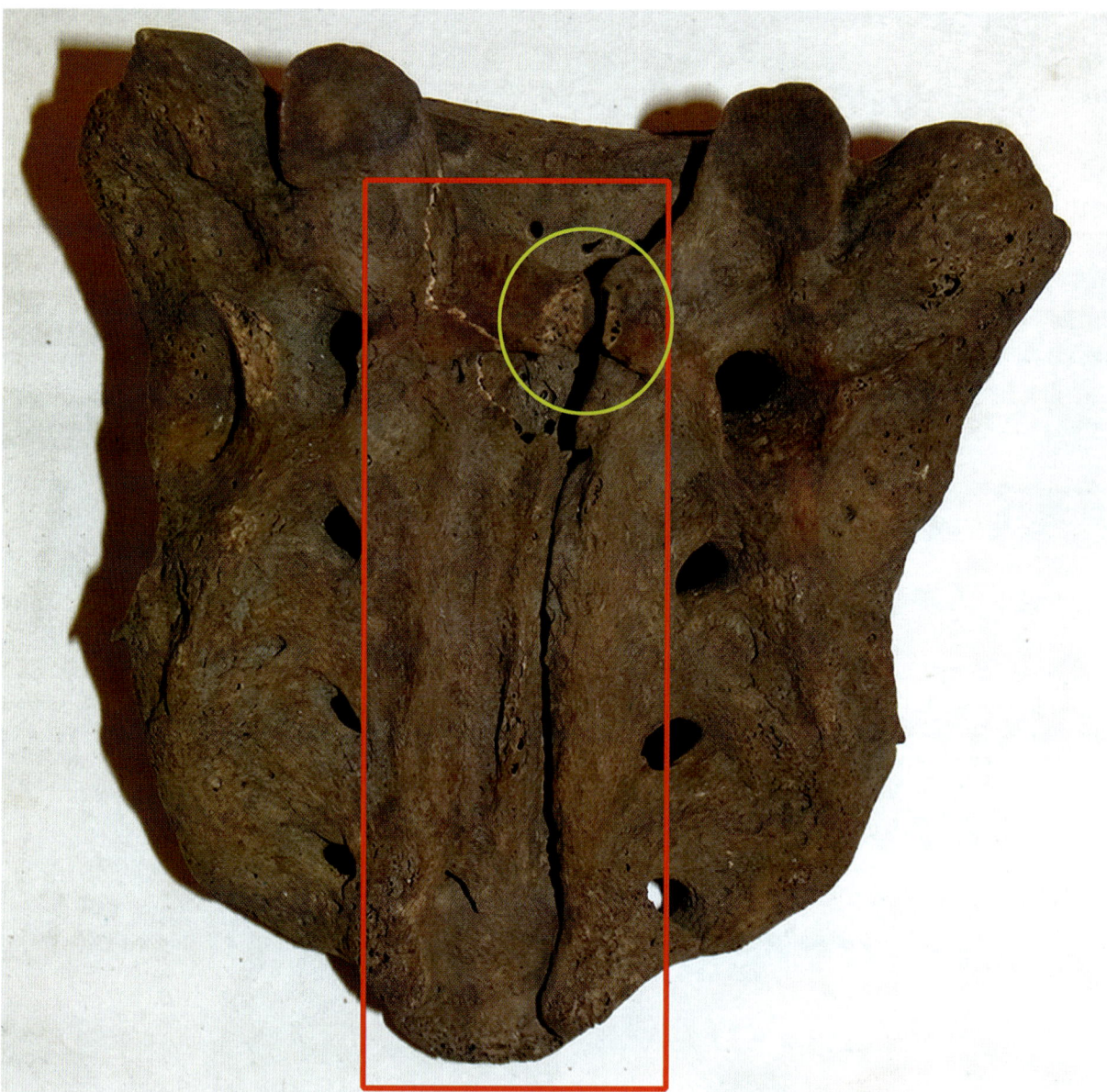

Figure 776. Complete spina bifida (rectangle) and cleft S1 neural arch (circle) of the sacrum resulting in a narrow slit-like cleft of the arches that gradually widens distally in an adult Asian. This is a developmental anomaly that is correctly classified as a pathological condition that may have been either symptomatic or asymptomatic.

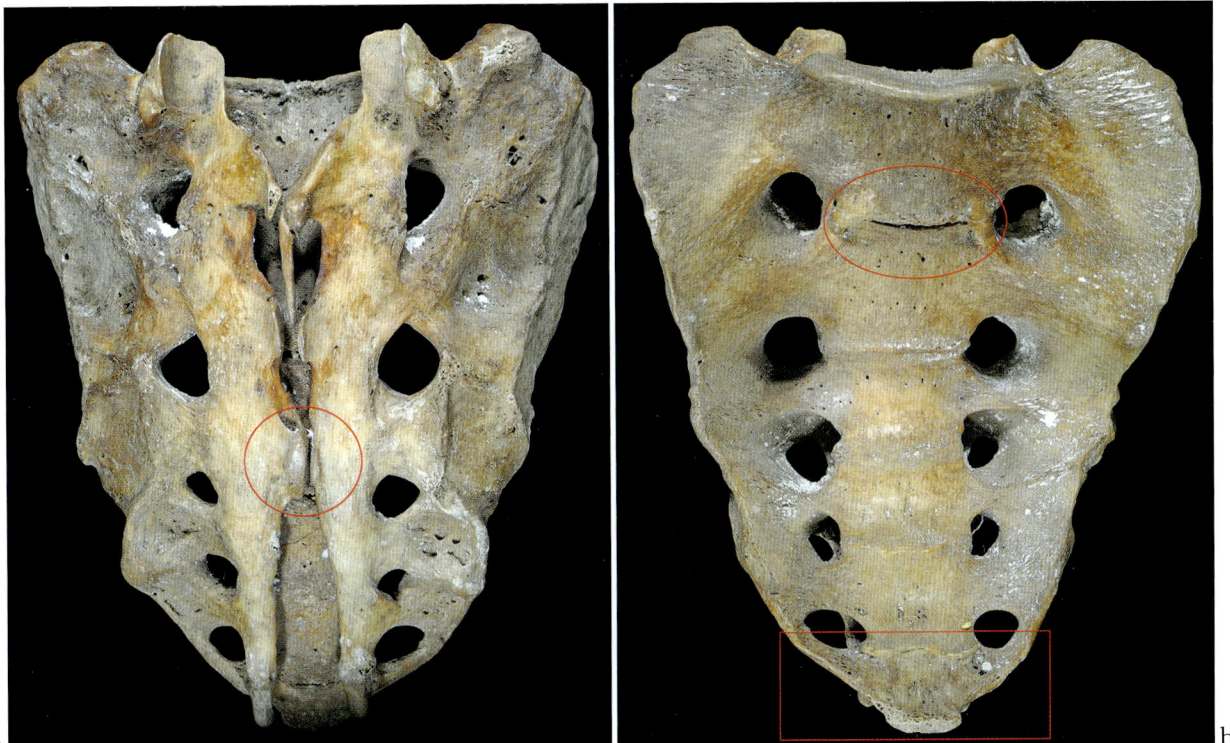

Figure 777a-b. Spina bifida in a six segmented sacrum sacrum with an irregular dorsal cleft and high sacral hiatus and incomplete fusion of S1 to S2. (a) Clefting/bifurcation/defect of posterior wall of the sacral canal (sometimes referred to as spina bifida) and sacrum. Note that a portion of the two halves (circle), almost achieving contact at midline. (b) Also note that the junction of S1 and S2 is still unfused (oval) and may remain open throughout the individual's life, as well as complete sacralization of the first segment (rectangle). Common finding. Cf. Barnes (1994); Mellado et al. (2011a).

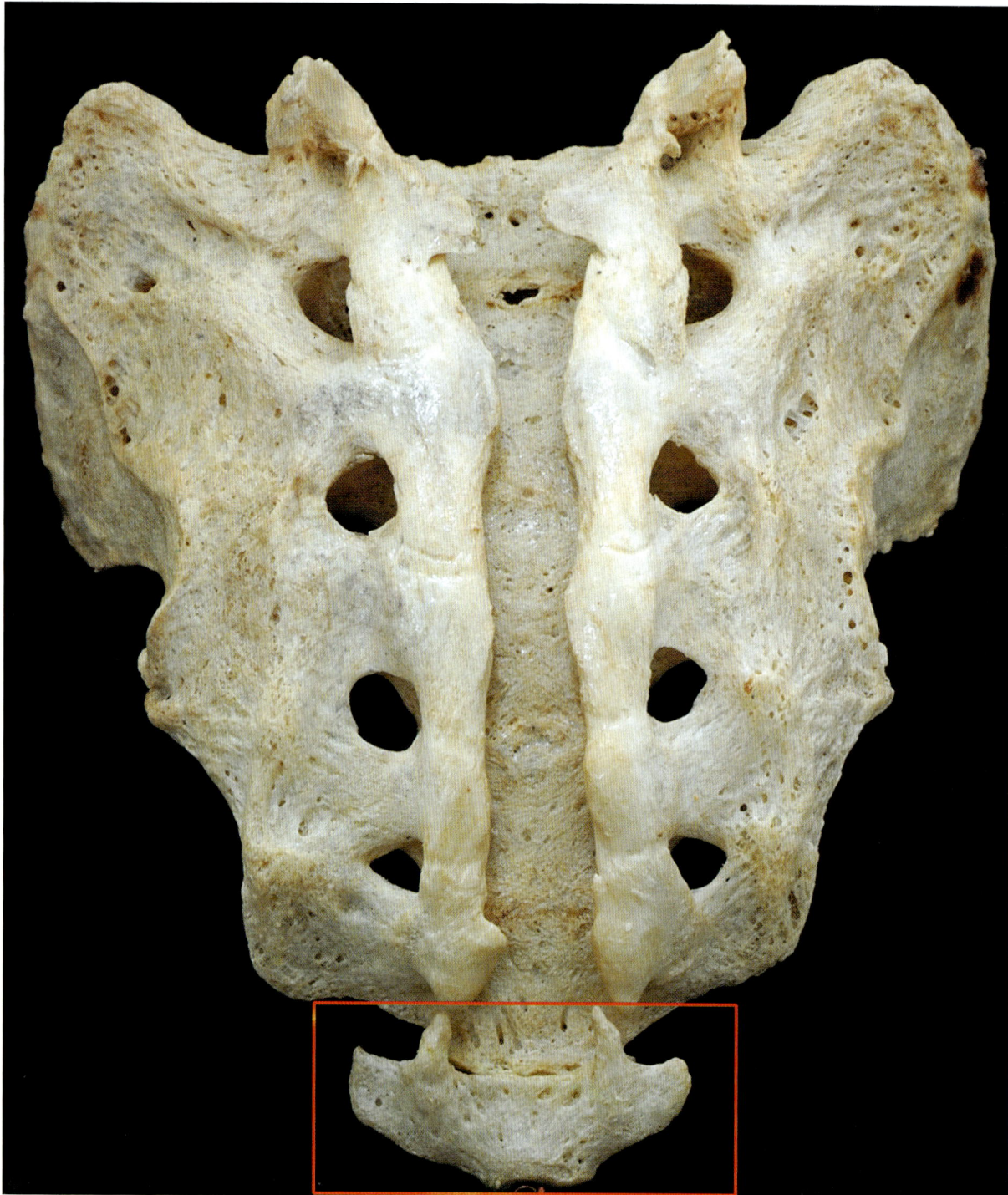

Figure 778. Complete neural arch cleft resulting in a wide opening of the sacrum with incomplete union of the coccyx (rectangle) in an adult (KKU) often referred to as spina bifida. Uncommon to rare finding. Cf. Barnes (1994, 2012); Mellado et al. (2011a).

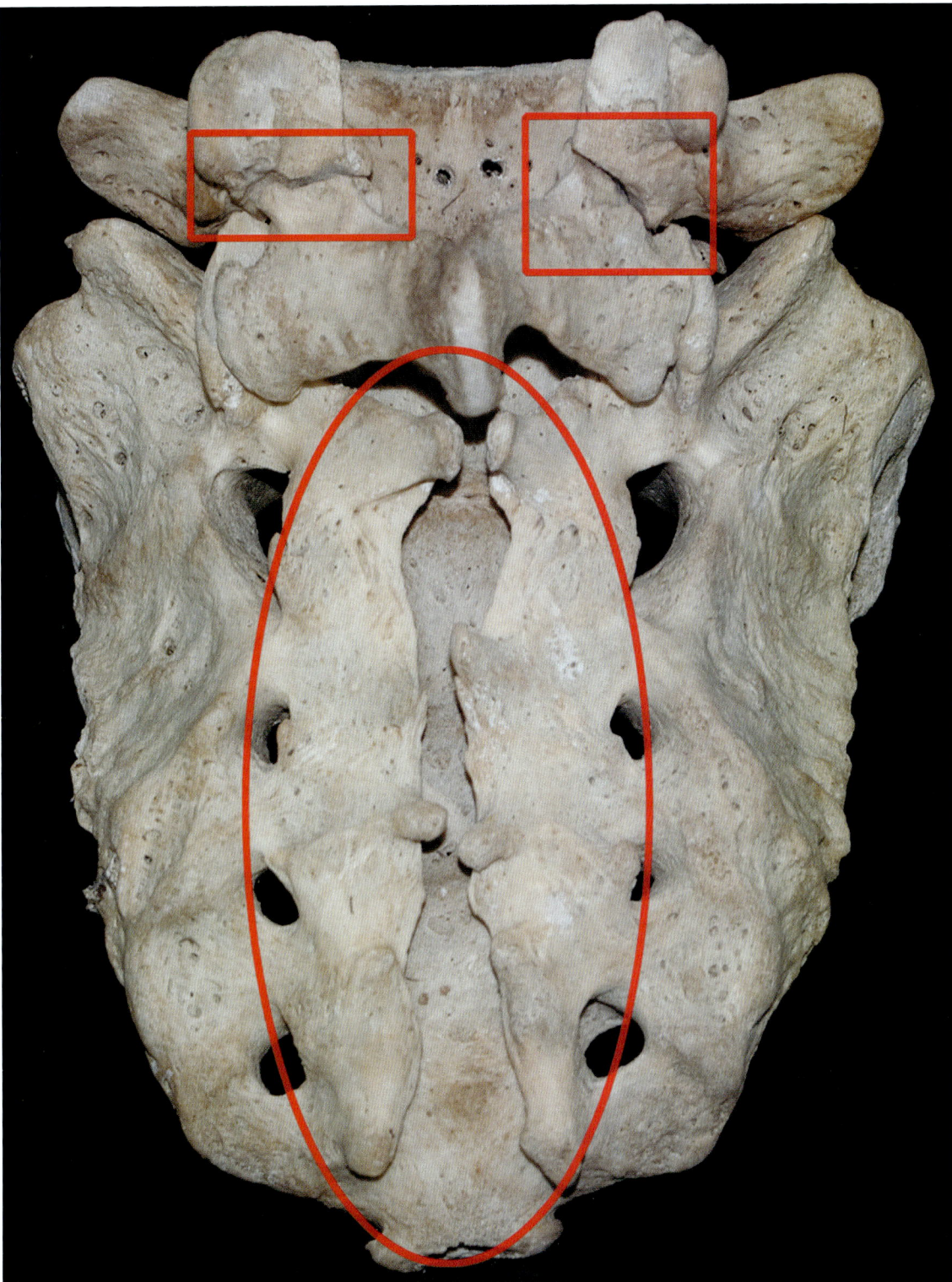

Figure 779. Bilateral spondylolysis of L5 through the pars interarticularis (rectangles) and cleft neural arch (oval) of the sacrum in an adult Thai male (KKU 0686). The cleft would have been spanned by a fibrous tissue in the extant individual. This condition represents incomplete closure of the neural arch rather than a notochord defect consistent with a diagnosis of spina bifida (personal communication, Ethne Barnes 2012). Cf. Barnes (1994, 2014); Mellado (2011a).

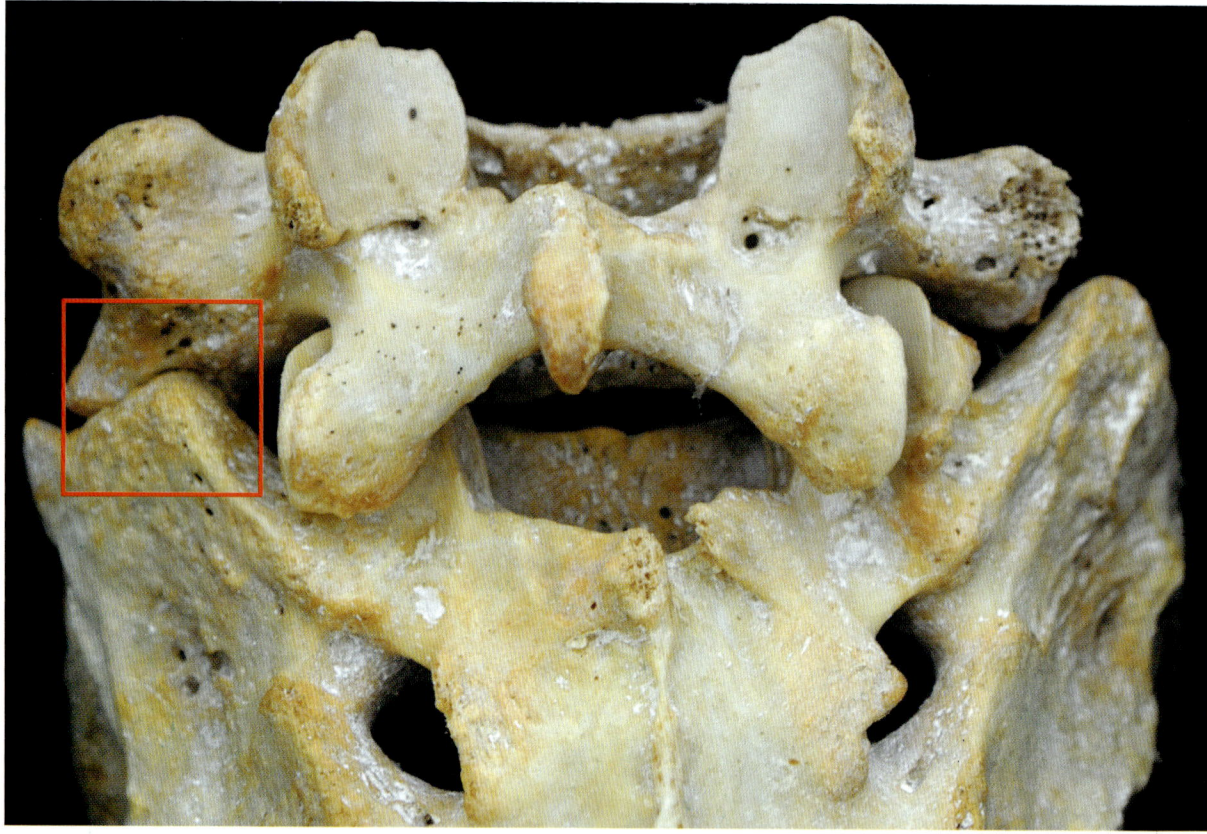

Figure 780. Partial sacralization (square) of the fifth lumbar (KKU). Uncommon finding. Cf. Barnes (1994, 2012). See Erken et al. (2002) for more on the relationship between sacralization and cervical ribs.

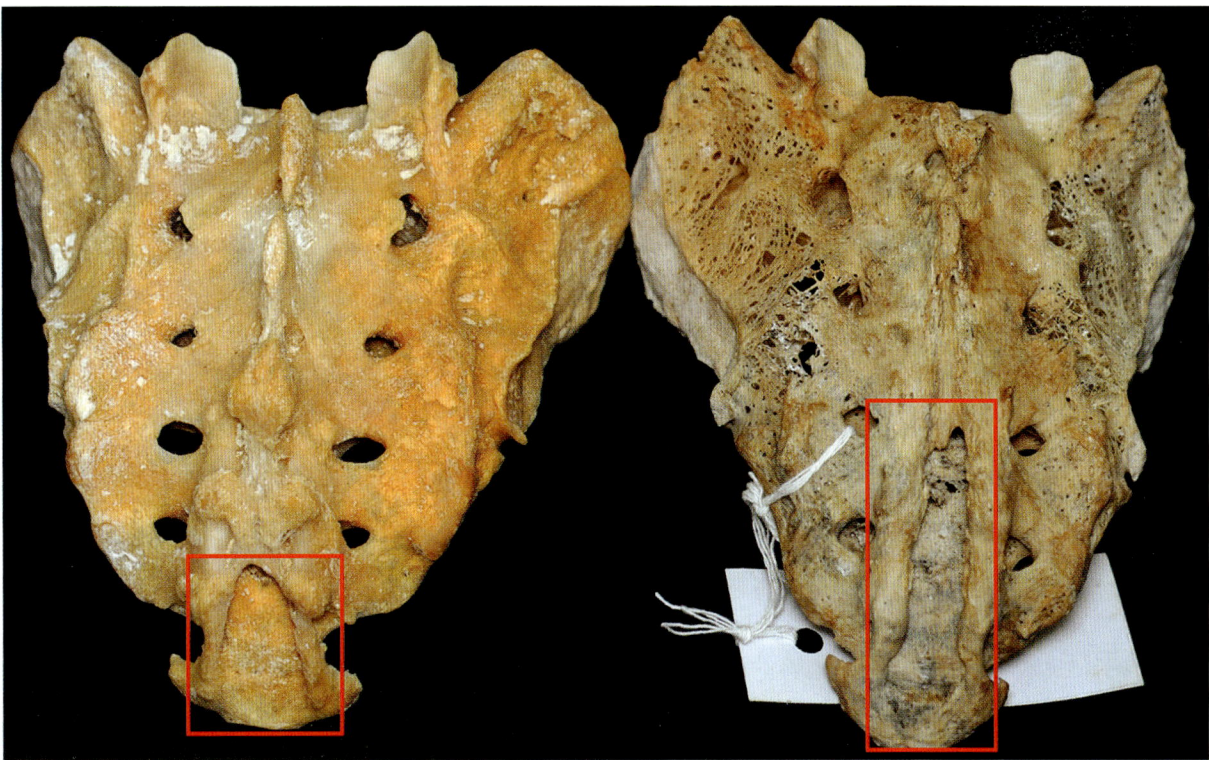

Figure 781. Normal variation of the sacral hiatus (square and rectangle) in two adults (**KKU**).

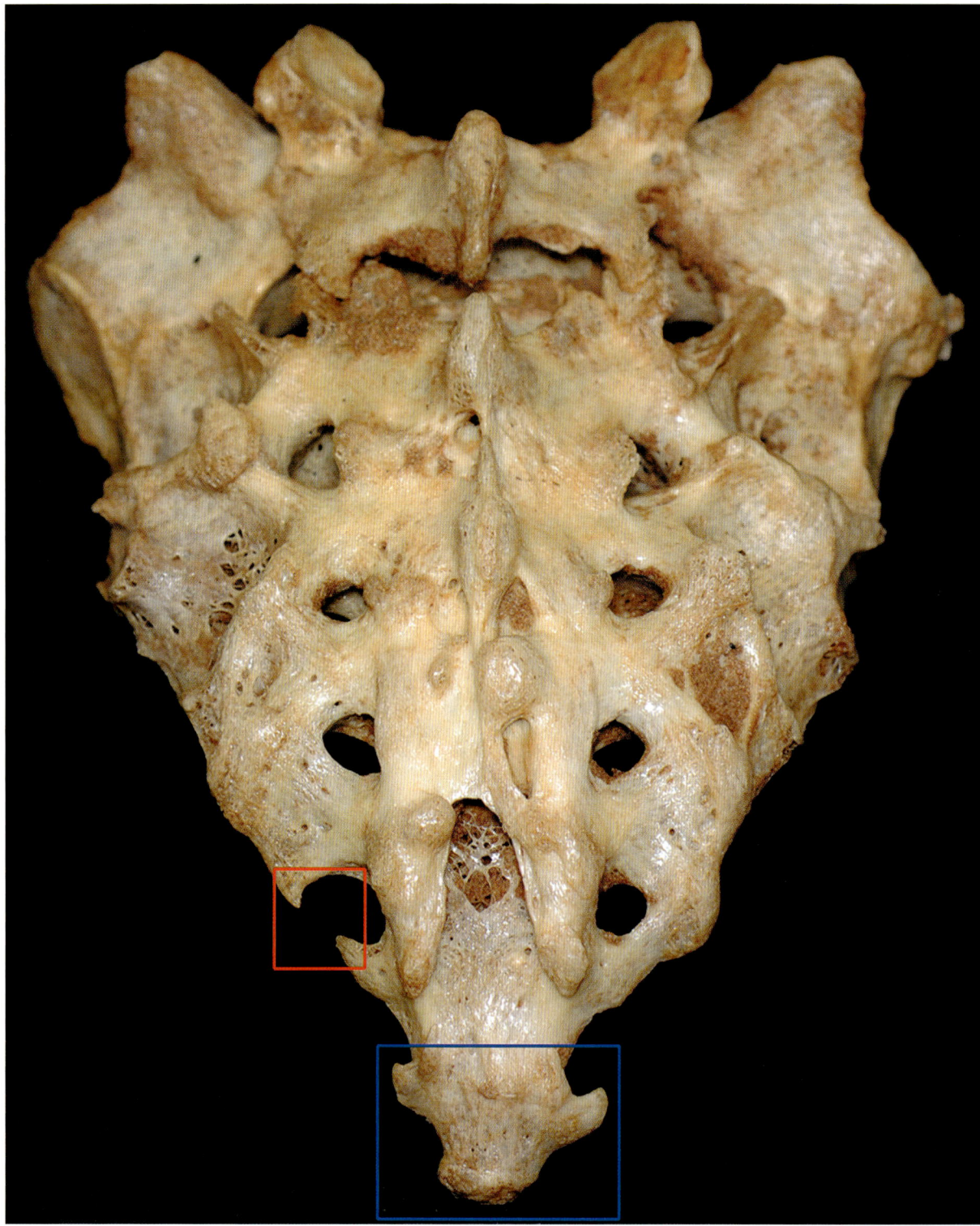

Figure 782. Unusually triangular sacrum with an incompletely formed left fifth sacral foramen (red square) and fused coccyx (blue rectangle). Cf. Barnes (1994, 2012).

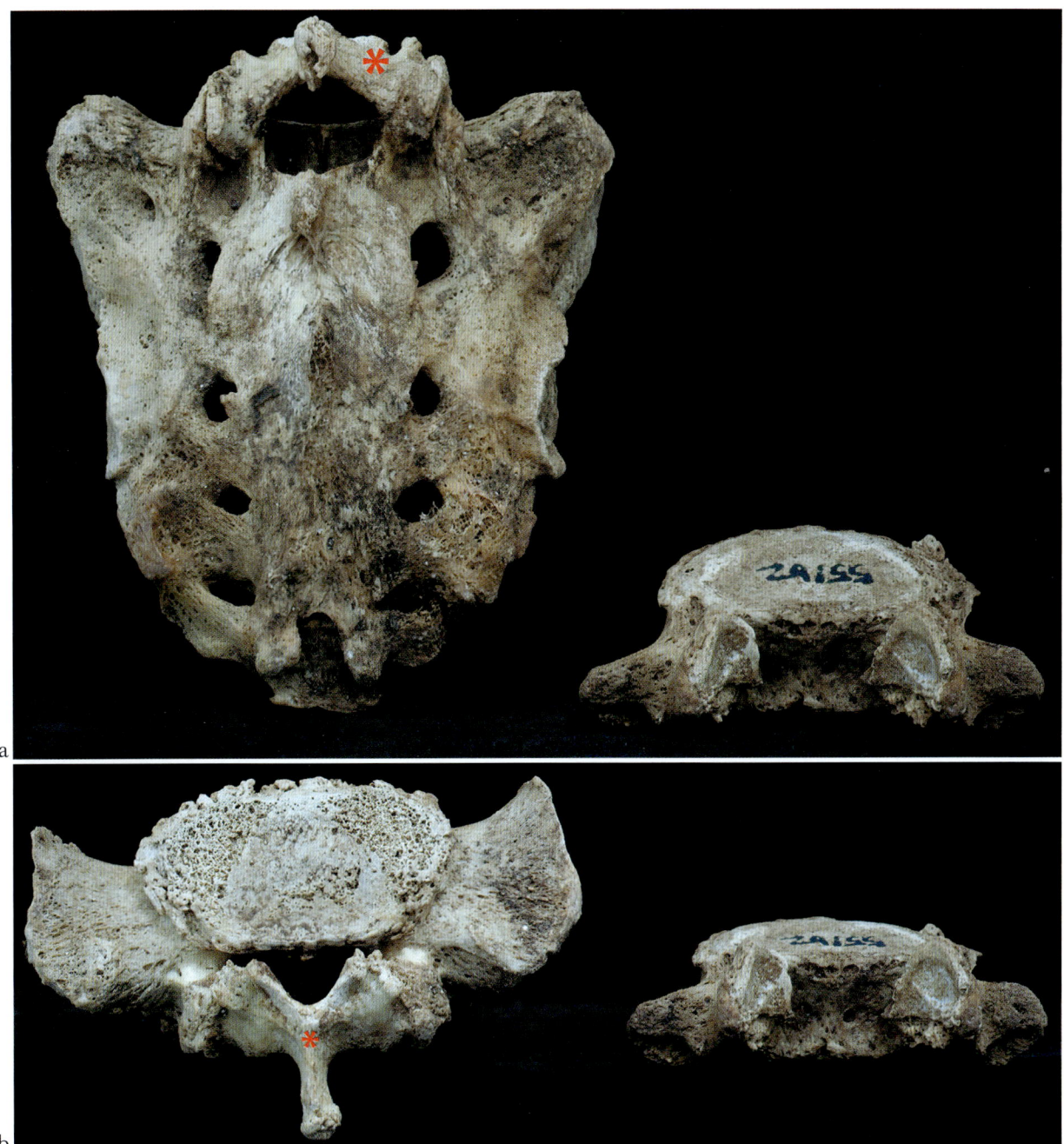

Figure 783a-b. Separate neural arch. (a) Dorsal view of separate neural arch (*) fused to the first sacral segment in an adult Thai (CMU 55/62). Cf. Barnes (1994, 2012). Fusion of the neural arch in this individual was likely the result of trauma or osteoarthritis. (b) Superior view illustrating the separate neural arch (*) fused to the sacrum.

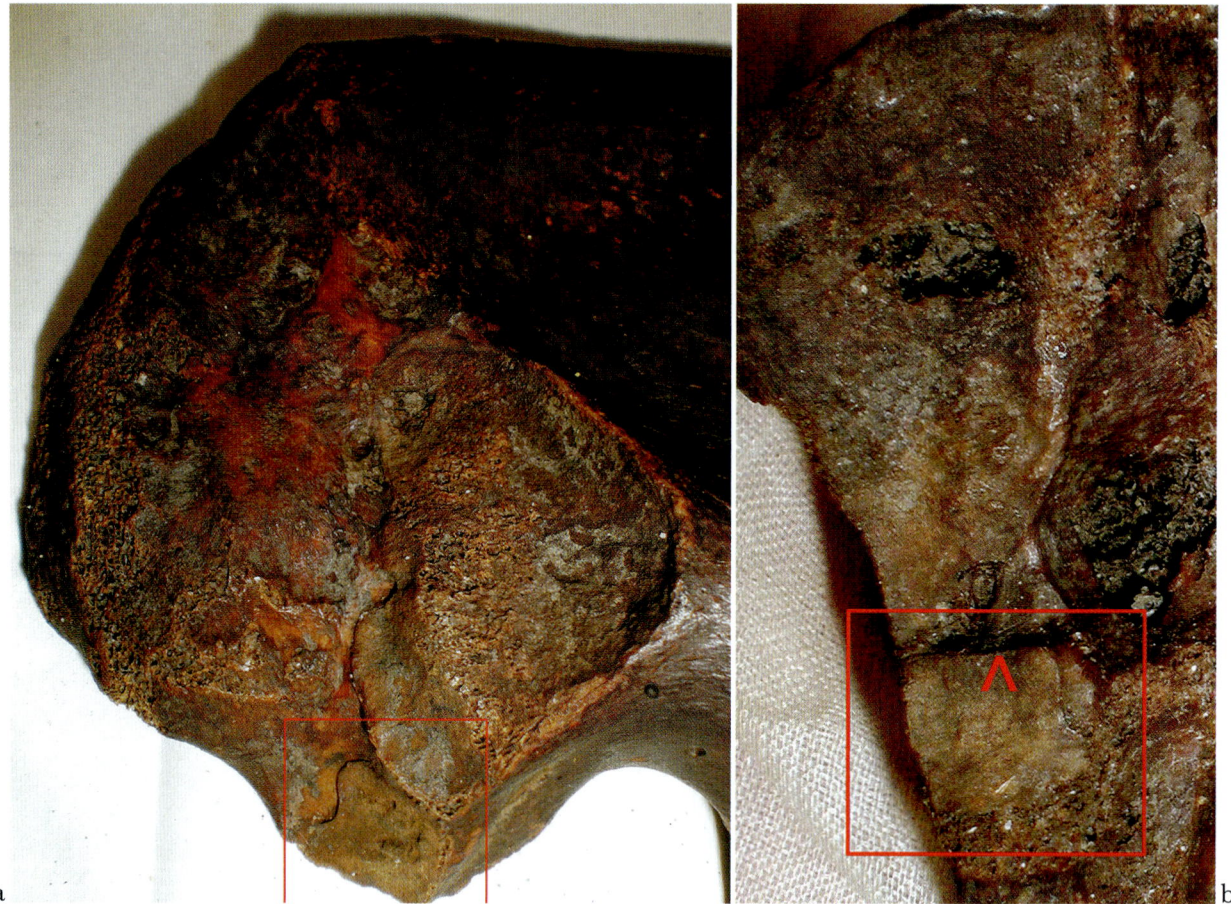

Figure 784a-b. Accessory articular facet of the sacrum. (a) Divided left auricular surface (square) resulting in an accessory articular facet, also known as the accessory sacroiliac joint, in an adult Asian male (Mann, unprovenienced). (b) Close-up showing the small inferior articular facet (square) separated from the superior portion of the auricular surface by a horizontal cleft (∧). It is not known whether this false joint, that is distal and independent from the synovial sacroiliac joint, is congenital or acquired (Fortin and Ballard 2009). However, Trotter (1937) reported an increased frequency of this trait with age, concluding that it was acquired. Cf. Barnes (1994, 2012); Derry (1911); Ehara et al. (1988).

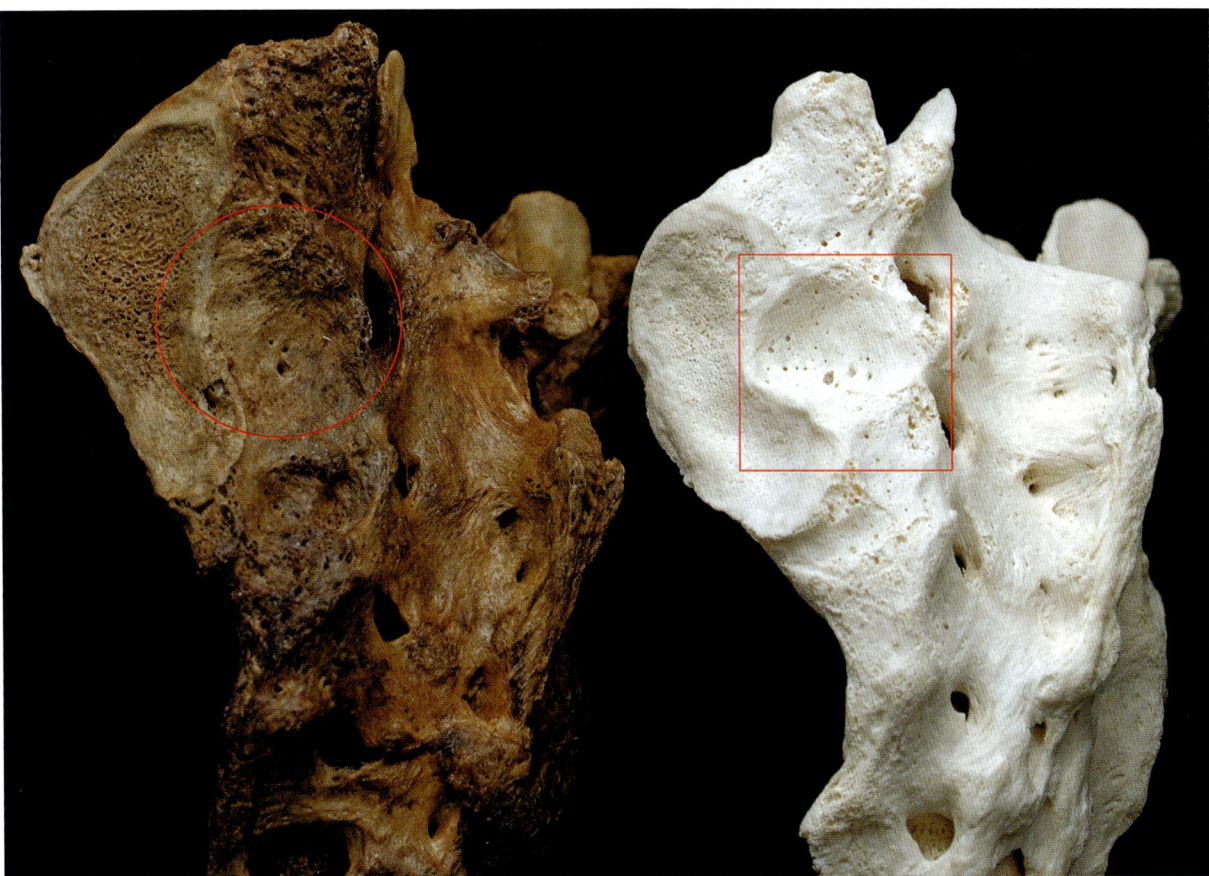

Figure 785. Adult sacra, one typical and without a a fossa cribrosa (circle; FSA CSC DS009) and the other with a fossa cribrosa (square) (FSA CSC DS033). This fossa accommodates a portion of the postauricular surface of the ilium and entrance of small anastomotic vessels into the sacrum. The craterlike depression of varying size and depth is usually located between the first and second sacral segments and it is found in approximately 30% of individuals (Kreyenbühl and Hessler 1973). Fossa cribrosa is usually accompanied by a transitional deformity of the spine.

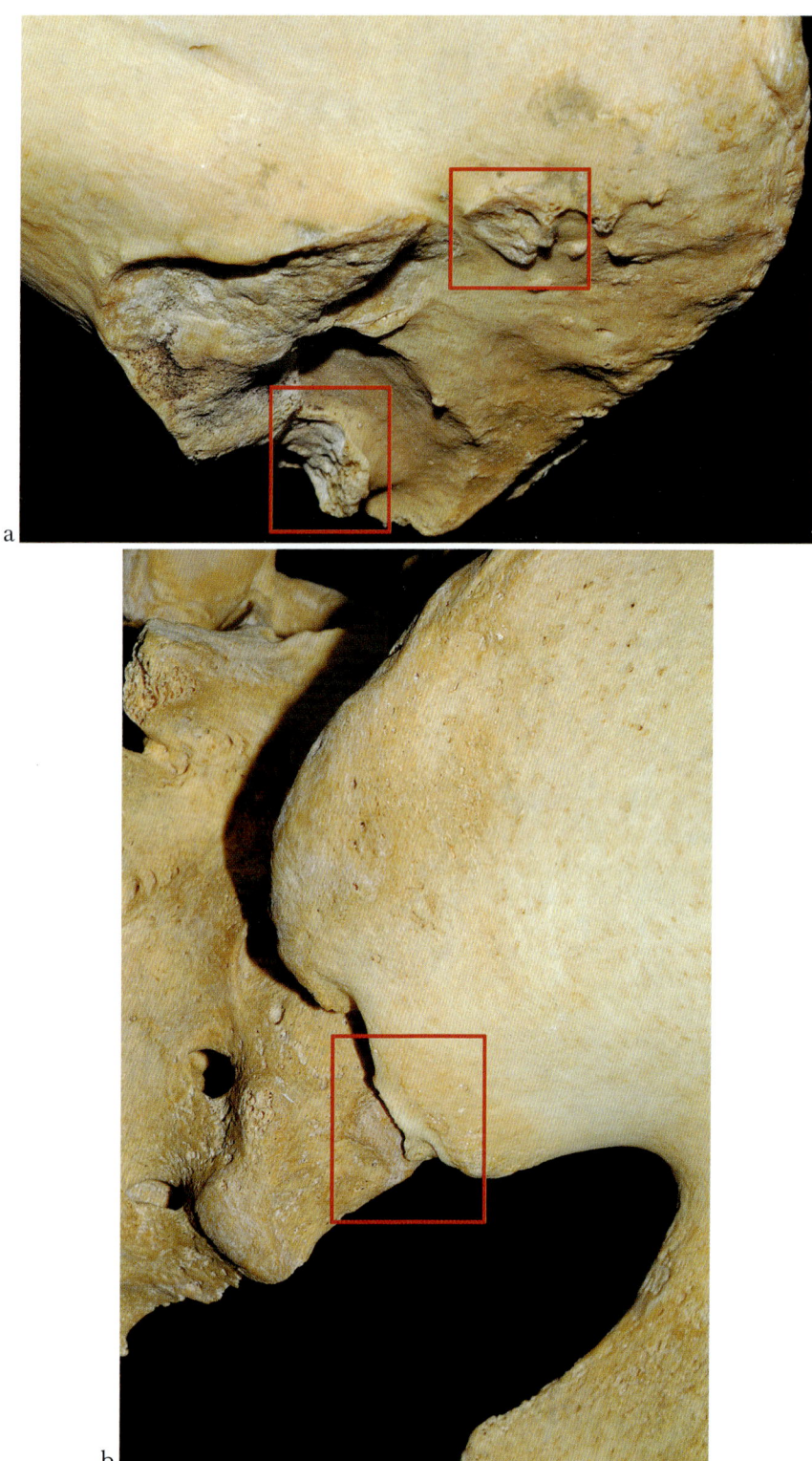

Figure 786a-b. Accessory articular facets in the right pelvis of an adult Thai. (a) Internal view demonstrating superior and inferior facets (square and rectangle) above the auricular surface for articulation with the sacrum (KKU). (b) External view showing the site of articulation of the inferior facet (rectangle). Common finding. Cf. Derry (1911); Ehara et al. (1988).

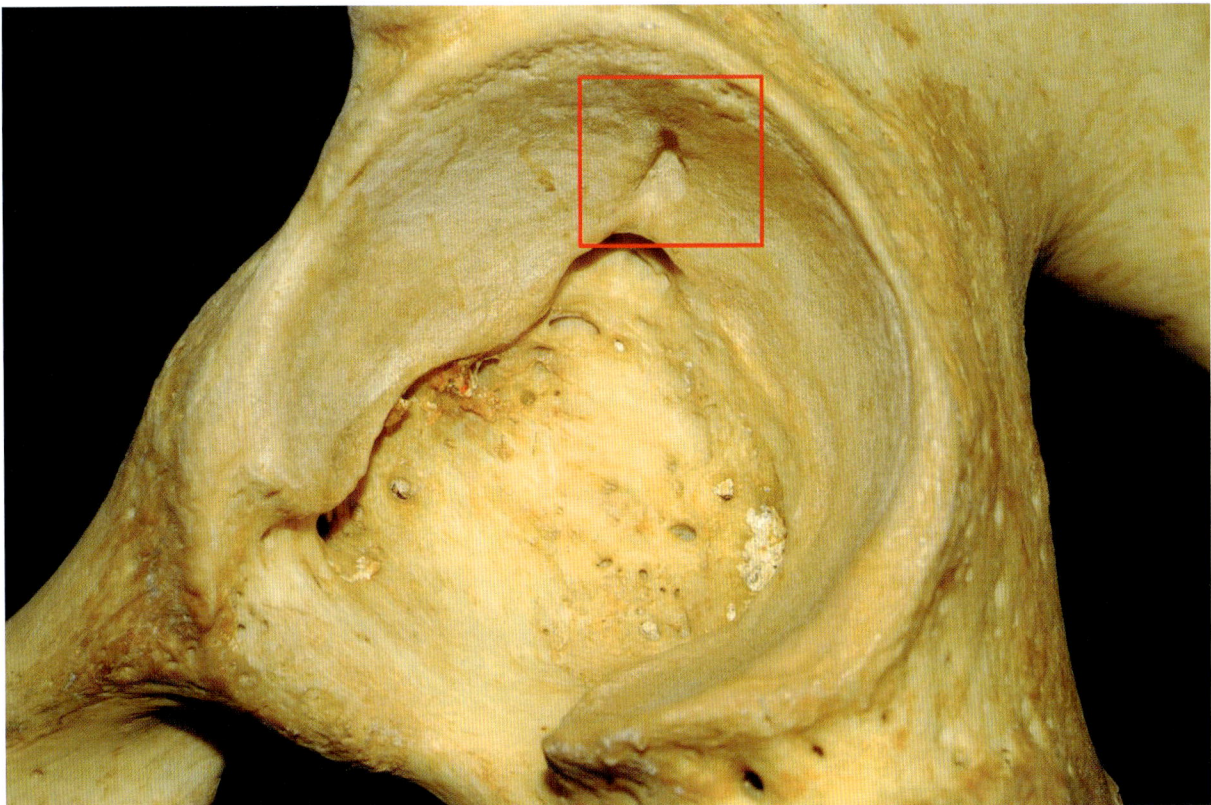

Figure 787. Left acetabulum with a deep tunnel, the supra-acetabular fossa (square) (SI Huntington). This individual exhibits a typical anatomical variant that occurs immediately inferior to the acetabular notch. Cf. Frayer (1987).

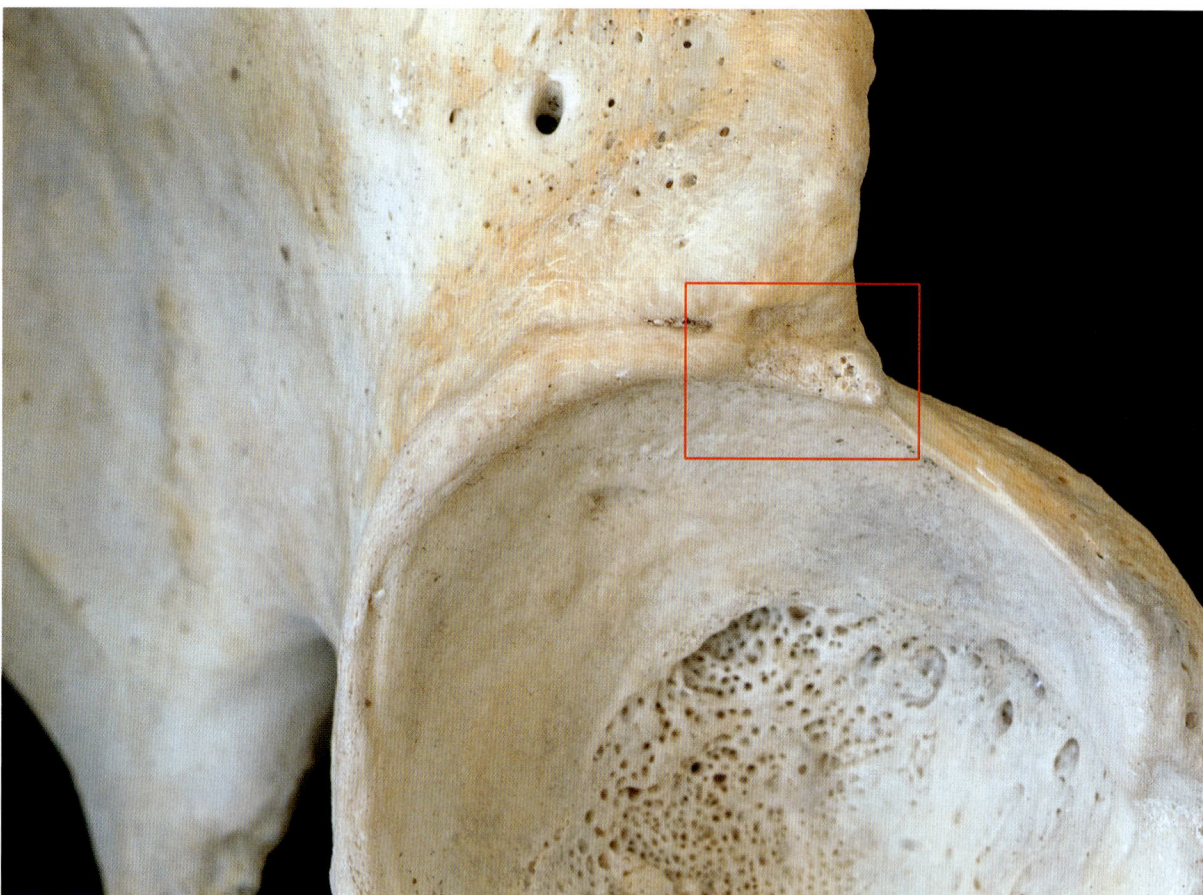

Figure 788. Site of articulation of a small accessory ossicle, likely a cotyloid bone or so-called flange lesion, in the right innominate of a 36-year-old Thai male (CMU 122 50). Whether this is a lesion or normal anatomical variant consisting of an accessory ossicle is unknown. The separate ossicle that is along the acetabular labrum, and in the region where the iliofemoral ligament attaches, was not recovered postmortem. The term "cotyloid bone" comes from the "cotyloid ligament" (in the older literature; see Frazer 1920), now known as the acetabular ligament that partially encircles the acetabulum. The rarity of this feature in osteological collections and the clinical literature renders its etiology difficult to interpret. The authors have seen only three examples of this accessory ossicle. Cf. Mann and Hunt (2005, 2012).

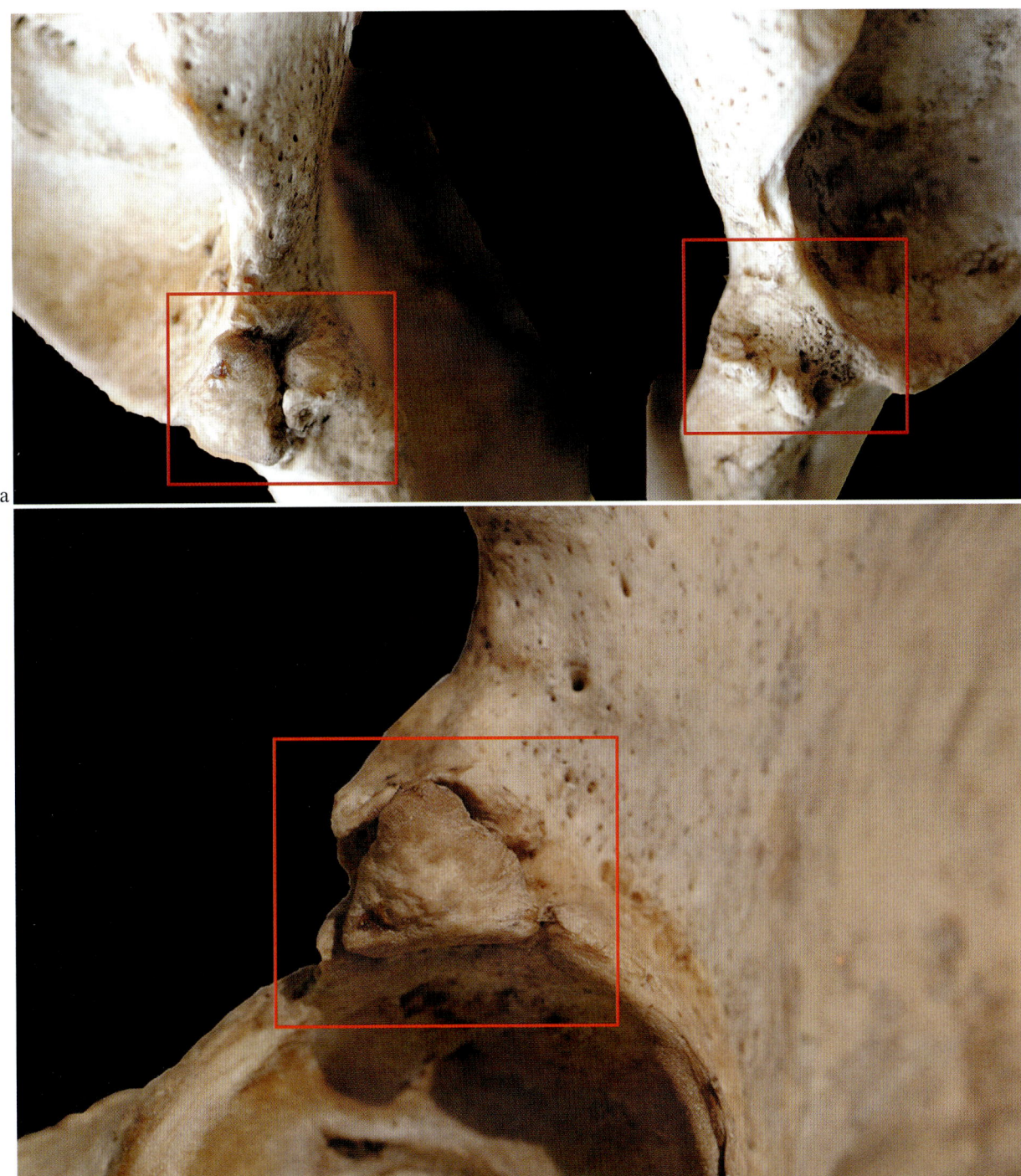

Figure 789a-b. Bilateral accessory ossicles (cotyloid bones) along the superior rim of the acetabulum in an adult African male (University of Pretoria). (a) While both innominates had accessory ossicles, that of the left innominate (b) is present and tightly-adhering, while the right is missing, leaving only a crescent-shaped defect along the acetabular rim. (b) Note that the pyramid-shaped ossicle on the left side does not fill the corresponding crescent defect precisely. The three examples that the authors have encountered were all present at this location along the acetabular rim in the region of the iliofemoral ligament and, possibly, the rectus femoris. Rare trait that involves the articular surface of the acetabulum. Cf. Mann and Hunt (2005, 2012).

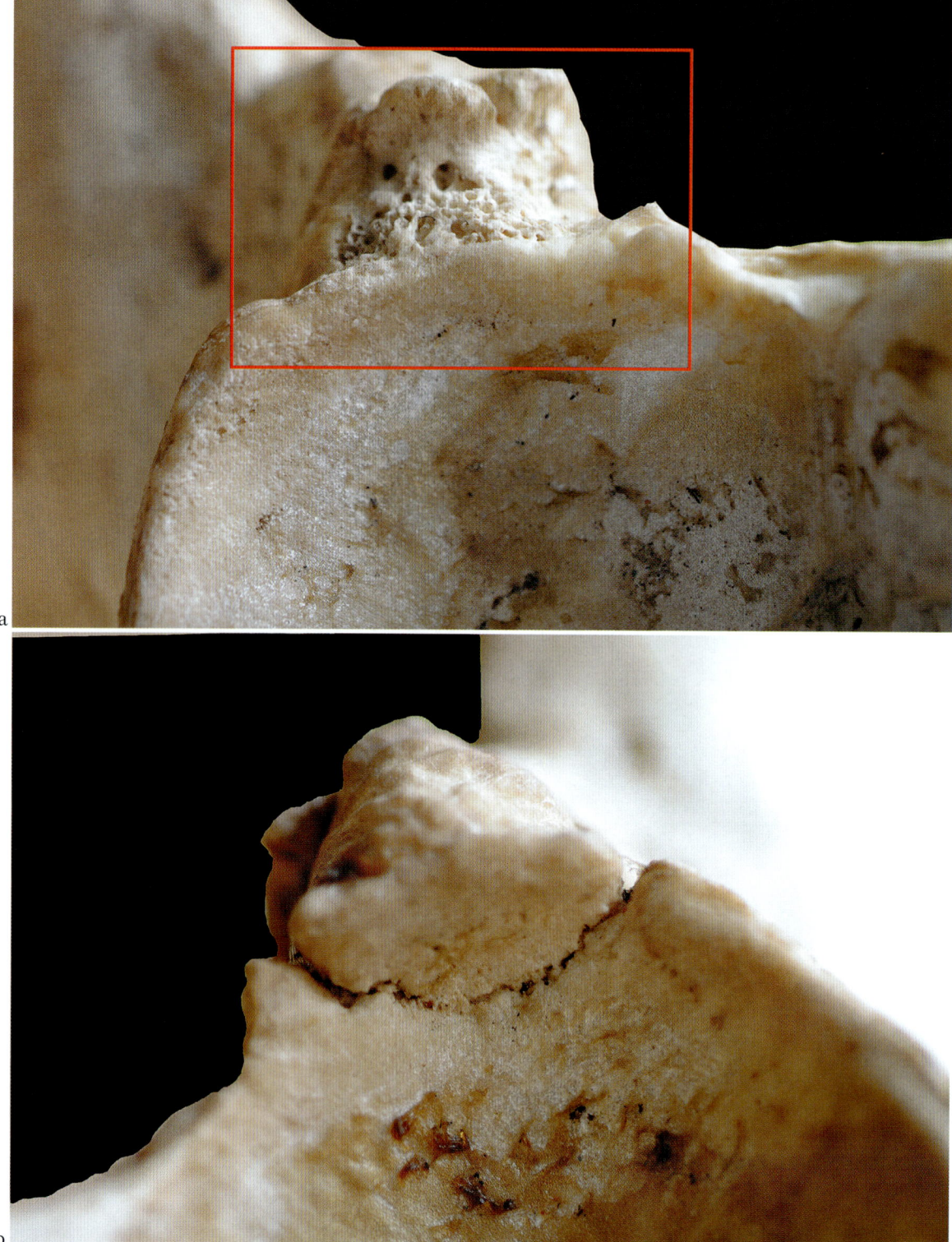

Figure 790a-b. Cotyloid bones. (a) Magnification of the right cotyloid bone notch without the accessory ossicle (rectangle). (b) Inferior view of the cotyloid bone along the superior rim of the left acetabulum showing that it is part of the articular lunate surface (University of Pretoria).

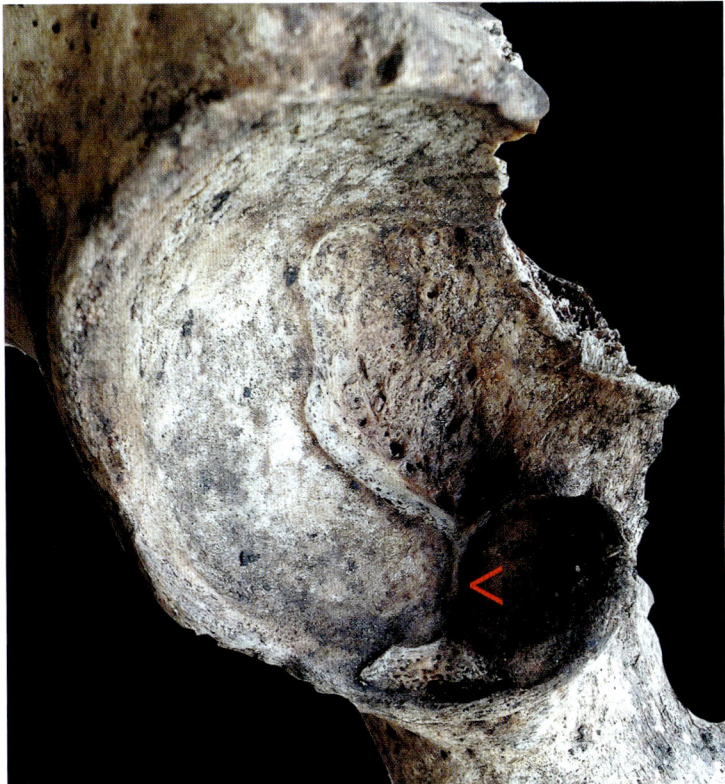

Figure 791. Divided (<) right acetabular surface in an adult male (LABANOF). Uncommon to rare trait of unknown etiology. Note what appears to be a triangular-shaped lesion inferior to the ridge of bone. These features were not present in the left acetabulum.

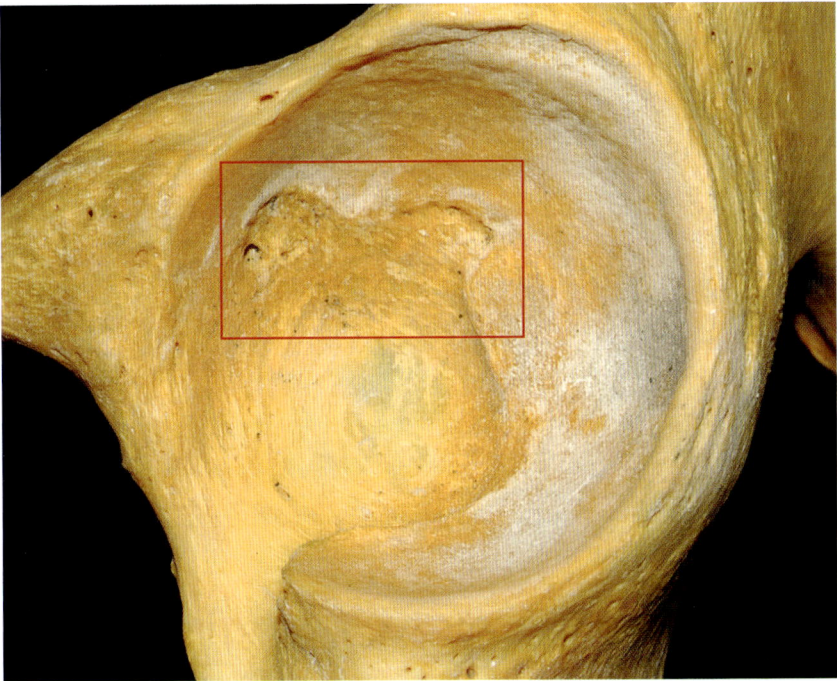

Figure 792. Variant of the acetabulum showing two indentations (rectangle) in the lunate surface (KKU).

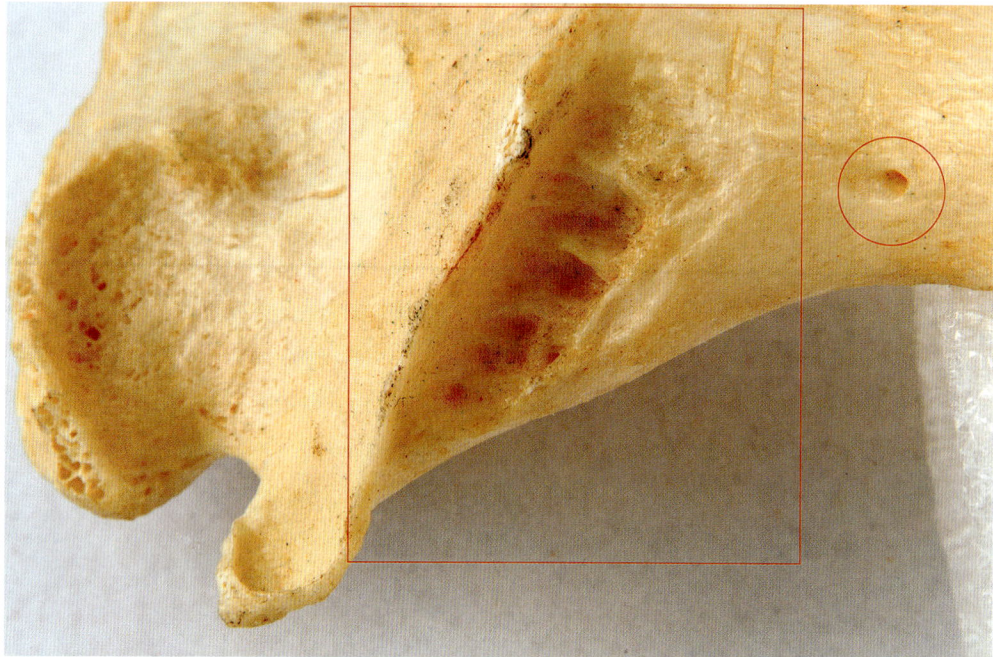

Figure 793. Preauricular sulcus (rectangle), a trait reportedly found only in females (23% of females examined radiographically), and a frequently occurring foramen (circle) in the left innominate of an adult female (KKU). See Cox and Scott (1992); Derry (1909); Gülekon and Turgut (2001) and Houghton (1977) for more on the preauricular sulcus.

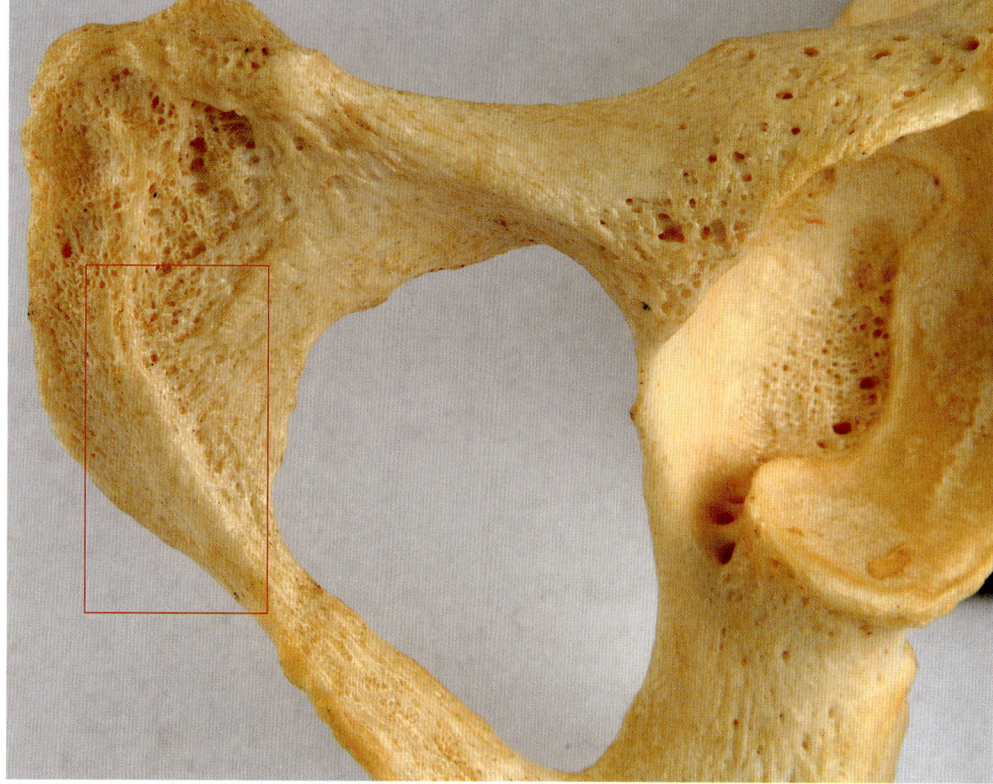

Figure 794. Ventral arc (rectangle) and wide pubic bone, attributes common in females (KKU). Cf. Phenice (1969); Sutherland and Suchey (1991).

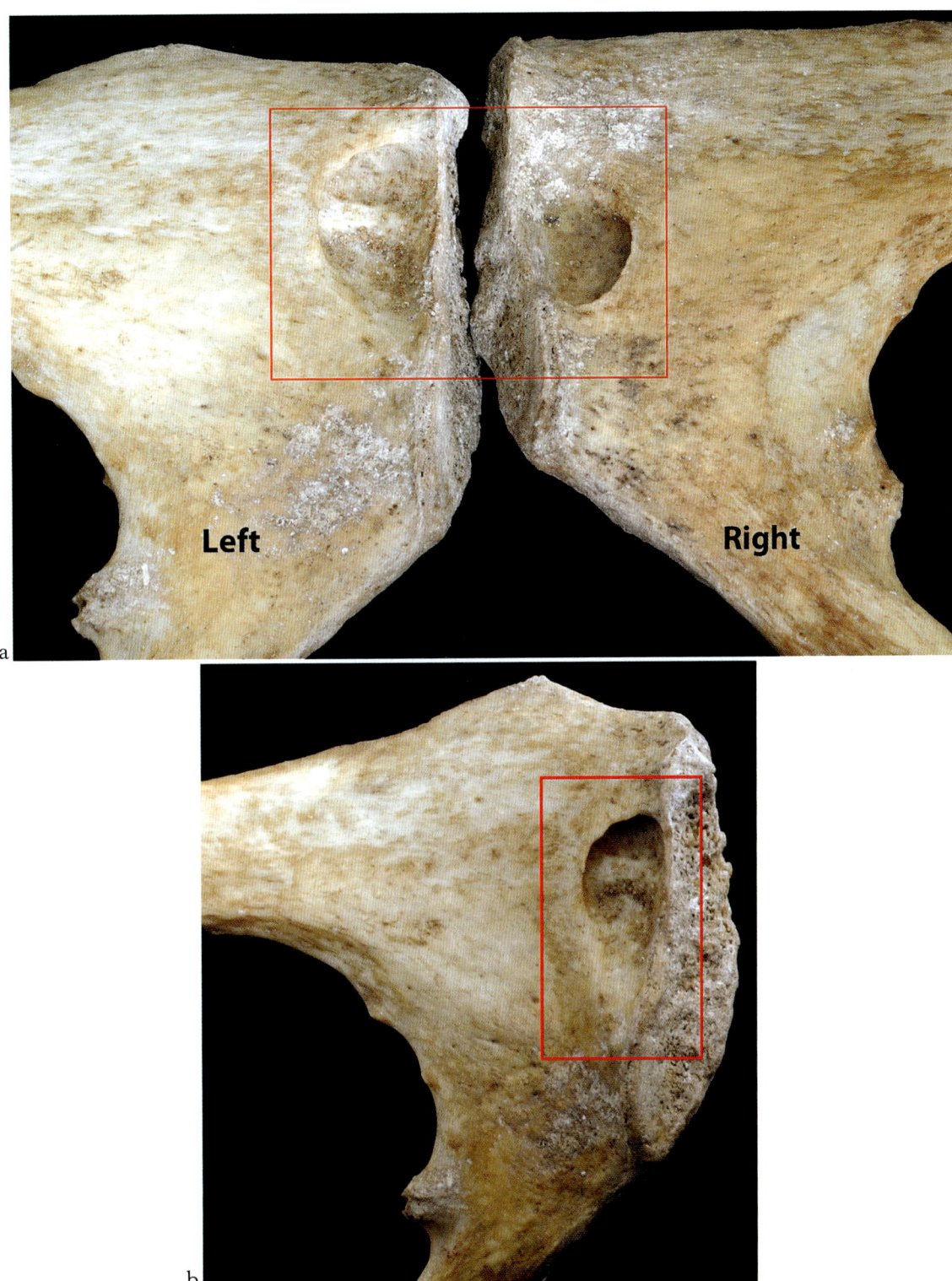

Figure 795a-b. Parturition pits of the pubes. (a) Parturition or parity pits (rectangle) in the dorsal surface of the pubic bones in an adult Asian female (KKU). (b) Higher magnification of the pit in the left pubic bone. There is disagreement on whether these pits, depressions and scars indicate pregnancy, are associated with the trauma of childbirth, reflect the number of births, or are caused by other factors. Cf. Cox and Scott (1992); Snodgrass and Galloway (2003).

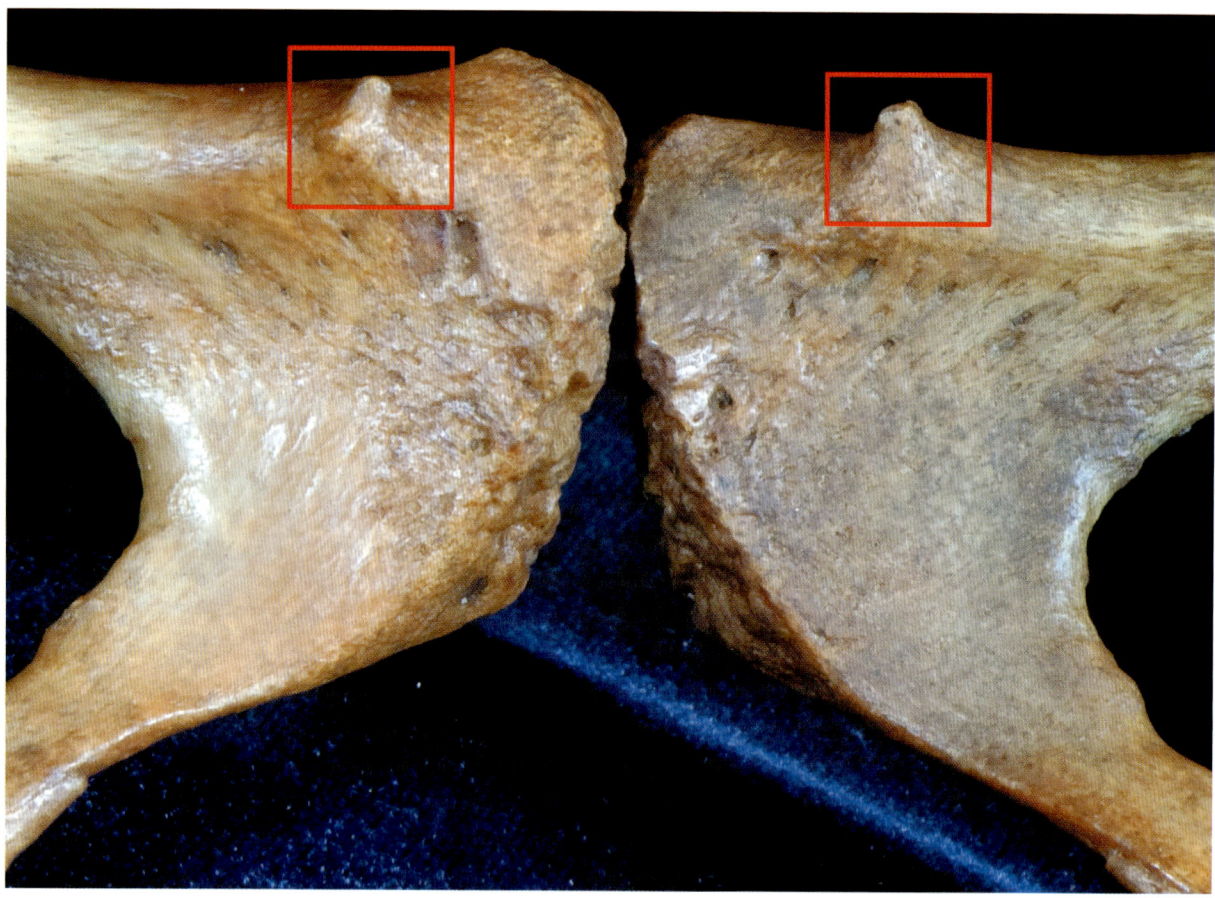

Figure 796. Large, pointed pubic tubercles/spine (squares) for attachment of the inguinal ligament in a subadult Black female (SI). The size of these tubercles corresponds to the distance from the pubic symphysis. Cf. Cox and Scott (1992); Snodgrass and Galloway (2003); Verna (2014).

Chapter 11

LEG AND FOOT
(FEMUR, TIBIA, FIBULA, PATELLA, TARSAL, METATARSAL, PHALANX)

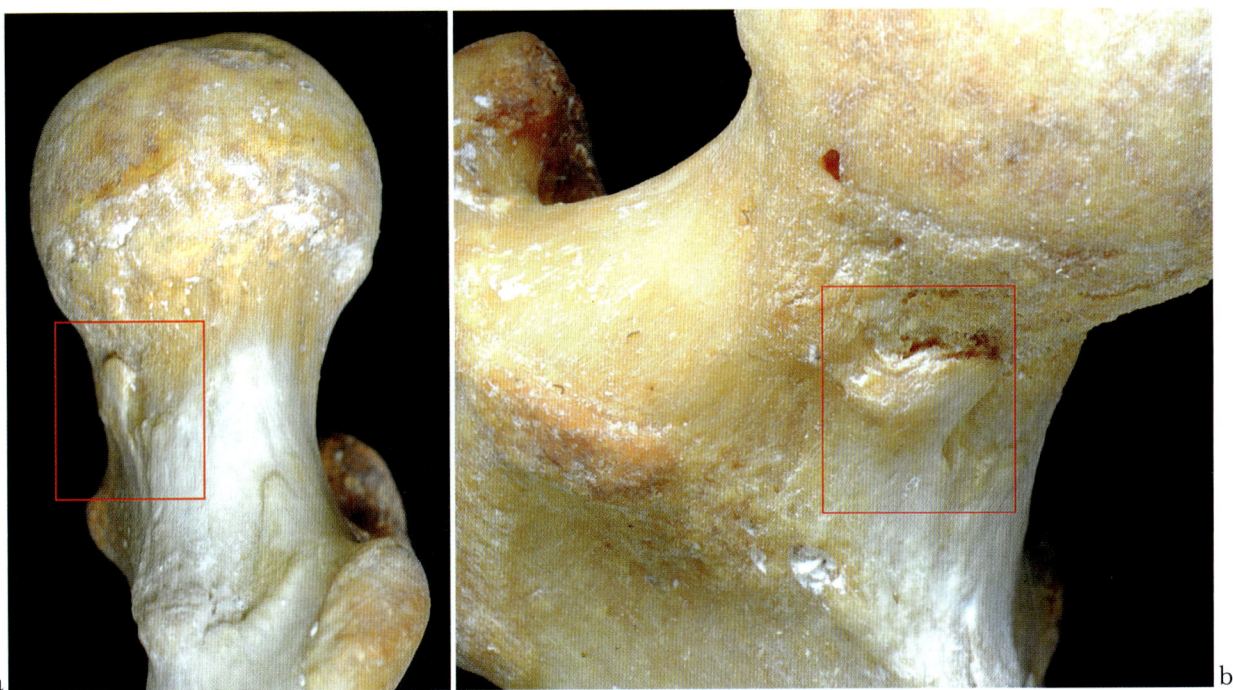

Figure 797a-b. Unilateral anterior femoral tubercle of the neck. (a) Superior view demonstrating an anterior tubercle (rectangle) in the right femur of an adult Thai (KKU). (b) Ventral view of the anterior femoral tubercle (rectangle). The tubercle lies along the margin where a Poirier's facet or plaque typically forms. However, this tubercle displays the characteristics of a enthesophyte that might have resulted from a muscular strain. It is one of only three specimens that the authors have observed and constitutes a rare finding that warrants more research to determine whether it is a non-metric trait, typical variant, or lesion.

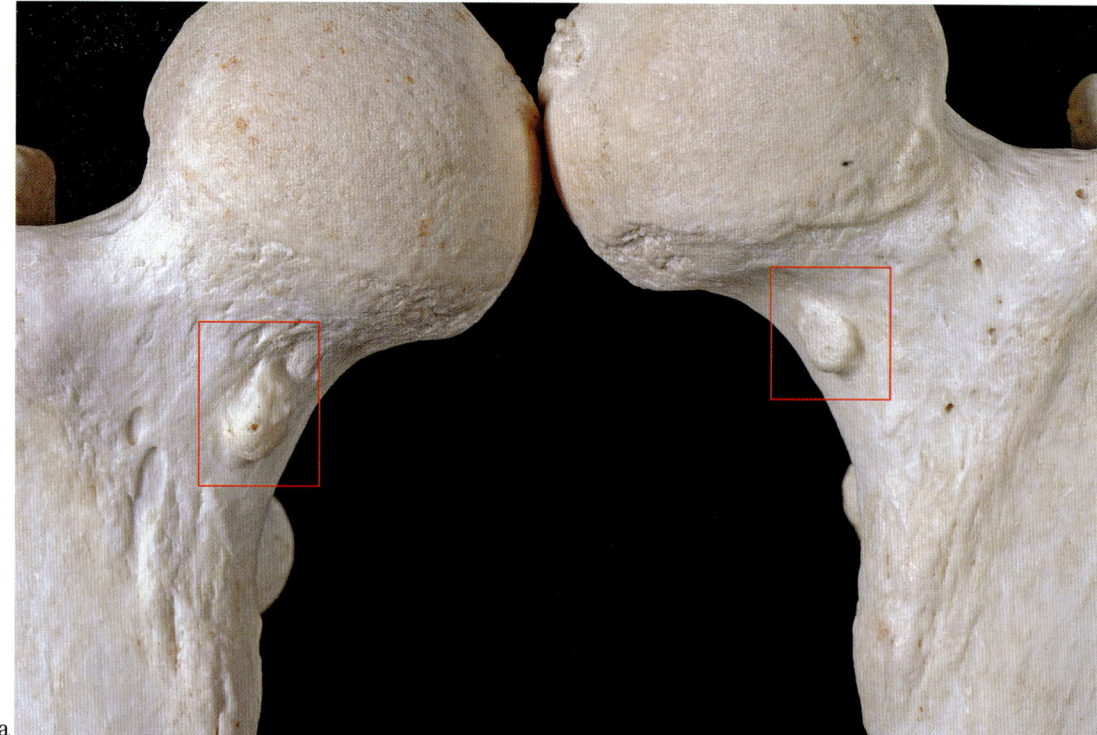
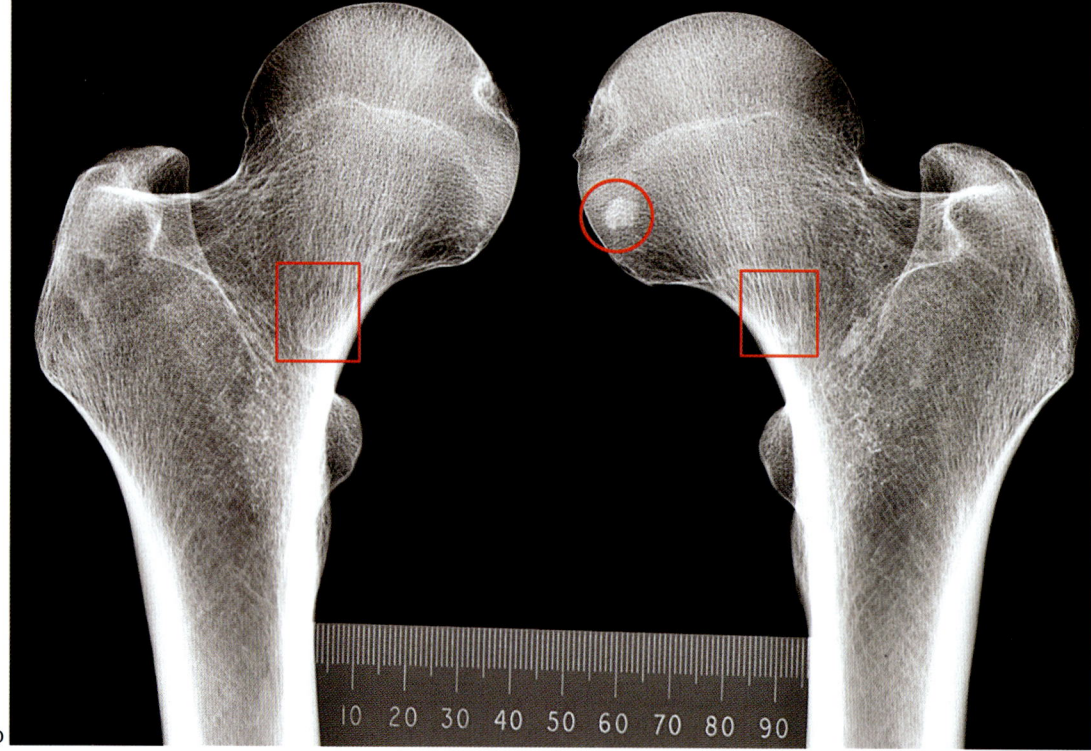

Figure 798a-b. Bilateral anterior femoral tubercles of the neck. (a) Ventral view showing anterior femoral tubercles (square and rectangle) in an elderly adult male (CSC). (b) Radiography of the same specimens reveals a thin cortex covering these tubercles. Note the enostosis or bone island (circle) in the left femur. Interestingly, these tubercles are not situated in the area where a Poirier's facet forms, which is more superior and lateral. Uncommon to rare finding that warrants further research.

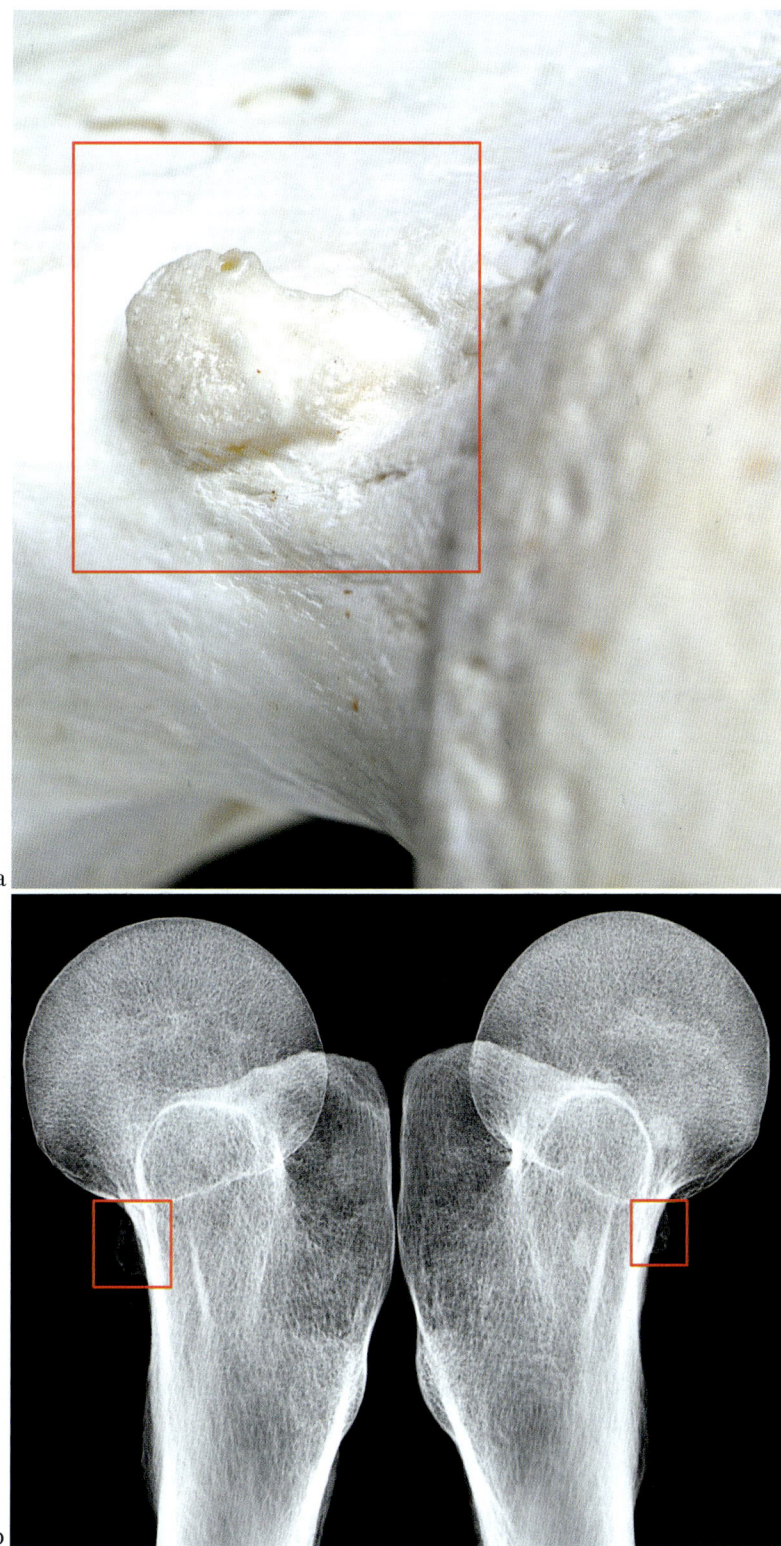

Figure 799a-b. Anterior tubercles in an elderly male (CSC). (a) Anterior view of the tubercle (square) on the right femur. (b) Radiograph showing the thin but normal cortex covering these tubercles (squares). See Figure 798a-b for more images in this individual. Uncommon to rare finding of unknown etiology and frequency.

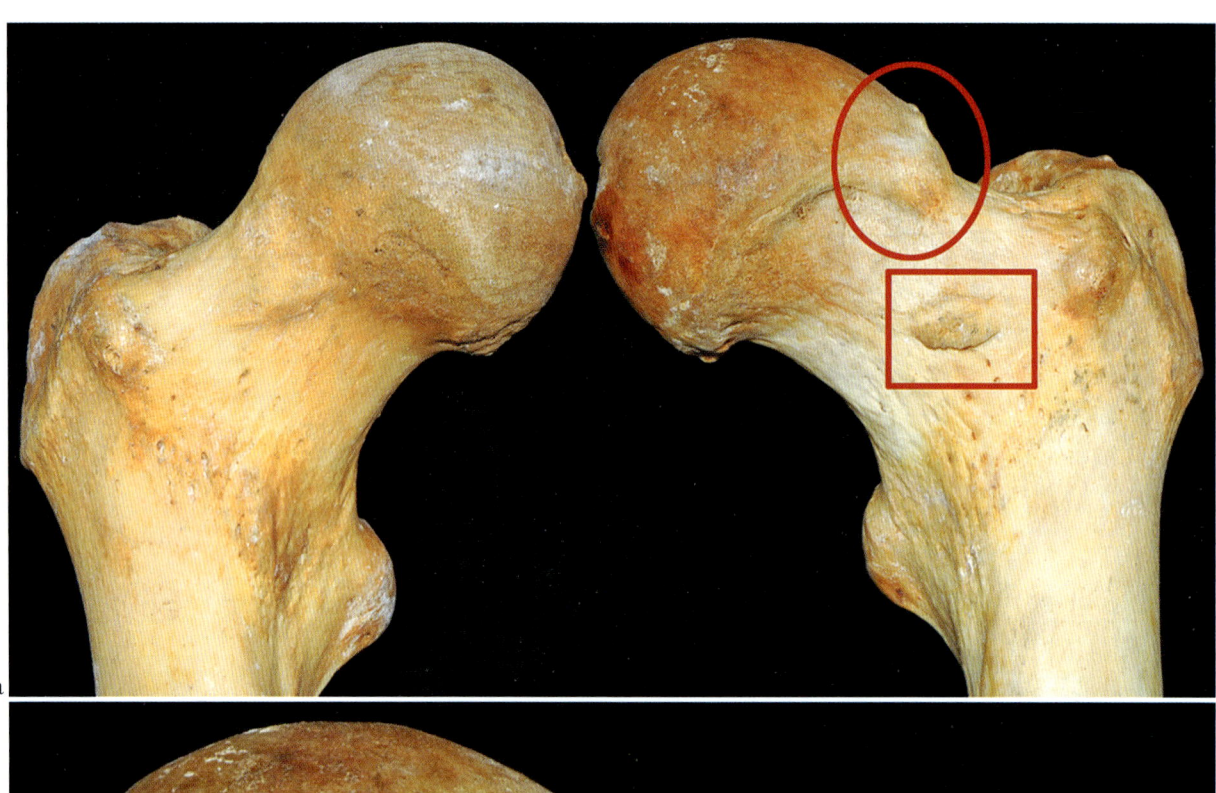

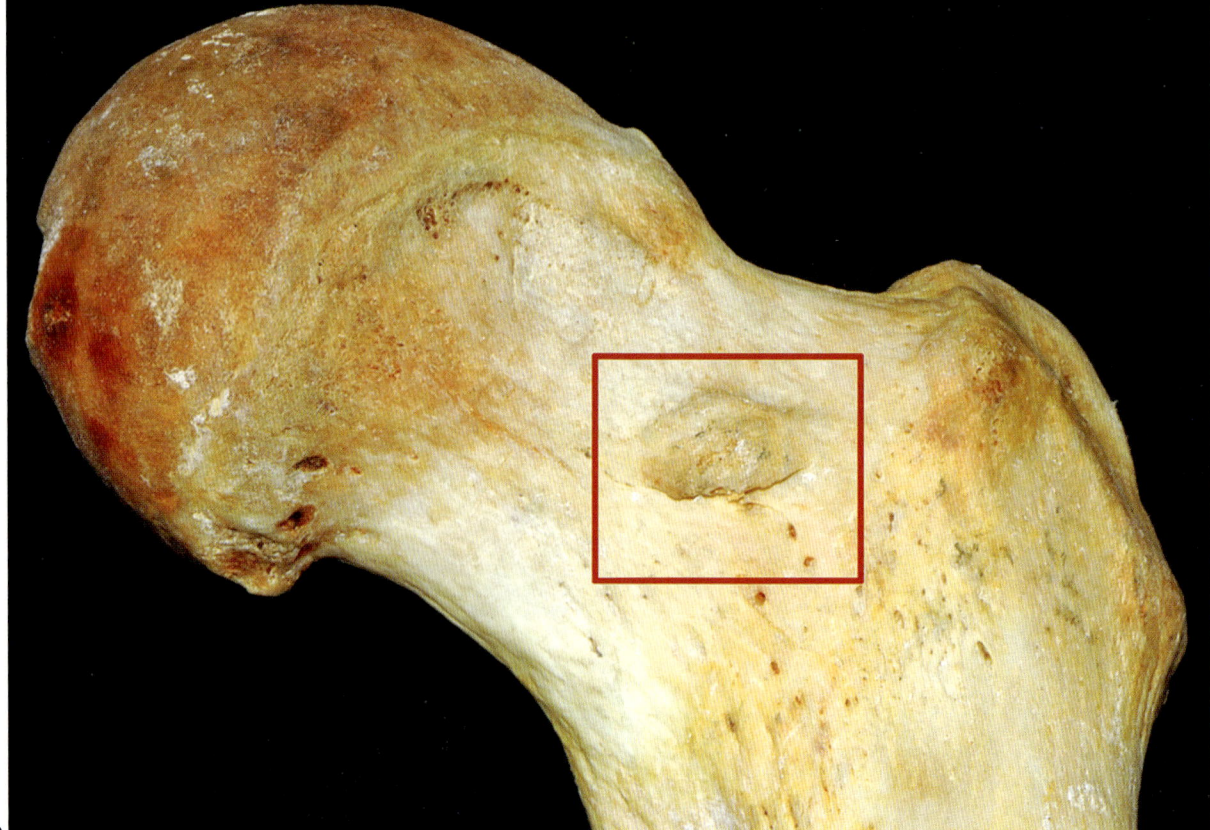

Figure 800a-b. Anterior femoral tubercle and Poirier's facet. (a) Poirier's facets (circle and oval) and unilateral femoral tubercle (square) on the left femur in an adult male (SI). Note that the Poirier's facet on the left femur is more prominent than the right. (b) Higher magnification of the anterior tubercle (rectangle) in the left femur. The tubercle is an uncommon to rare finding.

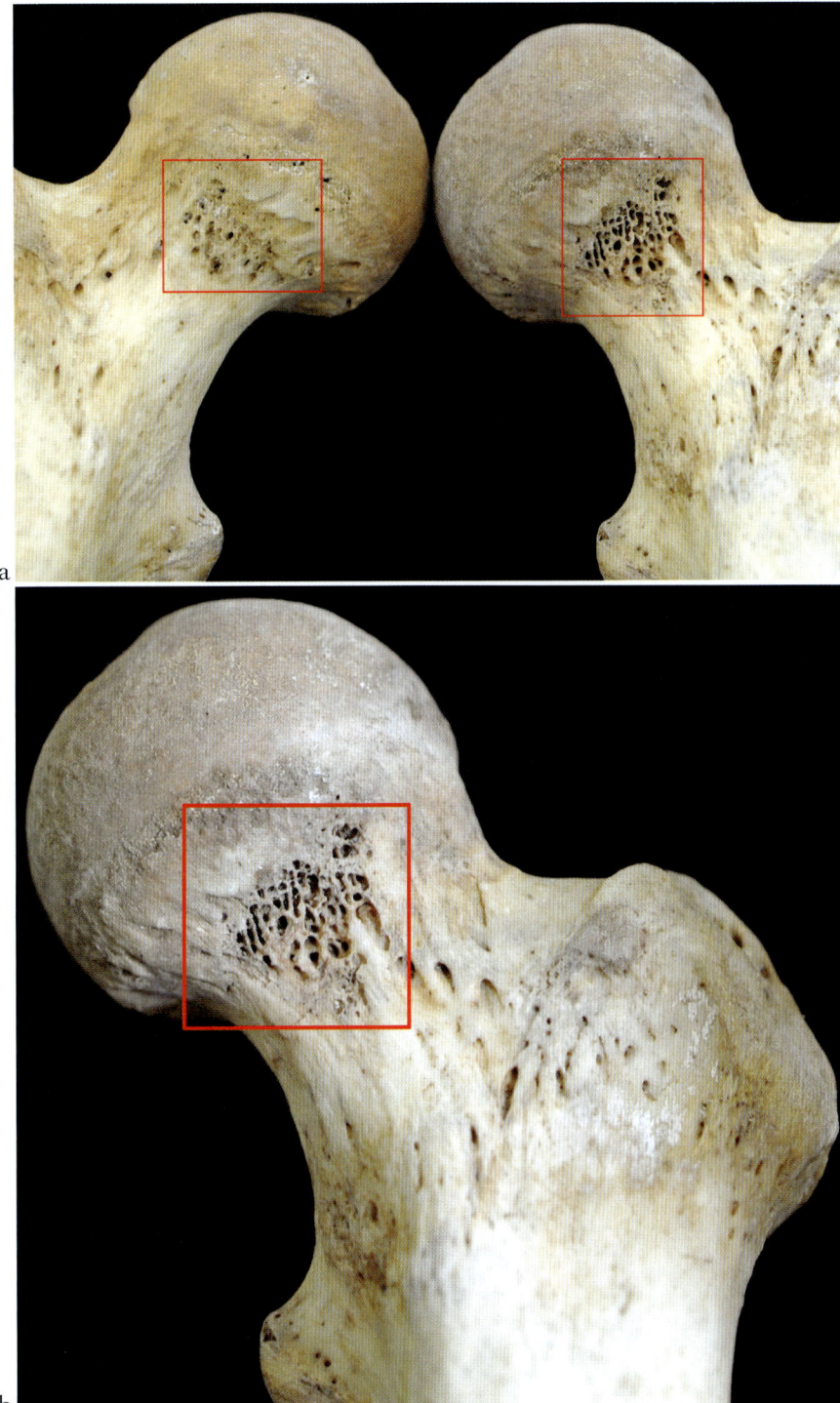

Figure 801a-b. Bilateral occurrence of fossa of Allen. (a) Fossa of Allen (square and rectangle), also known as "cervical fossa" of Allen, Allen's fossa, and cribra femoris. In an adult (KKU). (b) Note the porous and cribiform (sieve-like) appearance of the defect (square), revealing underlying trabeculae as well as the absence of a rimmed border. These features differentiate fossa of Allen from Poirier's or Kostick's facet. The cause of fossa of Allen has been attributed to biomechanical stresses and activities, soft-tissue insertions or vascular deficiencies. Horackova et al. (2005) found this fossa in 18% of adults. A review of the literature reveals considerable confusion in these defects. Common finding. Cf. Allen (1882); Kostick (1963); Odgers (1931); Pitt et al. (1982).

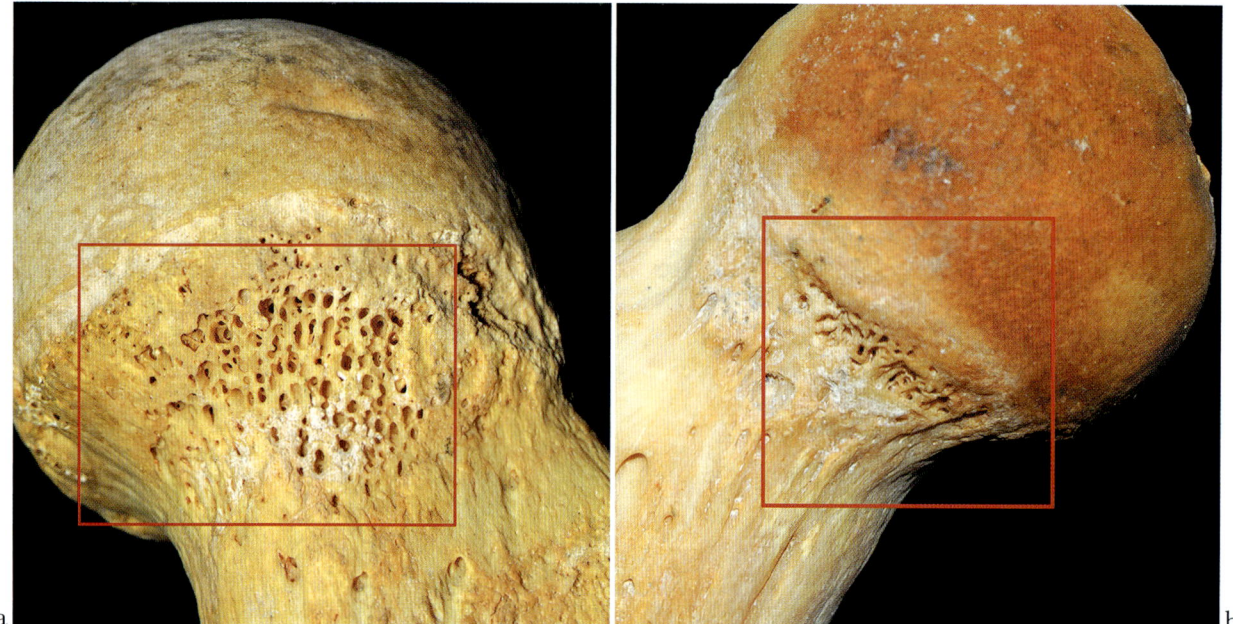

Figure 802a-b. Variants of the fossa of Allen. (a) Large fossa of Allen (rectangle) in a left femur (SI) and (b) a linear fossa of Allen (square) inferior to the right femoral head (SI Huntington), sometimes called "teenage imprint" (Kostick 1963). Common finding. Cf. Kostick (1963) and Odgers (1931) for examples.

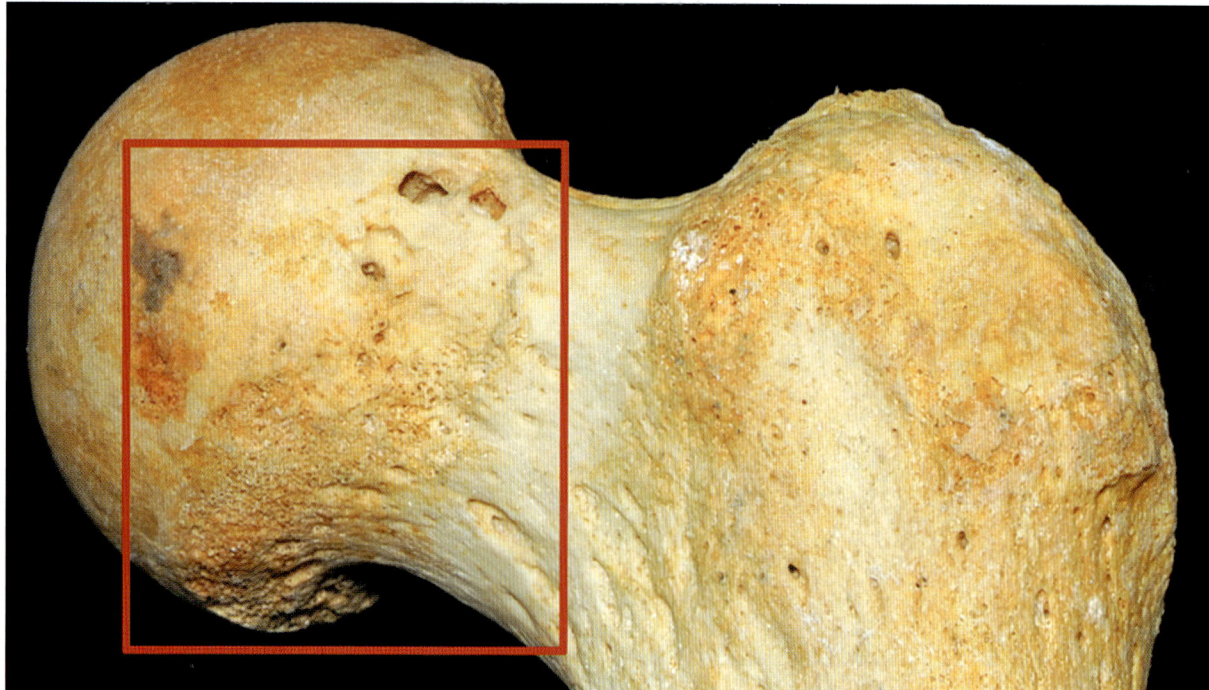

Figure 803. Fossa of Allen (square) revealing the underlying trabeculae and eroded, scalloped margin (SI, Huntington). Common finding. The fossa of Allen and Poirier's facet are not mutually exclusive and can occur simultaneously. Cf. Odgers (1931); Radi et al. (2013) for variation in a population.

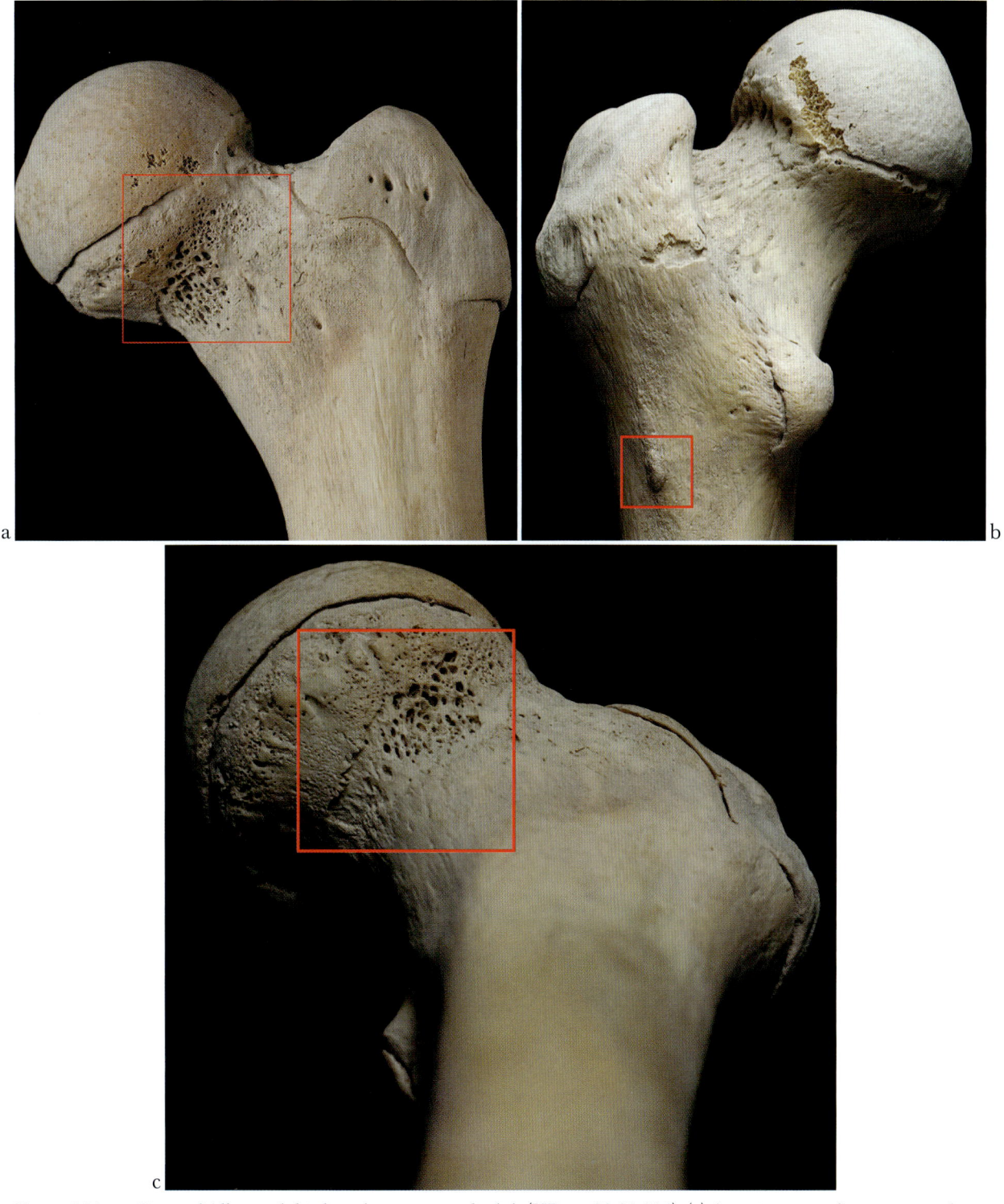

Figure 804a-c. Fossa of Allen and third trochanter in a subadult (UPenn 33-23-226). (a) Anterior view of a prominent fossa of Allen (square) and incomplete fusion of the femoral head and greater trochanter. (b) A small third trochanter (square) with visible lines of fusion of the femoral head, and greater and lesser trochanters. (c) Note position of fossa of Allen in relation to femoral head. Cf. Kostick (1963); Odgers (1931).

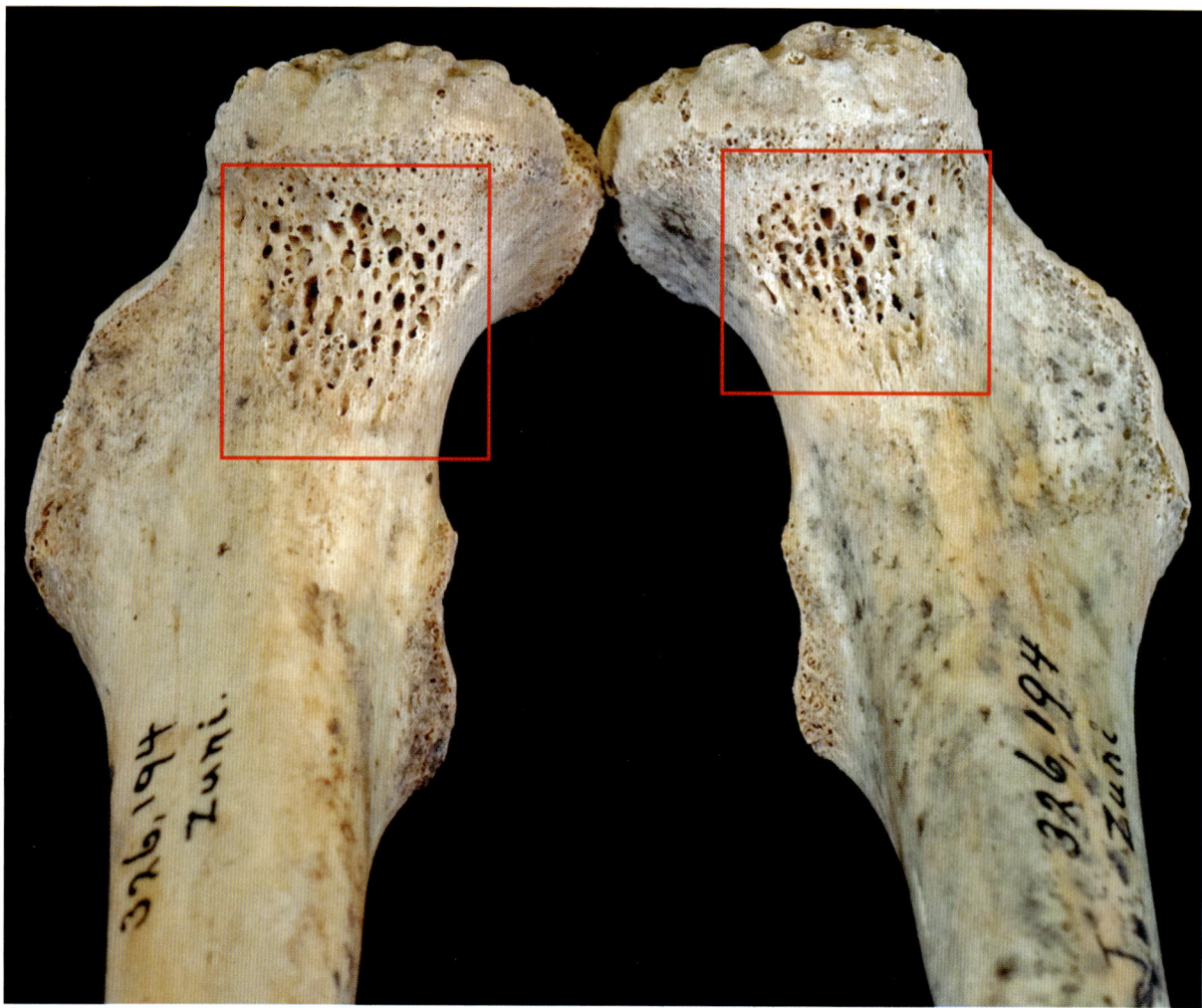

Figure 805. Unusually large fossa of Allen in a 5- to 6-year-old child from Zuni, New Mexico (SI 326194). These cribriform defects typically are present more frequently in subadults ("teenage imprint") compared with adults suggesting an etiology involving remodeling activity. Common finding. Cf. Kostick (1963); Odgers (1931).

Leg and Foot (Femur, Tibia, Fibula, Patella, Tarsal, Metatarsal, Phalanx) 615

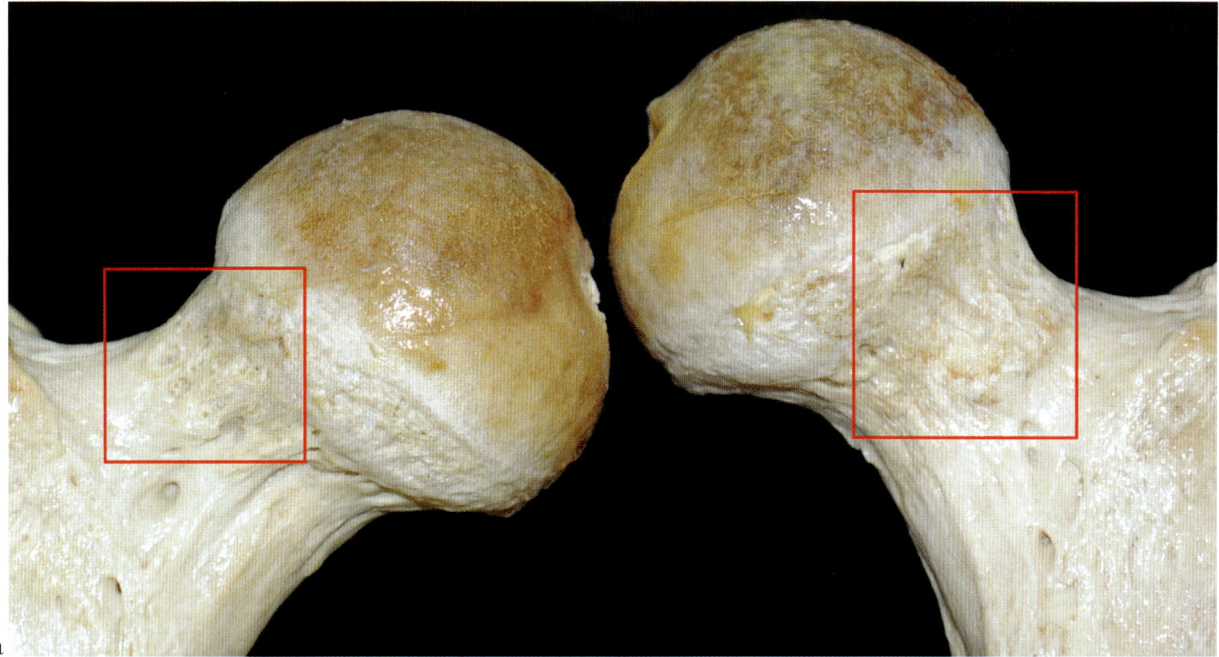

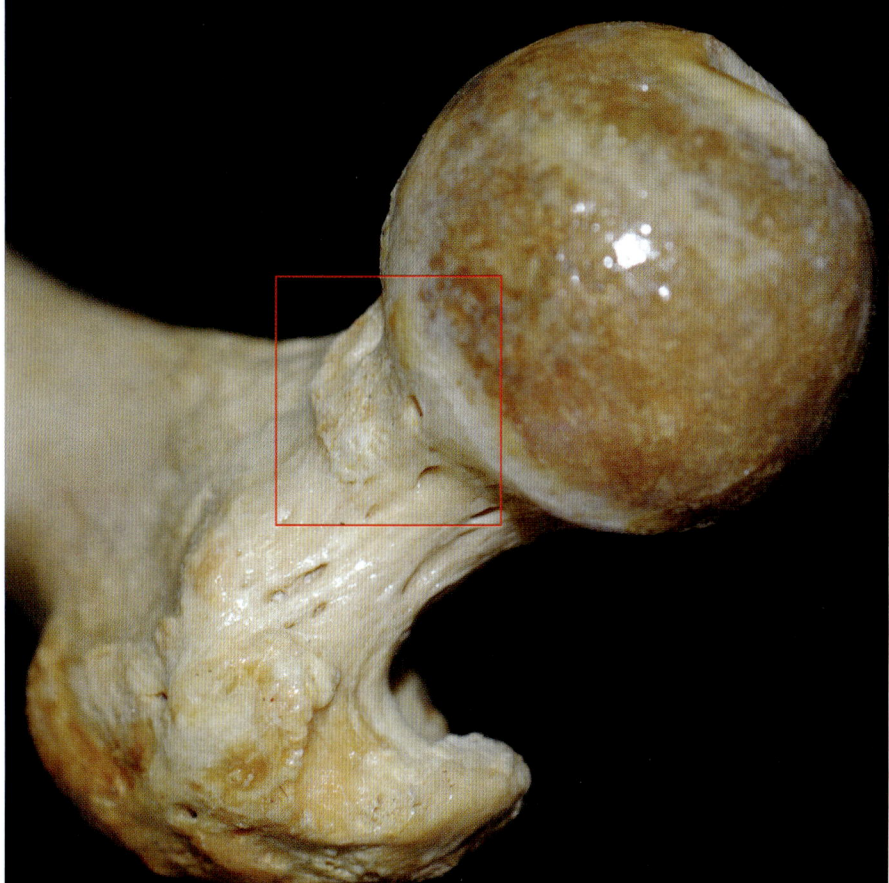

Figure 806a-b. Bilateral Poirier's facet in an adult Thai (KKU). (a) Raised margins delineating the feature squares) in both left and right femurs. (b) Higher magnification showing the size and shape of the Poirier's facet (square) in the left femur. Common findings. Cf. Kostick (1963); Odgers (1931).

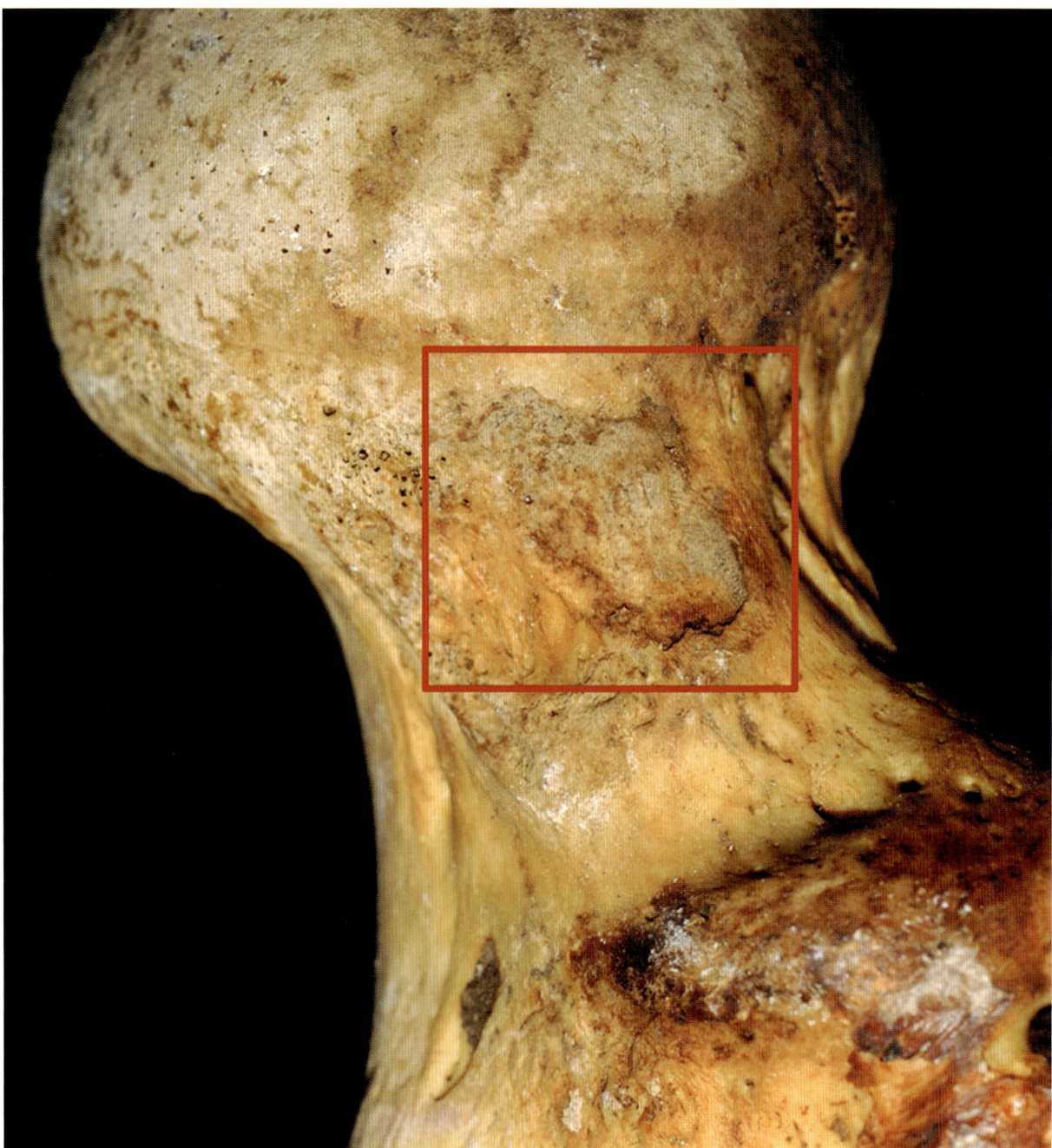

Figure 807. Walmsley's facet (square) along the posterior neck of the right femur in an adult (SI). Note the raised "plaque-like" bone with a rim that typically appears as an extension of the articular margin. Common to uncommon finding. See Odgers (1931) for a description and discussion of the "capsular ridge" of Walmsley, Cervical Fossa, the Eminentia, and "Empreinter Iliaque."

Leg and Foot (Femur, Tibia, Fibula, Patella, Tarsal, Metatarsal, Phalanx) 617

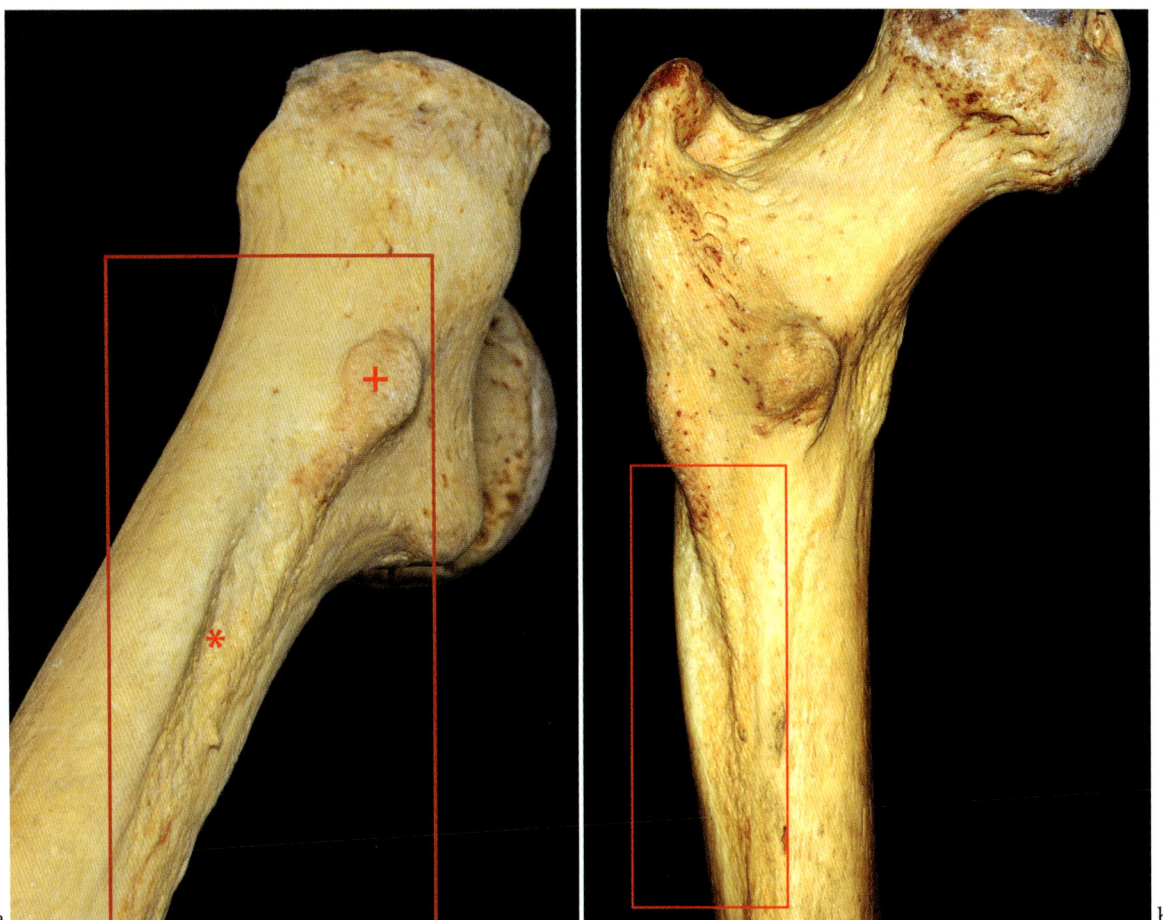

Figure 808a-b. Hypotrochanteric fossa and third trochanter in the left femur of an adult (SI, Huntington). (a) Inferior view illustrating a prominent fossa (* and rectangle) and third trochanter (+) positioned lateral to the gluteal ridge. (b) Posterior view of the fossa (rectangle) that may fill with bony projections in an adult that is related to platymeria, may be present in fetuses and begins as a flat, roughened area that later deepens. Cf. Hrdlička (1934) for extensive coverage of the fossa.

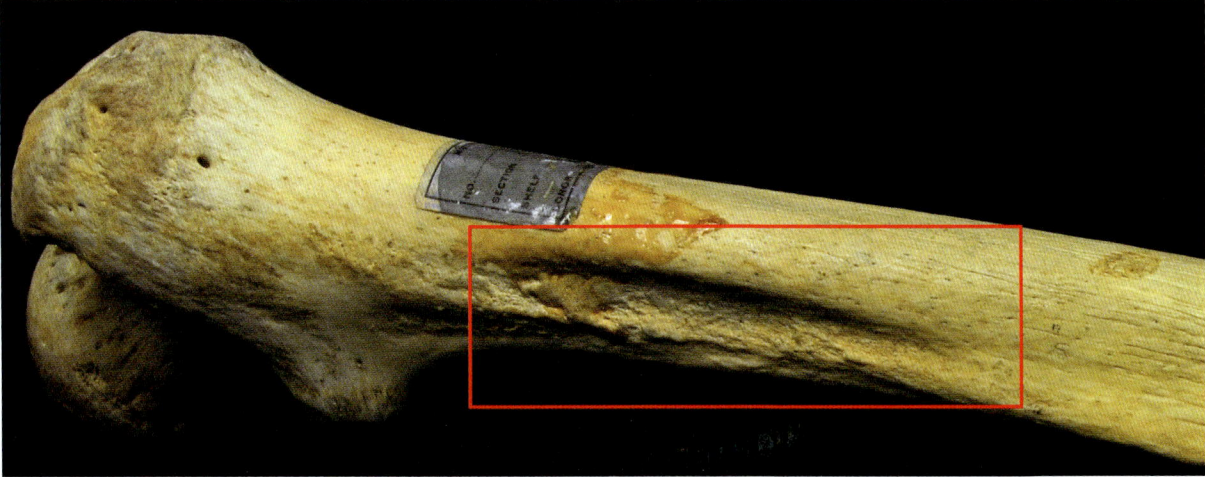

Figure 809. Hypotrochanteric fossa (rectangle) in the right femur of an adult (Mütter Museum, 1046 66). The frequency of this relatively common fossa varies by age and ancestral group.

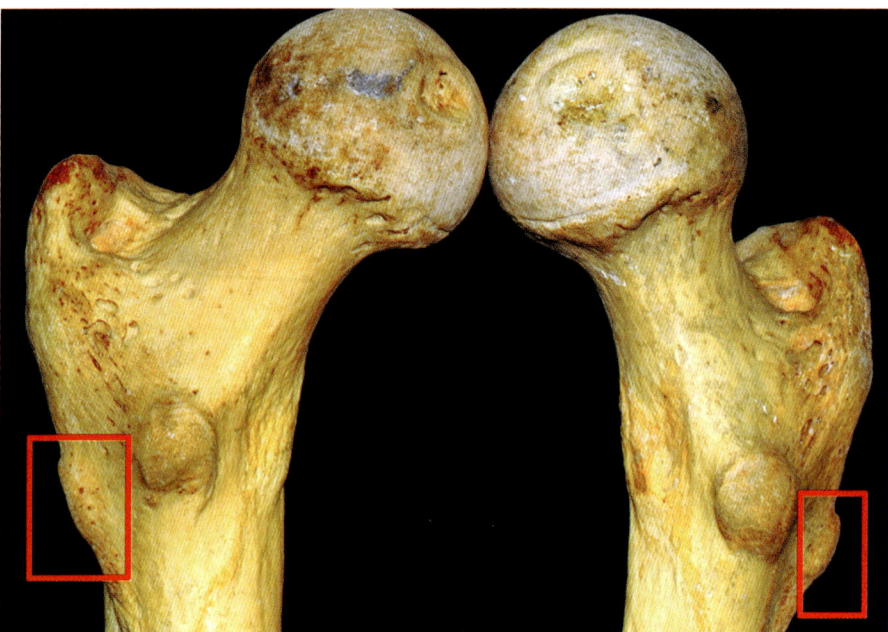

Figure 810. Bilateral third trochanters (rectangles) in an adult (SI Huntington). Cf. Bolanowski et al. (2005); Lozanoff et al. (1985).

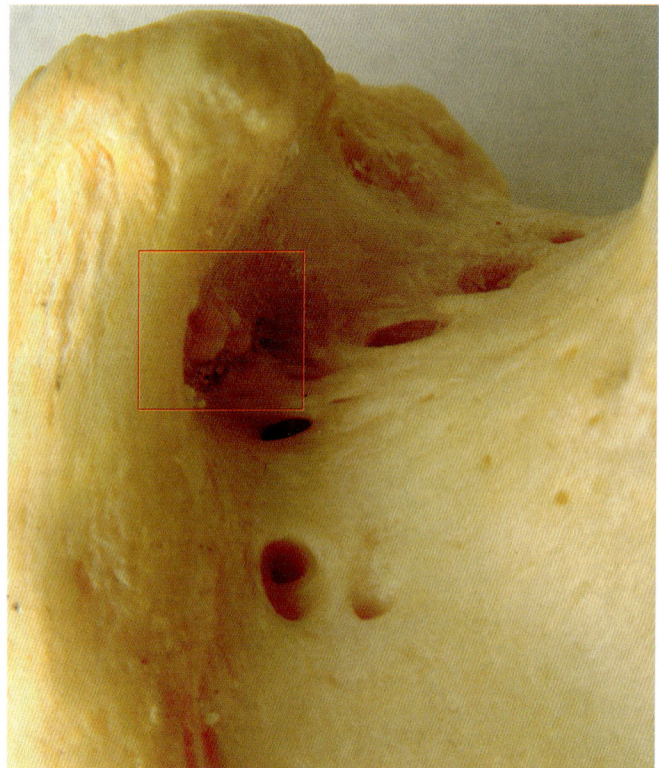

Figure 811. Trochanteric fossa spicules (square) that appear as single or multiple bony spikes (KKU) (see Mann and Hunt 2012). These spikes, likely reflecting enthesophytes, may prove useful as an indicator of middle-age and warrant further research (Pearlstein et al. 2007). Common finding in middle-aged and older adults.

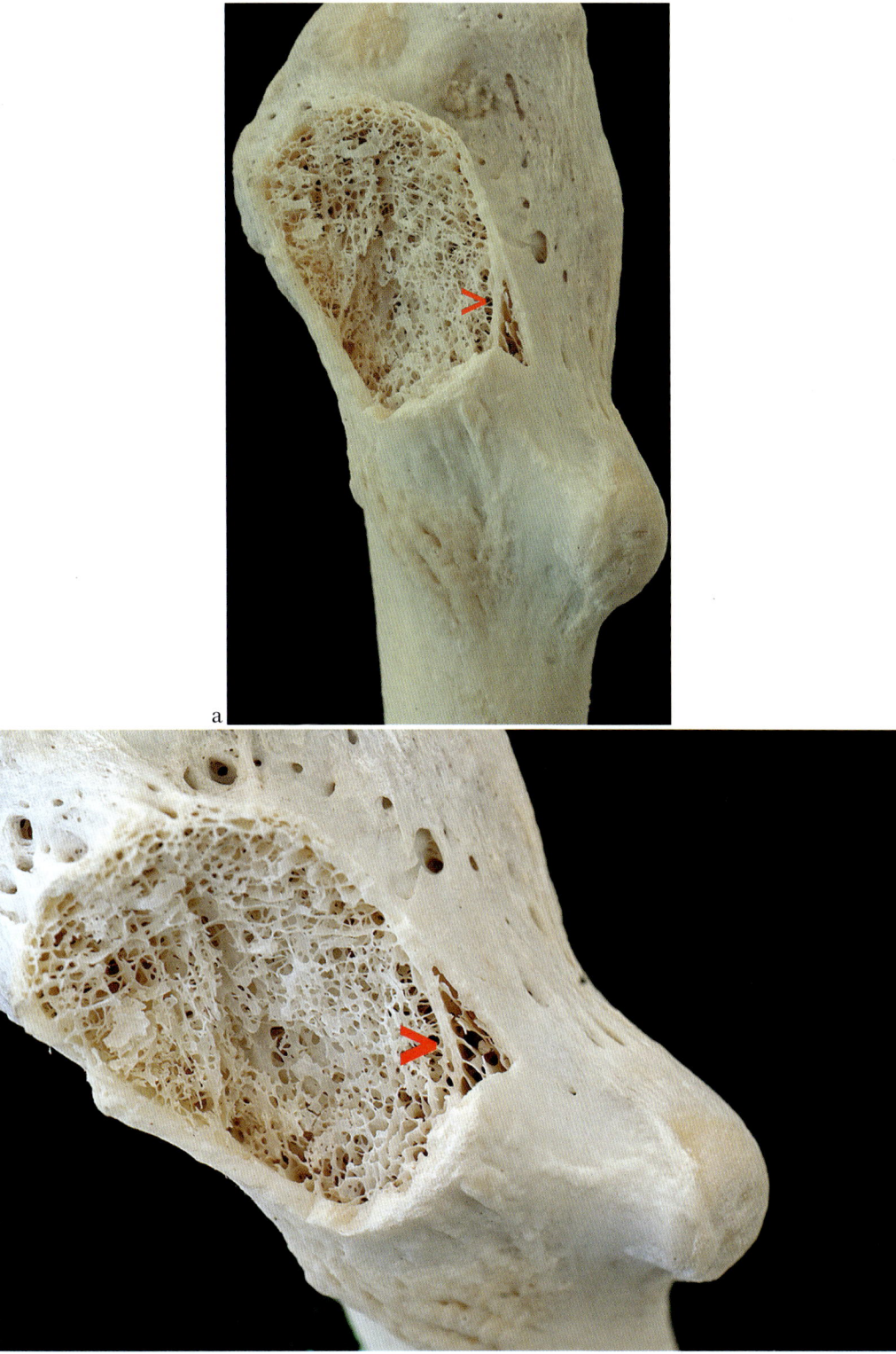

Figure 812a-b. Calcar femorale in a left femur. (a) Calcar femorale (>), a normally occurring bony plate or osseous wall extending into the cancellous bone near the lesser trochanter in the femoral neck. (b) Higher magnification of the calcar femorale (>). This vertical plate of bone is a radiographic landmark and serves to distribute stresses from the neck to the femoral diaphysis. Cf. Newell (1997).

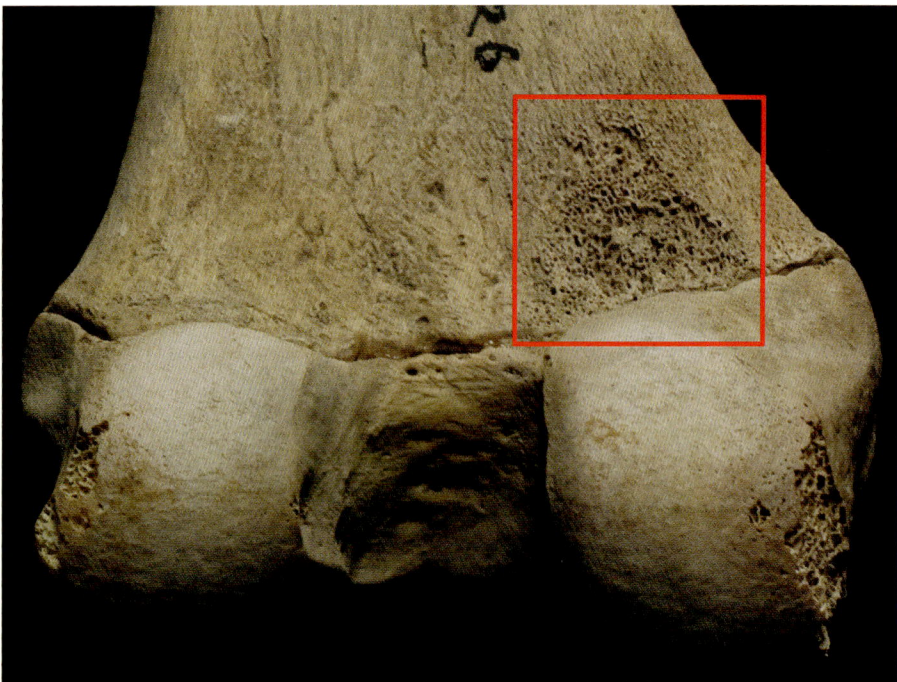

Figure 813. Shallow, distal femoral cortical excavation or Charles' facet in the femur of a subadult (UPenn 33-23-226). Note the location of the defect (square) adjacent to the metaphysis and its irregular and porous appearance. This lesion is commonly seen in children, attributed to stress at the insertion of the medial head of the gastrocnemius muscle, and usually remodels and disappears. Cf. Resnick and Greenway (1982); Hyman et al. (1995).

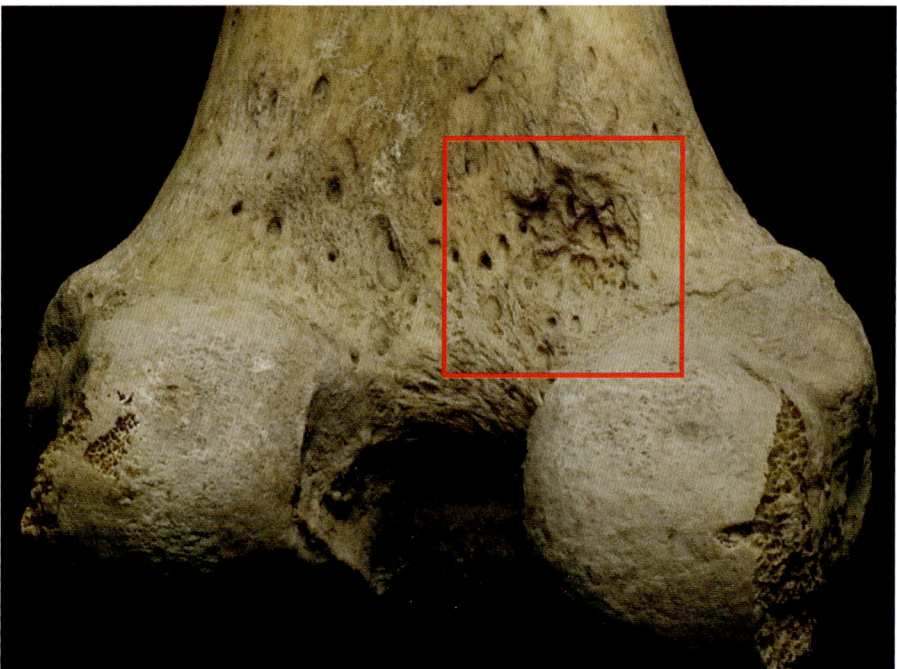

Figure 814. Deep distal femoral cortical defect or Charles' facet in an adult (UPenn 33-23-238C). This defect typically remodels and disappears completely during childhood.

Leg and Foot (Femur, Tibia, Fibula, Patella, Tarsal, Metatarsal, Phalanx) 621

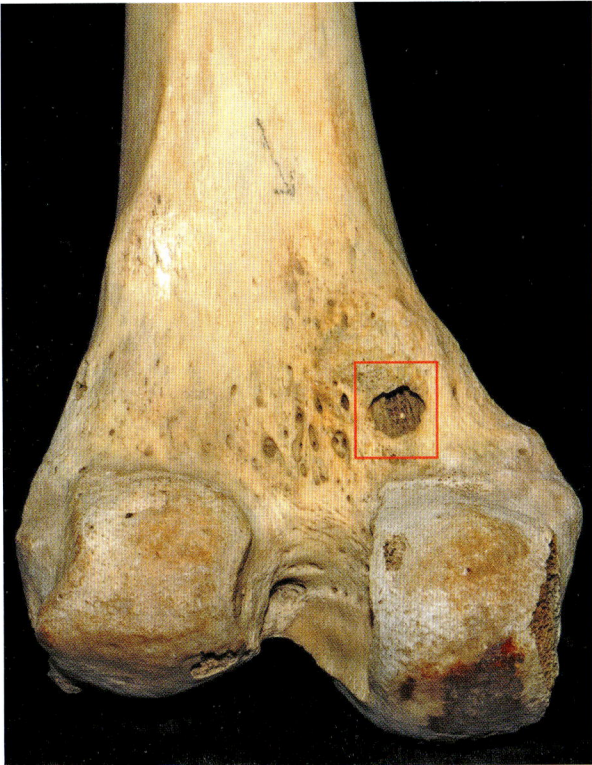

Figure 815. Small but well-defined and deep distal femoral cortical excavation (squarc), also known as Charles' facet, in the left femur of an elderly adult (SI).

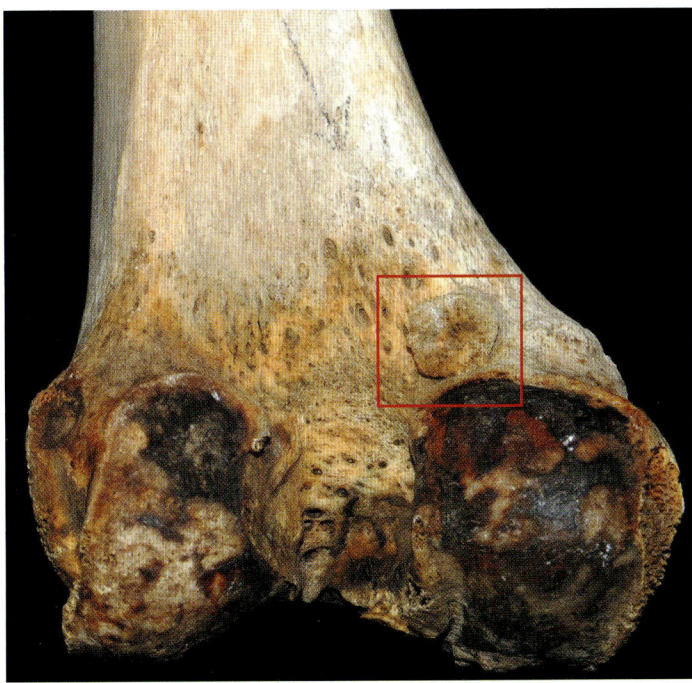

Figure 816. Raised variant of the distal femoral cortical excavation (Charles' facet) in the left femur of an elderly adult (SI). Note very severe alteration of the femoral condyles reflecting osteoarthritis.

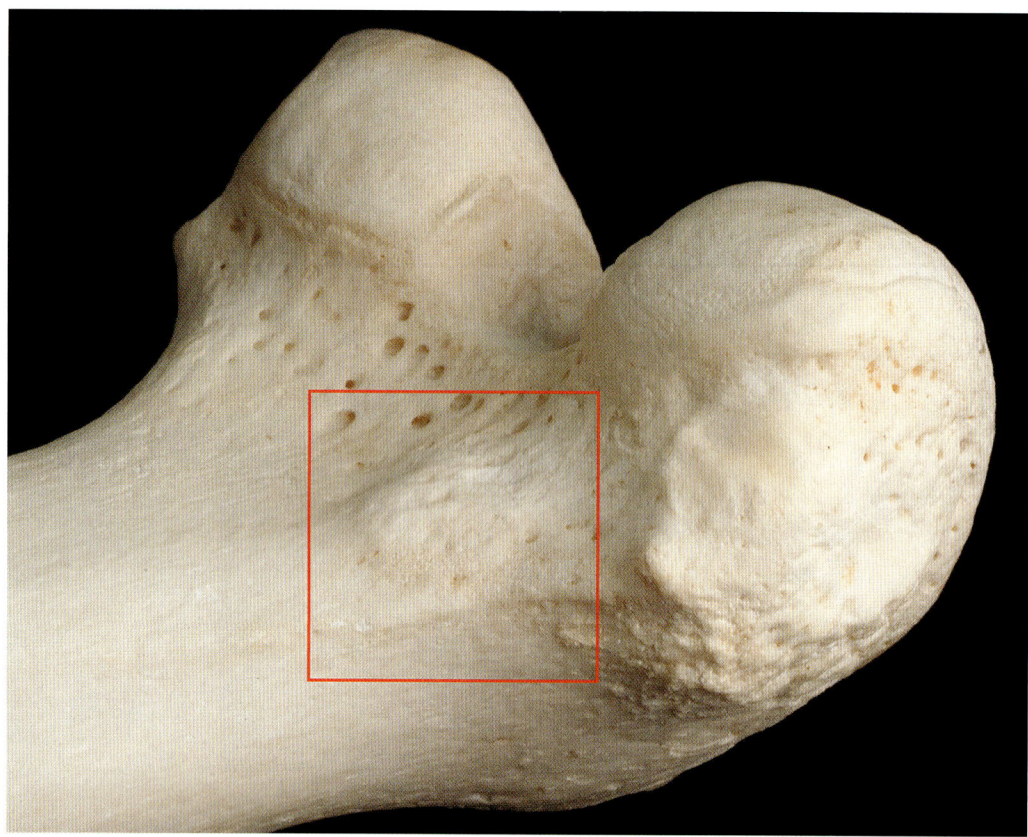

Figure 817. Raised variant (square) of the distal femoral cortical excavation or desmoid in the right femur of an elderly male (CSC). Common finding.

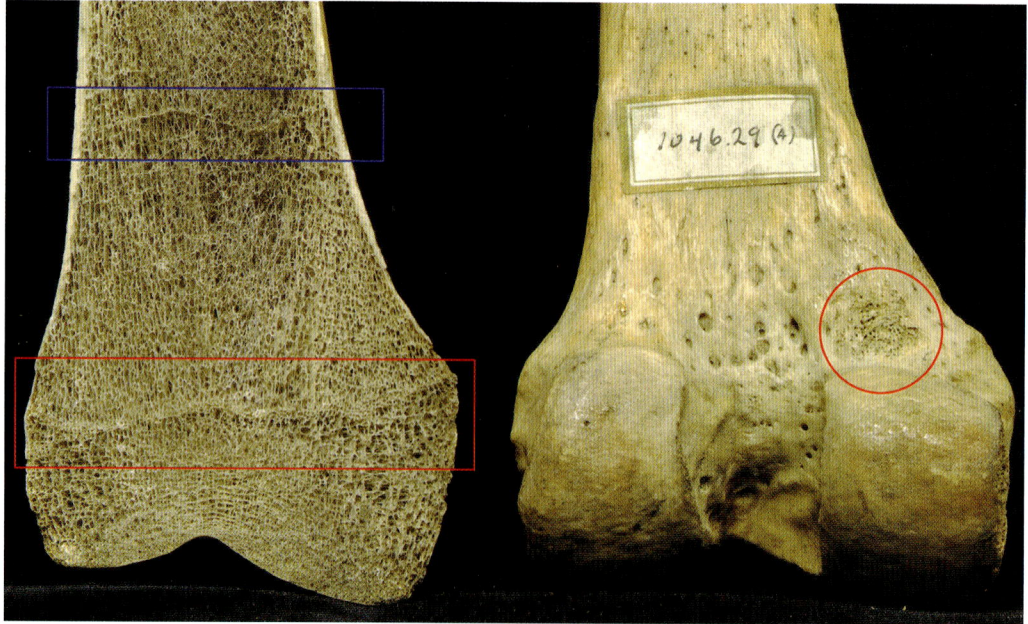

Figure 818. Distal femoral cortical excavation (circle) in the left femur (Mütter Museum, 1046 29(4). Note the growth arrest line (blue rectangle), also known as a Harris line and the normal epiphyseal line (red rectangle) that, on radiograph, would appear as a radiodense line.

Leg and Foot (Femur, Tibia, Fibula, Patella, Tarsal, Metatarsal, Phalanx)

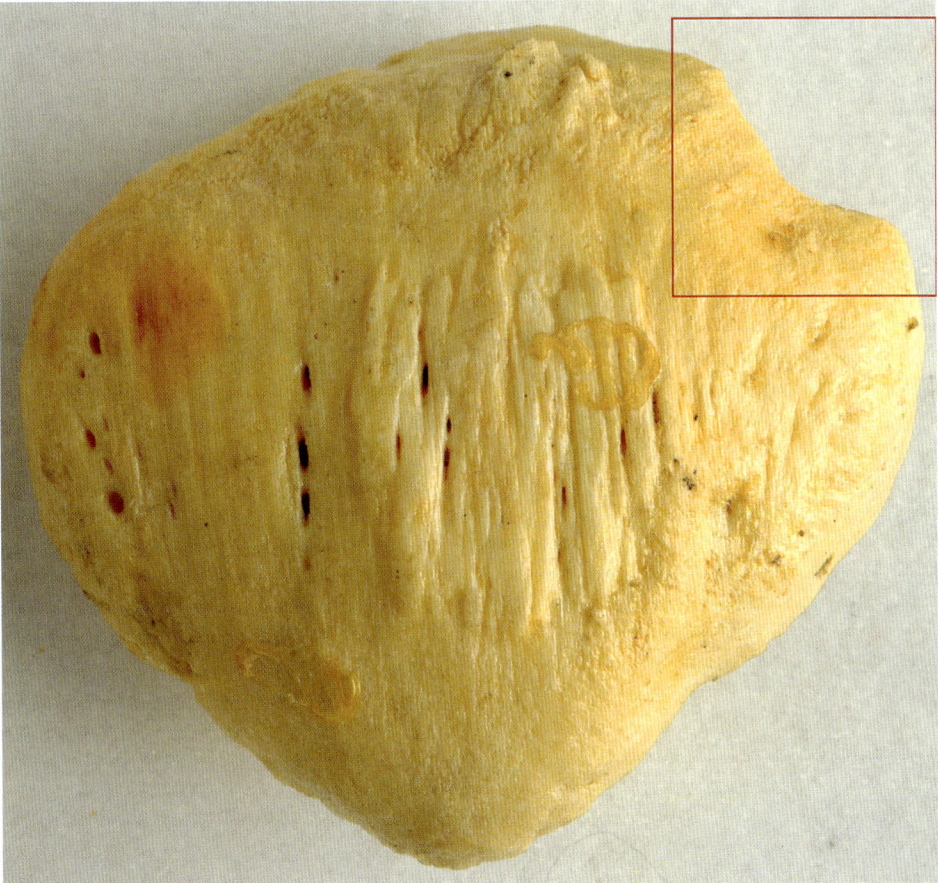

Figure 819. Vastus notch (square) in an adult patella. Note the smooth appearance of this notch distinguishing it from a bipartite patella that forms as a result of a secondary center of ossification. This notch merely reflects shape differences, not a center of ossification. Common finding.

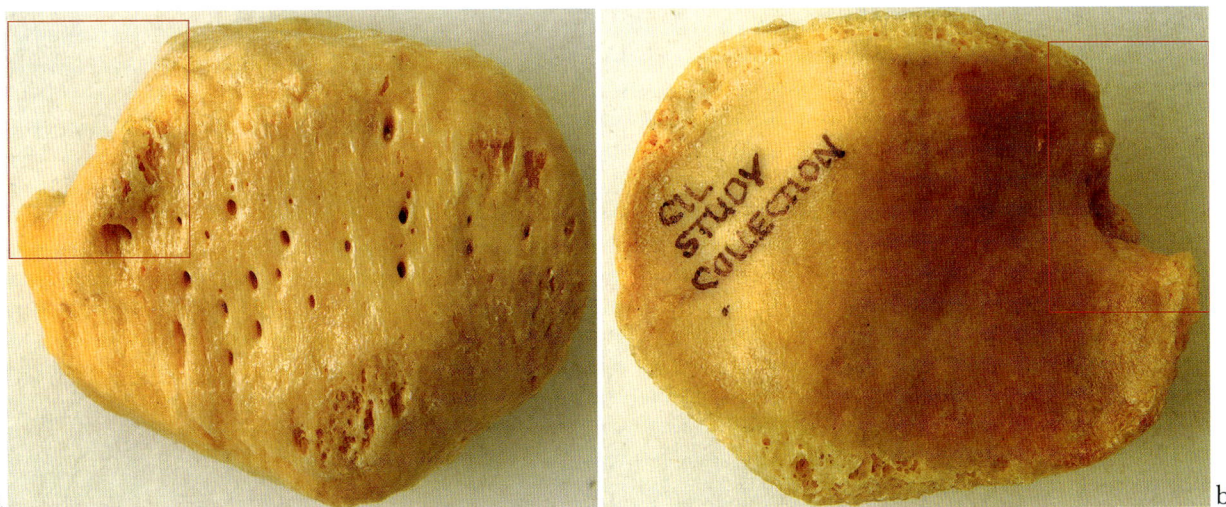

Figure 820a-b. Bipartite patella (CSC). (a) Ventral and (b) dorsal view of a bipartite right patella (rectangle). Note that the notch in this specimen, which would have served for attachment of a separate ossicle, is more irregular than the one in the figure above and that the trabeculae are visible. Common finding. Oetteking (1922) referred to this as emargination and the small ossicle as the patellula. Cf. Kempson (1902); Weckstrom et al. (2008); Wright (1903).

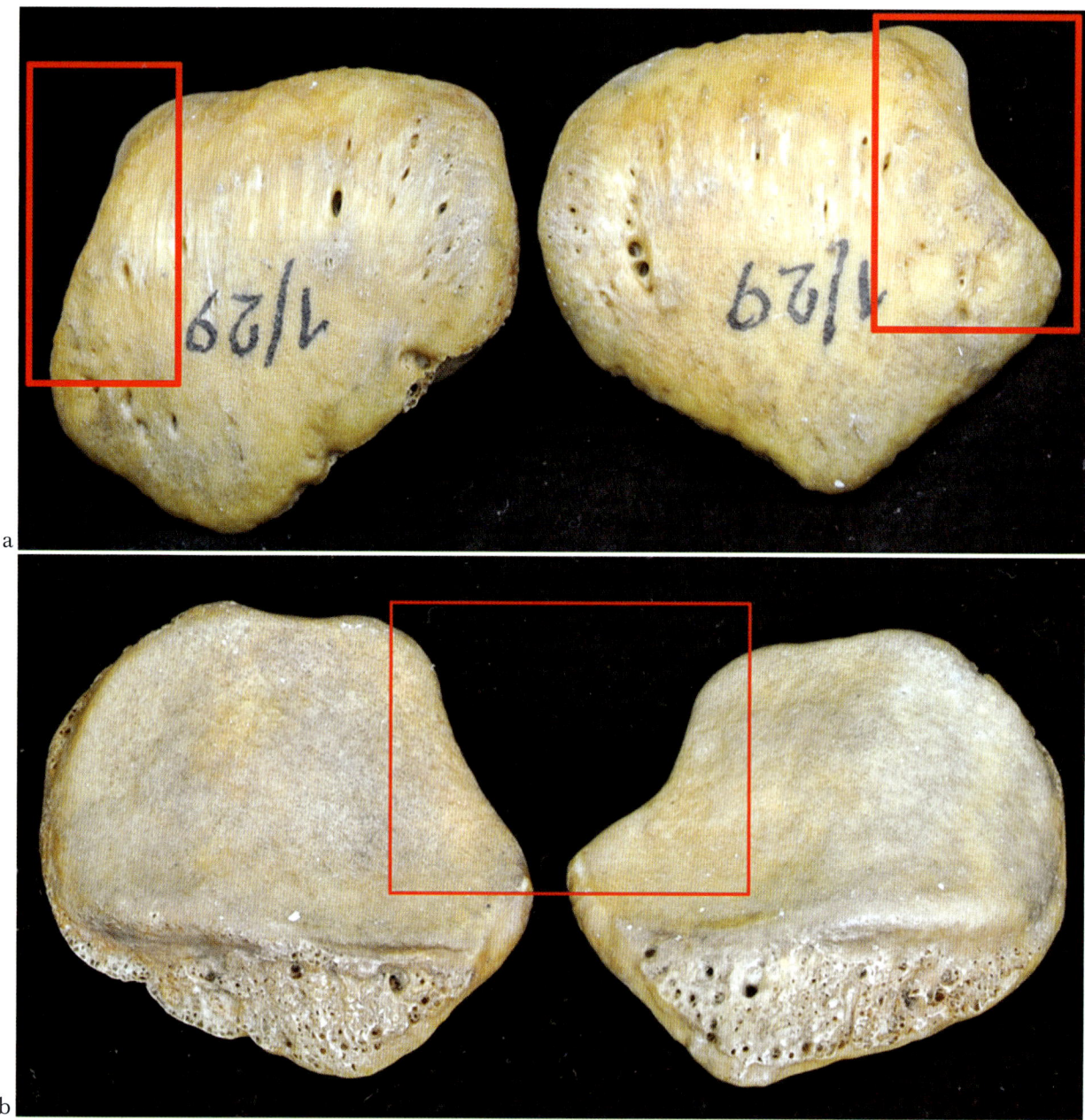

Figure 821a-b. Bilateral vastus notch. (a) Ventral and (b) dorsal views of bilateral vastus notches (rectangles) in an adult (KKU). Note that the surface of the indentations are smooth and compact consistent with the remaining articular surface of the patella. Common finding.

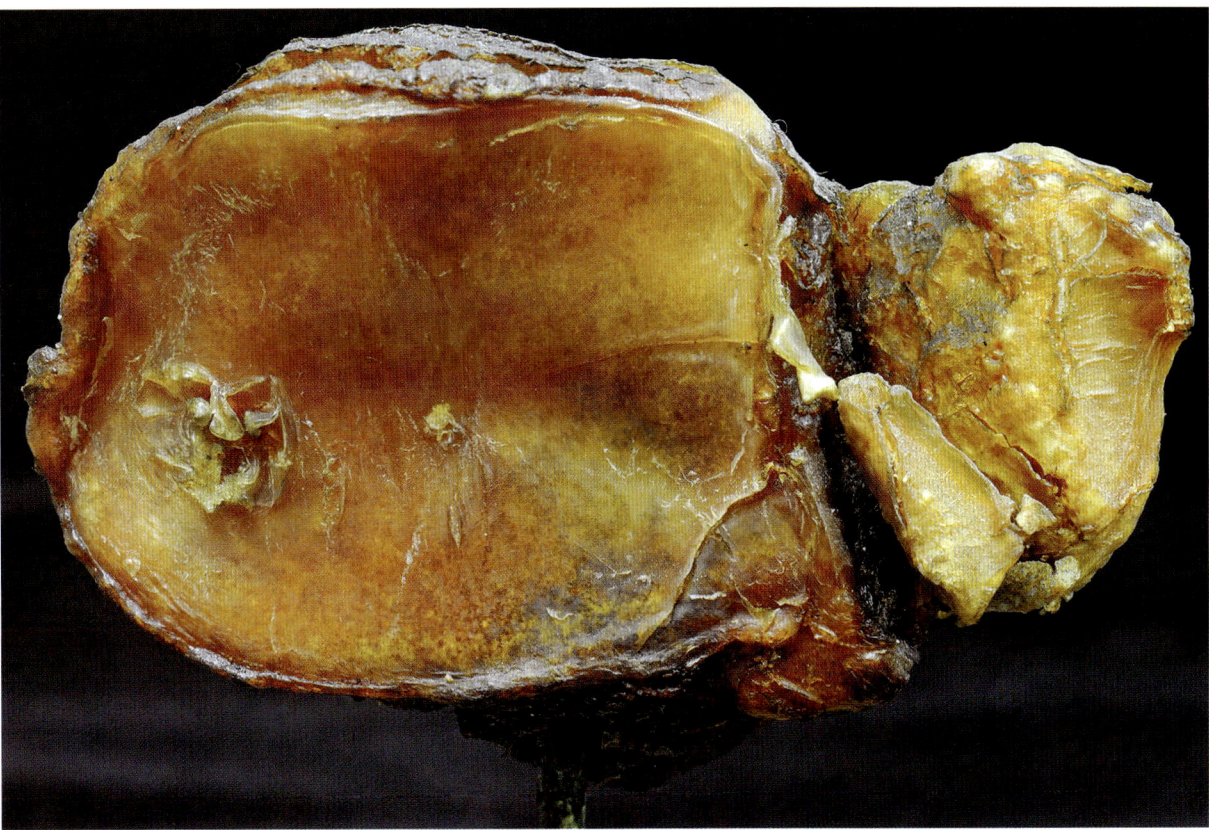

Figure 822. Congenital right bipartite patella, first described by Gruber (1883) and soft tissue holding the "loose bone" fragment (rectangle) to the main body of the patella (Mütter Museum 1412). Common finding with a much higher frequency in males. Cf. Kempson (1902); Oetteking (1922); Weckstrom (2008); Wright (1903).

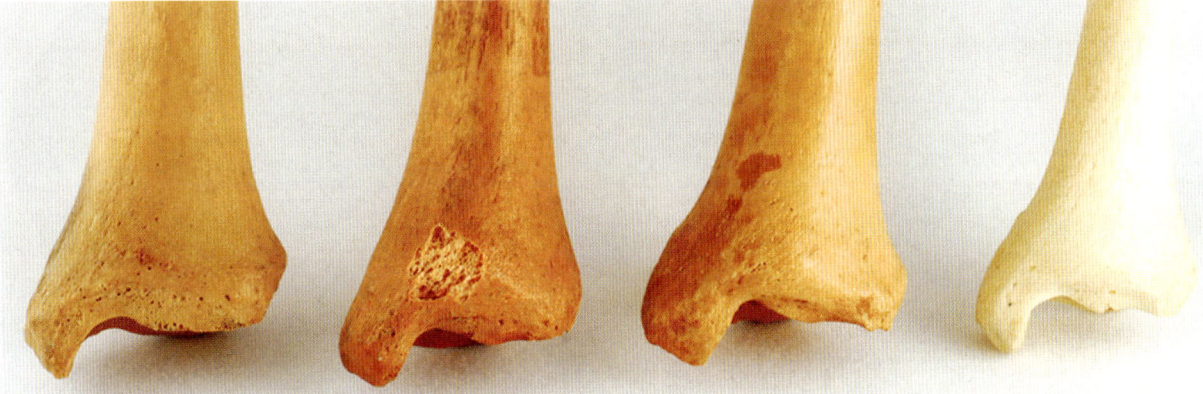

Figure 823. Continuum of lateral squatting facet expression (rectangles) ranging from absent (left) to large (right) viewed from the anterior perspective in left tibiae (KKU). Squatting facets are covered by hyaline cartilage in the living. Cf. Ari et al. (2003); Barnett (1954); Singh (1959).

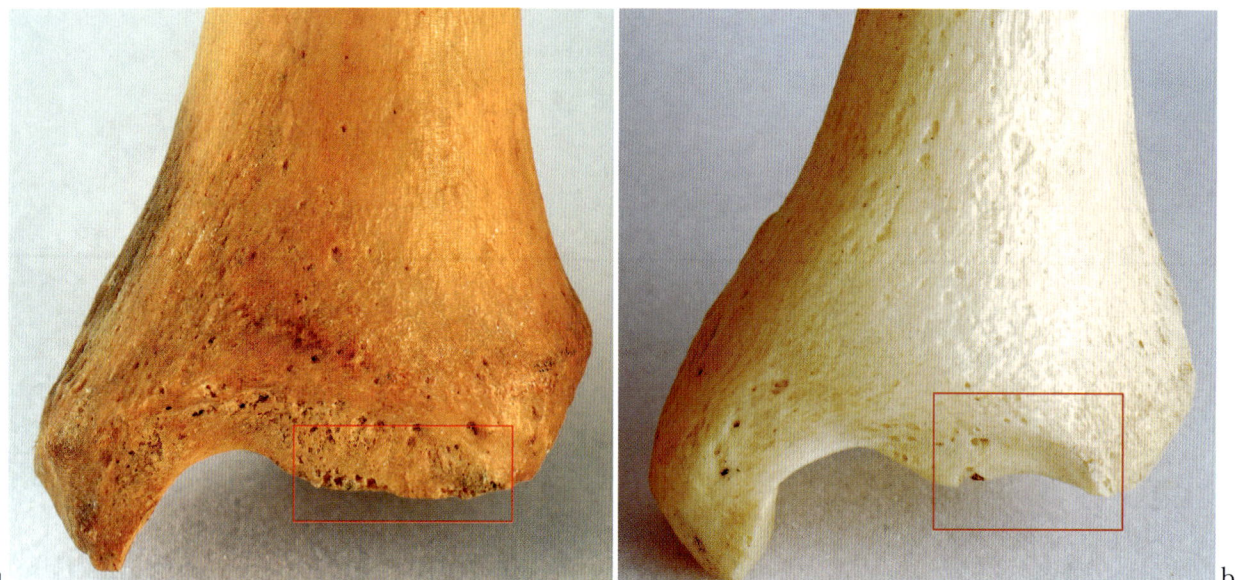

Figure 824a-b. Higher magnification of lateral squatting facets. (a) Left tibia showing absence of a lateral squatting facet (rectangle) compared to (b) distal tibia with a large squatting facet (rectangle) (KKU). Cf. Ari et al. (2003); Barnett (1954); Singh (1959).

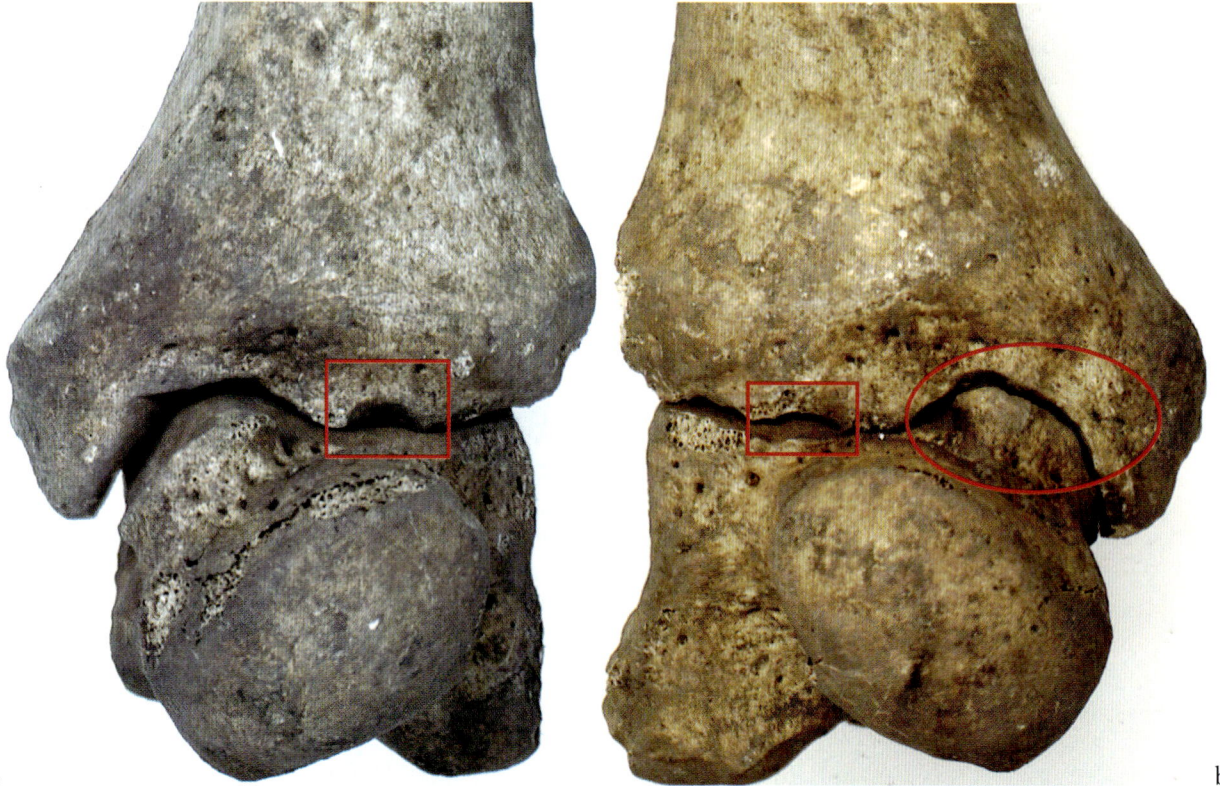

Figure 825a-b. Lateral squatting facets in two individuals. (a) Photographs of a left tibia and talus showing a well-defined lateral squatting facet (rectangle). (b) Right tibia and talus exhibiting a small lateral squatting facet in the distal tibia (rectangle) and a large irregular medial squatting facet (circle) that reflects the contour and morphology of the talar neck (CSC). Cf. Ari et al. (2003).

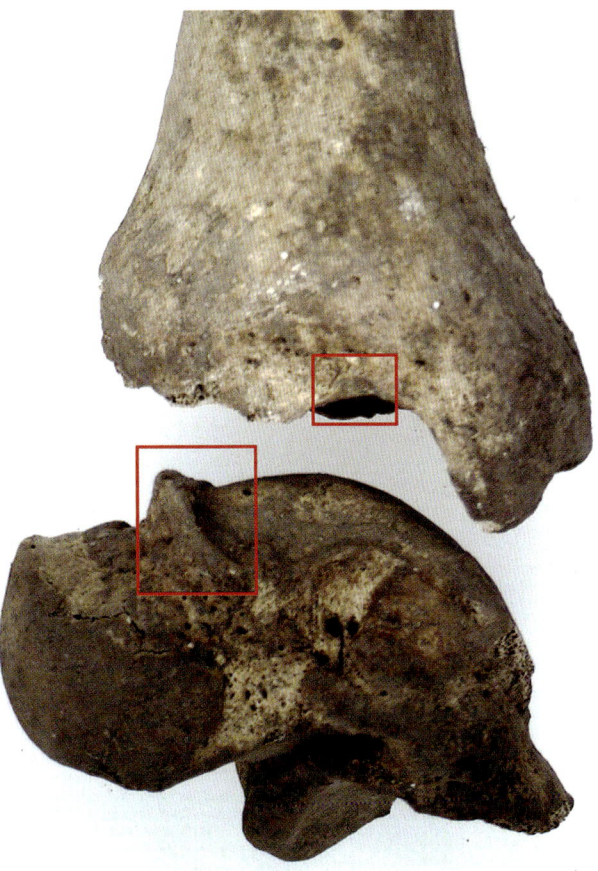

Figure 826. Medial squatting facet (small rectangle) in a right distal tibia that formed due to contact with the raised rim or beak of bone (large rectangle) (CSC). This feature is also known as a "footballer's" ankle.

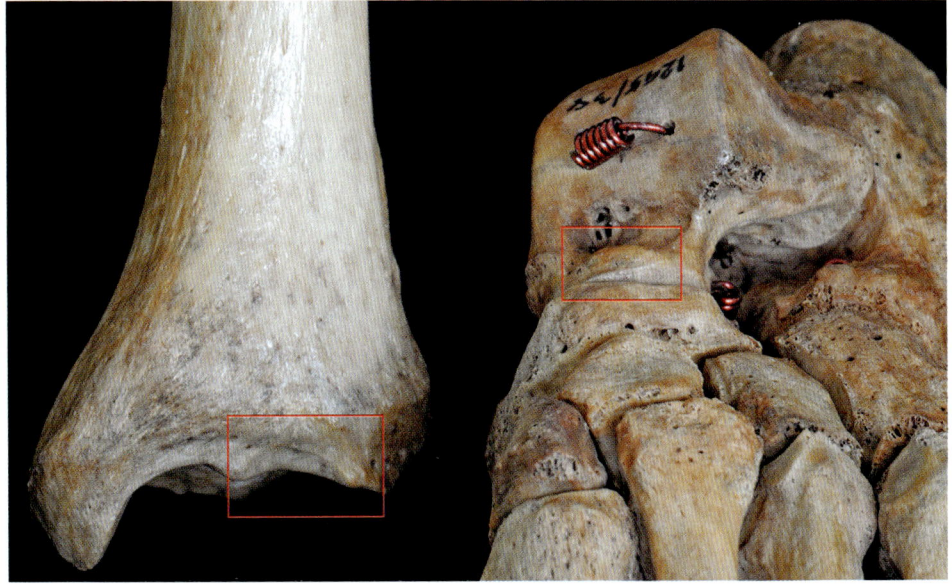

Figure 827. Large medial "facet" in the tibia that is congruent with the morphology of the talar neck (rectangles) (CIL). Cf. Barnett (1954).

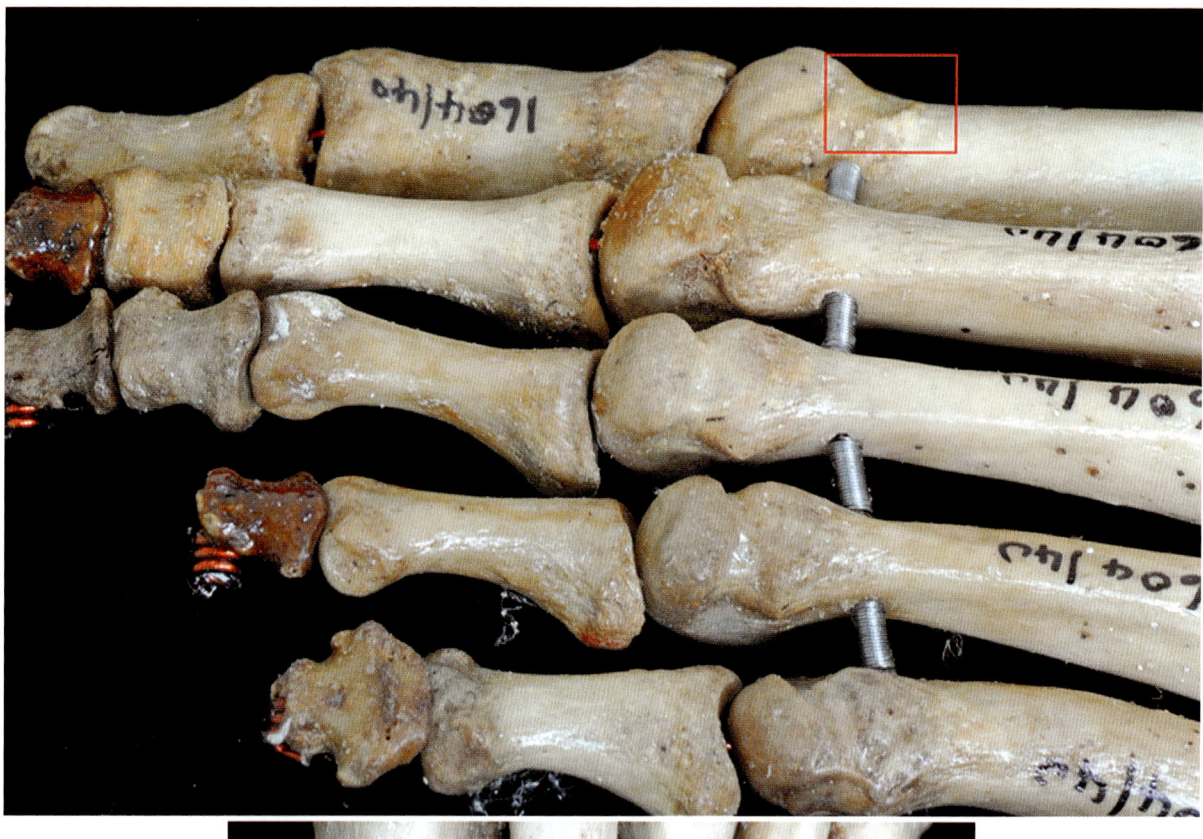
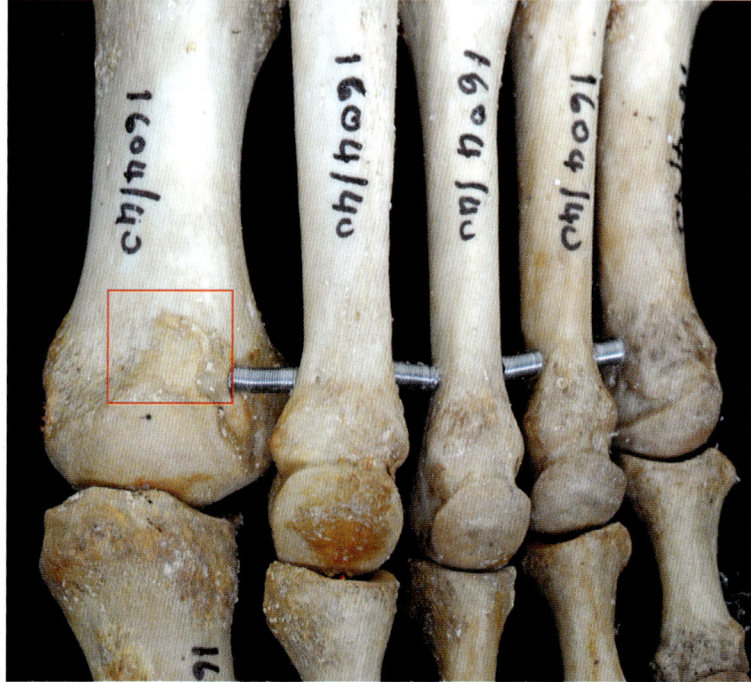

Figure 828a-b. Symphalangism. (a) Symphalangism or congenital fusion of the left distal and medial pedal phalanges and squatting facet (red rectangle) along the dorsal surface of the first metatarsal (KKU). (b) Dorsal squatting facet (square) on the left first metatarsal. Symphalangism is a common finding and this form of squatting facet is uncommon to common depending on the group studied. Fourth toe symphalangism is always accompanied by fifth toe involvement (Case and Heilman 2005) Cf. Borah et al. (2006); Geelhoed et al. (1969); Serrafian (1993).

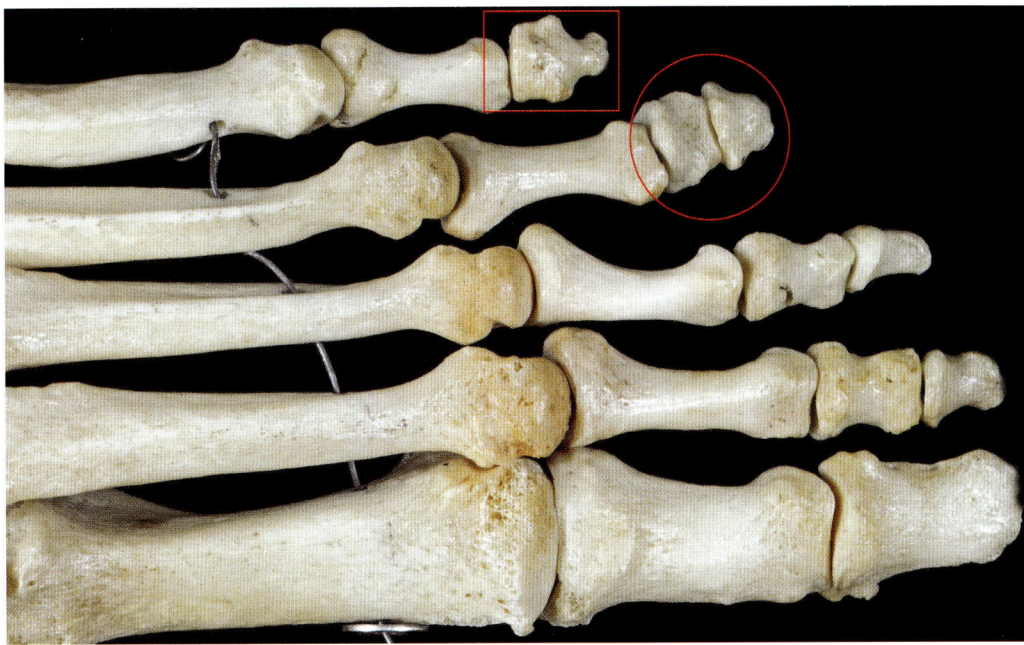

Figure 829. Pedal symphalangism of the left fifth toe (rectangle) and short, but normal medial and distal phalanges in the fourth digit (circle) of in an adult (CSC). Symphalangism is a common heritable anomaly. Common findings. Cf. Borah et al. (2006); Case and Heilman (2005); Geelhoed et al. (1969); Nakashima et al. (1995); Serrafian (1993).

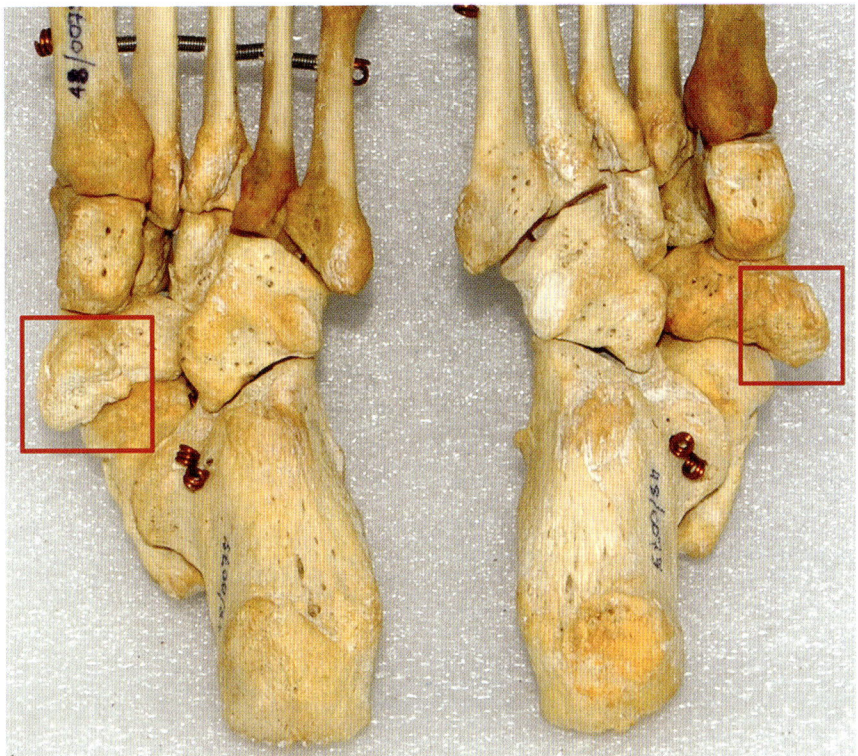

Figure 830. Bilateral os naviculare (squares) in an adult Thai (KKU). Coskun et al. (2009) noted 11.7% of 984 adult Turkish patients with os naviculare. While many consider the os naviculare a typical variant, it may become symptomatic and pathological (Bernaerts et al. 2004). Cf. Serrafian (1993); Silva (2010).

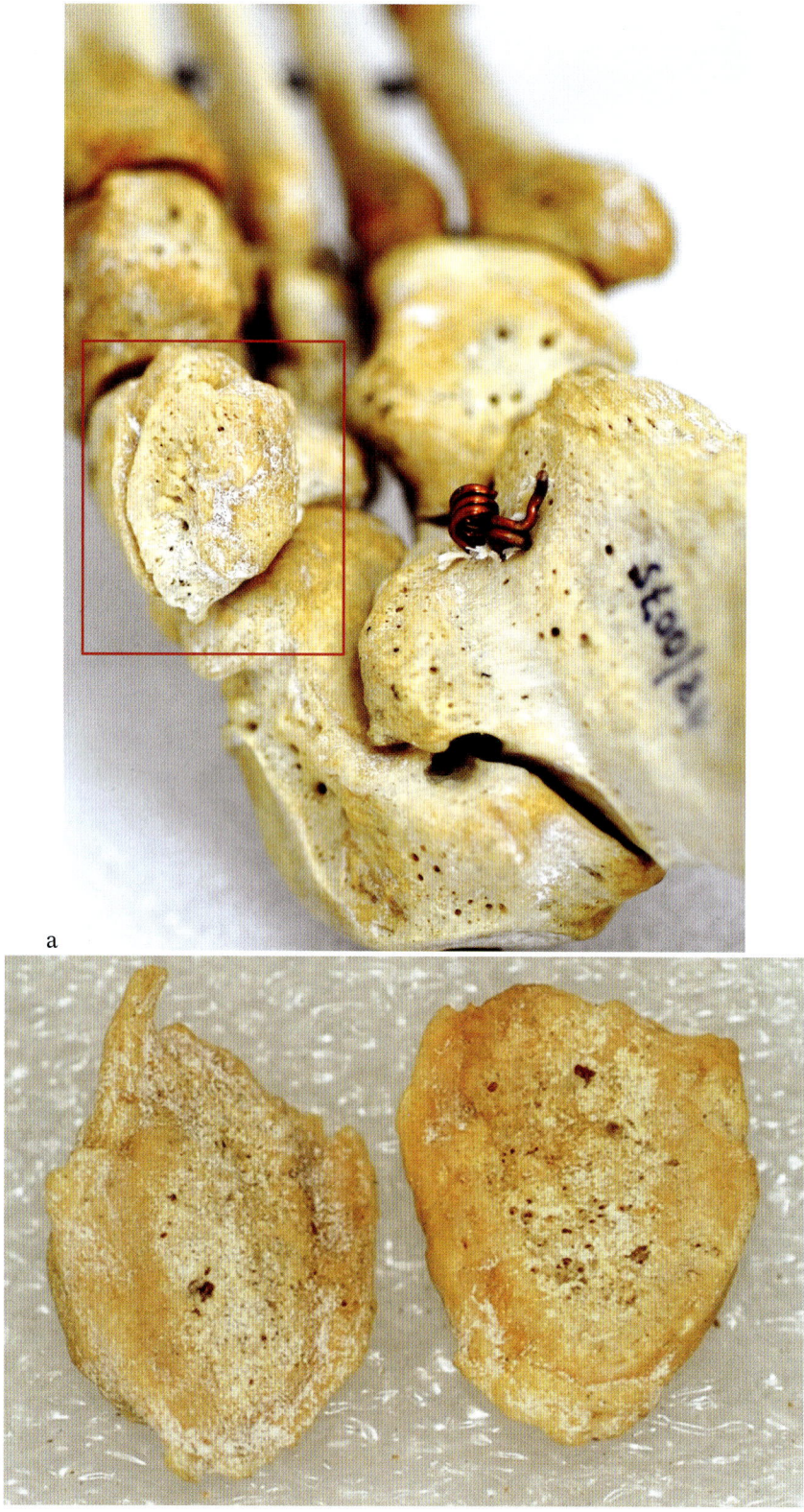

Figure 831a-b. Os naviculare. (a) Os naviculare (rectangle) of the left foot and (b) the two separate ossicles (KKU). Cf. Coskun et al. (2009); Dwight (1907); Serrafian (1993); Silva (2010).

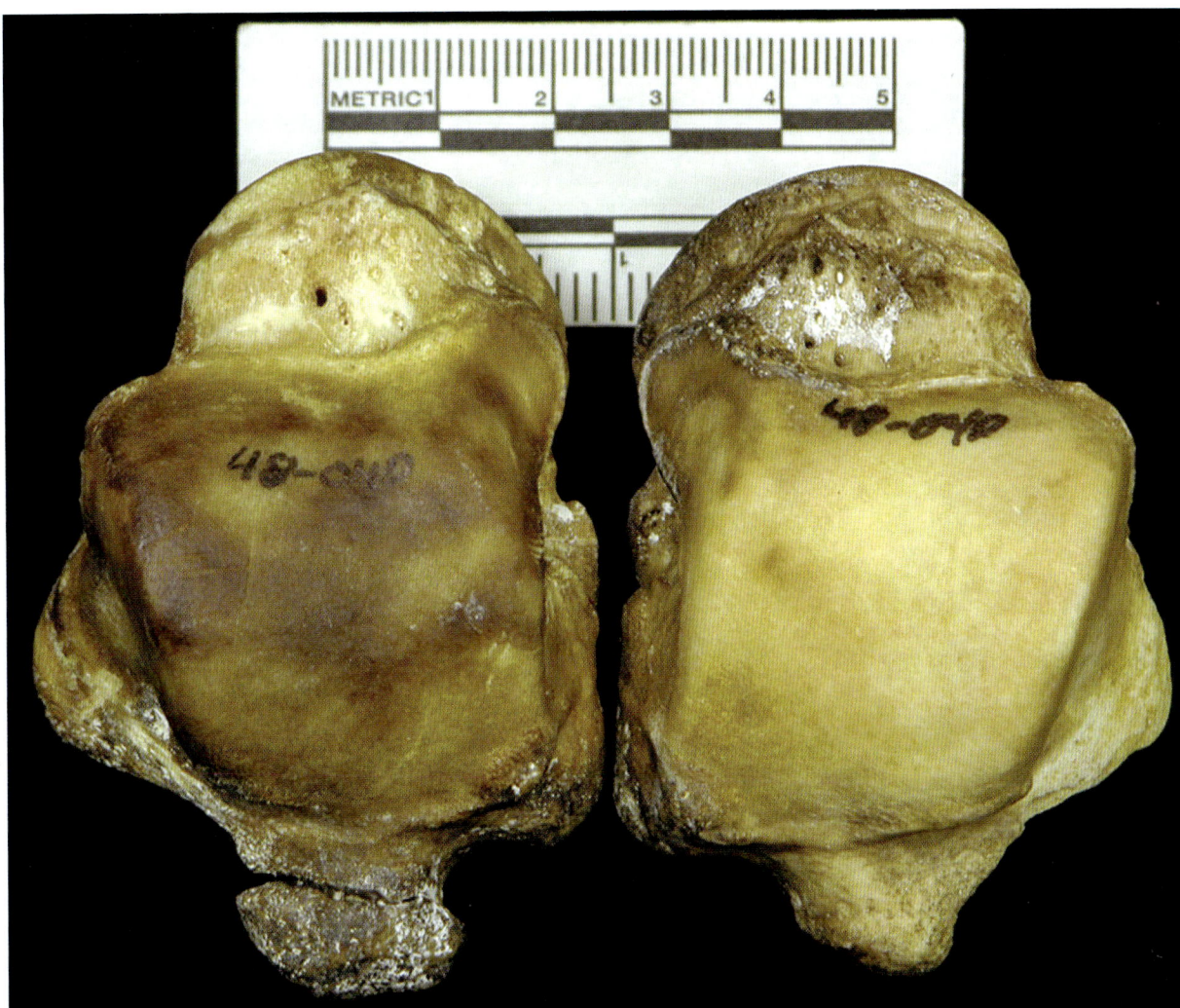

Figure 832. Separate but loosely attached os trigonum in the left talus and Steida's process in the right talus (UTK 48-040, Hefner). The os trigonum, a congenital developmental anomaly resulting from a separate center of ossification that fails to fuse, is present in 2.5% to 14% of typical feet (Wheeless' Anatomy, www.wheelessonline.com/ortho/anatomy_of_atlas). The os trigonum may be loosely attached to the talus or separated by cartilage and symptomatic. The separate ossicle often is overlooked or missed during recovery or misidentified as a sesamoid. Uncommon to common findings. Cf. Bennett (1886); Mann and Owsley (1990); Serrafian (1993); Silva (2010); Turner (1882). See McDougall (1955) and Sewell (1904) for comprehensive reviews of this condition.

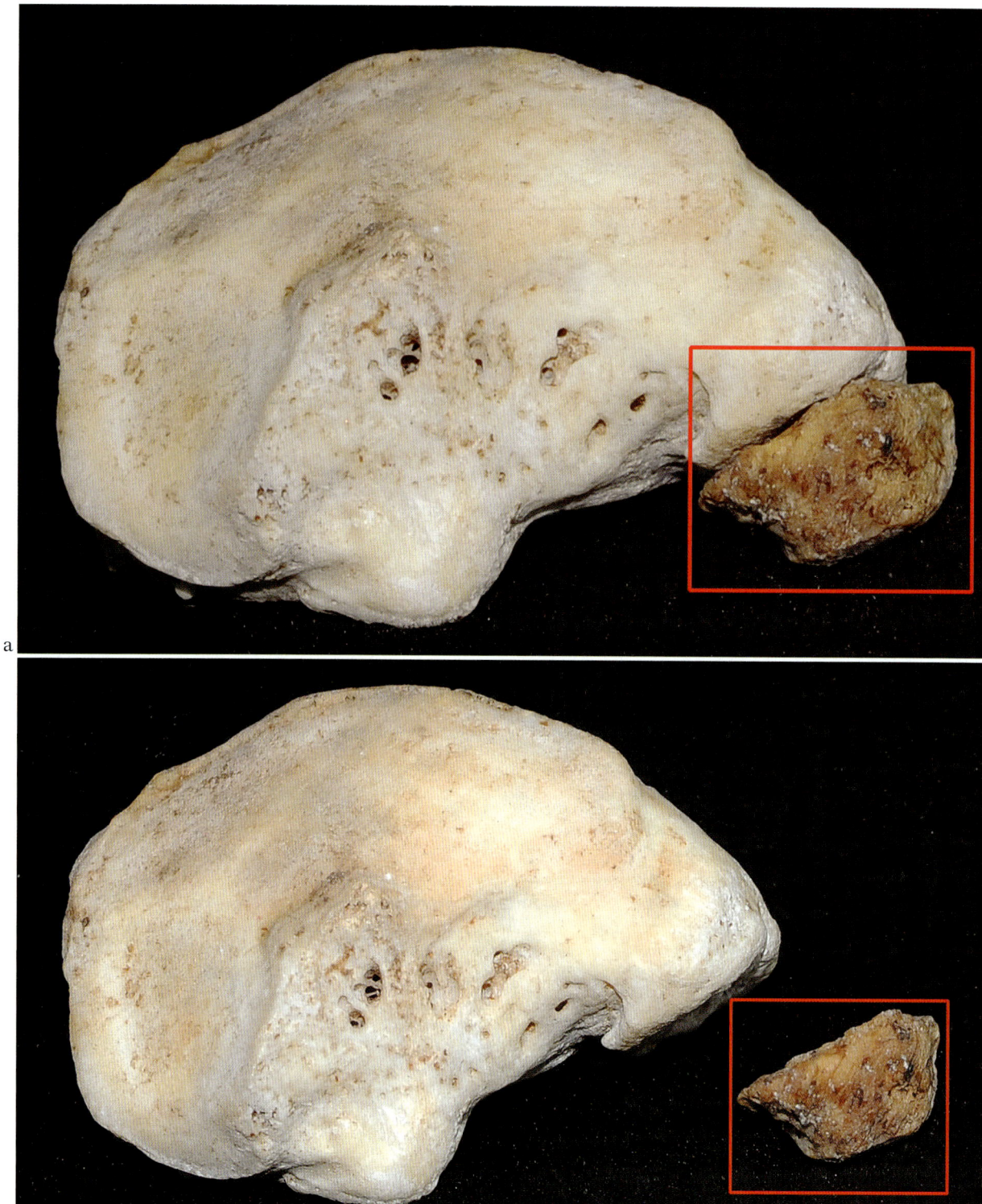

Figure 833a-b. Accessory navicular bone. (a) Attached and (b) separate accessory right navicular bone (os naviculare) (rectangles) in a 61-year-old Asian male (CMU 47/50). This trait was bilateral in this individual (Cf. Serrafian (1993). The accessory navicular, which is a common finding, is also known as os tibiale, os tibiale externum and os naviculare secundarium.

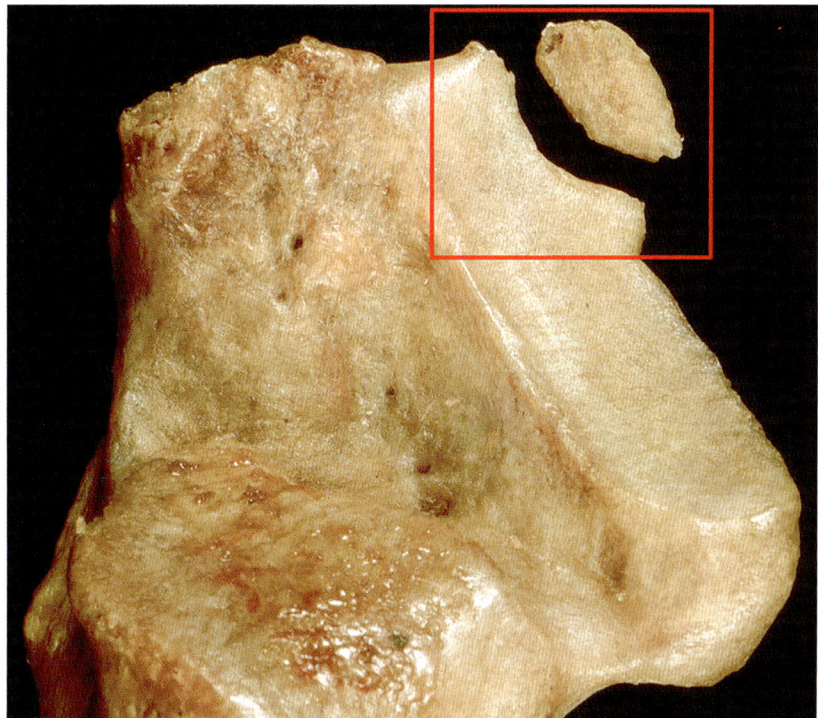

Figure 834. Calcaneus secundarius (square) and loose ossicle in the left calcaneus. Uncommon finding. Cf. Mann (1990). This feature should not be confused with the secondary os calcis (Cf. Mercer 1931). Cf. Silva (2010).

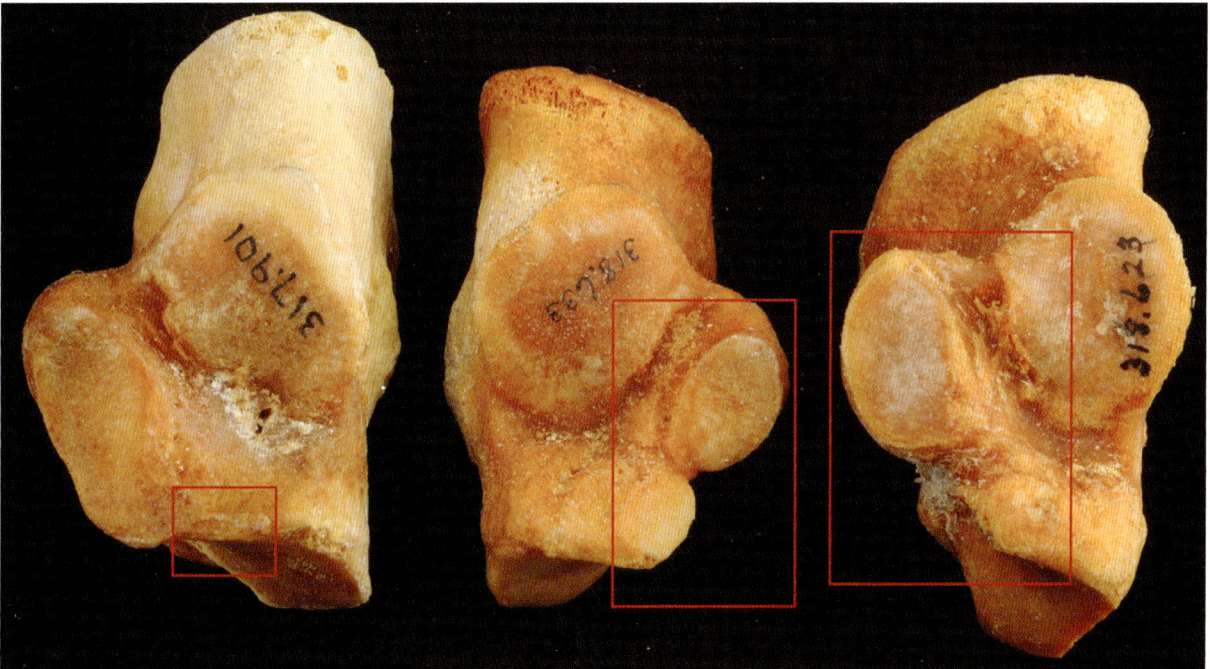

Figure 835. Variation of calcaneal facets in three adults. Single anterior and medial articular facets and a small beveled margin from contact with the talar neck (bone on left, small rectangle); double facets that are mildly separated (middle bone); and a large posterior and small anterior facet that is widely separated (right bone) (SI). Other variations include fused anterior, middle and posterior facets and absent anterior facets, among others. Cf. Bunning and Barnett (1965); Bidmos (2006).

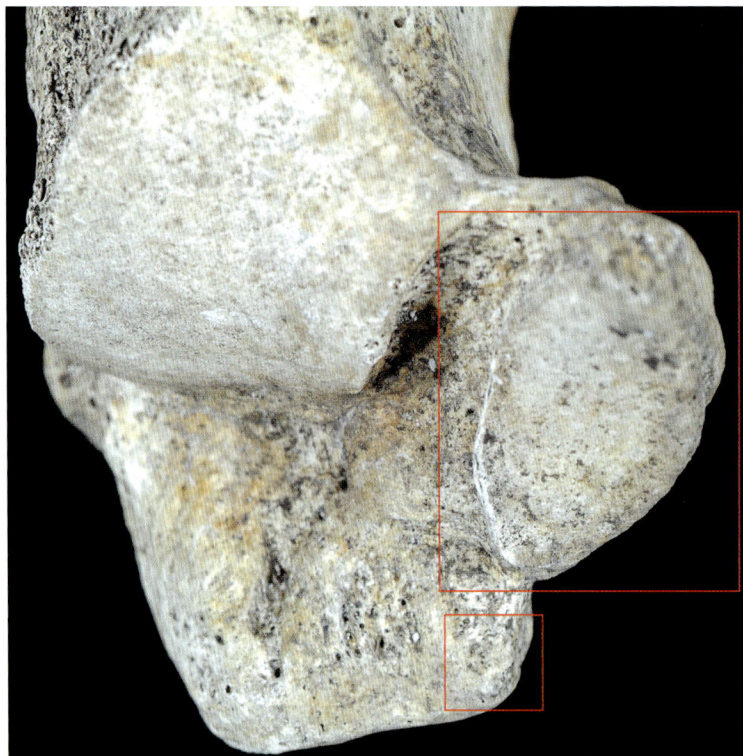

Figure 836. Large middle (rectangle) and tiny anterior facet (square) in the right calcaneus of an adult (CIL). The anterior facet may be absent (Ragab et al. 2003). Bunning and Barnett (1965).

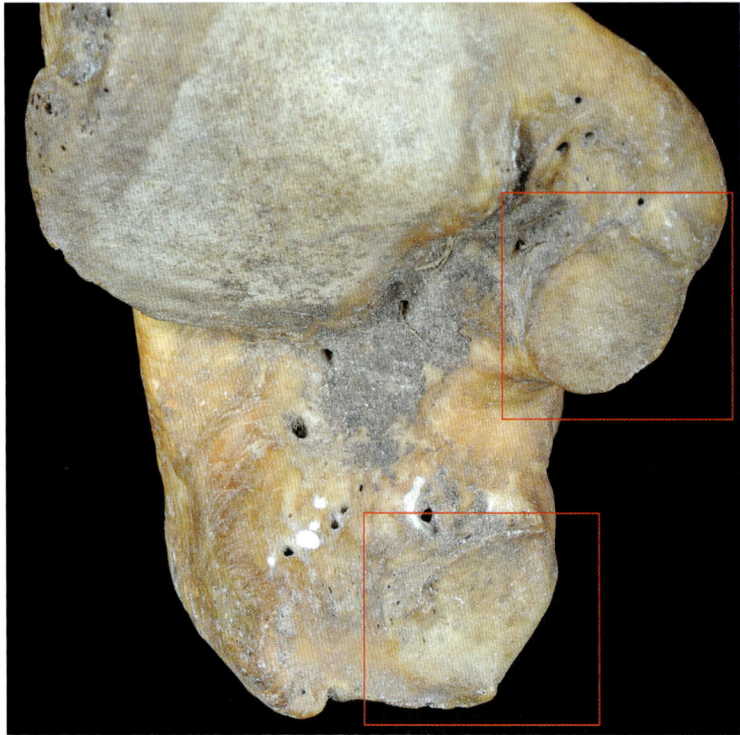

Figure 837. Small anterior and middle calcaneal facets (squares) that are widely separated (CIL).

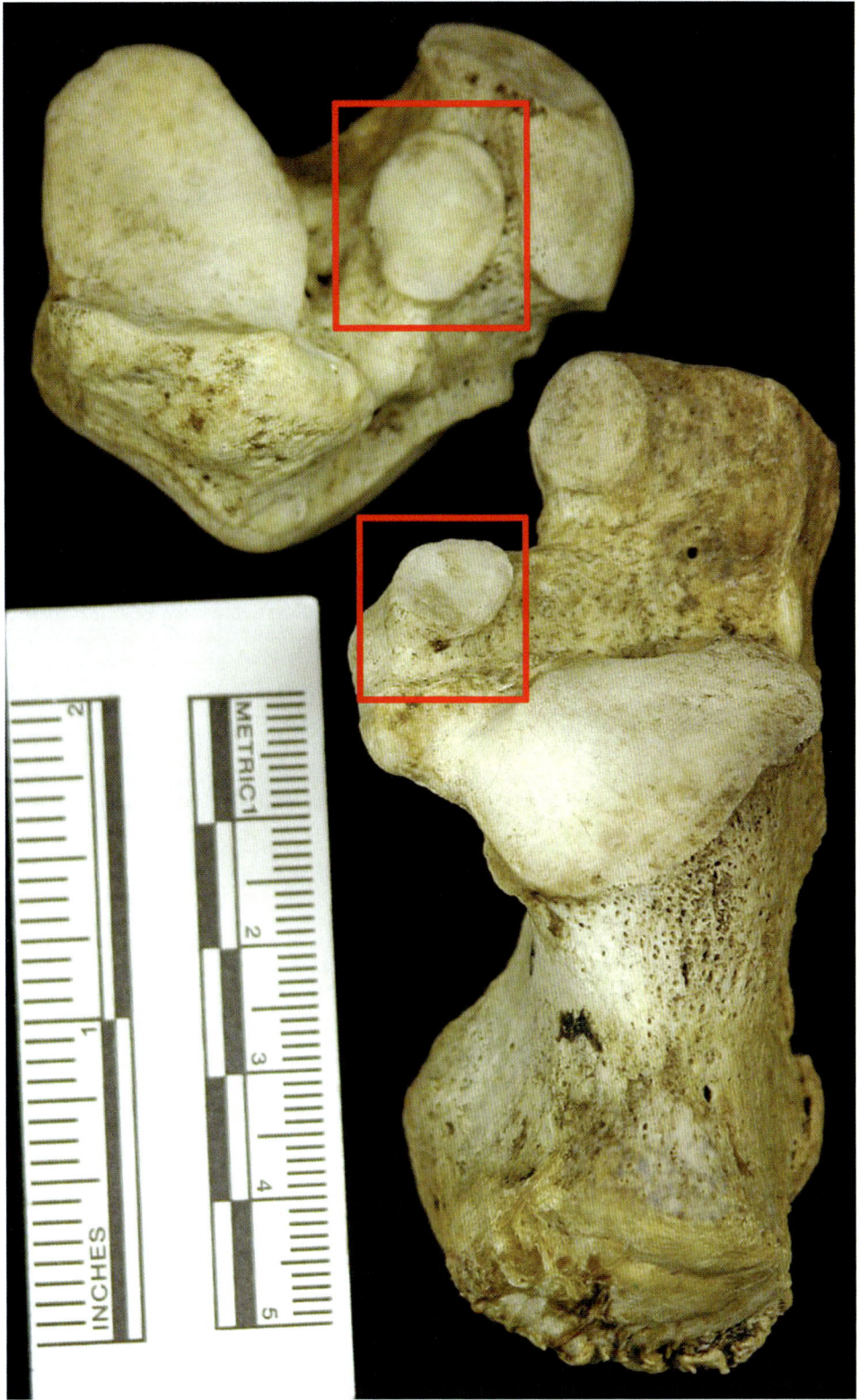

Figure 838. Separate anterior and middle facets (squares) resulting in large articular facets in an adult (Hefner, UTK 1999 09-99D). Typical variant and common finding. Cf. Bunning (1964); Bunning and Barnett (1965); Madhavi et al. (2008); Muthukumaravel et al. (2011); Padmanabhan (1986); Ragab et al. (2003).

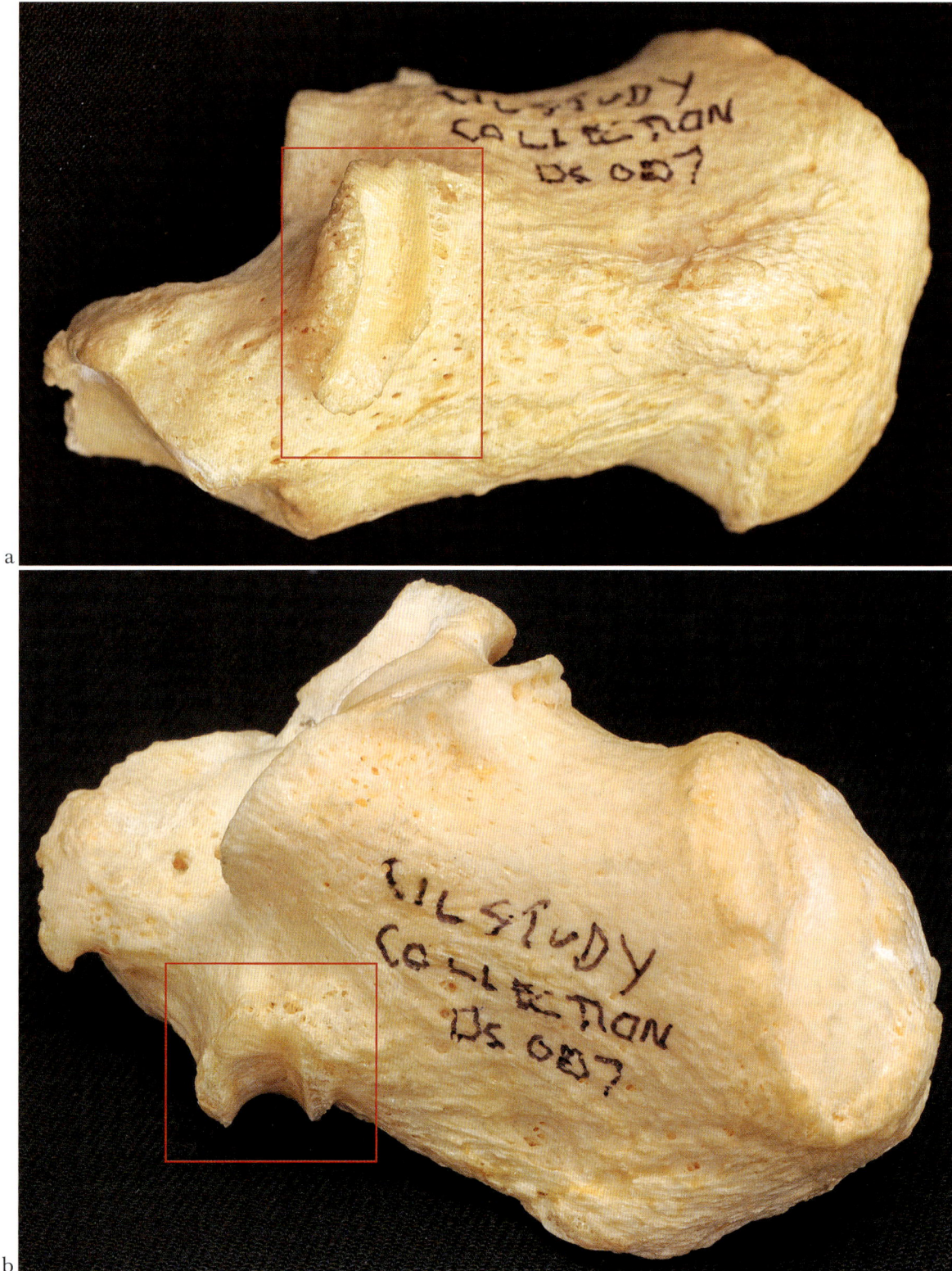

Figure 839a-b. Groove for peroneus longus. (a) Lateral view of the groove (rectangle) for the peroneus longus tendon in the left calcaneus of an adult (CSC DS 007). (b) Left oblique view of the peroneus longus groove (square).

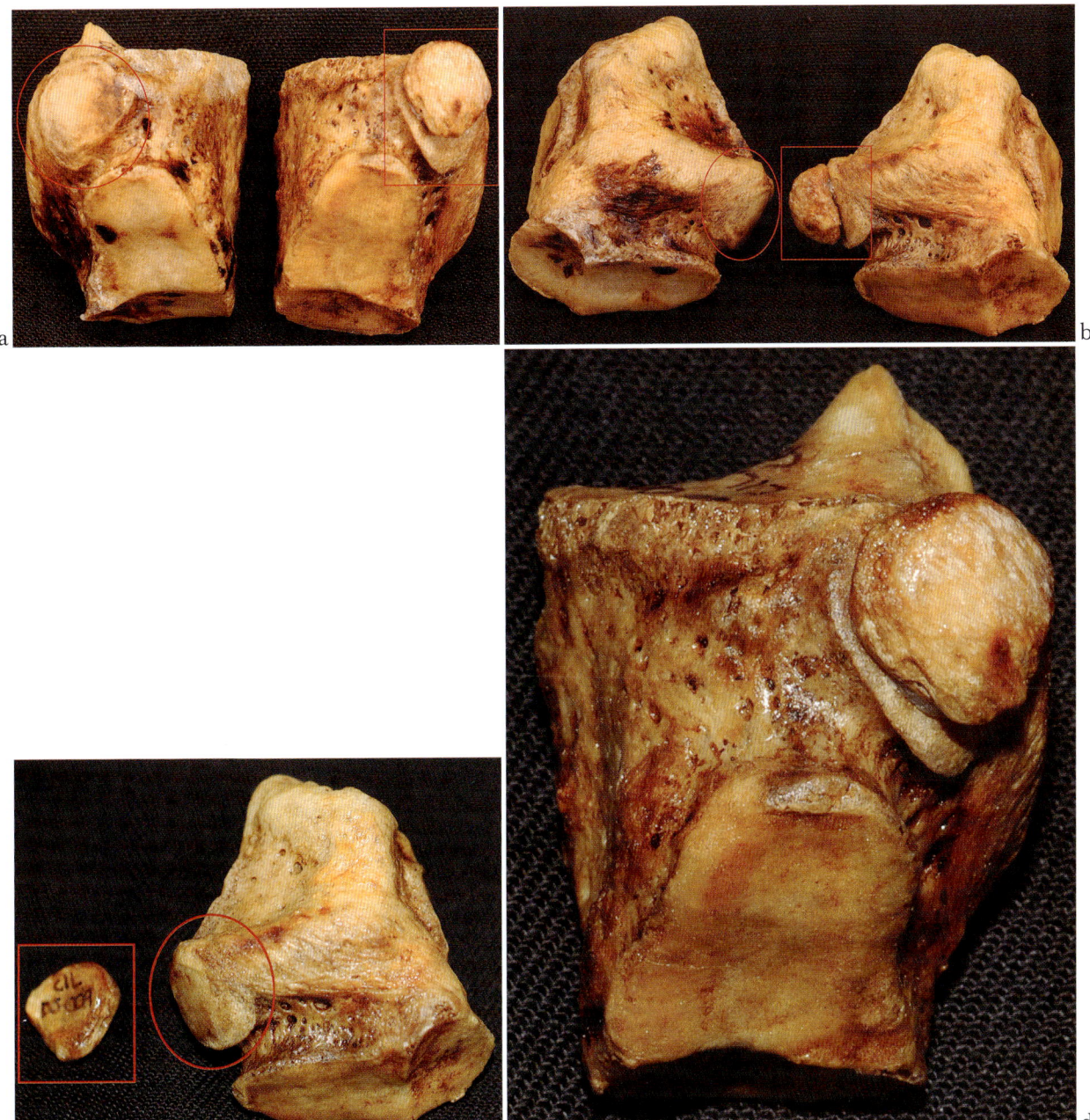

Figure 840a-d. Bilateral os peroneum in an adult (CSC DS 009). (a and b) Although the accessory ossicle for the right cuboid was not found with the remains, its articular facet is clearly visible (circles). (c) Left cuboid with separate os peroneum (square) showing the articular facet on the cuboid. (d) Higher magnification of the left cuboid showing the attached and articulated accessory bone. Due to their size, shape and rarity, these accessory ossicles may be misidentified as sesamoid bones of the hand or foot. Radiographic examination of 520 human feet (both sexes) revealed a frequency of os peroneum of 12.9% (64 of 520), was not always bilateral, showed no side or sex preference, may be bipartite or multipartite without any history of trauma, is quite variable in size and shape, and the size of the accessory bone is not related to the age of the individual (Le Minor 1987). Common to uncommon finding. Cf. Sarrafian (1993).

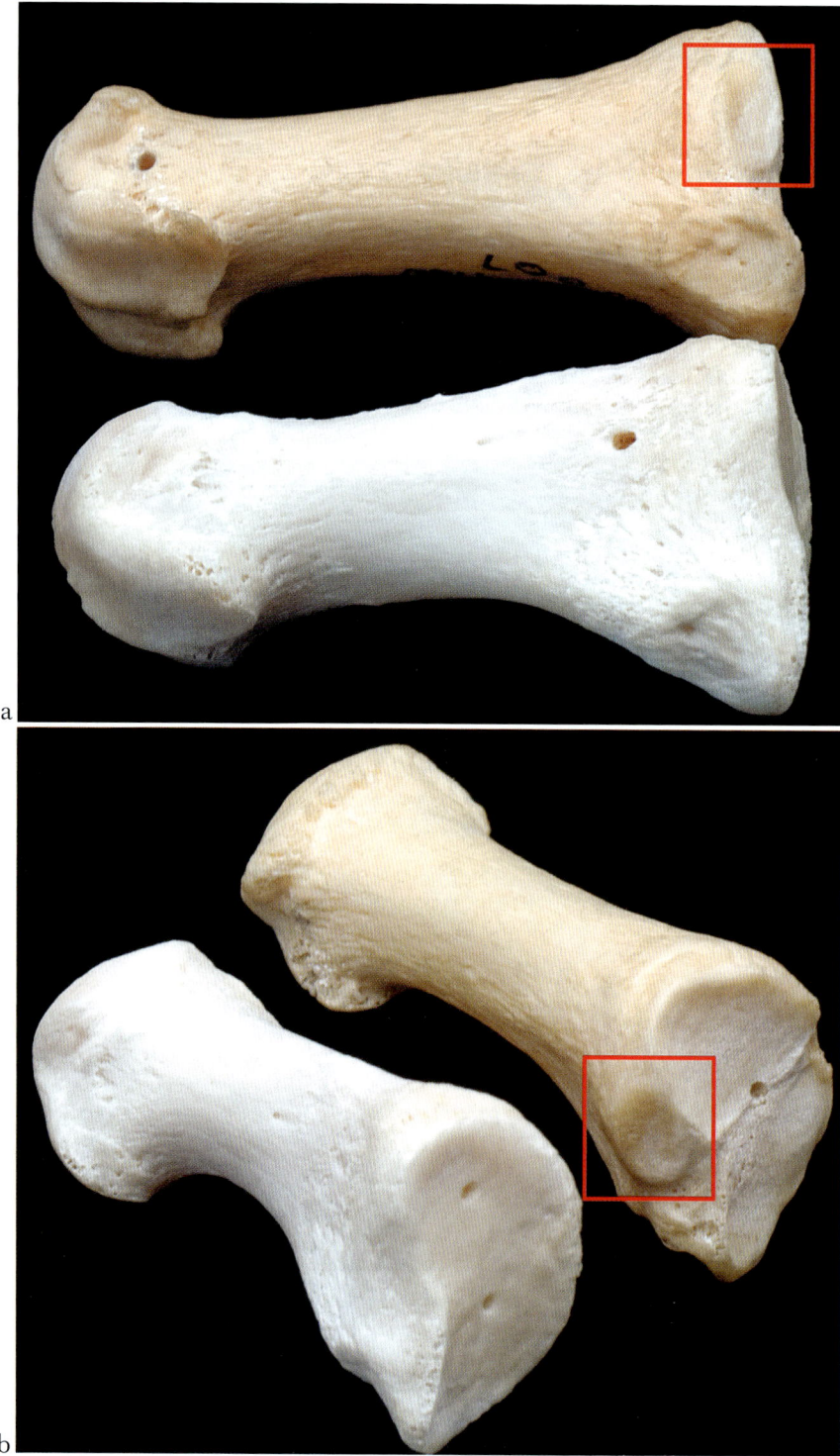

Figure 841a-b. Lateral intermetatarsal articular facet. (a) Lateral view of a lateral intermetatarsal articular facet of the left first metatarsal (square) compared to a left first metatarsal without an accessory facet (CSC DS007 with facet and CSC DS033 without facet). (b) Posterior oblique view of the left intermetatarsal facet (square) compared to a left first metatarsal without a facet. Le Minor and Winter (2003) noted this accessory facet in 127 of 412 bones (30.8%) and found no significant differences between right or left sides. This facet articulates with the medial surface of the second metatarsal (see 839a-b and 842a-b for more images of CSC DS007 individual's foot bones).

Leg and Foot (Femur, Tibia, Fibula, Patella, Tarsal, Metatarsal, Phalanx)

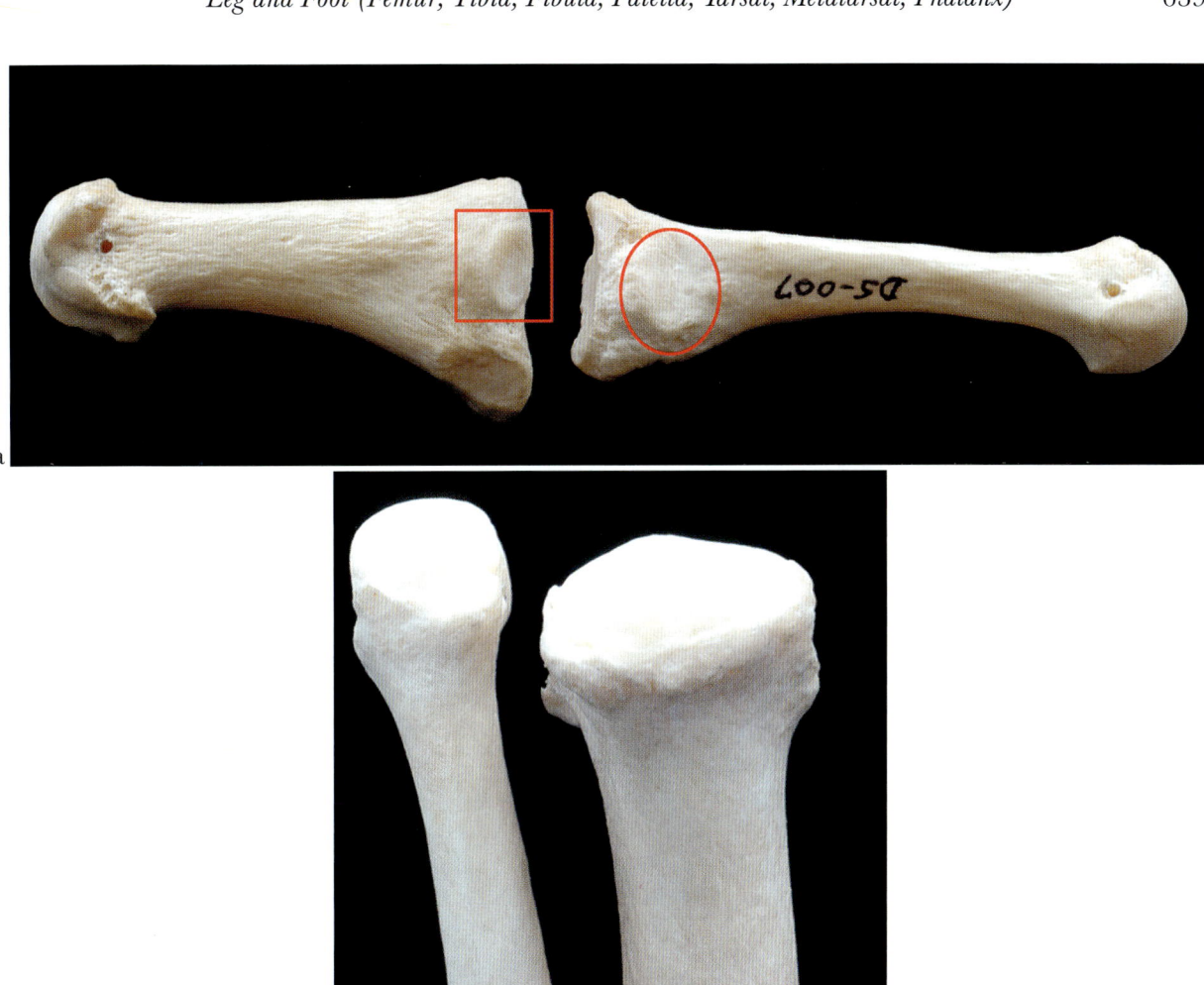

Figure 842a-b. Left lateral intermetatarsal articular facet. (a) Left first and second metatarsals showing the lateral intermetatarsal articular facet (bilateral in this individual) in an elderly male (CSC DS007). The accessory facet is situated near the proximal joint on the 1st metatarsal (square) and a corresponding oval-shaped facet (oval) is on the 2nd metatarsal. Note that the oval facet on the second metatarsal has a small non-articular area separating it from the proximal articular facet. (b) Site of articulation of the accessory intermetatarsal facet. Hyer et al. (2005) found this facet in 22 of 77 (29%) of first metatarsals in a cadaver sample and noted a relationship between this facet and metatarsus primus varus.

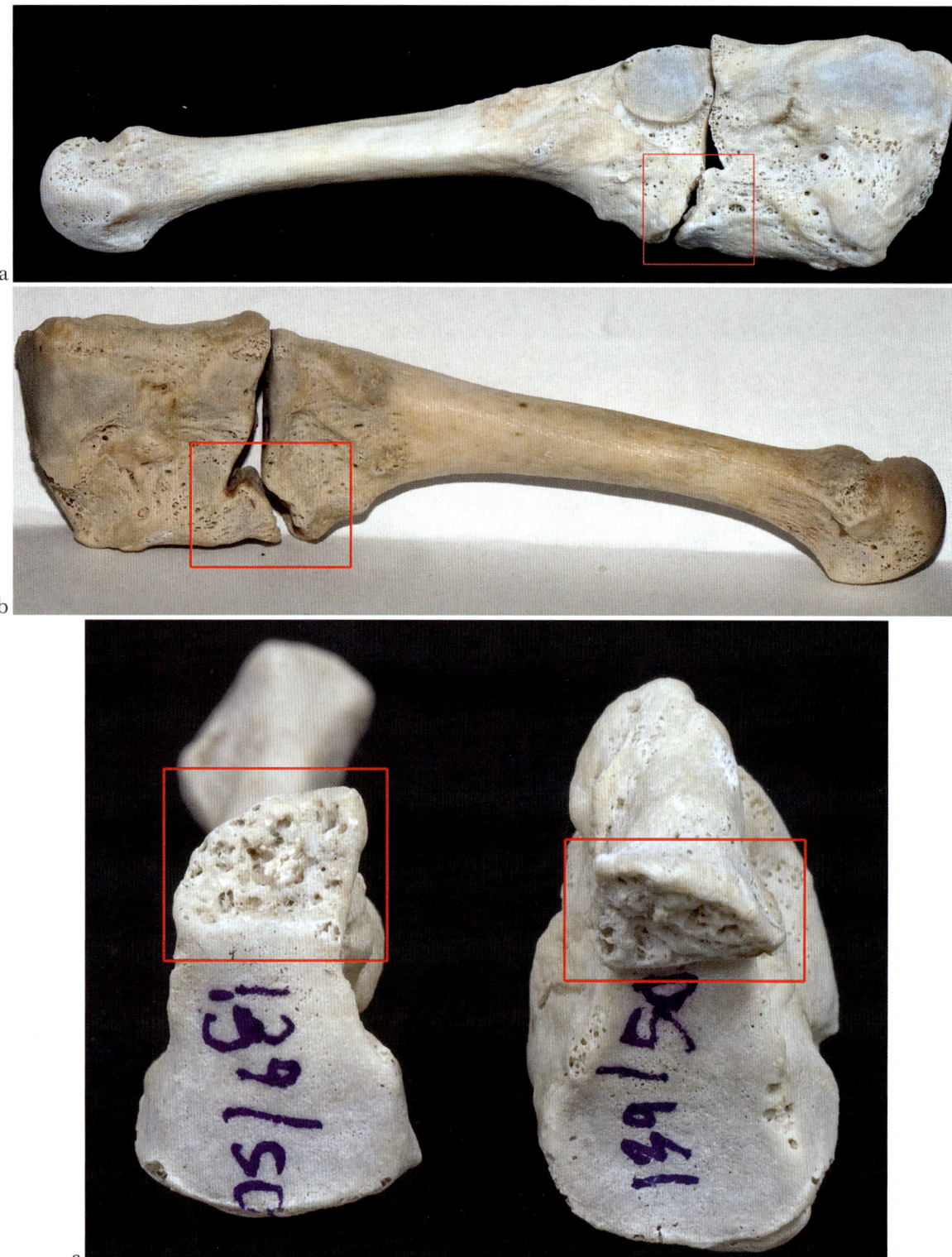

Figure 843a-c. Non-osseous tarsal coalition. (a) Lateral view of partial coalition (squares) of the third metatarsal and third cuneiform in a 57-year-old Thai male (CMU 139 50). (b) Medial view of the third metatarsal and cuneiform showing conformity of the articular and surfaces (rectangle). (c) Posterior view of the porous and roughened surfaces where the two bones partially coalesced (square and rectangle).

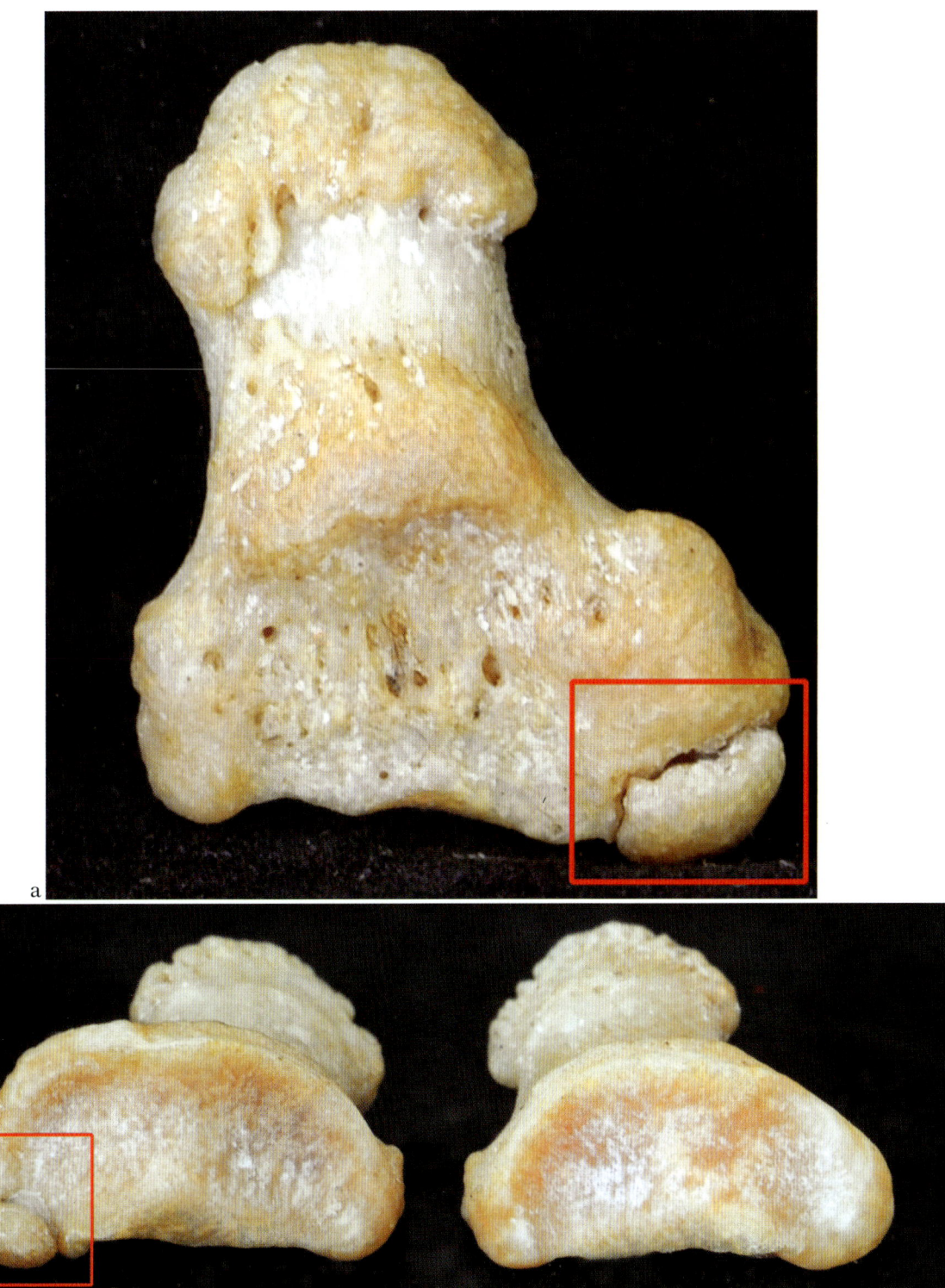

Figure 844a-b. Accessory or bipartite ossicle of the toe. (a) Inferior or plantar view of a small accessory ossicle (red square; the ossicle is held in place with wax) of the lateral portion of the left distal first phalanx of the foot in an adult Thai male (KKU). (b) Posterior view of the accessory ossicle (square) in the left phalanx compared to the articular surface of the right phalanx in the same individual. The morphology of this ossicle and site of attachment are consistent with an accessory bone and not trauma.

Chapter 12

A METHOD FOR REMOVING SOFT TISSUE FROM A HUMAN RIB CAGE WITH BLEACH

STEVEN LABRASH, ROBERT W. MANN AND SCOTT LOZANOFF

Removing the soft tissue from human remains, often the first step in preparation for skeletal analysis, whether a single bone or a complete body can be a laborious, time-consuming and complicated process. The methods for removing soft tissue vary and typically involve chemical or water-based maceration, gross and fine excision utilizing a scalpel, or, the method preferred by many commercial supply houses, natural decomposition utilizing dermestid (*Dermestidae*) "flesh-eating" beetles. Defleshing human remains is performed for a variety of reasons that include estimating the cause and time elapsed since death, determining age, sex, ethnicity, perimortem trauma and personal identity of an individual, and to address other medico-legal questions. This chapter reports a relatively rapid and reliable method for removing soft tissue from the human thorax with household bleach.

The method described here was modified by Mann and Berryman (2012) and involves immersing the rib cage in bleach. The technique not only keeps the bones and cartilage intact, but that maintains the overall size and shape of the thoracic cage. The bleach dissolves the perichondrium and some of the underlying cartilage matrix leaving a pattern of vertically-arranged plates, or "vertical plates" of collagen. The characteristic appearance of the ribs that occurs as a result of this technique has not been previously observed by the authors despite their cumulative examination of several thousand human skeletons spanning several decades. Therefore, this report details the gross and microscopic pattern of collagen in human costal cartilage that may be a feature of the aging thorax revealed by the process of bleaching. The authors are continuing to explore whether vertical plates is as an artifact of the bleaching process or a biological feature that may be of use as an indicator of age, sex, trauma or other physiological processes and is reported herein as a descriptive observation requiring additional research to better understand its composition and development.

The bleaching method reported herein was modified from Mann and Berryman (2012) and, depending on the condition and amount of adhering soft tissue, can take two to three days to complete. In the present study, bleach was first used to remove the soft tissue from a 72-year-old female and then tested and successfully utilized on a 55-year-old female, a 55-year-old male and a 107-year-old female as part of the Willed Body Program at the University of Hawaii John A. Burns School of Medicine (JABSOM) following standard operating procedures (Labrash and Lozanoff, 2007). In all four cases, the soft tissues were removed by the first author and rendered in an excellent state of preservation allowing examination of even the most fragile skeletal elements.

Removal of the soft tissue from the rib cage resulted in the appearance of a pattern of vertical plates within the costal cartilage. This pattern was an unexpected and incidental finding first noted in the thoracic region of a 72-year-old female. The finding prompted the authors to perform gross and histological analysis to ascertain its composition. The vertical plates may reflect the underlying structure of the costal cartilage after chemical removal of the overlying perichondrium.

Removal of the perichondrium (Figures 845 and 846) and some of the underlying tissues revealed a characteristic pattern of sequential vertical plates of what appears to be cartilage. Subsequent gross examination of the rib cage of a 55-year-old male revealed no evidence of vertical plates, but did reveal cracks in the perichondrium following complete immersion in bleach for 20 minutes. To test the hypothesis that all adult costal cartilage yield a similar pattern, if immersed in bleach, portions of right and left costal cartilage from a third adult, a 55-year-old female were excised and one side was immersed in bleach while the other was placed in tap water. Results showed that the pattern of vertical plates was present only in the costal cartilage after immersion in bleach (further research is needed to confirm). Household bleach (diluted and undiluted) is sometimes used during forensic inspection to remove adhering soft tissue to reveal stab marks in the bone and costal cartilage, as well as other trauma. A third rib cage was derived from a 107-year-old female and analyzed in a similar fashion. Some of the adhering soft tissue was removed by placing the rib cage in bleach (8.25%) for 20 minutes and subjected to radiographic visualization (80Kv at MA 200).

Removing soft tissue is also necessary if the goal is to render the human body to bone. Soft tissue removal may also be performed to reveal evidence of skeletal trauma or disease to the thoracic cage. While there are many methods available for removing soft tissue, regardless of the method used, it must be performed with care to avoid osseous damage (Onwuama et al. 2012). One potential drawback when skeletonizing remains results from the requirement of reassembly utilizing wires, springs, nuts and bolts and other fasteners if the goal is to produce an articulated skeleton. Additionally, when rearticulating the skeleton, brittle or badly damaged costal cartilage must be reconstructed or reinforced and reattached to the ribs with molded plastic or resin and wire.

While some researchers (McCormick 1980) found no evidence of destruction of the costal cartilage by insects under natural environmental conditions after several months, others (www.carolina.com) report that carrion beetles consume cartilage last, after other "soft" tissues are consumed. The present authors, however, note that a colony of carrion (dermestid) beetles housed in a common terrarium within a general anatomy laboratory can totally consume the costal cartilages in less than three days. Lastly, keeping the ribs articulated maintaining proper anatomical position and sequence facilitates methods for the rapid and reliable estimation of age.

Biological supply companies utilize a variety of chemical and mechanical methods to remove soft tissue to include removal of the plastron (chest plate) and adhering soft tissue. For example, the commercial website of "Skulls Unlimited©" (www.skullsunlimited.com) reveals that the bulk of soft tissue is mechanically excised and then fine removal is achieved through exposure to dermestid beetles. As a result, even the most fragile bones and calcified tissues are retained during this process. This step is followed by immersing the bones in hydrogen peroxide to remove pigments and cause them to lighten.

This chapter presents an effective method for removing the soft tissue from the human thoracic cage by immersion in water and chlorine bleach consisting of 8.25% sodium hypochlorite and 0.05% sodium hydroxide. Immersing remains in household bleach will render the bones devoid of soft tissue, and with little or no odor, fully articulated, and in correct anatomical position and alignment. Another advantage is that the method maintains natural articulations including ligaments, intervertebral discs and hyaline cartilage avoiding the unnecessary and time-consuming steps concerned with re-establishing skeletal element connectivity.

Due to the fragile and incompletely ossified nature of subadult remains, this method must be modified and adjusted to achieve optimal results. The following is an overview of the steps using household bleach (about 9 gallons):

1) The thoracic region is isolated and as much of the soft tissues as possible are removed mechanically using a scalpel, scissors and other routine gross anatomy dissection instruments.
   a) Excise the skin and subcutaneous tissues from the thorax as much as possible and remove internal organs. Immerse the intact and articulated thorax in a non-reactive container filled with household bleach (8.25% sodium hydroxide) for 20 minutes. Monitor the bones, ensuring that they do not remain too waxen or become overly bleached and brittle. The mixture will become rapidly warm to the touch; it will begin dissolving soft tissue,

indicated by the cloudy appearance with surface bubbles.

b) The reaction reaches equilibrium in approximately 20 minutes and the liquid is decanted. The specimen is placed on an absorbent towel and any remaining soft tissue is excised.

c) The specimen is immersed in a container and washed with slowly flowing tap water (12 hours).

d) The bleaching process is repeated with careful monitoring to achieve the desired degree of pigmentation. Exercise great caution to ensure that the bones are not becoming damaged or ashen since bones will appear whiter after they are removed from the bleach and begin to dry. Also, frequent inspection is necessary to ensure retention of intervertebral discs and costal cartilages.

e) A final wash is achieved for 24 hours to remove all bleach from the specimen. Care must be exercised when handling the fragile costal cartilage since it is brittle and prone to breakage.

f) The thoracic skeleton is dried by placing it in anatomical position on absorbent towels or a draining surface for a minimum of 24 hours.

g) The specimen is immersed in acetone for four to six weeks to degrease the bones.

h) Costal cartilage and other joints can be coated (saturated) with Super Glue® (cyanoacrylate adhesive) for hardening so that they can be handled. For better results the thoracic cage may be plastinated following standard methods provided by the International Society for Plastination (http://isp.plastination.org/silicone.html).

Expected results from this method include:

- The ribs remain fully attached and articulated to the spine and sternum.
- There is no need to rearticulate the rib cage with wire or other fasteners.
- The anatomical shape of the bones of the rib cage is maintained.
- Intervertebral discs are retained.
- The bones are clean, degreased and odor free.
- The costal cartilages are preserved in size, shape and detail.

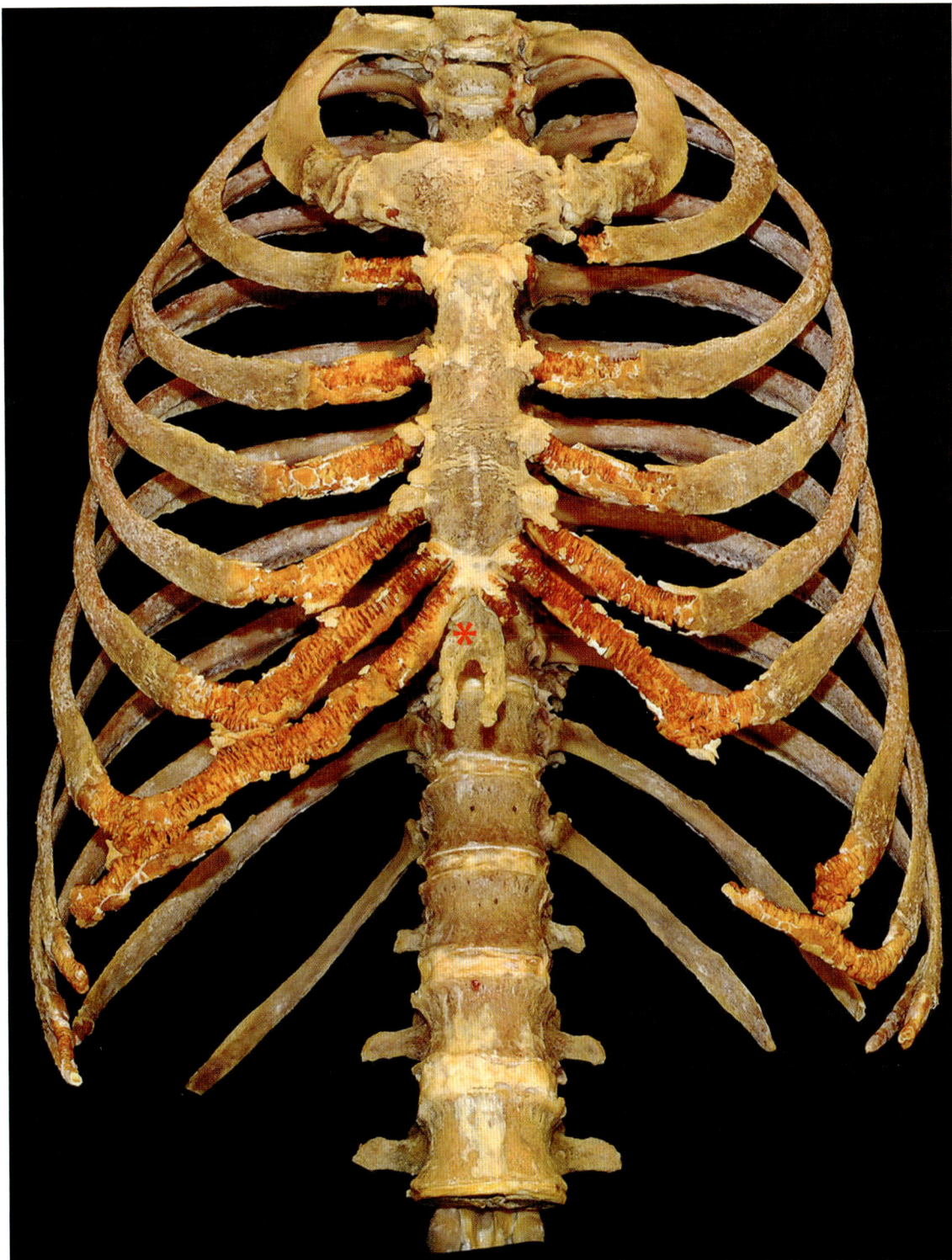

Figure 845. Ventral view of the thorax (rib cage) showing separation through T1 (superiorly) and L3/L4 (inferiorly) during the process of immersion in acetone (71-year-old female; JABSOM). Note the bifid xiphoid process (*), numerous calcifications and osteophytes joining the bars of costal cartilage to the sternum (as expected, most developed along the first ribs) and preservation of the costal cartilages and intervertebral discs. Also note that the right 11th and 12th ribs are longer than those on the left side.

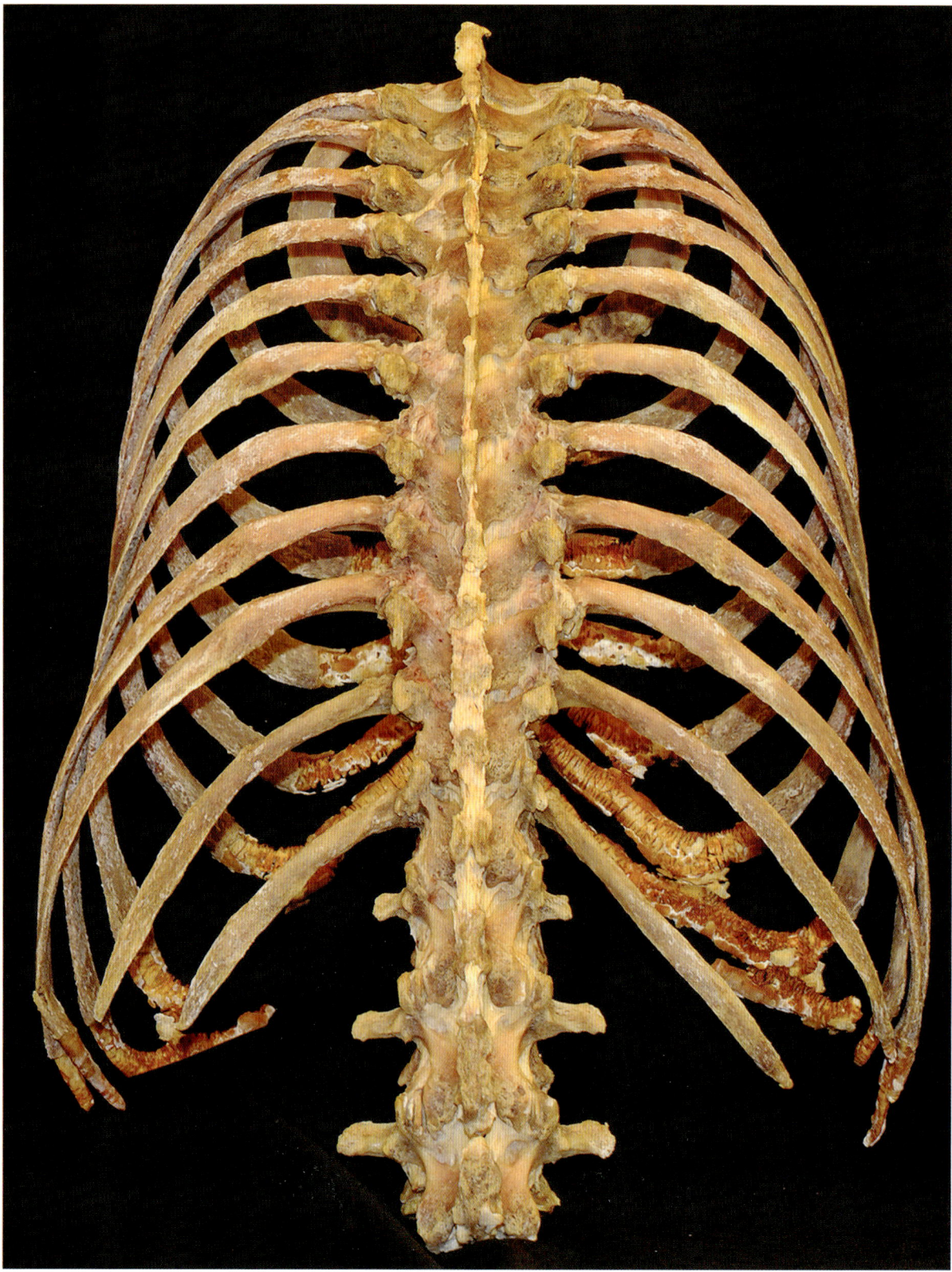

Figure 846. Dorsal view of the thorax showing preservation of the intervertebral ligaments. Note that immersion in bleach did not remove all of the soft tissue on the vertebral column in this 71-year-old female (JABSOM).

Chapter 13

UNUSUAL COMBINATION OF SKELETAL VARIANTS IN AN ADULT THAI MALE (KKU): A PHOTOGRAPHIC CASE REPORT

Robert Mann and Panya Tuamsuk

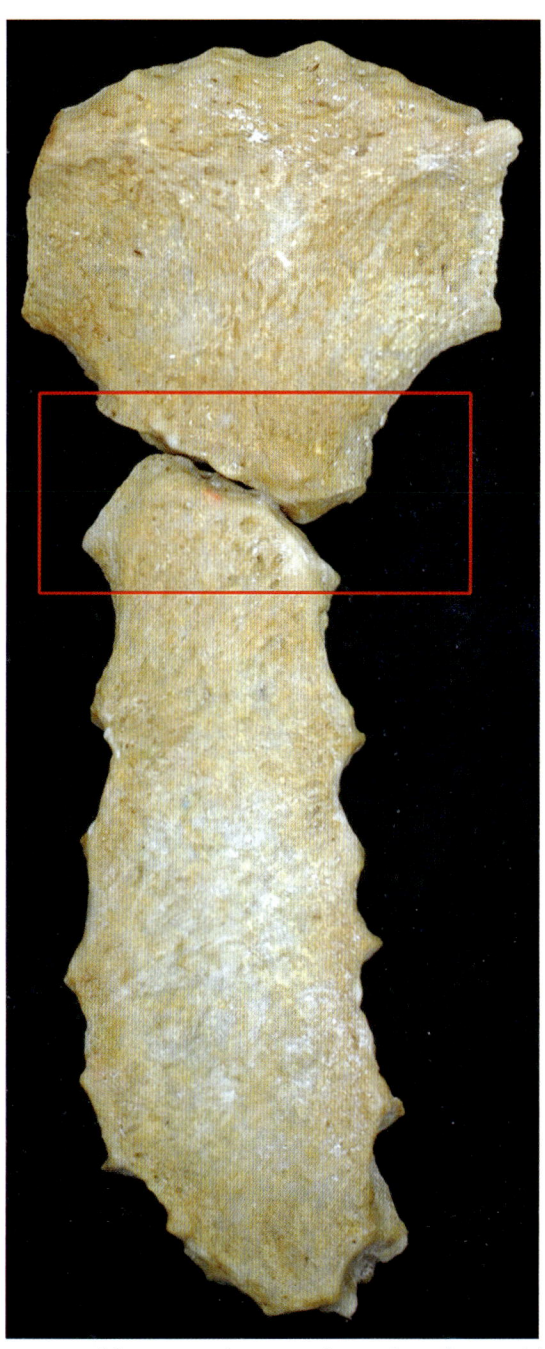

Figure 847. Sternum showing an oblique manubriosternal symphysis (rectangle) and misaligned notches for the second ribs. Common finding.

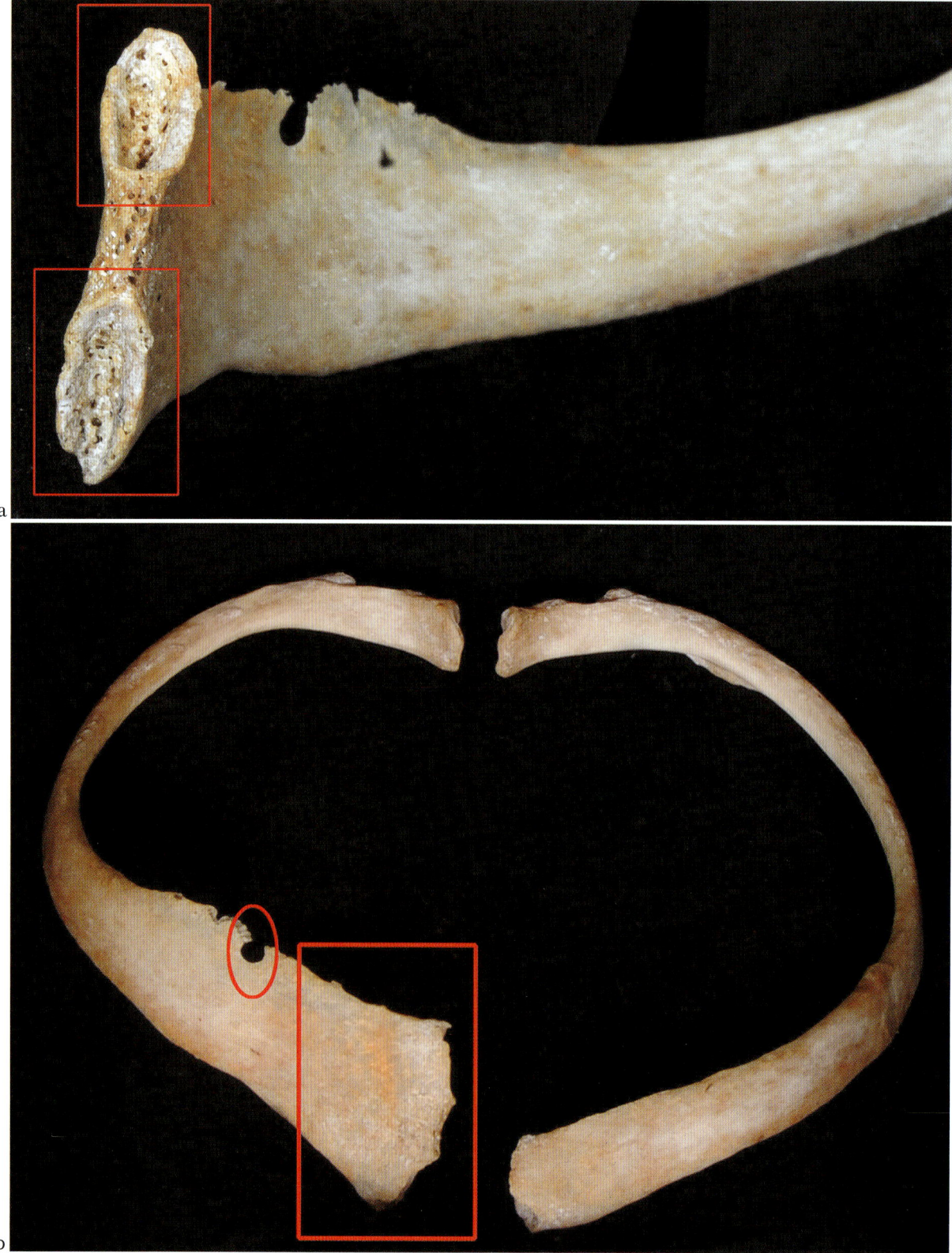

Figure 848a-b. Lushka's fourth right rib (rectangles). (a) Separate facets at the costal chondral joint with (b) wide, flat and mild bifurcation of the sternal end resulting in an additional costal facet on the right side.

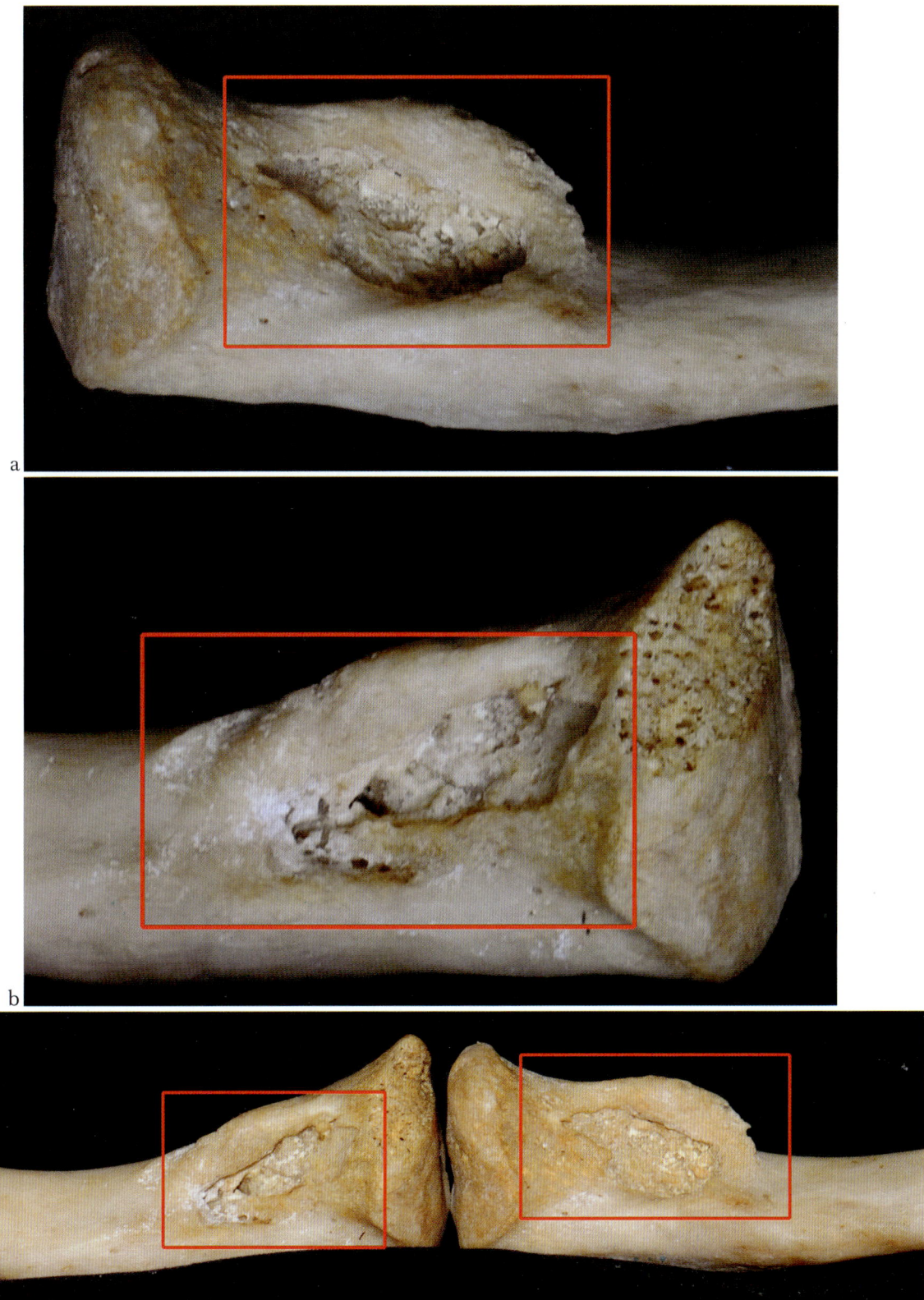

Figure 849a-c. Variants of rhomboid fossae (rectangles) showing large, deep concavities for the attachment of the costoclavicular ligament with large superoposterior rims on both clavicles.

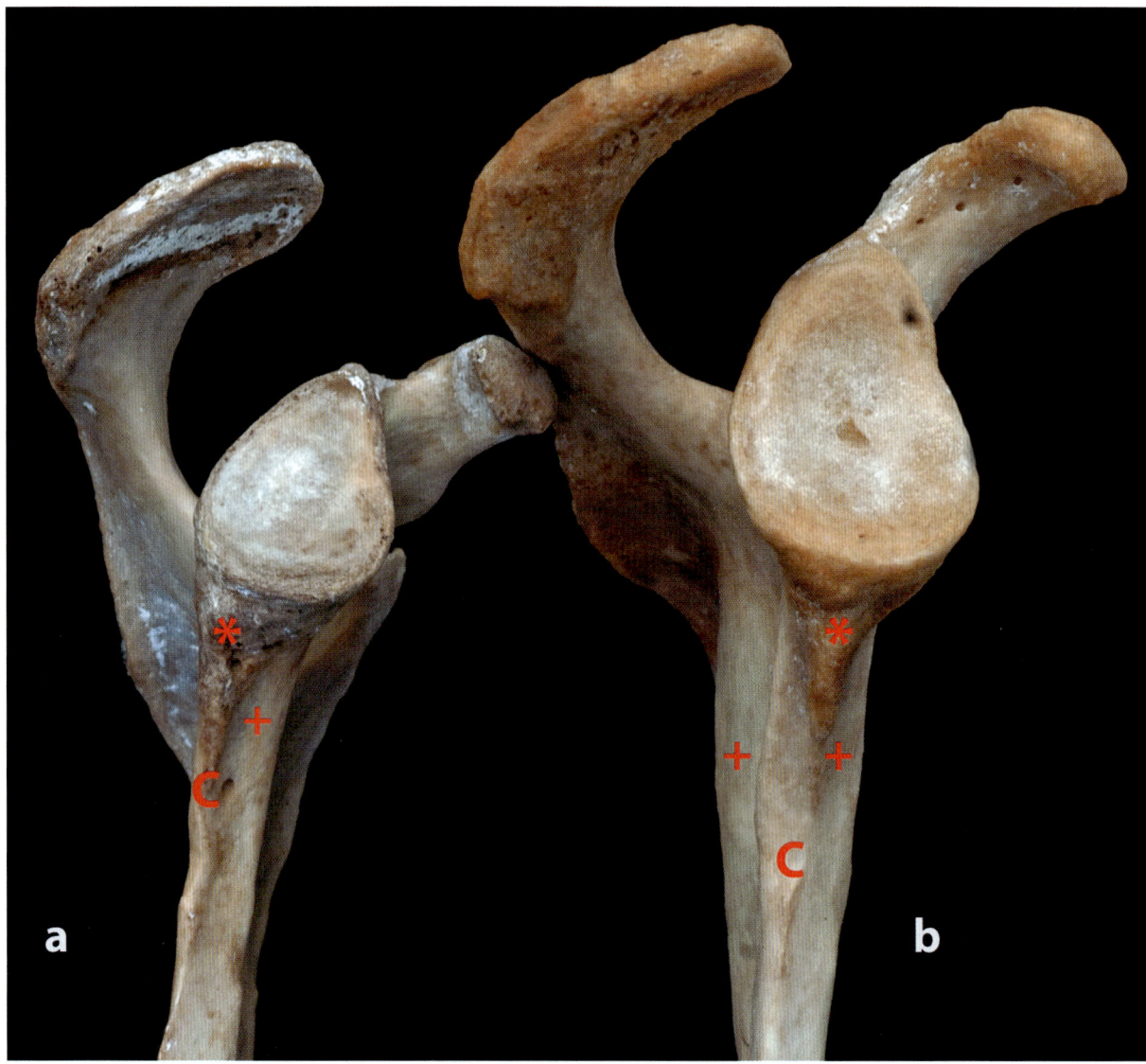

Figure 850. Prominent infraglenoid tubercle and crest (* and C) that is centrally located. Note the ridge in the right scapula of this individual (b) has a flat, step-like area (+) along either side of the crest, while in the comparative right scapula (a), the "step" (+) is only anterior, possibly reflecting muscularity and/or differing physical activity. (b) Prominent tubercle and crest (* and C) along the posterior or axillary border of the scapular body.

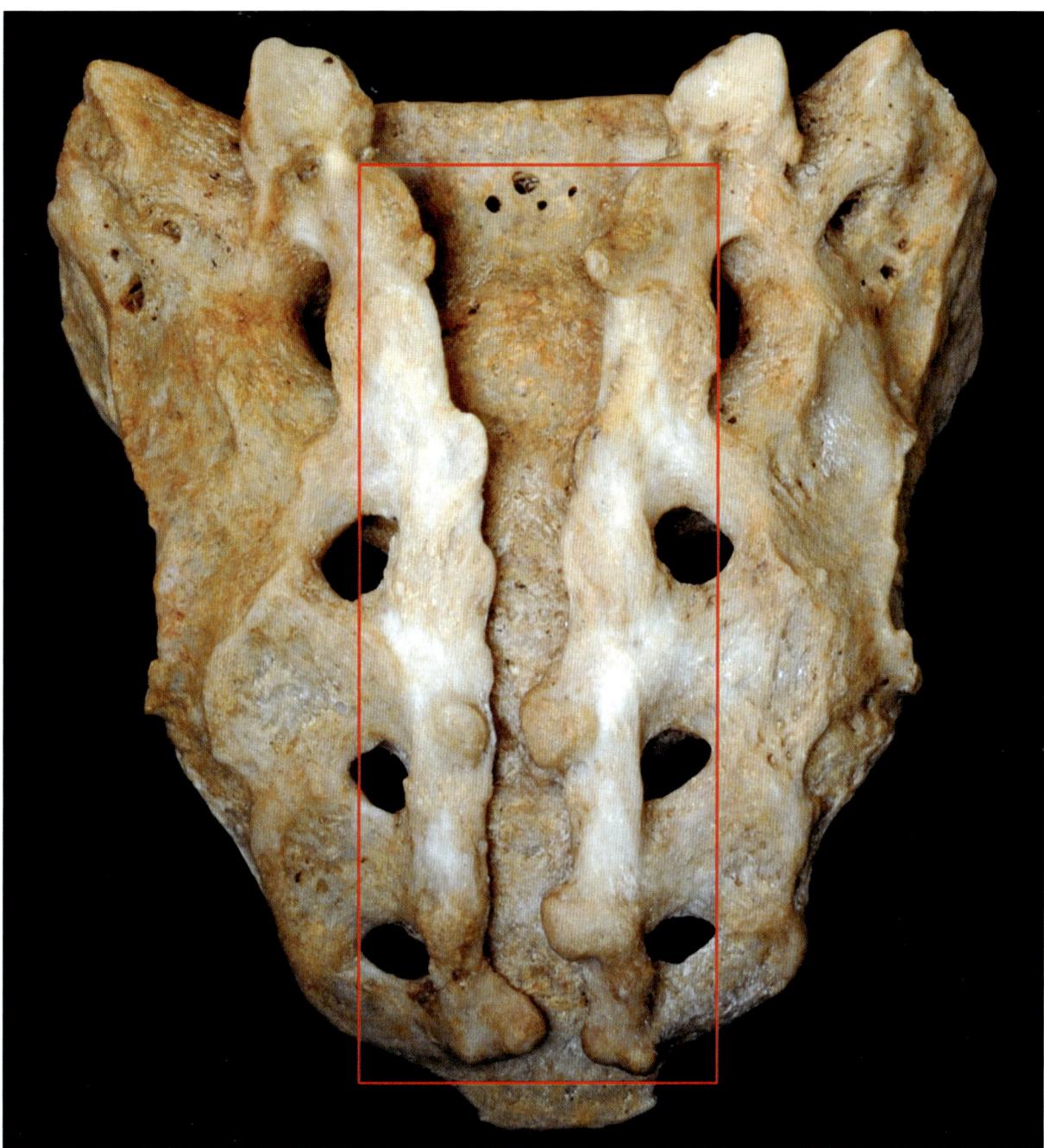

Figure 851 Complete sacral cleft or spina bifida of the sacrum.

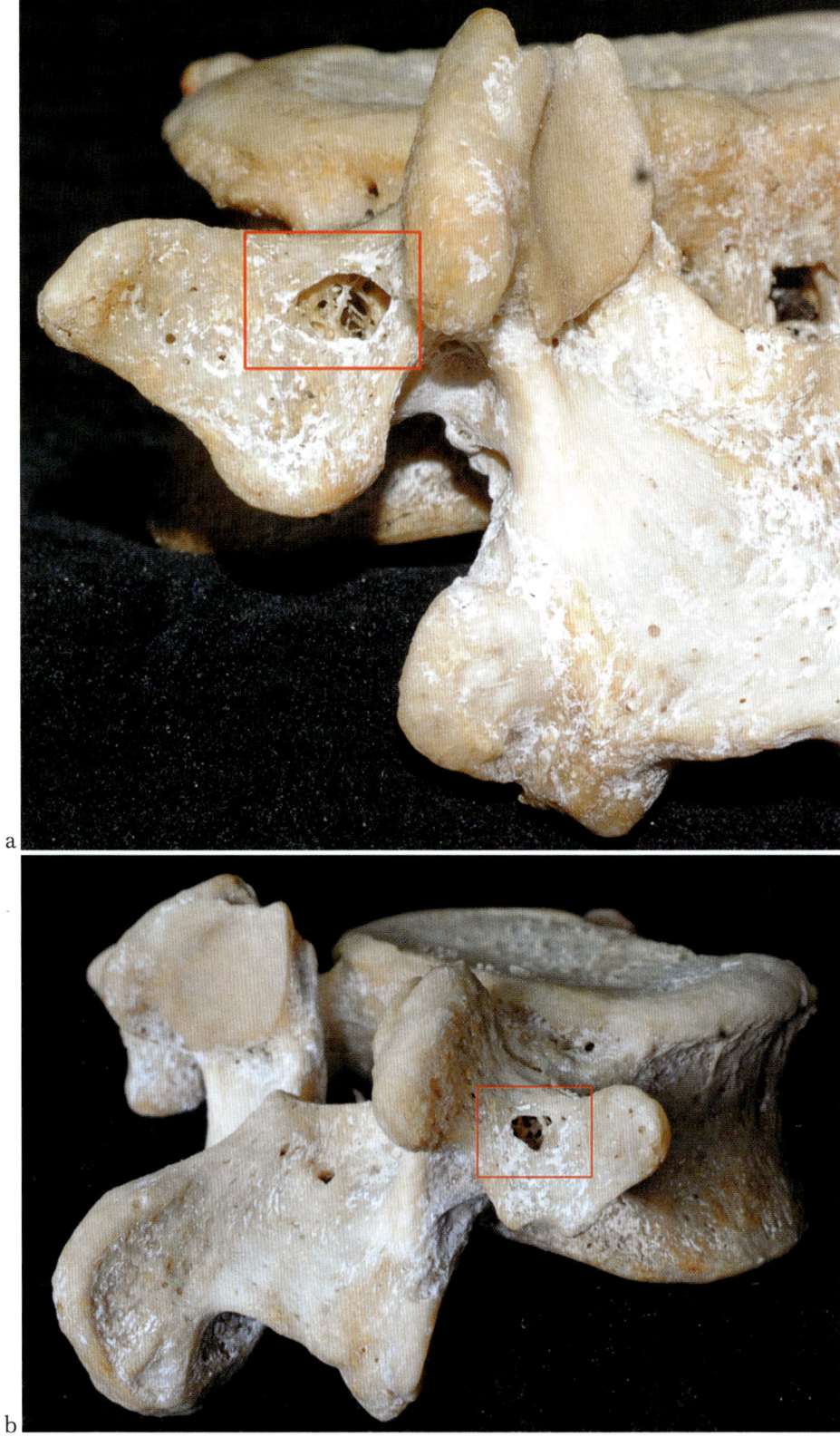

Figure 852a-b. Bilateral accessory vascular foramina or lytic lesions (rectangle) viewed from the postero-lateral aspect in the left (a) and right (b) transverse processes of a fourth lumbar vertebra.

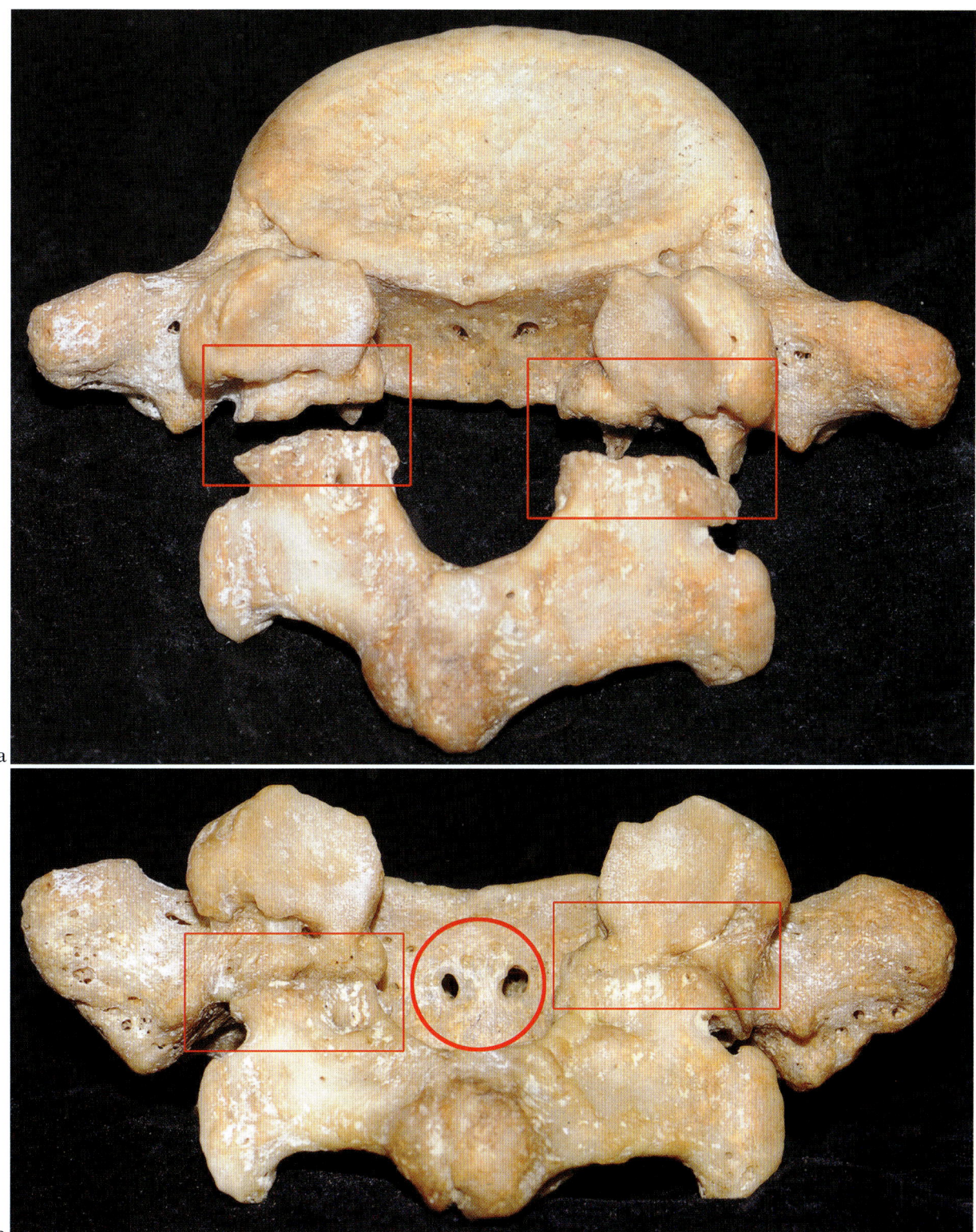

Figure 853a-b. Separate neural arch (spondylolysis, rectangles) in the fifth lumbar vertebra showing disarticulation of the arch and nutrient canals (circle) in the centrum.

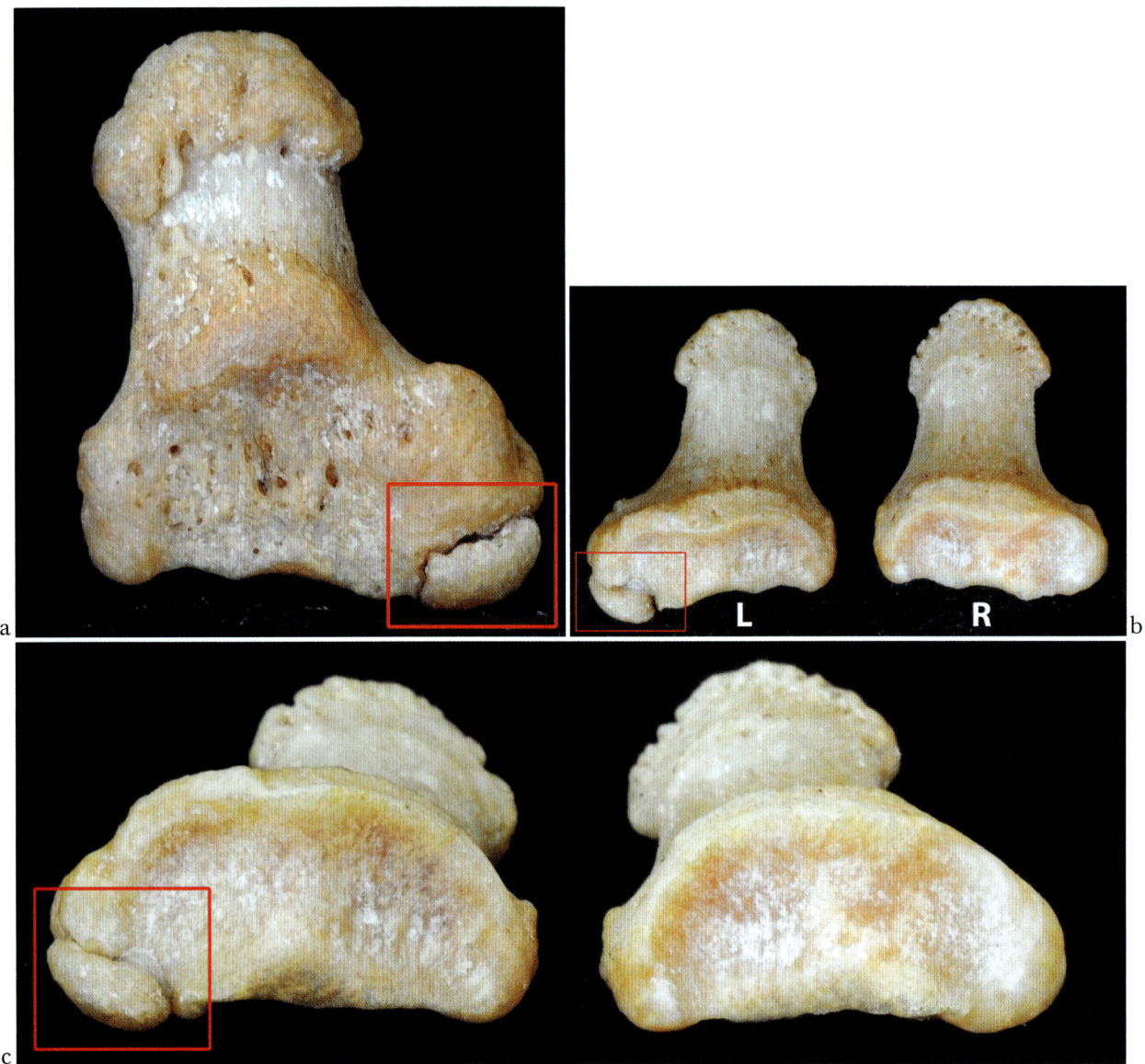

Figure 854a-c. Accessory ossicle or bipartite foot phalanx. (a) Plantar view of the separate ossicle (square) along the lateral surface of the left first foot phalanx. (b and c) Two views are demonstrated of this unilateral trait (squares) present only in the left phalanx. Rare finding.

APPENDIX: NON-METRIC TRAIT LIST

LIST OF FEATURES, TRAITS, ANATOMICAL VARIANTS AND SYNONYMS THAT AUTHORS HAVE IDENTIFIED AS NON-METRIC TRAITS IN THE HUMAN SKELETON

Non-metric Trait (as written)	Reference
Accessory apertures in the ramus (mandible)	Hauser and DeStefano 1989
Accessory foramen spinosum	Corruccini 1974
Accessory infrorbital foramen	Perizonius 1979
Accessory lesser palatine foramen	Perizonius 1979
Accessory mental foramen	Reed 2006
Accessory optic canal	Ossenberg et al. 2006
Accessory sacral facet present	Finnegan 1978
Accessory transverse foramina in cervical vertebrae	Rose et al. 1991
Acetabular crease	Anderson 1991; Finnegan 1978
Acetabular pit	Pietrusewsky 2002
Acromial articular facet present	Finnegan 1978
Acromion shape triangle	Pietrusewsky 2002
Alveolar prognathism	Gill 1998; Weinberg et al. 2005; L'Abeé et al. 2011
Anterior calcaneal facet absent	Finnegan 1978
Anterior ethmoid foramen exsutural	Perizonius 1979; Sutter and Mertz 2004; Reed 2006
Anterior and middle calcaneal facets (divided)	Bidmos 2006
Anterior Nasal Spine	Chunn 2008; Weinberg et al. 2005
Apertures in the tympanic plate	Hauser and DeStefano 1989
Apical bone	Buikstra and Ubelaker 1994
Ascending Ramus	Chunn 2008
Ascending ramus angle	Rhine 1990
Asterionic bone	Buikstra and Ubelaker 1994
Atlas bridging	Hauser and DeStefano 1989
Atlas bridging lateral	Rose et al. 1991
Atlas bridging posterior	Rose et al. 1991
Atlas double condylar facet	Anderson 1991
Double atlas facet	Veldman 2013
Atlas transverse foramen bipartite	Buikstra and Ubelaker 1994
Auditory exostosis (Aural exostosis; Dodo 1986)	Perizonius 1979; Rose et al. 1991; Buikstra and Ubelaker 1994; Ubelaker 1997
Auditory torus	Hauser and DeStefano 1989; Brasili et al. 1999

Note: This list does not include all non-metric traits in the literature.

Basal sphenoid bridges	Hauser and DeStefano 1989
Base angle	Rhine 1990
Biasterionic sutures	Hauser and DeStefano 1989
Bifaceted condyles	Corruccini 1974
Bipartite patella	Finnegan 1978
Bregmatic bone	Buikstra and Ubelaker 1994
Double calcaneal facet	Veldman 2013
Canine fossa	Rhine 1990
Chin prominence	Vitec 2012
Circumflex sulcus present	Finnegan 1978
Clinoid bridge (sellar bridge)	Saunders and Popovich 1978
Condylar canal	Rose et al. 1991; Buikstra and Ubelaker 1994; Hallgrimsson et al. 2005
Condylar canal patent	Dodo 1986
Condylar facet double	Hauser and DeStefano 1989; Perizonius 1979
Condylus tertius	Dodo 1974
Coronal ossicle	Buikstra and Ubelaker 1994
Cranial sutures	Gill 1998
Craniopharyngeal canal	Hauser and DeStefano 1989
Cribra orbitale	Khudaverdyan 2012
Depression at Nasion	Rhine 1990
Digastric groove	Finnegan and Ery 2000
Digastric fossa	Larnach and Macintosh 1966
Divided hypoglossal canal	Rose et al. 1991; Buikstra and Ubelaker 1994
Divided mastoid (sutura mastoideosquamosa)	Sternberg 1975
Divided parietal bone	Hauser and DeStefano 1989
Double hypoglossal canal	Spoilheap
Emarginate patella present	Finnegan 1978
Epipteric bone (pterionic ossicle, Wood 2012)	Buikstra and Ubelaker 1994; Hauser and DeStefano 1989
Epiteric bone	Sudha et al. 2013
Ethmoidal foramina	Hauser and DeStefano 1989
Exostosis in trochanteric fossa	Finnegan 1978
External occipital protuberance	Weinberg et al. 2005
Eye Orbit Shape	Chunn 2008
Facial prognathism	Gill 1998
Femoral bowing	Pietrusewsky 2002
Flexure of the sagittal sulcus	Buikstra and Ubelaker 1994
Foramen nasale	Perizonius 1979
Foramen of Huschke	Reed 2006

Foramen of Vesalius	Corruccini 1974; Hauser and DeStefano 1989; Rose et al. 1991
Foramen ovale incomplete	Perizonius 1979; Rose et al. 1991
Foramen pteryo-spinosum (pterygospinous)	MacCurdy 1914
Foramen spinosum incomplete	Rose et al. 1991
Foramen spinosum open	Perizonius 1979; Brasili et al. 1999
Foramen supraorbitalis	Perizonius 1979
Foramen zygomatico-faciale double	Perizonius 1979
Foramen zygomatico-faciale exsutural	Perizonius 1979
Foramen zygomatico-faciale absent	Perizonius 1979
Foramen zygomatico-orbitale	Perizonius 1979
Fossa faringea	Reed 2006
Fossa of Allen	Pietrusewsky 2002
Fovea capitis oval	Pietrusewsky 2002
Frontal foramen open	Reed 2006
Frontal groove(s)	Reed 2006; Hauser and DeStefano 1989; Perizonius 1979
Frontal notch or groove present	Larnach 1974
Frontal sinus	Hauser and DeStefano 1989
Fronto-temporal articulation	Hauser and DeStefano 1989; Perizonius 1979
Genial tubercles, median mental spine and genial pit	Hauser and DeStefano 1989
Glabella projection	Hefner 2007
Greater sciatic notch	Lavallo 2013
Highest nuchal line	Larnach 1974; Reed 2006; Hauser and DeStefano 1989; Perizonius 1979
Hyoid	Reed 2006
Hyoid Accessory	Reed 2006
Hypoglossal canal	Hauser and DeStefano 1989
Hypoglossal canal bridging	Perizonius 1979
Hypotrochanteric fossa	Finnegan 1978
Inca bone	Buikstra and Ubelaker 1994; Hauser and DeStefano 1989
Inca ossicle	Reed 2006
Incisor form	Gill 1998
Incisor shoveling	Rhine 1990
Incomplete foramen ovale	Buikstra and Ubelaker 1994
Incomplete foramen spinosum	Buikstra and Ubelaker 1994
Inferior talar articular surface	Finnegan 1978
Infraorbital foramen	Hauser and DeStefano 1989
Infraorbital suture	Hauser and DeStefano 1989; Perizonius 1979; Buikstra and Ubelaker 1994
Infraparietal foramen	Wood 2012

Inion hook	Rhine 1990; Hefner 2007; Vitec 2012
Inion salience	Corruccini 1974
Intermediate condylar canal	Hauser and DeStefano 1989
Interorbital Breadth	Chunn 2008; L'Abeé et al. 2011; Vitec 2012
Interorbital projection	Gill 1998
Interparietal division	Weinberg et al. 2005
Ischiopubic ramus ridge	Lavallo 2013
Jugular foremen bridging	Hauser and DeStefano 1989
Keeling	Arizona State Museum (Nonmetric Recording Form) (06/2011)
Lambdoidal ossicle	Buikstra and Ubelaker 1994
Lateral bridge present	Finnegan 1978
Lateral tibial exension present	Finnegan 1978
Lateral tibial squatting facet	Finnegan 1978
Lateral pterygoid perforation	Corruccini 1974
Lesser palatine foramina	Hauser and DeStefano 1989
Malar tubercle	Sternberg 1975
Malar form	Gill 1998
Mandible	Gill 1998
Mandibular torus	Corruccini 1974; Reed 2006; Hauser and DeStefano 1989; Rose et al. 1991
Manubrio-corpal synostosis	Barnes 1994
Marginal foramen of tympanic plate	Ossenberg et al. 2006
Marginal tubercle	Hauser and DeStefano 1989
Mastoid foramen	Buikstra and Ubelaker 1994; Hauser and DeStefano 1989
Mastoid foramen exsutural	Reed 2006
Mastoid foramen location	Rose et al. 1991
Mastoid foramen number	Rose et al. 1991
Mastoid form	Gill 1998
Maxillary prognathism	Rhine 1990
Maxillary sinus	Hauser and DeStefano 1989
Maxillary third molar	Perizonius 1979
Maxillary tori	Anderson 1991
Maxillary torus	Hauser and DeStefano 1989
Medial palatine canal	Hauser and DeStefano 1989
Medial talar facet present	Finnegan 1978
Medial tibial squatting facet	Finnegan 1978
Median basilar canal	Hauser and DeStefano 1989
Mendosal suture status	Weinberg et al. 2005
Mental foramen	Hallgrimsson et al. 2005; Hauser and DeStefano 1989; Rose et al. 1991

Appendix: Non-metric Trait List

Mental spine	Veldman 2013
Metopic fissure	Hauser and DeStefano 1989
Metopic suture	Hauser and DeStefano 1989
Metopism	Rhine 1990
Middle meningeal artery emissaries	Hauser and DeStefano 1989
Molar crenulations	Rhine 1990
Multiple infraorbital foramina	Hallgrimsson et al. 2005; Buikstra and Ubelaker 1994
Muscle Marks	Chunn 2008
Mylohyoid bridge	Buikstra and Ubelaker 1994; Hauser and DeStefano 1989
Mylohyoid bridge degree	Rose et al. 1991
Mylohyoid bridge location	Hallgrimsson et al. 2005; Rose et al. 1991
Nasal Aperture Width	Chunn 2008; Vitec 2012
Nasal bone size	Gill 1998
Nasal bridge form	Gill 1998
Nasal cavities	Hauser and DeStefano 1989
Nasal foramina	Hauser and DeStefano 1989
Nasal overgrowth	Vitec 2012
Nasal profile	Gill 1998
Nasal sill	Gill 1998
Nasal sill sharp	Corruccinni 1974
Nasal spine	Gill 1998
Nose form	Gill 1998
Occipital condyle double	Reed 2006
Occipital foramen	Hauser and DeStefano 1989
Occipital squamous convexity	Weinberg et al. 2005
Occipital squamous shape	Weinberg et al. 2005
Occipital third facet	Reed 2006
Occipital mastoid-wormians	Perizonius 1979
Occipitomastoid ossicle	Buikstra and Ubelaker 1994
Occipital protuberance	Hefner 2007; Vitec 2012
Open foramen spinosum	Corruccini 1974
Orbital form	Gill 1998; Hefner 2007; Vitec 2012
Orbital opening	Hauser and DeStefano 1989
Orbital osteoporosis	Corruccini 1974
Os acromiale	Veldman 2013
Os japonicum (Os Japon)	Reed 2006; Hauser and DeStefano 1989; Sutter and Mertz 2004
Os zygomaticum duplex	MacCurdy 1914
Os japonicum trace	Corruccini 1974; Perizonius 1979

Os trigonum present	Finnegan 1978
Ossicle at asterion and occipitomastoid wormians	Hauser and DeStefano 1989
Ossicle in occipito-mastoid suture	Rose et al. 1991
Oval window	Rhine 1990
Ovale-spinosum continuous	Corrccini 1974
Palatal form	Gill 1998; Weinberg et al. 2005
Palatine bridge	Reed 2006
Palatine bridging	Hauser and DeStefano 1989
Palatine suture	Gill 1998
Palatine torus	Corruccinni 1974; Hauser and DeStefano 1989; Hallgrimsson et al. 2005
Paracondylar process	Anderson 1991; Heard 2008; Hauser and DeStefano 1989
Paramastoid process	Sutter and Mertz 2004
Parietal foramen	Hauser and DeStefano 1989
Parietal foramen absent	Brasili et al. 1999
Parietal notch	Buikstra and Ubelaker 1994
Parietal notch bone	Hauser and DeStefano 1989; Perizonius 1979
Parietal process of the temporal squama	Hauser and DeStefano 1989; Ubelaker 1997
Parietal notch ossicle	Reed 2006
Partitioned temporal squama	Hauser and DeStefano 1989
Peroneal tubercle	Pietrusewsky 2002
Petrosquamous emissaries	Hauser and DeStefano 1989
Pharyngeal foveola	Hauser and DeStefano 1989
Pharyngeal tubercle	Hauser and DeStefano 1989
Plaque (femur)	Finnegan 1978
Porier's facet	Finnegan 1978
Post-bregmatic Depression	Chunn 2008
Post-condylar canal	Anderson 1991
Postcondylar tubercle	Corruccini 1974
Posterior bridge present	Finnegan 1978
Posterior ethmoid foramen absent	Perizonius 1979
Posterior ethmoid foramen exsutural	Reed 2006
Pre-auricular sulcus present	Finnegan 1978
Preauricular surface	Lavallo 2013
Precondylar tubercle	Reed 2006; Hauser and DeStefano 1989; Perizonius 1979
Processus marginalis	Perizonius 1979
Process of Kerckring	Weinberg et al. 2005
Prognathism	Vitec 2012
Protostylid of Lower Molars	Scott and Turner 1997; Wilson 2010

Appendix: Non-metric Trait List

Pterion form	Sutter and Mertz 2004
Pterygo-alar bridge	Rose et al. 1991; Hallgrimsson et al. 2005
Pterygo-basal bridge	Heard 2008; Perizonius 1979
Pterygoid spurs	Corruccini 1974
Pterygolar bridge	Buikstra and Ubelaker 1994
Pterygospinous bridge	Buikstra and Ubelaker 1994
Pterygo-spinous bridge	Perizonius 1979; Rose et al. 1991
Pterion X or K	Corruccini 1974
Ramus inversion (mandible)	Parr 2005
Retromastoid process	Hauser and DeStefano 1989
Retromolar foramen	Ossenberg 1987; von Arx et al. 2011; Rossi et al. 2012
Retropterygoid apertures in the greater wing	Hauser and DeStefano 1989
Robusticity of muscle attachment sites (mandible)	Parr 2005
Rocker (and non-rocker) jaw	Snow 1974
Sacralization of L6	Veldman 2013
Sagittal ossicle	Buikstra and Ubelaker 1994
Sella bridges	Hauser and DeStefano 1989
Septal aperture	Pietrusewsky 2002
Sternal aperture (foramen)	Veldman 2013
Squamomastoid suture	Hauser and DeStefano 1989
Squamous ossicles	Hauser and DeStefano 1989
Squamous-parietal ossicle	Reed 2006
Squatting facet (tibia, talus)	Pietrusewsky 2002
Sulcus supraorbitalis	Perizonius 1969
Sub-asterionic ossicle	Corruccini 1974
Subpubic concavity	Lavallo 2013
Subnasal margin definition	Weinberg et al. 2005
Superior sagittal sinus turns left	Rogers 2008
Supernumerary ossicles (category)	Heard 2008
Supernumerary rib on C7	Veldman 2013
Supra-acetabular fossa and groove	Frayer 1987
Supraclavicular foramen	Pietrusewsky 2002
Suprameatal spine and depression	Hauser and DeStefano 1989
Supranasal suture	Hauser and DeStefano 1989
Supraorbital foramen	Buikstra and Ubelaker 1994
Supraorbital nerve groove	Heard 2008
Supraorbital notch	Buikstra and Ubelaker 1994
Supraorbital osseous structures	Hauser and DeStefano 1989
Supratrochlear foramen	Perizonius 1979

Suprascapular notch	Pietrusewsky 2002
Sutures of the cranial vault	Hauser and DeStefano 1989
Suture complexity	Vitec 2012
Symmetrical thinness of the parietal bones	Hauser and DeStefano 1989; Phillips 2007
Talus squatting facet	Museum of London Code Expansions (LAARC 2007)
Taurodontism	Scott and Turner 1997; Wilson 2010
Temporal squamous shape	Weinberg et al. 2005
Third trochanter	Pietrusewsky 2002
Third occipital condyle	Dodo 1986
Tibia medial squatting facet	Museum of London Code Expansions (LAARC 2007)
Tibial bowing	Pietrusewsky 2002
Tibial squatting facets	Spoilheap Anderson 1991
Torus auditivi	Museum of London Code Expansions (LAARC 2007)
Torus auditivus	Anderson 1991
Torus palatinus	Anderson 1991; Khudaverdyan 2012
Transverse foramen bipartite	Finnegan 1978
Transverse palatine suture (shape)	Hauser and DeStefano 1989; L'Abeé et al. 2011
Transverse zygomatic suture vestige	Hanihara et al. 2012; Wood 2012
Trochlear spine (spur)	Hauser and DeStefano 1989; Veldman 2013
Tympanic dehiscence	Rose et al. 1991; Buikstra and Ubelaker 1994
Tympanic thickening (os tympanicum hyperostosis)	Oetteking 1930
Undulating lower border of mandible	Rhine 1990
Uto-Aztecan Upper Premolar	Scott and Turner 1997; Wilson 2010
Vastus facet	Pietrusewsky 2002
Vastus notch	Pietrusewsky 2002
Vault Sutures	Chunn 2008
Vomer shape	Weinberg et al. 2005
Venous markings	Rhine 1990
Ventral arc	Lavallo 2013
Wormian bones	Rhine 1990
Wormian osPtericum	Shivarama and Kumar 2015
Zygomatic foramen	Reed 2006
Zygomatico-facial foramen	Rose et al. 1991; Hallgrimsson et al. 2005; Hauser and DeStefano 1989
Zygomaticomaxillary foramina	Buikstra and Ubelaker 1994
Zygomaticomaxillary suture	Gill 1998
Zygomaxillary tubercle	Hauser and DeStefano 1989
Zygomaxillary tuberosity	Sutter and Mertz 2004

REFERENCES

Abd Latiff, A., Das, S., Sulaiman, I. M., Hlaing, K. P., Suhaimi, F. H., Ghazalli, H. and Othman, F. The accessory foramen ovale of the skull: An osteological study. *Clinica Terapeutica* 160(4):291–293, 2009.

Abed, S. F., Shams, P., Shen, S., Adds, P. J. and Uddin, J. M. A cadaveric study of ethmoidal foramina variation and its surgical significance in Caucasians. *British Journal of Opthalmology* published online March 22, 2011doi:10.1136/bjo.2010.197319 (accessed online October 4, 2011).

Adams, W. M., Jones, R. LO., Chavda, S. V. and Pahor, A. L. CT assessment of jugular foramen dominance and its association with hand preference. *The Journal of Laryngology & Otology* 111(3):290–292, 1997.

Aggarwal, B., Gupta, M. and Kumar, H. Ossified ligaments of the skull. *Journal of Anatomical Society of India* 61(1):37–40, 2012.

Agrawal, R., Ananthi, S. and Agrawal, S. Anomalies of the craniovertebral junction – a very rare case report. *European Journal of Anatomy* 14(1):43–47, 2010.

Agrawal, R., Ananthi, S. K., Agrawal, S. and Usha, K. Posterior arch of atlas with abnormal foramina in South Indians. *Journal of Anatomical Society of India* 61(1):30–32, 2012.

Aksu, F., Ceri, N. G., Arman, C., Zeybek, F. G. and Tetik, S. Location and incidence of the zygomaticofacial foramen: An anatomic study. *Clinical Anatomy* 22:559–562, 2009.

Allen, H. *A System of Human Anatomy Including its Medical and SurgicalRelations. Section II – Bones and Joints.* Lee, Philadelphia, 1882.

Allen, W. A. On the varieties of the atlas in the human subject, and the homologies of its transverse processes. *Journal of Anatomy and Physiology* 14(1):18–27, 1879.

Allen, W. On tertiary occipital condyle. *Journal of Anatomy and Physiology* 15(1):60–68, 1880.

Al-Motabagani, M. A. and Surendra, M. Total occipitalization of the atlas. *Anatomical Science International* 81(3):173–180, 2006.

Alsherhri, H., Alqahtani, B. and M Alqahtani, M. Dilated petrosquamosal sinus, mastoid emissary vein, and external jugular vein: A rare cause of pulsatile tinnitus, vertigo, and sensorineural hearing loss. *Indian Journal of Otology* 17(3):123–126, 2011.

Altug-Atac, A. T. and Erdem, D. Prevalence and distribution of dental anomalies in orthodontic patients. *American Journal of Orthodontics and Dentofacial Orthopedics* 131:510–514, 2007.

Amorim, M. M., Prado, F. B., Borini, C. B., Bittar, T. O., Volpato, M. C., Groppo, F. C. and Caria, P. H. F. The mental foramen position in dentate and edentulous Brazilian's mandible. *International Journal of Morphology* 26(4):981–987, 2008.

Anderson, S. *A Comparative Study of the Human Skeletal Material from Late First and Early Second Millennium Sites in the North-East of England.* Unpublished Thesis, University of Durham, 1991.

Anderson, L. C., Kosinski, T. F. and Mentag, P. J. A review of the intraosseous course of the nerves of the mandible. *Journal of Oral Implantology* 17(4):394–403, 1991.

Anderson, T. A medieval hypoplastic dens: A note on its discovery and a review of the previous literature. *OSSA* 2(6):13–37, 1987.

Anderson, T. Basilar clefting: A familial condition? *Annals of Anatomy* 182(6):583–587, 2000.

Anton, S. C. Intentional cranial vault deformation and induced changes of the cranial base and face. *American Journal of Physical Anthropology* 79:253–267, 1989.

Anton, S. C., Jaslow, C. R. and Swartz, S. M. Sutural complexity in artificially deformed human (Homo sapiens) crania. *Journal of Morphology* 214(3):321–332, 1992.

Antonopoulou, M., Piagou, M. and Anagnostopoulou, S. An anatomical study of the pterygospinous and pterygoalar bars and foramina. *Journal of Cranio-Maxillofacial Surgery* 36:104–108, 2008.

Apinhasmit, W., Chompoopong, S., Methathrathip, D., Sansuk, R. and Phetphunphiphat, W. Supraorbital notch/foramen, infraorbital foramen and mental foramen in Thais: Anthropometric measurements and surgical relevance. *Journal of the Medical Association of Thailand* 89(5):675–682, 2006.

Arey, L. B. *Developmental Anatomy: A Textbook and Laboratory Manual of Embryology*, Fourth Edition. W. B. Saunders Co., Philadelphia, 1946.

Ari, I., Oygucu, I. H. and Sendemir, E. The squatting facets on the tibia of Byzantine (13th) skeletons. *European Journal of Anatomy* 7(3):143–146, 2003.

Asala, S. A. and Mbajiorgu, F. E. Epigenetic variation in the Nigerian skull: Sutural pattern at the pterion. *East African Medical Journal* 73(7):484–486, 1996.

Ashley, G. T. The relationship between the pattern of ossification and the definitive shape of the mesosternum in man. *Journal of Anatomy* 90:87–105, 1956.

Ashley-Montagu, M. F. Medio-palatine bones. *American Journal of Physical Anthropology* 27(1):139–150, 1940.

Ashwini, L. S., Mohandas Rao, K. G., Saran, S. and Somayaji, S. N. Morphological and morphometric analysis of supraorbital foramen and supraorbital notch: A study on dry human skulls. *Oman Medical Journal* 27:129–133, 2012.

Aydinhoglu, A., Kavakh, A., and Erdem, S. Absence of frontal sinus in Turkish individuals. *Yonsei Medical Journal* 44(2):215–218, 2003.

Babu, K. Y., Sivanandan, R. and Saraswathy, P. Incidence of foramen meningo – Orbitale in South Indian population. *Recent Research in Science and Technology* 3(10):43–44, 2011.

Baert, A. L., Knauth, M. and Sartor, K. *Dural Cavernous Sinus Fistulas: Diagnosis and Endovascular Therapy.* Springer-Verlag, Berlin, 2010.

Bajaj, M., Jangid, H., Vats, A. K. and Meena M. L. Case report: Congenital absence of the dens. *Indian Journal of Radiology and Imaging* 20:109–111, 2010.

Baker, B. J., Dupras, T. L. and Tochieri, M. W. *The Osteology of Infants and Children*. Texas A&M University anthropology series; No. 12, College Station, 2005.

Balcioglu, H. A. and Kocaelli, H. Accessory mental foramen. *North American Journal of Medical Sciences* 1(6):314–315, 2009.

Barber, G., Shepstone, L. and Rogers, J. A methodology for estimating age at death using arachnoid granulation counts. *American Journal of Physical Anthropology* 20(Suppl.): 61, 1995.

Barberini, F., Bruner, E., Cartolari, R., Franchitto, G., Heyn, R., Ricci, F. and Manzi, G. An unusually-wide human bregmatic Wormian bone: Anatomy, tomographic description, and possible significance. *Surgical and Radiologic Anatomy* 30(8):683–687, 2008.

Barclay-Smith, E. A rare condition of wormian ossifications. *Journal of Anatomy and Physiology* 43(3):277–278, 1909.

Barclay-Smith, E. Two cases of Wormian bones in the bregmatic fontanelle. *Journal of Anatomy and Physiology* 44(4):312–314, 1910.

Barner, B. C. W. and Lockett, B. C. Multiple canals in the rami of a mandible. *Oral Surgery* 34:384–389, 1972.

Barnes, E. *Developmental Defects of the Axial Skeleton in Paleopathology*. University Press of Colorado, Niwot, 1994.

Barnes, E. Congenital anomalies. In R. Pinhasi and S. Mays (Eds.), *Advances in Human Paleopathology*. John Wiley & Sons, Ltd, West Sussex, 2008.

Barnes, E. *Atlas of Developmental Field Anomalies of the Human Skeleton: A Paleopathology Perspective*. Wiley-Blackwell, Hoboken, 2012.

Barnett, C. H. Squatting facets on the European talus. *Journal of Anatomy and Physiology* 88(4):509–513, 1954.

Basmajian, J. V. *Primary Anatomy*. Williams and Wilkins, Baltimore, 1964.

Bast, T. H. and Anson, B. J. *The Temporal Bone and the Ear*. Charles C Thomas, Springfield, 1949.

Bauer, L. Beitrage Zur Kraniologie der Baining (Neu Pommern). *Archiv Fur Anthropologie*, N.F. Band 14:145–202, 1915.

Bayaroğulları H, Yengil, E., Davran, R., Ağlagül, E., Karazincir, S. and Balci, A. Evaluation of the postnatal development of the sternum and sternal variations using multidetector CT. *Diagnostic and Interventional Radiology* 20:82–89, 2014.

Bayrak, A. H., Akay, H. O., Ozmen, C. A. and Senturk, S. Arachnoid granulations: Frequency and distribution in multi-detector row CT of dural sinuses. *Biotechnology and Biotechnology Equipment* 23/2009/2:1255–1258, 2009.

Becker, D. B., Cheverud, J. M., Govier, D. P. and Kane, A. A. Os Parietale Divisum. *Clinical Anatomy* 18:452–456, 2005.

Beers, G. J., Carter, A. P. and McNary, W. F. Vertical foramina in the lumbosacral region: CT appearance. *American Journal of Radiology* 143:1027–1029, 1984.

Belsky, J. L., Hamer, J. S., Hubert, J. E., Insogna, K. and Johns, W. Torus palatinus: A new anatomical correlation with bone density in postmenopausal women. *Journal of Clinical Endocrinology and Metabolism* 88(5):2081–2086, 2003.

Bennett, E. H. On the ossicle occasionally found on the posterior border of the astragalus. *Journal of Anatomy and Physiology* 21(1):59–65, 1886.

Berge, J. K. and Bergman, R. A. Variations in size and in symmetry of foramina of the human skull. *Clinical Anatomy* 14:406–413, 2001.

Bernaerts, A., Vanhoenacker, F. M., Van dee Perre, S., Schepper, A. M. and Parizel, P. M. Accessory navicular bone: Not such a normal variant. *Belgian Journal of Radiology* (JBR-BTR) 85(5):250–252, 2004.

Berry, R. J. A case of os bipartitum in an Australian aborigine skull. *Journal of Anatomy and Physiology* 44:73–82, 1910.

Berry R., and Berry A. Epigenetic Variation in the human cranium. *Journal of Anatomy* 101(2):361–379, 1967.

Beutler, W. J., Fredrickson, B. E., Murtland, A., Sweeney, C. A., Grant, W. D. and Baker, D. The natural history of spondylolysis and spondylolisthesis: 45-year follow-up evaluation. *Spine* 28(10):1027–1035, 2003.

Bhanu, P. S. and Sankar, K. D. Interparietal and pre-parietal bones in the population of south coastal Andhra Pradesh, India. *Folia Morphologica* 70(3):185–190, 2011.

Bidmos, M. Metrical and non-metric assessment of population affinity from the calcaneus. *Forensic Science International* 159(1):6–13, 2006.

Billmann, F., Le Minor, J-M. and Steinwachs, M. Bipartation of the superior articular facets of the first cervical vertebra (atlas or C1): A human variant probably specific among primates. *Annals of Anatomy-Anatomischer Anzeiger* 189(1): 79–85, 2007.

Birkby W., Fenton, T. and Anderson, B. Identifying Southwest Hispanics using nonmetric traits and the cultural profile. *Journal of Forensic Sciences* 53:29–33, 2008.

Bolanowski, W., Śmiszkiewicz-Skwarska, A., Polguj, M., and Jędrzejewski, K. S. The occurrence of the third trochanter and its correlation to certain anthropometric parameters of the human femur. *Folia Morphologica* 64(3): 168–175, 2005.

Bolk, L. On Metopism. *American Journal of Anatomy* 22(1):27–47, 1917.

Bongiovanni R., and Spradley, M. K. Estimating sex of the human skeleton based on metrics of the sternum. *Forensic Science International* 2012 Jun 10:219(1–3):290.e1-7. doi: 10.1016/j.forsciint.2011.11.034. Epub 2011 Dec 29. Accessed on-line January 2, 2013.

Bono, C. M. Low-back pain in athletes. *Journal of Bone and Joint Surgery* 86-A(2):382–396, 2004.

Boopathi, S., Chakravarthy, M. S., Dhalapahty, S. and Anupa, S. Anthropometric analysis of the infraorbital foramen in a South Indian population. *Singapore Medical Journal* 51(9):730–735, 2010.

Borah, D., Wadhwa, S., Singh, U. and Gupta, A. K. Symphalangism in an Indian family. *Indian Journal of Physical Medicine and Rehabilitation* 17(1):18–20, 2006.

Bots, J., Wijnaendts, L. C. D., Delen, S., Van Dongen, S., Heikinheimo, K. and Galis, F. Analysis of cervical ribs in a series of human fetuses. *Journal of Anatomy* 219(3):403–409, 2011.

Boyd, G. I. The emissary foramina of the cranium in man and the anthropoids. *Journal of Anatomy and Physiology* 65(1):1–121, 1930.

Brash, J. C. (editor). *Cunningham's Textbook of Anatomy*, Ninth Edition. Oxford University Press, London, 1953.

Brasili, P., Azccagni, L. and Gualdi-Russo, E. Scoring of nonmetric cranial traits: A population study. *Journal of Anatomy* 195:551–562, 1999.

Breathnach, A. S. *Frazer's Anatomy of the Human Skeleton*, Sixth Edition. J. & A. Churchill, London, 1965.

Bressan, C., Guena, S., Malerba, G., Giacobini, G., Giordano, M., Robecchi, M. G. and Vercellino, V. Descriptive and topographic anatomy of the accessory infraorbital foramen. Clinical implications in maxillary surgery. *Minerva Stomatologica* 53(9):495–505, 2004.

Brewin, J., Hill, M. and Ellis, H. The prevalence of cervical ribs in a London population. *Clinical Anatomy* 22(3):331–336, 2009.

Broman, G. E., Jr. Precondylar tubercles in American Whites and Negroes. *American Journal of Physical Anthropology* 15(1):125–136, 1957.

Brothwell D. R. *Digging Up Bones: The Excavation, Treatment, and Study of Human Skeletal Remains.* Cornell University Press, 1981.

Bryce, T. H. Observations on metopism. *Journal of Anatomy and Physiology* 51(2):153–166, 1917.

Buikstra, J. E. and Ubelaker, D. (Eds.). Standards for Data Collection from Human Skeletal Remains. Research Series, no. 44. Arkansas Archaeological Survey Press, Fayetteville, 1994.

Bunning, P. S. C. Some observations on the West African calcaneus and the associated talo-calcaneal interosseous ligamentous apparatus. *American Journal of Physical Anthropology* 22(4):467–472, 1964.

Bunning, P. S. C. and Barnett, C. H. A comparison of adult and foetal talocalacaneal articulations. *Journal of Anatomy* (London) 99(1):71–76, 1965.

Burdan, F., Umlawska, W., Dworzanski, W., Klepacz, R., Szumilo, J., Staroslawska E., and Drop, A. Anatomical variances and dimensions of the superior orbital fissure and foramen ovale in adults. *Folia Morphologica* (Warsz) 70(4):263–271, 2011.

Burgenen, F. A. and Kormano, M. *Differential Diagnosis in Chest X-rays*. Thieme, Stuttgart, 1997.

Butler, H. The development of certain human dural venous sinuses. *Journal of Anatomy* 91:510–526, 1957.

Butler, H. The development of mammalian dural venous sinuses with special reference to the post-glenoid foramen. *Journal of Anatomy* 102:33–52, 1967.

Caesar, R. H. and McNab, A. A. External dacryocystorhinostomy and local anesthesia: Technique to measure minimized blood loss. *Ophthalmic Plastic and Reconstructive Surgery* 20(1):57–59, 2004.

Campbell, J. A. Note of a case of abnormal union of several of the ribs. *Journal of Anatomy and Physiology* 4(20):245–246, 1870.

Canan, S., Asim, O. M., Okan, B., Ozek, C., and Alper, M. Anatomic variations of the infraorbital foramen. *Annals of Plastic Surgery* 43(6):613–617, 1999.

Cankal, F., Ugur, H. C., Tekdemir, I., Elhan, A. Karahan, T. and Sevim, A. Fossa navicularis: Anatomic variation at the skull base. *Clinical Anatomy* 17:118–122, 2004.

Carwardine, T. The suprasternal bones in man. *American Journal of Anatomy and Physiology* 27:231–234, 1893.

Case, D. T., Burnett, S. E. and Nielsen, T. Os aromiale: Population differences and their etiological significance. *HOMO* 57(1):1–18, 2006.

Case, D. T. and Heilman, J. Pedal symphalangism in modern American and Japanese skeletons. *Homo* 55(3):251–262, 2005.

Cave, A. J. E. The nature and morphology of the costoclavicular ligament. *Journal of Anatomy* 170–179, 1961.

Cave, A. J. E. The morphology of the mammalian cervical pleurapophysis. *Journal of Zoology* 177:377–393, 1975.

Cederberg, R. A., Benson, B. W., Nunn, M. and English, J. D. Calcification of the interclinoid and petroclinoid ligaments of sella turcica: A radiographic study of the prevalence. *Orthodontics and Craniofacial Research* 6(4):227–232, 2003.

Cederlund, C.-G., Andrén, L. and Olivecrona, H. Progressive bilateral thinning of the parietal bones. *Skeletal Radiology* 8:29–33, 1982.

Chaisuksunt, V., Kwathai, L., Namonta, K., Rungruang, T., Apinhasmit and Chompoopong, S. Occurrence of the Foramen of Vesalius and its morphometry relevant to clinical consideration. *The Scientific World Journal* Volume 2012, Article ID 817454, doi:10.1100/2012/817454 accessed online.reymond

Chauhan, N. S., Sharma, Y. P., Bhagra, T. and Sud, B. Persistence of multiple emissary veins of posterior fossa with unusual origin of left petrosquamosal sinus from mastoid emissary. *Surgical and Radiologic Anatomy* May 21, 2011. DOI 10.1007/00276-011-0822-x.

Cheatle, A. H. The petro-squamous sinus: Its anatomy and pathological importance. *Transactions of the 6th International Otological Conference* 160–170, 1899.

Chell, J. The squamoso-petrous sinus: A fetal remnant. *Journal of Anatomy* 175:269–271, 1991.

Cho, B. P. and Kang, H. S. Articular facets of the coracoclavicular joint in Koreans. *Acta Anat* (Basel) 163(1):56–62, 1998.

Choudhry, R., Anand, M., Choudhry, S., Tuli, A., Meenakshi, A. and Kalra, A. Morphologic and imaging studies of duplicate optic canals in dry adult human skulls. *Surgical and Radiologic Anatomy* 21:20201–20205, 1999.

Choudhry, R., Choudhry, S. and Anand, C. Duplication of optic canals in human skulls. *Journal of Anatomy and Physiology* 159:113–116, 1988.

Choudhry, S., Kalra, S., Choudhry, R., Choudhry, R., Tuli, A. and Kalra, N. Unusual features associated with cranial openings of optic canal in dry adult human skulls. *Surgical and Radiologic Anatomy* 27:455–458, 2005.

Chouke, K. S. On incidence of foramen of Civini and Porus crotaphitico – buccinatorius in American Whites and

Negroes I. *American Journal of Physical Anthropology* 4:203–225, 1946.

Chouke, K. S. On incidence of foramen of Civini and Porus crotaphitico – buccinatorius in American Whites and Negroes II. *American Journal of Physical Anthropology* 5:79–86, 1947.

Chouke, K. S. and Hodes, P. J. The pterygoalar bar and its recognition by Roentgen methods in Trigeminal neuralgia. *American Journal of Roentgenology* 65(2):180–182, 1951.

Chow, J. C. Y., Weiss, M. A. and Gu, Y. Anatomic variations of the hook of hamate and the relationship to carpal tunnel syndrome. *Journal of Hand Surgery* 30(6):1242–1247, 2005.

Christensen, A. M. The impact of Daubert: Implications for testimony and research in forensic anthropology (and the use of frontal sinuses in personal identification). *Journal of Forensic Sciences* 49(3):427–430, 2004.

Chung, M. S., Kim, H. J., Kang, H. S. and Chung, I. H. Locational relationship of the supraorbital notch or foramen and infraorbital and mental foramina in Koreans. *Acad Anat* (Basel) 154(2):162–166, 1995.

Chunn, B. L. *A Study of Non-metric Traits using the William M. Bass Donated Skeletal Collection.* University of Tennessee Honors Thesis Projects, 2008. Available on-line at http://trace.tennessee.edu/utk_chanhonoproj/1163

Church, A. The Neurology of Cervical Ribs. *The Journal of the American Medical Association* 73(1):1–4, 1919.

Clavelli, W. A., Romaris de Clavelli, S. S. and Jeanty, P. *The ultrasound detection of chromosomal anomalies.* Adapted from "The Ultrasound Detection of Chromosomal Anomalies – A multimedia Lecture" by Philippe Jeanty. ISBN (0-9667878-0-3) available at www.prenataldiagnosis.com and www.TheFetus.net, ND. Accessed online September 29, 2012.

Clegg, J. G. The optic foramen. *British Journal of Opthalmology* 20:667–673, 1936.

Cobb, W. M. The ossa suprasternalia in whites and American negroes and form of superior border of manubrium sterni. *Journal of Anatomy and Physiology* 71:245–291, 1937.

Cockshott, W. P. The coracoclavicular joint. *American Journal of Radiology* 131:313–316, 1979.

Cockshott, W. P. The geography of coracoclavicular joints. *Skeletal Radiology* 21:225–227, 1992.

Collins, H. B. The temporo-frontal articulation in man. *American Journal of Physical Anthropology* 9:343–348, 1926.

Cooper, P. D., Stewart, J. H., and McCormick, W. F. Development and morphology of the sternal foramen. *American Journal of Forensic Medicine and Pathology* 9(4):342–347, 1988.

Corner, E. M. The processes of the occipital and mastoid regions of the skull. *Journal of Anatomy and Physiology* 39(3):386–389, 1896.

Correll, R. W., Jensen, J. L., Taylor, J. B. and Rhyne, R. R. Mineralization of the stylohyoid-stylomandibular ligament complex: A radiographic incidence study. *Oral Surgery Oral Medicine Oral Pathology* 48:286–291, 1979.

Corruccini, R. S. An examination of meaning of cranial discrete traits for human skeletal biological studies. *American Journal of Physical Anthropology* 40:425–446, 1974.

Coskun, N., Yuksel, M., Cevener, M., Arican, R. Y., Ozdemir, H., Bircan, O., Sindel, T., Ilgi, S. and Sindel, M. Incidence of accessory ossicles and sesamoid bones in the feet: A radiographic study of the Turkish subjects. *Surgical and Radiologic Anatomy* 31(1):19–24, 2009.

Cousins, M. J., Carr, D. B., Horlacker, T. T. and Bridenbaugh, P.O. *Cousins & Bridenbaugh's Neural Blockade: In Clinical Anaesthesia and Pain Medicine,* 4th Edition. Philidelphia, 2009.

Cousins, M.J., Bridenbaugh, P.O., Carr, D.B., Horlocker,T.T. (eds) Cousins and Bridenbaugh's Neural Blockade in Clinical Anesthesia and Pain Medicine. Lippencott Williams & Wilkins, 2009.

Cox, M. and Scott, A. Evaluation of the obstetric significance of some pelvic characters in an 18th century British sample of known parity status. *American Journal of Physical Anthropology* 89(4):431–440, 1992.

Cukurova, I., Yaz, A., Gumussoy, M., Yigitbasi, O. G. and Karaman, Y. A patient presenting with concha bullosa in another concha bullosa: A case report. *Journal of Medical Case Reports* 6:87, 2012 doi:10.1186/1752-1947-6-87.

Cunningham, D. J. The connection of the os odontoideum with the body of the axis vertebra. *Journal of Anatomy and Physiology* 20(2):238–243, 1886.

Currarino, G. Normal variants and congenital anomalies in the region of the obelion. *American Journal of Roentgenology* 127:487–494, 1976.

Daimi, S. R., Siddiqui, A. U. and Gill, S. S. Analysis of foramen ovale with special emphasis on pterygoalar bar and pterygoalar foramen. *Folia Morphologica* 70(3):149–153, 2011.

Dauber, W. *Pocket Atlas of Human Anatomy,* Fifth Revised Edition. Georg Thieme Verlag, Stuttgart, 2007.

Davanzo, J., Samson, T., Tubbs, R. S. and Rizk, E. Bathrocephaly: A case report of a head shape associated with a persistent mendosal suture. *Italian Journal of Anatomy and Embryology* 119(3):263–267, 2014.

David, M. P. and Saxena, R. Use of frontal sinus and nasal septum patterns as an aid in personal identification: A digital radiographic pilot study. *Journal of Forensic Dental Sciences* 2(2):77–80, 2010.

de Freitas, V., Madeira, M. C., Toldeo Filho, J. L. and Chagas, C. F. Absence of the mental foramen in dry human mandibles. *Acta Anatomica (Basel)* 104(3):353–355, 1979.

de Graauw, N., Carpay, H. A. and Slooff, W. B. M. The paracondylar process: An unusual and treatable cause of posttraumatic headache. *Spine* 33(9):E283–E286, 2008.

Delashaw, J. B., Persing, J. A. and Jane, J. A. Cranial deformation in craniosynostosis: A new explanation. *Neurosurgery Clinics North America* 2(3):611–620, 1991.

Dereci, O. and Duran, S. Intraorally exposed anterior Stafne bone defect: A care report. *Oral Surgery Oral Medicine Oral Pathology and Oral Radiology* 113(5):e1-e3, 2012. Accessed online at http://dx.doi.org/10.1016/j.tripleo.2011.07.029 on 28 April 2012.

Derry, D. E. Note on the innominate bone as a factor in the determination of sex: with special reference to the sulcus preauricularis. *Journal of Anatomy and Physiology* 43:266–276, 1909.

Derry, D. E. Note on accessory articular facets between the sacrum and ilium, and their significance. *Journal of Anatomy* 45:204–210, 1911.

DeVilliers, H. *The Skull of the South African Negro: A Biomedical and Morphological Study.* Johannesburg: Witwatersrand University Press, 1968.

Dixon, A. F. On certain markings, due to nerves and blood-vessels, upon the cranial vault; their significance and the relative frequency of their occurrence in the different races of mankind. *Journal of Anatomy and Physiology* 38:25–398, 1904.

Dixon, A. F. Note on two cases of well-marked suprasternal bones. *Journal of Anatomy and Physiology* 48(3):219–221, 1914.

Dixon, A. F. *Dixon's Manual of Human Osteology*, Second Edition, revised by E. B. Jamieson. Oxford University Press, London, 1937.

Dodo, Y. Non-metrical cranial traits in the Hokkaido Ainu and the northern Japanese of recent times. *Journal of the Anthropological Society of Nippon* 82:31–51, 1974.

Dodo, Y. Metrical and non-metrical analyses of Jomon crania from eastern Japan. In T. Akazawa and C. M. Aikens (Eds.). *Prehistoric Hunter-gatherers in Japan.* The University Museum, The University of Tokyo, Bulletin No. 27, 1986, pp. 137–161.

Dorsey, G. A. Wormian bones in artificially deformed Kwakiutl crania. *The American Anthropologist* 10(6):169–173, 1897.

Duckworth, W. L. H. Note on an unusual anomaly in crania from the island of Kwaiawata, New Guinea. *Journal of Anatomy and Physiology* 41:1–5, 1906.

Dutton, J. J. *Atlas of Clinical and Surgical Orbital Anatomy*, Second Edition. Elsevier, 2011.

Dwight, T. A transverse foramen in the last lumbar vertebra. *Anatomischer Anzeiger* 20: 571–572, 1902.

Dwight, T. A bony supracondyloid oramen in man. *American Journal of Anatomy* 3:221–228, 1904.

Dwight, T. *Clinical Atlas: Variations of the Bones of the Hand and Foot.* J. B. Lippincott Company, Philadelphia, 1907.

Eagle, W. Elongated styloid process: Report of two cases. *Archives of Otolaryngology* 25:584–587, 1937.

Eagle, W. Elongated styloid process, further observations and a new syndrome. *Archives of Otolaryngology* 47:630–640, 1948.

Ehara, S., El-Khoury, G. Y. and Bergman, R. A. The accessory sacroiliac joint: A common anatomic variant. *American Journal of Roentgenology* 150:857–859, 1988.

Eisenstein, S. Spondylolysis: A skeletal investigation of two population groups. *Journal of Bone and Joint Surgery* 60(B):488–494, 1978.

Erdogmus, S., Pinar, Y. and Celik, S. A cause of entrapment of the lingual nerve: ossified pterygspinous ligament – a case report. *Neuroanatomy* 8:43–45, 2009.

Erken, E., Ozer, H. T. E., Gulek, B. and Durgun, B. The association between cervical rib and sacralization. *Spine* 27(15):1659–1664, 2002.

Erturk, M., Kayalioglu, G. and Govsa, F. Anatomy of the clinoidal region with special emphasis on the caroticoclinoid foramen and interclinoid osseous bridge in a recent Turkish population. *Neurosurgery Review* 27:22–26, 2004.

Erturk, M., Kayalioglu, G., Govsa, F., Varol, T. and Ozgur, T. The cranio-orbital foramen, the groove on the lateral wall of the human orbit, and the orbital branch of the middle meningeal artery. *Clinical Anatomy* 18(10):10–14, 2005.

Etter, L. E. Osseous abnormalities of the thoracic cage seen in forty thousand consecutive chest photoroentgenograms. *American Journal of Roentgenology and Radium Therapy* 51:359–363, 1944.

Fazekas, G. and Kosa, F. *Forensic Fetal Osteology.* Akademiai Kiado, Budapest, 1978.

Finnegan, M. Non-metric variation of the infracranial skeleton. *Journal of Anatomy* 125(1):23–37, 1978.

Finnegan, M. and Ery, K. Biological distance among six population samples excavated in the environs around Székesfehérvár, Hungary, as derived by non-metric trait variation. *Annales Historico-Naturales Musei Nationalis Hungarici*, Volume 92:455–476, Budapest, 2000.

Finnegan, M. and Marcsik A. Anomaly or pathology: The Stafne defect as seen in archaeological material and modern clinical practice. *Journal of Human Evolution* 9:19–31, 1980.

Finnegan, M. and Marcsik, A. The description and incidence of the Stafne idiopathic bone defect in six Avar period populations. *Acta Biological Szeged* 27:215–221, 1981.

Fisher, M. S. Eve's Rib (letter). *Radiology* 140:841, 1981.

Flecker, H. Observations upon cases of absence of lacrimal bones and of existence of perilacrimal ossicles. *Journal of Anatomy* 48(1):52–72, 1913.

Fortin, J. D. and Ballard, K. E. The frequency of accessory sacroiliac joints. *Clinical Anatomy* 22:876–877, 2009.

France D. L. *Sexual Dimorphism in the Human Humerus.* PhD dissertation, University of Colorado, Boulder, 1983.

Frayer, D. W. The supra-acetabular fossa and groove: A skeletal marker for Northwest European Mesolithic populations. *Human Evolution* 3(3):163–176, 1987.

Frazer, J. E. *The Anatomy of the Human Skeleton.* J & A Churchill, London, 1920.

Freire, A. R., Rossi, A. C., Prado, F. B., Caria, P. H. F. and Botacin, P. R. The caroticoclinoid foramen in the human skull and its clinical correlations. *International Journal of Anatomical Variations* 3:149–150, 2010.

Freire, A. R., Rossi, A. C., Prado, F. B., Groppo, F. C., Caria, P. H. F. and Botacin, P. R. Caroticoclinoid foramen in human skulls: Incidence, morphometry and its clinical implications. *International Journal of Morphology* 29(2): 427–431, 2011.

Freyschmidt, J. Brossman, J. Wiens, J. and Sternberg, A. *Freyschmidt's "Koehler/Zimmer" Borderlands of Normal and Early Pathological Findings in Skeletal Radiography*, Fifth Revised Edition. Georg Thieme Verlag, Stuttgart, 2002.

Galdames, I. S., Matamala, D. Z. and Luiz Smith, R. Anatomical study of the pterygospinous and pterygoalar bony bridges and foramens in dried crania and its clinical relevance. *International Journal of Morphology* 28(2):405–408, 2010.

Gallagher, E. R., Evans, K. N., Hing, A. V. and Cunningham, M. L. Bathrocephaly: A head shape associated with a persistent mendosal suture. *The Cleft Palate-Craniofacial Journal* 50(1):104–108, 2013. doi:10.1597/11-153. Epub 2011 Oct 4. Accessed online January 28, 2013.

Garcia-Garcia, A. S., Martinez-Gonzalez, J. M., Gomez-Font, R., Soto-Rivadeneira, A. and Oviedo-Roldan, L. Current status of the torus palatinus and torus mandibularis. *Medicina Oral Patologia Oral Y Cirugia Bucal* 1(15): e353-360, 2010 (accessed online www.medicinaoral.com on 27 December 2011).

Gayretli, O., Ali Gurses, I., Kale, A., Aksu, F., Ozturk, A., Bayraktar, B. and Sahinoglu, K. The mendosal suture. *British Journal of Neurosurgery*, Feb 23, 2011.

Geelhoed, G. W., Neel, J. V. and Davidson, R. T. Symphalangism and tarsal coalitions: A hereditary syndrome. *Journal of Bone and Joint Surgery* 51(B), No. 2:278–289, 1969.

Gershon-Cohen, J. and Delbridge, R. E. Pseudarthrosis, synchondrosis and other anomalies of the first ribs. *American Journal of Roentgenology and Radium Therapy* 53(1):49–54, 1945.

Ghai, R., Sinha, P., Rajguru, J. Jain, S., Khare, S. and Singla, M. Duplication of optic canals in human skulls. *Journal of Anatomical Society of India* 61(1):33–36, 2012.

Gill, G. W. Craniofacial Criteria in the Skeletal Attribution of Race. In K. J. Reichs (editor), *Forensic Osteology*. Charles C Thomas, Springfield, 1998.

Gill, G. W. and Rhine, S. (Eds.). *Skeletal Attribution of Race*. Anthropology Papers No. 4, Maxwell Museum of Anthropology, 1990.

Gilroy, A. M., MacPherson, B. R. and Ross, L. M. *Atlas of Anatomy*, Second Edition. Thieme Medical Publishers, New York, 2012.

Ginsberg, L. E. The Posterior Condylar Canal. *American Journal of Neuroradiology* 15:969–972, 1994.

Ginsberg, L. E., Pruett, S. W., Chen, M. Y. M. and Elster, A. D. Skull-base foramina of the middle cranial fossa: Reassessment of normal variation with high-resolution CT. *American Journal of Neuroradiology* 15:283–291, 1994.

Girdany, B. R. and Blank, E. Anterior fontanel bones. *American Journal of Radiology* 95(1):148–153, 1965.

Gladstone, R. J. and Erichsen-Powell, W. Manifestation of occipital vertebrae and fusion of the atlas with the occipital bone. *Journal of Anatomy and Physiology* 49(2):190–209, 1915.

Gladstone, R. J. and Wakeley, C. P. G. Variations of the occipito-atlantal joint in relation to the metameric structure of the cranio-vertebral region. *Journal of Anatomy and Physiology* 59(2):195–216, 1925.

Glassman, D. M. and Bass, W. M. Bilateral asymmetry of long arm bones and jugular foramen: implications for handedness. *Journal of Forensic Sciences* 31(2):589–595, 1986.

Gluncic, V., Lukic, I. K., Ivkic, G., Hat, J. and Marusic, A. Accessory foramen opticum, ovale, and spinosum. *Journal of Neurosurgery* 96:965, 2002.

Gopinathan, K. A rare anomaly of 5 ossicles in the pre-interparietal part of the squamous occipital bone in north Indians. *Journal of Anatomy* (Br) 180:201–202, 1992.

Gottlieb, K. Artificial cranial deformation and the increased complexity of the lambdoid suture. *American Journal of Physical Anthropology* 48(2):213–214, 1978.

Gözil, R., Yener, N., Çalguner, E., Araç, M., Tunç, E. and Bahcelioğlu, M. Morphological characteristics of styloid process evaluated by computerized axial tomography. *Annals of Anatomy* 183:527–535, 2001.

Graham, J. M., Jr. Skull. In Stevenson, R. G. and Hall J. G. (Eds.), *Human Malformations and Related Anomalies*, Second Edition. Oxford University Press, 2006.

Gray, H. *Anatomy Descriptive and Surgical*, Revised American, From the 15th English Edition. Originally published in 1901, Lea Brothers & Company, Philadelphia, 1901.

Green, H. L. H. H. An unusual case of atlanto-occipital fusion. *Journal of Anatomy and Physiology* 65(1):140–144, 1930.

Greene, M. H. and Hadied, A. M. Bipartite hamulus with ulnar tunnel syndrome – case report and literature review. *Journal of Hand Surgery* 6:605–609, 1981.

Greyling, L. M., Le Grange, F. and Meiring, J. H. Mandibular spine: A case report. *Clinical Anatomy* 10:416–418, 1997.

Grossman, C. B. and Potts, D. G. Arachnoid granulations: Radiology and anatomy. *Radiology* 113:95–100, 1974.

Gruber, W. In Bildungsanomalie mit Bildungshemmung begründete Bipartition beider Patellae eines jungen Subjectes. *Virchows Archives* 94:358–361, 1883.

Gülekon, I. N. and Turgut, H. B. The preauricular sulcus: Its radiologic evidence and prevalence. *Aibogaku Zasshi* 76(6):533–535, 2001.

Gumina, S., Salvatore, M., De Santis, P., Orsina, L. and Postacchini, F. Coracoclavicular joint: Osteologic study of 1020 human clavicles. *Journal of Anatomy* 201(6): 513–519, 2002.

Gunz, P. and Harvati, K. The Neanderthal "chignon": Variation, integration and homology. *Journal of Human Evolution* 52:262–274, 2007.

Gunz, P. and Harvati, K. Integration and Homology of "Chignon" and "Hemibun" Morphology, pp. 193–202. In S. Condemi and G.-C. Weniger (Eds.), *Continuity and Discontinuity in the Peopling of Europe: One Hundred Fifty Years of Neanderthal Study*. Vertebrate Paleobiology and Paleoanthropology, DOI 10.1007/978-94-007-0492-3_17, © Springer Science+Business Media B.V., 2011.

Gunzburg, R. and Szpalski, M. (Eds.). *Spondylolysis, Spondylolisthesis, and Degenerative Spondylolisthesis*. Lippincott, Williams & Wilkins, Philadelphia, 2005.

Gupta, S. C., Srivastava, A. K., Gupta, C. D. and Arora, A. K. Incidence of precondylar tubercle in crania of Uttar Pradesh. *Anthropologischer Anzeiger* 39(4):321–325, 1981.

Halpern, I. N. *A Comparative Analysis of Three Iroquoian Indian Populations Employing Non-Metrical Cranial Traits*. MA

Thesis, McMaster University, 1973.

Hallgrimmson, B., Donnabhain, B. O., Blom, D. E., Lozada, M. C. and Willmore, K. T. Why are rare traits unilaterally expressed? Trait frequency and unilateral expression for cranial nonmetric traits in humans. *American Journal of Physical Anthropology* 128:14–25, 2005.

Hanihara, T. and Ishida, H. Frequency variations of discrete cranial traits in major human populations. I. Supernumerary ossicle variations. *Journal of Anatomy* 198(6):689–706, 2001(a).

Hanihara, T. and Ishida, H. Frequency variations of discrete cranial traits in major human populations. IV. Vessel and nerve related variations. *Journal of Anatomy* 199(3): 273–287, 2001(b).

Hanihara, T. and Ishida, H. Os incae: variation in frequency in major human population groups. *Journal of Anatomy* 198(2):137–52, 2001(c).

Hanihara, T., Ishida, H., and Dodo, Y. Os zygomaticum bipartitum: Frequency distribution in major human populations. *Journal of Anatomy* 192:539–555, 1998.

Hanihara, T., Matsumura, H., Kawakubo, Y., Nguyen, L. C., Nguyen, K. T., Oxenham, M. F. and Dodo, Y. Population history of northern Vietnamese inferred from nonmetric cranial trait variation. *Anthropological Society of Nippon* published J-STAGE, published on line 9 February 2012. Accessed online at http://archanth.anu.edu.au/sites/default/files/documents/hanihara%20etal%202011.pdf on March 5, 2012.

Hart, B. L., Spar, J. A. and Orrison, W. W. Jr. Calcification of the trochlear apparatus of the orbit: CT Appearance and association with diabetes and age. *American Journal of Roentgenology* 159:1291–1294, 1992.

Hasan, M. and Pratap, P. *General Anatomy and Osteology of Head and Neck.* I. K. International Publishing House Pvt. Ltd., New Delhi, 2009.

Hasan, T., Fauzi, M. and Hasan, D. Bilateral absence of mental foramen – a rare variation. *International Journal of Anatomical Variations* 3:187–189, 2010.

Hassett, B. Torus Mandibularis: Etiology and Bioarchaeological Utility, EE Harris (ed.). In *Dental Anthropology* 19(1):1–16, 2006.

Hauser, G. and DeStefano, G. F. *Epigenetic Variants of the Human Skull.* Stuttgart, Verlag & Thieme, 1989.

Heathcote, G., Anderson, B., Bromage, T., Collins, S., Dean, D., Hanson, D., Knusel, C. Occupational Superstructures in Pacific Islanders: Occupational Markers? *Paper presented at the 19th Annual Meeting of the Paleopathology Association*, Las Vegas, Nevada, March 31–April 1, 1992.

Heathcote, G. M., Diego, V. P., Ishida, H. and Sava, V. J. Legendary Chamorro Strength: Skeletal Embodiment and the Boundaries of Interpretation, pp. 44–67. In L. W. Stodder and A. M. Palkovich (Eds.), *The Bioarchaeology of Individuals.* University Press of Florida, Gainesville, 2012.

Hefner, J. T. The *Statistical Determination of Ancestry Using Cranial Nonmetric Traits.* Doctoral Dissertation, The University of Florida, Gainesville, 2007.

Hefner, J. T. Cranial Morphoscopic Traits and the Assessment of American Black, American White, and Hispanic Ancestry, pp. 27–41. In G. E. Berg and S. C. Ta`ala (Eds.), *Biological Affinity in Forensic Identification of Human Skeletal Remains.* CRC Press, Boca Raton, 2015.

Hepburn, D. Anomalies in the supra-inial portion of the occipital bone, resulting from irregularities of its ossification, with consequent variations of the interparietal bone. *Journal of Anatomy and Physiology* 42(3):88–92, 1908.

Holden, L. and Langton, J. *Holden's Manual of the Dissection of the Human Body*, 4th Edition. J & A Churchill, London, 1879.

Horackova, L., Varegova, L., Krupa, P., Florian, Z., and Navrat, T. Proximal end of femur and problems of its superficial structure. *Slovenska Antropologia* 8(2):76–80, 2005.

Houghton, P. Human skeletal material from excavations in Eastern Coromandel. Records of the Auckland Institute and Museum 14:45–56, 1977.

Hrdlička, A. Divisions of parietal bone in man and other mammals. *Bulletin of the National Museum of Natural History* 19:231–386, 1903.

Hrdlička, A. Shovel-shaped teeth. *American Journal of Physical Anthropology* 3:429–465, 1920.

Hrdlička, A. The hypotrochanteric fossa of the femur. *The Smithsonian Miscellaneous Collections*, Volume 92, Issue 1. Smithsonian Institution, Washington, DC, 1934.

Hrdlička, A. The scapula: Visual observations. *American Journal of Physical Anthropology* 29:73–94, 1942.

Huanmanop, T., Agthong, S. and Chentanez, V. Surgical anatomy of fissures and foramina in the orbits of thai adults. *Journal of the Medical Association of Thailand* 90(11):2383–2391, 2007.

Humphrey, L. T. and Scheuer, L. Age of closure of the foramen of Huschke: An osteological study. *International Journal of Osteoarchaeology* 16(1):47–60, 2005.

Hunt, D. R. and Bullen, L. The frequency of os acromiale in the Robert J. Terry Collection. *International Journal of Osteoarchaeology* 17(3):309–317, 2007.

Hunter, R. H. An abnormal atlas. *Journal of Anatomy and Physiology* 58(2):140–141, 1924.

Hyer, C. F., Philbin, T. M., Berlet, G. C. and Lee, T. H. The incidence of the intermetatarsal facet of the first metatarsal and its relationship to metatarsus primus varus: A cadaveric study. *Journal of Foot and Ankle Surgery* 44(3): 200–202, 2005.

Hyman, A. A., Heiser, W. J., Kim, S. E. and Norfray, J. F. An excavation of the distal femoral metaphysis: A magnetic resonance imaging study. *The Journal of Bone and Joint Surgery* 77A (12):1897-1901, 1995.

Hyrtl, J. Ubder den prous crotaphitico-buccinatorius beim Menschen. *Sitzungsberichte d., Kaiserl, Akademia der Wissenschu Wien, Natur-mathem* 46:111–115, 1862.

Ilknur, A., Mustafa, K. I. and Sinan, B. A comparative study of variation of the pterion of human skulls from 13th and 20th century Anatolia. *International Journal of Morphology*

27(4):1921–1298, 2009.

Inoi, T. Estimation of sex and age by calcification pattern of costal cartilage in Japanese. *Nihon Hoigaku Zasshi* 51(2): 89–94, 1997.

International Society for Plastination. *The S10 Technique.* http://isp.plastination.org/silicone.html. Accessed May 23, 2015.

Isaac, B. and Holla, S. J. Variations in the shape of the coronoid process in the adult human mandible. *Journal Anatomical Society India* 50(2):137–139, 2001.

Isloor, S. D. *Lacrimal Drainage Surgery.* JP Medical Limited, London, 2014.

Jainkittivong, A., Apinhasmit, W. and Swasdison, S. Prevalence and clinical characteristics of oral tori in 1,520 Chulalongkorn University Dental School patients. *Surgical and Radiologic Anatomy* 29(2): 125–131, 2007.

Jamieson, E. B. *Dixon's Manual of Human Osteology*, 2nd Edition. E. B. Jamieson (Editor), Oxford University Press, London, 1937.

Jantz, R. L. *Change and Variation in Skeletal Populations of Arikara Indians.* Ph.D. dissertation, University of Kansas, Lawrence, 1970.

Jit, I., Jhingan, V., and Kulkarni, M. Sexing the human sternum. *American Journal of Physical Anthropology* 53(2):217–24, 1980.

Jivraj, L., Bhargava1, R., Aronyk, K., Quateen, A. and Walji, A. Diploic venous anatomy studied in-vivo by MRI. *Clinical Anatomy* 22(3):296–301, 2009.

Jovanovic, I., Vasovic, L., Ugrenovic, S., Zdravkovic, D., Vlajkovic, S., Dakovic-Bjelakovic, M. and Stojanovic, V. Variable foramen of Hyrtl of the human skull. *Acta Medica Medianae* 42(1):1–5, 2003.

Jurik, A. G. Bones and cartilage. In *Imaging of the Sternocostoclavicular Region*, A. G. Jurik (editor). Springer-Verlag, Berlin, 2007, pp. 13–26.

Kakizawa, Y., Abe, H., Fukushima, Y., Hongo, K., El-Khouly, H. and Rhoton, Jr., A. L. The course of the lesser petrosal nerve on the cranial fossa. *Operative Neurosurgery* 61(1): ONS-15-ONS-23, 2007. Accessed online DOI:10.1227/01.NEU.0000279977.17932.EB on 11 March 2012.

Kale, A., Aksu, F., Ozturk, A., Gurses, I. A., Garretli, O., Zeybek, F. G., Bayraktar, B., Ari, Z., and Onder, N. Foramen of Vesalius. *Saudi Medical Journal* 30(1):56–59, 2009a.

Kale, A., Ozturk, A., Aksu, F., Gurses, I. A., Garretli, O., Zeybek, F. G., Bayraktar, B., Taskara, N., Ari, Z. and Sahinoglu, K. Bony variations of the craniovertebral region. *Neurosciences* 14(3):296–297, 2009b.

Kale, A., Özturk, A., Aksu, F., Taskara, N., Bayraktar, B., Gurses, I. A., Zeybek, F. G., and Gayretli, O. *Vermian Fossa – An Anatomical Study.* Istanbul University, Arastirmalar/Research Articles 71(4):106–108, 2008.

Kassim, N. M., Latiff, L. L., Das, S., Ghafar, N. A., Suhaimi, F. H., Othman, F., Hussan, F. and Sulaiman, I. M. Atlantooccipital fusion: An osteological study with clinical implications. *Bratisl Lek Listy* 111(10):562–565, 2010.

Katsavrias, E. G. and Dibbets, J. M. The postglenoid tubercle: Prevalence and growth. *Annals of Anatomy* 184(2):185–188, 2002.

Kaur, H. and Jit, I. Coracoclavicular joint in northwest Indians. *American Journal of Physical Anthropology* 85(4):457–460, 1991.

Kempson, F. C. Emargination of the patella. *Journal of Anatomy and Physiology* 36(4):419–420, 1902.

Kennedy, G. E. The relationship between auditory exostoses and cold water: A latitudinal analysis. *American Journal of Physical Anthropology* 71(4):401–415, 1986.

Kennedy, K. A. Morphological variations in ulnar supinator crests and fossae as identifying markers of occupational stress. *Journal of Forensic Sciences* 28(4):871–876, 1983.

Keyes, J. E. L. Observations on four thousand optic foramina in human skulls of known origin. *Archives of Opthalmology* 13:538–568, 1935.

Khudaverdyan, A. Y. Nonmetric cranial variation in human skeletal remains from the Armenian Highland: Microevolutionary relations and an intergroup analysis. *European Journal of Anatomy* 16(2):134–149, 2012.

Knott, J. F. On the cerebral sinuses and their variations. *Journal of Anatomy* 16:27–42, 1881.

Ko, S. J. and Kim, Y-K. Incidence of calcification of the trochlear apparatus in the orbit. *Korean Journal of Opthalmology* 24(1):1–3, 2010.

Kodama, K., Inoue, K., Nagashima, M. Matsumura, G. Watanabe, S. and Kodame, G. Studies on the foramen Vesalius in the Japanese juvenile and adult skulls. *Hokkaido Igaku Zasshi* 72(6):667–674, 1997.

Köhler, A. and Zimmer, E. A. *Borderlands of the Normal and Early Pathologic in Skeletal Roentgenology.* Grune and Stratton Inc., New York, 1968.

Kohn, L. A. P., Vannier, M. W., Marsh, J. L. and Cheverud, J. M. Effect of premature sagittal suture closure on craniofacial morphology in a prehistoric male Hopi. *Cleft Palate-Craniofacial Journal* 31(5):385–396, 1994.

Kondrat, J. W. *Frontal Sinus Morphology: An Analysis of Craniometric and Environmental on the Morphology of Modern Human Frontal Sinus Patterns.* Master of Arts Thesis, Northern Illinois University, Dekalb, 1995.

Konigsberg, L. W., Kohn, L. A. P. and Cheverud, J. M. Cranial deformation and nonmetric trait variation. *American Journal of Physical Anthropology* 90:35–48, 1993.

Kosa, F. Characteristic morphological differences on "black and white" cranial fetal bones. In B. Jacob and W. Bonte (Eds.), *Forensic Odontology and Anthropology*, Koster, Berlin, pp. 104–111, 1995.

Kopsch, F. *Rauber's Lehrbuch der Anatomie des Menschen*, Abteilung 2: Knochen, Bänder. Verlag von Georg Thieme, Leipzig, 1914.

Kostick, E. L. Facets and imprints on the upper and lower extremities of femora from a Western Nigerian population. *Journal of Anatomy* 97(3):393–402, 1963.

Krayenbühl, N., Isolan, G.R. and Al-Mefty, O. The foramen spinosum. A landmark in middle fossa surgery. *Neurosurgery Review* 31:397–402, 2008.

Kreyenbühl, W. and Hessler, C. A variation of the sacrum

on the lateral view. *Radiology* 109:49–52, 1973.

Krishnamurthy, A., Nayak, S. R., Prabhu, L. V., Mansur, D. I., Ramanathan, L., Madhyastha, S. and Saralaya, V. The morphology of meningo-orbital foramen in south Indian population. *Bratislavski Lekarske Listy* 109(11):517–519, 2008.

Krmpotic-Nemanic, J., Vinter, I. and Jalsovec, D. Accessory oval foramen. *Annals of Anatomy* 183:293–295, 2001.

Kubikova, E. and Varga, I. A case of extremely long styloid process without clinical symptoms and complications. *Clinical Anatomy* 22:865–867, 2009.

Kwiatkowska, A., Gawlikowska-Sroka, A., Szczurowski, J. Nowakowski, D. and Dzieciolowska-Baran, E. A case of concha bullosa mucopyocele in a medieval human skull. *International Journal of Osteoarchaeology* 2009. DOI: 10.1002/0a.1137.

Kwiatkowski, J. Wysocki, J. and Nitek, S. The morphology and morphometry of the so-called "meningo-orbital foramen" in humans. *Folia Morphologica* (Warsz) 62(4): 323–325, 2003.

L'Abbé, E. N., VanRooyen, C., Nawrocki, S. P., and Becker, P. J. An evaluation of non-metric cranial traits used to estimate ancestry in a South African sample. *Forensic Science International* 209(1-3): 195.e1-7, 2001.

Labrash, S. and Lozanoff, S. Standards and guidlines for willed body donations at the John A. Burns School of Medicine. *Hawaii Medical Journal* 66(3):72–75, 2007.

Lacout, A., Marsot-Dupuch, K., Smoker, W. R. K. and Lasjaunias, P. Foramen tympanicum, or foramen of Huschke: Pathologic cases and anatomic CT study. *American Journal of Neuroradiology* 26:1317–1323, 2005.

Langlais, R. P., Miles, D. A., and Van Dis, M. L.: Elongated and mineralized stylohyoid ligament complex: A proposed classification and report of a case of Eagle's syndrome. *Oral Surgery Oral Medicine Oral Pathology* 61:527-532, 1986.

Lanzieri, C. F., Duchesneau, P. M., Rosenbloom, S. A., Smith, A. S. and Rosenbaum, A. E. The significance of asymmetry of the foramen of Vesalius. *American Journal of Neuroradiology* 9:1201–1204, 1988.

Larnach, S. L. An examination of the use of discontinuous cranial traits. *Archives and Physical Anthropology in Oceania* 9(3):217–225, 1974.

Larnach, S. L. and Macintosh, N. W. G. *The Craniology of the Aborigines of Coastal New South Wales*. Sydney, University of Sydney, 1966.

Last, R. J. (Editor). *Eugene Wolf's Anatomy of the Eye and Orbit*, 5th Edition. W. B. Saunders Company, Philadelphia, 1966.

Lavallo, G. *Variation in Non-metric Traits of the Pelvis Between White, Blacks, and Hispanics*. Master's thesis, Texas State University-San Marcos, 2013. Available on-line at https://digital.library.txstate.edu/handle/10877/4610.

Leach, J. L., Jones, B. V., Tomsick, T. A., Stewart, C. A. and Balko, M. G. Normal appearance of arachnoid granulations on contrast-enhanced CT and MR of the brain: Differentiation from dural sinus disease. *American Journal of Neuroradiology* 17:1523–1532, 1996.

LeDouble, A. F. *Traite des Variations des Os de la Face de l'Homme*. [Characteristics of the variations of the facial bones of man]: pp. 67, 116–124, 176. Paris, Vigot Freres, 1903.

LeDouble, A. F. *Traite des Variations de la Colonne Vertebrale de l'Homme. Anthropologique Zoologique*, Paris, 1912.

Lee, K. H, Lee, J. H. and Lee, H. J. Concurrence of torus mandibularis with multiple buccal exostoses. *Archives of Plastic Surgery* 40(4):466–468, 2013.

Lee, S. P., Paik, K. S. and Kim, M. K. Variations of the prominences of the bony palate and their relationship to complete dentures in Korean skulls. *Clinical Anatomy* 14:324–329, 2001.

Le Gros Clark, W. E. On the Pacchionian bodies. *Journal of Anatomy and Physiology* 55(1):40–48, 1920.

Le Minor, J-M. Comparative anatomy and significance of the sesamoid bone of the peroneus longus muscle (os peroneum). *Journal of Anatomy* 151:85–99, 1987.

Le Minor, J-M and Winter, M. The intermetatarsal articular facet of the first metatarsal bone in humans: A derived trait unique within primates. *Annals of Anatomy* 185:359–365, 2003.

Leng, L. A., Anand, V. K., Hartl, R. and Schwartz, T. H. Endonasal endoscopic resection of an os odontoideum to decompress the cervicomedullary junction. *Spine* 34(4):E139–E143, 2009.

Leo, J. T., Cassell, Martin I. D. and Bergman, R. A. Variation in human infraorbital nerve, canal and foramen. *Annals of Anatomy* 177:93–95, 1995.

Leonardi, R., Barbatob, E., Vichic, M. and Caltabianod, M. Skeletal anomalies and normal variants in patients with patally displaced canines. *The Angle Orthodontist* 79(4):727–732, 2009.

Lewis, O. J. The Coraco-clavicular joint. *Journal of Anatomy* 93(3):296–303, 1959.

Liang, L. Korogi, Y., Sugahara, T., Ikushima, I., Shigematsu, Y., Takahashi, M. and Provenzale, J. M. Normal structures in the intracranial dural sinuses: Delineation with 3D contrast-enhanced magnetization prepared rapid acquisition gradient-echo imaging sequence. *American Journal of Neuroradiology* 23:1739–1746, 2002.

Liang, X., Jacobs, R., Lambrichts, I. and Vandewalle, G. Lingual foramina on the mandibular midline revisited: A macroanatomical study. *Clinical Anatomy* 20:246–251, 2007.

Lindblom, K. A roentgenographic study of the vascular tumors and arteriorvenous aneurysms. *Acta Radiological* (Suppl.) (Stockholm) 30:1–146, 1936.

Liu, D. N., Guo, J. L., Luo, Q., Tian, Y., Xia, C. L., Li, Y. Q. and Su, L. Location of supraorbital foramen/notch and infraorbital foramen with reference to soft-and hard-tissue landmarks. *Journal of Craniofacial Surgery* 22(1):293–296, 2011.

Lockhart, R. D., Hamilton, G. F. and Fyfe, F. W. *Anatomy of the Human Body*. J. B. Lippincott Company, Philadelphia, 1965.

Lordan, J., Rauh, P. and Spinner, R. J. The clinical anatomy of the supracondylar spur and the ligament of Struthers. *Clinical Anatomy* 18:548–551, 2005.

Loukas, M., Owens, D. G., Tubbs, R. S., Spentzouris, G., Elochukwu, A. and Jordan, R. Zygomaticofacial, zygomaticoorbital and zygomaticotemporal foramina: Anatomical study. *Anatomical Science International* 83(2):77–82, 2008.

Lozanoff, S. P., Sciulli, P. and Schneider, K. N. Third trochanter incidence and metric trait covariation in the human femur. *Journal of Anatomy* 143:149–159, 1985.

Lu, C-X., Du, Y., Xu, X-X., Li, Y., Yang, H-F., Deng, S-Q., Xiao, D-M. and Tian Y-H. Multiple occipital defects caused by arachnoid granulations: Emphasis on T2 mapping. *World Journal of Radiology* 4(7):341–344, 2012.

Luboga, S. Supernumerary lumbar vertebrae in human skeletons at the Galloway Osteological Collection of Makerere University, Kampala. *East African Medical Journal* 77(1):16–19, 2000.

Lucas, M. F. (1) Two cases of cervical ribs (2) an anomalous arrangement of the vagi. *Journal of Anatomy and Physiology* 49(3):336–342, 1915.

Macalister, A. Notes on the Varieties and Morphology of the Human Lachrymal Bone and Its Accessory Ossicles. *Proceedings of the Royal Society of London* 37:229–250, 1884.

Macalister, A. Notes on the development and variations of the atlas. *Journal of Anatomy and Physiology* 27(4):519–542, 1893.

MacCurdy, G. G. *Human Skulls from Gazelle Peninsula.* University of Pennsylvania, The University Museum Anthropological Publications Vol. VI, No. 1, Philadelphia, 1914.

MacDonnell, R. L. Note on a case of bicipital rib. *Journal of Anatomy and Physiology* 20(3):405–406, 1886.

Macedo, V. C., Cabrini, R. R. and Faig-Leite, H. Infraorbital foramen location in dry human skulls. *Brazilian Journal of Morphological Sciences* 26(1):35–38, 2009.

Madeline, L. A. and Elster, A. D. Postnatal development of the central skull base: Normal variants. *Radiology* 196:757–763, 1995.

Madhavi, C. Madhuri, V., George, V. M. and Antonisamy, B. South Indian calcaneal talar facet configurations and osteoarthritic changes. *Clinical Anatomy* 21(6):581–586, 2008.

Mahato, N. K. Complete sacralization of L5 vertebrae: Traits, dimensions, and load bearing in the involved sacra. *The Spine Journal* 10:610–615, 2010.

Mahato, N. K. Foramen on the sacral ala and the lumbar transverse process: Reviewing not a very common observation. *International Journal of Anatomical Variations* 7:19–20, 2014.

Mangal, A., Choudhry, R., Tuli, A., Choudhry, S., Choudhry, R. and Khera, V. Incidence and morphological study of zygomaticofacial and zygomatico-orbital foramina in dry adult human skulls: The non-metrical variants. *Surgical and Radiologic Anatomy* 26:96–99, 2004.

Mangla, R., Singh, N., Dua, V., Padmanabhan, P. and Khanna, M. Evaluation of mandibular morphology in different facial types. *Contemporary Clinical Dentistry* 2(3):20–206, 2011.

Manjunath, K. Y. Paracondylar foramen – a new anomalous aperture of the occipital bone. *Indian Journal of Medical Sciences* 52(7):317–319, 1998.

Mann, R. W. Calcaneus secundarius: Description and frequency in six skeletal samples. *American Journal of Physical Anthropology* 81(1):17–25, 1990.

Mann, R. W. *Stafne's Defects of the Human Mandible.* Doctoral dissertation, University of Hawaii, Manoa, 2001.

Mann, R. W. and Berryman, H. E. A method for defleshing human remains using household bleach. *Journal of Forensic Sciences* 57(2):440–442, 2012.

Mann, R. W. and Hunt, D. R. *Photographical Regional Atlas of Bone Disease: A Guide to Normal and Pathologic Variation in the Human Skeleton,* Second Edition. Charles C Thomas, Springfield, 2005.

Mann, R. W. and Hunt, D. R. *Photographical Regional Atlas of Bone Disease: A Guide to Normal and Pathologic Variation in the Human Skeleton,* Third Edition. Charles C Thomas, Springfield, 2012.

Mann, R. W., Manabe, J. and Byrd, J. E. Relationship of the parietal foramen and complexity of the human sagittal suture. *International Journal of Morphology* 27(2):553–564, 2009.

Mann, R. W. and Owsley, D. W. Os trigonum: A common accessory ossicle of the talus. *Journal of the American Podiatric Medical Association* 80(10):536–539, 1990.

Mann, R. W. and Tsaknis, P. J. Cortical defects in the mandibular sulcus. *Oral Surgery Oral Medicine Oral Pathology* 71(4):514–516, 1991.

Manners-Smith, T. The variability of the last lumbar vertebra. *Journal of Anatomy and Physiology* 43(3):146–160, 1910.

Manning, K. P. and Singh, S. D. Hypoplasia of the nasal bones. *The Journal of Laryngology & Otology* 91:1085–1091, 1977.

Mardini, S. and Gohel, A. Exploring the Mandibular Canal in 3 Dimensions. An Overview of Frequently Encountered Variations in Canal Anatomy. Fall 2008 AADMRT Newsletter. Accessed online www.aadmrt.com/currents/mardinigohel fall 08 on December 8, 2011.

Marshall, D. S. Precondylar tubercle incidence rates. *American Journal of Physical Anthropology* 13(1):147–151, 1955.

Massler, M. and Schour, I. Growth patterns of the cranial vault in the albino rat. *Anatomical Record* 110:83–101, 1951.

Matsumura, G. Uchiumi, T., Kida, K., Ichikawa, R. and Kodama, G. Developmental studies on the interparietal part of the human occipital squama. *Journal of Anatomy* 182(2):197–204, 1993.

McCall, T., Coppens, J., Couldwell, W. and Dailey, A. Symptomatic occipitocervical paracondylar process. *Journal Neurosurgery Spine* 12:9–12, 2010.

McCormick W. F. Mineralization of the costal cartilages as an indicator of age: Preliminary observations. *Journal of Forensic Sciences* 25(4): 736–741, 1980.

McCormick, W. F. Sternal foramina in men. *American Journal of Medicine and Pathology* 2(3):249–252, 1981.

McCormick, W. F. and Stewart, J. H. Ossification patterns of costal cartilages as an indicator of sex. *Archives of Pathology and Laboratory Medicine* 107(4):206–210, 1983.

McCormick, W. F. and Stewart, J. H. Age related changes in the human plastron: A roentgenographic and morphologic study. *Journal of Forensic Sciences* 33(1):100–120, 1988.

McCormick, W. F., Stewart, J. H. and Langford, L. A. Sex determination from chest plate roentgenograms. *American Journal of Physical Anthropology* 68(2):173–195, 1985.

McDonnell, D., Nouri, M. R. and Todd, M. E. The mandibular lingual foramen: A consistent arterial foramen in the middle of the mandible. *Journal of Anatomy* 184:363–369, 1994.

McDougall, A. The os trigonum. *Journal of Bone and Joint Surgery* 37B(2):257–265, 1955.

Meier, L. N. Exploration Towards the Etiology of the Septal Aperture of the Humerus: A Non-metric Expression of Size, Environment, or Genetic Difference? MA Thesis, George Washington University, 2006.

Meier, L. N. and Hunt D. R. Incidence of humeral septal aperture and its relation to population and sex. *American Journal of Physical Anthropology* Supplement 42:106, 2006.

Mellado, J. M., Larrosa, R., Martin, J., Yanguas, N., Solanas, S. and Cozcolluela, M. R. MDCT of variations and anomalies of the neural arch and its processes: Part 1 – Pedicles, parts interarticularis, laminae, and spinous process. *American Journal of Roentgenology* 197(1):W104–W113, 2011(a).

Mellado, J. M., Larrosa, R., Martin, J., Yanguas, N., Solanas, S. and Cozcolluela, M. R. MDCT of variations and anomalies of the neural arch and its processes: Part 2 – Articular processes, transverse processes, and high cervical spine. *American Journal of Roentgenology* 197(2):W114–W121, 2011(b).

Melsen, B. and Ousterhout, D. K. Anatomy and development of the pterygopalatomaxillary region, studied in relation to Le Fort osteotomies. *Annals of Plastic Surgery* 19(1):16–28, 1987.

Mercer, J. The secondary os calcis. *Journal of Anatomy and Physiology* 66(1):84–97, 1931.

Mercer, S. R. and Bogduk, N. Clinical anatomy of ligamentum nuchae. *Clinical Anatomy* 16:484–493, 2003.

Moorrees, C. F. A, Osbourne, R. H. and Wilde, E. Torus mandibularis: Its occurrence in Aleut children and its genetic determinants. *American Journal of Physical Anthropology* 10:319–330, 1952.

More, C. B. and Asrani, M. K. Evaluation of the styloid process on digital panoramic radiographs. *Indian Journal of Radiology and Imaging* 20(4):261–265, 2010.

Morita, T., Ikata, T., Katoh, S., and Miyake, R. Lumbar spondylolysis in children and adolescents. *Journal of Bone and Joint Surgery* (Br.) 77(4):620–625, 1995.

Morris, H. *Morris's Human Anatomy: A Complete Systematic Treatise by English and American Authors*, Fourth Edition. Blakiston's Son and Company, Philadelphia, 1907.

Moseley, J. M. The paleopathologic riddle of "symmetrical osteoporosis." *American Journal of Roentgenology Radium Therapy and Nuclear Medicine* 95(1):135–142, 1965.

Murlimanju, B. V., Prabhu, L. V., Silpa, K., Rai, R., Dhananjaya, K. V. and Jiji, P. J. Accessory transverse foramina in the cervical spine: Incidence, embryological basis, morphology and surgical importance. *Turkish Neurosurgery* 21(3):384–387, 2011a.

Murlimanju, B. V., Prabhu, L. V., Prameela, M. D., Ashraf, C. M., Krishnamurthy, A. and Kumar, C. G. Accessory mandibular foramina: Prevalence, embryological basis and surgical implications. *Journal of Clinical and Diagnostic Research* (Suppl-1), 5(6):1137–1139, 2011b.

Murphy, T. The chin region of the Australian Aboriginal mandible. *American Journal of Physical Anthropology* 15:517–535, 1957.

Museum of London *Policy for the Care of Human Remains in Museum of London Collections.* Museum of London, London, 2006.

Mutalik, A., Kolagi, S., Hanji, C., Ugale, M. and Rairam, G. B. A morphometric anatomical study of the ethmoidal foramina on dry human skulls. *Journal of Clinical and Diagnostic Research* 5(1):28–30, 2011.

Muthukumaravel, N., Ravichandran, D. and Rajendran, M. Human calcaneal facets for the talus: Patterns and implications. *Journal of Clinical and Diagnostic Research* 5(4):791–794, 2011.

Naderi, S., Korman, E., Citak, G., Guvencer, M., Arman, C., Senoglu, M., Tetik, S. and Arda, M. N. Morphometric analysis of human occipital condyle. *Clinical Neurology and Neurosurgery* 107:191–199, 2005.

Nagar, M., Bhardwaj, R. and Prakash, R. Accessory lingual foramen in adult Indian mandibles. *Journal of Anatomical Society of India* 50(1):13–14, 2001.

Naik, S. M. and Naik S. S. Tonsillo-styloidectomy for Eagle's syndrome: A review of 15 Cases in KVG Medical College Sullia. *Oman Medical Journal* 26(2):122–126, 2011.

Nakashima, T., Hojo, T., Suzuki, K. and Ijichi, M. Symphalangism (two phalanges) in the digits of the Japanese foot. *Annals of Anatomy* 177(3):275–278, 1995.

Nalla, S. and Asvat, R. Incidence of the coracoclavicular joint in South African populations. *Journal of Anatomy* 186:645–649, 1995.

Nambiar, P., Naidu, M. D. K. and Subramaniam, K. Anatomical variability of the frontal sinuses and their application in forensic identification. *Clinical Anatomy* 12:16–19, 1999.

Napoli, M. L. and Birkby, W. H. Racial differences in the visibility of the oval window in the middle ear. In *Skeletal Attribution of Race*. Gill, G. W. and Rhine, S. (Eds.), Maxwell Museum of Anthropology, Anthropology Papers No. 4, 1990.

Natsis, K. Supracondylar process of the humerus: Study on 375 Caucasian subjects in Cologne, Germany. *Clinical Anatomy* 21:138–141, 2008.

Natsis, K., Didagelos, M, Totlis, T., Tsikaras, P. and Koebke, J. Intermediate supraclavicular nerve perforating the clavicle: A rare anatomical finding and its clinical significance. *Aristotle University Medical Journal* 34(1):61–63, 2007b.

Natsis, K., Totlis, T. Tsikaras, P., Appell, H. J., Skandalakis, P. and Koebke, J. Proposal for classification of the suprascapular nNotch: A study on 423 dried scapulas. *Clinical*

Anatomy 20(2):135–139, 2007a.

Navani, S., Shah, J. R. and Levy, P. S. Determination of sex by costal cartilage calcification. *American Journal of Roentgenology Radium Therapy and Nuclear Medicine* 108(4): 771–774, 1970.

Nayak, S. R., Saralaya, V., Prabhu, L. V., Pai, M. M., Vadgaonkar, R. and D'Costa, S. Pterygospinous bar and foramina in Indian skulls: Incidence and phylogenetic significance. *Surgical and Radiologic Anatomy* 29(1):5–7, 2007.

Nehme, A., Tricoire, J. L., Giordano, G., Chiron, P. and Puget, J. Coracoclavicular joints. Reflections upon incidence, pathophysiology and etiology of the different forms. *Surgical and Radiologic Anatomy* 26(1):33–38, 2004.

Neto, H. S., Penteado, C. V. and de Carvalho, V. C. Presence of a groove in the lateral wall of the human orbit. *Journal of Anatomy* 138:631–633, 1984.

Neves, F. S., Torres, M. G. G., Oliveira, C., Campos, P. S. F. and Crusoe-Rebello, I. Lingual accessory mental foramen: A report of an extremely rare anatomical variation. *Journal of Oral Science* 52(3):501–503, 2010.

Newell, R. L. M. The calcar femorale: A tale of historical neglect. *Clinical Anatomy* 10:27–33, 1997

Nickel, B. The parietal sagittal suture. *Neuroradiology* 3:36–40, 1971.

Nikolova, S. Y., Toneva, D. H., Yordanov, Y. A. and Lazarov, N. E. Absence of foramen spinosum and abnormal middle meningeal artery in cranial series. *Anthropologischer Anzeiger* 69(3):351–366, 2012.

Nolet, P. S., Friedman, L. and Brubaker, D. Paracondylar process: A rare cause of craniovertebral fusion – a case report. *The Journal of the Canadian Chiropractic Association* 43(4):229–235, 1999.

O'Brien, A. and McDonald, S. W. The meningo-orbital foramen in a Scottish population. *Clinical Anatomy* 20:880–885, 2007.

Odgers, P. N. B. Two details about the neck of the femur: (1) the eminentia. (2) the empreinte. *Journal of Anatomy and Physiology* 65(3):352–362, 1931.

Oetteking, B. Anomalous patellae. *Anatomical Record* 23(4):269–279, 1922.

Oetteking, B. On the morphological significance of certain cranio-vertebral variations. *Anatomical Record* 25(6):339–354, 1923.

Oetteking, B. Craniology of the North Pacific Coast. Memoirs of the American Museum of Natural History, Volume 15, Part 1, 1930.

Ogawa, K., Fukuda, H. and Omori, K. *Nihon Seikeigeka Gakkai Zasshi* 53(2):155–164, 1979. [Article in Japanese, abstract in English.]

Okumura, M. M. M., Boyadjian, C. H. C. and Eggers, S. Auditory exostoses as an aquatic activity marker: A comparison of coastal and inland skeletal remains from tropical and subtropical regions of Brazil. *American Journal of Physical Anthropology* 132:558–567, 2007.

Olotu, J. E., Oladipo, G. S., Eroje, M. A., and Edibamode, I. E. Incidence of coracoclavicular joint in adult Nigerian population. *Scientific Research and Essay* 3(4):165–167, 2008.

O'Loughlin, V. D. Effects of different kinds of cranial deformation on the incidence of wormian bones. *American Journal of Physical Anthropology* 123(2):146–155, 2004.

Ongkana, N. and M.D., and Sudwan, P. Morphologic indicators of sex in Thai mandibles. *Chiang Mai Medical Journal* 49(4):123–128, 2010.

Onwuama, K. T., Salami, S. O., Ali, M. and Nzalak, J. O. Effect of different methods of bone preparation on the skeleton of the African Giant Pouched Rat (*Cricetompy gamianus*). *International Journal of Morphology* 30(2):425–427, 2012.

Orban, B. J. *Orban's Oral History and Embryology*, 10th Edition, by S. N. Bhaskar (Editor). Mosby, St. Louis, 1986.

Ossenberg, N. S. *Discontinuous morphological variation in the human cranium.* University of Toronto, Ph.D. thesis, 1969.

Ossenberg, N. S. The influence of artificial cranial deformation on discontinuous morphological traits. *American Journal of Physical Anthropology* 33(3):357–371, 1970.

Ossenberg, N. S. Retromolar foramen of the human mandible. *American Journal of Physical Anthropology* 72(1):119–129, 1987.

Osunwoke, E. A., Mbadugha, C. C., Orish, C. N., Oghenemavwe, E. L., and Ukah, C. J. A morphometric study of foramen ovale and foramen spinosum of the human sphenoid bone in the southern Nigerian population. *Journal of Applied Biosciences* 26:1631–1635, 2010.

Ozcan, K. M., Selcuk, A., Ozcan, I., Akdogan, O. and Dere, H. Anatomical variations of nasal turbinates. *Journal of Craniofacial Surgery* 19(6):1678–1682, 2008.

Ozer, M. A., Celik, S. and Govsa, F. A morphometric study of the inferior orbital fissure using three-dimensional anatomical landmarks: Application to orbital surgery. *Clinical Anatomy* 22:649–654, 2009.

Padmanabhan, R. The talar facets of the calcaneus-an anatomical note. *Anatomischer Anzeiger* 161(5):389–92, 1986.

Pal, G. P. Variations of the interparietal bone in man. *Journal of Anatomy* 152:205–208, 1987.

Pang, D. and Thompson, D. N. P. Embryology and bony malformations of the craniovertebral junction. *Childs Nervous System* 27:523–564, 2011.

Parr, N. M. L. *Determination of Ancestry From Discrete Traits of the Mandible.* Master's Thesis, University of Indianapolis, 2005.

Parsons, F. G. The topography and morphology of the human hyoid bone. *Journal of Anatomy and Physiology* 43(4):279–290, 1909.

Patil, G. V., Kolagi, S., Padmavathi, G. and Rairam, G. B. The duplication of the optic canals in human skulls. *Journal of Clinical and Diagnostic Research* 5(3):536–537, 2011.

Patil, N., Karjodkar, F. R., Sontakke, S., Sansare, K. and Salvi, R. Uniqueness of radiographic patterns of the frontal sinus for personal identification. *Imaging Science in Dentistry* 42(4):213–217, 2012.

Pearlstein, K., Hunt, D. R. and Mann, R. W. The expression of femoral trochanteric spicules with reference to age. *American Journal of Physical Anthropology* Suppl. 44:90, 2007.

Peker, T., Karakose, M., Anil, A., Turgut, H. B. and Gulekon, N. The incidence of basal sphenoid bony bridges in dried crania and cadavers: Their anthropological and clinical relevance. *European Journal of Morphology* 40(3):171–180, 2002.

Perizonius, W. R. K. Non-metrical Cranial Traits: Sex difference and age dependence. *Journal of Human Evolution* 8:679–684, 1979.

Peuker, E. T., Fischer, G. and Filler, T. J. Entrapment of the lingual nerve due to an ossified pterygospinous ligament. *Clinical Anatomy* 14:282–284, 2001.

Phenice, T. W. 1969. A newly developed method of sexing the os pubis. *American Journal of Physical Anthropology* 30(2):297–302, 1969.

Phillips, S. R. *Cranial anomaly, pathology, or normal variant? Thin parietal bones in ancient Egyptian human remains.* PhD Dissertation, University of Pennsylvania, 2008.

Piagkou, M., Anagnostopoulou, S., Kouladouros, K. and Piagkos, G. Eagle's syndrome: A review of the literature. *Clinical Anatomy* 22(5):545–558, 2009.

Pick, M. G. *Cranial Sutures: Analysis, Morphology and Manipulative Strategies.* Eastland Press, Seattle, 1999.

Pietrusewsky, M. and Douglas, M. T. *Ban Chiang: A Prehistoric Village Site in Northeast Thailand I: The Human Skeletal Remains.* University of Pennsylvania, Pittsburgh, 2002.

Pillay, V. K. The coraco-clavicular joint. *Singapore Medical Journal* 8(3):207–213, 1967.

Pitt, M. J., Graham, A. R., Shipman, J. H. and Birkby, W. Herniation pit of the femoral neck. *American Journal of Roentgenology* 138:1115–1121, 1982.

Piyawinijwong, S., Sirisathira, N., Sricharoenvej, S. and Netvichit, S. Coracoclavicular joint: A preliminary report in Thai cadavers. *Siriraj Medical Journal* 58:1212–1215, 2006.

Polguj, M., Jędrzejewski, K., Podgórski, M., and Topol, M. Morphometric study of the suprascapular notch: Proposal of classification. *Surgical and Radiologic Anatomy* 33:781–787, 2011; DOI: 10.1007/s00276-011-0821-y.

Prabhu, L. V., Kumar, A., Nayak, S. R. Pai, M. M., Vadgaonkar, R., Krishnamurthy, A. and Madhan Kumar, S. J. An unusually lengthy styloid process. *Singapore Medical Journal* 48:e34–336, 2007.

Prakash, B. S., Padma, L. K., Mamatha, Y. and Ramesh, B. R. Left arteriae vertebralis canal in atlas – Kimmerle anomaly. *International Journal of Anatomical Variations* 3:130–131, 2010.

Prescher, A. The craniocervical junction in man, the osseous variations, their significance and differential diagnosis. *Annals of Anatomy* 179:1–19, 1997.

Prescher, A., Brors, D. and Adam, G. Anatomic and radiological appearance of several variants of the craniocervical junction. *Skull Base Surgery* 6(2):83–94, 1996.

Priya, R. Manjunath, K. Y. and Balasubramanyam, V. The varying shape of the coronoid process of the mandible. *Indian Journal of Dental Research* 15(3):96–98, 2004.

Quatrehomme, G., Fronty, P., Sapanet, M., Grévin, G., Bailet, P. and Ollier, A. Identification by frontal sinus pattern in forensic anthropology. *Forensic Science International* 83:147–153, 1996.

Radi, N., Mariotti, V., Rigi, A., Zampetti, S., Villa, C. and Belcastro, M.G. Variation of the anterior aspect of the femoral head-neck junction in a modern human identified skeletal collection. *American Journal of Physical Anthropology* 152:261–272, 2013.

Ragab, A. A., Stewart, S. L. and Cooperman, D. R. Implications of subtalar joint anatomic variation in calcaneal lengthening osteotomy. *Journal of Pediatric Orthopaedics* 23(1):79–83, 2003.

Ramadan, S. U., Gokharman, D., Tuncbilek, I., Kacar, M., Kosar, P. and Kosar, U. Assessment of the stylohyoid chain by 3D-CT. *Surgical and Radiologic Anatomy* 29:583–588, 2007.

Ramadhan, A., Messo, E. and Hirsch, J. M. Anatomical variation of mental foramen. A case report. *Stomatologija, Baltic Dental and Maxillofacial Journal* 12:93–96, 2010.

Rani, A., Chopra, J., Rani, A., Mishra, S. R., Srivastava, A. K., Sharma, P. K., and Diwan, R. A study of morphological features of attachment area of costoclavicular ligament on clavicle and first rib in Indians and its clinical relevance. *Biomedical Research* 22(3):349–354, 2011.

Rani, A., Mishra, S. R., Chopra, J., Rani, A., Manik, P., Kumar, N. and Dewan, R. K. Coracoclavicular and costoclavicular joints at a common juncture: A rare phenomenon. *International Journal of Morphology* 27(4):1089–1092, 2009.

Rau, R. K. Supra condylar process. *Journal of Anatomy and Physiology* 65(3):392–394, 1931.

Rauber-Kopsch. *Rauber's der Anatomie des Menschen* von Prof. Dr. Fr. Kopsch. Abteilungen 2: Knochen, Bänder. Leipzig, Georg Thieme, 1914.

Redlund-Johnell, I. The costoclavicular joint. *Skeletal Radiology* 15:25–26, 1986.

Reed, J. C. *The Utility of Cladistic Analysis of Nonmetric Skeletal Traits for Biodistance Analysis.* Doctoral Dissertation, Pittsburgh, University of Pittsburgh, 2006.

Rejtarova, O., Hejna, P., Rejtar, P., Bukac, J., Slizova, D. and Krs, O. Sexual dimorphism of ossified costal cartilage. Radiograph scan study on Caucasian men and women (Czech population). *Forensic Science International* 191, 110. e1–110.e5, 2009.

Remmelick, H-J. Orientation of maxillary sutural surfaces. *European Journal of Orthodontics* 10:223–226, 1988.

Remmelick, H-J. Letters, Orthopedic headgear forces. *The Angle Orthodontist* 63(4):245, 1993.

Rengachary, S. S., Neff, J. P., Singer, P. A. and Brackett, C. F. Suprascapular nerve entrapment neuropathy: A clinical, anatomical and comparative study. Part 1. Clinical study. *Neurosurgery* 5:441–446, 1979.

Resnick, D. and Greenway G. Distal femoral cortical defects, irregularities and excavations. *Radiology* 143(2):345–354, 1982.

Restrepo, C. S., Martinez, S., Lemos, D. F., Washington, L., McAdams, H. P., Vargas, D., Lemos, J. A., Carrillo, J. A. and Diethelm, L. Imaging appearances of the sternum and sternoclavicular joints. *Radiographics* 29:839–859, 2009.

Reymond, J., Charuta, A. and Wysocki, J. The morphology

and morphometry of the foramina of the greater wing of the human sphenoid bone. *Folia Morpholia* 64(3):188–193, 2005.

Rhine, S. Nonmetric skull racing. In Gill, G., and Rhine, S. (Eds.). *Skeletal Attribution of Race*. Maxwell Museum of Anthropological papers No. 4. Albuquerque, NM: University of New Mexico, 1990.

Riesenfeld, A. Multiple infraorbital, ethmoidal and mental foramina in the races of man. *American Journal of Physical Anthropology* 14:85–100, 1956.

Roche, J. and Warner, D. Arachnoid granulations in the transverse and sigmoid sinuses: CT, MR, and MR angiographic appearance of a normal anatomic variation. *American Journal of Neuroradiology* 17:677–683, 1996.

Roche, M. B. and Rowe, G. G. The incidence of separate neural arch and coincident bone variations: A Summary. *Journal of Bone and Joint Surgery* 34-A(2):491–493, 1952.

Rogers, M. An analysis of discrete cranial traits of Northwestern Plains Indians. In G. W. Gill and R. L. Weathermon (Eds.), S*keletal Biology and Bioarchaeology of the Northwestern Plains*. University of Utah Press, Salt Lake City, 2008.

Rogers, N. L., Flournoy, L. E., and McCormick, W. F. The rhomboid fossa of the clavicle as a sex and age estimator. *Journal of Forensic Sciences* 45(1):61–67, 2000.

Rosa, R. R., Faig-Leite, H., Faig-Leite, F. S., Moraes, L. C., Moraes, M. E. L. and Filho, E. M. Radiographic study of ossification of the pterygospinous and pterygoalar ligaments by the Hirtz axial technique. *Acta Odontologica Latinoamericana* 23(1):63–67, 2010.

Rose, J. C., Anton, S. C., Aufderheide, A. C., Buikstra, J. E., Eisenberg, L., Gregg, J. B., Hunt, E. E., Neiburger, E. J. and Rothschild, B. *Skeletal Database Committee Recommendations*. Paleopathology Association, Detroit, 1991.

Rossi, A. C., Freire, A. R., Manoel, C., Prado, F. B., Botacin, P. R. and Caria, P. H. F. Incidence of the ossified pterygoalar ligament in Brazilian human skulls and its clinical implications. *Journal of Morphological Science* 28(1):69–71, 2011.

Rossi, A. C., Freire, A. R., Prado, F. B., Caria, P. H. F. and Botacin, P. R. Morphological characteristics of foramen of Vesalius and its relationship with clinical implications. *Journal of Morphological Science* 27(1):26–29, 2010.

Rossi, A. C., Freire, A. R., Prado, G. B., Prado, F. B., Botacin, P. R. and Caria, P. H. F. Incidence of retromolar foramen in human mandibles: Ethnic and clinical aspects. *International Journal of Morphology* 30(30): 1074–1078, 2012.

Rouas, P., Nancy, J. and Bar, D. Identification of double mandibular canals: Literature review and three case reports with CT scans and cone beam CT. *Dentomaxillofacial Radiology* 36:34–38, 2007.

Saheb, H. S., Mavishetter, G. F., Thomas, S. T., Prasanna, L. C., Muralidhar, P. and Magi, P. A study of sutural morphology of the pterion and asterion among human adult Indian skulls. *Biomedical Research* 22(1):73–75, 2011.

Sahin, B., Ozkan, H. S. and Gorgu, M. An anatomical variation of mental nerve and foramen in a trauma patient. *International Journal of Anatomical Variations* 3:165–166, 2010.

Saifuddin, A., White, J., Tucker, S. and Taylor, B.A. Orientation of lumbar pars defects: implications for radiological detection and surgical management. *The Journal of Bone and Joint Surgery* 80-B (2): 208-211, 1998.

Sammarco, V. J. Os acromiale: Frequency, anatomy, and clinical implications. *Journal of Bone and Joint Surgery* (Am) 82(3):394–400, 2000.

Sampson, H. W., Montgomery, J.L. and Henryson, G. K. *Atlas of the Human Skull*. Texas A&M Press, College Station, 1991.

Sanchis, J. M., Peñarrocha, M., and Soler, F. Bifid mandibular canal. *Journal of Oral and Maxillofacial Surgery* 61(4):422–424, 2003.

Sanders, C. F. Sexing by costal cartilage calcifications. *British Journal of Radiology* 39(459): 233, 1966.

Sant'Ana Castilho, M. A., Oda, J. Y. and Goncales Sant'Ana, D. M. Metopism in adult skulls from Southern Brazil. *International Journal of Morphology* 24(1):1–13, 2006. Accessed online http://www.scielo.cl/scielo.php.

Saran, R. S., Ananthi, K. S., Subramaniam, A., Balaji, M. S. T., Vinaitha, D. and Vaithianathan, G. Foramen of Civinini: A new anatomical guide for maxillofacial surgeons. *Journal of Clinical and Diagnostic Research* 7(7):1271–1275, 2013.

Sarrafian, S. K. *Anatomy of the Foot and Ankle: Descriptive, Topographic, Functional*. Lippincott Williams and Wilkins, Philadephia, 1993.

Saunders, S. R. and Popovich, F. A family study of two skeletal variants: Atlas bridging and clinoid bridging. *American Journal of Physical Anthropology* 49(2):193–203, 1978.

Saunders, S. R. and Rainey, D. L. Nonmetric trait variation in the skeleton: Abnormalities, anomalies, and atavisms. In M. A. Katzenberg and S. R. Saunders (Eds.), *Biological Anthropology of the Human Skeleton*, Second Edition. Wiley and Sons, Hoboken, 2008.

Savage, C. *Lumbosacral Transitional Vertebrae: Classification of Variation and Association with Low Back Pain*. Master's thesis, University of Missouri-Columbia, 2005.

Saxena, S. K., Chowdhary, D. S. and Jain, S. P. Interparietal bones in Nigerian skulls. *Journal of Anatomy* 144:235–237, 1986.

Schaefer, M., Black, S. and Scheuer, L. *Juvenile Osteology: A Laboratory and Field Manual*. Elsevier Academic Press, San Diego, 2009.

Scheuer, L. Application of osteology to forensic medicine. *Clinical Anatomy* 15:297–312, 2002.

Scheuer, L. and Black, S. *Developmental Juvenile Osteology*. Elsevier Academic Press, San Diego, 2000.

Scheuer, L. and Black, S. *The Juvenile Skeleton*. Elsevier Academic Press, San Diego, 2004.

Schiel, J. A. UMFC #66 A Comprehensive Forensic Analysis Case Report. Professional paper as part of master of arts degree. University of Montana, Missoula, 2007.

Schiwy-Bochat, K.H. The roughness of the supranasal region – A morphological sex trait. *Forensic Science International* 117:7–13, 2001.

Schultz, A. H. The fontanella metopica and its remnants in

an adult skull. *American Journal of Anatomy* 23(2):259–272, 1918.

Schultz, A. H. The metopic fontanelle, fissure, and suture. *American Journal of Anatomy* 44(3):475–499, 1929.

Schwalbe, G. Uber die Fontanella metopica und ihre Bildungen. *Zeitschrift fur Morphologie und Anthropologie* 3:93–129, 1901.

Scott, G. R. Dental morphology. In M. A. Katzenberg and S. R. Saunders (Eds.), *Biological Anthropology of the Human Skeleton*, Second Edition. Wiley and Sons, Hoboken, 2008.

Scott, G. R. and Turner, C. G. II. *The Anthropology of Modern Human Teeth: Dental Morphology and its Variation in Recent Human Populations.* Cambridge University Press, Cambridge, 1997.

Segall, J., Mikity, V. G., Rumbaugh, C. L., Bergeron, R. T., Teal, J. S., Richmond J. and Wu, P. Y. The radiology of the normal anterior fontanelle. *Radiology* 107:105–107, 1973.

Serman, N. J. The mandibular incisive foramen. *Journal of Anatomy* 167:195–198, 1989.

Serrafian, S. K. *Anatomy of the Foot and Ankle: Descriptive, Topographic, Functional*, Second Edition. J. B. Lippincott Company, Philadelphia, 1993.

Sewell, R. B. A study of the astragalus. *Journal of Anatomy and Physiology* 38(3):423–434, 1904.

Shankar, L., Evans, K., Hawke, M. and Stammberger, H. *An Atlas of Imaging of the Paranasal Sinuses.* JB Lippincott Company, Philadelphia, 1993.

Shapiro, R. Anomalous parietal sutures and the bipartite parietal bone. *American Journal of Roentgenology* 115(3):569–577, 1972.

Shapiro, R. and Robinson, F. The foramina of the middle fossa: a phylogenetic, anatomic and pathologic study. *The American Journal of Roentgenology* 101(4):779–794, 1967.

Shapiro, R. and Robinson, F. Embryogenesis of the human occipital bone. *American Journal of Roentgenology* 126:1063–1068, 1976.

Sharma, M., Singh, B., Abhaya, A. and Kumar, H. Occipitalization of atlas with other associated anomalies of skull. *European Journal of Anatomy* 12(3):159–167, 2008.

Shaw, J.P. Pterygospnous and pterygoalar foramina: A role in the etiology of Trigeminal Neuralgia. *Clinical Anatomy* 6(3): 173-178, 1993.

Sheehy, J. J. Diffuse exostoses and osteomata of the external auditory canal: A report of 100 operations. *Otolaryngology Head and Neck Surgery* 90:337–340, 1982.

Shinohara, A. L., de Souza Melo, C. G., Silveira, E. M. V., Lauris, J. R. P., Andreo, J. C. and de Castro Rodrigues, A. Incidence, morphology and morphometry of the foramen of Vesalius: Complementary study for a safer planning and execution of the trigeminal rhizotomy technique. *Surgical and Radiologic Anatomy* 32:159–164, 2010.

Shivarama, C. and Kumar, S. A. The Wormian os ptericum (epipteric bone). *International Journal of Scientific Research and Education* 3(1): 2834–2837, 2015.

Sholts, S. B. and Wärmländer, S. K. T. S. Zygomaticomaxillary suture shape analyzed with digital morphometrics: Reassessing patterns of variation in American Indian and European populations. *Forensic Science International* 217:234e1–234.36, 2012.

Shore, L. R. Abnormalities of the vertebral column in a series of skeletons of Bantu Natives of South Africa. *Journal of Anatomy* 64(2):206–238, 1930.

Silva, A. M. Foot anomalies in the Late Neolithic/Chalcolithic population exhumed from the rock cut cave of São Paulo 2 (Almada, Portugal). *International Journal of Osteoarchaeology* 2010. DOI: 10.1002/0a.1148

Simsek, S., Yigitkanli, K., Comert, A., Acar, H. I., Seckin, H., Er, U., Belen, D., Tekdemir, I. and Elhan, A. Posterior osseous bridging of CD1. *Journal of Clinical Neuroscience* 15:686–688, 2008. PMCID: PMC1244546.

Singh, I. Squatting facets on the talus and tibia in Indians. *Journal of Anatomy* 93(4):540–550, 1959.

Singh, M. Duplication of optic canal in adult Japanese human skulls. *Journal of Anatomical Society of India* 54:1–9, 2005.

Singh, R. A new foramen on posterior aspect of ala of first sacral vertebra. *International Journal of Anatomical Variations* 5:29–31, 2012.

Singh, J. and Chavali, K. H. Age estimation from clavicular epiphyseal union sequencing in a Northwest Indian population of the Chandigarh region. *Journal of Forensic and Legal Medicine* 18(2):82–87, 2011.

Singh, M. and Anand, M. Varying positions of foramen spinosum in relation to spine of sphenoid. *Journal of Anatomical Society of India* 58(2):144–148, 2009.

Singh, S. K., Prabhu, R., Mamatha, G. P., Gupta, A. and Jain, M. Morphologic variations in the mandibular canal: A retrospective study of panoramic radiographs. *Journal of Oral Health Research* 1(3):106–112, 2010.

Singh, V., Anand, M. K. and Dinesh, K. Variations in the pattern of mental spines and spinous mental foramina in dry adult human mandibles. *Surgical and Radiologic Anatomy* 22:169–173, 2000.

Singhal, S. and Rao, V. Supratrochlear foramen of the humerus. *Anatomical Science International* 82:105–107, 2007.

Sinkeet, S. R., Awori, K. O., Odula, P. O., Ogeng'o, J. O. and Mwachaka, P. M. The suprascapular notch: Its morphology and distance from the glenoid cavity in a Kenyan population. *Folia Morphologica* 69(4):241–245, 2010.

Sisman, Y., Ertas, E. T., Gokce, C. and Akgunlu, F. Prevalence of torus palatinus in Cappadocia Region population of Turkey. *European Journal of Dentistry* 2:269–275, 2008.

Skrzat, J. and Walocha, J. Application of fractal dimension in evaluation of cranial suture complexity. *Harmonic and Fractal Image Analysis* 2003:39–41, 2003a.

Skrzat, J. and Walocha, J. Fractal dimensions of the sagittal (interparietal) sutures in humans. *Folia Morphologica* 62:119–122, 2003b.

Skrzat, J., Walocha, J. and Srodek, R. An anatomical study of the pterygoalar bar and the pterygoalar foramen. *Folia Morphoogica* 64:92–96, 2005.

Skrzat, J. Walocha, J. and Zawilinski, J. Accessory spine of the foramen ovale. *Folia Morphologica* 71(4):263–266, 2012.

Skrzat, R., Szewczyk, R. and Walocha, J. The ossified

interclinoid ligament. *Folia Morphologica* 65(3):242–245, 2006a.

Skrzat, R., Walocha, J., Srodek, R. and Nizankowska, A. An atypical position of the foramen ovale. *Folia Morphologica* 65(4):396–399, 2006b.

Smoker, W. R. K. Craniovertebral junction: Normal anatomy, craniometry, and congenital anomalies. *Radiographics* 14:255–277, 1994.

Snodgrass, J. J. and Galloway, A. Utility of dorsal pits and pubic tubercle height in parity assessment. *Journal of Forensic Sciences* 48(6):940–948, 2003. Accessed online at www.astm.org on January 27, 2012.

Snow, C. E. *Early Hawaiians: An Initial Study of Skeletal Remains from Mokapu.* University of Kentucky Press, Lexington, 1974.

Sperber, G. H. *Craniofacial Development.* B. C. Decker, Ontario, 2001.

Sperber, G. H., Sperber, S. M. and Guttmann, G. D. *Craniofacial Embryogenetics and Development.* Peoples Medical Publishing House, Beijing, 2010.

Srivastava, H. C. Development of ossification centres in the squamous portion of the human occipital bone in man. *Journal of Anatomy* 124(3):643–649, 1977.

Stafne, E. C. Bone cavities situated near the angle of the mandible. *Journal of the American Dental Association* 29:1969–1972, 1942.

Stark, P., Watkins, G. E., Hildebrandt-Stark, H. E. and Dunbar, R. D. Episternal ossicles. *Radiology* 165:143–144, 1987.

Stathis, G., Economopoulos, N., Mavraganis, D., Kelekis, N. and Alexopoulou, E. Paracondylar process, a rare normal variant: The value of MRI in the diagnosis. *Surgical and Radiologic Anatomy* 26 July 2011. DOI 10.1007/s00276-011-0857-z accessed online October 14, 2011.

Steele, D. G. and Bramblett, C. A. *The Anatomy and Biology of the Human Skeleton.* Texas A&M University Press, College Station, 1988.

Sternberg, L. E. Biological Divergence Between Six Western European Populations as Determined by Non-Metrical Cranial Variants. Open Access Dissertations and Theses (1975). Paper 5380. Accessed online at http://digital commons.mcmaster.ca/opendissertations/5380 on January 9, 2012.

Stewart, J. H. and McCormick, W. F. A sex- and age-limited ossification pattern in human costal cartilages. *American Journal of Clinical Pathology* 81(6):765–769, 1984.

Stewart, T. D. The tympanic plate and external auditory meatus in the Eskimo. *American Journal of Physical Anthropology* 17(4):481–496, 1933.

Stewart, T. D. Are supra-inion depressions evidence of prophylactic trephination? *Bulletin of the History of Medicine* 50:413–434, 1976.

Stibbe, E. P. Skull showing exaggerated grooving of temporal region. *Journal of Anatomy* 63(2):278–279, 1929.

Stilianos, E., Kountakis, B. A. Sr., and Draf, W. *The Frontal Sinus.* Springer-Verlag, Heidelberg, 2005.

Straus, W. L. Jr., and Temkin, O. Vesalius and the problem of variability. *Bulletin of the History of Medicine* 14:609–633, 1943.

Sudha, R., Sridevi, C. and Ezhilarasi, M. Anatomical variations in the formation of pterion and asterion in South Indian population. *International Journal of Current Research and Review* 5(9): 92–101, 2013.

Sutherland, L. D. and Suchey, J. M. Use of the ventral arc in pubic sex determination. *Journal of Forensic Sciences* 36(2):501–11, 1991.

Sutter, R. C. and Mertz, L. Nonmetric cranial trait variation and prehistoric biocultural change in the Azapa Valley, Chile. *American Journal of Physical Anthropology* 123:130–145, 2004.

Sutton, J. B. On the relation of the orbito-sphenoid to the region pterion in the side wall of the skull. *Journal of Anatomy and Physiology* 18(2):219–222, 1884.

Szawlowski, J. Ueber einige seltene varationen an der wirbelsaeule beim menschen. *Anatomischer Anzeiger* 20:305–320, 1901.

Taitz, C. Bony observations of some morphological variations and anomalies of the craniovertebral region. *Clinical Anatomy* 13:354–360, 2000.

Tappen, N. C. The development of the vermiculate pattern in the brow region of crania from Indian Knoll, Kentucky. *American Journal of Physical Anthropology* 60(4):523–537, 1983.

Tavassoli, M. M. Metopism: As an indicator of cranial pathology; A good example from Iranian Plateau. *Acta Medica Iranica* 49(6):331–335, 2011.

Taveras, J. M. and Wood, E. H. *Diagnostic Neuroradiology*, 5th Edition. Williams and Wilkins, Baltimore, 1964.

Tebo, H. G. The pterygospinous bar in panoramic roentgenography. *Oral Surgery Oral Medicine Oral Pathology* 26:654–657, 1968.

Tekdemir, I., Deda, H., Karahan, S. T. and Arinci, K. The intracranial course of the abducens nerve. *Turkish Neurosurgery* (6):96–102, 1996.

Tetradis, S., and Kantor, M. L. Prevalence of skeletal and dental anomalies and normal variants seen in cephalometric and other radiographs of orthodontic patients. *American Journal of Orthodontics and Dentofacial Orthopedics* 116:572–577, 1999.

Tharp, A. and Jason, D. R. Anomalous parietal suture mimicking skull fracture. *American Journal of Forensic Medicine and Pathology* 30(1):49–51, 2009.

Todd, T. "Cervical" rib: Factors controlling its presence and its size. Its bearing on the morphology and development of the shoulder. *Journal of Anatomy and Physiology* 46(3):244–288, 1912.

Toldt, C. *An Atlas of Human Anatomy for Students and Physicians,* 2nd Edition, Volume 1. The Macmillan Company, New York, 1928.

Toldt, C. U. Die entwickelung der scheitelbeins des menschen. *Zeitschr. f. Heilkunde,* Bd. IV: 83-86, Taf. II, Figs. 10 and 11, 1883.

Travan, L., Sabbadini, G., Saccheri, P. and Crivellato, E. Unusual case of occipital vertebra in a medieval skeleton. *Anatomical Science International* 83:286–290, 2008.

Trivedi, D. J., Shrimankar, P. S., Kariya, V. B., and Pensi, A. A study of supraorbital notches and foramina in Gujarati human skulls. *National Journal of Integrated Research in Medicine* 1(3):1–6, 2010.

Trotter, M. Septal apertures in the humerus of American Whites and Blacks. *American Journal of Physical Anthropology* 19(2):213–227, 1934.

Trotter, M. Accessory sacroiliac articulations. *American Journal of Physical Anthropology* 22:247–261, 1937.

Truumees, E. Os odontoideum. *Emedicine Orthopedic Surgery*, 2008. Accessed online at http://emedicine.medscape.com/article/1265065 on May 29, 2010.

Tubbs, R. S., May, W. R., Jr., Apaydin, N., Shoja, M. M., Shokouhi, G., Loukas, M. and Cohen-Gadol, A. A. Ossification of ligaments near the foramen ovale: An anatomic study with potential clinical significance regarding transcutaneous approaches to the skull base. *Neurosurgery* 65(6 Suppl):60–64, 2009.

Tubbs, R. S., Nechtman, C., D'Antoni, A. V., Shoja, M. M., Mortazavi, M. M., Loukas, M., Rozzelle, C. J. and Spinner, R. J. Ossification of the suprascapular ligament: A risk factor for suprascapular nerve compression? *International Journal of Shoulder Surgery* 7(1):19–22, 2013b.

Tubbs, R. S., Salter, E. G. and Oakes, W. J. Duplication of the Occipital Condyles. *Clinical Anatomy* 18:92–95, 2005.

Tubbs, R. S., Salter, E. G. and Oakes, W. J. Does the mendosal suture exist in the adult? *Clinical Anatomy* 20(2): 124–125, 2007.

Tubbs, R. S., Sharma, A., Loukas, M. and Cohen-Gadol, A. A. Ossification of the petrosphenoidal ligament: Unusual variation with the potential for abducens nerve entrapment in Dorello's canal at the skull base. *Surgical and Radiologic Anatomy*, 23 July 2013a, DOI 10.1007/x00276-013-1171-8.

Tubbs, R. S., Smith, M. D. and Oakes, W. J. Parietal foramina are not synonymous with giant parietal foramina. *Pediatric Neurosurgery* 39(4):216–217, 2003.

Turner, W. On Supernumerary cervical ribs. *Journal of Anatomy and Physiology* 4(1):130–139, 1869.

Turner, W. On exostoses within the external auditory meatus. *Journal of Anatomy and Physiology* 13(2):200–293, 1879.

Turner, W. A secondary astragalus in the human foot. *Journal of Anatomy and Physiology* 17(1):82–83, 1882.

Turner, W. Cervical ribs, and the so-called bicipital ribs in man, in relation to corresponding structures in the cetacea. *Journal of Anatomy and Physiology* 17(3):384–400, 1883.

Turner, W. The Infra-orbital suture. *Journal of Anatomy and Physiology* 19(2):218–220, 1885.

Turner, W. Human neck with the odontoid process distinct from the body of the axis vertebra. *Journal of Anatomy and Physiology* 24(3):358–359, 1890.

Turner, W. Double right parietal bone in an Australian skull. *Journal of Anatomy and Physiology* 25(4):473–474, 1891.

Turner, W. Double left parietal bone in a Scottish skull. *Journal of Anatomy and Physiology* 35(4):496, 1901.

Ubelaker, D. H. *Skeletal Biology of Human Remains from La Tolita, Esmeraldas Province, Ecuador.* Smithsonian Contributions to Anthropology, Number 41. Smithsonian Institution Press, Washington, D.C., 1997.

Unlu, Z., Orguc, S. Eskiizmir, G., Aslan, A. and Bayindir, P. Elongated styloid process and cervical spondylosis. *Clinical Medicine Case Reports* I:57–64, 2008.

Vacher, C., Onolfo, J. P., and Barbet, J. P. Is the pterygopalato-maxillary suture (*sutura sphenomaxillaris*) a growing suture in the fetus? *Surgical Radiology and Anatomy* 32:689–692, 2010.

Van Arsdale, A. P. and Clark, J. L. Re-examining the relationship between cranial deformation and extra-sutural bone formation. *International Journal of Osteoarchaeology* 22:119–126, 2012.

van Buggenhout, G. and Bailleul-Forestier, I. Mesiodens. *European Journal of Medical Genetics* 51(2):178–181, 2008.

Vastine, J. H., Vastine, M. F. and Arango, O. Genetic influence on osseous development with particular reference to the deposition of calcium in the costal cartilages. *American Journal of Roentgenology, Radium Therapy and Nuclear Medicine* 59(2): 213–221, 1948.

Vasudeva, N. and Choudhry, R. Precondylar tubercles on the basiocciput of adult human skulls. *Journal of Anatomy and Physiology* 188:207–210, 1996.

Vaziri A, Nayeb-Hashemi H and Akhavan-Tafti. B. 2009. Computational model of rib movement and its application in studying the effects of age-related thoracic cage calcification on respiratory system. *Computer Methods in Biomechanics and Biomedical Engineering*. Vol. 00, No. 0, 1–8. Accessed online April 3, 2015.

Vázquez, J. F. P., Verona, J. A. G., Fernández, F. J. De Paz and Cachorro, M. B. *Atlas De Variaciones Epigenéticas Craneales.* Medicina Manuales Y Textos Universitarios No. 22. Universidad De Valladolid, 2001.

Vayvada, H., Demirdover, C., Yilmaz, M. and Barutcu, A. An anatomic variation of the mental nerve and foramina. *Clinical Anatomy* 19:700–701, 2006.

Veldman, J. K. *Non-Metric Traits. An Assessment of Cranial and Post-Cranial Non-Metric Traits in the Skeletal Assemblage from the 17th-19th Century Churchyard of Middenbeemster, the Netherlands.* Msc Thesis, Leiden University, Netherlands, 2013. Available online at http://hdl.handle.net/1887/21705

Verna, E. Les Variations Osseuses Asymptomatiques Du Squelette Postcranien: Leur Contribution A L'Identification En Anthropologie Mesico-Legale. Doctorat d'Aix-Marseille Universite, Anthropologie Biologique. Aix-Marseille Université, December 2014.

Verna, G. L., Agarwal, G. R. and Hiran, S. Sex determination by costal cartilage calcification. *Indian Journal of Radiology* 34: 22–25, 1980.

Vodanovic, M., Slaus, M., Galic, I., Marotti, M. and Brkic, H. Stafne's defects in two mandibles from archaeological sites in Croatia. *International Journal of Osteoarchaeology* 21:119–126, 2011.

von Arx, T., Hänni, A., Sendi, P., Buser, D. and Bornstein, M. M. Radiographic study of the mandibular retromolar canal: An anatomic structure with clinical importance. *Journal of Endodontics* 37(12):1630–1635, 2011.

von Arx, T. Location and dimensions of the mental foramen: A radiographic analysis by using cone-beam computed tomography. *Journal of Endodontics* 39(12):1522–1528, 2013.

von Ludinghausen, M., Fahr, M., Prescher, A., Schindler, G., Kenn, W., Weiglein, A., Yoshimura, K., Kageyama, I., Kobayashi, K. and Tsuchimochi, M. Accessory joints between basiocciput and atlas/axis in the median plane. *Clinical Anatomy* 18:558–571, 2005.

Vu, H. L., Panchal, J., Parker, E. E., Levine, N. S. and Francel, P. The timing of physiologic closure of the metopic suture: A review of 159 patients using reconstructed 3D CT scans of the craniofacial region. *Journal of Craniofacial Surgery* 12(6):527–532, 2001.

Wackenheim, A. Hypoplasia of the basi-occipital bone and persistence of the spheno-occipital synchondrosis in a patient with transitory supplementary fissure of the basi-occipital. *Neuroradiology* 27(3):226–231, 1985.

Wahby, B. Abnormal nasal bones. *Journal of Anatomy and Physiology* 38:49–51, 1903.

Wang, H-J., Chen, C., Wu, L. P., Pan, C. Q. and Zhang, W. J. Variable morphology of the suprascapular notch: An investigation and quantitative measurements in Chinese population. *Clinical Anatomy* 24(1):47–55, 2011.

Wang, R. G., Bingham, B., Hawke, M., Kwok, P. and Li, J. R. Persistence of the foramen of Huschke in the adult: An osteological study. *Journal of Otolaryngology* 29(4):251–253, 1991.

Wang, Y., Videman, T., and Battie, Michele C., Lumbar Vertebral endplat lesions: Prevalence, classification and association with age. *Spine* 37(17):1432-1439. 2012.

Wartmann, C. T. and Loukas, M. Letter to the editor: Zygomaticofacial, zygomaticoorbital, and zygomaticotemporal foramina. *Clinical Anatomy* 22:637–638, 2009.

Warwick, R. A juvenile skull exhibiting duplication of the optic canals and subdivision of the superior orbital fissure. *Journal of Anatomy* 85(3):289–291, 1951.

Warwick, R. *Eugene Wolff's Anatomy of the Eye and Orbit: Including the Central Connexions, Development, and Comparative Anatomy of the Visual Apparatus*, 7th Edition. W. B. Saunders Company, Philadelphia, 1976.

Wasterlain, S. N. and Silva, A. M. Study of Stafne's defects on Late Neolithic, Late Roman, Medieval and Modern skeletal samples from Portugal. *International Journal of Osteoarchaeology* 22:423–434, 2012.

Weber, J., Collman, A., Czarnetzki, A., Spring, C. and Pusch, M. Morphometric analysis of untreated adult skulls in syndromic and nonsyndromic craniosynostosis. *Neurosurgical Review* 31:179–188, 2008.

Weckström, M., Parviainen, M. and Pihlajamäki, H.K. Excision of painful bipartite patella: Good long-term outcome in young adults. *Clinical Orthopaedics and Related Research* 466(11):2848–2855, 2008.

Weinberg, S. M., Putz, D. A., Mooney, M. P. and Siegel, M. I. Evaluation of non-metric variation in the crania of black and white perinates. *Forensic Science International* 151:177–185, 2005.

Weinzweig, J., Kirschner, Farley, A., Reiss, P., Hunter, J., Whitaker, L. A. and Bartlett, P. Metopic synostosis: Defining the temporal sequence of normal suture fusion and differentiating it from synostosis on the basis of computed tomography images. *Plastic and Reconstructive Surgery* 112(5):1211–1218, 2003.

Werb, A. Surgery of the lacrimal sac. *Royal College of Surgeons of England* 54:236–243, 1974.

White, T. D. and Folkens, P. A. *Human Osteology*. New York, Academic Press, 2005.

White, T. D. and Folkens, P. A. *The Human Bone Manual*. Academic Press, Burlington, MA, 2005.

Whitnall, S. E. On a tubercle on the malar bone, and on the lateral attachments of the tarsal plates. *Journal of Anatomy* 45(4):426–432, 1911.

Whitnall, S. E. *The Anatomy of the Human Orbit and Accessory Organs of Vision*. Henry Frowde and Hodder and Stoughton, Strand, London, 1921.

Wilczak, C. A. and Ousley, S. D. Test of the relationship between sutural ossicles and cultural cranial deformation: Results from Hawikuh, New Mexico. *American Journal of Physical Anthropology* 139(4):483–493, 2009.

Willis, T. A. The separate neural arch. *Journal of Bone and Joint Surgery* 13(4)A:709–721, 1931.

Wilson, C. The relationship between size and expression of nonmetric traits on the human skull. *The Arbitus Review* 1:81–97, 2010.

Wiltse, L. L., Widell, E. H. and Jackson, D. W. Fatigue fracture: The basic lesion in isthmic spondylolisthesis. *Journal of Bone and Joint Surgery* (Am) 57(A):17–22, 1975.

Wobig, J. L. and Dailey, R. A. *Oculofacial Plastic Surgery: Face, Lacrimal System, and Orbit*. Thieme Medical Publishers, New York, 2004.

Woo, J. K. Anterior and posterior medio-palatine bones. *American Journal of Physical Anthropology* 6(2): 209–224, 1948.

Woo, J. K. Racial and sexual differences in the frontal curvature and its relation to metopism. *American Journal of Physical Anthropology* 7:215–226, 1949.

Wood, C. C. E. *The Influence of Growth and Development in the Expression of Human Morphological Variation*. Doctoral thesis, University of Toronto, 2012. Available online at http://hdl.handle.net/1807/43402.

Wood-Jones, F. The non-metrical morphological characters of the skull as criteria for racial diagnosis. Part I. General discussion of the morphological characters employed in racial diagnosis. *Journal of Anatomy and Physiology* 65:179–195, 1931.

Wong, M. and Carter, D. R. Mechanical stress and morphogenetic endochondrial ossification of the sternum. *Journal of Bone and Joint Surgery* 70(A)7:992–1000, 1988.

Wright, W. A case of accessory patellae in the human subject, with remarks on emargination of the patella. *Journal of Anatomy and Physiology* 38(1):65–67, 1903.

www.carolina.com 2008. Accessed online March 6, 2015.

www.skullsunlimited.com. Accessed online on October 2, 2014.

Wysocki, J. Morphology of the temporal canal and postglenoid foramen with reference to the size of the jugular foramen in man and selected species of animals. *Folia Morphologica* 61(4):199–208, 2002.

Wysocki, J., Kobryn, H., Bubrowski, M. and Kwiatkowski, J. The morphology of the hypoglossal canal and its size in relation to skull capacity in man and other animal species. *Folia Morphologica* 63(1):11–17, 2004.

Yaczi, A. B., Kiroglu, Y., Ozdemir, B. and Kara, C. O. Three-dimensional computed tomography of a complete stylohyoid ossification with articulation. *Surgical and Radiologic Anatomy* 30:167–169, 2008.

Yadav, A., Kumar, V. and Srivastava, R. K. Study of metopic suture in the adult human skulls of North India. *Journal of Anatomical Society of India* 59(2):232–236, 2010.

Yazar, F. and Acar, H. I. Supracondylar process with a high origin of the radial artery. *Clinical Anatomy* 19:730–731, 2006.

Yekeler, E., Tunaci, M., Tunaci, A., Dursun, M. and Acunas, G. Frequency of sternal variations and anomalies evaluated by MDCT. *American Journal of Roentgenology* 186:956–960, 2006.

Yochum, T. R. and Rowe, L. J. *Essentials of Skeletal Radiology*, 3rd Edition. Lippincott Williams & Wilkins, Baltimore, 2005.

Yoshioka, N., Rhoton, A. L., Jr. and Abe, H. Scalp to meningeal arterial anastomosis in the parietal foramen. *Operative Neurosurgery* 58:123–126, 2006. Accessed online at www.neurosurgery-online.com in 2012.

Zografos, J. and Mutzuri, A. Incidence of double mental foramen in a sample of Greek population. *Odontostomatol Proodos* 43(6):521–523, 1989.

Zona, A. Le suture abnormi della volta palatine. *La Stomatologia* 33:223–244, 1935.

NAME INDEX

A

Abd Latiff, A., 337
Abe, H., 198, 211, 216, 218, 364
Abed, S. F., 91
Abhaya, A., 408
Acar, H. I., 536, 568
Acunas, G., 542, 543, 545, 547, 550, 551
Adam, G., 310, 326, 339, 381, 382, 383, 384
Adams, W. M., 345
Adds, P. J., 91
Agarwal, G. R., 542, 551
Aggarwal, B., 280, 291
Ağlagül, E., 549
Agrawal, R., 338, 390, 567
Agrawal, S., 338, 390, 567
Agthong, S., 91
Akay, H. O., 269
Akdogan, O., 20
Akgunlu, F., 498
Akhavan-Tafti. B., 542, 551
Aksu, F., 113, 114, 142, 153, 253, 283, 284, 285, 292, 297, 298, 320, 338, 339
Alexopoulou, E., 310
Ali, M., 643
Ali Gurses, I., 142, 253
Allen, H., 611
Allen, W., 401
Allen, W. A., 408
Al-Mefty, O., 283, 292, 337
Al-Motabagani, M. A., 390, 408
Alper, M., 56
Alqahtani, B., 161
Alqahtani, M., 161
Alsherhri, H., 161
Amorim, M. M., 478
Anagnostopoulou, S., 163, 180, 290, 346, 348, 352, 355, 357, 358, 379
Anand, C., 92, 354, 357, 359, 360, 369, 372, 374, 377
Anand, M. K., 452, 481, 483, 484
Anand, V. K., 564
Ananthi, K. S., 312, 313, 334, 390, 567
Ananthi, S., 338
Anderson, B., 148, 219
Anderson, L. C., 655
Anderson, T., 325, 565
Andrén, L., 215, 236
Andreo, J. C., 284, 285, 321, 364
Anil, A., 163, 352, 404, 431, 433
Anson, B. J., 363

Anton, S. C., 65, 194, 231, 656, 659, 661
Antonisamy, B., 635
Antonopoulou, M., 163, 290, 346, 348, 352, 355, 357, 358, 379
Anupa, S., 53, 56, 73, 100
Apaydin, N., 312, 346, 354, 355, 357, 358
Apinhasmit, W., 3, 9, 323, 494, 495, 496, 498
Appell, H. J., 529, 533, 534
Araç, M., 180
Arango, O., 551
Arda, M. N., 307, 340, 422, 423, 424, 425
Arey, L. B., 557, 574
Ari, I., 625, 626
Ari, Z., 283, 284, 285, 292, 320, 338, 339
Arican, R. Y., 629, 630
Arinci, K., 291
Arman, C., 113, 114, 153, 307, 340, 422, 423, 424, 425
Aronyk, K., 219
Arora, A. K., 325, 338
Asala, S. A., 129
Ashley, G. T., 546
Ashley-Montagu, M. F., 505, 506, 507, 508
Ashraf, C. M., 460, 462
Ashwini, L. S., 49, 50
Asim, O. M., 56
Aslan, A., 180
Asrani, M. K., 119
Asvat, R., 524
Aufderheide, A. C., 656, 657, 658, 661
Awori, K. O., 529
Aydinhoglu, A., 26
Azccagni, L., 655, 658, 659

B

Babu, K. Y., 95, 97
Baert, A. L., 285
Bahcelioğlu, M., 180
Bailet, P., 27
Bailleul-Forestier, I., 503
Bajaj, M., 565
Baker, B. J., 430
Baker, D., 576, 577
Balaji, M. S. T., 312, 313, 334
Balasubramanyam, V., 480
Balci, A., 549
Balcioglu, H. A., 473
Balko, M. G., 269
Ballard, K. E., 596
Bar, D., 463

Barbatob, E., 291, 568
Barberini, F., 7, 209, 210, 212
Barbet, J. P., 388
Barclay-Smith, E., 190, 209, 210
Barner, B. C. W., 462
Barnes, E., 326, 328, 329, 333, 338, 339, 345, 546, 555, 556, 557, 564, 565, 569, 574, 575, 576, 578, 584, 587, 589, 590, 591, 592, 594, 595, 596, 655
Barnett, C. H., 625, 626, 627, 633, 634, 635
Bartlett, P., 6, 9, 17
Barutcu, A., 470
Bass, W. M., 345
Bast, T. H., 363
Bauer, L., 129, 179
Bayaroğullari, H., 549
Bayindir, P., 180
Bayrak, A. H, 269
Bayraktar, B., 142, 253, 283, 284, 285, 292, 297, 298, 320, 338, 339
Becker, B. J., 655, 657, 658
Becker, D. B., 121
Beers, G. J., 585
Belcastro, M.G., 612
Belen, D., 568
Belsky, J. L., 494
Bennett, E. H., 631
Benson, B. W., 286
Berge, J. K., 3, 243, 258, 283, 292, 294, 324, 342, 343, 344, 364, 398, 417, 418, 419, 422, 423, 424, 425, 490
Bergeron, R. T., 8
Bergman, R. A., 3, 74, 100, 243, 258, 283, 292, 294, 324, 342, 343, 344, 364, 398, 417, 418, 419, 422, 423, 424, 425, 490, 596, 598
Berlet, G. C., 639
Bernaerts, A., 629
Berry, A., 172, 438
Berry, R., 172, 438
Berry, R. J. A., 121
Berryman, H. E., 642
Beutler, W. J., 576, 577
Bhagra, T., 127, 167, 169, 176
Bhanu, P. S., 238, 243, 247, 248, 250, 251, 255
Bhardwaj, R., 452, 453
Bhargaval, R., 219
Bidmos, M., 633, 655
Billmann, F., 569
Bingham, B., 165
Bircan, O., 629, 630
Birkby, W., 148, 611
Birkby, W. H., 148
Bittar, T. O., 478
Black, S., 3, 4, 58, 62, 238, 259, 325
Blank, E., 7, 8, 212
Blom, D. E., 656, 657, 661
Bogduk, N., 228, 230
Bolanowski, W., 618
Bolk, L., 62
Bongiovanni R., 542, 543
Bono, C. M., 576
Boopathi, S., 53, 56, 73, 100
Borah, D., 628, 629
Borini, C. B., 478
Bornstein, M. M., 463, 465, 467, 659
Botacin, P. R., 163, 283, 289, 290, 315, 346, 347, 348, 352, 355, 357, 358, 404, 431, 433, 659
Bots, J., 573
Boyadjian, C. H. C., 138, 139
Boyd, G. I., 127, 161, 162, 165, 166, 169, 170, 176, 198, 200, 201, 222, 243, 258, 283, 303, 343, 344, 398, 411, 434, 439
Brackett, C. F., 533
Bramblett, C. A., 285
Brash, J. C., 4, 58, 128, 169, 230
Brasili, P., 655, 658, 659
Breathnach, A. S., 198
Bressan, C., 55, 56
Brewin, J., 558, 573, 574
Bridenbough, P. O., 412
Brkic, H., 454, 458
Bromage, T., 219
Broman, G. E., Jr., 325, 333, 338, 382, 386, 416
Brors, D., 310, 326, 339, 381, 382, 383, 384
Brossman, J., 62, 91, 184, 259, 260, 271, 290, 303, 325, 385, 401, 529, 536, 537, 538, 546, 551
Brothwell D. R., 505, 506, 507, 508
Brubaker, D., 403, 409
Bruner, E., 7, 209, 210, 212
Bryce, T. H., 6
Bubrowski, M., 422, 423, 424, 425
Buikstra, J. E., 404, 655, 656, 657, 658, 659, 661–662
Bukac, J., 542, 551
Bullen, L., 528
Bunning, P. S. C., 633, 634, 635
Burch, Ashley, 579
Burdan, F., 337
Burgenen, F. A., 568
Burnett, S. E., 528
Buser, D., 463, 465, 467, 659
Butler, H., 127, 165
Byrd, J. E., 194, 198, 199, 200, 201, 220, 228, 237, 253

C

Cabrini, R. R., 75
Cachorro, M. B., 81, 92, 100, 103, 127, 129, 165, 167, 169, 222, 256, 258, 297, 307, 310, 364, 369, 386, 387, 391, 398, 439, 487
Caesar, R. H., 54
Çalguner, E., 180
Caltabianod, M., 291, 568
Campbell, J. A., 555
Campos, P. S. F., 473, 475

Canan, S., 56
Cankal, F., 390, 391, 392, 435
Caria, P. H. F., 163, 283, 289, 290, 315, 346, 347, 348, 352, 355, 357, 358, 404, 431, 433, 478, 659
Carpay, H. A., 310, 409
Carr, D. B., 412
Carrillo, J. A., 550
Carter, A. P., 585
Carter, D. R., 546
Cartolari, R., 7, 209, 210, 212
Carwardine, T., 550
Case, D. T., 528, 628, 629
Cassell, Martin I. D., 74, 100
Cave, A. J. E., 521, 574
Cederberg, R. A., 286
Cederlund, C.-G., 215, 236
Celik, S., 65, 290
Ceri, N. G., 113, 114, 153
Cevener, M., 629, 630
Chagas, C. F., 473, 479
Chaisuksunt, V., 284, 323
Chakravarthy, M. S., 53, 56, 73, 100
Charuta, A., 321, 364, 367, 370
Chauhan, N. S., 127, 167, 169, 176
Chavali, K. H., 522
Chavda, S. V., 345
Cheatle, A. H., 434
Chell, J., 434
Chen, C., 529, 531, 533, 582
Chen, M. Y. M., 360, 363, 364, 367
Chentanez, V., 91
Cheverud, J. M., 121, 143, 205
Chiron, P., 524
Cho, B. P., 524
Chompoopong, S., 3, 9, 323
Chopra, J., 521, 524, 525, 526
Choudhry, R., 92, 113, 114, 153, 325, 338, 341
Choudhry, S., 92, 113, 114, 153
Chouke, K. S., 163, 312, 346, 348, 350, 352, 353, 354, 355, 357, 358
Chow, J. C. Y., 541
Chowdhary, D. S., 250, 255
Christensen, A. M., 27
Chung, I. H., 3, 9, 45, 49
Chung, M. S., 3, 9, 45, 49
Chunn, B. L., 655
Church, A., 574
Citak, G., 307, 340, 422, 423, 424, 425
Clark, J. L., 194, 202, 250
Clavelli, W. A., 547
Clegg, J. G., 92
Cobb, W. M., 550, 551
Cockshott, W. P., 524
Cohen-Gadol, A. A., 280, 312, 346, 354, 355, 357, 358
Collins, H. B., 129
Collins, S., 219

Collman, A., 205
Comert, A., 568
Cooper, P. D., 545, 547
Cooperman, D. R., 634, 635
Coppens, J., 310, 401, 402, 410
Corner, E. M., 310, 342
Correll, R. W., 180
Corruccini, R. S., 655–656
Coskun, N., 629, 630
Couldwell, W., 310, 401, 402, 410
Cousins, M. J., 412
Cox, M., 604, 605, 606
Cozcolluela, M. R., 576, 577, 579, 589, 590, 591
Crivellato, E., 333
Crusoe-Rebello, I., 473, 475
Cukurova, I., 97, 99
Cunningham, D. J., 564
Cunningham, M. L., 184
Currarino, G., 198
Czarnetzki, A., 205

D

Dailey, A., 310, 401, 402, 410
Dailey, R. A., 53
Daimi, S. R., 312, 350, 353, 354, 355
Dakovic-Bjelakovic, M., 81, 95, 97
D'Antoni, A. V., 529
Das, S., 337, 408
Dauber, W., 388, 389
Davanzo, J., 184
David, M. P., 24
Davidson, R. T., 628, 629
Davran, R., 549
D'Costa, S., 163, 352
Dean, D., 219
de Carvalho, V. C., 81
de Castro Rodrigues, A., 284, 285, 321, 364
Deda, H., 291
de Freitas, V., 473, 479
de Graauw, N., 310, 409
Delashaw, J. B., 231
Delbridge, R. E., 555, 556
Delen, S., 573
Demirdover, C., 470
Deng, S-Q., 268
Dere, H., 20
Dereci, O., 457
Derry, D. E., 596, 598, 604
De Santis, P., 523, 524
de Souza Melo, C. G., 284, 285, 321, 364
DeStefano, G. F., 3, 10, 13, 14, 35, 39, 40, 45, 48, 49, 53, 55, 56, 57, 58, 60, 63, 73, 74, 76, 78, 80, 103, 105, 118, 121, 123, 127, 129, 131, 132, 134, 137, 138, 139, 141, 142, 143, 144, 151, 161, 164, 165, 167, 168, 170, 172, 176, 178, 179, 201, 208, 209, 210, 211, 218, 222,

233, 237, 240, 243, 246, 248, 250, 253, 255, 258, 265, 294, 307, 310, 311, 312, 315, 319, 324, 333, 337, 338, 342, 346, 347, 348, 350, 353, 355, 357, 358, 359, 360, 374, 379, 382, 386, 387, 390, 391, 398, 402, 403, 404, 411, 416, 417, 418, 419, 422, 423, 424, 425, 430, 438, 439, 459, 460, 494, 567, 655, 656, 657–658, 660, 661, 662
DeVilliers, H., 126, 475
Dewan, R. K., 521, 524
Dhalapahty, S., 53, 56, 73, 100
Dhananjaya, K. V., 462, 567
Didagelos, M., 525, 529, 531
Diego, V. P., 218, 219, 228, 233
Diethelm, L., 550
Dinesh, K., 452, 481, 483, 484
Diwan, R., 521, 525, 526
Dixon, A. F., 10, 16, 200, 550, 551
Dodo, Y., 77, 78, 152, 153, 656, 657
Donnabhain, B. O., 656, 657, 661
Dorsey, G. A., 155, 159, 194, 248, 250
Douglas, M. T., 58, 73, 659–660
Draf, W., 26
Drop, A., 337
Du, Y., 268
Dua, V., 472
Duchesneau, P. M., 283, 317, 321, 323, 334, 360, 367
Duckworth, W. L. H., 105, 107
Dunbar, R. D., 550, 551
Dupras, T. L., 430
Duran, S., 457
Durgun, B., 558
Dursun, M., 542, 543, 545, 547, 550, 551
Dutton, J. J., 3, 17, 49, 53, 60, 79, 80, 91
Dwight, T., 537, 585, 630
Dworzsanski, W., 337
Dzieciolowska-Baran, E., 95, 97, 98

E

Eagle, W., 180
Economopoulos, N., 310
Edibamode, I. E., 524
Eggers, S., 138, 139
Ehara, S., 596, 598
Eisenberg, L., 656, 657, 659, 661
Eisenstein, S., 577, 579
Elhan, A., 390, 391, 392, 435, 568
El-Khouly, H., 364
El-Khoury, G. Y., 596, 598
Ellis, H., 558, 573
Elster, A. D., 259, 260, 326, 328, 329, 360, 363, 364, 367, 385, 400
English, J. D., 286
Er, U., 568
Erdem, S., 26
Erdogmus, S., 290

Erichsen-Powell, W., 129
Erken, E., 558, 587, 592
Eroje, M. A., 524
Ertas, E. T., 498
Erturk, M., 289, 290
Ery, K., 656
Eskiizmir, G., 180
Etter, L. E., 558, 574
Evans, K., 26
Evans, K. N., 184
Ezhilarasi, M., 661

F

Fahr, M., 382, 401
Faig-Leite, F. S., 290, 346, 347, 348, 355, 357, 358
Faig-Leite, H., 75, 290, 346, 347, 348, 355, 357, 358
Farley, A., 6, 9, 17
Fauzi, M., 473
Fazekas, G., 238, 253, 259, 260, 385
Fenton, T., 148
Fernández, F. J. De Paz, 81, 92, 100, 103, 127, 129, 165, 167, 169, 222, 256, 258, 297, 307, 310, 364, 369, 386, 387, 391, 398, 439, 487
Filho, E. M., 290, 346, 347, 348, 355, 357, 358
Filler, T. J., 312, 346, 347, 348, 354, 357, 358
Finnegan, M., 454, 655, 656
Fischer, G., 312, 346, 347, 348, 354, 357, 358
Fisher, M. S., 573
Flecker, H., 53, 54, 66, 68
Florian, Z., 611
Flournoy, L. E., 525, 526
Folkens, P. A., 146
Fortin, J. D., 596
France, D. L., 537
Francel, P., 6, 9, 11, 17, 39, 40
Franchitto, G., 7, 209, 210, 212
Frayer, D. W., 599, 656
Frazer, J. E., 600
Fredrickson, B. E., 576, 577
Freire, A. R., 35, 163, 283, 289, 290, 315, 346, 347, 348, 352, 355, 358, 404, 431, 433, 659
Freyschmidt, J., 5, 62, 92, 184, 259, 260, 271, 290, 303, 325, 385, 401, 529, 536, 537, 538, 546, 551
Friedman, L., 403, 409
Fronty, P., 27
Fukuda, H., 550
Fukushima, Y., 364
Fyfe, F. W., 144, 182

G

Galdames, I. S., 163, 290, 346, 352, 355, 357, 358, 379, 431
Galic, I., 454, 458
Galis, F., 573
Gallagher, E. R., 184

Galloway, A., 605, 606
Garcia-Garcia, A. S., 494
Garretli, O., 283, 284, 285, 292, 320, 338, 339
Gawlikowska-Sroka, A., 95, 97, 98
Gayretli, O., 142, 238, 253, 297, 298
Geelhoed, G. W., 628, 629
George, V. M., 635
Gershon-Cohen, J., 555, 556
Ghafar, N. A., 408
Ghai, R., 92
Ghazalli, H., 337
Giacobini, G., 55, 56
Gill, G. W., 148, 656–657
Gill, S. S., 312, 350, 353, 354, 355
Gilroy, A. M., 544
Ginsberg, L. E., 258, 343, 344, 360, 363, 364, 367
Giordano, G., 524
Giordano, M., 55, 56
Girdany, B. R., 7, 8, 212
Gladstone, R. J., 129, 390, 408
Glassman, D. M., 345
Gluncic, V., 337
Gohel, A., 463
Gokce, C., 498
Gokharman, D., 180
Gomez- Font, R., 494
Goncales Sant'Ana, D. M., 60
Gopinathan, K., 205, 246, 250
Gorgu, M., 463
Gottlieb, K., 194, 231
Govier, D. P., 121
Govsa, F., 65, 289, 290
Gözil, R., 180
Graham, A. R., 611
Graham, J. M., Jr., 184
Grant, W. D., 576, 577
Gray, H., 121, 169, 259, 260, 581
Green, H. L. H. H., 129
Greene, M. H., 541
Greenway G., 620
Gregg, J. B., 656, 657, 659, 661
Grévin, G., 27
Greyling, L. M., 483
Groppo, F. C., 289, 478
Grossman, C. B., 268, 271
Gruber, W., 625
Gu, Y., 541
Gualdi-Russo, E., 655, 658, 659
Guena, S., 55, 56
Gulek, B., 558
Gülekon, N., 163, 352, 404, 431, 433, 604
Gumina, S., 523, 524
Gumussoy, M., 97, 99
Gunz, P., 184
Gunzburg, R., 576
Guo, J. L., 13

Gupta, A. K., 628, 629
Gupta, C. D., 325, 338, 463
Gupta, M., 280, 291, 325
Gupta, S. C., 338
Gurses, I. A., 283, 284, 285, 292, 297, 298, 320, 338, 339
Guttman, G.D., 3
Guvencer, M., 307, 340, 422, 423, 424, 425

H

Hadied, A. M., 541
Hallgrimmson, B., 656, 657, 661
Halpern, I. N., 126
Hamer, J. S., 494
Hamilton, G. F, 144, 182
Hanihara, T., 13, 54, 55, 56, 60, 77, 78, 143, 151, 152, 153, 201, 238, 239, 243, 246, 247, 248, 250, 251, 294, 333, 338, 344, 382, 383, 417, 418, 419, 422, 423, 424, 425, 430, 460, 657
Hanji, C., 91
Hänni, A., 463, 465, 467, 659
Hanson, D., 219
Hart, B. L., 80
Hartl, R., 564
Harvati, K., 184
Hasan, D., 473
Hasan, M., 364
Hasan, T., 473
Hassett, B., 486, 498
Hat, J., 337
Hauser, G., 3, 10, 13, 14, 35, 39, 40, 45, 48, 49, 53, 55, 56, 57, 58, 60, 63, 73, 74, 76, 78, 80, 103, 105, 118, 121, 123, 127, 129, 131, 132, 134, 137, 138, 139, 141, 142, 143, 144, 151, 161, 164, 165, 167, 168, 170, 172, 176, 178, 179, 201, 208, 209, 210, 211, 218, 222, 233, 237, 240, 243, 246, 248, 250, 253, 255, 258, 265, 294, 307, 310, 311, 312, 315, 319, 324, 333, 337, 338, 342, 346, 347, 348, 350, 353, 355, 357, 358, 359, 360, 374, 379, 382, 386, 387, 390, 391, 398, 402, 403, 404, 411, 416, 417, 418, 419, 422, 423, 424, 425, 430, 438, 439, 459, 460, 494, 567, 655, 656, 657–658, 660, 661, 662
Hawke, M., 26, 165
Heathcote, G., 219
Heathcote, G. M., 218, 219, 228, 233
Hefner, J. T., 140, 187, 254, 551, 555, 557, 558, 559, 574, 575, 580, 581, 635, 657, 658, 661
Heikinheimo, K., 573
Heilman, J., 628, 629
Heiser, W. J., 620
Hejna, P., 542, 551
Henryson, G. K., 369
Hepburn, D., 238
Hessler, C., 597
Heyn, R., 7, 209, 210, 212
Hildebrandt-Stark, H. E., 550, 551

Hill, M., 558, 573
Hing, A. V., 184
Hiran, S., 542, 551
Hirsch, J. M., 463, 471, 473, 474, 475
Hlaing, K. P., 337
Hodes, P. J., 312, 346, 348, 350, 353, 354, 355, 357, 358
Hojo, T., 629
Holden, L., 62
Holla, S. J., 480
Hongo, K., 364
Horackova, L., 611
Horlacker, T. T., 412
Houghton, P., 604
Hrdlička, A., 253, 511, 519, 533, 617
Huanmanop, T., 91
Hubert, J. E., 494
Humphrey, L. T., 165
Hunt, D. R., 236, 528, 536, 538, 600, 601, 618
Hunt, E. E., 656, 657, 659, 661
Hunter, J., 6, 9, 17
Hunter, R. H., 564
Hussan, F., 408
Hyer, C. F., 639
Hyman, A. A., 620

I

Ichikawa, R., 238, 246, 250
Ijichi, M., 629
Ikata, T., 576
Ikushima, I., 269
Ilgi, S., 629, 630
Ilknur, A., 179
Inoi, T., 542, 551
Inoue, K., 283
Insogna, K., 494
International Society for Plastination, 644
Isaac, B., 480
Ishida, H., 13, 54, 55, 56, 60, 77, 78, 143, 151, 152, 153, 201, 218, 219, 228, 233, 238, 239, 243, 246, 247, 248, 250, 251, 294, 333, 338, 344, 382, 383, 417, 418, 419, 422, 423, 424, 425, 430, 460
Isloor, S. D., 53
Isolan, G.R., 283, 292, 337
Ivkic, G., 337

J

Jackson, D. W., 576
Jacobs, R., 452
Jain, M., 463
Jain, S., 92
Jain, S. P., 250, 255
Jainkittivong, A., 494, 495, 496, 498
Jalsovec, D., 337
Jamieson, E. B., 500, 502
Jane, J. A., 231
Jangid, H., 565
Jaslow, C. R., 231
Jason, D. R., 121
Jeanty, P., 547
Jędrzejewski, K., 531
Jędrzejewski, K. S., 618
Jensen, J. L., 180
Jhingan, V., 542
Jiji, P. J., 462, 567
Jit, I., 523, 524, 542
Jivraj, L., 219
Johns, W., 494
Jones, B. V., 269
Jones, R. LO., 345
Jovanovic, I., 81, 95, 97
Jurik, A. G., 549

K

Kacar, M., 180
Kageyama, I., 382, 401
Kakizawa, Y., 364
Kale, A., 142, 253, 283, 284, 285, 292, 297, 298, 320, 338
Kane, A. A., 121
Kang, H. S., 3, 9, 45, 49, 524
Kantor, M. L, 17, 20, 286
Kara, C. O., 119, 180, 181
Karahan, S. T., 291
Karahan, T., 390, 391, 392, 435
Karakose, M., 163, 352, 404, 431, 433
Karaman, Y., 97, 99
Karazincir, S., 549
Kariya, V. B., 13
Kassim, N. M., 408
Katoh, S., 576
Kaur, H., 523, 524
Kavakh, A., 26
Kawakubo, Y., 657
Kayalioglu, G., 289, 290
Kelekis, N., 310
Kempson, F. C., 623, 625
Kenn, W., 382, 401
Kennedy, G. E., 138, 139
Kennedy, K. A., 539
Keyes, J. E. L., 92, 286
Khanna, M., 472
Khare, S., 92
Khera, V., 113, 114, 153
Khudaverdyan, A. Y., 655, 658
Kida, K., 238, 246, 250
Kim, H. J., 3, 9, 45, 49
Kim, M. K., 500, 515
Kim, S. E., 620
Kim, Y-K., 79, 80
Kiroglu, Y., 119, 180, 181

Kirschner, R., 6, 9, 17
Klepacz, R., 337
Knauth, M., 285
Knott, J. F., 434
Knusel, C., 219
Ko, S. J., 79, 80
Kobayashi, K., 382, 401
Kobryn, H., 422, 423, 424, 425
Kocaelli, H., 473
Kodama, G., 238, 246, 250, 283
Koebke, J., 525, 529, 531, 533, 534
Köhler, A., 271, 555
Kohn, L. A. P, 143, 205
Kolagi, S., 27, 91, 92
Kondrat, J. W., 26
Kongisberg, L. W., 143
Korman, E., 307, 340, 422, 423, 424, 425
Kormano, M., 568
Korogi, Y., 269
Kosa, F., 238, 253, 259, 260, 385
Kosar, P., 180
Kosar, U., 180
Kosinski, T. F., 655
Kostick, E. L., 611, 612, 613, 614, 615
Kouladouros, K., 180
Kountakis, B. A. Sr., 26
Kövári, Ivett, 121
Krayenbühl, N., 283, 292, 337
Kreyenbühl, W., 597
Krishnamurthy, A., 81, 95, 97, 180, 460, 462
Krmpotic-Nemanic, J., 337
Krs, O., 542, 551
Krupa, P., 611
Kubikova, E., 180
Kulkarni, M., 542
Kumar, A., 180
Kumar, C. G., 460, 462
Kumar, H., 280, 291, 408
Kumar, N., 521, 524
Kumar, S. A., 661
Kumar, V., 17, 62, 63
Kwathai, L., 284, 323
Kwiatkowska, A., 95, 97, 98, 424, 425
Kwiatkowski, J., 97, 422, 423
Kwok, P., 165

L

L'Abeé, E. N., 655, 657, 658
Lacout, A., 165
Lambrichts, I., 452
Langford, L. A., 542, 551, 552
Langlais, R. P., 119
Langton, J., 62
Lanzieri, C. F., 283, 317, 321, 323, 334, 360, 367

Larnach, S. L., 658
Larrosa, R., 576, 577, 579, 589, 590, 591
Lasjaunias, P., 165
Last, R. J., 53, 54
Latiff, L. L., 408
Lauris, J. R. P., 284, 285, 321, 364
Lavallo, G., 659
Lazarov, N. E., 324
Leach, J. L., 269, 271
LeDouble, A., 578
LeDouble, A. F., 165
Lee, H. J., 498
Lee, J. H., 498
Lee, K. H., 498
Lee, S. P., 500, 515
Lee, T. H., 639
Le Grange, F., 483
Le Gros Clark, W. E., 9, 268, 271
Le Minor, J-M., 569, 637, 638
Lemos, D. F., 550
Lemos, J. A., 550
Leng, L. A., 564
Leo, J. T., 74, 100
Leonardi, R., 291, 568
Levine, N. S., 6, 9, 11, 17, 39, 40
Levy, P. S., 542, 551
Lewis, O. J., 524
Li, J. R., 165
Li, Y., 268
Li, Y. Q., 13
Liang, L., 269
Liang, X., 452
Lindblom, K., 324
Liu, D. N., 13
Lockett, B. C., 462
Lockhart, R. D., 144, 182
Lordan, J., 536
Loukas, M., 113, 153, 280, 312, 346, 354, 355, 357, 358, 529
Lozada, M. C., 656, 657, 661
Lozanoff, Beth, 79
Lozanoff, S. P., 618
Lu, C-X., 268
Luboga, S., 584
Lucas, M. F., 558
Luiz Smith, R., 163, 290, 346, 352, 355, 357, 358, 379, 431
Lukic, I. K., 337
Luo, Q., 13

M

Macalister, A., 66, 67, 68, 69, 70, 71, 72, 390, 566, 567
MacCurdy, G. G., 151, 659
MacDonnell, R. L., 557, 559
Macedo, V. C., 75
Macintosh, N. W. G., 658
MacPherson, B. R., 544

Madeira, M. C., 473, 479
Madeline, L. A., 259, 260, 326, 328, 329, 385, 400
Madhan Kumar, S. J., 180
Madhavi, C., 635
Madhuri, V., 635
Madhyastha, S., 81, 95, 97
Magi, P., 179, 238
Mahato, N. K., 585, 587
Malerba, G., 55, 56
Mamatha, G. P., 463
Mamatha, Y., 568
Manabe, J., 194, 198, 199, 200, 201, 220, 228, 237, 253
Mangal, A., 113, 114, 153
Mangla, R., 472
Manik, P., 521, 524
Manjunath, K. Y., 330, 480
Mann, R. W., 194, 198, 199, 200, 201, 220, 228, 236, 237, 253, 454, 457, 458, 465, 506, 536, 596, 600, 601, 618, 631, 633, 642
Manners-Smith, T., 576
Manning, K. P., 31
Manoel, C., 290, 315, 346, 347, 348, 352, 355, 357, 358, 404, 431, 433, 659
Mansur, D. I., 81, 95, 97
Manzi, G., 7, 209, 210, 212
Marcsik A., 454
Mardini, S., 463
Mariotti, V., 612
Marotti, M., 454, 458
Marsh, J. L., 205
Marshall, D. S., 325, 333, 338
Marsot-Dupuch, K., 165
Martin, J., 576, 577, 579, 589, 590, 591
Martinez, S., 550
Martinez-Gonzalez, J. M., 494
Marusic, A., 337
Massler, M., 3
Matamala, D. Z., 163, 290, 346, 352, 355, 357, 358, 379, 431
Matsumura, G., 238, 246, 250
Matsumura, H., 657
Mavishetter, G. F., 179, 238
Mavraganis, D., 310
May, W. R., Jr., 312, 346, 354, 355, 357, 358
Mbadugha, C. C., 337
Mbajiorgu, F. E., 129
McAdams, H. P., 550
McCall, T., 310, 401, 402, 410
McCormick, W. F., 525, 526, 542, 545, 547, 551, 552, 643
McDonald, S. W., 81, 95
McDonnell, D., 452
McDougall, A., 631
McNab, A. A., 54
McNary, W. F., 585
Meena M. L., 565
Meier, L. N., 538

Meiring, J. H., 483
Mellado, J. M., 576, 577, 579, 589, 590, 591
Melsen, B., 389
Mentag, P. J., 655
Mercer, J., 631
Mercer, S. R., 228, 230
Mertz, L., 656, 659, 660, 661
Messo, E., 463, 471, 473, 474, 475
Methathrathip, D., 3, 9
Mikity, V. G., 8
Miles, D. A., 119
Mishra, S. R., 521, 524, 525, 526
Miyake, R., 576
Mohandas Rao, K. G., 49, 50
Montgomery, J. L., 369
Mooney, M. P., 246, 253, 259, 260, 385, 655, 657, 662
Moorrees, C. F. A., 486
Moraes, L. C., 290, 346, 347, 348, 355, 357, 358
Moraes, M. E. L., 290, 346, 347, 348, 355, 357, 358
More, C. B., 119
Morita, T., 576
Morris, H., 500, 502, 516
Mortazavi, M. M., 529
Moseley, J. M., 236
Muralidhar, P., 179, 238
Murlimanju, B. V., 460, 462, 567
Murphy, T., 475
Murtland, A., 576, 577
Museum of London, 659
Mustafa, K. I., 179
Mutalik, A., 91
Muthukumaravel, N., 635
Mutzuri, A., 473
Mwachaka, P. M., 529

N

Naderi, S., 307, 340, 422, 423, 424, 425
Nagar, M., 452, 453
Nagashima, M., 283
Naidu, M. D. K., 19, 26
Naik, S. M., 180
Naik, S. S., 180
Nakashima, T., 629
Nalla, S., 524
Nambiar, P., 19, 26
Namonta, K., 284, 323
Nancy, J., 463
Napoli, M. L., 148
Natsis, K., 525, 529, 531, 533, 534, 536
Navani, S., 542, 551
Navrat, T., 611
Nawrocki, S. P., 655, 657, 658
Nayak, S. R., 81, 95, 97, 163, 180, 352, 404, 431, 433
Nayeb-Hashemi H., 542, 551
Nechtman, C., 529

Neel, J. V., 628, 629
Neff, J. P., 533
Nehme, A., 524
Neiburger, E. J., 656, 657, 659, 661
Neto, H., 81
Netvichit, S., 524
Neves, F. S., 473, 475
Newell, R. L. M., 619
Nguyen, K. T., 657
Nguyen, L. C., 657
Nickel, B., 121
Nielsen, T., 528
Nikolova, S. Y., 324
Nitek, S., 97
Nizankowska, A., 315, 349, 404, 431, 433
Nolet, P. S., 403, 409
Norfray, J. F., 620
Nouri, M. R., 452
Nowakowski, D., 95, 97, 98
Nunn, M., 286
Nzalak, J. O., 643

O

Oakes, W. J., 142, 220, 238, 246, 253, 259, 395
O'Brien, A., 81, 95
Oda, J. Y., 60
Odgers, P. N. B., 611, 612, 613, 614, 615, 616
Odula, P. O., 529
Oetteking, B., 126, 325, 333, 338, 339, 341, 343, 382, 383, 384, 386, 416, 431, 432, 623, 625, 659
Ogawa, K., 550
Ogeng'o, J. O., 529
Oghenemavwe, E. L., 337
Okan, B., 56
Okumura, M. M. M., 138, 139
Oladipo, G. S., 524
Olivecrona, H., 215, 236
Oliveira, C., 473, 475
Ollier, A., 27
Olotu, J. E., 524
O'Loughlin, V. D., 203, 207, 231, 250
Omori, K., 550
Onder, N., 283, 284, 285, 320
Ongkana, M.D., 471
Ongkana, N., 471
Onolfo, J. P., 388
Onwuama, K. T., 643
Orban, B. J., 500, 502, 516
Orguc, S., 180
Orish, C. N., 337
Orrison, W. W. Jr., 80
Orsina, L., 523, 524
Osbourne, R. H., 486
Ossenberg, N. S., 80, 194, 465, 467, 659
Osunwoke, E. A., 337

Othman, F., 337, 408
Ousley, S. D., 194, 250
Ousterhout, D. K., 389
Oviedo-Roldan, L., 494
Owsley, D. W., 631
Oxenham, M. F., 657
Oygucu, I. H., 625, 626
Ozcan, I., 20
Ozcan, K. M., 20
Ozdemir, B., 119, 180, 181
Ozdemir, H., 629, 630
Ozek, C., 56
Ozer, H. T. E., 558
Ozer, M. A., 65
Ozkan, H. S., 463
Ozmen, C. A., 269
Öztürk, A., 142, 253, 283, 284, 292, 298, 320, 338, 339

P

Padma, L. K., 568
Padmanabhan, P., 472
Padmanabhan, R., 635
Padmavathi, G., 27, 92
Pahor, A. L., 345
Pai, M. M., 163, 180, 352, 431, 433
Paik, K. S., 500, 515
Pal, G. P., 250, 255
Pan, C. Q., 529, 531, 533
Panchal, J., 6, 9, 11, 17, 39, 40
Pang, D., 381, 383, 564, 565
Parizel, P. M., 629
Parker, E. E., 6, 9, 11, 17, 39, 40
Parr, N. M. L., 659
Parsons, F. G., 491
Parviainen, M., 623
Patil, G. V., 27, 92
Pearlstein, K., 618
Peker, T., 163, 352, 404, 431, 433
Peñarrocha, M., 463
Pensi, A., 13
Penteado, C. V., 81
Perizonius, W. R. K., 656, 658, 659, 660
Persing, J. A., 231
Peuker, E. T., 312, 346, 347, 348, 354, 355, 357, 358
Phenice, T. W., 604
Phetphunphiphat, W., 3, 9
Philbin, T. M., 639
Phillips, S. R., 215, 236, 658
Piagkos, G., 180
Piagkou, M., 180
Piagou, M., 163, 290, 346, 348, 352, 355, 357, 358, 379
Pick, M. G., 388, 389
Pietrusewsky, M., 58, 73, 659–660
Pihlajamäki, H.K., 623
Pillay, V. K., 523

Pinar, Y., 290
Pitt, M. J., 611
Piyawinijwong, S., 524
Podgórski, M., 531
Polguj, M., 531, 618
Popovich, F., 290, 292, 294, 661
Postacchini, F., 523, 524
Potts, D. G., 268, 271
Prabhu, L. V., 81, 95, 97, 163, 180, 352, 404, 431, 433, 460, 462, 463, 567
Prado, F. B., 163, 283, 289, 290, 315, 346, 347, 348, 352, 355, 357, 358, 404, 431, 433, 478, 659
Prakash, R., 452, 453, 568
Prameela, M. D., 460, 462
Prasanna, L. C., 179, 238
Pratap, P., 364
Prescher, A., 310, 325, 326, 329, 339, 340, 381, 382, 383, 384, 401, 410, 564
Priya, R., 480
Provenzale, J. M., 269
Pruett, S. W., 360, 363, 364, 367
Puget, J., 524
Pusch, M., 205
Putz, D. A., 246, 253, 259, 260, 385, 655, 657, 662

Q

Quateen, A., 219
Quatrehomme, G., 27

R

Radi, N., 612
Ragab, A. A., 634, 635
Rai, R., 462, 567
Rainey, D. L., 141, 142
Rairam, G. B., 27, 91, 92
Rajendran, M., 635
Rajguru, J., 92
Ramadan, S. U., 180
Ramadhan, A., 463, 471, 473, 474, 475
Ramanathan, L., 81, 95, 97
Ramesh, B. R., 568
Rani, A., 521, 524, 525, 526
Rao, V., 536, 537, 538
Rau, R. K., 536
Rauh, P., 536
Ravichandran, D., 635
Redlund-Johnell, I., 521
Reed, J. C., 656, 658, 659, 660
Reiss, P., 6, 9, 17
Rejtar, P., 542, 551
Rejtarova, O., 542, 551
Remmelick, H-J., 388, 389
Rengachary, S. S., 533
Resnick, D., 620

Restrepo, C. S., 550
Reymond, J., 321, 364, 367, 370
Rhine, S., 148, 660–661
Rhoton, A. L., Jr., 198, 211, 216, 218
Rhoton, Jr., A. L., 364
Rhyne, R. R., 180
Ricci, F., 7, 209, 210, 212
Richmond J., 8
Riesenfeld, A., 100
Rigi, A., 612
Rizk, E., 184
Robecchi, M. G., 55, 56
Robinson, F., 238, 246, 253, 259, 260, 283, 299, 334, 385
Roche, J., 268, 269, 271
Roche, M. B., 576, 577, 581
Rogers, M., 661
Rogers, N. L., 525, 526
Romaris de Clavelli, S. S., 547
Rosa, R. R., 290, 346, 347, 348, 355, 357, 358
Rose, J. C., 656, 657, 659, 661
Rosenbaum, A. E., 283, 317, 321, 323, 334, 360, 367
Rosenbloom, S. A., 283, 317, 321, 323, 334, 360, 367
Ross, L. M., 544
Rossi, A. C., 163, 190, 283, 289, 315, 346, 347, 348, 352, 355, 357, 358, 404, 431, 433, 465, 659
Rothschild, B., 656, 657, 659, 661
Rouas, P., 463
Rowe, G. G., 576, 577, 581
Rowe, L. J., 555, 557, 559
Rozzelle, C. J., 529
Rumbaugh, C. L., 8
Rungruang, T., 284, 323

S

Sabbadini, G., 333
Saccheri, P., 333
Saheb, H. S., 179, 238
Sahin, B., 463
Sahinoglu, K., 142, 253, 292, 338, 339
Saifuddin, A., 576
Salami, S. O., 643
Salter, E. G., 142, 238, 246, 253, 259, 395
Salvatore, M., 523, 524
Sammarco, V. J., 528
Sampson, H. W., 369
Samson, T., 184
Sanchis, J. M., 463
Sanders, C. F., 542, 551
Sankar, K. D., 238, 243, 247, 248, 250, 251, 255
Sansuk, R., 3, 9
Sant'Ana Castilho, M. A., 60
Sapanet, M., 27
Saralaya, V., 81, 95, 97, 163, 352, 404, 431, 433
Saran, S., 49, 50, 312, 313, 334
Saraswathy, P., 95, 97

Sarrafian, S. K., 637
Sartor, K., 285
Saunders, S. R., 141, 142, 290, 292, 294, 661
Sava, V. J., 218, 219, 228, 233
Savage, C., 587
Saxena, R., 24, 250, 255
Schaefer, M., 3, 4, 238, 259
Schepper, A. M., 629
Scheuer, L., 3, 4, 58, 62, 165, 238, 259, 325, 542, 552
Schiel, J. A., 388, 389
Schindler, G., 382, 401
Schiwy-Bochat, K.H., 40
Schneider, K. N., 618
Schour, I., 3
Schultz, A. H., 57, 63, 190
Schwalbe, G., 57
Schwartz, T. H., 564
Sciotto, Christopher, 223, 365, 577
Sciulli, P., 618
Scott, A., 604, 605, 606
Scott, G. R., 492, 493, 661
Seckin, H., 568
Segall, J., 8
Selcuk, A., 20
Sendemir, E., 625, 626
Sendi, P., 463, 465, 467, 659
Senoglu, M., 307, 340, 422, 423, 424, 425
Senturk, S., 269
Serman, N. J., 470, 490
Serrafian, S. K., 628, 629, 630, 631, 632
Sevim, A., 390, 391, 392, 435
Sewell, R. B., 631
Shah, J. R., 542, 551
Shams, P., 91
Shankar, L., 26
Shapiro, R., 121, 238, 246, 253, 259, 260, 283, 299, 334, 385
Sharma, A., 280, 408
Sharma, P. K., 521, 525, 526
Sharma, Y. P., 127, 167, 169, 176
Shaw, J. P., 346
Sheehy, J. J., 138, 139
Shen, S., 91
Shigematsu, Y., 269
Shinohara, A. L., 284, 285, 321, 335, 364
Shipman, J. H., 611
Shivarama, C., 661
Shoja, M. M., 312, 346, 354, 355, 357, 358, 529
Shokouhi, G., 312, 346, 354, 355, 357, 358
Sholts, S. B., 45
Shore, L. R., 573, 576, 587
Shrimankar, P. S., 13
Siddiqui, A. U., 312, 350, 353, 354, 355
Siegel, M. I., 246, 253, 259, 260, 385, 655, 657, 662
Silpa, K., 462, 567
Silva, A. M., 454, 458, 629, 630, 631, 633

Silveira, E. M. V., 284, 285, 321, 364
Simsek, S., 568
Sinan, B., 179
Sindel, M., 629, 630
Sindel, T., 629, 630
Singer, P. A., 533
Singh, B., 408
Singh, I., 625, 626
Singh, J., 522
Singh, M., 92, 354, 357, 359, 361, 369, 372, 374, 377
Singh, N., 472
Singh, R., 586
Singh, S. D., 31
Singh, S. K., 463
Singh, U., 628, 629
Singh, V., 452, 481, 483, 484
Singhal, S., 536, 537, 538
Singla, M., 92
Sinha, P., 92
Sinkeet, S. R., 529, 531
Sirisathira, N., 524
Sisman, Y., 498
Sivanandan, R., 95, 97
Skandalakis, P., 529, 533, 534
Skrzat, J., 163, 194, 302, 312, 315, 346, 352, 354, 357, 358, 404, 431
Skrzat, R., 290, 315, 349, 404, 431, 433
Slaus, M., 454, 458
Slizova, D., 542, 551
Slooff, W. B. M., 310, 409
Śmiszkiewicz-Skwarska, A., 618
Smith, A. S., 283, 317, 321, 323, 334, 360, 367
Smith, M. D., 220
Smoker, W. R. K., 165, 382, 383, 384, 564, 565
Snodgrass, J. J., 605, 606
Snow, C. E., 661
Solanas, S., 576, 577, 579, 589, 590, 591
Soler, F., 463
Somayaji, S. N., 49, 50
Soto-Rivadeneira, A., 494
Spar, J. A., 80
Sperber, G. H., 3, 259
Sperber, S. M., 3
Spinner, R. J., 529, 536
Spradley, M. K., 542, 543
Spring, C., 205
Sricharoenvej, S., 524
Sridevi, C., 661
Srivastava, A. K., 521, 525, 526
Srivastava, R. K., 17, 62, 63, 238, 246, 248, 250, 325, 338
Srodek, R., 163, 249, 312, 315, 346, 349, 352, 354, 357, 358, 404, 431, 433
Stafne, E. C., 454, 458
Stammberger, H., 26
Stark, P., 550, 551
Staroslawska E., 337

Stathis, G., 310
Steele, D. G., 285
Steinwachs, M., 569
Sternberg, A., 62, 92, 143, 184, 259, 260, 271, 290, 303, 325, 385, 401, 529, 536, 537, 538, 546, 551
Sternberg, L. E., 163, 172, 661
Stewart, C. A., 269
Stewart, J. H., 542, 545, 547, 551, 552
Stewart, S. L., 634, 635
Stewart, T. D., 126, 227
Stibbe, E. P., 183
Stilianos, E., 26
Stojanovic, V., 81, 95, 97
Straus, W. L., Jr., xiii
Su, L., 13
Subramaniam, A., 312, 313, 334
Subramaniam, K., 19, 26
Sud, B., 127, 167, 169, 176
Sudha, R., 661
Sudwan, P., 471
Sugahara, T., 269
Suhaimi, F. H., 337, 408
Sulaiman, I. M., 337, 408
Surendra, M., 390, 408
Sutherland, L. D., 604
Sutter, R. C., 656, 659, 660, 661
Sutton, J. B., 134, 178
Suzuki, K., 629
Swartz, S. M., 231
Swasdison, S., 494, 495, 496, 498
Sweeney, C. A., 576, 577
Szawlowski, J., 585
Szczurowski, J., 95, 97, 98
Szewczyk, R., 290, 315, 404, 431, 433
Szpalski, M., 576
Szumilo, J., 337

T

Taitz, C., 303, 382, 401, 431
Takahashi, M., 269
Tappen, N. C., 40, 80
Taskara, N., 292, 297, 298, 338
Tavassoli, M. M., 58
Taveras, J. M., 271
Taylor, B. A., 576
Taylor, J. B., 180
Teal, J. S., 8
Tebo, H. G., 348, 354, 355
Tekdemir, I., 291, 390, 391, 392, 435, 568
Temkin, O., xiii
Tetik, S., 113, 114, 153, 307, 340, 422, 423, 424, 425
Tetradis, S., 17, 20, 286
Tharp, A., 121
Thomas, S. T., 179, 238
Thompson, D. N. P., 381, 383, 564, 565

Tian, Y., 13
Tian Y-H., 268
Tochieri, M. W., 430
Todd, M. E., 452
Todd, T., 558
Toldeo Filho, J. L., 473, 479
Toldt, C., 80, 105, 297
Toldt, C. U., 121
Tomsick, T. A., 269
Toneva, D. H., 324
Topol, M., 531
Torres, M. G. G., 473, 475
Totlis, T., 525, 529, 531, 533, 534
Travan, L., 333
Tricoire, J. L., 524
Trivedi, D. J., 13
Trotter, M., 537, 538, 596
Truumees, E., 564, 565
Tsaknis, P. J., 465
Tsikaras, P., 525, 529, 531, 533, 534
Tsuchimochi, M., 382, 401
Tubbs, R. S., 142, 184, 220, 238, 246, 253, 259, 280, 312, 346, 354, 355, 357, 358, 395, 529
Tucker, S., 576
Tuli, A., 113, 114, 153
Tuller, H., 57
Tunaci, A., 55, 542, 543, 545, 547, 550
Tunaci, M., 542, 543, 545, 547, 550, 551
Tunç, E., 180
Tuncbilek, I., 180
Turgut, H. B., 163, 352, 404, 431, 433, 604
Turner, C. G. II, 661
Turner, W., 53, 73, 121, 138, 139, 556, 559, 564, 573, 574, 631

U

Ubelaker, D., 404, 655, 657, 658, 659, 661–662
Uchiumi, T., 238, 246, 250
Uddin, J. M., 91
Ugale, M., 91
Ugrenovic, S., 81, 95, 97
Ugur, H. C., 390, 391, 392, 435
Ukah, C. J., 337
Umlawska, W., 337
Unlu, Z., 180
Usha, K., 567

V

Vacher, C., 388, 389
Vadgaonkar, R., 163, 180, 352
Vaithianathan, G., 312, 313, 334
Van Arsdale, A. P., 194, 203, 250
van Buggenhout, G., 503

Van dee Perre, S., 629
Vandewalle, G., 452
Van Dis, M. L., 119
Van Dongen, S., 573
Vanhoenacker, F. M., 629
Vannier, M. W., 205
Van Rooyen, C., 655, 657, 658
Varegova, L., 611
Varga, I., 180
Vargas, D., 550
Vasovic, L., 81, 95, 97
Vastine, J. H., 551
Vastine, M. F., 551
Vasudeva, N., 325, 338, 341
Vats, A. K., 565
Vayvada, H., 470
Vaziri A., 542, 551
Vázquez, J. F. P., 81, 92, 100, 103, 127, 129, 165, 167, 169, 222, 256, 258, 297, 307, 310, 364, 369, 386, 387, 391, 398, 439, 487
Veldman, J. K., 658, 662
Vercellino, V., 55, 56
Verna, E., 537, 606
Verna, G. L., 542, 551
Verona, J. A. G., 81, 92, 100, 103, 127, 129, 165, 167, 169, 222, 256, 258, 297, 307, 310, 364, 369, 386, 387, 391, 398, 439, 487
Vesalius, Andreas, xiii
Vichic, M., 291, 568
Villa, C., 612
Vinaitha, D., 312, 313, 334
Vinter, I., 337
Vlajkovic, S., 81, 95, 97
Vodanovic, M., 454, 458
Volpato, M. C., 478
von Arx, T., 463, 465, 467, 473, 474, 475, 476, 477, 478, 659
von Ludinghausen, M., 382, 401
Vu, H. L., 6, 9, 11, 17, 39, 40

W

Wackenheim, A., 329
Wadhwa, S., 628, 629
Wahby, B., 31
Wakeley, C. P. G., 129, 390, 408
Walji, A., 219
Walocha, J., 163, 194, 247, 290, 302, 312, 315, 346, 349, 352, 354, 358, 404, 431, 433
Wang, J. J., 529, 531, 533, 582
Wang, R. G., 165
Wärmländer, S. K. T. S., 45
Warner, D., 268, 269, 271
Wartman, C. T., 113, 153
Warwick, R., 54, 92
Washington, L., 550
Wasterlain, S. N., 454, 458
Watkins, G. E., 550, 551
Weber, J., 205
Weckström, M., 623, 625
Weiglein, A., 382, 401
Weinberg, S. M., 246, 253, 259, 260, 385, 655, 662
Weinzweig, J., 6, 9, 17
Weiss, M. A., 541
Werb, A., 54
Whitaker, L. A., 6, 9, 17
White, J., 576
White, T. D., 146
Whitnall, S. E., 54, 90
Widell, E. H., 576
Wiens, J., 62, 92, 184, 259, 260, 271, 290, 303, 325, 385, 401, 529, 536, 537, 538, 546, 551
Wijnaendts, L. C. D., 573
Wilczak, C. A., 194, 250
Wilde, E., 486
Willis, T. A., 576, 577
Willmore, K. T., 656, 657, 661
Wilson, C., 143, 661
Wiltse, L. L., 576
Winter, M., 638
Wobig, J. L., 53
Wong, M., 546
Woo, J. K., 57, 505, 506, 507, 508
Wood, C. C. E., 39, 310, 433, 434, 656, 657, 662
Wood, E. H., 271
Wood-Jones, F., 126, 283, 285, 337, 343
Wright, W., 623, 625
Wu, L. P., 529, 531, 533, 582
Wu, P. Y., 8
www.carolina.com, 643
www.skullsunlimited.com, 643
Wysocki, J., 97, 165, 321, 364, 367, 370, 422, 423, 424, 425

X

Xia, C. L., 13
Xiao, D-M., 268
Xu, X-X., 268

Y

Yaczi, A. B., 119, 129, 180, 181
Yadav, A., 17, 62, 63
Yang, H-F., 268
Yanguas, N., 576, 577, 579, 589, 590, 591
Yaz, A., 97, 99
Yazar, F., 536
Yekeler, E., 542, 543, 545, 547, 550, 551
Yener, N., 180
Yengil, E., 549
Yigitbasi, O. G., 97, 99
Yigitkanli, K., 568
Yilmaz, M., 470

Yochum, T. R., 555, 557, 559
Yordanov, Y. A., 324
Yoshimura, K., 382, 401
Yoshioka, N., 198, 211, 216, 218
Yuksel, M., 629, 630

Z

Zampetti, S., 612
Zawilinski, J., 302

Zdravkovic, D., 81, 95, 97
Zeybek, F. G., 113, 114, 153, 283, 284, 285, 292, 297, 298, 320, 338, 339
Zhang, W. J., 529, 531, 533, 582
Zimmer, E. A., 271, 555
Zografos, J., 473
Zona, A., 506, 507, 508

SUBJECT INDEX

A

accessory ossicle(s), 134, 600, 601, 654
accessory suture, 121
accessory teeth, 503
acetabular crease, 655
acetabular labrum, ossicle along, 600
acetabular ligament (term), 600
acetabular notch, 599
acetabular pit, 655
acetabulum, 601, 603
acetabulum, left, 599
acetone, immersing remains in, 645
acromial articular facet, 655
acromium shape triangle, 655
adolescent
    anterior fontanelle in, 195
    basilar synchondrosis in, 302
    Bregma and Lamda features in, 204
    cranial base alar ligament in, 304
    cranial modification (deformation) in, 261
    lambdoidal ossicle in, 247
    nasofrontal suture in, 38
    occipital crest and occipital fossa sulcus absence in, 298
    paracondylar process, right in, 409
    supernumerary tooth in, 494
    supranasal suture in, 37, 38
    trochlear spur in, 85, 88
adulthood, tympanic dehiscence persistence into, 147
adult(s)
    clavicle, left, nutrient foramen in, 527
    cranium, flattened in, 430
    interclinoid ligament calcification in, 294
    maxilla and mandible, sectioned in, 464
    Mendosal sutures in, 259
    metopic and supranasal sutures in, 39, 61
    nasal rim spine in, 107–108
    ossification centers in, 3
    sternal foramina in, 545
    supra-bregmatic ossicle/bone in, 244
    See also under ethnic group and gender
African adult
    basilar bone, hard palate and nasolacrimal canal in, 140
    foramen ovale in, 361
    frontal sinuses in, 28
    hard palate in, 140
    mental foramen/foramina, right, triple in, 476
    nasal guttering in, 51
    pars tympanica in, 127
    petrosal ridge in, 296

African American male, elderly, 278, 279
African Americans, 188
African child, 224, 313, 314, 318
African female, 110, 221, 303
African male, 340, 393, 601
Africans, lumbar vertebra(e) in, 584
African subadult, 333, 340
African young adult, 508
age indicators (at death)
    arachnoid granulations as potential, 271
    coronal suture extensions as, 208
    nasal bone suture obliteration pattern as, 35
    overview, 642
    sphenomaxillary suture and junction as possible, 388
    synchondrosis as, 288
    vault suture role as, 232
agujero retrojugular de Serrano, 386
alar cartridges, 106–107
alar ligament, 304, 305, 314, 431
Allen's fossa (term), 611
    See also fossa of Allen
alveolar prognathism, 655
anatomical traits, identifying and labeling, xiii
anatomical variants, xiii, xiv
ancestry, indicators of, 45
Angle of Sandifort (term), 487
anomaly, clarity concerning, xiv
antegonial notch, 471, 472
antemortem and postmortem features, difficulty of distinguishing, 122
anterior fontanelle
    in adolescent, 195
    bones, 7, 212
    characteristics of, 4
    closure of, 4, 8
    comparisons of, 5
    in female adult, 210
    in newborn, 196–197
anterior medio-palatine bones, 505, 506, 508
anterior-posterior X-rays, 27
apical bone, 655
apical ligament, 431, 432
apical odontoid ligament, 402
Apofsis Lemuriana de Albrecht (term), 487
arachnoid granulations, 188, 214, 215, 269, 271
arcuate foramen (term), 568
arteries (face, left side and temporal region), 53
articular facet(s)
    acromial, 655
    anterior and middle facets, separate, 635

atlas, 390, 563
    calcification and formation of, 523
    intermetatarsal, 638, 639
    of os peroneum, bilateral, 637
    pelvis, right, 598
    sacrum/sacra, 596
artificial cranial modification (deformation)
    in child, 203
    childhood head binding causing, 155–156
    coronal ossicles associated with, 159
    cultural (asymmetrical), 203
    in Peruvian, 231
    in Peruvian adolescent, 261
    in Peruvian adult, 157, 179, 194, 220, 430
    in Peruvian child, 207
    in Peruvian subadult, 158
    sagittal/parietal groove in, 192
    suprainion depression associated with, 227
Asian adult
    atlas and atlanto-occipitalization in, 408
    basilar transverse cleft, unilateral in, 325
    basi-occipital segmentation, incomplete in, 326
    digastric muscles, anterior, accessory foramina and
        roughened areas in, 481
    ethmoidal foramina in, 95
    foramen ovale and other foramina in, 365, 370, 443
    frontal grooves, accessory in, 15
    frontal sinuses in, 24, 26
    hypoglossal canal, left in, 417
    Inca bone in, 249
    infraorbital foramina in, 74
    lacrimal ossicle and foramen in, 68
    left upper orbital plate of, 96
    lumbar vertebra(e) foramina in, 582
    mandibular canal, bifid/bifurcated in, 463
    maxilla, Carabelli's trait, bilateral in, 492
    maxillary incisors in, 493
    meningo-orbital foramina in, 95
    nasal bones, asymmetrically sized in, 31
    occipital crest and occipital foramen in, 411
    orbit, right of, 15, 65
    parietal notch bone, left and petrosquamous suture in,
        172
    postcondylar depressions (basilar invaginations) in, 436
    postcondylar fossa/canal, right in, 342
    precondylar tubercle in, 431
    pterygosphenoid bridge and foramen of Civinini in, 347
    sagittal suture ossicle and parietal foramen, left in, 211
    spina bifida in, 588
    styloid process absence in, 412
    stylomastoid foramen in, 398
    temporal bone, right in, 82, 407
    temporal squama parietal process in, 145
    trochlear pulley/spur in, 86
    zygomaticofacial foramina in, 150
    zygomaticofrontal suture in, 96
Asian child, 132, 175, 489
Asian female, 46, 71, 543
Asian female, adolescent, 247, 298
Asian female, adult
    antegonial notch absence in, 472
    clinoid processing, partial in, 292
    foramen of Vesalius in, 284, 300, 319
    foramen spinosum in, 359
    lacrimal ossicles in, 69
    mastoid foramen and sigmoid sinus in, 257
    occipitomastoid ossicle in, 256
    occipitomastoid suture of, 439
    pterygospinous bridiging, partial in, 348
    pubic bones in, 605
Asian female, elderly, 236, 392, 498
Asian female, young adult, 283, 299
Asian fetus, cranial anatomy of, 178
Asian male, 191, 228, 344
Asian male, adolescent, 409
Asian male, adult
    antegonial notch in, 472
    calcifications in, 280
    emissary occipital foramina, double in, 222
    ethmoidal foramina in, 92
    exostoses in, 375
    foramen spinosum in, 374, 375
    metopic and supranasal sutures in, 11
    metopic fissure, metopism and sulcus of Gustav
        Schwalbe in, 154
    metopism and metopic/frontal/interfrontal fissure in, 63
    nuchal superstructure in, 234
    occipital superstructure, nuchal spike and retromastoid
        tubercles/processes in, 233
    occipital superstructure and Inion spike in, 234
    occipital view of skull, 218
    optic foramen in, 92, 94
    orbital rim spurs in, 82
    palatine crest, tag along, 502
    palatine groove bridging in, 501
    pterion, H-shaped in, 129
    pterygoalar bridge, left trace in, 407
    sacroiliac joint, accessory in, 596
    skull superior view in, 193
    supraorbital notches and orbital rim spurs in, 82
Asian male, elderly, 632
Asian male, young adult, 152, 289, 335, 514
Asian(s)
    foramen spinosum in, 443
    lambdoidal ossicles in, 241
    nasal guttering in, 50, 103
    post-bregmatic depression frequency in, 188
    zygomaticulomaxillary tubercles, prominent in, 45
Asian young adult, 369, 380
Asterion, 142, 143, 252
asterionic ossicles/bones, 248, 655, 659
atlanto-occipital assimilation (term), 408

atlanto-occipitalization, 129, 390, 408
atlas
    apical ligament of, 431, 432
    articular facets of, 563
    bridging in, 567, 655
    dens, congenital separation of, 564, 565
    facets in, 655
    inferior facets of, 390
    superior condyles, divided/double in, 569
atlas, bifid, 408
atlas process, 410
atresia, 510
auditory canal, right, 138, 139
auditory/ear ossicle, right, 149
auditory exostosis, xii, 138, 139, 655
auditory meatus
    anterosuperior portion of, 137
    external, 127, 149
    internal left, 281
    right, 139
auditory torus, 655
Australian adult, 385
axis, odontoid process of, 572

B

base angle, 656
basilar bone, 140, 287, 328
basilar canal, medial, 658
basilar cleft/clefting, 325, 326
basilar depression, 399
basilar fissures, 326, 327, 328
basilar process(es), 325, 339
basilar synchondrosis
    closed, 326
    in female adolescent, 302
    in female young adult, 303
    in fetus, 429
    formation of, 429
    in Hungarian subadult, 337
    open, 287, 302
    in Peruvian child, ancient, 429
    of petrous bone, 288
    in subadult, 442
    in Thai subadult, 302
    trace of, 303
basilar transverse cleft, unilateral, 325
basilar transverse fissure, 329
basilar tubercles/wings, 416
basioccipital segmentation, incomplete of, 326
basioccipital synchondrosis, 394
bathrocephaly, 184
betel nuts, 129, 452, 485
biasterionic sutures, 656
bicipital rib (term), 559
bifaceted condyles, 656

bifid parietal (intraparietal suture) (term), 121
bifid rib. *See* Luschka's rib
bifid spinous process. *See* spina bifida
bifurcated rib. *See* Luschka's rib
bilobate mandible, 451
biomechanical stresses, 41, 61, 483, 611
bipartate bone, 134
bipartite occipital bone (term), 243
bipartite patella, xii, 623, 624, 656
black adult(s), 50, 91, 510
black female, adolescent, 494
black female, elderly, 188, 291, 292
black female, subadult, 606
black male, 201
black male, adult, 126, 226, 230, 255
black male, young adult, 277, 290, 299
black/Negroid traits, 50
black perinatal individuals, 385
blacks, 188
blasterionic suture (term), 142
bleach, immersing remains in, 642, 643–644, 646
bone, rendering human body to, 643
bone islands, 293
bone spur, xii
bony ossification (exostosis), 277
brachycephaly, 179
Brazilian skulls, 289
breech position, 184
Bregma, foramina at, 201
Bregma, ossicles at, 204, 209, 264
"Bregma-like" junction, 121
bregmatic bone, 202, 656
bregmatic fontanelle, 8, 190
bregmatic fontanelle bone, 7
bridge of bone, calcified, 387
broken nose, healed, 12
buccal foramina, 469, 474

C

C1 (cervical vertebra), 568
C7 (cervical vertebra), 573, 574, 661
calcaneal facets, 633, 634, 655, 656
calcaneus, left, 633, 636
calcaneus, right, 634
calcaneus secundarius, xii, 633
calcar femorale, 619
calcification
    foramen formed by, 415
    in inferior oblique muscle attachment area, 102
    magnification of, 279, 280
    in male, elderly, 277
calcified ligaments, exostosis/es as, 375
calotte, 206
canaliculus innominatus (foramen of Arnold)
    in Asian adult, 370, 443

and foramen of Vesalius, 369
  magnification of, 365
  in male adult, 329
  position of, 364, 370
  possible, 363, 365, 371
  precondylar tubercles and, 324
  in Thai female, elderly, 368
  variant of, 364
canaliculus innominatus, right, 371
canalis hypoglossi biparrtitus (term), 325
cancellous bone (mandible), 458
canines
  accessory, 513
  agenesis of, 517
  ectopic, 118, 503, 520
  fossa, 656
Carabelli's cusp, 493
Carabelli's trait, 492
Carabelli's trait, bilateral, 492
caroticoclinoid foramen, 289
carrion beetles, 643
Caucasoid adult, 23
Caucasoid male, 72
Caucasoid male, elderly, 281
cavernous foramen/foramina, 321, 322, 367, 370
cerebral ridges, 273
cervical fossa of Allen, xii, 611
  See also fossa of Allen
cervical ribs, 558, 573, 574
cervical vertebrae, 567, 655
  first, 568
  seventh, 573, 574, 661
Charles' facet (term), 620, 621
chest plate, 543, 544
chewing, 41, 61, 151, 483
"chignon" (term), 184
childhood head binding, 155–156
child(ren)
  anatomy, normal in, 25
  Bregma, ossicles in, 264
  craniosynostosis, premature in, 190
  diploic area in, 216
  epiteric bone in, 177
  ethmoid bone and vomer in, 21
  fossa of Allen in, 614
  frontal bone in, 6
  frontal suture in, 30
  frontonasal ossicle in, 5
  "frozen waves" in, 9
  inferior squamous foramen in, 168
  interfrontal suture in, 30, 270
  interparietal/lambdoidal ossicle, left in, 262
  jaws, developing anatomy in, 115
  lambdoidal ossicles in, 226
  mandibular canal, mental foramina and tooth root developmental stages in, 490

maxilla and mandible anatomy, 116
medial sutures in, 504
median frontal suture in, 30
Mendosal sutures in, 436
mesiodens in, 503
metopic suture in, 30, 270
nasal rim spine in, 106
nasofrontal suture in, 59
optic foramina in, 93
orbital plates in, 9
palatal sutures, accessory in, 505
palate of, 503
parietal bones in, 199
parietal foramen, left in, 198
petrous bones in, 287
positional plagiocephaly in, 203
postglenoid foramen in, 186
pterygoalar bridging, partial in, 346
skull, frontal view of, 6
sutures in, 59
teeth, developing in, 25, 115
trochlear spurs in, 83–84, 87
See also under ethnic group
chin, square, 451
chin prominence, 656
chin shape, xi
circumflex artery, 528
circumflex sulcus, 528, 655
clavicle, right, 522, 523
clavicular foramen, left, 527
cleft. *See* spina bifida
cleft spinous process, 578
clinoid bridge/bridging, 290, 656
clinoid process(es)
  anterior, bridging of, 292
  anterior and middle, bridging of, 289
  anterior and posterior, bridging of, 286, 292, 429
  posterior, anatomy of, 291
coccyx, 590, 594
cold water, pathological lesion/growth associated with, 138
compressive stresses, 9
concha bullosa, 97, 98, 99
condylar canal, 656, 657
condylar dysplasia, 303
condylar facet (atlas), 655
condylar facet, double, 656
condyle, two-portioned, 317
condylus tertius, 382, 656
coraclavicular/conoid joint, 523, 524
coronal ossicle(s)
  cranial modification (deformation), association with, 159
  location of, 176
  in Peruvian child, ancient, 78
  references, 656
  sutures, obliteration of, 141
  in Thai adult, 141, 208

coronal suture
- in Asian male, adult, 218
- closure of, 125, 232
- complexity of, 62
- coronal ossicle positioned along, 176
- craniosyntosis of, 125, 190
- endocranial and ectocranial morphology comparison, 141
- epiteric bone terminating into, 136
- extensions along, 208
- in male adult, 209
- obliteration of, 125
- simple *versus* complex, 194
- sutures, other differentiated from, 217
- thickened bone along, 193

coronoid process, 480, 533

costal cartilage
- attachment sites of, 543
- calcification of, 542, 551, 552
- collagen pattern in, 642
- excision of, 642–643
- in female, elderly, 553, 554
- preserving, 644
- reconstructing and reinforcing, 643

costal chondral joint, facets at, 648
costal joints, attachment of, 560
costoclavicular joint, congenital unilateral, 521
costoclavicular ligament, attachment of, 526, 649
cotyloid bones (term), 600, 601, 602

cranial base
- alar ligament of, 304
- developmental anomaly of, 506
- foramina in, 316, 367
- lateral pterygoid plate of, 380
- thickness of, 301

cranial modification (deformation), artificial. *See* artificial cranial modification (deformation)
cranial nerve VII, 281, 398
cranial shift/ing, 325, 328, 395
cranial sutures, 656, 662
cranial vault, sutures of, 662
craniomandibular joint, disease of, 482
craniopharyngeal canal, 656
craniopharyngeal foramen, possible, 310

craniosynostosis, premature
- in adult, 125
- in black male, adult, 230
- in child, 190
- keeling independent of, 189
- sagittal/parietal groove in, 192
- of sagittal suture, 205, 230

cranium, growth of, 3
cribiform plate, 40
cribra femoris (term), 611
cribra orbitale, 656
crista galli, 21, 274

D

death, age at. *See* age indicators (at death)
death, estimating cause and time elapsed since, 642
deciduous teeth, 115
dental appliance, 495
dental crowding, 483
dermestid beetles, 643
desmoid (term), 622
developing teeth, 25, 115
deviated septum. *See* nasal septum: deviated
digastric fossa, 656
digastric groove, 656
digastric muscles, anterior, 481
diploë
- areas, 216
- areas where lacking, 301
- exposure of, 195, 219, 236
- and metopic suture, 273
- veins, 120

distal femoral cortical excavation, xii, 620, 621, 622
"divided mastoid" (sutura mastoideosquamosa) (term), 172
dolicocephalic skulls, 62
Dorello's canal, 291
dura mater, 5, 195, 197, 275, 279

E

Eagle's syndrome, 180
ectocranium, 188
ectopic canine, 118, 503, 520
Egyptians, 12th Dynastic, 537
Egyptians, ancient, 7, 8, 235
elderly
- basilar synchrondrosis trace in, 303
- bony ossification (exostosis) in, 277, 278
- costal cartilage calcification in, 551
- distal femoral cortical excavation in, 621
- lingual foramina in, 453
- median basioccipital canal in, 308, 309
- occipital condyles and paracondylar foramen/bridge in, 396
- parietal bone out plate perforation in, 214
- postglenoid tubercle and spine of Henle in, 448
- supraorbital or frontal foramina in, 43
- *See also under ethnic group and gender*

elongated processes, frequency of, 180
emissary vein of Santorini, 229
enamel pearl (mandibular molar), 491
endocranial tubercles, 400
epiphyseal endplates, 583
epiphyseal line, 622
episternal bones, 550
epiteric bone(s)
- in child, 177
- and frontomalar suture, 131

parietal extension and, 135
in Peruvian child, 132
references, 656
in right side of skull, 146
squamosal ossicle and, 136
squamosal suture of, 134
in subadult, 177
in Thai female, 124
in Thai male, 133, 134
ethmoidal foramina
anterior, 102, 655
in Asian adult, 92, 95
in Asian male, 92
in Indian crania, 91
posterior, 102, 660
references, 655, 656
ethmoidal sinus(es), 20, 266
ethmoid bone, 21
ethnicity, determining, 642
European males, adult, 58
exostosis/es
as calcified ligaments, 375
lingual, 483
maxillary torus/tori or, 498
palatal (torus palatinus), xii
petrosal, 290
terminology, 138
in trochanteric fossa, 656
in white male, adult, 376
exosutural posterior ethmoid foramen, 660
extracranial vessels, foramina for, 64
eye orbit shape, 656

F

facial arteries, 53
facial nerve, motor branch of, 398
facial prognathism, 656
facial region, 19, 20, 99
"false" jugular foramen (term), 165
falx cerebri, 275
female adolescent, 88, 302, 304
female adult
anterior fontanelle/fonticular bone in, 210
axis odontoid process in, 572
buccal foramina, bilateral in, 469
coraclavicular/conoid joint clavicular facets in, 524
foramen of Vesalius in, 285, 367
precondylar tubercles in, 338
female elderly adult
costal cartilage in, 553, 554
hypoglossal canal, left in, 426
mental foramen/foramina, left in, 477
rib cage, deriving in, 643
sagittal/parietal groove in, 192
soft tissue, removing from, 642, 645–646

thoracic region of, 642, 645–646
vertebral column of, 646
females, 117, 604
See also under ethnic group
female young adult, 303, 508
femoral bowing, 656
femoral condyles, 621
femoral tubercle, 607, 608, 609, 610
femur (plaque), 660
femur, left, 617, 619, 621
femur, right, 616, 617, 622
fetus
basilar synchondrosis in, 429
clavicles, left, age and size increase in, 525
occipital bone, 259
postglenoid foramen in, 165
skull, 4, 5, 73, 253
squama, 260
flange lesion, 600
folded sutures, 48
fontanelle, 195, 197
See also anterior fontanelle
fontanelle bones, 7
fonticular bone, 210
foot, left, 630
"footballer's ankle" (term), 627
foramen (left upper orbital plate), 96
foramen cecum, 274
foramen jugulare spurium of Luschka, 165
foramen magnum, 340, 397, 400, 415, 432
foramen meningo-orbitale (term), 95
foramen nasale, 656, 659
foramen of Arnold (term), 364, 371
See also canaliculus innominatus (foramen of Arnold)
foramen of Civinini
formation of, 355, 433
pterygosphenoid bridge, right and, 347, 352
pterygosphenoid bridge and, 355
term, 147
foramen of Huschke (term), 147, 166, 447, 656
foramen of Hyrtl
formation of, 95, 347, 358
in left orbit, 81
overview of, 350, 449
term, 95
foramen of Vesalius
absence of, 325
in African child, 318
in Asian adult, 370, 443
in Asian female, adult, 284, 300, 319
in Asian female, young adult, 283
bilateral, 283, 319
canaliculus innominatus and, 369
divided, 320, 335, 362
double, 300, 320
double left, 323

ectocranial views of, 334
in female adult, 285, 367
foramina, other positions relative to, 321
frequency of, 284
left, 322, 325
long, slit-like, 319
in male adult, 317, 323
references, 657
right, 285, 320, 364
size of, 318
in Thai adult, 320, 360
in Thai female, adult, 362
foramen ovale
in African adult, 361
in African child, 318
in Asian adult, 370, 443
bilateral, 337
divided, 325, 335, 360, 361, 362, 385
in female young adult, 303
foramen of Vesalius and, 325, 364
foramina, other in area of, 365
in Hungarian subadult, 337
incomplete, 657
left, 385
ligament positions relative to, 313, 315
in Malaysian adult, 337
overview of, 283, 350
position of, 323
pterygoalar and pterygospinous bridging positions relative to, 314
references, 657
right, 303, 317, 385
in Thai adult, 360
in Thai female, adult, 362
in white male, adult, 377
foramen petrosum (term), 364
foramen rotundum, 283
foramen spinosum
accessory, 655
in African child, 318
in Asian adult, 326, 370, 443
in Asian female, adult, 359
in Asian male, adult, 375
bilateral partial bridging of, 374, 375
bridging of, 299, 353, 359, 372, 404, 405, 406
double, 443
in female young adult, 303
and foramen ovale, 303, 317
in Hungarian subadult, 337
incomplete, 657
left, 353, 372, 374
in male elderly adult, 334
open, 659
overview of, 283
position of, 323
references, 657, 659

right, 324, 342, 404
in Thai adult, 360, 372
foramen tympanicum (term), 147
forked rib. *See* Luschka's rib
Fosita Torcular (term), 297
fossa cribrosa, 597
fossa navicularis (term), 390, 391
fossa of Allen
bilateral occurrence of, 611
in child, 614
origin and development of, xii
and Poirier's facet, 612
references, 657
and trochanter, third, 613
variants of, 612
fovea capitis oval, 657
fracture(s), 121, 157
frontal bone(s)
anterior fontanelle bone in, 212
keeled/steepled, 18
maturation in males, 39
in newborn skull, 3
in one-year-old child's skull, 6
Pacchionian pits in, 268
pits and lines in, 12
pitting in, 29
thin areas in, 193
vertical fracture/breakage in, 16
frontal foramen and grooves (newborn), 43
frontal foramina
in elderly, 43
frequency of, 64
in Hungarian adult, 16
open, 657
right orbit pierced by, 15
in Thai adult, 13
frontal grooves, 10, 16, 657
frontal grooves, accessory, xii, 15
frontal notch, 657
frontal sinus, right, 25
frontal sinuses
in African adult, 28
in Asian adult, 24, 26
bilateral aplasia (absence) of, 24, 25
in child, 25
exposed, 19, 20
in male, elderly, 275
morphology of, 26
pattern variations, 27, 28
references, 657
symmetry and asymmetry of, 24
in Thai male, adult, 266
unilateral aplasia of, 24
frontal suture, 4, 6
frontoethmoidal suture, 102
frontomalar suture, 131

frontonasal ossicle, 5
frontonasal suture, 30
frontotemporal articulation, 129, 179, 657
"frozen waves," 9
fusion (left first and second ribs), 555

G

gastrocnemius muscle, 620
genial pit, 657
genial tubercles, 453, 483, 484, 657
German male, adult, 521, 522
glabella projection, 657
glabellar region (term), 58
Glaserian fissure, 379, 380
gonial eversion, 487
gonial flaring, 117
Greek mandibles, 473
growth arrest line, 622
Gruber's ligament, 278, 279, 280, 291
gubernacular canals, 502, 516

H

hamartoma (term), 138
hamulus, bipartite, 541
hard palate, 140
Harris line, 622
human body, viewing and interpreting, xiii
human remains, removing soft tissue from, 642–644
humerus, left, 538
humerus, right, 536, 537
Hungarian adult, 7, 16
Hungarian subadult, 337
Hungarian young adult, 328
hydrogen peroxide, immersing bones in, 643
hyoid bone, 491, 657
hyperdontia (term), 494
hyperostosis frontalis interna (HFI), 281
hypertrophied turbinates, 99
hypochordal arch, 381
hypocone, 493
hypoglossal canal, left
    divided, 422
    double bridging of, 426
    in female, elderly, 426
    internally divided, 417
    in Thai male, elderly, 424
    triple, 421
hypoglossal canal, right
    accessory foramen adjacent to, 427
    calcified spicules forming in, 419
    divided or accessory, 428
    fibrous bar/septum across, calcification of, 419
    internally and externally divided, 418
    non-divided, 446

triple, 420, 425
vertically grooved, 420
in Vietnamese adult, 428
hypoglossal canals
    bridging, 657
    demonstration of, 445
    divided, 656
    divided/double left, 294
    double, 656
    foramina lateral to, 330
    non-divided, 418
    openings, lateral of, 332
    paracondylar foramina communication with, 331
    partial bridging of, 423
    references, 657
    triple, 421
    variants of, 424
hypoglossal nerve, 330
hypoplastic nasal bones, 31
hypotrochanteric fossa, 617, 657

I

idiopathic bone cavity (term), 454
Inca bone
    in Asian adult, 249
    asymmetric/bipartite, 243
    in black male, adult, 255
    formation of, 246
    with lambdoidal ossicles, 248
    in male adult, 239
    references, 657
    in Thai male, adult, 238
    type II, 251
    variations in, 250
Inca ossicle, 657
incisive canal, 517
incisive fossa, 22, 510
incisive suture, 510
incisors
    cementoenamel junction of, 115
    central, 103, 109
    form, 657
    lateral, 487, 488, 511, 512, 519
    maxillary, 493, 511, 512, 519
    shoveling, 657
incus attachments, 149
Indian crania, 91
Indian female, 391
Indian mandibles, 453
Indian patients, frontal sinuses in, 24
infant, Obelion (region) defects in, 213
inferior squamousal foramen (term), 161
inferior squamous foramen/foramina, 167, 168, 169, 170
infraglenoid tubercle and crest, 650
infraorbital foramen/foramina

accessory, 56, 655
　　direction, position and size of, 56
　　double, 103
　　"folded"/overhanging margin of, 74
　　infraorbital sutures into, 53, 55
　　left, 25, 74
　　lessor, 75
　　multiple, 659
　　neurovascular bundle through, 25
　　references, 657, 659
　　right, 100
　　sutures extending into, 73
　　triple left, 56
infraorbital foramina, 56
infraorbital suture(s)
　　bilateral, 73
　　folding of, 48
　　into infraorbital foramen, 53, 55
　　path of, 73
　　references, 657
infraparietal foramen, 657
inguinal ligament attachment, 606
Inion, 193, 222, 657, 658
Inion spike, 218, 228, 234, 266
innominate, left, 604
innominate, right, 600
interclinoid ligaments, calcification of, 286, 290, 294
interfrontal/frontal/metopic suture, 57, 270
interfrontal/metopic suture, 59, 64
intermetatarsal articular facet, lateral, 638, 639
internasal suture, 64
interorbital breadth, 658
interorbital projection, 658
interparietal bones (term), 243
interparietal division, 658
interparietal/lambdoidal ossicle, left, 262
intervertebral disc, 583
ischiopubic ramus ridge, 658

J

Japanese adult, 525
Japanese male, adult, 57
Japanese male, elderly, 181
jaw, rocker and non-rocker, 661
jaws, developmental anatomy in child, 115
jugal bone (term), 45
jugal point (term), 45
jugular foramen, 283, 330, 345, 658
jugular fossa, 345

K

keeling, 18, 189, 205, 658
Kerckring's center, 259
Kerckring's process
　　in Australian adult, 385
　　in fetal occipital bone, 259
　　in fetal squama, 260
　　in perinatal individuals, 385
　　references, 660
　　in Thai female, elderly, 386
Kilgore International skull collection, 21, 25, 116
Kimmerle's anomaly, 566, 568, 570
Klippel-Feil, 555
Korean patients, 79
Kostick's facet, 611
Kreckring's process, probable, 385

L

L2 vertebra, 579
L4 vertebra, 652
L5 vertebra, 575, 576, 577, 582, 585, 653
L6 vertebra, 661
labia foraminis magni (term), 339
lacrimal canal, 66, 69, 71
lacrimal foramen, 70, 71, 72, 81, 95
lacrimal ossicles, 66, 67, 68, 69, 219
lacrimal sac, 66
lambdoidal ossicle(s)
　　in adult, 223
　　in African child, 224
　　alternative classifications for, 246
　　in Asian child, 175
　　Asian female, adolescent, 247
　　bregmatic ossicles and, 204, 244
　　in child, 226
　　complex, 240, 252
　　defined, 247
　　ectrocranial view of, 242
　　in fetal skull, 253
　　Inca bone with, 248
　　large, 240, 243
　　in male adult, 241
　　morphology of, 245
　　in Peruvian child, ancient, 238
　　references, 658
　　right, identification of, 246
　　trace of, 205
lambdoidal suture
　　accessory ossicles in, 225
　　in adult, 223
　　in African child, 224
　　closure of, 125
　　complex, 252
　　exposure of, 219
　　in newborn, 225
　　obliteration of, 125
　　ossicles along, xii, 247
　　with parietal foramina, asymmetrical, 237
　　in Peruvian, ancient, 231

in Peruvian child, ancient, 240
sagittal suture and, 229
sutures, other along, 244
sutures, other differentiated from, 217, 255
in Thai adult, 231
in Thai female, elderly, 232
variations in, 250
lateral bridge, 658
lateral incisors, 487, 488, 511, 512, 519
lateral orbital tubercle, 89
lateral pre-interparietal bone (term), 243
lateral pterygoid plate, 380
lateral rectus muscle, attachment of, 90
lateral union (of left first and second ribs), 555
ligament of Struthers, attachment of, 536
lingual exostoses, 483
lingual foramina, 452, 453
lingual plate, 458
lingual sphenoidialis, 300
lingual staining, 485
lingula sphenoidalis, 285
lumbar vertebra(e)
    in African skeletons, 584
    endplate concavities in, 582
    fifth, 565, 566, 567, 582, 585, 653
    foramina in, 582, 652
    fourth, 652
    ossification in, 583
    sacralization, partial of, 592
    second, 579
    sixth, 661
    spondylolysis in, 581, 653
    in Thai male, 584
    transverse processes of, 581, 652
Luschka's rib
    anterior and internal view of, 560
    bilateral, 557
    first and second ribs, left, 555, 562
    fourth, left, 561
    fourth, right, 560, 648
    left, 559
    term usage, 559
lytic lesions, 652

M

macrocephaly, 206
malar bone. *See* zygomatic (malar) bone
Malaysian adult, 337
male adolescent, 85
male adult
    acetabulum in, 603
    atlas articulation with occipital condyles in, 563
    basilar fissure and pharyngeal tubercle in, 329
    basilar process(es), bilateral in, 339
    bone, single in, 389

bregmatic ossicle in, 209
canaliculus innominatus in, 329
costoclavicular ligament attachment in, 526
foramen of Vesalius in, 317, 323
foramen ovale in, 317
hypoglossal canal, left in, 422, 423
hypoglossal canals in, 332
Inca bone in, 239
inferior malar tubercle in, 76
infraorbital foramina, multiple in, 56
lambdoidal ossicles in, 241
mastoid process, left and suprameatal crest in, 174
maxillary/infraorbital foramina and zygomaxillary
    tubercles in, 74
mental foramen/foramina, right, triple in, 476
occipital bun in, 184
occipital condyles and foramen of Vesalius in, 317
os odontoideum in, 345
palatine foramen/foramina, lesser in, 514
paracondylar foramen, left in, 331
paracondylar process in, 403
parietal notch bones, trace Mendosal suture and
    petrosquamosal suture in, 174
in Paris catacombs, 41
pterygoalar bridge, trace right in, 379
pterygospinous bridge in, 315
rib, right cervical on 7th cervical vertebra in, 573
sagitally sectioned cranium in, 267
sphenoid spine in, 373
supernumerary tooth in, 519
male Caucasian, elderly, 318
male elderly adult
    atlas superior condyles, divided/double in, 569
    calcification in, 277
    distal femoral cortical excavation in, 622
    falx cerebri and frontal sinuses in, 275
    femoral tubercles in, 608, 609
    foramen spinosum, left in, 334
    hamulus, bipartite in, 541
    metatarsals, left, first and second in, 639
    odontoid facet extension in, 572
    retromolar fossa cavitation defect in, 466
males
    costal cartilage calcification in, 552
    gonial flaring in, 117
    nasal rim spine in, 105
    See also under ethnic group
male vermiculate pattern, 10, 12, 40, 80
male young adult
    anterior fontanelle bone in, 212
    clavicle, right, medial epiphysis in, 522
    lumbar vertebrae in, 585
    mental foramen/foramina, left, internally divided in,
        473
    nasal bone, tripartite in, 33
    neural arch, congenital articulating in, 579

malleous, 149
mandible
   anatomy of, 116
   cancellous bone, 458
   developing teeth in, 25
   foramina in, 453
   lingual plate, left of, 458
   lower border, undulating of, 662
   with mental eminence, rounded, 471
   mental foramen/foramina in (see mental foramen/foramina)
   references, 658
   sectioned, 458, 464
   of Thai female, elderly, 458
mandibular canal, 463, 474, 490
mandibular condyle, 451
mandibular condyle fossa, 482
mandibular foramen/foramina, 460, 462, 475
mandibular incisors, 115, 487, 488
mandibular molar, 491
mandibular sulcus, left, defect in, 465
mandibular tori, 486, 658
manubrial aperture, 547, 548
manubrio-corpal symphysis, 658
manubriosternal symphysis (sternum), 647
manubrium, 549, 556
marginal sinus, 297
marginal tubercle (tuberculum marginale), 118, 658
masseter muscle, 74, 150
mastication, 41, 61, 151, 483
mastoid, 120, 656, 658
mastoid foramen/foramina
   bilateral, 173
   ectocranial and endocranial views of, 257
   location of, 265
   occipitomastoid ossicle and, 439
   references, 658
   sutural and temporal, 243
   in Thai male, adult, 438
   in Thai male, elderly, 440
   vertically divided, 256
mastoid notch, 143
mastoid notch bone, 142
mastoid processes, 172, 174, 437, 441
maxilla, 25, 68, 116, 464
maxillary antrum (MA), 20, 22, 118, 120
maxillary canines, 517
maxillary incisors, 493, 511, 512, 519
maxillary/infraorbital foramina, accessory, 74
maxillary molar, third, 493, 658
maxillary/palatal bridging, 499, 513
maxillary prognathism, 658
maxillary sinus, 20, 658
maxillary sutures, 518
maxillary torus/tori
   cross-section through, 515
   long and divided, 497
   or exostoses, 498
   references, 658, 662
   in Thai, elderly, 495
   in Thai adult, 494, 515
   in Thai female, 496
   in Thai male, adult, 266
medial orbit, 79
medial sutures, 504
median basioccipital canal, 307, 308, 309, 310
median canal, 402
median foramina, 311, 444
median palatine suture, posterior, 506
medio-palatine bone, posterior, 509
medio-palatine bones, anterior, 506, 508
Mendosal/asterionic suture, 246
Mendosal/biasterionic suture, 238, 253
Mendosal suture(s)
   in adult male, 174
   in child, 436
   in fetal occipital bone, 259
   occipital bun caused by persistent, 184
   status, 658
   in Thai adult, 142
meningeal artery emissaries, middle, 659
meninges, canal carrying, 92
meningo-orbital foramen, 81, 95, 97
mental eminence, rounded, 471
mental foramen/foramina
   absence of, 479
   accessory, 655
   and accessory foramen, 471
   double, 479
   external and internal, 479
   in newborn skull, 3
   references, 658
   superior and inferior, 480
   in Thai adult, 469
   in Thai young adult, 470
   vertically divided, 473
mental foramen/foramina, left, 473, 474, 477, 480
mental foramen/foramina, right
   in child, 490
   double, 470, 475, 481
   horizontally divided, 481
   partial bridging of, 478
   triple, 476, 477
   vertically divided, 478
mental spine, 657, 658
mental symphysis, 3
mesiodens, 503
metacone, 493
metatarsals, left, 639
metopic fissure, 57, 63, 154, 218
metopic/frontal/interfrontal suture, 63
metopic ossicle, 34, 59

metopic suture
    in adult male, 11, 41
    in adults, 39, 61
    in child, 9, 30, 59
    complexity of, 58
    developmental misalignment of, 64
    in fetal skull, 5
    in frontal bone, 6
    frontal view of, 63
    hypoplastic nasal bones and, 31
    keeled/steepled frontal bone along, 18
    keeling along, 189
    misalignment of, 210, 215
    in newborn, 3, 43
    obliteration of, 39
    open, 62, 273
    overview of, 60
    references, 659
    remnant of, 59
    simple, 61
    in Thai adult, 14
    in white male, adult, 40
metopism
    in Asian male, adult, 63, 154
    frequency of, 11, 62
    in male adult, 209
    in Peruvian child, 207
    references, 659
    in Thai adult, 17
middle-age indicator, 618
middle cranial fossa, foramina of, 366
middle turbinate bones, 22
molars
    bilateral presence of, 517
    cremulations, 659
    horizontally impacted, 489
    mandibular, 491
    maxillary, 493, 658
    protostylid of lower, 660
    right third, 489
    roots, 22
    six-year, eruption of, 502
morphoscopic characteristics, xi, xiv
muscle attachment sites, robusticity of, 661
muscle marks, 659
muscle trauma and calcification, 523
mylohyoid bridge
    along mylohyoid canal, 459
    degree, 659
    location, 659
    references, 659
    Stafne's defect and, 458
    in Thai adult, 459
    in white female, adult, 461
mylohyoid canal, 459, 460
myositis ossificans, 523

N

narrow (dolicocephalic) skulls, 62
nasal aperture, 19, 22, 103, 105, 659
nasal bones
    in Asian adult, 31
    asymmetrically sized, 31
    in fetal skull, 4
    foramen, xii, 36
    fractured and healed, 32, 64
    fractures, absence of, 32
    overhang, 138, 140, 187
    references, 659
    sutures, obliteration of, 35
    tripartite, 33
nasal bridge form, 659
nasal cavity/ies, 104, 659
nasal foramina, 656, 659
nasal form, 659
nasal fracture, healed, 12
nasal guttering, 50, 51, 52, 103
nasal margin, 103
nasal overgrowth, 659
nasal profile, 659
nasal region, transverse section through, 517
nasal rim spine, 105, 106, 107–108
nasal septum
    deviated, 20, 45, 97, 99, 103, 117
    in fetal skull, 4
    inferior-superior view through facial region showing, 22
nasal shape, xi
nasal sill, 659
nasal sill sharp, 659
nasal spine/nasal spinalis
    anterior, 22, 23, 140, 187, 655
    bone extending inferiorly from, 109
    divided anterior, 110
    of frontal bone, 29
    in Peruvian male, 138
    posterior, 515
    references, 659
Nasion, depression at, 656
Nasion, region superior to, 58
nasofrontal ossicle, 34
nasofrontal suture, 38, 59
nasolacrimal canal, 140
nasolacrimal ducts, 22
Native American adult, 227
navicular bone, accessory, 632
Negroid ancestry, 266
Negroid individuals, 103
neural arch
    cleft, 588, 590, 591
    congenital articulating, 579
    defects, 579
    disarticulation of, 653

fusion of, 595
  incomplete closure of, 591
  separate, 577, 595
neurovascular bundle(s)
  through left infraorbital foramen, 25
  transmission of, 473, 474, 476, 477, 481
newborn
  anterior fontanelle in, 196–197
  frontal foramen and grooves in, 43
  lambdoial suture in, 225
  metopic suture, supraorbital foramina and frontal foramen and grooves in, 43
  Obelion (region) defects in, 213
  ossification centers in, 3
  skull anatomy in, 3, 196
New Guinea skulls, 105
non-metric traits, xi, xii, xiii, xiv
nose, broken, healed, 12
nose form, 659
nuchal crest
  in Asian male, 228
  in Asian male, adult, 234
  in Egyptian male, ancient, 235
  foramina along, 220
  muscle attachments along, 219, 258
  in Thai male, adult, 235
nuchal foramina, 220
nuchal ligament attachment, 411
nuchal line, highest, 657
nuchal spike, 233
nuchal superstructure, 227, 234, 235
nutrient foramen, 525, 527

O

Obelion (region)
  artery at, 229
  biomechanics of, 253
  in black male, adult, 226
  in child, 199
  defects in, 213
  depression at, 193
  faulty ossification in, xii
  magnification of, 237
  overview of, 200, 213
  parietal foramen formation at, 198
  parietal foramina at, 220
  in Peruvian, ancient, 253
  sagittal ossicle superior to, 209
  sagittal/parietal groove in, 192
  sagittal suture at, 217, 228, 251, 263
  suture, simple at, 240
oblique muscle, inferior, attachment of, 79, 101–102
oblique muscle, superior, 79
occipital base, 336
occipital bone, 22, 255

occipital bun, 184
occipital condyle, left, 306, 340, 401
occipital condyle, third. See tertiary occipital condyle
occipital condyles
  asymmetrical, 395, 442
  atlas articulation with, 563, 569
  basilar processes anterior to, 339
  condylar dysplasia encroaching on, 303
  divided, 318, 395, 396
  double, 659
  extension of, 385
  in male Caucasian, elderly, 318
  medial tubercles of, 305
  median foramina medial to, 444
  partially divided, 393
  precondylar tubercles or pedestals continuous with, 324
  in Thai adult, 442
occipital crest, external, 411
occipital crest, internal, 298
occipital emissary foramen, 222, 411
occipital facet, third, 659
occipital foramen, xii, 432, 659
occipital fossa, 297, 298
occipital mastoid wormians, 659
occipital protuberance, 656, 659
occipital region, left, 231
occipital squamous convexity, 659
occipital squamous shape, 659
occipital superstructure, 218, 230, 233, 234
occipital vertebra, 403
occipitocervical border, somites of, 328
occipitomastoid ossicle, 243, 256, 439, 659
occipitomastoid suture, 243, 257, 265, 660
occipitomastoid wormians, 659
odontoid facet, extension of, 572
odontoid process (axis), 572
odontoma, 503, 520
older individuals. See elderly
ophthalmic artery, 92
optic canal, accessory, 655
optic foramen/foramina, 92, 93, 94, 283, 429
optic nerve, 92
orbicularis occuli, 90
orbit, left, 70, 83, 101, 114, 122
orbit, right
  anatomy of, 79
  calcification and bony projection absence in, 101
  foramen of unknown etiology in, 70
  foramen perforating lateral wall of, 128
  lacrimal foramen absence in, 71, 72
  lacrimal ossicle along, 67
  lateral rectus muscle, attachment of, 90
  medial shelf in, 65
  ossiculus canalis and ossiculus hamuli in, 69
orbital border, lower, 75
orbital fissure, superior, 97, 283

orbital foramina, 81, 91, 97
orbital form, 659
orbital opening, 659
orbital ossicles, 70
orbital osteoporosis, 659
orbital plates, 96, 270, 273, 276
orbital rim spurs, 82
orbital tubercle of malar bone (term), 89
orbits
    floor of, 73
    frontal porosity (porotic hyperostosis) above, 60
    male vermiculate pattern above, 10, 40
    pits and lines above, 10
    porosity above and medial to, 45
    soft-tissue attachment of, 19, 20
os acromiale, 528, 529, 659
os bipartite divisum (term), 121
os japonicum (Os zygomaticum bipartitum)
    in Asian male young adult, 152
    frequency of, 78
    lack of evident, 153–154
    partially obliterated, 152
    in Peruvian child, ancient, 77, 78
    references, 659
    in Thai female, 164
    trace, 185, 659
os japonicum, bilateral, 77
os japonicum, left, 164, 185
os japonicum, right, 152
os japonicum, trace, 151, 153, 185
os naviculare, 629, 630
os naviculare secondarium (term), 632
os odontoideum, 564, 565, 566
os odontoideum, congenital, 345, 564
os parietale bipartitum (term), 121
os parietale divisum (term), 121
os peroneum, bilateral, 637
osseous projections, 81
ossicle at asterion, 248, 655, 659
Ossicle of Infraorbital Margin (term), 66
Ossicle of Lacrimal Groove (term), 66
ossicle of Riolano, 243, 256, 439, 659
ossiculum canalis naso-lachrymalis, 68
ossiculus canalis, 69, 70
ossiculus hamuli, 69, 70
ossification, centers of, 3
ossified trochlear pulley, xii
osteoarthritis, 482, 595, 621
osteoma (term), 138
osteoporosis, 29, 236, 321, 659
os tibiale (term), 632
os tibiale externum (term), 632
os trigonum, xii, 631, 659
os zygomaticum duplex, 151, 659
ovale spinosum, continuous, 660
oval window
    demonstration of, 166, 447
    in external auditory meatus, 149
    references, 660
    in Thai male adult, 148
    tympanic dehiscence revealing, 147

P

Pacchionian bodies (term), 214
Pacchionian pits
    in child's skull, 9
    distribution of, 272
    encocast of, 272
    examples of, 62
    frozen waves of, 270
    in Thai, elderly, 269
    in Thai adult, 268
Pacific Islander groups, 219
Pacific Northwest aboriginal crania, 126
palatal bridge/bridging, 499, 500, 513, 660
palatal exostosis (torus palatinus), xii
palatal form, 660
palatal sutures
    in child, 505
    in female young adult, 508
    partial obliteration of, 506
    references, 660
    superior aspects of, 517
    transverse, 662
    in white male, adult, 506
palatal sutures, accessory, 505, 506, 508
palate, 41, 140, 515
palatine crest, 502
palatine foramen/foramina, 335, 514, 655, 658
palatine groove bridging, 501
palatine nerve, lesser, transmission of, 514
palatine torus, 495, 660
paracondylar foramina, 330, 331, 396
paracondylar process, 310, 340, 403, 660
paracondylar process, left, 410, 571
paracondylar process, right, 409
paracondylar tubercles, 342, 401, 402
paramastoid process, 310, 660
parasagittal plane, 310
parietal bone(s)
    bipartite, xii, 121
    bregmatic bone confined to, 202
    divided, 656
    growth of, 145
    left, 214, 262
    Pacchionian pits in, 268
    thin areas in, 193, 662
parietal extension, 135
parietal foramen, left, 211, 229, 261
parietal foramen/foramina
    in adult, 263

in adult cranium from Samoa, 202
anatomical position of, 201
in Asian male, adult, 218
asymmetrical, 237
bilateral, 193, 228, 240, 249, 253
in black male, adult, 230
enlarged, xii, 221
formation of, 198
Obelion with, 220
Obelion without, 199
in Peruvian, ancient, 253
references, 660
vessels transmitted by, 211, 216
parietal grooves, 198
parietal notch, 660
parietal notch bone(s), 172, 174, 175, 660
parietal notch ossicle, 175, 660
parietal process, 160, 660
parietal sagittal suture (term), 121
parietal striae, 146
parietal suture, accessory (bipartite), 122
Paris, catacombs of, 41
pars tympanica (bilateral), 126, 127
patella, 623, 656
patella, bipartite, xii, 623, 624, 656
pathological lesion/growth, cold water association of, 138
pathological symptoms, xi
pedal phalanges, left distal and medial, 628
pelvis, right, articular facets in, 598
perichondrium, removal of, 642
perilacrimal ossicles, 66
perimortem trauma (facial region), 99
perimortem trauma, determining, 642
perinatal individuals, 385
periosteum, 54, 63
permanent anterior teeth, 516
peroneal tubercle, 660
peroneus longus groove, 636
personal identity, determining, 642
Peruvian, ancient
cranial modification (deformation) in, 160
dental crowding and genial tubercles in, 483
frontal grooves in, 10
metopic suture in, 18
parietal foramina, bilateral in, 253
postcondylar tubercles in, 435
pterygospinous bridge and foramen of Civinini in, 355
sagittal and lambdoidal sutures in, 231
Peruvian adolescent, 204, 261
Peruvian adult
auditory exostosis in, 139
cranial deformation in, 157
parietal foramina in, 221
sagittal suture in, 254
Peruvian adult, ancient
basilar tubercles/wings and precondylar tubercles/

processes in, 416
coronal ossicle in, 176
cranial modification (deformation) in, 194, 430
early childhood head binding in, 155
paracondylar tubercles and apical odontoid ligament in, 402
supraglenoid foramen and suprameatal pit in, 186
suprainion depression in, 227
Peruvian child
epiteric bone in, 132
tertiary occipital condyle in, 384
trochlear spur in, 84
Peruvian child, ancient
basilar synchondrosis in, 429
coronal ossicles in, 159
cranial modification (deformation) and metopism in, 207
cranial modification (deformation) in, 156
lambdoidal suture and porotic hyperostosis in, 240
Mendosal/biasterionic suture in, 238
occipital emissary foramen in, 222
os japonicum, bilateral in, 77, 78
palatal bridging, bilateral in, 500
Peruvian female, adult, 383, 384, 402
Peruvian male, 138, 140, 189
Peruvian male, adult
auditory exostosis in, 138
parietal extension and epiteric bone/squamosal ossicle in, 135
Peruvian male, adult, ancient
cranial modification (deformation) in, 179
suprameatal pit and postglenoid/inferior squamosal foramen in, 162
supranasal suture and metopism in, 60
Peruvian male, ancient, 451
Peruvian subadult, 158, 165
petroclinoid bridging, bilateral, 299
petrosal exostosis, 290
petrosal nerves, 371
petrosal sinus, superior, 278, 279, 280, 281
petrosphenoid ligament (of Gruber), 279, 280, 291
petrosquamosal suture, persistent, 174
petrosquamous emissaries, 168, 170, 660
petrosquamous suture, 143, 172, 173
petrous bone, left, 371
petrous bone, right, 277
petrous bones
basilar synchondrosis and bony islands of, 288
bilateral calcifications along, 296
in child, 287
foramen entering, 161
ossification along apex of, 442
overhanging appearance of, 295
petrous ridge, 279, 280, 282, 300
phalanx, bipartite foot, 654
phalanx, left, 641, 654

pharyngeal fossa (fossa faringea), 657
pharyngeal foveola (fossa navicularis)
    in African male, adult, 393
    in Asian female, elderly, 392
    in Indian female, 391
    overview of, 435
    references, 660
    in Thai adult, 390, 391
pharyngeal tubercle, 326, 329, 660
physiological notch, 537, 538
piriform aperture, 22
pitting, 63, 321
plaque (femur), 660
Poirier's facet, 610, 611, 612, 615, 660
Polynesian adult, 378
ponticulus posticus (term), 568
porotic hyperostosis, 10, 63, 240
Porus crotaphitico-buccinatorium foramen, 212
postbregmatic depression, 188, 266, 660
postcondylar canals, 343, 344, 660
postcondylar depressions (basilar invaginations), 436
postcondylar foramina, 344
postcondylar fossa/canal, right, 342
postcondylar process, 340
postcondylar tubercles, 435, 660
postcondyloid canal, 414
postcondyloid foramina, 303, 413
posterior arch, bifid, 390
posterior bridge, 660
posterior foramen, 102, 400, 660
postglenoid foramen
    in child, 186
    in fetus, 165
    inferior, 165
    left, 161
    location of, 169
    term, 434
    in Thai adult, 169
    in Thai child, 167
postglenoid/inferior squamosal foramen, 162
postglenoid/supraglenoid foramen, 127
postglenoid tubercle/process, 137, 176, 448
postmortem breakage, 29, 122, 157
postmortem damage, 198
preauricular sulcus, 604, 660
preauricular surface, 660
precondylar pit, 434
precondylar processes, 416
precondylar tubercle(s)
    along midline, 382
    in Asian adult, 431
    basilar tubercles/wings and, 416
    bilateral and asymmetrical, 338
    and canaliculus innominatus, 324
    formation of, 431
    frequency of, 325

    overview of, 336
    pedestaled, 333
    references, 660
    in Thai adult, 343
    in Thai female, elderly, 386
    in Thai male, adult, 341
    pre-interparietal bone, 249, 251
    see also Inca bone
premolars, 513, 662
premolars, bilateral accessory, 485
procerus muscle attachments, 64
Process of Kerckring. *See* Kerckring's process
processus marginalis, 660
prognathism, 655, 656, 658, 660
pseudoarthritis, 523
pseudoarthroses, 558
pterion, 129, 130, 660
pterionic ossicle, 656
pterion X or K, 661
pterygoalar bar, 449
pterygoalar bridge
    in African child, 313, 314
    in Asian male, adult, 407
    and foramen, 312, 346
    formation of, 302
    in male adult, 379
    pterygospinous bridge and, 354
    references, 660, 661
    in Thai adult, male, 347
pterygoalar bridging, 346, 347, 350, 351, 433
pterygoalar ligament, 313, 350, 357, 375, 380
pterygoalar ligament, left, 358
pterygoalar ligament, right, 353, 358
pterygoalar spine, 315
pterygo-basal bridge, 661
pterygoid perforation, lateral, 658
pterygoid plate, 355
pterygoid plate, lateral, 380
pterygoid spurs, 661
pterygomaxillary suture (term), 388
pterygopalatine suture (term), 388
pterygopalatomaxillary suture (term), 388
pterygospinous bridge
    and foramen of Civinni, 247, 352, 355
    formation of, 355
    incompletely formed, 163
    partial, 404
    pterygoalar bridge and, 354
    references, 661
pterygospinous bridging, partial, 215, 348
pterygospinous foramen, 313, 431, 657
pterygospinous ligament, 313, 375, 380
pterygospinous ligament, right, 349, 378
pubes, parturition pits of, 605
pubic bone, 604
pubic tubercles/spine, 606

Q

qualitative terms, use of, xiii
quantitative methods, xiii

R

radial tuberosity, dimpled, 540
radiodense line, 622
ramus, 489, 655
ramus angle, ascending, 655
ramus inversion (mandible), 661
rectus lateralis muscle attachment, 94
rectus muscle, lateral, attachment of, 90
retroglenoid foramen, left, 434
retromastoid tubercles/processes, 218, 233, 661
retromolar canals, left, 467, 468
retromolar foramen, 467, 661
retromolar fossa, 466
retromolar process, 661
retropterygoid apertures, 661
rhomboid fossa/e, xii, 525, 526, 649
rib cage, 642, 645, 646
ribs
    first and second, bridging of, 555
    first and second, synostosis of, 559
    fusion of left first and second, 555
    supernumerary, 661
    See also Luschka's rib
ribs, cervical, 558, 573, 574
ribs, left, first and second, synostosis of, 555, 562
ribs, lumbar, 580, 581
ribs, lumbar, left, 585
ribs, right, 555
rocker (and non-rocker) jaw, 661
round window/fenestra cochleae, 148

S

S1 vertebra, 588, 589
sacral cleft, 651
sacral facet, accessory, 655
sacral foramen, 594
sacral hiatus, 593
sacralization, 587, 592, 661
sacral segment, 595
sacroiliac joint, accessory, 596
sacrum/sacra
    accessory foramen in, 586
    articular facet, accessory in, 596
    cleft neural arch in, 591
    segmented, 589
    spina bifida of, 651
    triangular, 594
    variations in, 587
    wide opening of, 590
    with and without fossa cribrosa, 597
sagitally sectioned cranium, 26, 267, 275
sagittal ossicle(s)
    in adult, 223
    in Asian, elderly, 215
    references, 661
    in Thai adult, 208
    in Thai male, elderly, 209
    in young adult, 244
sagittal/parietal groove, 192
sagittal sulcus, flexure of, 656
sagittal suture
    in black male, adult, 226, 230
    craniosyntosis of, 190, 205
    in Egyptian adult, ancient, 8
    keeling along, 189
    misalignment of, 210, 215
    at Obelion, 200, 217, 251, 253, 263
    obliteration of, 231
    ossicles along, xii
    with parietal foramen, left, 229
    parietal foramen on, 220
    with parietal foramina, asymmetrical, 237
    in Peruvian, ancient, 231
    in Peruvian adolescent, ancient, 261
    in Peruvian adult, 254
    sutures, other differentiated from, 121, 217
    in Thai adult, 228
    in Thai female, elderly, 232
    thickened bone along, 193
sagittal suture ossicle, 211
salivary gland depression (term), 454
Samoa, adult cranium from, 202
Sauser's fissure (term), 325
scaphocephaly, 205
scapula, left, 528, 530, 534
scapula, right, 523, 529, 535, 650
scapular body, 533
sciatic notch, greater, 657
scoliosis, 555
secondary os calcis, 633
sectioned adult cranium, 22
sella bridges, 661
septal aperture(s), 537, 538, 661
sex, determining, 472, 642
shoulder, trauma to, 523
sigmoid sinus, 257
sinuses, 28
siphoid foramen, 545
size, normal *versus* pathological nature determined based on, xii
skeletal trauma or disease, evidence of, 643
skeleton collections, xvi
skeletons, intra- and inter-variability of, xiv
Skulls Unlimited, 643
soft tissues, periorbital calcification of, 65

Sömmering, processus marginalis of, 118
South Indians, 56
sphenobasilar syncondrosis (term), 302
sphenofrontal suture, 95, 123
sphenoidal emissary foramen (term), 284
sphenoidal tubercle, 287
sphenoid bone
    angular spine of, 353
    calcified spines in, 356
    clinoid process bridging in, 429
    clivus of, 279
    elevations, 183
    epiteric bone joining with, 133
    foramen in, 285
    temporal bone, joining to, 293
    unilateral ossicle along upper portion of, 132
sphenoid bone, left, 176, 321, 370
sphenoid ligament. partial bridging of, 350
sphenoid spine, 355, 373, 376, 377
sphenomaxillary suture, 388, 389
sphenooccipital syncondrosis (term), 302
sphenotemporal sulcus of Gustav Schwalbe, 183
spheroid bridges, basal, 655
spina bifida
    in Asian adult, 588
    conditions, other differentiated from, 591
    definition and overview of, 590
    in sacrum, 589, 651
    in Thai male, elderly, 575
spina recti lateralis, 94
spina trochlearis (term), 80
spina zygomatica, 118
spine of Civinini, right, 334
spine of Henle, 137, 171, 187, 448
spinous ligament, 431
spondylolysis
    bilateral, 578, 591
    bilateral lumbar, 576, 577
    in lumbar vertebra, fifth, 653
    neural arch defects, other differentiated from, 579
    unilateral, 581
squamomastoid suture (term), 143, 661
squamosal foramen
    location of, 165, 169
    parietal extension of, 185
    term, 434
    in Thai adult, 176
squamosal foramen, inferior
    emissary vein transmitted by, 127
    in Peruvian male, adult, 162
    zygomatic arch, superior to, 170
squamosal ossicle
    in ancient Peruvian child, 78
    and epiteric bone, 136
    parietal extension and, 135
    references, 661

    in Thai adult, 178
    in Thai male, adult, 133
squamosal suture, 122, 125, 182, 243
squamosopetrous foramen (term), 434
squamosopetrous foramen and sinus, 165
squamousal glenoid foramen (term), 161
squamous bones, 161
squamous-parietal ossicle, 661
squatting facets, 625, 626, 627, 661
Srb's anomaly, 555, 556, 559
Stafne's defects
    anterior, 457, 485
    classic, 457
    early-stage, 456
    features resembling, 465
    and mylohyoid bridge, 458
    overview of, 455
    sublingual fovea misidentified as, 485
    in Thai male mandible, 454, 456, 457
stapes, attachments, 149
stapes, base of, 148
static bone cavity (term), 454
Steida's process, 631
sternal foramen, 545, 661
sterno-manubrial junction, 549
sternum, 546, 549, 560, 647
"stylalgia" (term), 180
styloid process
    absence of, 412
    bilateral in Thai female, adult, 129
    left, 181
    right, 397, 448
    in Thai male, adult, 180
    variants of, 119
stylomastoid foramen, 398
subadult(s)
    basilar synchondrosis in, 442
    Bregma foramina in, 201
    coronal suture extensions in, 208
    epiteric bone in, 177
    femur, distal femoral cortical excavation in, 620
    foramen spinosum, left and pterygoalar ligament, right in, 353
    foramina, right in, 313
    fossa of Allen in, 613, 614
    lumbar vertebrae ossification in, 583
    metopic and supranasal suture formation in, 39
    nuchal crest and muscle attachments in, 258
    os japonicum, trace in, 151
    remains, removing soft tissue from, 643
    sagittal section of, 275
    septal aperture(s) in, 538
    sternum in, 546
    temporal and parietal bone growth in, 146
    trace os japonicum in, 151
    trochanter, third in, 613

trochlear spurs in, 85
See also under ethnic group and gender
sub-asterionic ossicle, 661
subdural ossifications, 278
sublingual arteries, 453
sublingual fovea, 485
subnasal margin (defined), 661
subpublic concavity, 661
subsagittal suture, 121
Subsagittal Suture of Pozzi, 198
sulcus, variant for, 297
sulcus of Gustav Schwalbe, 154
sulcus supraorbitalis, 661
superciliary arches, 39, 58
supernumerary ossicles, 661
supernumerary rib, 661
supernumerary teeth, 494, 511, 519
supinator crest, 539
supra-acetabular fossa, 599
supra-acetabular fossa and groove, 661
supra-bregmatic ossicle/bone, 244
supraclavicular foramen, 661
supracondyloid foramen, 537
supraglenoid foramen, 161, 167, 186
suprainion depression, 227
supramastoid foramen, 243
suprameatal crest, 174
suprameatal pit, 137, 162, 176, 186
suprameatal spine and depression, 661
suprameatal spine of Henle (term), 171
supranasal notches, 45
"supranasal" region (term), 58
supranasal suture
    in adults, 39, 61
    breakage, postmortem resembling, 29
    complexity of, 58
    formation of, 41
    in frontal bone, 6
    horizontally oriented, 61
    inferior view of, 80
    with lateral extensions, 58
    in male adult, 11, 41, 42
    morphology of, 42, 61
    obliteration of, 39
    overview of, 60
    prominent, 10
    references, 661
    remnants of, 12
    in teenager, 37, 38
    in Thai adult, 17, 80
    in white male, adult, 40
supraorbital bridge, right, 14
supraorbital canals, 13
supraorbital foramen, right, 17
supraorbital foramen/foramina
    above left orbit, 55
    in black adult, 50
    in elderly, 43
    in newborn, 43
    in newborn skull (bilateral), 3
    references, 657, 661
    in Thai female, adult, 14
    variants, 13
supraorbital nerve groove, 661
supraorbital notch
    above left orbit, 55
    in Asian male adult, 82
    and foramen, xii, 60
    references, 661
    in Thai female, adult, 14
supraorbital notch, left, 14, 50
supraorbital osseous structures, 661
supraorbital region, striations/grooves in, 40
suprascapular bridging, early-stage, 534
suprascapular foramen, 529, 531, 533
suprascapular (transverse) ligament, calcified, 529, 531, 532, 534, 535
suprascapular notch, 534, 662
suprasternal bones, 550
suprasternal tubercle, unilateral, 551
supratrochlear foramen, 661
supratrochlear/supracondylar spur/supracondyloid process, 536
"surfer's ear" (term), 138
sutura mastoideosquamosa (term), 143
sutura notha (false suture), 53, 54
suture-like bone, 175
sutures, 9, 29, 122, 196, 662
symphalangism, pedal, 628, 629
synchondroses, 293
synodontia, 487, 488
synostosis(es), 125, 555, 559, 562
    See also craniosynostosis, premature

T

talar articular surface, inferior, 657
talar facet, medial, 658
talar neck, 627
talus, left, os trigonum in, 631
talus, right, Steida's process in, 631
talus, squatting facet in, 626, 662
tarsal component of orbicularis occuli, 90
tarsal condition, non-osseous, 640
taurodontism, 662
teaching skeleton, chest plate in, 544
"teenage imprint" (term), 612, 614
teenager. *See* adolescent
teeth
    accessory, 503
    alveolar neurovascular bundles supplying, 464
    blackened, 129

canines, 118, 503, 513, 517, 520, 656
   crowding of, 483
   developing, 25, 115
   loss, antemortem, remodeling after, 335
   loss of, 478
   occlusal surfaces, dental attrition of, 103
   permanent anterior, 516
   roots, developmental stages of, 490
   stresses transmitted from, 41
   supernumerary, 494, 511, 519
tegman tympani (defined), 380
tegum dehiscence, 276
temporal artery, superficial, 144
temporal bone
   exostosis along ridge of right, 290
   Glaserian fissure, left, foramen in, 379
   growth of, 145
   inferior squamousal/postglenoid foramen in, 169
   petrous portions of, 287
   sphenoidal bone, joining to, 293
   styloid process of, 119, 397
   superior petrosal sinus of, 277, 280
   vaginal process of, 450
temporal bone, left, 162, 175
temporal bone, right, 133, 137, 148, 282, 407
temporal extension, 124
temporalis muscles, attachment of, 193, 198
temporal lines, superior, 191, 218
temporal region, arteries of, 53
temporal squama, 123, 133, 144–145, 660
temporal squamous portion, left, 160
temporal squamous shape, 662
temporal styloid process, 119, 353, 450
tensile stresses, 9
tentorium cerebelli, 277
tertiary occipital condyle
   as abnormal non-metric trait and anatomical variant, xii
   and accessory foramen, 401
   as occipital condyle extension, 385
   peg-shaped, 386
   in Peruvian child, 384
   in Peruvian female, adult, 383, 384
   references, 662
   in Thai adult, 382, 386
   in Thai male, adult, 341
   variants of, 434
Thai, 47, 53, 284, 286, 560
Thai adult
   antegonial notch in, 471
   asterionic ossicles/bones in, 248
   atlanto-occipitalization, bifid posterior arch and atlas articular facets in, 390
   atlas in, 432
   basilar depression in, 399
   bone/ossicle and petrosquamous suture trace/remnant in, 143

   canines, accessory in, 513
   concha bullosa in, 98
   condylar dysplasia in, 303
   coronal ossicle(s) in, 141, 208
   coronal suture extensions in, 208
   episternal bones in, 550
   femur, right of, 607
   foramen magnum in, 297, 415
   foramen of Vesalius, foramen ovale and foramen spinosum in, 360
   foramen of Vesalius, right in, 320
   foramen spinosum, left in, 372
   foramen spinosum and pterygospinous bridge in, 404
   foramina and sutures in, 142
   frontotemporal articulation in, 179
   hypoglossal canal divided/double left in, 294
   inferior oblique muscle attachment area calcification in, 102
   inferior squamous foramen in, 169
   infraorbital suture and zygomaticomaxillary tubercles in, 48
   infraorbital sutures and foramina in, 73
   lacrimal or perilacrimal ossicles in, 66
   lambdoidal suture in, 231
   lateral incisors in, 511, 512
   lingual foramina in, 452
   malar bones in, 128
   male vermiculate pattern in, 80
   mandibular sulcus, left in, 465
   maxillary canine agenesis and molar presence in, 517
   maxillary incisors, lateral in, 512, 519
   maxillary/palatal bridging in, 499, 513
   maxillary torus/tori in, 494, 515
   median basioccipital canals, bilateral in, 307
   mental foramen/foramina in, 469
   metopic suture and Pacchionian pits in, 62
   metopism, supranasal suture and zygomaxillary tubercles in, 17
   mylohyoid bridge in, 459
   nasal bone foramina absent in, 36
   nasal guttering in, 103
   nasofrontal or metopic ossicle, 34
   nuchal crest muscle attachment nodules in, 219
   occipital condyles in, 306, 442
   orbit, left, calcification along inferior border of, 101
   os naviculare, bilateral in, 629
   Pacchionian pits in, 268
   with parietal foramina, bilateral and sagittal suture, 228
   petrous and basilar bones in, 287
   pharyngeal foveola in, 390, 391
   Poirier's facet, bilateral in, 615
   postcondyloid canal in, 414
   postcondyloid foramen and condylar dysplasia in, 303
   postglenoid foramen in, 169
   precondylar pit in, 434
   precondylar tubercle in, 343, 382

procerus muscle attachments in, 64
pterygoalar ligament in, 357
pterygospinous bridge, incompletely formed in, 163
pterygospinous bridge and foramen of Civinini in, 352, 433
pterygospinous foramen in, 431
retroglenoid foramen, left in, 434
sacral segment, neural arch fused to first in, 595
sagittal and coronal ossicles in, 208
sphenoid and temporal styloid process in, 353
squamosal foramen and postglenoid/supreglemoid foramen in, 127
squamosal ossicles, multiple in, 178
suprameatal pit, Spine of Henle and postglenoid tubercle/process in, 137
suprameatal pit (squamosal foramen) and postglenoid tubercle/process in, 176
supranasal triangle in, 58
supraorbital canals and foramina in, 13
suprascapular (transverse) ligament, calcified in, 532, 535
suprasternal bones in, 550
sutura notha, possible in, 54
temporal bone, left of, 175
temporal squama bony extension in, 144
tertiary occipital condyle in, 382, 386
trochelar apparatus in, 80
trochlear spurs, bilateral in, 86
zygomatic foramina, multiple in, 111
zygomaticofacial foramen in, 114
zygomaticomaxillary suture tubercles in, 46
Thai adult mandible
  gonial eversion in, 487
  mandibular incisor, lateral in, 488
  mental foramen/foramina, double in, 479
  mental foramen/foramina, right, partial bridging in, 478
  mental foramen in, 473
  molar, right third in, 489
  mylohyoid canal, left in, 460
  mylohyoid canal perforation in, 459
  premolars, bilateral accessory in, 485
Thai child
  gubernacular canals in, 502, 516
  inferior squamous foramen in, 167
  lacrimal ossicle in, 67
  normal morphology of, 45
  permanent anterior teeth in, 516
  postglenoid foramen in, 167
  sphenomaxillary suture in, 388
  tertiary occipital condyle and accessory foramen in, 401
Thai elderly, 188, 269, 475, 495, 542
Thai female, 164, 478, 496, 569, 571
Thai female, adult, 14, 95, 123, 129, 362
Thai female, elderly, 109, 124, 232, 368, 458
Thai male
  epiteric bone in, 133, 134
  lumbar vertebra(e) in, 584
  malar tubercle in, 128
  mandible in, 454, 456, 457, 480
  os odontoideum in, 345, 565, 566
  parietal or squamosal suture in, 122
  tarsal condition, non-osseous in, 640
  temporal bone in, 397
Thai male, adult
  ethmoidal sinus(es) in, 266
  hypochordal arch in, 381
  hypoglossal canal, right in, 418, 419
  innominate, right in, 600
  mandibular foramen, triple in, 462
  marginal tubercle in, 118
  mastoid foramen/foramina in, 438
  mastoid processes in, 441
  Mendosal/biasterionic sutures in, 238
  nasal bones in, 32, 35
  nasal cavity, left, bony projects on floor of, 104
  nasal guttering in, 52
  nuchal crest in, 220
  nuchal superstructure in, 235
  occipital superstructure in, 230
  os odontoideum in, 565, 566
  petrosquamous suture in, 172
  phalanx, left distal first, ossicle in, 641
  precondylar tubercle and occipital condyle, third in, 341
  pterygoalar bridge in, 347
  sacrum, cleft neural arch in, 591
  sinuses, maxillary torus and Inion spike in, 266
  squamosal suture obliteration in, 182
  styloid process, elongated in, 180
  vermian fossa in, 298
Thai male, elderly
  cavernous foramen in, 321
  hypoglossal canal, left in, 424
  hypoglossal canal, right in, 419, 420
  lumbar vertebra(e) in, 585
  mastoid foramina in, 440
  median basioccipital canal in, 308
  osteoporosis in, 236
  sagittal ossicle in, 209
  sphenomaxillary suture in, 388
  spina bifida in, 575
  temporal styloid process in, 119
Thai subadult
  basilar synchondrosis in, 302
  foramen magnum in, 400
  frontal bone in, 29
  maxillary incisor, lateral in, 511
  median basioccipital canal and paracondylar process in, 310
  parietal grooves in, 198
  petrous bone and basilar in, 288
  postcondyloid foramina in, 413

Thai young adult, 346, 470
thoracic cage, 643
thoracic region, soft tissue, removing from, 643–644
thoracic vertebra, 575
tibia(e)
    bowing, 662
    extension, lateral, 658
    medial squatting facet, 662
    squatting facet in, 625, 626, 627, 658, 662
toe, left fifth, 629
toe, ossicle, accessory or bipartite, 641
tori mandibular, 486, 658
torus auditivi, 662
torus occipitalis transversus (term), 228, 230
torus palatinus. See maxillary torus/tori
transverse accessory suture, 123
transverse foramen, bipartite, 662
transverse palatine suture, 22, 503
trauma, 198, 595
trisomy, 31
trochanter, third, xii, 613, 617, 618, 662
trochanteric fossa, exostosis in, xii, 656
trochanteric fossa spicules, 618
trochlear apparatus (pulley), xii, 79, 80, 86
trochlear fossa, 79, 84, 85, 89
trochlear mound, 87
trochlear projection, 91
trochlear spine, 80, 662
trochlear spur, right, 80
trochlear spur(s)
    in adolescent female, 88
    in adolescent male, 85
    in Asian adult, 86, 89
    bilateral, 86, 88
    calcified, 81, 88
    in children, 83–84, 87
    frequency of, 83, 84, 85, 89
    microscopy of, 86
    term, 80
    variant of, 82
tubercles, 48
Turkish adults, 629
Turkish children, 487
Turkish skulls, 317
tympanic dehiscence
    in ancient Peruvian child, 78
    bilateral, 430
    demonstration of, 166, 447
    oval window revealed by, 147
    references, 662
tympanic dehiscense/foramen of Huschke/foramen tympanicum, 165
tympanic plate, 162, 655, 658
tympanic thickening (os tympanicum hyperostosis), 126, 662

U

ulna, right, 539
U-shaped ligament, 88

V

vaginal process, 450
"vascular foramen" (term), 71, 652
vastus notch, xii, 623, 624
venous markings, 662
ventral arc, 604, 662
vermian fossa, 298
vertebral artery, 567
vessel foramen, 533
vessel grooves, 9, 16
vessels "twiggs," 54
Vietnamese adult, 405, 406, 428
vomer, 21

W

Walmsley's facet, xii, 616
water, cold, pathological lesion/growth associated with, 138
white female, 345
white female, adult, 395, 461
white female, elderly, 81
white female, newborn, 43
white male, adult
    anterior nasal spine and nasal bones in, 187
    exostosis/es in, 376
    metopic and supranasal sutures in, 40
    palatal sutures, accessory in, 506
    petrous bone overhanging appearance in, 295
    sagittal section through skull of, 42
    sphenoid spine, left, foramen ovale and exostosis in, 377
    sphenoid spine, left in, 376
    squamosal ossicles and sphenoparietal suture in, 136
    styloid, left non-segmented in, 181
white male, elderly, 297, 503
white male, young adult, 171
white perinatal individuals, 385
Whitnall's tubercle (term), 89
wide (brachycephalic) skulls, 62
Willed Body Program, 642
wormian bones, 662
wormian os ptericum, 662

Y

young adult(s)
    anterior fontanelle bones in, 212
    interclinoid ligament calcification in, 294
    maxilla and mandible, sectioned in, 464
    nasal rim spine in, 107–108

sternal foramina in, 545
supra-bregmatic ossicle/bone in, 244
See also under ethnic group and gender

Z

Zuni, New Mexico, child from, 614
zygoma, left, 112
zygoma, right, 65, 150, 152, 154
zygomatic arch, 170
zygomatic (malar) bone, left, 163
zygomatic (malar) bone, right, 128, 150, 151
zygomatic foramina, 111, 662
zygomatic (malar) form, 658
zygomaticofacial foramen, Type I, 114
zygomaticofacial foramen, Type II, 113
zygomaticofacial foramen/foramina, 113, 150, 153, 657, 662
zygomaticofacial nerve, 114
zygomaticofrontal suture, 96, 151
zygomaticomaxillary foramina, 112, 662
zygomaticomaxillary suture, 46, 47, 73, 662
zygomaticomaxillary tubercles, 48
zygomatico-orbital foramina, 114, 657
zygomaticotemporal foramen, 128
zygomatic process, 167
zygomatic suture, 152, 662
zygomatic (malar) tubercle, 47, 48, 128, 658
zygomatic (malar) tubercle, inferior, 76
zygomaticulomaxillary sutures, 45, 66, 76, 101
zygomaxillary/malar tubercle, 46
zygomaxillary tubercles, 17, 74, 662
zygomaxillary tuberosity, 662
zygomic bone, 76, 101